Schizophrenia

Dedication

This Third Edition of *Schizophrenia* is dedicated to the founding editor, Steven R. Hirsch, M.D., whose vision and devotion to schizophrenia research launched the first edition of this book and was instrumental in the success of the second, and whose legendary persistence and commitment to this field, to his students and his colleagues, nurtured a generation of researchers and clinicians interested in understanding patients with schizophrenia and in helping them.

Schizophrenia

Daniel R. Weinberger MD

Director, Genes, Cognition and Psychosis Program,
Clinical Studies Section,
Clinical Brain Disorders Branch,
National Institute of Health,
Bethesda,
MD, USA

Paul J. Harrison MA, BM, BCh, DM(Oxon), FRCPsych

Department of Psychiatry,
University of Oxford,
Warneford Hospital,
Oxford, UK

THIRD EDITION

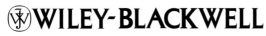

A John Wiley & Sons, Ltd., Publication

This edition first published 2011, © 1995, 2003, 2011 by Blackwell Publishing Ltd

Blackwell Publishing was acquired by John Wiley & Sons in February 2007. Blackwell's publishing program has been merged with Wiley's global Scientific, Technical and Medical business to form Wiley-Blackwell.

Registered office: John Wiley & Sons Ltd, The Atrium, Southern Gate, Chichester, West Sussex, PO19 8SQ, UK

Editorial offices: 9600 Garsington Road, Oxford, OX4 2DQ, UK
The Atrium, Southern Gate, Chichester, West Sussex, PO19 8SQ, UK
111 River Street, Hoboken, NJ 07030-5774, USA

For details of our global editorial offices, for customer services and for information about how to apply for permission to reuse the copyright material in this book please see our website at www.wiley.com/wiley-blackwell

The right of the author to be identified as the author of this work has been asserted in accordance with the Copyright, Designs and Patents Act 1988.

Library of Congress Cataloging-in-Publication Data

Schizophrenia / [edited by] Daniel R. Weinberger, Paul J. Harrison. – 3rd ed.
    p. ; cm.
  Includes bibliographical references and index.
  ISBN 978-1-4051-7697-2
1. Schizophrenia. I. Weinberger, Daniel R. (Daniel Roy) II. Harrison, P. J. (Paul J.), 1960–
  [DNLM: 1. Schizophrenia. WM 203 S33721 2010]
  RC514.S33413 2010
  616.89'8--dc22
                                                        2010015115

A catalogue record for this book is available from the British Library.

This book is published in the following electronic formats: ePDF 9781444327304; Wiley Online Library 9781444327298

Set in 9.25 on 12 pt Palatino by Toppan Best-set Premedia Limited
Printed and bound in Singapore by Fabulous Printers Pte Ltd

1 2011

Contents

Contributors

A. Abi-Dargham, MD
Professor of Clinical Psychiatry and Radiology, Chief, Division of Translational Imaging, Chief of Clinical and Imaging Research, Lieber Center, Department of Psychiatry, Columbia University & New York State Psychiatric Institute, New York, NY, USA

J. Addington, PhD
Professor, Department of Psychiatry, Alberta Mental Health Centennial Research Chair, Novartis Chair in Schizophrenia Research, University of Calgary, Canada

W. an der Heiden, DIPL-PSYCH PhD
Deputy Head, Schizophrenia Research Unit, Central Institute of Mental Health, Mannheim, Germany

N.C. Andreasen, MD PhD
Andrew H. Woods Chair of Psychiatry, Department of Psychiatry, Roy J. and Lucille A. Carver College of Medicine, The University of Iowa, Iowa City, IA, USA

C. Arango, MD PhD
Head, Adolescent Unit, Department of Psychiatry, Hospital General Universitario Gregorio Marañon, Cibersam, Madrid, Spain

T.R.E. Barnes, MD FRCPsych DSc
Professor of Clinical Psychiatry, Centre for Mental Health, Imperial College, Charing Cross Campus, London, UK

P.E. Bebbington, MA PhD FRCP FRCPsych
Professor of Social and Community Psychiatry, UCL, London, UK

E.T. Bullmore, PhD FRCP FRCPsych FMedSci
Professor, Department of Psychiatry, University of Cambridge, Cambridge, UK

T. Burns, DSc FRCPsych
Professor of Social Psychiatry, Department of Psychiatry, University of Oxford, Warneford Hospital, Oxford, UK

T.D. Cannon, PhD
Staglin Family Professor, Departments of Psychology and Psychiatry and Biobehavioral Sciences Director, Staglin Center for Cognitive Neuroscience Associate Director, Semel Institute for Neuroscience and Human Behavior, University of California, Los Angeles, Los Angeles, CA, USA

W.T. Carpenter, MD
Professor of Psychiatry & Pharmacology, University of Maryland School of Medicine, Director, Maryland Psychiatric Research Center, University of Maryland School of Medicine, Baltimore, MD, USA

E. Chemerinski, MD
Assistant Professor of Psychiatry, Mount Sinai School of Medicine, New York, NY, and James J. Peter Veterans Affairs Medical Center, Bronx, NY, USA

C.U. Correll, MD
Medical Director, Recognition and Prevention (RAP) Program, The Zucker Hillside Hospital, Glen Oaks, NY; Associate Professor of Psychiatry, Albert Einstein College of Medicine; and The Feinstein Institute for Medical Research, Manhasset, NY, USA

N.H. Covell, PhD
Assistant Professor, Division of Mental Health Services & Policy Research, College of Physicians and Surgeons, Columbia University, New York State Psychiatric Institute, New York, NY, USA; Connecticut Department of Mental Health and Addiction Services, Hartford, CT, USA

A.S. David, MD FRCP FRCPsych MSc
Professor of Cognitive Neuropsychiatry, Institute of Psychiatry, King's College, London, London, UK

B. Drake, MD, PhD
Professor of Psychiatry and of Community and Family Medicine, Director, Dartmouth Psychiatric Research Center, Lebanon, New Hampshire, USA

M.F. Egan, MD
Senior Director, Clinical Neurosciences, Merck & Co Inc, North Wales, PA, USA

S.M. Essock, PhD
Edna L. Edison Professor of Psychiatry, Director, Division of Mental Health Services & Policy Research, College of Physicians and Surgeons, Columbia University, New York State Psychiatric Institute, New York, NY, USA

L.K. Frisman, PhD
Director of Research, Connecticut Department of Mental Health and Addiction Services, University of Connecticut School of Social Work, Hartford, CT, USA

J.R. Geddes, MD FRCPsych
Professor of Epidemiological Psychiatry, Department of Psychiatry, University of Oxford, Warneford Hospital, Oxford, UK

J.A. Gogos, MD PhD
Professor, Department of Physiology and Department of Neuroscience, Columbia University Medical School, New York, NY USA

J.M. Gold, PhD
Associate Professor, Maryland Psychiatric Research Center, University of Maryland School of Medicine, Crownsville, MD, USA

T.E. Goldberg, PhD
Professor, Psychiatry and Behavioral Science, Albert Einstein College of Medicine Zucker Hillside Hospital/Litwin Zucker Alzheimer's Disease Research Center Feinstein Institute for Medical Research Manhasset, NY, USA

A.A. Grace, PhD
Professor of Neuroscience, Psychiatry and Psychology, Department of Neuroscience, University of Pittsburgh, Pittsburgh, PA, USA

P.M. Haddad, MD FRCPsych
Consultant Psychiatrist and Honorary Senior Lecturer, Neuroscience and Psychiatry Unit, School of Psychiatry and Behavioral Sciences, University of Manchester, Manchester, UK

G. Haddock, BSc MClinPPsychol PhD
Professor of Clinical Psychology, School of Psychological Sciences, University of Manchester, Manchester, UK

H. Häfner, MD PhD Dres.h.c.
Professor of Psychiatry, Head, Schizophrenia Research Unit, Central Institute of Mental Health, Mannheim, Germany

P.J. Harrison, MA BM BCh DM(Oxon) FRCPsych
Professor of Psychiatry, Department of Psychiatry, University of Oxford, Warneford Hospital, Oxford, UK

C. Hollis, MBBS, BSc PhD DCH MRCPsych
Professor of Child and Adolescent Psychiatry, Division of Psychiatry, University of Nottingham, Queen's Medical Centre, Nottingham, UK

R. Howard, MD MRCPsych
Professor of Old Age Psychiatry and Psychopathology, Department of Old Age Psychiatry, Institute of Psychiatry, King's College London, London, UK

T.M. Hyde, MD PhD
Chief Operating Officer, Lieber Institute for Brain Development, Baltimore, Maryland MD, USA

A. Jablensky, MD DMSc FRCPsych FRANZCP
Professor of Psychiatry, School of Psychiatry and Clinical Neurosciences, The University of Western Australia, Perth, WA, Australia

D.V. Jeste, MD
Estelle and Edgar Levi Chair in Aging, Professor of Psychiatry and Neurosciences, Chief, Division of Geriatric Psychiatry, University of California; VA San Diego Healthcare System, San Diego, CA, USA

P.B. Jones, MD FRCPsych
Head, Department of Psychiatry, University of Cambridge, Cambridge, UK

J.M. Kane, MD
Chairman, Department of Psychiatry, The Zucker Hillside Hospital, Psychiatry Research, North Shore—Long Island Jewish Health System, Glen Oaks, NY, Albert Einstein College of Medicine, Bronx, NY, and The Feinstein Institute for Medical Research, Manhasset, NY, USA

K.S. Kendler, MD
Rachel Brown Banks Distinguished Professor of Psychiatry, Professor of Human Genetics, Departments of Psychiatry and Human and Molecular Genetics, and Director, Virginia Institute for Psychiatric and Behavioral Genetics, Virginia Commonwealth University, Richmond, VA, USA

J.B. Kirkbride, PhD
Postdoctoral Research Fellow, Department of Psychiatry, University of Cambridge, Cambridge, UK

J.E. Kleinman, MD PhD
Chief, Section on Neuropathology, Clinical Brain Disorders Branch, Genes, Cognition and Psychosis Program, Intramural Research Program, National Institute for Mental Health, National Institute for Health, Bethesda, MD, USA

I. Kooyman, MBBS, MA, MRCPsych
Specialist Registrar in Forensic Psychiatry, North London Forensic Service, and Department of Forensic Mental Health Science, Institute of Psychiatry, London, UK

J.H. Krystal, MD
Robert L. McNeil, Jr. Professor of Clinical Pharmacology and
Deputy Chairman for Research, Department of Psychiatry, Yale
University School of Medicine, New Haven, CT; Schizophrenia
Biological Research Center (151-D), VA Connecticut Healthcare
System, West Haven, CT, USA

E. Kuipers, BSc MSc PhD FBPsS
Professor of Clinical Psychology, Head of Department of
Psychology, Institute of Psychiatry, King's College London,
London, UK

S.M. Lawrie, MD FRCPsych Hon.FRCP(Edin)
Professor of Psychiatry and Head of Psychiatry, University of
Edinburgh Division of Psychiatry, Royal Edinburgh Hospital,
Edinburgh, UK

S. Leucht, MD
Vice-Chairman, Department of Psychiatry and Psychotherapy,
Technische Universität München, Klinikum rechts der Isar,
Munich, Germany

P. Levitt, PhD
Director, Zilkha Neurogenetic Institute, Chair, Department of Cell
& Neurobiology, Keck School of Medicine of University of
Southern California, Los Angeles, CA, USA

D.A. Lewis, MD
UPMC Professor in Translational Neuroscience and Chair,
Department of Psychiatry, University of Pittsburgh, Medical
Director and Director of Research, Western Psychiatric Institute
and Clinic, Pittsburgh, PA, USA

S. Lewis, MD FMedSci
Professor of Adult Psychiatry, University of Manchester,
Manchester, UK

J.A. Lieberman, MD
Chairman, Department of Psychiatry, College of Physicians &
Surgeons, Columbia University; Director, New York State
Psychiatric Institute; Director, Lieber Center for Schizophrenia
Research; Psychiatrist-in-Chief at New York Presbyterian Hospital
& Columbia University Medical Center, New York, NY, USA

B.K. Lipska, PhD
Staff Scientist, Genes, Cognition and Psychosis Program,
Intramural Research Program, National Institute of Mental Health,
National Institutes of Health, Bethesda, MD, USA

S.R. Marder, MD
Professor and Director, Section on Psychosis Semel Institute for
Neuroscience at UCLA, Veterans Affairs Mental Illness Research,
Education, and Clinical Center, Los Angeles, CA, USA

V.S. Mattay, MD
Director, Neuroimaging Core, Genes, Cognition and Psychosis
Program, National Institutes of Mental Health, National Institutes
of Health, Bethesda, MD, USA

R.W. McCarley, MD
Professor and Head, Harvard Department of Psychiatry; and
Associate Director, Mental Health Service, VA Boston Healthcare
System, Brockton, MA, USA

J.J. McGrath, AM MBBS MD PhD FRANZCP
Professor and Director, Queensland Centre for Mental Health
Research and Department of Psychiatry, Queensland Brain
Institute, University of Queensland, Australia

A. Meyer-Lindenberg, MD PhD MSc
Director, Central Institute of Mental Health, Mannheim, Professor
and Chair of Psychiatry and Psychotherapy, University of
Heidelberg, Medical Faculty, Mannheim, and Chairman,
Department of Psychiatry and Psychotherapy, Central Institute of
Mental Health, Mannheim, Germany

B. Moghaddam, PhD
Professor of Neuroscience, Psychiatry and Pharmacy, Center for
Neuroscience, University of Pittsburgh, Pittsburgh, PA, USA

R.M. Murray, MD M Phil MRCP MRC Psych FRS
Professor of Psychiatric Research, Institute of Psychiatry at the
Maudsley, King's College, University of London; Honorary
Consultant Psychiatrist, Maudsley Hospital, London, UK

J.W. Newcomer, MD
Gregory B. Couch Professor of Psychiatry, Psychology and
Medicine; Medical Director, Center for Clinical Studies at
Washington University School of Medicine, St. Louis, MO, USA

M.C. O'Donovan, FRCPsych PhD
Professor of Psychiatric Genetics, UKMRC Centre for
Neuropsychiatric Genetics and Genomics, Department of
Psychological Medicine and Neurology, School of Medicine,
Cardiff University, Cardiff, UK

C.M.P. O'Tuathaigh, PhD
Senior Research Fellow, Molecular & Cellular Therapeutics, Royal
College of Surgeons in Ireland, Dublin, Ireland

M.J. Owen, FRCPsych PhD
Head, Department of Psychological Medicine, UKMRC Centre for
Neuropsychiatric Genetics and Genomics, Department, of
Psychological Medicine and Neurology, School of Medicine,
Cardiff University, Cardiff, UK

C. Pantelis, MB BS MD MRCPsych FRANZCP
Associate Professor and Head, Cognitive Neuropsychiatry
Research and Academic Unit, Department of Psychiatry; Co-
ordinator, Applied Schizophrenia Division, Mental Health
Research Institute; Principal Fellow, Centre for Neuroscience, The
University of Melbourne, Melbourne, Australia

J. Rapoport
Chief, Child Psychiatry Branch, National Institute of Mental
Health, National Institutes of Health, Bethesda, MD, USA

G.J. Remington, MD PhD FRCPC

Director, Medication Assessment Program for Schizophrenia (MAPS) Clinic and Professor of Psychiatry, Schizophrenia Division, Centre for Addiction and Mental Health, Faculty of Medicine, University of Toronto, Toronto, Canada

B. Riley, PhD

Director of Molecular Genetics, Departments of Psychiatry and Human and Molecular Genetics, and Virginia Institute for Psychiatric and Behavioral Genetics, Virginia Commonwealth University, Richmond, VA, USA

M.A. Ron, MD PhD FRCP FRCPsych

Professor of Neuropsychiatry, Institute of Neurology, University College London, London, UK

L.J. Siever, MD

Professor of Psychiatry, Department of Psychiatry, Mount Sinai School of Medicine New York, NY, and James J. Peter Veterans Affairs Medical Center, New York, NY, USA

W. Spaulding, PhD

Professor of Psychology, University of Nebraska, Lincoln, USA

T.S. Stroup, MD

Department of Psychiatry, Columbia University College of Physicians and Surgeons and the New York State Psychiatric Institute, New York, NY, USA

J.L. Waddington, PhD DSc

Professor of Neuroscience, Molecular & Cellular Therapeutics, Royal College of Surgeons in Ireland, Dublin, Ireland

E. Walsh, MB BCh BAO MSc MRCPsych MD

Consultant in General Adult and Forensic Psychiatry, South London and Maudsley NHS Trust, London, UK

D.R. Weinberger, MD

Director, Genes, Cognition and Psychosis Program, Clinical Brain Disorders Branch, National Institute of Mental Health, Bethesda, MD, USA

G. Winterer, MD PhD

Head, Translational Neurogenetics Group, Cologne Center for Genomics (CCG), University of Cologne, Germany

Editor's Note

The Third Edition of *Schizophrenia* represents a milestone in the evolution of this textbook. It is an extensive revision and update on dramatic new developments in research about schizophrenia and its therapeutics. But it also marks the end of Steven Hirsch's tenure as a founding editor. Professor Hirsch was the visionary figure behind the creation of this volume. His idea was that we would assemble a team of prominent basic and clinical scientists and scholars at the leading edge of schizophrenia research from both sides of the Atlantic—and beyond—to collaborate in producing this comprehensive review of the field. His retirement has not compromised this vision or its implementation, but his participation has been missed. In keeping with the goal of trans-Atlantic cooperation in assembling the faculty for this new volume, and in seeking a translational scientist in the tradition of Professor Hirsch to co-edit this project with me, I invited Professor Paul Harrison of the University of Oxford to pick up the mantle and step into Professor Hirsh's shoes. Professor Harrison brings a unique background in basic molecular neuroscience and extensive clinical experience to serve in this capacity. I could not have done this without his help, dedication, and insight. I look forward to the next volume and the ones after that in partnership with Professor Harrison.

Daniel. R. Weinberger, M.D.

Preface to the 3rd edition

In the eight years since the previous edition of this book, the pace and breadth of research into schizophrenia has increased dramatically, generating much light but also heat. There have been dramatic new findings, concepts, and interpretations across the whole spectrum—from biological to social, and from aetiology to therapeutics: the prodrome, genes, cannabis, cognition, brain oscillations, and metabolic syndrome, to name but a few. And older debates continue, not least concerning the relative merits of atypical versus typical antipsychotics—and how schizophrenia should be classified.

We have attempted to capture the progress, the excitement, and the controversies in the field. Reflecting the developments, as well as the retirement of some experts and the emergence of others, substantial revisions have been made to the content and authorship of this edition; in reality, this is not a revision but a new volume. Seven new chapters have been introduced, eleven chapters dropped, and many of the surviving chapters have new authors or co-authors. The new chapters focus on areas that are particularly topical, or where there has been significant research developments since the last edition; equally, chapters were not retained if there had been little new research findings, or if their key elements were better subsumed within another chapter. Overall this has led to significant changes to all four parts of the book. In Part 1, there is a new chapter on the prodrome (Chapter 6). In Part 2, the

dramatic increase in genetic research is reflected in a second genetics chapter (Chapter 13), and the chapter on brain imaging has been divided into separate chapters on structural (Chapter 16) and functional (Chapter 17) modalities. Part 3, covering physical treatments, has been reorganised, with chapters now focusing on psychopharmacological principles (Chapter 24), typical versus atypical antipsychotics (Chapter 25) and on their metabolic effects (Chapter 28). Part 4 has also been updated and reorganised, in line with the increasing focus on psychosocial treatments and societal outcomes.

We are fortunate that so many leading experts have again contributed to this volume, ensuring that every chapter is an authoritative, up-to-date, and cutting edge review. Chapters are comprehensively referenced, and a detailed index is provided, allowing the book to be used as a standard reference text and also to serve as an entrée to the primary literature. We worked with the authors to remove unnecessary redundancy between chapters, but some overlap has been retained where it allows for complementary perspectives. We thank our colleagues for their important and authoritative contributions and our families for their extraordinary patience and support.

Daniel R. Weinberger
Paul J. Harrison
January 2011

For Sandra, Rosie, Charlie and Grace
Paul J Harrison

For Leslie and Collin
Daniel R Weinberger

Preface to the First Edition

Schizophrenia has been a controversial topic since the term was first proposed by Eugen Bleuler to describe a uniquely human syndrome of profoundly disturbed behaviour. In the years following Bleuler's original work the controversies have continued at least as vigorously, but their content has changed. The debate is no longer about the nature of intra-psychic mechanisms, or whether schizophrenia really exists, or whether it is an illness as opposed to a life choice, or whether it is an important public health concern. Indeed, a recent editorial in *Nature* reified the current status of schizophrenia in the biomedical research establishment by declaring, 'Schizophrenia is arguably the worst disease affecting mankind, even AIDS not excepted' (*Nature* Editorial, 1988). In the United States alone it is estimated to cost over $40 billion each year in economic terms: the price that is paid by affected individuals and their families is inestimable.

The debate has shifted away from the view that schizophrenia is caused by a fault in the infant–mother psychological relationship. This had gained the status of orthodoxy during the late/middle part of this century and has been radically revised. Early parenting as a aetiologic factor never stood up to scientific scrutiny (Hirsch & Leff, 1975). The evidence that schizophrenia is associated with objective changes in the anatomy and function of the brain and has a genetic predisposition is incorporated in a major revision of the concept of schizophrenia encompassed in this book.

Schizophrenia has assumed an increasingly important place in neuroscience and molecular biological research programs around the world. Provocative evidence has suggested that aberrations of complex molecular processes responsible for the development of the human brain may be responsible for this illness. The possibility of finding a specific genetic defect that may participate in the liability to develop this disease has never seemed brighter. At the same time, the pharmaceutical industry has revitalized the search for effective new medical treatments. Where it was believed for almost three decades that all antipsychotic drugs were equally effective, it has now been shown that

this is not the case. Moreover, it is clear that more effective drugs can be developed which are safer and have fewer side effects.

This textbook of schizophrenia represents a major shift of thinking influenced by the recent changes in our understanding of the brain, the developments in methodology which have influenced scientifically informed notions of our clinical practice, and the changes in our culture which have led to new concepts of management and treatment and a new understanding of the factors which are likely to affect relapse.

While we have asked the authors to make their chapters up to date and comprehensive, we have also worked with them to maintain a "textbook" orientation so that students and researchers from other disciplines, as well as clinical and research specialists in the field, may be intelligibly informed about schizophrenia.

Promising as some of the basic science may seem, schizophrenia is still a disease whose diagnosis depends on clinical acumen and careful assessment. Therefore all the traditional subject areas are covered. This includes a series of chapters that discuss current issues in the phenomenological characterization of the illness, from its history to the ongoing debate about clinical subtypes, modifying factors, spectrum disorders, and the very nature and prognostic implications of the fundamental symptoms. The increased recognition of the importance of neuropsychological deficits in the chronic disability and outcome of this illness is highlighted by several contributors.

The series of chapters focused around the theme of aetiological factors emphasizes the dramatic shift in thinking on the medical aspects of schizophrenia. The application of new methods for studying the brain during life and at postmortem examination has provided compelling data that subtle abnormalities are associated with the illness. The precise nature of the fundamental pathological process is unknown, and many uncertainties about it need to be answered. Is brain development disturbed in a characteristic way? Is there a common aetiology, or can schizophrenia arise from a myriad of causes, any of which affect a final common path of brain disturbance? Could the developmental abnormality result solely from environmental causes, or is a genetic factor essential? What is the correspondence between pathological changes and clinical manifestations? Does everyone with the pathological change manifest the illness, or is it possible to have the defect but compensate for it? What makes decompensation happen? What factors encourage clinical recovery?

The application of recombinant DNA technology involves a new language in asking the old question of how and what genetic factors play a role in the illness. While it is widely believed that a simple Mendelian genetic defect does not account for schizophrenia, what does it take in genetic terms? How many genes could be involved in liability? Are the genes likely to be recognizable as having anything to do with the phenotype as we have traditionally perceived it? What should relatives of a patient be advised about genetic risk? The straightforward dopamine hypothesis that had guided most researchers for the seventies and eighties has become much more sophisticated and enlightened. It is still important in understanding how the illness is treated, but it clearly has much less explanatory power than it seemed to have in the past. Is dopamine really involved in schizophrenia, or is it simply a way of modulating symptoms by affecting neurotransmission in a relatively unimportant but peripherally connected brain system? Can the illness be treated with drugs that do not touch the dopamine system?

Intensive, insight oriented psychotherapy on an individual basis is no longer used to treat patients with schizophrenia. Indeed, controlled outcome studies indicate that doing so is potentially harmful. However, more rationally based cognitive behavioural methods have shown real gains in symptom control and are becoming increasingly important in modern management. There is solid evidence that therapy aimed at altering the family environment significantly reduces the risk of relapse. The value of community rather than hospital based treatment is a modern trend, but the evidence from carefully controlled research leaves many questions unanswered: yet, a consensus is beginning to emerge on several of the basic issues.

We have invited leading experts to review established knowledge of the major fields of study in schizophrenia. This inevitably leads us to include new topical areas of interest including homelessness, the risk of violence and the relationship of depression to schizophrenia, as well as brain imaging studies and the treatment of refractory states which would not have appeared in texts a decade ago. The result is a radical revision of our concepts and understanding which we believe justifies the effort of our authors whom we gratefully thank for their contribution.

Steven R. Hirsch
Daniel R. Weinberger
1995

References

Editorial (1988) Where next with psychiatric illness? *Nature* **336**, 95–96.

Hirsch, S.R. & Leff, J. (1975) *Abnormalities in Parents of Schizophrenics: Review of the Literature and an Investigation of Communication Defects and Deviances.* Maudsley Monograph Services, No. 22. Oxford: Oxford University Press.

PART 1

Descriptive Aspects

Concept of schizophrenia: past, present, and future

Nancy C. Andreasen

Roy J. and Lucille A. Carver College of Medicine, The University of Iowa, Iowa City, IA, USA

Schizophrenia is one of the most important public health problems in the world. A survey by the World Health Organization ranks schizophrenia among the top ten illnesses that contribute to the global burden of disease (Murray, 1996). Because of its early age of onset and its subsequent tendency to persist chronically, often at significant levels of severity, it produces great suffering for patients and also for their family members. It is also a relatively common illness. Although estimates of rates in the general population vary, it appears to affect from 0.5% to 1% of people worldwide. Furthermore, it is an illness that affects the essence of a person's identity—the brain and the most complex functions that the brain mediates. It affects the ability to think clearly, to experience and express emotions, to read social situations and to have normal interpersonal relationships, and to interpret past experiences and plan for the future. Some of its symptoms, such as delusions and hallucinations, produce great subjective psychological pain. Other facets of the illness produce great pain as well, such as the person's recognition that they are literally "losing their mind" or being controlled or tormented by forces beyond personal control. Consequently, it can be fatal—a substantial number of its victims either attempt or complete suicide.

It is also an illness that is conceptually challenging, because its manifestations are so diverse. Over the past several centuries various attempts have been made to formulate a consensus about the definition and essence of schizophrenia. This introduction will review this conceptual history in order to provide a foundation for the later chapters in this book. Even at present, creating a consensus about how best to define the phenotype(s) of schizophrenia is a task that has not yet been successfully achieved. And yet the definition of the concept and its phenotype must provide a foundation for both the study of disease mechanisms and for the development of improved approaches to treatment and prevention.

The past: early concepts of psychosis

The term "schizophrenia" was only coined in the last century, and therefore it is sometimes assumed that it is a "new disease", perhaps a consequence of the development of a complex highly-industrialized world and resultant stresses in lifestyle. Although the name for this illness is relatively new, the concept of psychosis is very old. Based on portrayals of similar psychotic states in early history and literature and on early medical descriptions, we know that schizophrenia-like psychoses have been recognized since at least the first millenium BC.

One of the earliest descriptions of a psychotic condition occurs in the book of Samuel in the Old Testament. After David successfully defends the Israelites against the Philistines by killing Goliath and then wins several subsequent battles, King Saul becomes increasingly paranoid about David's military prowess, to the point of repeatedly making plans to murder David, and even attempting to do it himself:

Schizophrenia, 3rd edition. Edited by Daniel R. Weinberger and Paul J Harrison © 2011 Blackwell Publishing Ltd.

… the evil spirit from God came upon Saul, and he prophesied in the midst of the house: and David played [music] with his hand, as at other times; and there was a javelin in Saul's hand. And Saul cast the javelin; for he said, I will smite David even to the wall with it. And David avoided out of his presence twice. And Saul was afraid of David, because the Lord was with him, and was departed from Saul.

(1 Samuel 10–12)

In fact, Saul eventually begins to have hallucinatory-like experiences, seeking help from the witch of Endor, and also having visions of his former advisor, the deceased prophet Samuel.

If we move on to the classical era in Greece and Rome, there are many descriptions of paranoid schizophrenia-like psychotic states. Greek tragedy is filled with portrayals of individuals who are tormented by psychosis, and are often driven to committing horrendous acts while insane. In *The Bacchae*, Agave murders her son Pentheus with her own hands, driven by the delusional belief that he is a lion. In *Medea*, after Jason abandons his wife Medea, she falls into a psychotic rage that drives her to murder their two children with a sword, also murdering King Creon and his daughter by giving them a poisoned robe and chaplet that consumes them in a fiery painful death. In *The Oresteia*, Orestes is pursued by the Furies until he finally loses his reason and lapses into madness. And there are many more examples.

In the 16th and 17th centuries Elizabethan and Jacobean drama are similarly filled with portrayals of individuals who experience schizophrenia-like psychotic states. Some of the best known are in the plays of Shakespeare. Hamlet, Lear, Othello, and Lady Macbeth all experience psychosis. *King Lear* is a vivid and powerful example. Three main characters are all "mad": Lear himself, Gloucester, and Edgar (pretending to be a "bedlam beggar"—an escapee from the Bethleham Hospital for the insane in London). As Gloucester says of Lear:

Thou say'st the King grows mad; I'll tell thee, friend,
I am almost mad myself. I had a son,
Now outlaw'd from my blood; he sought my life. …
The grief hath craz'd my wits

(King Lear III.iv.169–174)

In addition to these historical and literary portrayals, which document that schizophrenia-like illnesses have been present for at least three millennia, the "medical" literature of these early times provides parallel evidence that psychotic disorders similar to schizophrenia were recognized as important medical illnesses. They are described in the writings of our early medical forefathers, such as Hippocrates, Galen, or Soranus of Ephesus. The disorders described by these forefathers do not map perfectly on to modern classification systems, but they have surprising similarities. Mental illnesses were clearly seen as "physical"

in origin, deriving either from an imbalance of humors (yellow bile, black bile, phlegm, and blood) or to an imbalance in the brain. In general, five groups of illnesses were described: melancholia, phrenitis, mania, hysteria, and epilepsy. Mania was essentially equivalent to our concept of psychosis. Psychotic disorders were not, however, further subdivided until the late 19th century.

The past: further delineation of psychoses and early definitions of schizophrenia

Kraepelin (1919) gave us the conceptual framework that created the modern concept of schizophrenia. One of Kraepelin's many great contributions was to take the general concept of psychosis and to subdivide it into two major groups, based on his observation of differences in course and outcome. One group of patients who were psychotic had an episodic course, typically with a full remission of symptoms. A second group of psychotic patients had a chronic course and typically progressed to a deteriorated state. He named these two groups "manic-depression" and "dementia praecox". Although this distinction is so familiar today that we scarcely think about it, it was a major intellectual achievement at the time, and it has influenced psychiatric classification and the concept of schizophrenia for more than a century.

Kraepelin did not, however, consider psychotic symptoms to be the most important features of dementia praecox. When he spoke of symptoms, those that he considered to be most fundamental were what we today would call negative symptoms. Negative symptoms include abnormalities in cognition and emotion: alogia, avolition, anhedonia, affective blunting, and (in some conceptualizations) attentional impairment. Kraepelin said:

There are apparently two principal groups of disorders that characterize the malady. On the one hand we observe a weakening of those emotional activities which permanently form the mainsprings of volition. … Mental activity and instinct for occupation become mute. The result of this highly morbid process is emotional dullness, failure of mental activities, loss of mastery over volition, of endeavor, and ability for independent action. … The second group of disorders consists in the *loss of the inner unity* of activities of intellect, emotion, and volition in themselves and among one another. … The near connection between thinking and feeling, between deliberation and emotional activity on the one hand, and practical work on the other is more or less lost. Emotions do not correspond to ideas. The patient laughs and weeps without recognisable cause, without any relation to their circumstances and their experiences, smile as they narrate a tale of their attempted suicide.

(Kraepelin, 1919, pp. 74–75)

Such passages in Kraepelin's textbook indicate that he perceived negative symptoms to be the most important symptoms of schizophrenia. Nevertheless, his comprehensive description of schizophrenia covered a broad range of symptoms, including delusions and hallucinations.

Bleuler (1950), on the other hand, tried to clarify the group of schizophrenias by very explicitly attempting to identify what he considered to be the underlying fundamental abnormality. Consequently, he divided the symptoms of schizophrenia into two broad categories: fundamental and accessory symptoms. Bleuler believed that the fundamental symptoms were present in all patients, tended to occur only in schizophrenia, and therefore were pathognomonic. The accessory symptoms, on the other hand, could occur in a variety of different disorders. Depending how one interprets and summarizes his writings, one can argue that Bleuler identified four, five, or six fundamental symptoms of schizophrenia. These included the loss of the continuity of associations, loss of affective responsiveness, loss of attention, loss of volition, ambivalence, and autism. These symptoms correspond relatively closely to those we currently refer to as negative symptoms. They reflect abnormalities in basic cognitive and emotional processes, which (in Bleuler's thinking) provided the basis for other types of symptoms observed in the illness. Accessory symptoms, on the other hand, include phenomena such as delusions and auditory hallucinations. Bleuler wrote:

> Certain symptoms of schizophrenia are present in every case and in every period of the illness even though, as with every other disease symptom, they must have attained a certain degree of intensity before they can be recognized with any certainty. ... Besides the specific permanent or fundamental symptoms, we can find a host of other, more accessory manifestations such as delusions, hallucinations, or catatonic symptoms. ... As far as we know, the fundamental symptoms are characteristic of schizophrenia, while the accessory symptoms may also appear in other types of illness.
>
> (Bleuler, 1950, p. 13)

When Kraepelin called the disorder "dementia praecox", he intended to highlight the fact that it had an early ("praecox") onset and therefore differed from another type of dementia described by his friend and colleague, Alois Alzheimer. However, in choosing the term "dementia", he wished to highlight the fact that the illness had a chronic and deteriorating course. His contemporary Swiss colleague, Eugen Bleuler, admired many of Kraepelin's ideas, but he took exception to the fact that chronicity and deterioration were inevitable. Therefore, he chose to rename the illness in order to highlight his own view that a fragmenting of thinking, sometimes referred to as "thought disorder", was the most important feature, and also to eliminate the concept that deterioration was inevitable. He chose the name "schizophrenia" (schiz = fragmenting, splitting; phren = mind, Gk). Bleuler's name eventually prevailed over Kraepelin's. Today many feel that either is an unfortunate choice, because each leads to misunderstanding about the nature of the illness by the general public. Too often people assume that the name refers to a "split personality". However, to date no good substitute has been identified.

Since Bleuler's fundamental symptoms involve cognition and emotion, since negative symptoms (a related but also slightly different concept) also involve cognition and emotion, and since "cognitive dysfunction" in schizophrenia is currently a topic of considerable interest, some clinicians and investigators find the interface between cognition and negative symptoms confusing. The word "cognition" has multiple meanings in cognitive psychology and clinical usage (Andreasen, 1997). Sometimes it refers to all activities of "mind", including emotion and language. Sometimes it refers to "rational" as opposed to "emotional" processes. Sometimes it is used very narrowly to refer to performance on objective neuropsychological tests or experimental cognitive psychology tests. Heuristically, the term "cognition" is probably most useful in the context of schizophrenia when it is used to refer to the broadest meaning (activities of mind). Since negative symptoms are closely tied to defects in basic cognitive processes (e.g., volition, ability to think abstractly, initiation of thoughts and language, attributing affects to experiences), assessing them at the clinical level may provide a relatively direct "window" into cognitive impairments in schizophrenia. While Kraepelin and Bleuler did not refer to their clusters of fundamental symptoms by calling them "negative", this appears to be the point that they were making. In a sense, therefore, negative symptoms may be the most fundamental and clinically important symptoms of schizophrenia.

Neither Kraepelin nor Bleuler actually used the terms "positive symptoms" or "negative symptoms". While various sources for these terms can be cited (Berrios, 1985), one of the earliest and most prominent was Hughlings-Jackson (1931). Although Hughlings-Jackson's work was not published until much later, in the late 19th century Jackson speculated about the mechanisms that might underlie psychotic symptoms:

> Disease is said to "cause" the symptoms of insanity. I submit that disease only produces negative mental symptoms, answering to the dissolution, and that all elaborate positive mental symptoms (illusions, hallucinations, delusions, and extravagant conduct) are the outcome of activity of nervous elements untouched by any pathological process; that they arise during activity on the lower level of evolution remaining.
>
> (Hughlings-Jackson, 1931)

Thus Hughlings-Jackson believed that some symptoms represented a relatively pure loss of function (negative symptoms answer to the dissolution), while positive symptoms such as delusions and hallucinations represented an exaggeration of normal function and might represent release phenomena. Hughlings-Jackson presented these ideas at a time when Darwinian evolutionary theories were achieving ascendance, and his concepts concerning the mechanisms that produced the various symptoms were clearly shaped by a Darwinian view that the brain is organized in hierarchical evolutionary layers. Positive symptoms represent aberrations in a primitive (perhaps limbic) substrate that is for some reason no longer monitored by higher cortical functions. Thus Huglings-Jackson's concept of negative and positive symptoms rather closely resembles those which are currently discussed. Although most investigators do not necessarily embrace the specific mechanism that he proposed, they accept his view that they must be understood in terms of brain mechanisms, as well as his basic descriptive psychopathology.

The writings of Kraepelin, Bleuler, and Huglings-Jackson laid down a descriptive and conceptual foundation for contemporary thinking about the symptoms and definition of schizophrenia. Both Kraepelin and Hughlings-Jackson attempted to understand symptoms in terms of their underlying neural mechanisms. While Hughlings-Jackson stressed the importance of the interplay between brain regions that were hierarchically organized, Kraepelin discussed the possible localization of the various symptoms in the prefrontal, motor, and temporal cortex. Kraepelin and Bleuler both stressed the importance of a *loss* of cognitive, affective, volitional, and attentional function in schizophrenia. Kraepelin clearly believed that these could be the most debilitating and central symptoms of the disorder, while Bleuler stated that they were pathognomonic. Throughout most of the 20th century, Bleuler's perspective predominated. Clinicians all over the world were taught to define and diagnose schizophrenia based on the symptoms Bleuler saw as fundamental, such as associative loosening and affective blunting.

The present: Schneiderian symptoms, psychosis, and the dominance of diagnostic criteria

For a variety of historical reasons, this emphasis shifted in the 1960s and 1970s. This change in emphasis arose primarily from an interest in improving diagnostic precision and reliability. Because they are essentially "all or none" phenomena, which are relatively easy to recognize and define, florid psychotic symptoms such as delusions and hallucinations were steadily given greater prominence and indeed even placed at the forefront of the definition of schizophrenia.

The emphasis on florid psychotic symptoms arose because of the influence of Kurt Schneider and the inter-pretation of his thinking by influential British psychiatrists. Schneider was greatly influenced by the work of Karl Jaspers, who explored phenomenology and created a bridge between psychiatry and philosophy. Jaspers believed that the essence of psychosis was the experience of phenomena that were "non-understandable", i.e., symptoms that a "normal" person could not readily imagine experiencing. Schneider, like Bleuler, wished to identify symptoms that were fundamental. He concluded that one critical component was an inability to find the boundaries between self and not-self and a loss of the sense of personal autonomy. This led him to discuss various "first-rank" symptoms that were characterized by this loss of autonomy, such as thought insertion or delusions of being controlled by outside forces (Schneider, 1959; Fish, 1962; Mellor, 1970).

Schneiderian ideas were introduced to the English-speaking world by British investigators and began to exert a powerful influence on the concept of schizophrenia. An emphasis on Schneiderian first-rank symptoms satisfied the fundamental need to find an anchor in the perplexing flux of the phenomenology of schizophrenia. Schneiderian symptoms were incorporated into the first major structured interview developed for use in the International Pilot Study of Schizophrenia (IPSS), the Present State Examination (PSE) (Wing *et al.*, 1974). From this major base, they were thereafter introduced into other standard diagnostic instruments such as the Schedule for Affective Disorders and Schizophrenia (SADS) (Endicott & Spitzer, 1978), Research Diagnostic Criteria (RDC) (Spitzer *et al.*, 1978), and the Diagnostic and Statistical Manual (DSM-III) (American Psychiatric Association, 1980).

The emphasis on positive symptoms, and especially Schneiderian symptoms, derived from several concerns. The first was that Bleulerian symptoms were difficult to define and rate reliably. They are often continuous with normality, while positive symptoms are clearly abnormal. In addition to concerns about reliability, work with the IPSS and the US/UK Study also indicated that in the US the concept of schizophrenia had broadened to an excessive degree, particularly in the North-eastern parts of the US (Kendell *et al.*, 1971; Wing *et al.*, 1974). Thus, in the US there was clearly a need to narrow the concept of schizophrenia. Stressing florid psychotic symptoms, particularly Schneiderian symptoms, was a useful way to achieve this end, since it appeared that schizophrenia was often being diagnosed on the basis of mild Bleulerian negative symptoms. When diagnostic criteria such as the RDC and later DSM-III were written, these placed a substantial emphasis on positive symptoms and essentially ignored negative symptoms.

While there have been many good consequences of this progression and of the interest in Schneider's work, there have also been problems.

From a Schneiderian perspective, Schneider's work and point of view have been oversimplified and even misunderstood. As a Jasperian phenomenologist, Schneider was in fact deeply interested in the subjective experience of schizophrenia—in understanding the internal psychological processes that troubled his patients. For him, the fundamental core of the illness was not the specific first-rank symptoms themselves, but rather the internal cognitive and emotional state that they reflected. It is somewhat ironic that he has become the symbol of objective quantification and reductionism. He himself was a complex thinker who was concerned about individual patients.

The development of diagnostic criteria has also had both advantages and disadvantages. When DSM-III was originally developed, it was intended only as a "provisional consensus agreement" based on clinical judgment. The criteria were created by a small group of individuals who reached a decision about what to include based on a mixture of clinical experience and research data available up to that point. The criteria were chosen to serve as a gatekeeper that would include or exclude individual cases, and they were not intended to be a full description of the illness. Unfortunately, they are now sometimes treated as a textbook of psychiatry. Further, the criteria have become reified and given a power that they originally were never intended to have.

Diagnostic criteria have substantial and undeniable advantages: they improve reliability, provide a basis for cross-center standardization both nationally and internationally, improve clinical communication, and facilitate research. However, they may also have potential disadvantages and even abuses: they provide an oversimplified and incomplete view of the clinical picture, discourage clinical sensitivity to individual patients and comprehensive history-taking, lead students and even clinicians to believe that "knowing the criteria is enough", reify an agreement that was only intended to be provisional, and discourage creative or innovative thinking about the psychological and neural mechanisms of schizophrenia.

The future: beyond diagnostic criteria and the search for fundamental mechanisms

As the present moves toward the future, corrective readjustments are already beginning to occur. Paradoxically, these often occur by returning to the past and coming back full circle to the work of Kraepelin, Bleuler, Jackson, and Schneider.

Clinically, the emphasis on negative as well as psychotic symptoms is leading to increased interest in the full range of symptoms of schizophrenia and in developing methods for treating that full range. The development of atypical antipsychotics, which may affect a broader range of symptoms than the older "typicals", has been helpful in effecting this change (Green et al., 1997; Tollefson & Sanger, 1997).

The interest in negative symptoms has been complemented by a return to an interest in cognitive aspects of schizophrenia. Many negative symptoms are cognitive in nature—alogia (poverty of thought and speech), avolition (inability to formulate plans and pursue them), and attentional impairment. While their assessment may emphasize objective aspects of behavior in order to achieve reliability, their underlying essence is in the domains of thought and emotion. Increasingly, therefore, investigators are returning to the original insights of Kraepelin and Bleuler that the core symptoms of schizophrenia represent a fundamental deficit in cognition and emotion. This in turn has led to recent initiatives to incorporate assessments of cognitive function into clinical drug trials (Green & Neuchterlein, 2004).

Several prominent investigators have turned from a focus on explaining and "localizing" the specific symptoms of schizophrenia to a search for more fundamental underlying cognitive mechanisms (Andreasen, 1997). Examples include Frith's (1992) hypotheses concerning an inability to think in "metarepresentations", Goldman-Rakic's (1994) studies of working memory, our descriptions of cognitive dysmetria (Andreasen et al., 1996), or the work of Holzman et al. (1976), Braff (1993), Swerdlow and Geyer (1993), and Freedman et al. (1991) on information processing and attention. These cognitive models provide a general theory of the disease that is consistent with its diversity of symptoms, permit testing in human beings with a variety of convergent techniques (e.g., imaging, neurophysiology), and even permit modeling in animals. This efficient and parsimonious approach offers considerable hope for the future because it facilitates the search both for improved treatments and for molecular mechanisms.

Finally, the growing maturation of the field of complex genetics offers many potential opportunities for understanding the mechanisms of schizophrenia at the molecular level and hope for improved pre-emption, prevention, and personalization of care. The most pressing need facing those engaged in this work is to identify more meaningful ways to define the phenotype of schizophrenia. The success of the Human Genome Project has conceptually revolutionized our thinking about the ways in which the search for phenotypes must be guided. It has created a new discipline that is sometimes referred to as "phenomics" (Freimer & Sabatti, 2003). The primary task of this new discipline is to delineate the various phenotypic components that comprise the phenome—in this case the phenome of a disease, schizophrenia. Phenomics takes a broad approach to defining the concept of the phenotype. That is, the phenotype includes not just clinical symptoms and other "behavioral" measures, but also morphological, biochemical, and physiological characteristics. What will eventually emerge from a phenomic approach is a more valid and etiologically-based definition of disease phenotypes that may be quite different from those created by using the clinical level alone, as has been the tradition in psychiatry and the rest of medicine for the past century. These improved phenotypes will advance the field in several ways. One is to assist in the identification of individualized treatment strategies that are more rationally based and data-driven. A second is to improve our knowledge of disease mechanisms at the neural and genomic levels so that more targeted treatment strategies can be developed.

References

American Psychiatric Association Committee on Nomenclature and Statistics (1980) *Diagnostic and Statistical Manual of Mental Disorders*; 3rd edn. Washington, DC: American Psychiatric Association.

Andreasen, N.C. (1997) Linking mind and brain in the study of mental illnesses: A project for scientific psychopathology. *Science* **275**, 1586–1593.

Andreasen, N.C., O'Leary, D.S., Cizadlo, T. *et al.* (1996) Schizophrenia and cognitive dysmetria: A positron-emission tomography study of dysfunctional prefrontal-thalamic-cerebellar circuitry. *Proceedings of the National Academy of Sciences USA* **93**, 9985–9990.

Berrios, G.E. (1985) Positive and negative symptoms and Jackson. *Archives of General Psychiatry* **42**, 95–97.

Bleuler, E.P. (1950) *Dementia Praecox of the Group of Schizophrenias* (translated by Zinkin, J.). New York: International Universities Press.

Braff, D.L. (1993) Information processing and attention dysfunctions in schizophrenia. *Schizophrenia Bulletin* **19**, 233–259.

Endicott, J. & Spitzer, R.L. (1978) A diagnostic interview: The schedule for affective disorders and schizophrenia (SADS). *Archives of General Psychiatry* **35**, 837–844.

Fish, F.J. (1962) *Schizophrenia*. Bristol: John Wright & Sons, Ltd.

Freedman, R., Waldo, M., Bickford-Wimer, P. & Nagamoto, H. (1991) Elementary neuronal dysfunctions in schizophrenia. *Schizophrenia Research* **4**, 233–243.

Freimer, N. & Sabatti, C. (2003). "The human phenome project". *Nature Genetics* **34**, 15–21.

Frith, C.D. (1992). *The Cognitive Neuropsychology of Schizophrenia*. East Sussex: Lawrence Erlbaum.

Goldman-Rakic, P.S. (1994) Working memory dysfunction in schizophrenia. *J. Journal of Neuropsychiatry and Clinical Neurosciences* **6**, 348–357.

Green, M.F. & Neuchterlein, K.H. (2004) The MATRICS initiative: developing a consensus cognitive battery for clinical trials. *Schizophrenia Research* **72**, 1–3.

Green, M.F., Marshall Jr, B.D., Wirshing, W.C. *et al.* (1997) Does risperidone improve verbal working memory in treatment-resistant schizophrenia? *American Journal of Psychiatry* **154**, 799–804.

Holzman, P.S., Levy, D.L. & Proctor, L.R. (1976) Smooth pursuit eye movements, attention, and schizophrenia. *Archives of General Psychiatry* **45**, 641–647.

Kendell, R.E., Cooper, J.R., Gourlay, A.J. *et al.* (1971) Diagnostic criteria of American and British psychiatrists. *Archives of General Psychiatry* **25**, 123–130.

Kraepelin, E. (1919) *Dementia Praecox and Paraphrenia* (tranlstated by Barclaym, R.M. & Robertson, G.M). Edinburgh: ES Livingstone.

Mellor, C.S. (1970) First-rank symptoms of schizophrenia. *British Journal of Psychiatry* **117**, 15–23.

Murray, C.J.L. (1996) The global burden of disease: a comprehensive assessment of mortality and disability from diseases, injuries, and risk factors in 1990 and projected to 2020. Cambridge, MA: Harvard School of Public Health on behalf of the World Health Organization and the World Bank; distributed by Harvard University Press.

Schneider, K. (translated by Hamilton, M.W.) (1959) *Clinical Psychopathology*. New York: Grune & Stratton, Inc.

Spitzer, R.L., Endicott, J. & Robins, E. (1978) Research diagnostic criteria: Rationale and reliability. *Archives of General Psychiatry* **35**, 773–782.

Swerdlow, N.R. & Geyer, M.A. (1993) Clozapine and haloperidol in an animal model of sensorimotor gating deficits in schizophrenia. *Pharmacology, Biochemistry, and Behaviour* **44**, 741–744.

Taylor, J. ed. (1931) *Selected writings of J.Hughlings-Jackson*. London: Hodder & Stoughton, Ltd.

Tollefson, G.D. & Sanger, T.M. (1997) Negative symptoms: A path-analytic approach to the double-blind, placebo- and haloperidol-controlled clinical trial experience with olanzapine. *American Journal of Psychiatry* **154**, 457–465.

Wing, J.K., Cooper, J.E. & Sartorius, N. (1974) *The Measurement and Classification of Psychiatric Symptoms*. Cambridge: Cambridge University Press.

CHAPTER 2

The schizophrenia construct: symptomatic presentation

Celso Arango[1] and William T. Carpenter[2]

[1]Hospital General Universitario Gregorio Marañon, Cibersam, Madrid, Spain
[2]University of Maryland School of Medicine, Baltimore, MD, USA

Introduction

The syndrome schizophrenia is composed of a broad collection of symptoms from all domains of mental function. Most persons who have this diagnosis experience delusions and hallucinations. Many, but not all, manifest disorganization of thought. These psychotic experiences are most commonly associated with the syndrome, but other pathological features are critical to the concept. These include avolitional and restricted affect pathologies, motor signs, and impaired basic cognitive functions. There is considerable variation between cases. Heterogeneity is a hallmark of schizophrenia.

The concept of schizophrenia as a disease entity as described by Kraepelin and Bleuler has been badly compromised by evidence that schizophrenia syndrome may comprise a number of specific disease entities (Kendell,

1987; Carpenter, 2007). The diagnostic criteria currently used (ICD-10 and DSM-IV-TR) can be considered provisional and arbitrary constructs with some face validity that meet the objective of facilitating international communication and research. A good example of this is the classical subtypes of schizophrenia (paranoid, catatonic, disorganized or hebephrenic in ICD-10, residual and undifferentiated) that have been shown to have low validity. Dividing patients into mutually exclusive categorical subgroups is the classical procedure in the disease model in medicine and may help to reduce heterogeneity and enhance research. However, for clinical purposes and based on epidemiological data, many authors support the clinical usefulness of psychopathological dimensions. There are some studies showing a continuous distribution of psychosis-like symptoms (Rössler *et al.*, 2007) and even of dimensions of positive, negative, and depressive symptoms (Stefanis *et al.*, 2002) in the general population. Diagnostic models using both categorical and dimensional representations of psychosis may have better predictive validity than either model independently (Allardyce *et al.*, 2007).

Schizophrenia, 3rd edition. Edited by Daniel R. Weinberger and Paul J Harrison © 2011 Blackwell Publishing Ltd.

Description of pathological manifestations associated with the diagnosis of schizophrenia

Reality distortion: delusions and hallucinations

A delusion is an unshakable, false idea or belief that cannot be attributed to the patient's educational, social, or cultural background, which is held with extraordinary conviction and subjective certainty, and is not amenable to logic. Delusions have been divided into primary and secondary delusions. Primary delusions, which are more characteristic of schizophrenia, do not occur in response to another psychopathological form, such as mood disorder or hallucinations. Jaspers (1946/1963) considered that the perception of reality is a primary event not determined by the sense organs. Secondary delusions can be understood in terms of a person's background culture or emotional state. Kurt Schneider (1959) posited that "first-rank symptoms", which reflect an inability to define boundaries between the self and non-self and which mainly include delusions and hallucinations (see below), were the defining characteristics of schizophrenia. As a result of this influential view, diagnostic criteria mainly used those symptoms for the diagnosis of schizophrenia. In fact, it was not until DSM-IV that negative symptoms have been included among the symptoms for diagnosing schizophrenia.

Primary delusions include delusional perceptions and delusional intuitions. Delusional perceptions are normal perceptions that are interpreted with a delusional meaning, usually with personal significance. They were described by Kurt Schneider as one of the first-rank symptoms in schizophrenia (see Table 2.1).

Table 2.1 First-rank symptoms of schizophrenia as defined by K. Schneider.

Delusions
Delusional perception

Auditory hallucinations
Audible thoughts
Voices arguing or discussing
Voices commenting on the patient's action

Thought disorder: passivity of thought
Thought withdrawal
Thought insertion
Thought broadcasting (diffusion of thought)

Passivity experiences
Passivity of affect
Passivity of impulse
Passivity of volition
Somatic passivity

Delusions are extremely variable in content. The most common delusions with respect to type of content are shown in Table 2.2. The most common content of delusion in schizophrenia is persecution. Unlike the form of the delusion, the content is determined by the maturational, emotional, social, educational, and cultural background of the patient.

Kretschmer (1927) stressed the importance of the underlying personality for the explanation of some delusional

Table 2.2 Content of delusion.

Content	Example
Delusions of persecution	"No matter wherever I go, there are cameras filming me to know what I do"
Delusions of influence/control	"My brain has no bricks and my feelings are controlled from the outside because they are accessible to everyone"
Thought withdrawal	"My thoughts are removed from my mind by strangers when I pass them in the street"
Thought insertion	"They put thoughts in my mind that are not mine"
Thought broadcasting	"Everyone knows what I am thinking because my brain is transparent"
Morbid jealousy	"My wife cheats on me with everyone, even our neighbors and friends"
Delusions of love (erotomania)*	"I would give my life for my loved one who, although he makes others believe he does not know me, is truly and deeply in love with me"
Delusional misidentification	
Capgras syndrome	"My sister has been replaced by a double"
Fregoli syndrome	"You [to an stranger] are my sister, do not try to pretend you are not"
Grandiose delusions	"I have the mission to save this world"
Religious delusions	"I am the Virgin Mary and cannot have contact with men"

*de Clerambault described a variant of erotomania in which a woman believes that a man, who is usually older and of higher social status that she, is in love with her. The person who is supposed to be in love has done nothing to deserve her attention and is usually quite unaware of her existence, and sometimes is even a famous person.

experiences. He described the sensitive personality in people who retain affect-laden complexes and have a limited capacity for emotional self-expressions. This type of person is usually rigid and paranoid, and has sensitive ideas of reference. A trigger experience may happen in life circumstances and the ideas are structured as delusions of reference.

Patients with schizophrenia experience abnormal perceptions, mainly in the form of sensory distortions, where real objects are perceived to be distorted, and false perceptions, where a new perception occurs that may or may not be in response to an external stimulus. In false perceptions, we have illusions and hallucinations, which were separated phenomenologically by Esquirol (1838). Illusions are transformations of perceptions, with a mixing of the reproduced perceptions of the subject's fantasy with the real perceptions. An hallucination is a perception without object and the most common, although not at all specific, hallucinations in schizophrenia are auditory. Kandinsky (1890) described pseudohallucinations as a separate form of perception, as they are recognized by the subject as having no external correlate. Another abnormality of perception experienced by patients with schizophrenia is autoscopy, the experience of seeing oneself and knowing that it is oneself (also called phantom mirror image).

Hallucinations can occur in any sensory modality (auditory, visual, olfactory, gustatory and tactile, somatic or kinesthetic). Around 50% of patients with schizophrenia experience auditory hallucinations, 15% visual, and 5% tactile (DeLeon et al., 1993). These anomalous experiences are usually present at the time of the first psychotic episode. The most common hallucinatory experiences are voices talking to the patient or among themselves. On many occasions, the voice, which can be identified as male or female, is not associated with anyone known by the patient. The voice is usually clear, objective, and definite, and experienced as coming from the outside. Sometimes these experiences are pleasurable and patients feel comfort when hearing reassuring comments by the voices. Occasionally, patients experience command hallucinations that, in most instances, are not obeyed. Particularly characteristic of schizophrenia are voices that repeat the patient's thoughts aloud, give commentaries on the patient's actions or thoughts, or argue with one another and talk to the patient in the third person. The three types of auditory hallucinations described as first-rank symptoms by Kurt Schneider are given in Table 2.1.

The neural correlates of auditory hallucinations have been studied with functional imaging showing activations associated with auditory hallucinations in a network of cortical and subcortical areas, some of which match those activated during normal hearing (Silbersweig et al., 1995; Shergill et al., 2000).

The different mechanisms used by patients with schizophrenia to cope with hallucinations are related to changes in behavior (e.g., seeking someone to talk to or change in environment), changes in sensory/affective state (e.g., exercise, thinking about pleasurable moments) or changes in cognition (e.g., control of attention) (Falloon & Talbot, 1981).

Disorganization: thought and behavior

Most patients with schizophrenia have different degrees of impairment in the thought process. Formal thought disorders can be assessed from manifestations present in speech and from the patient's subjective awareness of disturbed thought patterns.

The most prominent formal thought disorders in schizophrenia are retardation, circumstantiality, tangentiality, derailment, thought blocking, and perseveration. Patients with retardation take a long time before answering questions, showing a delay before producing any speech. Mutism would be the extreme form of retardation. In circumstantiality, patients give unnecessary details, obscuring and decorating the answers before getting to the point. Unlike tangentiality, where the patient never gets to the point, in circumstantiality, the question is eventually answered. In derailment, there is a breakdown in association with no logical connection in the chain of thoughts. The patient is unable to link the flow of ideas, and there are illogical and unconnected changes in the direction of thinking. In thought blocking, the patient experiences a sudden breaking of the train of thought, without an explanation for this. Illogicality is the tendency to offer bizarre explanations for things and events. It is present where there are erroneous conclusions or internal contradictions in thinking. Illogicality is a difficult category that survives in disputed territory between disorders of thought form and content. Neologism is the creation of new words. Some patients also distort words or use real words in an idiosyncratic manner. Paraphasia is the use of a word with a new meaning. A remarkable feature of neologism and paraphasia is that patients with schizophrenia usually seem unaware that they lack meaning for the listener. Finally, in perseveration, the patient repeats an idea or an answer that has become inappropriate.

Abnormal thought processes in schizophrenia usually result in concrete thinking with literalness of expression and understanding. Concrete thinking is a tendency to select one aspect of a concept or thing at the expense of the overall meaning. It is usually tested with interpretation of proverbs and similitudes between things or categories. These patients also have problems with abstraction and symbolism.

Andreasen (1979) studied the incidence of 18 varieties of thought disorders in patients with diagnoses of mania, depression, and schizophrenia. She argued against the pathognomonic characteristic that Eugen Bleuler had given to these symptoms in schizophrenia. In the study, derailment was the most common variety in patients with schizophrenia (56%), but it did not discriminate between patients with mania and schizophrenia. Other symptoms, such as neologism or blocking, were very rare.

Negative symptoms

In general, negative symptoms are conceptualized as disorders of omission, or things patients do not do. In schizophrenia, disturbances of volition are more at the level of motivation or will than at the level of need.

The distinction between positive and negative symptoms was originally introduced by Reynolds (1828–1896) and Jackson (1834–1911) (see Berrios, 1985). Jackson described positive symptoms as an exaggeration of normal brain processes, whereas negative symptoms were conceptualized as a diminution or negation of normal processes. Jackson's concept of hierarchical organization of the brain was that negative symptoms were secondary to tissue destruction and that positive symptoms were disinhibiting consequences for that tissue destruction. Kraepelin (1919) provided a compelling framework to distinguish between positive and negative symptoms, referring to two groups of maladies within dementia praecox:

> There are apparently two principal groups of disorders which characterize the malady. On one hand we observe a weakening of those emotional activities which permanently form the mainsprings of volition. The results of this part of the morbid process is emotional dullness, failure of mental activities, loss of mastery over volition, of endeavour, and ability for independent action. The essence of personality is thereby destroyed, the best and most precious part of its being, as Griesinger once expressed it, torn from her.

Strauss et al. (1974) reintroduced negative symptom terminology, supporting the advantages of using three different types of psychopathological manifestations: positive symptoms, negative symptoms, and disorders of relating. Subsequently, Crow (1985) described Type I and Type II schizophrenia, with various criteria, one being the presence of negative symptoms in Type II schizophrenia. Andreasen and Olsen (1982) conceptualized positive and negative symptoms as different ends of the same continuum and described patients as either predominantly positive or negative, and subsequently introducing a third mixed group.

In many instances, negative symptoms are present before the onset of positive symptomatology. They are present through the psychotic phase, when they are usually obscured by florid positive symptoms, and usually persist to varying degrees once the positive symptoms remit. Negative symptoms vary depending on the scale used to

Table 2.3 Most common negative symptoms and definitions.

Alogia	Marked poverty of speech, or poverty of content of speech
Affective flattening or blunted affect	Reduction in emotional expressiveness
Anhedonia	Inability to experience pleasure
Asociality	Lack of interest in social contacts
Avolition	Lack of motivation
Apathy	General lack of interest

assess them. The most commonly used assessment scales have been the Scale for the Assessment of Negative Symptoms (SANS; Andreasen, 1983), the Positive and Negative Syndrome Scale (PANSS; Kay et al., 1987), Negative Symptom Assessment (NSA; Alphs et al., 1989), and the Schedule for the Deficit Syndrome (SDS) (Kirkpatrick et al., 1989). The generally accepted negative symptoms are shown in Table 2.3.

Negative symptoms are more important for prognosis than positive symptoms. It is important to distinguish between primary and secondary negative symptoms, as these may be due to positive symptoms (e.g., not wanting to go into the street for fear of being killed), medication (e.g., parkinsonism), depression (e.g., anhedonia) or institutionalization. If negative symptoms are to be useful in the etiopathophysiology of schizophrenia, they should be direct expressions of such processes (Carpenter et al., 1988). Enduring, primary negative symptoms have been distinguished from negative symptoms in general and are used to define deficit syndrome in schizophrenia (Carpenter et al., 1988). The validity of deficit syndrome has been demonstrated using brain imaging, neuropsychological, neurological, illness outcome, and developmental history data, temporal stability, and treatment response (Kirkpatrick et al., 2001). The distinction between primary and negative symptoms is also important at the level of drug treatment and drug discovery, and novel approaches such as antipsychotics have not proven effective in primary negative symptoms (Arango et al., 2004, Kirkpatrick et al., 2006).

Cognition

Cognitive deficits, discussed in detail in Chapter 8, have been considered core features of schizophrenia since the original descriptions by Kraepelin (1919) and Bleuler (1911). It has been consistently shown that patients with schizophrenia have cognitive deficits right from the onset of psychotic symptoms (Good et al., 2004) and even in the prodromal period (Simon et al., 2007) or well before showing any kind of symptomatology (Reichenberg et al., 2006).

Post-psychotic deterioration does not seem to occur as duration of illness has not been significantly related to cognitive level (Gold *et al.*, 1999) and most longitudinal studies do not show further deterioration (Nopoulos *et al.*, 1994; Hoff *et al.*, 2005). However, deterioration or a developmental arrest may account for reduced cognitive capacity during childhood and early adolescence.

One problem in the assessment of cognition in schizophrenia has been the lack of standard assessment scales. The assessment scales used differ in domains assessed, time requirements, repeatability, ease of administration, face validity, and availability of co-normative data (Kraus & Keefe, 2007). Under the name of Measurement and Treatment Research to Improve Cognition in Schizophrenia (MATRICS), a consensus cognitive battery has been developed for clinical trials of cognition-enhancing treatments for schizophrenia through a broadly based scientific evaluation of measurements. MATRICS has recently been validated (Nuechterlein *et al.*, 2008; Kern *et al.*, 2008). Seven separable cognitive factors were replicable across studies and represent fundamental dimensions of cognitive deficit in schizophrenia that may be amenable to change (Verbal Comprehension was not included, as it was thought to be resistant to change): Speed of Processing, Attention/Vigilance, Working Memory, Verbal Learning and Memory, Visual Learning and Memory, Reasoning and Problem Solving, and Social Cognition.

Cognitive impairment is associated with poorer prognosis and functional outcome (Bowie *et al.*, 2008), negative symptoms (O'Leary *et al.*, 2000); more specifically to deficit syndrome (Buchanan *et al.*, 1994), and disorganized symptoms (Bilder *et al.*, 1985; Cuesta & Peralta, 1995), but not with positive symptoms (Cuesta & Peralta, 1995; O'Leary *et al.*, 2000). Patients with deficit syndrome seem to do more poorly in social cognition, global cognition, and language (Cohen *et al.*, 2007).

Motor/neurological signs

Movement disorders are characteristic of catatonia, in which the patient may become immobilized in a retarded–stuporous way or, on the contrary, with hyperactivity in an excited–delirious variety of catatonia. Karl Ludwig Kahlbaum (1973) characterized catatonia as a specific disturbance in motor functioning that represents a phase in a progressive illness that typically ends in dementia. Later, Emil Kraepelin incorporated the features of catatonia into his concept of dementia praecox. Bleuler followed Kraepelin's conceptual model for catatonia and, although numerous authors have argued against this view (Taylor & Fink, 2003), catatonia has been considered a subtype of schizophrenia in all DSM and ICD editions.

The most common signs are posturing, mutism, stupor, negativism, staring, rigidity, and echophenomena, but the

Table 2.4 Diagnostic criteria for schizophrenia, catatonic type [DSM-IV 295.20] (from *Diagnostic and Statistical Manual of Mental Disorders*, 4th edn. American Psychiatric Association, 1994.).

A type of schizophrenia in which the clinical picture is dominated by at least two of the following:

1. Motoric immobility as evidenced by catalepsy (including waxy flexibility) or stupor

2. Excessive motor activity (that is apparently purposeless and not influenced by external stimuli)

3. Extreme negativism (an apparently motiveless resistance to all instructions or maintenance of rigid posture against attempts to be moved) or mutism

4. Peculiarities of voluntary movement as evidenced by posturing (voluntary assumption of inappropriate or bizarre postures), stereotyped movements, prominent mannerisms or prominent grimaces

5. Echolalia or echopraxia

presence of two prominent signs is sufficient for the patient to meet the current DSM criteria (Table 2.4).

The two most common abnormal movements in schizophrenia are mannerisms and stereotypy. Mannerisms are idiosyncratic voluntary movements that are odd and stilted, although they seem to have a purpose. Grimacing, for instance, is a common feature in schizophrenia. Stereotypy is a constant repetition of certain meaningless gestures or movements that are not goal-directed. The posture may be retained for a long time.

Patients may be stuporous with a virtual absence of movements and speech while fully conscious. Some patients with schizophrenia show abnormalities in the execution of movements. This can take the form of negativism, automatic obedience, or ambitendency in which there is an alternation of cooperation and opposition. Other abnormal movements are mitgehen (the patient's limbs can be moved by slight pressure, despite being told to resist the pressure) and echopraxia (imitating the movements of another person). Finally, waxy flexibility, now rarely seen, describes a posture maintained indefinitely after being manipulated into that attitude by the observer.

Patients with schizophrenia, healthy relatives, and patients at risk of developing schizophrenia also show neurological soft signs. These signs have been described as non-localizing neurological abnormalities that cannot be related to impairment of a specific brain region or are not believed to be part of a well-defined neurological syndrome (signs elicited through graphesthesia, stereoagnosis, motor coordination assessment, go/no go test, or primitive reflexes). Their occurrence is independent of demographic variables and most medication variables. Neurological signs are strongly associated with negative symptoms and cognitive impairment, and have been used in some studies as prognostic markers (Bombin *et al.*, 2005).

Phenotypes

In addition to symptomatic manifestations, schizophrenia is associated with a number of information processing and neuroanatomic variables that distinguish the syndrome from normal control cohorts. These include electrophysiological measures related to sensory gating phenomena (e.g., P50 and PPI; Braff & Light, 2005; Javitt *et al.*, 2008), to early and late components of evoked response potentials, and to differences in functional anatomy measured with neuroimaging techniques during task performance.

Considered intermediate between symptomatic manifestations and pathophysiology, such measures may reduce heterogeneity, provide more decisive assessment of genetic associations, and contribute to the understanding of pathophysiology. The use of endophenotypes is an alternative method for measuring phenotypic variation that may facilitate the identification of susceptibility genes for complexly inherited traits, rather than the use of more heterogeneous diagnostic groups, such as the schizophrenia phenotype (Braff *et al.*, 2007). Endophenotypes are now hypothesized to be treatment targets for drug development (Thaker, 2007).

Other aspects critical to clinical evaluation and treatment

Developmental history and prognostic indicators

Accurate diagnosis of psychotic disorders at early stages of the disease has critical clinical relevance, since the importance of early treatment implementation has been demonstrated using different measures of outcome (Keshavan & Amirsadri, 2007).

This variable has been conceptualized mainly as the level of social functioning prior to the onset of illness, and it has been suggested that it may be an important factor related to diagnosis, disease progression, and outcome (Addington *et al.*, 2007). It has also been reported that there is an association between premorbid adjustment and certain aspects of illness. Negative symptoms have been related to poorer premorbid adjustment in patients with first-episode schizophrenia (Buchanan *et al.*, 1990). Poor premorbid adjustment in schizophrenia has been associated with male sex, earlier age at onset, illness severity, negative symptoms, worse response, poor outcome (Schmael *et al.*, 2007), and worse response to treatment after a first episode (Rabinowitz *et al.*, 2006).

Emotion and suicide

Emotion is a non-specific term covering feeling, affect and mood. Different languages have different descriptions that are not equal when translated. Feeling is used to describe a positive or negative reaction to an experience, in Jaspers' words, "an individual unique and radical commotion of the psyche" (Jaspers, 1946/1963). Affect is used to describe a momentary differentiated specific emotional process directed towards objects; in Jaspers words, "a momentary and complex emotional process of great intensity with conspicuous bodily accompaniment and sequelae" (Jaspers, 1946/1963). Mood is a more pervasive state or disposition describing the state of the self in relation to its environment; in Jaspers' words, "states of feeling of frames of mind that come about with prolonged emotion" (Jaspers, 1946/1963).

All feelings, affect, mood, and motivation have different phenomenological varieties and can be abnormal in schizophrenia (Table 2.5). Some of those symptoms are regarded as part of the dimensions of disorganization (inappropriate affect) or negative symptoms (blunted affect, apathy, or loss of motivation). Some of the affective symptoms may in turn be reactive to the stress of the primary schizophrenia experiences.

The rate of depression in schizophrenia varies greatly in the published studies (Koreen *et al.*, 1993; Bressan *et al.*, 2003). Depression has been found to be more prevalent in women and patients with first-episode schizophrenia (Emsley *et al.*, 1999). People with comorbid schizophrenia and depressive symptoms have poorer long-term functional outcomes in terms of poorer quality of life, greater use of mental health services, higher risk of problems with the law, and higher risk of suicide (Siris *et al.*, 2001; Conley *et al.*, 2007). Post-schizophrenic depression is defined as depression occurring following or in conjunction with psy-

Table 2.5 Disturbances of emotion [reproduced with permission from Cutting, J. (2003) Descriptive psychopathology. In: Hirsch, S.R. & Weinberger, D., eds. *Schizophrenia*, 2nd edn. Oxford: Blackwell Science].

Normal aspects	Main psychopathological varieties
Feeling	Loss of feeling—anhedonia
	Heightened feeling
Affect	Inappropriate affect
	Flattened, blunted affect
Mood	Depression
	Elation
	Anxiety
Motivation	Apathy

chotic symptoms in a person with schizophrenia and is included as a subtype in the ICD-10. Depression-like symptoms may also be confounded with antipsychotic side effects, neuroleptic-induced dysphoria, or negative symptoms (Van Putten & May, 1978; Carpenter, 1995).

Suicide is unfortunately one of the leading causes of death in people with schizophrenia. Up to 40% of people who have schizophrenia will attempt suicide at least once. Males with schizophrenia attempt suicide at a much higher rate than females; approximately 60% of males will make at least one attempt. The result of these attempts is that between 5% and 13% of people with schizophrenia die by suicide (Pompili et al., 2007). Risk factors for suicide in schizophrenia are comorbid depression and substance abuse, feelings of hopelessness and loss, fear of mental disintegration, a first episode, especially in previously high-functioning patients, and periods of exacerbation of psychotic symptoms (Caldwell & Gottesman, 1990; Drake et al., 1984). Suicide ideation and planning, as well as a prior history of suicide ideation and attempts, should always be part of the clinical history when assessing patients with schizophrenia. Protective factors (e.g., social and family support) also play an important role in assessing suicide risk and should also be carefully evaluated.

Substance abuse

Substance use disorder is very common in patients with schizophrenia as half of patients are also substance abusers at some time during their illness (Buckley, 1998). Drug use, abuse, and dependence drastically worsen the outcome. Substance use in patients with schizophrenia has been associated with poor social adjustment, more hospitalizations and relapses, medication non-compliance, and poor treatment response (Dixon et al., 1990; Brady & Sinha, 2005; see also Chapter 31).

All patients with schizophrenia should be assessed and monitored carefully regarding their substance use. As acute intoxication and withdrawal from drugs of abuse can mimic symptoms of schizophrenia disorders, the overlap of symptoms can be problematic in making an accurate diagnosis. Therefore, a thorough examination about use of drugs and the temporal relationship with symptoms is necessary for the differential diagnosis between schizophrenia and a drug-induced psychosis.

A thorough physical exploration may be done in patients with schizophrenia and comorbid substance abuse, especially if symptoms related to the most common comorbid medical conditions are present [e.g., cardiovascular disease, liver complications, lung cancer, human immunodeficiency virus (HIV) and hepatitis B or C infections; Ziedonis et al., 2005].

Physical health

Mortality due to all causes has been shown to be considerably greater among patients with chronic schizophrenia than in the general population in different settings (Brown et al., 2000; Morgan et al., 2003). The reasons for this excess mortality include patients' lifestyle, increased suicidality, premature development of cardiovascular disease, and high prevalence of metabolic syndrome (MS) and carbohydrate and lipid metabolic disorders (Bobes et al., 2007a). The heightened health risks in schizophrenia are associated with the medications used in its treatment (Marder et al., 2004; see also Chapters 27 and 28.).

Patients with schizophrenia show a higher rate of tobacco smoking than the general population, which has been related to the effect of nicotine on the neurobiology of schizophrenia and to sociocultural factors (Srinivasan & Thara, 2002; DeLeon & Diaz, 2005; Martin & Freedman, 2007). In turn, compared with general population subjects, people with schizophrenia also have more respiratory symptoms and poorer lung function (Filik et al., 2006).

In patients with schizophrenia, the prevalence of diabetes has been reported to be between 9% and 14% (Lindenmayer et al., 2003; Kabinoff et al., 2003), and of dyslipidemia and hypertension to be 43% and 30%, respectively (Gupta et al., 2003). The Clinical Antipsychotic Trials of Intervention Effectiveness (CATIE), which included patients receiving antipsychotic treatment matched for age, race, and gender, compared with subjects from the National Health and Nutrition Examination Study (NHANES) study (McEvoy et al., 2005; Meyer et al., 2005; Goff et al., 2005a, Stroup et al., 2006), estimated the mean risk of serious fatal and non-fatal coronary heart disease (CHD) within 10 years, according to the Framingham function, at 9.4% in males and 6.3% in females (Goff et al., 2005a). These figures are higher than those reported for the general population in the US, i.e., 7.0% in males and 4.2% in females (Plan and Operation of the Third National Health and Nutrition Examination Survey, 1988–1994). Clinicians treating patients with schizophrenia should monitor their metabolic and cardiovascular status. Patients with schizophrenia on antipsychotics are more prone to obesity than the general population (Allison et al., 1999). Overweight and obesity not only increase cardiovascular and metabolic morbidity and mortality but also have important effects on an individual's adjustment in the community, adherence to prescribed medication, and self-image (Marder et al., 2004). Intervention programs targeted to reducing smoking (Goff et al., 2005a) and to improving diet and fostering healthy lifestyles, including efforts to combat general and abdominal obesity (Goff et al., 2005b), as well as to choosing an appropriate antipsychotic treatment that does not cause or worsen these variables are of the utmost importance in the integral treatment of patients with schizophrenia.

Patients with schizophrenia also have a higher rate of hepatitis C, osteoporosis, altered pain sensitivity, sexual dysfunction, obstetric complications, dental problems, and polydipsia than the general population (Carney *et al.*, 2006, Leucht *et al.*, 2007). The relationship with HIV is controversial: some studies find a higher rate of HIV, but one recent study found that those with a concomitant substance use disorder were 22% more likely to have HIV, and those with schizophrenia but no concomitant substance use disorder were 50% less likely to have HIV (Himelhoch *et al.*, 2007).

Despite this vulnerability to different physical illnesses, persons with schizophrenia are at risk for failure to receive medical services. Patients with schizophrenia should have routine physical examinations and their physical symptoms should be explored no differently from those of the general population, even if they have fewer complaints about them. Both psychiatrists and physicians in medical specialties other than psychiatry should be aware of the frequent comorbidity between schizophrenia and physical illness. Health promotion is especially important in this patient population (Marder *et al.*, 2004).

Other critical issues, including sexual dysfunction, sleep problems, and eating disorders

Sexual dysfunctions are not uncommon in patients with schizophrenia. These can be secondary to the disease itself or an adverse event of antipsychotic medication (Malik, 2007). Prevalences for sexual dysfunctions in schizophrenia are as high as 54% for low sexual desire or 42% for problems in having an orgasm (Uçok *et al.*, 2007). In the same study, erectile dysfunction and ejaculation problems were seen in 48.1% and 64.2% of the men, respectively; amenorrhea was seen in 24.9% of the women (Uçok *et al.*, 2007). Examination of sexual dysfunction is important as it not only results in a reduction of the quality of life but is also associated with medication non-adherence (Smith *et al.*, 2002; see also Chapter 31).

Sleep disturbances are common in patients with schizophrenia and include long sleep-onset latencies, poor sleep efficiency, slow wave sleep deficits, and reduction in stage 4 sleep and rapid eye movement (REM) latencies (Benson, 2006). Schizophrenia can also be associated with comorbid sleep disorders, and insomnia is one of the prodromal symptoms associated with psychotic relapse. Aggressive treatment seems to be important in patients with schizophrenia suffering from insomnia as it has been related to poor outcome and suicidal ideation (Singareddy & Balon, 2001).

Some patients with schizophrenia suffer form different types of eating disorders. In an analysis of 119 long-term outcome studies of anorexia nervosa, covering 5590 patients, a mean of 4.6% of patients with anorexia nervosa

were diagnosed with schizophrenia in the long run (Steinhausen, 2002). However, other studies have not found an association between the two disorders (Halmi *et al.*, 1991). In any case, as previously mentioned, many patients with schizophrenia suffer from obesity or starvation due to poor control of food habits. Therefore, patients with schizophrenia are in need of supervised dietetic counseling, close monitoring, and stabilization of their nutritional status.

Social and occupational role performance

Deficits in social functioning are a hallmark phenomena in schizophrenia. Impairments in adaptive life skills are a major source of disability in patients with schizophrenia. Any interview with patients with schizophrenia must assess issues such as socioeconomic status, social difficulties, life skills, occupational role, problems with previous jobs, social and family support. Differential predictors of functional competence and performance have been found to be related to discrete neuropsychological domains. The attention/working memory domain has been related to work skills, executive functions to interpersonal behaviors, and processing speed to many real-world behaviors (Bowie *et al.*, 2008). In this study, all neuropsychological domains predicted functional competence, but only processing speed and attention/working memory predicted social competence. Cognitive performance was shown to be a better predictor of job tenure than job attainment in a clinical trial of two vocational rehabilitation approaches (Gold *et al.*, 2002).

Quality of life

Quality of life is defined by the World Health Organization as, "Individuals' perceptions of their position in life in the context of the culture and value systems in which they live, and in relation to their goals, expectations, standards, and concerns" (WHOQOL Group, 1995). Patients with schizophrenia have a worse quality of life than that of the general population and usually worse that that of other physically ill patients (see Chapter 7). A longer length of the illness, more psychopathology, especially negative and depressive symptoms, and more side effects are related to a worse quality of life. On the other hand, family support and integration in community support programs are related to a better quality of life (Bobes *et al.*, 2007b).

Assessment of quality of life should be explored in patients with schizophrenia although this may be a controversial issue. Despite the fact that assessment of quality of life has to take into account patients' right of autonomy, which necessarily includes their opinion, symptoms of schizophrenia may affect the mental, emotional, and social judgments on which patients' responses to quality of life instruments are based. This would translate into a distortion of self-report ratings of both quality of life and the impact of health-related life events (Atkinson *et al.*, 1997). Some authors suggest that in patients with prominent perceptual distortions, lack of insight, delusions or response bias, self-report instruments should be discarded in favor of assessment made by treatment professionals or proxy report measures based on observable or descriptive data (Jenkins, 1992).

Paradigm shift

Kraepelin joined putative disease entities of paranoia, catatonia, and hebephrenia into one disease (dementia praecox) and observed that avolition and dissociative pathology were the two primary defining attributes. This disease was separated from the manic-depressive psychoses and formed the basis for the two illnesses of the dichotomy for psychosis. Blueler hypothesized that the dissociative pathology was the core feature for all cases of what he termed schizophrenia. For more than a century the dominant paradigm has been schizophrenia as a disease entity. However, the key evidence for a disease (rather than a syndrome) has not been established at the level of etiopathophysiology, and it has not been documented that all cases meeting schizophrenia criteria share the dissociative pathology hypothesized by Bleuler. In all other regards (e.g., onset, course, treatment response, biomarkers, quality of life, function, genes, epidemiological risk factors), substantial heterogeneity is observed. At the definitional level, schizophrenia is a syndrome rather than a single disease entity: more compatible with Bleuler's "the group of schizophrenias" than with a unifying pathophysiology manifest as dissociative pathology.

The concept of nuclear schizophrenia, based on the work of Schneider and Langfeldt, evolved the definition of schizophrenia with far greater emphasis on reality distortion pathology. This concept was incorporated in the DSM-III and has been influential. The result has been a de-emphasis on dissociative pathology (disorganization of thought and behavior in the DSM-III and -IV terminology) and a disconnection between psychosis and avolition—the critical link in Kraepelin's concept. In fact, the only criteria related to avolition (i.e., restricted affect) was omitted in DSM-III and included only as an optional criteria in DSM-IV. Reality distortion symptoms (i.e., hallucinations and delusions) are caused by many diverse pathological processes, such as temporal lobe epilepsy, affective disorders, and drugs, and are not uncommon in normal populations (van Os, 2003). Heterogeneity of the syndrome is assured with current diagnostic criteria. A major challenge in understanding schizophrenia and in study designs is the reduction of this heterogeneity. The studies that led to the rejection of the nuclear schizophrenia concept and the paradigm shifts described below have been briefly summarized (Carpenter, 2006).

Disease entity *versus* domains of pathology

There are two conceptual approaches to reducing heterogeneity of syndromes: defining separate disease entities within the syndrome or defining separate pathological processes. The first approach has had minimal success. The traditional subtyping of schizophrenia began with paranoid, catatonic, hebephrenic, and simple (added by Bleuler) and have not proven heuristic in this regard. Too many cases are mixed, and subtype designation changes too often for a case over the course of illness. Current subtypes in ICD-10 and DSM-IV-R receive little attention. An alternative approach involves reconceptualizing subtypes. New subtype hypotheses include the Kraepelinian type (Keefe *et al.*, 1996), Type I/II (1985), and deficit schizophrenia (Carpenter *et al.*, 1988; Kirkpatrick *et al.*, 2001).

The second approach has been considered as dimensions or domains of pathology. This paradigm emerged from work in the Washington Center of the International Pilot Study of Schizophrenia. At the time it was expected that symptoms defining nuclear schizophrenia would reduce heterogeneity and identify cases with a progressive course and poor outcome. First-rank symptoms of Schneider and characteristic symptoms of true schizophrenia as proposed by Langfeldt were used to define nuclear schizophrenia. However, when separating broadly defined schizophrenia into two groups (i.e., nuclear or true schizophrenia and non-nuclear or pseudoschizophrenia), the hypothesized prognostic significance was not confirmed. Outcome was composed of several areas such as course of psychosis, social outcomes, and occupational functioning. These areas were only weakly related to each other over time, and nuclear symptoms had little predictive validity. A far stronger relationship was found between measures of function prior to the onset of psychosis and the outcome measures. Also, outcome domain was best predicted by functioning in the same area during the developmental, pre-psychotic era. Strauss *et al.* (1974) interpreted these data as representing domains of pathology observed within the schizophrenia syndrome and proposed that each domain represented the target for etiological, pathophysiological, and therapeutic discovery. The weak correlation between psychosis measures and outcome measures suggested that schizophrenia defined by psychotic symptoms was a poor object for study. The continuity over time of the premorbid or prognostic factors with the outcome factors suggested that these features were early morbid manifestations rather than premorbid features. The question of age of onset of schizophrenia was thus transformed.

These studies and subsequent work support a new paradigm based on deconstructing schizophrenia into discrete

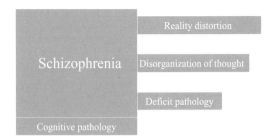

Fig. 2.1 The tripartite model.

pathological processes. The initial proposal defined three domains: positive psychotic symptoms (i.e., disorganization of thought, delusions, and hallucinations); negative symptoms (reduction of normal functions observed as restricted affect, alogia, and anergia); and pathology that is best observed in the interpersonal sphere (poor rapport, low social drive). It was later observed by Andreasen and Olsen (1982) that hallucinations and delusions form a separate factor from disorganization of thought and behavior.

The importance of these symptom domains would not surprise Kraepelin or Bleuler, but the emphasis in this paradigm is different. Rather than viewing these domains as varied expressions of a single latent structure or secondary manifestation, the domains paradigm views each pathological domain as having its own latent structure, different from the other domains. Another domain of interest relates to basic cognitive processes. Long observed to be impaired in schizophrenia, current emphasis results from the more extensive neuropsychological data and the robust association of cognition impairment with functional outcomes (Green, 2006). Just as the symptom domains are weakly correlated, neuropsychological test scores are relatively independent of the symptom domains (Heinrichs & Zakzanis, 1998; Harvey *et al.*, 2006). A common view of the domains paradigm at present is represented in Figure 2.1 including impaired cognition.

Onset of illness in each paradigm

When viewing schizophrenia as a disease entity, onset is usually depicted as late adolescence/early adulthood in males and adulthood in females. The data supporting this view are based on psychotic symptoms and initiation of diagnosis and treatment.

When viewing schizophrenia as a syndrome deconstructed into domains of pathology, the onset of illness question is more complex. The above view fits for the psychotic domains of reality distortion and disorganization. Even here there is substantial variation with childhood-onset cases at one extreme and late age onset at the other. The negative symptoms of schizophrenia are pathological

traits and often precede the onset of psychosis by years. Developmental history suggests that some cases may have the pathological traits from birth with a schizoid developmental trajectory. Cognitive pathology may be impaired at birth, and may be further reduced between the ages of about 5 and 15 (Seidman *et al.*, 2006; Woodberry *et al.*, 2008). Much of the data are based on IQ testing where future patients with schizophrenia lose ground to their peers during developmental years and plateau at a lower IQ level than predicted from parental sociodemographic variables. Cognitive capacity appears as a stable trait thereafter and does not manifest as a progressive disease beyond the early years. The average loss in IQ points is estimated to be in the 5–10 point range.

Onset of illness must be determined separately for each pathological domain, and questions of progression addressed for each.

Therapeutic implications of the paradigm shift

The single disease paradigm with the underlying assumption that psychosis is the latent disease structure has been effective in developing therapeutic approaches to psychosis, but these have not proven to be broadly efficacious for the range of pathology observed in patients with this diagnosis. For over 50 years dopamine antagonists have been marketed for schizophrenia, but no drugs have proven to be efficacious for primary negative symptoms or cognitive pathology. The focus on domains places drug discovery on an entirely different path (Carpenter & Koenig, 2008). Rather than seeking molecular targets for the primary pathological process underlying the various manifestations, discovery is based on the assumptions of multiple pathological processes. Each domain is a target for clinical assessment, and each merits therapeutic emphasis. This paradigm shift has occurred in a major National Institute for Mental Health (NIMH) initiative and the Food and Drug Administration (FDA) has agreed on clinical trial designs that would support an indication for therapeutic efficacy for cognition or for negative symptoms (Buchanan *et al.*, 2005; Kirkpatrick *et al.*, 2006).

Anticipating DSM-V and ICD-11

The next addition of DSM-V is scheduled for 2013 and ICD-11 is due some time after that. It is expected that the two manuals will have extensive similarity. The following is based on the authors' personal view of likely developments relating to schizophrenia in DSM-V.

There is little doubt that the current diagnostic classes associated with psychosis will be radically revised when etiology and pathophysiology are detailed for the various diseases associated with psychosis. This has already been achieved to a degree in diagnostic distinctions between temporal lobe epilepsy, syphylitic psychosis, phencyclidine psychosis, etc. However, among the major psychotic conditions that remain at the syndrome level, there is insufficient progress to base a radical revision on an etiological footing. Although caseness in classification will continue to be based principally on pattern and type of symptomatic manifestation, it is hoped that biomarkers might clarify the classification structure. These intermediate manifestations are based on genotype and phenotype information drawn from genetics, imaging, electrophysiological and other biomarkers. Data from these fields have increased knowledge regarding the porous and imperfect boundaries between current classes of psychoses. But they have not yet established new putative disease entities, nor are these data sufficient to redesign the classification of psychoses. We therefore anticipate that classes such as schizophrenia and bipolar disorders will be present in the next editions of the diagnostic manuals.

Nosological classes for DSM-V and ICD-11

At the level of diagnostic class, the following issues, in addition with to those described in the introduction to the diagnostic category, Attenuated Psychotic Symptoms Syndrome, will be considered.

Should schizoaffective schizophrenia exist as a class?

And, if so, should it be grouped with bipolar disorders instead of schizophrenia? Is schizoaffective disorder with mania different from schizoaffective disorder with depression?

Schizoaffective disorder has not been documented as a separate syndrome. Study designs are badly flawed in that criteria and concept will capture some patients who have schizophrenia and some who have affective disorders with psychosis. It has not been possible to determine if a third separate group truly exists. If there is a superordinate category of psychosis associated with affective disturbance, then schizoaffective disorder will disappear from the nomenclature and these cases will join those drawn from depression with psychosis, bipolar with psychosis, and schizophrenia with affective disturbance (Cheniaux *et al.*, 2008).

Are cases of bipolar I with psychosis more similar to cases with schizophrenia than they are to bipolar II without psychosis?

A number of studies support this proposition, but the question remains as to whether there are valid syndrome distinctive measures and, if so, are these being used to test for similarities and differences. For example, bipolar patients' neurocognitive scores are impaired compared to non-ill controls and the pattern appears similar to schizophrenia except less severe. But in schizophrenia the cognition impairments are early onset traits while in bipolar they appear more state dependent. Both syndromes are associated with reality distortion symptoms, but also with anxiety and depression. These may be general psychopathological manifestations associated with many disorders. The avolitional pathology described by Kraepelin may be more informative, but this domain has not been the focus of studies comparing the two syndromes. Patients with a diagnosis of schizophrenia can be divided into a subgroup with avolitional pathology (i.e., primary negative symptoms), referred to as deficit schizophrenia; and into a subgroup without this pathologic domain (i.e., non-deficit schizophrenia) (see above). The former group has restricted affect and low drive and is unlikely to experience depression. Comparison of patients with bipolar disorder with psychosis to the deficit group may show critical differences, while comparisons to the non-deficit group may maximize similarities. Because these types of specific comparisons have not been made, it is unlikely that there will sufficient evidence to determine if the diagnostic classes for major psychoses should be merged, rearranged, or remain in their current status.

An important aspect of the DSM-V process is to achieve a comprehensive review of data on these and other questions to enable the work groups to make recommendations where evidence is compelling.

Spectrum concepts

The schizophrenia spectrum concept is based on the following:
• Similarity in pathological manifestations in cluster A personality disorders (i.e., paranoid, schizoid, and schizotypal and schizophrenia);
• Studies of biological relatives of schizophrenia probands document an increase in traits considered similar to pathology manifest in schizophrenia (e.g., suspiciousness, perceptual aberrations, magical ideation, low sociality, modestly reduced cognitive capacity, and impaired social cognition);
• Tendency for sibs of schizophrenia probands to be intermediate on imaging, cognition, and other measures; intermediate between their schizophrenia sib and healthy controls;
• Family history studies provided stronger evidence for genetic transmission when broader criteria for schizophrenia were used for probands, and when schizophrenia spectrum traits were used to define caseness in the pedigree.
A presentation of 11 potential validating criteria for spectra pathology was given by the Diagnostic Spectra Study Group (Memorandum to workgroup chairs and workgroups. Unpublished data, American Psychiatric Association, 2007).

DSM-V will have to address the question of whether cluster A personality disorders (or, at least, schizotypal personality disorder) should be grouped together with schizophrenia in classification and considered minor versions of the same psychotic syndrome.

The fact that spectrum pathology tends to join schizophrenia with certain personality disorders, while reality distortion pathology combined with affective disturbance tends to erode the boundary between schizophrenia and affective disorders reveals the degree of uncertainty at the level of nosological class. The principle approach to resolving these vexing issues is likely to be derived from the domains of the pathology paradigm and the institution of a system of dimensions to compensate for the lack of knowledge conveyed by diagnostic class.

Introduction of dimensions

The discussion above suggests that dimensions will represent domains of pathology, but this is only one option. Several critical questions will have to be resolved. These include whether dimensions are independent of diagnostic criteria or highly related. Is a patient located at a place on each dimension or located in multidimensional space? Do dimensions replace or complement typology? Are dimensions closely related to defining features of the class and therefore should each be expected to be highly correlated with diagnostic class? Should dimensions be drawn from pathology, function, quality of life, or other attributes relevant to understanding each patient? Should dimensions be selected to guide research, clinical care, or some other purpose?

The position advance here is based on the presumed syndrome status of diagnostic class of schizophrenia. Pathological domains are selected which provide critical information that is not conveyed by the diagnosis *per se*. The dimensions are selected in part to understand the syndrome and guide investigations, and in part to call attention to assessment factors critical to clinical management and therapeutic discovery. Examples of each will illustrate this, together with potential candidates to be used as dimensions.

Persons who receive a diagnosis of schizophrenia may or may not have avolitional pathology. This is not required for the diagnosis, but is an important domain in a subgroup. A negative symptom dimension can be scaled from normal to severe pathology with each patient located somewhere on that scale. This would facilitate finding genes for negative symptoms and call the clinician's attention to this aspect of pathology for management. It would also encourage therapeutic discovery for this specific domain. If this dimension is used in other psychotic classes, it will help clarify points of similarity and difference.

Insomnia is a frequent problem in persons with schizophrenia, but is not part of the diagnostic construct. It is critical for clinical management. Systematic assessment as a dimension may facilitate detection and treatment. This dimension may not be compelling for etiological study.

DSM-V will need to make dimensions "mandatory", user friendly, and their relevance must be clear to the clinician. One implication is that the number needs to be small, and clinicians understand the clinical assessment relevance. A short list might include the following: reality distortion, disorganization, negative symptoms, cognition impairment, depression, mania, anxiety, substance abuse, and suicidality.

Conclusions

Schizophrenia is a major public health problem and a leading cause of suffering and disability. We conceptualise schizophrenia as a syndrome comprising several pathological domains with substantial variability across cases. Manifestations are described and the syndrome is deconstructed. A new paradigm provides a more heuristic guide for discovery.

References

Addington, J., Cadenhead, K.S., Cannon, T.D., *et al.*; North American Prodrome Longitudinal Study (2007) North American Prodrome Longitudinal Study: a collaborative multisite approach to prodromal schizophrenia research. *Schizophrenia Bulletin* **33**, 665–672.

Allardyce, J., McCreadie, R.G., Morrison, G. & van Os, J. (2007) Do symptom dimensions or categorical diagnoses best discriminate between known risk factors for psychosis? *Social Psychiatry Psychiatric Epidemiology* **42**, 429–437.

Allison, D.B., Fontaine, K.R., Heo, M. *et al.* (1999) The distribution of body mass index among individuals with and without schizophrenia. *Journal of Clinical Psychiatry* **60**, 215–220.

Alphs, L.D., Summerfelt, A., Lann, H. & Muller, R.J. (1989) The negative symptom assessment: a new instrument to assess negative symptoms of schizophrenia. *Psychopharmacological Bulletin* **25**, 159–163.

Andreasen, N.C. (1979) Thought, language, and communication disorders. II. Diagnostic significance. *Archives of General Psychiatry* **36**, 1325–1330.

Andreasen, N.C. (1983) *The Scale for the Assessment of Negative Symptoms (SANS)*. Iowa City: University of Iowa.

Andreasen, N.C. & Olsen, S. (1982) Negative v positive schizophrenia. Definition and validation. *Archives of General Psychiatry* **39**, 789–794.

Arango, C., Buchanan, R.W., Kirkpatrick, B. & Carpenter, W.T. (2004) The deficit syndrome in schizophrenia: implications for the treatment of negative symptoms. *European Psychiatry* **19**, 21–26.

Atkinson, M., Zibin, S. & Chuang, H. (1997) Characterizing quality of life among patients with chronic mental illness: A critical examination of the self-report methodology. *American Journal of Psychiatry* **154**, 99–105.

Benson, K.L. (2006) Sleep in schizophrenia: impairments, correlates, and treatment. *Psychiatric Clinics of North America* **29**, 1033–1045.

Berrios, G.E. (1985) Positive and negative symptoms and Jackson. A conceptual history. *Archives of General Psychiatry* **42**, 95–97.

Bilder, R.M., Mukherjee, S., Rieder, R.O. & Pandurangi, A.K. (1985) Symptomatic and neuropsychological components of defect states. *Schizophrenia Bulletin* **11**, 409–419.

Bleuler, E.P. (1911/1959) *Dementia Praecox or the Group of Schizophrenias*. New York: International Universities Press (translated by Zinkin, J.). New York: International Universities Press.

Bobes, J., Arango, C., Aranda, P., Carmena, R., Garcia-Garcia, M. & Rejas, J.; CLAMORS Study Collaborative Group (2007a) Cardiovascular and metabolic risk in outpatients with schizophrenia treated with antipsychotics: results of the CLAMORS Study. *Schizophrenia Research* **90**, 162–73.

Bobes, J., Garcia-Portilla, M.P., Bascaran, M.T., Saiz, P.A. & Bousoño, M. (2007b) Quality of life in schizophrenic patients. *Dialogues in Clinical Neuroscience* **9**, 215–226.

Bombin, I., Arango, C. & Buchanan, R.W. (2005) Significance and meaning of neurological signs in schizophrenia: two decades later. *Schizophrenia Bulletin* **31**, 962–977.

Bowie, C.R., Leung, W.W., Reichenberg, A. *et al.* (2008) Predicting schizophrenia patients' real-world behavior with specific neuropsychological and functional capacity measures. *Biological Psychiatry* **63**, 505–511.

Braff, D.L. & Light, G.A. (2005) The use of neurophysiological endophenotypes to understand the genetic basis of schizophrenia. *Dialogues in Clinical Neuroscience* **7**, 125–135.

Braff, D.L., Freedman, R., Schork, N.J. & Gottesman, I.I. (2007) Deconstructing schizophrenia: an overview of the use of endophenotypes in order to understand a complex disorder. *Schizophrenia Bulletin* **33**, 21–32.

Brady, K.T. & Sinha, R. (2005) Co-occurring mental and substance use disorders: The neurobiological effects of chronic stress. *American Journal of Psychiatry* **162**, 1483–1493.

Bressan, R.A., Chaves, A.C., Pilowsky, L.S., Shirakawa, I. & Mari, J.J. (2003) Depressive episodes in stable schizophrenia: critical evaluation of the DSM-IV and ICD-10 diagnostic criteria. *Psychiatry Research* **117**, 47–56.

Brown, S., Inskip, H. & Barraclough, B. (2000) Causes of the excess mortality of schizophrenia. *British Journal of Psychiatry* **177**, 212–217.

Buchanan, R.W., Kirkpatrick, B., Heinrichs, D.W. & Carpenter, W.T., Jr. (1990) Clinical correlates of the deficit syndrome of schizophrenia. *American Journal of Psychiatry* **147**, 290–294.

Buchanan, R.W., Strauss, M.E., Kirkpatrick, B., Holstein, C., Breier, A. & Carpenter, W.T., Jr. (1994) Neuropsychological impairments in deficit vs nondeficit forms of schizophrenia. *Archives of General Psychiatry* **51**, 804–811.

Buchanan, R.W., Davis, M., Goff, D. *et al.* (2005) A summary of the FDA-NIMH-MATRICS workshop on clinical trial design for neurocognitive drugs for schizophrenia. *Schizophrenia Bulletin* **31**, 5–19.

Buckley, P.F. (1998) Substance abuse in schizophrenia: a review. *Journal of Clinical Psychiatry* **59** (Suppl. 3), 26–30.

Caldwell, C.B. & Gottesman, I.I. (1990) Schizophrenics kill themselves too: a review of risk factors for suicide. *Schizophrenia Bulletin* **16**, 571–589.

Carney, C.P., Jones, L. & Woolson, R.F. (2006) Medical comorbidity in women and men with schizophrenia: a population-based controlled study. *Journal of General Internal Medicine* **21**, 1133–1137.

Carpenter, W.T., Jr. (1995) Serotonin-dopamine antagonists and treatment of negative symptoms. *Journal of Clinical Psychopharmacology* **15** (1 Suppl 1), 30S–35S.

Carpenter W.T., Jr. (2006) The schizophrenia paradigm: A hundred year challenge. *Journal of Nervous and Mental Disease* **194**: 639–643.

Carpenter, W.T., Jr. (2007) Schizophrenia: disease, syndrome, or dimensions? *Family Process* **46**, 199–206.

Carpenter, W.T. & Koenig, J.I. (2008) The evolution of drug development in schizophrenia: past issues and future opportunities. *Neuropsychopharmacology* **33**, 2061–2079.

Carpenter, W.T., Jr, Heinrichs, D.W. & Wagman, A.M. (1988) Deficit and nondeficit forms of schizophrenia: the concept. *American Journal of Psychiatry* **145**: 578–583.

Cheniaux, E., Landeira-Fernandez, J., Lessa Telles, L. *et al.* (2008) Does schizoaffective disorder really exist? A systematic review of the studies that compared schizoaffective disorder with schizophrenia or mood disorders. *Journal of Affective Disorders* **106**, 209–217.

Cohen, A.S., Saperstein, A.M., Gold, J.M., Kirkpatrick, B., Carpenter, W.T., Jr & Buchanan, R.W. (2007) Neuropsychology of the deficit syndrome: new data and meta-analysis of findings to date. *Schizophrenia Bulletin* **33**, 1201–1212.

Conley, R.R., Ascher-Svanum, H., Zhu, B., Faries, D.E. & Kinon, B.J. (2007) The burden of depressive symptoms in the long-term treatment of patients with schizophrenia. *Schizophrenia Research* **90**, 186–197.

Crow, T.J. (1985) The two-syndrome concept: origins and current status. *Schizophrenia Bulletin* **11**, 471–486.

Cuesta, M.J. & Peralta, V. (1995) Cognitive disorders in the positive, negative, and disorganization syndromes of schizophrenia. *Psychiatry Research* **58**, 227–235.

DeLeon, J., Cuesta, M.J. & Peralta, V. (1993) Delusions and hallucinations in schizophrenic patients. *Psychopathology* **26**, 286–291.

DeLeon, J. & Diaz, F.J. (2005) A meta-analysis of worldwide studies demonstrates an association between schizophrenia and tobacco smoking behaviors. *Schizophrenia Research* **76**, 135–157.

Dixon, L., Haas, G., Weiden, P., Sweeney, J. & Frances, A. (1990) Acute effects of drug abuse in schizophrenic patients: clinical observations and patients' self-reports. *Schizophrenia Bulletin* **16**, 69–79.

Drake, R.E., Gates, C., Cotton, P.G. & Whitaker, A. (1984) Suicide among schizophrenics. Who is at risk? *Journal of Nervous and Mental Disease* **172**, 613–617.

Emsley, R.A., Oosthuizen, P.P., Joubert, A.F., Roberts, M.C. & Stein, D.J. (1999) Depressive and anxiety symptoms in patients with schizophrenia and schizophreniform disorder. *Journal of Clinical Psychiatry* **60**, 747–751.

Esquirol, J.E.D. (1838) *Des Maladies Mentales Considérééś dous les Rapports Médical, Hygiénique et Médiq-légal.* Paris: Ed. Balliere. Librarie de l'Academie de Médicine.

Falloon, I.R. & Talbot, R.E. (1981) Persistent auditory hallucinations: coping mechanisms and implications for management. *Psychological Medicine* **11**, 329–339.

Filik, R., Sipos, A., Kehoe, P.G. *et al.* (2006) The cardiovascular and respiratory health of people with schizophrenia. *Acta Psychiatrica Scandinavica* **113**, 298–305.

Goff, D.C., Sullivan, L.M., McEvoy, J.P. *et al.* (2005a) A comparison of ten-year cardiac risk estimates in schizophrenia patients from the CATIE study and matched controls. *Schizophrenia Research* **80**, 45–53.

Goff, D.C., Cather, C., Evins, A.E. *et al.* (2005b) Medical morbidity and mortality in schizophrenia: guidelines for psychiatrists. *Journal of Clinical Psychiatry* **66**, 183–194.

Gold, S., Arndt, S., Nopoulos, P., O'Leary, D.S. & Andreasen, N.C. (1999) Longitudinal study of cognitive function in first-episode and recent-onset schizophrenia. *American Journal of Psychiatry* **156**, 1342–1348.

Gold, J.M., Goldberg, R.W., McNary, S.W., Dixon, L.B. & Lehman, A.F. (2002) Cognitive correlates of job tenure among patients with severe mental illness. *American Journal of Psychiatry* **159**, 1395–1402.

Good, K.P., Rabinowitz, J., Whitehorn, D., Harvey, P.D., DeSmedt, G. & Kopala, L.C. (2004) The relationship of neuropsychological test performance with the PANSS in antipsychotic naïve, first-episode psychosis patients. *Schizophrenia Research* **68**, 11–19.

Green, M.F. (2006) Cognitive impairment and functional outcome in schizophrenia and bipolar disorder. *Journal of Clinical Psychiatry* **67**, e12.

Gupta, S., Steinmeyer, C., Frank, B. *et al.* (2003) Hyperglycemia and hypertriglyceridemia in real world patients on antipsychotic therapy. *American Journal of Therapy* **10**, 348–355.

Halmi, K.A., Eckert, E., Marchi, E.P. & Sampugnaro V. (1991) Comorbidity of psychiatric diagnosis in anorexia nervosa. *Archives of General Psychiatry* **48**, 712.

Harvey, P.D., Koren, D., Reichenberg, A. & Bowie, C.R. (2006) Negative symptoms and cognitive deficits: what is the nature of their relationship? *Schizophrenia Bulletin* **32**, 250–258.

Heinrichs, R.W. & Zakzanis, K.K. (1998) Neurocognitive deficit in schizophrenia: a quantitative review of the evidence. *Neuropsychology* **12**, 426–445.

Himelhoch, S., McCarthy, J.F., Ganoczy, D., Medoff, D., Dixon, L.B. & Blow, F.C. (2007) Understanding associations between serious mental illness and HIV among patients in the VA Health System. *Psychiatric Services* **58**, 1165–1172.

Hoff, A.L., Svetina, C., Shields, G., Stewart, J. & DeLisi, L.E. (2005) Ten year longitudinal study of neuropsychological functioning subsequent to a first episode of schizophrenia. *Schizophrenia Research* **78**, 27–34.

Jaspers, K. (1946/1963) *General Psychopathology.* Manchester: Manchester University Press. Translated by Hoenig, J. & Hamilton, M. from *Allgemeine Psychopathologie.* Heidelberg: Springer Verlag.

Javitt, D.C., Spencer, K.M., Thaker, G.K., Winterer, G. & Hajós, M. (2008) Neurophysiological biomarkers for drug development in schizophrenia. *Nature Reviews Drug Discovery* **7**: 68–83.

Jenkins, C.D. (1992) Assessment of outcomes of health intervention. *Social Science and Medicine* **35**, 367–375.

Kabinoff, G.S., Toalson, P.A., Healey, K.M., McGuire, H.C. & Hay, D.P. (2003) Metabolic issues with atypical antipsychotics in primary care: dispelling the myths. *Primary Care Companion Journal of Clinical Psychiary* **5**, 6–14.

Kandinsky, V.Kh. (1890) *O psevdohallucinatsiakh. Kritiko-klinicheskii etud [About pseudohallucinations. Critical clinical study].* Sanct-Petersburg: Izdanie EK Kandinskoi.

Kahlbaum, K.L. (translated by Levi, Y. & Pridon, T.) (1973) *Catatonia.* Baltimore: Johns Hopkins University Press.

Kay, S.R., Fiszbein, A. & Opler, L.A. (1987) The positive and negative syndrome scale (PANSS) for schizophrenia. *Schizophrenia Bulletin* **13**, 261–276.

Keefe, R.S., Frescka, E., Apter, S.H. *et al.* (1996) Clinical characteristics of Kraepelinian schizophrenia: replication and extension of previous findings. *American Journal of Psychiatry* **153**, 806–811.

Kendell, R.E. (1987) Diagnosis and classification of functional psychoses. *British Medical Bulletin* **43**, 499–513.

Kern, R.S., Nuechterlein, K.H., Green, M.F. *et al.* (2008) The MATRICS Consensus Cognitive Battery, Part 2: Co-Norming and Standardization. *American Journal of Psychiatry* **165**, 214–220.

Keshavan, M.S. & Amirsadri, A. (2007) Early intervention in schizophrenia: current and future perspectives. *Current Psychiatry Reports* **9**, 325–328.

Kirkpatrick, B., Buchanan, R.W., McKenney, P.D., Alphs, L.D. & Carpenter, W.T., Jr. (1989) The schedule for the deficit syndrome: an instrument for research in schizophrenia. *Psychiatry Research* **30**, 119–123.

Kirkpatrick, B., Buchanan, R.W., Ross, D.E. & Carpenter, W.T., Jr. (2001) A separate disease within the syndrome of schizophrenia. *Archives of General Psychiatry* **58**, 165–171.

Kirkpatrick, B., Fenton, W.S., Carpenter, W.T. Jr & Marder, S.R. (2006) The NIMH-MATRICS consensus statement on negative symptoms. *Schizophrenia Bulletin* **32**, 214–219.

Koreen, A.R., Siris, S.G., Chakos, M., Alvir, J., Mayerhoff, D. & Lieberman, J. (1993) Depression in first-episode schizophrenia. *American Journal of Psychiatry* **150**, 1643–1648.

Kraepelin, E. (1913/1919) *Psychiatrie,* 8th edn, Vol. **3**, Part 2. (translated by Barclay, R.M. as *Dementia Praecox and Paraphrenia*). Edinburgh: ES Livingstone.

Kraus, M.S. & Keefe, R.S. (2007) Cognition as an outcome measure in schizophrenia. *British Journal of Psychiatry* **50** (Suppl), s46–51.

Kretschmer, E. (1966) *The Sensitive Delusion of Reference* Berlin: Springer; 4. erw.Aufl.edition.

Leucht, S., Burkard, T., Henderson, J., Maj, M. & Sartorius, N. (2007) Physical illness and schizophrenia: a review of the literature. *Acta Psychiatrica Scandinavica* **116**, 317–333.

Lindenmayer, J.P., Czobor, P., Volavka, J. *et al.* (2003) Changes in glucose and cholesterol levels in patients with schizophrenia treated with typical or atypical antipsychotics. *American Journal of Psychiatry* **160**, 290–296.

Malik, P. (2007) Sexual dysfunction in schizophrenia. *Current Opinion in Psychiatry* **20**, 138–142.

Marder, S.R., Essock, S.M., Miller, A.L. *et al.* (2004) Physical health monitoring of patients with schizophrenia. *American Journal of Psychiatry* **161**, 1334–1349.

Martin, L.F. & Freedman, R. (2007) Schizophrenia and the alpha7 nicotinic acetylcholine receptor. *International Review of Neurobiology* **78**, 225–246.

McEvoy, J.P., Meyer, J.M., Goff, D.C. *et al.* (2005) Prevalence of the metabolic syndrome in patients with schizophrenia: baseline results from the Clinical Antipsychotic Trials of Intervention Effectiveness (CATIE) schizophrenia trial and comparison with national estimates from NHANES III. *Schizophrenia Research* **80**, 19–32.

Meyer, J.M., Nasrallah, H.A., McEvoy, J.P. *et al.* (2005) The Clinical Antipsychotic Trials of Intervention Effectiveness (CATIE) schizophrenia trial: clinical comparison of subgroups with and without the metabolic syndrome. *Schizophrenia Research* **80**, 9–18.

Morgan, M.G., Scully, P.J., Youssef, H.A., Kinsella, A., Owens, J.M. & Waddington, J.L. (2003) Prospective analysis of premature mortality in schizophrenia in relation to health service engagement: a 7.5-year study within an epidemiologically complete, homogeneous population in rural Ireland. *Psychiatry Research* **117**, 127–135.

Nopoulos, P., Flashman, L., Flaum, M., Arndt, S. & Andreasen, N. (1994) Stability of cognitive functioning early in the course of schizophrenia. *Schizophrenia Research* **14**: 29–37.

Nuechterlein, K.H., Green, M.F., Kern, R.S. *et al.* (2008) The MATRICS Consensus Cognitive Battery, Part 1: Test selection, reliability, and validity. *American Journal of Psychiatry* **165**, 203–213.

O'Leary, D.S., Flaum, M., Kesler, M.L., Flashman, L.A., Arndt, S. & Andreasen, N.C. (2000) Cognitive correlates of the negative, disorganized, and psychotic symptom dimensions of schizophrenia. *Journal of Neuropsychiatry and Clinical Neurosciences* **12**, 4–15.

Pompili, M., Amador, X.F., Girardi, P. *et al.* (2007) Suicide risk in schizophrenia: learning from the past to change the future. *Annals of General Psychiatry* **6**, 10.

Rabinowitz, J., Harvey, P.D., Eerdekens, M. & Davidson, M. (2006) Premorbid functioning and treatment response in recent-onset schizophrenia. *British Journal of Psychiatry* **189**, 31–35.

Reichenberg, A., Weiser, M., Rapp, M.A. *et al.* (2006) Premorbid intra-individual variability in intellectual performance and risk for schizophrenia: a population-based study. *Schizophrenia Research* **85**, 49–57.

Rössler, W., Riecher-Rössler, A., Angst, J. *et al.* (2007) Psychotic experiences in the general population: a twenty-year prospective community study. *Schizophrenia Research* **92**, 1–14.

Schmael, C., Georgi, A., Krumm, B. *et al.* (2007) Premorbid adjustment in schizophrenia—an important aspect of phenotype definition. *Schizophrenia Research* **92**, 50–62.

Schneider, K. (1959) *Clinical Psychopathology*. Translated by Hamilton, M.W. New York: Grune & Stratton.

Seidman, L.J., Giuliano, A.J., Smith, C.W. *et al.* (2006) Neuropsychological functioning in adolescents and young adults at genetic risk for schizophrenia and affective psychoses: Results from the Harvard and Hillside Adolescent High Risk Studies. *Schizophrenia Bulletin* **32**, 507–524.

Shergill, S.S., Brammer, M.J., Williams, S.C., Murray, R.M. & McGuire, P.K. (2000) Mapping auditory hallucinations in schizophrenia using functional magnetic resonance imaging. *Archives of General Psychiatry* **57**, 1033–1038.

Silbersweig, D.A., Stern, E., Frith, C. *et al.* (1995) A functional neuroanatomy of hallucinations in schizophrenia. *Nature* **378**, 176–179.

Simon, A.E., Cattapan-Ludewig, K., Zmilacher, S. *et al.* (2007) Cognitive functioning in the schizophrenia prodrome. *Schizophrenia Bulletin* **33**, 761–771.

Singareddy, R.K. & Balon, R. (2001) Sleep and suicide in psychiatric patients. *Annals of Clinical Psychiatry* **13**, 93–101.

Siris, S.G., Addington, D., Azorin, J.M., Falloon, I.R., Gerlach, J. & Hirsch, S.R. (2001) Depression in schizophrenia: recognition and management in the USA. *Schizophrenia Research* **47**, 185–197.

Smith, S.M., O'Keane, V. & Murray, R. (2002) Sexual dysfunction in patients taking conventional antipsychotic medication. *British Journal of Psychiatry* **181**, 49–55.

Srinivasan, T.N. & Thara, R. (2002) Smoking in schizophrenia —all is not biological. *Schizophrenia Research* **56**, 67–74.

Stefanis, N.C., Hanssen, M., Smirnis, N.K. *et al.* (2002) Evidence that three dimensions of psychosis have a distribution in the general population. *Psychological Medicine* **32**, 347–358.

Steinhausen, H.C.H. (2002) The outcome of anorexia nervosa in the 20th century. *American Journal of Psychiatry* **159**, 1284–1293.

Strauss, J.S., Carpenter, W.T. & Jr, Bartko, J.J. (1974) The diagnosis and understanding of schizophrenia. Part III. Speculations on the processes that underlie schizophrenic symptoms and signs. *Schizophrenia Bulletin* **11**, 61–69.

Stroup, T.S., Lieberman, J.A., McEvoy, J.P. *et al.* CATIE Investigators (2006) Effectiveness of olanzapine, quetiapine, risperidone, and ziprasidone in patients with chronic schizophrenia following discontinuation of a previous atypical antipsychotic. *American Journal of Psychiatry* **163**, 611–622.

Taylor, M.A. & Fink, M. (2003) Catatonia in psychiatric classification: a home of its own. *American Journal of Psychiatry* **160**: 1233–1241.

Thaker, G.K. (2007) Schizophrenia endophenotypes as treatment targets. *Expert Opinion on Therapeutic Targets* **11**, 1–18.

Uçok, A., Incesu, C., Aker, T. & Erkoç, S. (2007) Sexual dysfunction in patients with schizophrenia on antipsychotic medication. *European Psychiatry* **22**, 328–333.

van Os, J. (2003) Is there a continuum of psychotic experiences in the general population? *Epidemiology, Psychiatry and Sociology* **12**, 242–252.

Van Putten, T. & May, R.P. (1978) "Akinetic depression" in schizophrenia. *Archives of General Psychiatry* **35**, 1101–1107.

WHOQOL Group (1995) The World Health Organization Quality of Life Assessment (the WHOQOL): position paper from the World Health Organisation. *Social Science and Medicine* **41**, 1403–1409.

Woodberry, K., Giuliano, A.J. & Seidman, L.J. (2008) Premorbid IQ in schizophrenia: A meta-analytic review. *American. Journal of. Psychiatry* **165**, 579–587.

Ziedonis, D.M., Smelson, D., Rosenthal, R.N. *et al.* (2005) Improving the care of individuals with schizophrenia and substance use disorders: consensus recommendations. *Journal of Psychiatric Practice* **11**, 315–339.

CHAPTER 3

Child and adolescent schizophrenia

Chris Hollis[1] and Judith Rapoport[2]

[1]Division of Psychiatry, University of Nottingham, Queen's Medical Centre, Nottingham, UK
[2]NIMH, Bethesda, MD, USA

Schizophrenia, 3rd edition. Edited by Daniel R. Weinberger and
Paul J Harrison © 2011 Blackwell Publishing Ltd.

Introduction

Schizophrenia is one of the most devastating psychiatric disorders to affect children and adolescents. Although extremely rare before the age of 10, the incidence of schizophrenia rises steadily though adolescence to reach its peak in early adult life. The clinical severity, impact on development, and poor prognosis of child and adolescent-onset schizophrenia reinforces the need for early detection, prompt diagnosis, and effective treatment.

The current concept of schizophrenia in children and adolescents evolved from a different perspective held during much of the 20th century. Until the early 1970s, the term childhood schizophrenia was applied to children who would now be diagnosed with autism. Kolvin's landmark studies distinguished early-onset (autistic) cases from children with a relatively "late-onset" psychosis which closely resembled schizophrenia (Kolvin, 1971; Kolvin et al., 1971). Importantly, in DSM-III and ICD-9 the separate category of childhood schizophrenia was removed, and the same diagnostic criteria for schizophrenia were applied across the age range. Major additional evidence for the validity of the diagnosis of schizophrenia in childhood and adolescence comes from the Maudsley Child and Adolescent Psychosis Follow-up Study (Hollis, 2000). First, a DSM-IIIR diagnosis of schizophrenia in childhood and adolescence predicted a significantly poorer adult outcome compared to other non-schizophrenic psychosis. Second, the diagnosis of schizophrenia showed a high level of stability, with 80% having the same diagnosis recorded at adult follow-up (see also Jarbin et al., 2003).

Clinical phases

Premorbid social and developmental impairments

Child and adolescent-onset schizophrenia is associated with poor premorbid functioning and early developmental delays, particularly striking for patients with onset before adolescence (Alaghband-Rad et al., 1995; Hollis, 1995, 2003). Similar developmental and social impairments in childhood have been reported in adult-onset schizophrenia, but premorbid impairments appear to be more common and severe in the child and adolescent-onset forms of the disorder. In the Maudsley study (Hollis, 2003) significant early delays were particularly common in the areas of language (20%), reading (30%), and bladder control (36%). Just over 20% of cases of adolescent schizophrenia had significant early delays in either language or motor development. In contrast, language and motor developmental delays have been reported in only about 10% of individuals who develop schizophrenia in adult life (Jones et al., 1994). A consistent characteristic in the premorbid phenotype is impaired sociability. For example, in the Maudsley study of child and adolescent-onset psychoses (Hollis, 2003), about a third of cases with schizophrenia had significant difficulties in social development, affecting the ability to make and keep friends.

Premorbid IQ in child and adolescent-onset schizophrenia is in the mid to low 80s, some 10–15 points lower than in the adult form of the disorder (Alaghband-Rad et al., 1995; Asarnow et al., 1994b; Hollis, 2000). In the Maudsley study (Hollis, 2000), a third of child and adolescent-onset cases had an IQ below 70, with the whole distribution of IQ shifted down compared to both adolescent affective psychoses and adult schizophrenia.

Cannon et al. (2002) reported a specific association between adult schizophreniform disorder and an antecedent pattern of childhood pan-developmental impairments involving motor development, receptive language, and IQ. These findings are consistent with the view that premorbid impairments are manifestations of a genetic/developmental liability to schizophrenia. It seems clear that the premorbid phenotype does not just represent non-specific psychiatric disturbance. Looking backward from schizophrenia to early impairment, subtle problems of language, attention, and social relationships are typical, while in contrast, conduct problems are rare. However, looking forward from childhood impairments to later schizophrenia, prediction is much weaker. In addition, premorbid social and behavioral difficulties are not unique to schizophrenia and do occur in other psychiatric disorders.

Are premorbid impairments a risk or precursor of psychosis?

Premorbid impairments could lie on a causal pathway for psychosis or, alternatively, they could be markers of an underlying neuropathological process, such as aberrant neural connectivity, which may be the cause of both premorbid social impairment and psychosis. Frith (1994) has speculated on the possible cognitive mechanisms that might link deficits in social cognition or "theory of mind" in a causal pathway to both positive and negative psychotic symptoms. If these characteristics are causally related, then modifying the "primary" cognitive or social deficits may reduce the risk of psychosis. Alternatively, cognitive and social deficits, although often present, may not be necessary in the pathogenesis. The fact that individuals can develop schizophrenia without obvious premorbid impairments supports this view. Ideally, a high-risk longitudinal intervention study is needed to adequately address the issue of causality, and this would require an intervention that had benefits for all individuals who had the premorbid phenotype, including those phenocopies at low risk of developing psychosis. Alternatively, presence of premorbid impairments may represent a subgroup associated with, for example, particular genetic risks (Addington & Rapoport, 2009).

Premorbid psychopathology

A diverse range of clinical diagnoses, including attention deficit hyperactivity disorder (ADHD), conduct disorder, anxiety, depression, and autism spectrum disorders (ASDs), may precede the diagnosis of schizophrenia in children and adolescents (Schaeffer & Ross, 2002) and in adults (Kim-Cohen *et al.*, 2003). However, there is a lack of any specific premorbid diagnosis that could practically aid early clinical identification of those at high risk for schizophrenia. A more promising line of research has demonstrated a strong link between self-reported psychotic symptoms in childhood and later schizophrenia (Poulton *et al.*, 2000). In the Dunedin cohort study in New Zealand, psychotic symptoms at age 11 increased the risk of schizophreniform disorder at age 26 but not other psychiatric diagnoses. Relative to the rest of the cohort, those identified at age 11 with "strong" psychotic symptoms also had significant impairments in motor development, receptive language, and IQ (Cannon *et al.*, 2002). While none of these cases met criteria for a diagnosis of schizophrenia during adolescence, it appears that isolated or attenuated psychotic symptoms in combination with pan-developmental impairment constitute a significant high-risk premorbid phenotype.

Prodromal symptoms and onset of psychosis

People who develop schizophrenia typically enter a prodromal phase characterized by a gradual but marked decline in social and academic functioning that precedes that onset of active psychotic symptoms (see Chapter 6). An insidious deterioration prior to onset of psychosis is typical of the presentation of schizophrenia in children and adolescents (Werry *et al.*, 1994), and is more common in schizophrenia than in affective psychoses (Hollis, 1999). Non-specific behavioral changes, including social withdrawal, declining school performance, uncharacteristic and odd behavior, began, on average, over a year before the onset of positive psychotic symptoms. In retrospect, non-specific behavioral changes were frequently early negative symptoms, which had their onset well before positive symptoms such as hallucinations and delusions.

Early recognition of the disorder is difficult, as premorbid cognitive and social impairments gradually shade into prodromal symptoms before the onset of active psychotic symptoms (Hafner & Nowotny, 1995). Prodromal symptoms can include odd ideas, eccentric interests, changes in affect, unusual experiences, and bizarre perceptual experiences. While these are also characteristic features of schizotypal personality disorder, in a schizophrenic prodrome there is usually progression to more severe dysfunction.

Diagnosis in childhood and adolescence

Clinical characteristics

Even if strict adult definitions of schizophrenia (DSM-IIIR/DSM-IV or ICD-10) are applied, there are age-dependent variations in phenomenology. Child and adolescent-onset cases are characterized by a more insidious onset, negative symptoms, hallucinations in different modalities, and, for relatively fewer patients, systematized or persecutory delusions (Green *et al.*, 1992; Werry *et al.*, 1994). Early-onset schizophrenia is characterized by greater disorganization (incoherence of thought and disordered sense of self) and more negative symptoms, while in later-onset cases there is a higher frequency of systematized and paranoid delusions (Hafner & Nowotny, 1995).

A wide variety of anomalous perceptual experiences may occur at the onset of an episode of schizophrenia, leading to a sense of fear or puzzlement which may constitute a delusional mood and herald a full psychotic episode. These anomalous experiences may include the sense that familiar places and people and their reactions have changed in some subtle way. These experiences may result from a breakdown between perception and memory (for familiar places and people) and associated affective responses (salience given to these perceptions). For example, a young person at the onset of illness may study their reflection in the mirror for hours because it looks strangely unfamiliar, misattribute threatening intent to an innocuous comment, or experience family members or friends as being unfamiliar, leading to a secondary delusional belief that they have been replaced by doubles or aliens.

In summary, some clinical phenomena in schizophrenia can be understood in terms of a loss of normal contextualization and coordination of cognitive and emotional processing.

Course and outcome

Short-term course

Child and adolescent-onset schizophrenia characteristically runs a chronic course, with only a minority of cases making a full symptomatic recovery from the first psychotic episode. Hollis (1999) found that only 12% of cases with schizophrenia were in full remission at discharge compared to 50% of cases with affective psychoses. The short-term outcome for schizophrenia presenting in early life appears to be worse than that for first-episode adult patients (Robinson *et al.*, 1999). If full recovery does occur, then it is most likely within the first 3 months of onset of psychosis. In the Maudsley study, those adolescent-onset patients who were still psychotic after 6 months had only a 15% chance of achieving full remission, while over half of all cases who made a full recovery had active psychotic symptoms for less than 3 months (Hollis, 1999). The clinical implication is that the early course over the first 6 months is the best predictor of remission and that longer observation over 6 months adds relatively little new information.

Long-term outcome

A number of long-term follow-up studies of child and adolescent-onset schizophrenia all describe a typically chronic, unremitting long-term course with severely impaired functioning in adult life (Werry *et al.*, 1991; Schmidt *et al.*, 1995; Eggers & Bunk, 1997; Hollis, 2000; Lay *et al.*, 2000; Jarbin *et al.*, 2003; Fleischhaker *et al.*, 2005). Referral bias towards selecting more severe cases is a potential problem in clinical follow-up studies. However, population-based studies have yielded similar results (Hollis, 2000). Several common themes emerge from these studies. First, the generally poor outcome of early-onset schizophrenia conceals considerable heterogeneity. About one-fifth of patients in most studies have a good outcome with only mild impairment, while at the other extreme about a third of patients are severely impaired, requiring intensive social and psychiatric support. Second, after the first few years of illness there is little evidence of further progressive decline. Third, child and adolescent-onset schizophrenia has a worse outcome than either adolescent-onset affective psychoses or adult-onset schizophrenia. Fourth, social functioning, in particular the ability to form friendships and love relationships, appears to be very impaired in early-onset schizophrenia. Taken together, these findings confirm schizophrenia presenting in childhood and adolescence lies at the extreme end of a continuum of phenotypic severity.

Prognostic factors

The predictors of poor outcome in adolescent-onset affective psychoses include premorbid social and cognitive impairments (Hollis, 1999; Fleischhaker *et al.*, 2005), a prolonged first psychotic episode (Schmidt *et al.*, 1995), extended duration of untreated psychosis (Hollis, 1999), and the presence of negative symptoms (Hollis, 1999). Premorbid functioning and negative symptoms at onset provide better prediction of long-term outcome than categorical diagnosis (Hollis, 1999; Fleischhaker *et al.*, 2005).

Mortality

The risk of premature death is increased in child and adolescent-onset psychoses. In the Maudsley study (Hollis, 1999), there were nine deaths among the 106 cases followed-up (8.5%), corresponding to a 12-fold increase in the risk of death compared to an age- and sex-matched general UK population over the same period. Of the nine deaths in the cohort, seven were male and seven had a diagnosis of schizophrenia. Three subjects suffered violent deaths, two died from self-poisoning, and three had unexpected deaths due to previously undetected physical causes (cardiomyopathy and status epilepticus), possibly associated with high-dose antipsychotic medication.

Epidemiology

Incidence and prevalence

Good population-based incidence figures for child and adolescent-onset schizophrenia are lacking, though there are data for broader categories of psychosis, with diagnoses made without the benefit of standardized assessments. Gillberg *et al.* (1986) calculated age-specific prevalence for all psychoses (including schizophrenia, schizophreniform, affective psychosis, atypical psychosis, and drug psychoses) in the age range 13–18 years using case-register data from Goteborg, Sweden. Of the cases, 41% had a diagnosis of schizophrenia. At age 13 years, the prevalence for all psychoses was 0.9 in 10 000, showing a steady increase during adolescence, reaching a prevalence of 17.6 in 10 000 at age 18 years.

Sex ratio

Males are over-represented in many clinical studies of childhood-onset schizophrenia (Russell *et al.*, 1989; Spencer & Campbell, 1994). However, other studies of predominantly adolescent-onset schizophrenia have described an equal sex ratio (Werry *et al.*, 1994; Gordon *et al.*, 1994; Hollis, 2000). The interpretation of these studies is complicated by the possibility of referral biases to clinical centers. In an epidemiological study of first admissions for schizophrenia and paranoia in children and adolescents, there was an equal sex ratio for patients under the age of 15 (Galdos *et al.*, 1993). The finding of an equal sex distribution with adolescent-onset schiziophrenia is intriguing as it differs from the consistent male predominance (ratio 2:1) reported in incident samples of early adult-onset schizophrenia (Castle & Murray, 1991). Clearly, future studies require population-based samples free from potential referral biases.

Etiology and risk factors

Pregnancy and birth complications

Pregnancy and birth complications (PBC) have long been implicated as a risk factor in schizophrenia, though the evidence is mixed (Geddes & Lawrie, 1995; Kendell *et al.*,

2000; see Chapter 11). In two independent case–control studies of childhood-onset schizophrenia, Matsumoto *et al.* (1999, 2001) reported an odds ratio of 3.2–3.5 for PBC, suggesting a greater risk in very early-onset cases. However, in the National Institute of Mental Health (NIMH) study of childhood-onset schizophrenia, PBCs were no more common in cases than in sibling controls (Nicholson *et al.*, 1999). Insofar as there is a significant association, it seems likely that PBCs are *consequences* rather than *causes* of abnormal neurodevelopment (Goodman, 1988). This view is supported by the finding that people with schizophrenia have smaller head size at birth than controls (McGrath & Murray, 1995), which is likely to be a consequence of either defects in genetic control of neurodevelopment or prenatal environmental factors such as viral exposure, nutritional stress, etc.

Prenatal famine

Severe maternal intrauterine nutritional deficiency may increase the risk for schizophrenia in adult life. Evidence of a two-fold increase for schizophrenia in children born to the most malnourished mothers comes from studies of the 1944–1945 Dutch Hunger Winter (Susser & Lin, 1992) and the Chinese Famine of 1959–1961 (St Clair *et al.*, 2005). (This subject is discussed in detail in Chapter 11.)

Cannabis

There is little doubt that acute intoxication with cannabis and other illicit substances such as stimulants and hallucinogens can precipitate psychotic symptoms, or exacerbations of existing psychotic illness. However, there is controversy whether cannabis use in particular is a risk factor for the development of schizophrenia. A meta-analysis of four well-conducted longitudinal population-based studies from Sweden (Swedish conscript cohort), the Netherlands (NEMESIS), and New Zealand (Dunedin and Christchurch cohorts) concluded that, at an individual level, cannabis confers an overall two-fold increased risk for later schizophrenia (Arseneault *et al.*, 2004). In the Dunedin cohort, Arseneault *et al.* (2002), showed that the association was strongest for the youngest cannabis users (after controlling for prior psychotic symptoms), with 10.3% of the cannabis users at age 15 developing schizophreniform disorder at age 26. So far, cannabis use has not been directly implicated in child and adolescent-onset schizophrenia—possibly because of the relatively lower prevalence of cannabis use in younger adolescents and a short duration between exposure and psychotic outcome. However, cannabis use is associated with earlier age of onset of schizophrenia in adults (Arendt *et al.*, 2005).

The mechanism and causal direction for this association remains unclear. It is possible that subtle social and developmental impairments that precede schizophrenia are also risk factors for cannabis use (reverse causality or a third factor). Perhaps a more plausible explanation is a gene–environment interaction effect whereby cannabis exposure causes schizophrenia only in those with a pre-existing susceptibility. Caspi *et al.* (2005) provided evidence for such a gene–environment interaction specific to adolescent cannabis exposure: the catechol-O-methyltransferase (*COMT*) Val158Met polymorphism moderated the link between psychosis and adolescent-onset cannabis use, but not adult-onset cannabis use. The *COMT* Val allele is associated with greater COMT activity (relative to the COMT Met allele) and reduced dopamine transmission in the prefrontal cortex. These results, taken together with human (Dean *et al.*, 2003) and animal (Pistis *et al.*, 2004) neuropharmacological studies, suggest that cannabis may enhance the risk of schizophrenia in vulnerable individuals during a critical period of adolescent brain development.

Psychosocial risks

Expressed emotion

High levels of expressed emotion (EE) among relatives of adults with schizophrenia predict psychotic relapse and poor outcome (Leff & Vaughn, 1985), raising the question of whether high EE might act to "bring forward" the onset of the disorder in a vulnerable individual. Goldstein (1987) reported that measures of parental criticism and over-involvement taken during adolescence were associated with an increased risk of schizophrenia spectrum disorders in young adulthood. However, a causal link was not proven, and the association may reflect either an expression of some common underlying trait or a parental response to premorbid disturbance in the pre-schizophrenic adolescent. More direct comparisons between the parents of adult- and childhood-onset cases of schizophrenia fail to support the hypothesis of higher parental EE in childhood-onset cases. Asarnow *et al.* (1994a) used the Five Minute Speech Sample to measure parental EE and found that people with childhood-onset schizophrenia were no more likely to have "high EE" parents than normal controls. It appears that, on average, the parents of children with schizophrenia generally express *lower* levels of criticism and hostility than parents of adult-onset patients, due to a greater tendency to attribute their children's behavior to an illness which is beyond their control (Hooley, 1987).

Childhood abuse and neglect

A causal link between child abuse and psychosis, in particular hallucinations, in adult life has been proposed (Read *et al.*, 2005). While strong claims have been made for this link, the evidence to date remains inconclusive, with most studies supporting the link having serious methodological weaknesses (Morgan *et al.*, 2006).

Concepts of schizophrenia

The neurodevelopmental model

Over the last two decades the concept of schizophrenia as a neurodevelopmental disorder has been the dominant explanatory model, with a tension between "early" and "late" versions of the model. However, more recently, these positions have converged as it has been recognized that both early events (during pre- and peri-natal brain development) and late events (during adolescent brain maturation) contribute to schizophrenia (Hollis & Taylor, 1997; Rapoport et al., 2005).

The "early" neurodevelopmental model views the primary cause of schizophrenia as a static "lesion", either neurogenetic or environmental in origin, occurring during fetal brain development (Weinberger, 1987). Two main lines of evidence support this model. First, Roberts et al. (1986) reported an absence of gliosis, suggesting aberrant neurodevelopment rather than neurodegeneration. Second, schizophrenia is associated with premorbid social and cognitive impairments (Jones et al., 1994), pregnancy and birth complications (Lewis & Murray, 1987), and minor physical anomalies (Gualtieri et al., 1982). According to this "early" model, during childhood this lesion is relatively silent, giving rise only to subtle social and cognitive impairments. However, in adolescence, or early adult life, the lesion interacts with the process of *normal* brain maturation (e.g., myelination of cortico-limbic circuits and/or synaptic pruning and remodelling) and leads to psychotic symptoms.

A limitation of the "early" model is that a neurodevelopmental insult on its own cannot account for the finding of increased extracerebral (sulcal) cerebral spinal fluid (CSF) space in schizophrenia. Diffuse loss of brain tissue limited to the pre- or peri-natal periods would result in enlargement of the lateral ventricles but not increased extracerebral CSF space (Woods, 1998).

The "late" neurodevelopmental model, first proposed by Feinberg (1983), argues that the key neuropathological events in schizophrenia occur as a result of *abnormal* brain development during adolescence. The current formulation of the "late" neurodevelopmental model proposes that *excessive* synaptic and/or dentritic elimination occurring during adolescence produces aberrant neural connectivity (Woods, 1998; McGlashen & Hoffman, 2000). This "late" model characterizes schizophrenia as a *progressive* late-onset neurodevelopmental disorder and predicts that progressive structural brain changes and cognitive decline will be seen in adolescence around the onset of psychosis. Excessive synaptic pruning is regarded as an amplification of the normal process of progressive pruning and elimination of synapses that begins in early childhood and extends through late adolescence (Purves & Lichtmen, 1980). In the "late" model, premorbid abnormalities in early childhood are viewed as non-specific risk factors rather than early manifestations of an underlying schizophrenic neuropathology.

Both the "early" and "late" models suppose that there is a direct and specific expression of the eventual brain pathology as schizophrenic disorder. A third viewpoint, the neurodevelopmental "risk" model, proposes that early and/or late brain pathology acts as a risk factor rather than a sufficient cause, so that its effects can only be understood in the light of an individual's exposure to other risk and protective factors (Hollis & Taylor, 1997). This latter formulation provides a probabilistic model of the onset of schizophrenia in which aberrant brain development is expressed as neurocognitive impairments that interact with environmental risk factors to produce psychotic symptoms.

Over the last decade, further evidence has emerged to refine the neurodevelopmental model of schizophrenia. Data from premorbid social and developmental impairments, brain morphology, neuropsychology, and genetics all suggest an aberrant neurodevelopmental process resulting from an interplay of genetic and environmental factors that is set in train before the onset of psychotic symptoms and continues into late adolescence. This formulation of schizophrenia is discussed in greater detail in Chapter 19.

Neurobiology

Structural brain abnormalities

The brain changes reported in childhood-onset schizophrenia appear to be very similar to those described in adult schizophrenia (see Chapter 16), supporting the idea of an underlying neurobiological continuity. In the NIMH study of childhood-onset schizophrenia (onset at younger than 13 years of age), subjects had smaller brains than normals, with larger lateral ventricles and reduced prefrontal lobe volume (Jacobsen & Rapoport, 1998). As in adult studies, reduced total cerebral volume is associated with negative symptoms (Alaghband-Rad et al., 1997). Midsagittal thalamic area is decreased while midsagittal area of the corpus callosum is increased (Giedd et al., 1996), suggesting that the reduction in total cerebral volume in childhood-onset schizophrenia is due to relative reduction in gray matter with relative sparing of white matter. Childhood-onset patients have a higher rate of developmental brain abnormalities than controls, including an increased frequency of cavum septum pelucidum (Nopoulos et al., 1998). Abnormalities of the cerebellum have also been found, including reduced volume of the vermis, midsagital area, and inferior posterior lobe (Jacobsen et al., 1997a). Associated with reports of reduced cortical thickness are gyrification abnormalities, including more flattened curvature in the sulci and more peaked or steep curvature in the gyri (White *et al.*, 2003), consistent with a neurodevelopmental origin of cortical abnormalities. In patients with adolescent-onset schizophrenia, there is evidence of ventricular enlargement and reduced volume of the prefrontal cortex and reduced thalamic volume (Dasari *et al.*, 1999; James *et al.*, 2004).

Progressive brain changes

Two different types of progressive brain change have been described in schizophrenia. First, treatment with traditional antipsychotics appears to cause progressive enlargement of the basal ganglia, with these structures returning to their original size when patients are transferred to the atypical antipsychotic clozapine (Frazier *et al.*, 1996). Second, there is evidence of progressive volume reductions in the temporal and frontal lobes during the first 2–3 years after the onset of schizophrenia (Gur *et al.*, 1998). In the NIMH study of childhood-onset schizophrenia, longitudinal repeated magnetic resonance imaging (MRI) scans through adolescence revealed a progressive increase in ventricular volume and progressive decrease in cortical volume with frontal (11% decrease), parietal (8.5%), and temporal lobes (7%) disproportionately affected (Rapoport *et al.*, 1999; Sporn *et al.*, 2003). Overall, this represents a four-fold greater reduction in cortical volume than in healthy adolescents. A similar progressive loss in cerebellar volume has been reported in the NIHM childhood-onset schizophrenia sample (Keller *et al.*, 2003). Most strikingly, the pattern of the exaggerated gray matter loss is identical to the pattern of normal development, suggesting that the "gain is up" for some normal developmental process (Rapoport & Gogtay, 2007). Age-related volume reduction across adolescence has also been reported for the anterior cingulate gyrus (Marquardt *et al.*, 2005). Progressive changes appear to be time-limited to adolescence, with the rate of volume reduction in frontal and temporal structures associated with premorbid developmental impairment and baseline symptom severity (Sporn *et al.*, 2003) declining as subjects reach adult life (Giedd *et al.*, 1999). The pattern of progressive cortical volume reduction described in the NIMH childhood-onset schizophrenia sample appears to be an exaggeration of the normal "back-to-front" pattern of cortical volume reduction seen during adolescence (Gogtay *et al.*, 2004). At present, it is unclear whether the dramatic findings from the NIMH childhood-onset schizophrenia sample, which is atypical in terms of very early onset (<13 years) and neuroleptic-treatment resistance, can be generalized to other samples of children and adolescents with schizophrenia (James *et al.*, 2002). It should be noted, however, that by adulthood, the NIMH childhood-onset sample pattern resembles that of typical adult patients with primarily superior temporal and dorso-lateral prefrontal cortical deficits as the healthy controls "catch up" over the years (Greenstein *et al.*, 2006), suggesting that the abnormal loss represents in part a "shift to the left" of cortical development (Greenstein *et al.*, 2006; Rapoport & Gogtay, 2007).

Because progressive brain changes have been described *after* the onset of psychosis, it is possible that they are a consequence of psychosis or of the treatment of psychosis. Evidence that progressive brain changes precede the onset of psychosis is very limited. Pantelis *et al.* (2003) have reported brain MRI findings in high-risk subjects scanned before and after the transition into psychosis. The baseline cross-sectional comparison found that those about to develop psychosis had reduced cortical gray matter in the right temporal, inferior frontal cortex, and cingulate bilaterally. When re-scanned, those subjects who developed psychosis had further volume reductions in gray matter in the left parahippocampal, fusiform, orbito-frontal and cerebellar cortices, and cingulate gyri. The only significant longitudinal changes in cases who remained non-psychotic were in the cerebellum. These are important findings, and if replicated, provide strong support for the idea that excessive developmental reductions in gray matter both predate and accompany the onset of psychotic symptoms. Moreover, recent twin studies in adult patients suggest that these brain changes are at least in part genetically determined (Brans *et al.*, 2008a,b).

Functional brain imaging

In a positron emission tomography (PET) study in childhood-onset schizophrenia using the Continuous Performance Test (CPT), Jacobsen *et al.* (1997b) reported reduced activation compared to healthy controls in the mid and superior frontal gyrus, and increased activation in the inferior frontal, supramarginal gyrus, and insula. Clearly, a simple description of "hypofrontality" does not capture the complex pattern of changes involving interconnected frontal areas. Older, localizationist models based on focal cerebral dysfunction in schizophrenia have tended to give way to models of cerebral disconnectivity (Bullmore *et al.*, 1997) that fit well with both neuropathological and functional neuroimaging findings. This may be one reason for inconsistent neuroanatomical findings in schizophrenia, as "lesions" in different areas of a widely distributed neural system could produce similar functional disturbance.

Magnetic resonance spectroscopy: abnormal neuronal metabolism

Magnetic resonance spectroscopy (MRS) is an imaging technique that can be used to extract *in vivo* information on dynamic biochemical processes at a neuronal level. Proton (^{1}H) MRS focuses on changes in the neuronal marker *N*-acetyl aspartate (NAA). Studies in adult patients with schizophrenia have shown reductions in NAA in the hippocampal area and dorso-lateral prefrontal cortex (DLPFC).

Similar reductions in NAA ratios specific to the hippocampus and DLPFC (Bertolino *et al.*, 1998) and frontal gray matter (Thomas *et al.*, 1998) have been reported in childhood-onset schizophrenia, suggesting neuronal damage or malfunction in these regions.

Pettegrew *et al.* (1991) used ^{31}P MRS with non-medicated patients during a first episode of schizophrenia and found reduced phosphonoester (PME) resonance and increased phosphodiester (PDE) resonance in the PFC. This result is compatible with reduced synthesis and increased breakdown of connective processes in the PFC. A similar finding of reduced PME and increased PDE resonance has been reported in adults with autism, although they showed increased prefrontal metabolic activity, which was not seen in people with schizophrenia (Pettegrew *et al.*, 1991). Keshavan *et al.* (2003) reported reduced PME moieties (e.g., synaptic vesicles and phosphorylated proteins) in the PFC using ^{31}P MRS in a sample of children and adolescents at genetic high risk for schizophrenia. These findings suggest abnormal synaptic structure and function in the PFC is a marker of schizophrenia risk. Further follow-up is required to determine if these findings have predictive value.

Implications for neurodevelopmental models of schizophrenia

Taken together, the neuropathological and brain imaging findings provide considerable support for the idea of progressive neurodevelopmental changes in schizophrenia, including excessive synaptic elimination resulting in aberrant neural connectivity. The progressive nature of brain volume reductions in adolescence, and the fact that reduced brain volume is not accompanied by reduced intracranial volume, suggests that a static pre- or peri-natal brain insult is insufficient to account for this process. While early random events in fetal neurodevelopment (e.g., hypoxia, viruses, etc.) may affect baseline synaptic density, genetically determined excessive synaptic elimination (or alternatively a "shift to the left" of a normal developmental process), as proposed by the "late" neurodevelopmental model, may be the neurobiological process underlying disorders in the schizophrenia spectrum (McGlashen & Hoffman, 2000). The support for a premature process in cortical development is suggested by the diminution in differences between childhood-onset schizophrenia and controls with age; by age 25, patients with childhood-onset schizophrenia have the same pattern as seen in adults (Greenstein *et al.*, 2006). What is unclear is whether excessive synaptic elimination in the PFC (and possibly other brain regions) is a sufficient cause for psychosis to occur, or whether it provides a vulnerable neurocognitive substrate that must interact with environmental stressors (e.g., cannabis exposure or cognitive/social stressors) to produce psychotic symptoms. Abnormal synaptic elimination remains one hypothesis that may account for structural brain changes seen on MRI. However, most of the postmortem evidence does not suggest synaptic elimination abnormalities in schizophrenia nor neurotoxicity, nor even evidence of cortical thinning at post-mortem examination (see Chapter 18). So, the interpretation of changes seen with MRI is not clear.

Genetics

Multigene models of risk

Twin studies have suggested the heritability of schizophrenia to be as high as 83% (Cannon *et al.*, 1998). However, one of the most significant implications of twin, adoption, and family studies in schizophrenia has been the challenge the results pose to traditional qualitatively distinct categories of the disorder (Rutter & Plomin, 1997). Quantitative genetic studies have shown that the genetic liability to schizophrenia extends to schizoptypal personality disorders and other conditions viewed as lying on the broader schizophrenia spectrum (Kendler *et al.*, 1995; Erlenmeyer-Kimling *et al.*, 1995). These results suggest that in schizophrenia quantitative traits that determine liability to disorder are likely to be inherited.

While the mode of inheritance in schizophrenia remains unknown, most evidence supports a multilocus or multifactorial threshold model. This model proposes that schizophrenia results from the combined action of multiple genes of small effect which confer susceptibility to the schizophrenic phenotype, with the disorder being expressed above a particular liability threshold. Susceptibility to the disorder is expressed as a dimension in the population, i.e., the risk of schizophrenia in the population is distributed normally, not bimodally. Because there are likely to be multiple genes involved, the genetics of schizophrenia is moving away from the rather simplistic notion of finding a single major gene for the disorder, towards a search for genes that confer susceptibility traits. Susceptibility alleles may be quite common in the population and hence the predictive value of any individual allele alone will be low. These concepts are discussed in greater detail in Chapters 12 and 13.

It is sometimes assumed that genes that affect brain development in schizophrenia are only expressed during fetal neurodevelopment. However, it is likely that some susceptibility genes for schizophrenia affect both fetal and later processes such as synaptic pruning (Feinberg, 1997).

Candidate genes in childhood-onset schizophrenia

The D-amino acid oxidase activator (DAOA) polymorphism (13q33.2) was associated with childhood-onset schizophrenia in the NIMH sample (Addington *et al.*, 2004). Interestingly, in the same NIMH sample, DAOA was associated with *later* age of onset and *lower* scores for pre-morbid autism symptoms. Another intriguing finding in the NIMH childhood-onset schizophrenia sample is an association between dysbindin (*DTNBP1*, 6p22.3) and poor premorbid social and academic adjustment (Rapoport *et al.*, 2005). Additionally, polymorphisms of the *GAD1* (glutamic acid decarboxylase) gene have been associated with both childhood-onset schizophrenia and abnormal frontal gray matter loss (Addington *et al.*, 2005). Finally, neuroregulin 1 (*NRG1*) susceptibility haplotypes have been associated with abnormal developmental trajectories for both gray and white matter in this population (Addington *et al.*, 2007). Effects differed for the childhood schizophrenia and control groups, suggesting unique epistatic effects for the patient sample.

Cytogenetic abnormalities

The association between schizophrenia and chromosomal deletions offers another possible route to locating candidate genes (Hennah *et al.*, 2006). The velocardiofacial syndrome (VCFS) microdeletion on chromosome 22q11 (which includes the *COMT* gene plus two candidates, *PRODH* and *ZDHHC8*) is associated with adult schizophrenia, occurring at a rate of up to 2% compared to 0.02% in the normal population (Karayiorgou *et al.*, 1995). The association with schizophrenia is not specific, as the VCFS microdeletion is also linked with higher rates of other psychiatric disorders (e.g., affective disorder, ADHD, autism). In the NIMH study of childhood-onset schizophrenia, a high rate of previously undetected cytogenetic abnormalities was found, including 4 of 80 (5%) with VCFS (Sporn *et al.*, 2004b). The 22q11DS is associated with progressive cortical gray matter loss in children and adolescents who are not yet psychotic, suggesting that a gene or genes mapping to 22q11 is responsible for a high-risk phenotype (Sporn *et al.*, 2004b). The overall high rate of various cytogenetic abnormalities (seen in 10% of the NIMH sample) suggests the possibility of more subtle genomic instability similar to that seen in autism (Rapoport *et al.*, 2005). This idea is supported by the high rate of small structural deletions/duplications that disrupt genes seen in early-onset cases (Walsh *et al.*, 2008).

Neuropsychology

Pattern of cognitive deficits

There is growing awareness that cognitive deficits in schizophrenia are a core feature of the disorder and cannot simply be dismissed as secondary consequences of psychotic symptoms (Breier, 1999; see also Chapter 8). As noted above, the degree of cognitive impairment is greater in child and adolescent-onset than in adult-onset patients. These findings raise several important questions: First, are the cognitive deficits specific or general, i.e., are some aspects of cognitive functioning affected more than others? Second, which deficits precede the onset of psychosis and could be causal, and which are consequences of psychosis? Third, is the pattern of deficits specific to schizophrenia or shared with other developmental and psychotic disorders? Fourth, are cognitive impairments progressive or static after the onset of psychosis?

Children with schizophrenia have specific difficulties with cognitive tasks that make demands on short-term, working memory, selective and sustained attention, and speed of processing (Asarnow *et al.*, 1995). These deficits are similar to those reported in adult schizophrenia (Saykin *et al.*, 1994). Deficits of attention and short-term and recent long-term memory have also been reported in adolescents with schizophrenia (Friedman *et al.*, 1996). In contrast, well-established "over learned" rote language and simple perceptual skills are unimpaired in child and adolescent-onset schizophrenia. Asarnow *et al.* (1991, 1995) have shown that children with schizophrenia have impairments in the span of apprehension task (a target stimulus has to be identified from an array of other figures when displayed for 50 ms). Performance on the task deteriorates markedly when increasing demands are made on information processing capacity (e.g., increasing the number of letters in the display from 3 to 10). Furthermore, event-related potential (ERP) studies using the span of apprehension task in both children and adults with schizophrenia, when compared to age-matched controls, show less negative endogenous activity measured between 100 and 300 ms after the stimulus. Similar findings of reduced ERPs (processing negativity Np and P2 components) have been found during the CPT in both childhood- and adult-onset schizophrenia (Strandburg *et al.*, 1999). These findings indicate a deficit in the allocation of attentional resources to a stimulus (Asarnow *et al.*, 1995). As with adults, children and adolescents with schizophrenia show high basal autonomic activity and less autonomic responsivity than controls (Gordon *et al.*, 1994), with attenuated increases in skin conductance following the presentation of neutral sounds (Zahn *et al.*, 1997). Childhood-onset patients, like adults, show increased reaction times with a loss of ipsimodal advantage compared to healthy controls (Zahn *et al.*, 1998). Eye tracking dysfunction (ETD)—a putative proxy of frontal lobe dysfunction—as indexed by abnormalities in smooth pursuit eye movements (SPEM), has also been found in childhood-onset schizophrenia (Kumra *et al.*, 2001). Similar ETD has been reported in adult schizophrenia (Iacono & Koenig, 1983). ETD is also a potential genetic endophenotype trait marker for schizophrenia, which has been detected in healthy siblings of childhood-onset schizophrenia and parents of adult-onset patients (Sporn *et al.*, 2005). Non-psychotic relatives of patients with schizophrenia also show eye-tracking deficits that correlate with subtle frontal lobe dysfunction (O'Driscoll *et al.*, 1999). Finally, children with schizophrenia also show similar impairments to adult patients on tests of frontal lobe executive function, such as the Wisconsin Card Sorting Test (WCST) (Asarnow *et al.*, 1994b). Hence, reduced prefrontal activation may be one expression of a genetic susceptibility to schizophrenia

In summary, while basic sensorimotor skills, associative memory, and simple language abilities tend to be preserved in children with schizophrenia, deficits are most marked on tasks which require focused and sustained attention, flexible switching of cognitive set, high information processing speed, and suppression of prepotent responses (Asarnow *et al.*, 1995). The diverse cognitive processes described here have been integrated under the cognitive domain of "executive functions" which are presumed to be mediated by the PFC system. Executive function skills are necessary to generate and execute goal-directed behavior, especially in novel situations. Goal-orientated action requires that information in the form of plans and expectations are held "on-line" in working memory and flexibly changed in response to feedback. Similar deficits have also been found in children genetically at "high risk" for schizophrenia (Erlenmeyer-Kimling & Cornblatt, 1978) and non-psychotic relatives of probands with schizophrenia (Park *et al.*, 1995). This strengthens the argument that cognitive deficits cannot be simply dismissed as non-specific consequences of schizophrenic symptoms, but rather are likely to be indicators of underlying genetic and neurobiological risk. Several candidate susceptibility genes (*dysbindin-1* and *COMT*) have been linked to impaired working memory and may provide molecular mechanisms underlying this intermediate (endo) phenotype of schizophrenia (Egan *et al.*, 2001). However, executive function deficits are probably not a primary or sufficient cause of schizophrenia given that they also occur in other neurodevelopmental disorders, including autism and ADHD (Pennington, 1997).

Course of cognitive deficits

Kraepelin's term "dementia praecox" implied a progressive cognitive decline as part of the disease process. Jones *et al.* (1994) described how academic performance becomes progressively more deviant during adolescence in those individuals destined to develop schizophrenia in adult life. A similar finding of IQ decline from childhood through adolescence that precedes the onset of schizophrenia in adult life has been reported from a large Israeli population-based cohort (Reichenberg *et al.*, 2005). There is some tentative evidence for a small decline in IQ following the onset of psychosis in childhood-onset schizophrenia (Alaghband-Rad *et al.*, 1995), followed by a stabilization of cognitive function despite progressive cortical gray matter loss during adolescence (Gochman *et al.*, 2005). However,

without longitudinal control data, this is difficult to evaluate, given that, in typically-developing samples, most IQ tests will show improved scores with repeated administration. Furthermore, the small drop in IQ after the onset of psychosis could possibly be due to the effect of psychotic symptoms on performance or the effect of treatment. Insofar as there is an effect, it looks like premature arrest, or slowing, of normal cognitive development in child and adolescent-onset schizophrenia, rather than a progressive dementia.

Assessment

The assessment of a child or adolescent with possible schizophrenia should include a detailed history, mental state and physical examination, and laboratory tests. In addition, a baseline psychometric assessment is desirable. A detailed understanding of specific cognitive deficits in individual cases of adolescent schizophrenia can be particularly helpful in guiding education and rehabilitation. In the physical examination, particular attention should be given to detecting dysmorphic features that may betray an underlying genetic syndrome. The neurological examination should focus on abnormal involuntary movements and other signs of extrapyramidal dysfunction. Spontaneous, abnormal involuntary movements have been detected in a proportion of drug-naïve first-episode schizophrenic or schizophreniform patients, as well as in those receiving typical antipsychotics (Gervin *et al.*, 1998).

Physical investigations

Physical investigations and laboratory tests in suspected cases of child and adolescent-onset schizophrenia are listed in Table 3.1. It is usual to obtain a full blood count and biochemistry, including liver and thyroid function and a drug screen (urine or hair analysis). The high yield of cytogenetic abnormalities reported in childhood-onset schizophrenia (Nicholson *et al.*, 1999) suggests the value of cytogenetic testing, including karyotyping for sex chromosome aneuploidies and fluorescent *in situ* hybridization (FISH) for 22q11DS (VCFS). The evidence of progressive structural brain changes (Rapoport *et al.*, 1999) indicates the value of obtaining a baseline and annual follow-up brain MRI scans. Although structural MRI does not provide a diagnostic test for schizophrenia, it can be helpful in ruling out occult central nervous system (CNS) disease.

Assessment interviews and rating scales

Structured diagnostic investigator-based interviews that cover child and adolescent psychotic disorders include the Schedule for Affective Disorders and Schizophrenia for School-Age Children (K-SADS; Ambrosini, 2000), the CAPA (Child and Adolescent Psychiatric Assessment;

Table 3.1 Physical investigations in child and adolescent-onset psychoses.

Investigation	Target disorder
Urine drug screen	Drug-related psychosis (amphetamines, ecstasy, cocaine, LSD and other psychoactive compounds)
EEG	Complex partial seizures/TLE
MRI brain scan	Ventricular enlargement, structural brain anomalies (e.g., cavum septum pellucidum)
	Enlarged caudate (typical antipsychotics)
	Demyelination (metachromatic leukodystrophy)
	Hypodense basal ganglia (Wilson disease)
Serum copper and ceruloplasmin	Wilson disease
Urinary copper	
Arylsulfatase A (white blood cell)	Metachromatic leukodystrophy
Karyotype/cytogentics (FISH)	Sex chromosome aneuploides, velocardiofacial syndrome (22q11 microdeletion)

EEG, electroencephalogram; FISH, fluorescent *in situ* hybridization; LSD, lysergic acid diethylamine; MRI, magnetic resonance imaging; TLE, temporal lobe epilepsy.

Angold & Costello, 2000), and the DICA (Diagnostic Interview for Children and Adolescents; Reich, 2000). The DSM and ICD definitions of schizophrenia do not provide symptom definitions so the detailed glossaries that accompany these interviews are particularly useful.

Rating scales give quantitative measures of psychopathology and functional impairment. Scales to assess psychotic symptoms include the Scale for Assessment of Positive Symptoms (SAPS; Andreasen, 1984), the Scale for Assessment of Negative Symptoms (SANS; Andreasen, 1983), and the Positive and Negative Syndrome Scale (PANSS; Kay *et al.*, 1987). The 30-item Kiddie-PANSS has been developed for use in children and adolescents, and contains three subscales: positive syndrome, negative syndrome, and general psychopathology (Fields *et al.*, 1994). The Children's Global Assessment Scale (C-GAS) provides a rating of functional impairment on a 0–100 scale (Shaffer *et al.*, 1983). These scales can be used to record the longitudinal course of illness and treatment response. The Kiddie Formal Thought Disorder Story Game and Kiddie Formal Thought Disorder Scale (Caplan *et al.*, 1989) are research instruments produced for the assessment of thought disorder in children. Assessments of extrapyramidal symptoms

and involuntary movements can be made using the Abnormal Involuntary Movements Scale (AIMS; Rapoport *et al.*, 1985) and the Simpson–Angus Neurological Rating Scale (Simpson & Angus, 1970).

Developmental issues

The cognitive level of the child will influence their ability to understand and express complex psychotic symptoms, such as passivity phenomena, thought alienation, and hallucinations. In younger children, careful distinctions have to be made between developmental immaturity and psychopathology. For example, distinguishing true hallucinations from normal subjective phenomena like dreams and communication with imaginary friends may be difficult for young children. Developmental maturation can also affect the localization of hallucinations in space. Internal localization of hallucinations is more common in younger children and makes these experiences more difficult to subjectively differentiate from inner speech or thoughts (Garralda, 1984). Formal thought disorder may also appear very similar to the pattern of illogical thinking and loose associations seen in children with immature language development. Negative symptoms can appear very similar to non-psychotic language and social impairments, and can also be easily confused with anhedonia and depression.

Differential diagnosis

Psychotic symptoms in children and adolescents are diagnostically non-specific, occurring in a wide range of functional psychiatric and organic brain disorders. A summary of physical investigations in children and adolescents with suspected schizophrenia is listed in Table 3.2. Referral for a neurological opinion is recommended if neurodegenerative disorder is suspected (see below).

Affective, schizoaffective, and "atypical" psychoses

The high rate of positive psychotic symptoms found in adolescent-onset major depression and mania can lead to diagnostic confusion (Joyce, 1984). Affective psychoses are most likely to be misdiagnosed as schizophrenia if a Schneiderian concept of schizophrenia is applied with its emphasis on first-rank symptoms. Because significant affective symptoms also occur in about one-third of first-episode patients with schizophrenia, it may be impossible to make a definitive diagnosis on the basis of a single cross-sectional assessment. In DSM-IV the distinction between schizophrenia, schizoaffective disorder, and affective psychoses is determined by the relative predominance and temporal overlap of psychotic symptoms (hallucinations and delusions) and affective symptoms (elevated or

Table 3.2 Differential diagnosis of schizophrenia in childhood and adolescence.

Psychoses	Affective psychoses (bipolar/major depressive disorder)
	Schizoaffective disorder
	Atypical psychosis
Developmental disorders	Autism spectrum disorders (Asperger syndrome)
	Developmental language disorder
	Schizotypal personality disorder
	"Multidimensionally impaired" disorder
Organic conditions	Drug-related psychosis (amphetamines, ecstasy, LSD, PCP)
	Complex partial seizures (temporal lobe epilepsy)
	Wilson disease
	Metachromatic leukodystrophy

LSD, lysergic acid diethylamine; PCP, phencyclidine.

depressed mood). Given the difficulty in applying these rules with any precision, there is a need to identify other features to distinguish between schizophrenia and affective psychoses. Irrespective of the presence of affective symptoms, the most discriminating symptoms of schizophrenia are an insidious onset and the presence of negative symptoms (Hollis, 1999). Similarly, complete remission from a first psychotic episode within 6 months of onset is the best predictor of a diagnosis of affective psychosis (Hollis, 1999). Schizoaffective and atypical psychoses are diagnostic categories with low predictive validity and little longitudinal stability (Hollis, 2000).

Autistic spectrum and developmental language disorders

Some children on the autistic spectrum or with Asperger syndrome have social and cognitive impairments that overlap closely with the premorbid phenotype described in schizophrenia. Furthermore, children on the autistic spectrum can also develop psychotic symptoms in adolescence (Volkmar & Cohen, 1991). Towbin *et al.* (1993) have labeled another group of children who seem to belong within the autistic spectrum as having "multiplex developmental disorder". An increased risk for psychosis has also been noted in the adult follow-up of childhood developmental receptive language disorders (Clegg *et al.*, 2005). In the NIMH childhood-onset schizophrenia sample, 19 cases

(25%) had a lifetime diagnosis of ASD; one had autism, two had Asperger syndrome and 16 had pervasive developmental disorder-not otherwise specified (PDD-NOS; Sporn *et al.*, 2004a). The childhood-onset schizophrenia–ASD subgroup did not differ from the rest of the childhood-onset schizophrenia sample on a range of measures including age of onset, IQ, response to medications, and familial schizotypy. However, the rate of cortical gray matter loss was greater in the ASD group. While the authors concluded that ASD was more likely to be a severe form of premorbid social impairment rather than true comorbidity, an unexplained finding was the occurrence of two cases of autism in the siblings of the childhood-onset schizophrenia –ASD subgroup. While some children on the autistic spectrum can show a clear progression into classic schizophrenia, others show a more episodic pattern of psychotic symptoms without the progressive decline in social functioning and negative symptoms characteristic of child and adolescent-onset schizophrenia. These unexpected connections between ASD and schizophrenia are intriguing as several of the rare copy number variations (CNVs) reported for schizophrenia have also been reported for autism (Rapoport *et al.*, 2009), linking at least a subgroup etiologically.

Often it is only possible to distinguish between schizophrenia and disorders on the autistic spectrum by taking a careful developmental history that details the age of onset and pattern of autistic impairments in communication, social reciprocity, and interests/behaviors. According to DSM-IV, schizophrenia cannot be diagnosed in a child with autism/PDD unless hallucinations/delusions are present for at least 1 month. DSM-IV does not rank the active-phase symptoms of thought disorder, disorganization or negative symptoms as sufficient to make a diagnosis of schizophrenia in the presence of autism. In contrast, ICD-10 does not include autism/PDD as exclusion criteria for diagnosing schizophrenia.

"Multidimensionally impaired syndrome" and schizotypal personality disorder

"Multidimensionally impaired syndrome" (MDI) is a label applied to children who have brief, transient, psychotic symptoms, emotional lability, poor interpersonal skills, normal social skills, and multiple deficits in information processing (Kumra *et al.*, 1998c). The diagnostic status of this group remains to be fully resolved. Short-term follow-up suggests that they do not develop full-blown schizophrenic psychosis. However, they have an increased risk of schizophrenia-spectrum disorders among first-degree relatives and the neurobiological findings (e.g., brain morphology) are similar to those in childhood-onset schizophrenia (Kumra *et al.*, 1998c). At 11-year follow-up, 38% of patients met criteria for bipolar 1 disorder, 12% (4 of 23) for major depressive disorder (MDD), and 3% (1 of 32) for schizoaffective disorder. The remaining 47% (15 of 32) were divided into two groups on the basis of whether they were in remission and neuroleptic-free ("good outcome", n = 5) or still severely impaired and/or psychotic regardless of pharmacotherapy ("poor outcome", n = 10) (Stayer *et al.*, 2005).

Children with schizotypal personality disorder (SPD) lie on a phenotypic continuum with schizophrenia, have similar cognitive and social impairments, and are prone to magical thinking, mood disturbances, and non-psychotic perceptual disturbances. Distinction from the prodromal phase of schizophrenia is particularly difficult when there is a history of social and academic decline without clear-cut or persisting, psychotic symptoms. A follow-up of children with SPD found that 25% developed schizophrenia spectrum disorders (schizophrenia and schizoaffective disorder), suggesting that SPD may be a precursor of schizophrenia (Asarnow, 2005). It has been reported that negative symptoms and attention in SPD improve with a low dose of risperidone (0.25–2.0 mg) (Rossi *et al.*, 1997).

Epilepsy

Psychotic symptoms can occur in temporal and frontal lobe partial seizures (see Chapter 9). A careful history is usually sufficient to reveal an aura followed by clouding of consciousness and the sudden onset of brief ictal psychotic phenomena accompanied often by anxiety, fear, derealization or depersonalization. However, longer-lasting psychoses associated with epilepsy can occur in clear consciousness during postictal or interictal periods (Sachdev, 1998). In epileptic psychoses, hallucinations, disorganized behavior, and persecutory delusions predominate, while negative symptoms are rare. Children with complex partial seizures also have increased illogical thinking and use fewer linguistic-cohesive devices, which can resemble formal thought disorder (Caplan *et al.*, 1992). A PET study showed hypoperfusion in the frontal, temporal, and basal ganglia in psychotic patients with epilepsy compared to non-psychotic epileptic patients (Gallhofer *et al.*, 1985).

Epilepsy and schizophrenia may co-occur in the same individual, so that the diagnoses are not mutually exclusive. The onset of epilepsy almost always precedes psychosis unless seizures are secondary to antipsychotic medication. In a long-term follow-up of 100 children with temporal lobe epilepsy, 10% developed schizophrenia in adult life (Lindsay *et al.*, 1979).

An electroencephalogram (EEG) should be performed if a seizure disorder is considered in the differential diagnosis or arises as a side effect of antipsychotic treatment. Ambulatory EEG monitoring and telemetry with event recording may be required if the diagnosis remains in doubt.

Neurodegenerative disorders

Rare neurodegenerative disorders with onset in late childhood and adolescence can mimic schizophrenia (see Chapter 9). The most important examples are Wilson disease (hepato-lenticular degeneration) and metachromatic leukodystrophy. These disorders usually involve significant extrapyramidal symptoms (e.g., tremor, dystonia, bradykinesia) or other motor abnormalities (e.g., unsteady gait) and a progressive loss of skills (dementia) that can aid the distinction from schizophrenia. Suspicion of a neurodegenerative disorder is one of the clearest indications for brain MRI in adolescent psychoses. Adolescents with schizophrenia show relative gray matter reduction with white matter sparing. In contrast, metachromatic leukodystrophy is characterized by frontal and occipital white matter destruction and demyelination. In Wilson disease, hypodense areas are seen in the basal ganglia, together with cortical atrophy and ventricular dilatation. The pathognomonic Kayser–Fleisher ring in Wilson disease begins as a greenish-brown crescent-shaped deposit in the cornea above the pupil (this is most easily seen during slit lamp examination). In Wilson disease there is increased urinary copper excretion, and reduced serum copper and serum ceruloplasmin levels. The biochemical marker for metachromatic leukodystrophy is reduced arylsulfatase-A (ASA) activity in white blood cells. This enzyme deficiency results in a deposition of excess sulfatides in many tissues including the CNS.

Drug psychoses

Illicit drug use is increasingly common among young people, so the frequent co-occurrence of drug use and psychosis is to be expected. Psychotic symptoms can occur as a direct pharmacological effect of intoxication with stimulants (amphetamine, ecstasy, cocaine), hallucinogens [lysergic acid diethylamide (LSD), phencyclidine, psilocybin "magic mushrooms",, mescaline), cannabis (Poole & Brabbins, 1996), and ketamine, an *N*-methyl-D-aspartic acid (NMDA) receptor antagonist and anesthetic (Krystal *et al.*, 2006). The psychotic symptoms associated with drug intoxication are usually short-lived and resolve within a few days of abstinence from the drug. These drugs can have surprisingly long half-lives with cannaboids still measurable up to 6 weeks after a single dose. Psychotic symptoms in the form of "flashbacks" can also occur after cessation of chronic cannabis and LSD abuse. These phenomena are similar to alcoholic hallucinosis and typically involve transient, vivid, auditory hallucinations occurring in clear consciousness.

It is often assumed that there is a simple causal relationship between drug use and psychosis, with any evidence of drug use excluding the diagnosis of a functional psychosis. However, this is a naïve approach, as drug use can both be a consequence of psychosis with patients using drugs to "treat" their symptoms in the early stages of a psychotic relapse, or with cannabis, a cause of schizophrenia in susceptible individuals (Arseneault *et al.*, 2004). Overall, there is very little evidence to invoke a separate entity of "drug-induced" psychosis in cases where psychotic symptoms arise during intoxication but then persist after the drug is withdrawn (Poole & Brabbins, 1996). Patients whose so-called "drug-induced" psychoses last for more than 6 months appear to have more clear-cut schizophrenic symptoms, a greater familial risk for psychosis, and greater premorbid dysfunction (Tsuang *et al.*, 1982). DSM-IV takes the sensible position that a functional psychosis should not be excluded unless there is compelling evidence that symptoms are uniquely associated with drug use.

Treatment approaches

General principles

While antipsychotic drugs remain the cornerstone of treatment in child and adolescent schizophrenia, all young patients with schizophrenia require a multimodal treatment package that includes pharmacotherapy, family and individual counseling, education about the illness, and provision to meet social and educational needs (Clark & Lewis, 1998; American Academy of Child and Adolescent Psychiatry, 2001).

Prevention and early detection

In theory at least, the onset of schizophrenia could be prevented if an intervention reduced the premorbid "risk" status or exposure to causative risk factors. The difficulty with the premorbid phenotype as currently conceived (i.e., subtle social and developmental impairments) is its extremely low specificity and positive predictive value for schizophrenia in the general population. The premorbid psychopathology in childhood-onset schizophrenia is equally non-specific with a range of diagnoses, e.g., conduct disorder, ADHD, anxiety states, depression, and ASD, preceding schizophrenia (Schaeffer & Ross, 2002). Future refinement of the premorbid phenotype is likely to move from the traditional phenomenological approach to include genetic and neurocognitive markers in order to achieve greater sensitivity and specificity.

An alternative approach is to target putative environmental risk factors such as cannabis exposure. If a direct causal relationship between cannabis and schizophrenia is assumed, then the population attributable fraction for the Dunedin cohort is 8% (Arseneault *et al.*, 2004). Put another way, removal of cannabis use from 15 year olds in the Dunedin cohort would have resulted in an 8% reduction in the incidence of schizophrenia. Given the rising prevalence of cannabis use in younger adolescents—a group who may be particularly sensitive to its effects—an important public policy intervention would be to delay the onset of cannabis use in young people.

In contrast to primary prevention, the aims of early detection are to identify the onset of deterioration in vulnerable individuals with a high predictive validity. Follow-up of the Australian EPPIC "ultra-high-risk" sample over 12 months found 40.8% developed a psychotic disorder. Significant predictors of transition to psychosis included long duration of prodromal symptoms, poor functioning at intake, low-grade psychotic symptoms, depression, and disorganization (Yung *et al.*, 2003). A key question is whether early intervention in an "ultra-high-risk" or prodromal group can prevent the transition to psychosis. The EPPIC group conducted a randomized controlled trial of combined low-dose risperidone (mean 1.3 mg/day) and cognitive–behavioral therapy (CBT) compared to standard needs-based intervention in the "ultra high risk" (McGorry *et al.*, 2002). The risperidone/CBT intervention significantly reduced transition to psychosis at 6 months (3 of 31 *vs.* 10 of 28 developed psychosis) but there was no significant difference by 12 months. These findings suggest that aggressive early intervention in a population presenting with high-risk mental states and attenuated psychotic symptoms may delay the onset of frank psychosis (prevalence reduction) but may not necessarily reduce the incidence of psychosis. A pragmatic stance would be to monitor children and adolescents with a strong family history and/or suggestive prodromal symptoms to ensure prompt treatment of psychosis.

A key argument used to support early intervention in psychosis has been the finding that a long duration of untreated psychosis is associated with poor long-term outcome in schizophrenia (Loebel *et al.*, 1992; Wyatt, 1995). A similar association has been found in child and adolescent-onset psychoses (Hollis, 1999). While the association between duration of untreated psychosis and poor outcome seems secure, the causal connection is far less certain. A long duration of untreated psychosis is also associated with insidious onset and negative symptoms which could confound links with poor outcome. While there are good *a priori* clinical reasons for the early treatment of symptoms to relieve distress and prevent secondary impairments, as yet, it remains unproven whether early intervention actually alters the long-term course of schizophrenia and there is significant concern about "false-positive" diagnosis and over-treatment with antipsychotic medication.

Pharmacological treatments

Because of the very small number of antipsychotic trials conducted with child and adolescent patients, it is necessary to extrapolate most evidence on drug efficacy from studies in adults. This seems a reasonable approach given that schizophrenia is similar in many respects whether it has onset in childhood or adulthood. However, it should be noted that children and adolescents show a greater sensitivity to a range of antipsychotic-related adverse events, including extrapyramidal side effects (EPS), treatment resistance with traditional antipsychotics (Kumra et al., 1998b), and weight gain, obesity, and metabolic syndrome with the newer atypical antipsychotics (Ratzoni et al., 2002).

Antipsychotics can be broadly divided into the traditional "typical" and newer "atypical" drugs. The typical drugs include haloperidol, chlorpromazine, and trifluperazine, which block D_2 receptors, produce catalepsy in rats, raise plasma prolactin, and induce EPS. The newer atypical drugs are effective antipsychotics that are "atypical" in the sense that they do not produce catalepsy, do not raise prolactin levels, and produce significantly fewer EPS. Not all atypicals neatly fit this definition; for example, risperidone raises prolactin levels and may cause EPS at higher doses (>4 mg/day) with "atypicality" resulting from antagonism of 5-HT receptors rather than reduced D_2 receptor blockade. The atypicals were introduced during the 1990s and currently include clozapine, risperidone, olanzapine, quetiapine, zotepine, and amisulpride. More recently, aripiprazole, a partial dopamine agonist, has been introduced. The pharmacological profile of the atypicals is diverse, involving various combinations of 5-HT and dopamine receptor blockade. Apripipazole acts as dopamine antagonist at hyperdopaminergic sites (e.g., mesolimbic system in schizophrenia) and as a dopamine agonist at hypodopaminergic sites (e.g., PFC in schizophrenia). Interestingly, the therapeutic effects of clozapine (potent affinity for D_4 and 5-HT$_{1,2,3}$ receptors) is independent of D_2 receptor occupancy, previously thought to be essential for antipsychotic action. The pharmacology of antipsychotic drugs is discussed in Chapter 23.

The typical antipsychotic haloperidol has been shown to be superior to placebo in two double-blind controlled trials of children and adolescents with schizophrenia (Pool et al., 1976; Spencer & Campbell, 1994). It is estimated that about 70% of patients show a good or partial response to antipsychotic treatment, although this may take 6–8 weeks to be apparent (Clark & Lewis, 1998; American Academy of Child and Adolescent Psychiatry, 2001). The main drawbacks concerning the use of high-potency typicals such as haloperidol in children and adolescents is the high risk of EPS (produced by D_2 blockade of the nigrostriatal pathway), tardive dyskinesia, and the lack of effect against negative symptoms and cognitive impairment. Clozapine (the prototypic atypical) has been shown to be superior to haloperdol in a double-blind trial of 21 cases of childhood-onset schizophrenia (Kumra et al., 1996). Larger open clinical trials of clozapine confirm its effectiveness in child and

adolescent-onset schizophrenia (Remschmidt et al., 1994). Similar, though less marked, benefits of olanzapine over typical antipsychotics in childhood-onset schizophrenia have been reported (Kumra et al., 1998a). The dopamine partial agonist aripiprazole has been shown to be effective and well tolerated in a short-term (6-week) double-blind randomized placebo controlled trial in adolescents (age 13–17 years) with schizophrenia (Findling et al., 2008).

Recent head-to-head comparisons of atypicals (risperidone and olanzapine) *versus* typicals (haloperidol) in adolescents with schizophrenia have reported broadly similar efficacy against psychotic symptoms (with a non-significant trend in favor of atypicals) but a differing profile of adverse effects (Gothelf et al., 2003; Sikich et al., 2008). These finding broadly replicate results from the large NIMH CATIE pragmatic trial that found no overall difference in effectiveness between typical and atypical antipsychotics in adults, whereas there were differences in tolerability and side effect profiles (Lieberman et al., 2005). The UK CUtLASS study compared effects after randomization to either typical or atypical antipsychotics following a clinical decision to change medication in adults with chronic schizophrenia (Jones et al., 2006). There were no differences in outcome (quality of life, symptoms, and adverse events) measured at 1 year when comparing the broad classes of typical and atypical antipsychotics. While similar pragmatic clinical effectiveness studies are needed in children and adolescents with schizophrenia, it is known that younger and first-episode patients are more sensitive to both therapeutic and adverse effects of antipsychotics. Furthermore, individual drugs within both classes differ importantly in terms of tolerability and side effect profiles when prescribed to children and adolescents. In younger patients (children and adolescents), EPS are more common with haloperidol and high-dose risperidone than with olanzapine. Weight gain and obesity are most common with olanzapine (most), then with risperidone, and least with haloperidol. Sedation is greater with olanzapine and haloperiol than with risperidone (Toren et al., 2004). Further evidence is emerging that children and adolescents experience more rapid and serious weight gain on olanzapine and risperidone than do adults (Ratzoni et al., 2002). Morbid obesity [body mass index (BMI) > 90th percentile] is found in up to 50% of adolescents and young people chronically treated with atypical antipsychotics (Theisen et al., 2001). Complications of obesity include hyperglycemia (Type 2 diabetes), hyperlipidemia, and hypercholesterolemia. It is recommended that dietary advice (reducing carbohydrate intake) combined with regular exercise should be prescribed before initiating atypicals in children and adolescents.

Baseline investigations and monitoring

Before starting treatment with antipsychotic medication, a physical examination should include height, weight

(BMI), cardiovascular system examination, including pulse and blood pressure, and a neurological examination for evidence of abnormal movements. Baseline laboratory investigations include full blood count, liver function and electrolytes, prolactin, fasting blood glucose, and plasma lipids. Physical examination, laboratory investigations, and review of adverse effects should be repeated 6 monthly while a young person is receiving antipsychotic medication.

Summary

Drawing this evidence together, a strong case can be made for the first-line use of atypicals in child and adolescent schizophrenia (clozapine is licensed in the UK only for treatment-resistant schizophrenia). Treatment resistance in child and adolescent patients should be defined as follows: (1) non-response with at least two antipsychotics (drawn from different classes and at least one being an atypical) each used for at least 4–6 weeks, and/or (2) significant adverse effects with conventional antipsychotics. The recommended order of treatment for first-episode schizophrenia in children and adolescents is: atypical as first line; if inadequate response, change to a different atypical or conventional antipsychotic; if response is still inadequate or side effects are intolerable, then initiate clozapine.

While atypicals reduce the risk of EPS, they can produce other troublesome side effects (usually dose related), including weight gain (olanzapine, clozapine, risperidone), hyperlipidemia (olanzapine), sedation, hypersalivation, and seizures (clozapine, olanzapine, quetiapine), and hyperprolactinemia (risperidone, amisulpride). The risk of blood dyscrasias on clozapine is effectively managed by mandatory routine blood monitoring. However, knowledge about potential adverse reactions with the newest atypicals is still limited in child and adolescent patients. Baseline investigations and follow-up monitoring every 6 months is recommended when prescribing antipsychotics. Baseline monitoring should include height, weight, blood pressure, full blood count, liver function and creatine kinase, fasting glucose, prolactin (risperidone, amisulpride), lipids (olanzapine, clozapine), and electrocardiogram (ECG) (zotepine). A further consideration is the greater cost of the newer atypicals compared to traditional antipsychotics. Although economic studies of cost-effectiveness have suggested that the costs of the atypicals are recouped in reduced inpatient stays and indirect social costs (Aitchison & Kerwin, 1997; see Chapter 33), the high cost of these drugs may limit availability, particularly in developing countries.

The UK National Institute for Health and Clinical Excellence (2002) has recommended the use of atypicals (risperidone, olanzapine, quetiapine, amisulpride, and zotepine) in all first-episode, newly diagnosed patients with schizophrenia and those on established therapy showing resistance to typical antipsychotics. Clinical trial evidence suggests that clozapine is the most effective antipsychotic in child and adolescent-onset schizophrenia, although its use is restricted to treatment-resistant cases. Atypicals such as olanzapine or risperidone should be used as a first-line treatment given that child and adolescent-onset schizophrenia is characterized by negative symptoms, cognitive impairments, sensitivity to EPS, and relative resistance to traditional antipsychotics. However, a growing awareness of adverse-effect profiles of different drugs and greater sensitivity to these effects in children and adolescents means drug choice should be a collaborative exercise, tailored to the needs and preferences of the young person and their family.

Psychosocial interventions

Psychosocial interventions range from CBT targeted at symptoms, problem-solving skills, and stress reduction, to patient and family psychoeducation, family therapy, counseling and support, social skills training, and remedial education (see Chapter 32).

Psychoeducation and family interventions

The rationale for psychosocial family interventions follows from the association between high expressed emotion (EE) and the risk of relapse in schizophrenia (Dixon & Lehman, 1995). The overall aim is to prevent relapse (secondary prevention) and improve the patient's level of functioning by modifying the family atmosphere. Psychosocial family interventions have a number of principles in common (Lam, 1991). First, it is assumed that it is useful to regard schizophrenia as an illness as patients are then less likely to be seen as responsible for their symptoms and behavior. Second, the family is not implicated in the etiology of the illness. Instead, the burden borne by the family in caring for a disturbed or severely impaired young person is acknowledged. Third, the intervention is offered as part of a broader multimodal package including drug treatment and outpatient clinical management.

An important issue when working with parents of children and adolescents with schizophrenia is to recognize that the illness typically results in a bereavement process for the loss of their "normal" child. Parents will often value a clear diagnosis of schizophrenia as it can provide an explanation for previously unexplained perplexing and disturbed behavior. Understanding schizophrenia as a disorder of the developing brain can also relieve commonly expressed feelings of guilt among parents and carers.

Lam (1991) conducted a systematic review of published trials of psychoeducation and more intensive family interventions in schizophrenia and drew the following conclusions. First, education packages on their own increase knowledge about the illness but do not reduce the risk of relapse. Second, more intensive family intervention studies with high EE relatives have shown a reduction in relapse rates linked to a lowering of EE. Third, family interventions tend to be costly and time-consuming with most clinical trials employing highly skilled research teams. Whether these interventions can be transferred into routine clinical practice is uncertain. Fourth, interventions have focused on the reduction of EE in "high-risk" families. Whether low-EE families would also benefit from these interventions is less clear. This is particularly relevant to the families of children and adolescents with schizophrenia as, on average, these parents express *lower* levels of criticism and hostility than parents of adult-onset patients (Asarnow *et al.*, 1994a).

Cognitive–behavioral therapy

In adult patients, cognitive therapy has been used to reduce the impact of treatment-resistant positive symptoms (Tarrier *et al.*, 1993). CBT has been shown to improve the short-term (6-month) outcome of adult patients with schizophrenia with neuroleptic-resistant positive symptoms (Turkington & Kingdon, 2000). Whether CBT is equally effective with younger patients, or those with predominant negative symptoms, remains to be established.

Cognitive remediation

Cognitive remediation is a relatively new psychological treatment which aims to arrest or reverse the cognitive impairments in attention, concentration, and working memory associated with negative symptoms and poor functional outcome in schizophrenia (Greenwood *et al.*, 2005). The results of an early controlled trial in adults are promising, with gains found in the areas of memory and social functioning (Wykes *et al.*, 2000). The severity of cognitive executive impairments in child and adolescent patients suggests that early remediation strategies may be particularly important interventions in younger patients. Helpful advice can also be offered to parents, teachers, and professionals, such as breaking down information and tasks into small, manageable parts to reduce demands on working memory and speed of processing.

Organization of treatment services

It is a paradox that patients with very early-onset schizophrenia have the most severe form of the disorder, yet they often receive inadequate and poorly coordinated services. Possibly this is because the responsibility for schizophrenia is seen to lie with adult psychiatric services with a remit that typically does not extend to patients under age 18. In the UK, community-based child and adolescent mental health services (CAMHS) provide the first-line assessment and care for child and young adolescent psychoses, with only about half of these cases referred to inpatient units (Slaveska *et al.*, 1998). While adolescent inpatient admis-

sion is often inappropriate, generic CAMHS services are usually unable to provide the mix of assertive outreach, early intervention, and crisis resolution services that have developed over the last decade in UK adult mental health services for psychoses and severe mental illness. Young people with schizophrenia are not generally well served by a separation of services and professional responsibilities at age 16 or 18. An alternative model is a community-based young person's psychosis service spanning ages 14–25 with access to dedicated adolescent and young adult beds. Such a service would provide early intervention, assertive outreach, intensive home treatment, and crisis resolution. It would integrate professional expertise from CAMHS (in particular addressing family, developmental, and educational issues) and adult mental health services.

Conclusions

The last decade has seen a dramatic growth in our understanding of the clinical course and neurobiological underpinnings of schizophrenia presenting in childhood and adolescence. It is now clear that adult-based diagnostic criteria have validity in this age group and the disorder has clinical and neurobiological continuity with schizophrenia in adults. Childhood-onset schizophrenia is a severe variant of the adult disorder associated with greater premorbid impairment, a higher familial risk, and more severe clinical course and poorer outcome. The poor outcome of children and adolescents with schizophrenia has highlighted the need to target early and effective treatments, and develop specialist services for this high-risk group. Unraveling neurocognitive and clinical heterogeneity should lead to improvements in our ability to deliver individually targeted treatments, as well as the ability to identify those "at risk" in order to prevent the onset of psychosis.

References

Addington A.M. & Rapoport J.L. (2009) The genetics of childhood-onset schizophrenia: when madness strikes the prepubescent. *Current Psychiatry Reports* **11**, 156–161.

Addington, A.M., Gornick, M., Sporn, A.L. *et al.* (2004) Polymorphisms in the 13q33.2 gene G72/G30 are associated with childhood-onset schizophrenia and psychosis not otherwise specified. *Biological Psychiatry* **55**, 976–980.

Addington, A.M., Gornick, M., Duckworth, J. *et al.* (2005) GAD1 (2q31.1), which encodes glutamic acid decarboxylase (GAD67), is associated with childhood-onset schizophrenia and cortical gray matter loss. *Molecular Psychiatry* **10**, 581–588.

Addington, A.M., Gornick, M.C., Shaw, P. *et al.* (2007) Neuregulin 1 (8p12) and childhood-onset schizophrenia: susceptibility haplotypes for diagnosis and brain development trajectories. *Molecular Psychiatry* **12**, 195–205.

Aitchison, K.J. & Kerwin, R.W. (1997) The cost effectiveness of clozapine. *British Journal of Psychiatry* **171**, 125–130.

Alaghband-Rad, J., McKenna, K., Gordon, C.T. *et al.* (1995) Childhood-onset schizophrenia: The severity of premorbid course. *Journal of the American Academy of Child Adolescent Psychiatry* **34**, 1273–1283.

Alaghband-Rad, J., Hamburger, S.D., Giedd, J., Frazier, J.A. & Rapoport, J.L. (1997) Childhood-onset schizophrenia: Biological markers in relation to clinical characteristics. *American Journal of Psychiatry* **154**, 64–68.

Ambrosini, P.J. (2000) Historical development and present status of the Schedule for Affective Disorders and Schizophrenia for School-Age Children (K-SADS). *Journal of the American Academy of Child Adolescent Psychiatry* **39**, 49–58.

American Academy of Child and Adolescent Psychiatry (2001) Practice parameter for the assessment and treatment of children and adolescents with schizophrenia. *Journal of the American Academy of Child Adolescent Psychiatry* **40** (Suppl.), 4S–23S

Andreasen, N.C. (1983) *Scale for the Assessment of Negative Symptoms (SANS)*. Iowa City: University of Iowa.

Andreasen, N.C. (1984) *Scale for the Assessment of Positive Symptoms (SAPS)*. Iowa City: University of Iowa.

Angold, A. & Costello, J.E. (2000) The Child and Adolescent Psychiatric Assessment (CAPA). *Journal of the American Academy of Child Adolescent Psychiatry* **39**, 39–48.

Arendt, M., Rosenberg, R., Foldager, L., Perto, G. & Munk-Jorgensen, P. (2005). Cannabis induced psychosis and subsequent schizophrenia-spectrum disorders: follow-up study of 535 incident cases. *British Journal of Psychiatry* **187**, 510–515.

Arseneault, L., Cannon, M., Poulton, R. *et al.* (2002) Cannabis use in adolescence and risk of adult psychosis: longitudinal prospective study. *British Medical Journal* **325**, 1212–1213.

Arseneault, L., Cannon, M., Witton, J. & Murray, R. (2004) Causal association between cannabis and psychosis: examination of the evidence. *British Journal of Psychiatry* **184**, 110–117.

Asarnow, J.R. (2005) Childhood-onset schizotypal disorder: a follow-up study and comparison with childhood-onset schizophrenia. *Journal of Child and Adolescent Psychopharmacology* **15**, 395–402.

Asarnow, R., Granholm, E. & Sherman, T. (1991) Span of apprehension in schizophrenia. In: Steinhauer, S.R., Gruzelier, J.H., Zubin, J., eds. *Handbook of Schizophrenia, Vol. 5: Neuropsychology, Psychophysiology and Information Processing*. Amsterdam: Elsevier, pp. 335–370.

Asarnow, J.R., Thompson, M.C., Hamilton, E.B., Goldstein, M.J. & Guthrie, D. (1994a) Family expressed emotion, childhood onset depression, and childhood onset schizophrenic spectrum disorders. Is expressed emotion a non-specific correlate of psychopathology or a specific risk factor for depression? *Journal of Abnormal Psychology* **22**, 129–146.

Asarnow, R., Asamen, J., Granholm, E., Sherman, T., Watkins, J.M. & William, M.E. (1994b) Cognitive/neuropsychological studies of children with schizophrenic disorder. *Schizophrenia Bulletin* **20**, 647–669.

Asarnow, R., Brown, W. & Stranberg R. (1995) Children with schizophrenic disorder: Neurobehavioural studies. *European Archives of Psychiatry and Clinical Neuroscience* **245**, 70–79.

Bertolino, A., Kumra, S., Callicott, J.H. *et al.* (1998) Common pattern of cortical pathology in childhood-onset and adult-onset schizophrenia as identified by proton magnetic resonance spectroscopic imaging. *American Journal of Psychiatry* **155**, 1376–1383.

Brans, R.G., van Haren, N.E., van Baal, G.C., Schnack, H.G., Kahn, R.S. & Hulshoff Pol, H.E. (2008) Heritability of changes in brain volume over time in twin pairs discordant for schizophrenia. *Archives of General Psychiatry* **65**, 1259–1268.

Brans, R.G., van Haren, N.E., van Baal, G.C. *et al.* (2008). Longitudinal MRI study in schizophrenia patients and their healthy siblings. *British Journal of Psychiatry* **193**, 422–423.

Breier, A. (1999) Cognitive deficit in schizophrenia and its neurochemical basis. *British Journal of Psychiatry* **174** (Suppl. 37), 16–18.

Bullmore, E.T., O'Connell, P., Frangou, S. & Murray, R.M. (1997) Schizophrenia as a developmental disorder or neural network integrity: the dysplastic net hypothesis. In: Keshavan, M.S. & Murray, R.M., eds. *Neuorodevelopment and Adult Psychopathology*. Cambridge: Cambridge University Press, pp. 253–266.

Cannon, T.D., Kaprio, J., Lonnqvist, J. *et al.* (1998) The genetic epidemiology of schizophrenia in a Finnish twin cohort. A population-based modelling study. *Archives of General Psychiatry* **55**, 67–74.

Cannon, M., Caspi, A., Moffitt, T.E. *et al.* (2002) Evidence for early childhood, pan-developmental imparment specific to schizophreniform disorder: results from a longitudinal birth cohort. *Archives of General Psychiatry* **59**, 449–456.

Caplan, R., Guthrie, D., Tanguay, P.E., Fish, B. & David-Lando, G. (1989) The Kiddie Formal Thought Disorder Scale (K-FTDS): clinical assessment reliability and validity. *Journal of the American Academy of Child and Adolescent Psychiatry* **28**, 408–416.

Caplan, R., Guthrie, D., Shields, W.D. & Mori, L. (1992) Formal thought disorder in paediatric complex partial seizure disorder. *Journal of Child Psychology and Psychiatry* **33**, 1399–1412.

Caspi, A., Moffitt, T.E., Cannon, M. *et al.* (2005) Moderation of the effect of adolescent-onset cannabis use on adult psychosis by a functional polymorphism in the catechol-O-methyltransferase gene: Longitudinal evidence of a gene X environment interaction. *Biological Psychiatry* **57**, 117–127.

Castle, D. & Murray, R. (1991) The neurodevelopmental basis of sex differences in schizophrenia. *Psychological Medicine* **21**, 565–575.

Clark, A. & Lewis, S. (1998) Treatment of schizophrenia in childhood and adolescence. *Journal of Child Psychology and Psychiatry* **39**, 1071–1081.

Clegg, J., Hollis, C. & Rutter, M. (2005) Developmental language disorders—A follow–up in later adult life: Cognitive, language and psychosocial outcomes. *Journal of Child Psychology and Psychiatry* **46**, 128–149.

Dasari, M., Friedman, L., Jesberger, J. *et al.* (1999) A magnetic resonance study of thalamic area in adolescent patients with either schizophrenia or bipolar disorder as compared to healthy controls. *Psychiatry Research* **91**, 155–162.

Dean, B., Bradbury, R. & Copolov, D.L. (2003) Cannabis-sensitive dopaminergic markers in post mortem central nervous system: changes in schizophrenia. *Biological Psychiatry* **53**, 585–592.

Dixon, L.B. & Lehman, A.F. (1995) family interventions for schizophrenia. *Schizophrenia Bulletin* **21**, 631–643.

Egan, M.F., Goldberg, T.E., Kolanchana, B.S. *et al.* (2001) Effect of COMT Val108/158Met genotype on frontal lobe function and risk for schizophrenia. *Proceedings of the National Academy of Sciences USA* **98**, 6917–6922.

Eggers, C. & Bunk, D. (1997) The long-term course of childhood-onset schizophrenia: A 42-year follow-up. *Schizophrenia Bulletin* **23**, 105–117.

Erlenmeyer-Kimling, L. & Cornblatt, B. (1978) Attentional measures in a study of children at high risk for schizophrenia. In: Wynne, L.C., Cromwell, R.L. & Matthysse, S., eds. *The Nature of Schizophrenia: New Approaches to Research and Treatment.* New York: Wiley.

Erlenmeyer-Kimling, L., Squires-Wheeler, E., Adamo, U.H. *et al.* (1995) The New York High Risk Project: Psychoses and cluster A personality disorders in offspring of schizophrenic parents at 23 years of follow-up. *Archives of General Psychiatry* **52**, 857–865.

Feinberg, I. (1983) Schizophrenia: Caused by a fault in programmed synaptic elimination during adolescence. *Journal of Psychiatric Research* **17**, 319–344.

Feinberg, I. (1997) Schizophrenia as an emergent disorder of late brain maturation. In: Keshavan, M.S. & Murray, R.M., eds. *Neuorodevelopment and Adult Psychopathology.* Cambridge: Cambridge University Press, pp. 237–252.

Fields, J.H., Grochowski, S. & Lindenmayer, J.P. *et al.* (1994) Assessing positive and negative symptoms in children and adolescents. *American Journal of Psychiatry* **151**, 249–253.

Findling, R.L., Robb, A., Nyilas, M. *et al.* (2008) A multi-centre, randomised, double-blind, placebo-controlled study of oral aripiprazole for treatment of adolescents with schizophrenia. *American Journal of Psychiatry* **165**, 1432–1441.

Fleischhaker, C., Schulz, R., Tepper, K., Martin, M., Hennighausen, K. & Remschmidt, H. (2005) Long-term course of adolescent schizophrenia. *Schizophrenia Bulletin* **31**, 769–780.

Frazier, J.A., Giedd, J.N., Kaysen, D. *et al.* (1996) Childhood-onset schizophrenia: Brain magnetic resonance imaging rescan after two years of clozapine maintenance. *American Journal of Psychiatry* **153**, 564–566.

Friedman, L., Finding, R.L., Buch, J. *et al.* (1996) Structural MRI and neuropsychological assessments in adolescent patients with either schizophrenia or affective disorders. *Schizophrenia Research* **18**, 189–190.

Frith, C.D. (1994) Theory of mind in schizophrenia. In: David, A. & Cutting, J.S., eds. *The Neuropsychology of Schizophrenia.* Hove: Lawrence Erlbaum, pp. 147–161.

Galdos P.M., van Os J. & Murray, R. (1993) Puberty and the onset of psychosis. *Schizophrenia Research* **10**, 7–14.

Gallhofer, B., Trimble, M.R., Frackowiak, R., Gibbs, J. & Jones, T. (1985) A study of cerebral blood flow and metabolism in epileptic psychosis using positron emission tomography and oxygen. *Journal of Neurology, Neurosurgery and Psychiatry* **48**, 201–206.

Garralda, M.E. (1984) Hallucinations in children with conduct and emotional disorders; I. The clinical phenomena. *Psychological Medicine* **14**, 589–596.

Geddes, J.R. & Lawrie, S.M. (1995) Obstetric complications and schizophrenia: a meta-analysis. *British Journal of Psychiatry* **167**, 786–793.

Gervin, M., Browne, S., Lane, A. *et al.* (1998) Spontaneous abnormal involuntary movements in first-episode schizophrenia and schizophreniform disorder: baseline rate in a group of patients from an Irish catchment area. *American Journal of Psychiatry* **155**, 1202–1206.

Giedd, J.N., Castellanos, F.X., Rajapaske, J.C. *et al.* (1996) Quantitative analysis of grey matter volumes in childhood-onset schizophrenia and attention deficit/hyperactivity disorder. *Society for Neuroscience Abstracts* **22**, 1166.

Giedd, J.N., Jefferies, N.O., Blumenthal, J. *et al.* (1999) Childhood-onset schizophrenia: progressive brain changes during adolescence. *Biological Psychiatry* **46**, 892–898.

Gillberg, C., Wahlstrom, J., Forsman, A., Hellgren, L. & Gillberg, J.C. (1986) Teenage psychoses—epidemiology, classification and reduced optimality in the pre-, peri- and neonatal periods. *Journal of Child Psychology and Psychiatry* **27**, 87–98.

Gochman, P.A., Greenstein, D., Sporn, A. *et al.* (2005) IQ stabilisation in childhood-onset schizophrenia. *Schizophrenia Research* **77**, 271–277.

Gogtay, N., Sporn, A., Clasen, L.S. *et al.* (2004) Comparison of progressive cortical gray matter loss in childhood-onset schizophrenia and that in childhood-onset atypical psychoses. *Archives of General Psychiatry* **61**, 17–22.

Goldstein, M.J. (1987) The UCLA High Risk Project. *Schizophrenia Bulletin* **13**, 505–514.

Goodman, R. (1988) Are complications of pregnancy and birth causes of schizophrenia? *Developmental Medicine and Child Neurology* **30**, 391–406.

Gordon, C.T., Frazier, J.A., McKenna, K. *et al.* (1994) Childhood-onset schizophrenia: A NIMH study in progress. *Schizophrenia Bulletin* **20**, 697–712.

Gothelf, D., Apter, A., Reidman, J. *et al.* (2003) Olanzapine, risperidone and haloperidol in the treatment of adolescent patients with schizophrenia. *Journal of Neural Transmission* **110**, 545–560.

Green, W., Padron-Gayol, M., Hardesty, A. & Bassiri, M. (1992) Schizophrenia with childhood onset: a phenomenological study of 38 cases. *Journal of the American Academy of Child and Adolescent Psychiatry* **31**, 968–976.

Greenstein, D., Lerch, J., Shaw, P. *et al.* (2006). Childhood onset schizophrenia: cortical brain abnormalities as young adults. *Journal of Child Psychology and Psychiatry* **47**, 1003–1012.

Greenwood, K.E., Landau, S. & Wykes, T. (2005) Negative symptoms and specific cognitive impairments as combined targets for improved functional outcome within cognitive remediation therapy. *Schizophrenia Bulletin* **31**, 910–921.

Gualtieri, C.T., Adams, A. & Chen, C.D. (1982) Minor physical abnormalities in alcoholic and schizophrenic adults and hyperactive and autistic children. *American Journal of Psychiatry* **139**, 640–643.

Gur, R.E., Cowell, P., Turetsky, B.I. *et al.* (1998) A follow-up magnetic resonance imaging study of schizophrenia. Relationship of neuroanatomical changes to clinical and neurobehavioural measures. *Archives of General Psychiatry* **55**, 145–152.

Hafner, H. & Nowotny, B. (1995) Epidemiology of early-onset schizophrenia. *European Archives of Psychiatry and Clinical Neuroscience* **245**, 80–92.

Hennah, W., Thompson, P., Peltonen, L. & Porteous, D. (2006). Beyond schizophrenia: The role of DISC1 in major mental illness. *Schizophrenia Bulletin* **32**, 409–416.

Hollis, C. (1995) Child and adolescent (juvenile onset) schizophrenia: a case control study of premorbid developmental impairments. *British Journal of Psychiatry* **166**, 489–495.

Hollis, C. (1999) *A Study of the Course and Adult Outcomes of Child and Adolescent-Onset Psychoses.* PhD Thesis, University of London.

Hollis, C. (2000) The adult outcomes of child and adolescent-onset schizophrenia: diagnostic stability and predictive validity. *American Journal of Psychiatry* **157**, 1652–1659.

Hollis, C. (2003) Developmental precursors of child- and adolescent-onset schizophrenia and affective psychoses: diagnostic specificity and continuity with symptom dimensions. *British Journal of Psychiatry* **182**, 37–44.

Hollis, C. & Taylor, E. (1997) Schizophrenia: a critique from the developmental psychopathology perspective. In: Keshavan, M.S. & Murray, R.M., eds. *Neurodevelopment and Adult Psychopathology.* Cambridge: Cambridge University Press, pp. 213–233.

Hooley, J.M. (1987) The nature and origins of expressed emotion. In: Hahlweg, K. & Goldstein, M.J., eds. *Understanding Major Mental Disorder: The Contribution of Family Interaction Research.* New York: Family Process, pp. 176–194.

Iacono, W.G. & Koenig, W.G.R. (1983). Features that distinguish smooth pursuit eye tracking performance in schizophrenic, affective disordered and normal individuals. *Journal of Abnormal Psychology* **92**, 29–41.

Jacobsen, L. & Rapoport, J. (1998) Research update: Childhood-onset schizophrenia: Implications for clinical and neurobiological research. *Journal of Child Psychology and Psychiatry* **39**, 101–113.

Jacobsen, L., Giedd, J.N., Berquin, P.C. *et al.* (1997a) Quantitative morphology of the cerebellum and fourth ventricle in childhood-onset schizophrenia. *American Journal of Psychiatry* **154**, 1663–1669.

Jacobsen, L., Hamburger, S.D., Van Horn, J.D. *et al.* (1997b) Cerebral glucose metabolism in childhood-onset schizophrenia. *Psychiatry Research* **75**, 131–144.

James, A.C.D., Javaloyes, J.S. & Smith D.M. (2002) Evidence of non-progressive changes in adolescent-onset schizophrenia. *British Journal of Psychiatry* **180**, 339–344.

James, A.C.D., Smith, D.M. & Jayaloes, J.S. (2004) Cerebellar, prefrontal cortex, and thalamic volumes over two time points in adolescent-onset schizophrenia. *American Journal of Psychiatry* **161**, 1023–1029.

Jarbin, H., Ott, Y. & Von Knorring, A.L. (2003) Adult outcome of social function in adolescent-onset schizophrenia and affective psychosis. *Journal of the American Academy of Child and Adolescent Psychiatry* **42**, 176–183.

Jones, P., Rogers, B., Murray, R. & Marmot, M. (1994) Child development risk factors for adult schizophrenia in the British 1946 birth cohort. *Lancet* **344**, 1398–1402.

Jones, P., Barnes, T.R.E., Davies, L. *et al.* (2006) Randomised controlled trial of effect on quality of life of second vs. first-generation antipsychotic drugs in schizophrenia. *Archives of General Psychiatry* **63**, 1079–1087.

Joyce, P.R. (1984) Age of onset in bipolar affective disorder and misdiagnosis of schizophrenia. *Psychological Medicine* **14**, 145–149.

Karayiorgou, M., Morris, M.A., Morrow, B. *et al.* (1995) Schizophrenia susceptability associated with interstitial deletions of chromosome 22q11. *Proceedings of the National Academy of Sciences USA* **92**, 7612–7616.

Kay, S.R., Opler, L.A. & Lindenmayer, J.P. (1987) The positive and negative syndrome scale (PANSS) for schizophrenia. *Schizophrenia Bulletin* **13**, 261–276.

Keller, A., Castellanos, F.X., Vaituzis, A.C., Jeffries, N.O., Giedd, J.N. & Rapoport, J.L. (2003) Progressive loss of cerebellar volume in childhood-onset schizophrenia. *American Journal of Psychiatry* **160**, 128–133.

Kendell, R.E., McInneny, K., Juszczak, E. & Bain, M. (2000) Obstetric complications and schizophrenia. Two case-control studies based on structured obstetric records. *British Journal of Psychiatry* **176**, 516–522.

Kendler, K.C., Neale, M.C. & Walsh, D. (1995) Evaluating the spectrum concept of schizophrenia in the Roscommon Family Study. *American Journal of Psychiatry* **152**, 749–754.

Keshavan, M.S., Stanley, J.A., Montrose, D.M., Minshew, N.J. & Pettigrew, J.W. (2003) Prefrontal membrane phospholipids metabolism of child and adolescent offspring at risk for schizophrenia or schizoaffective disorder: an *in vivo* MRS study. *Molecular Psychiatry* **8**, 316–323.

Kim-Cohen, J., Caspi, A., Moffitt, T.E., Harrington, H., Milne, B.J. & Poulton, R. (2003) Prior juvenile diagnosis in adults with mental disorder: developmental follow-back of a prospective longitudinal cohort. *Archives of General Psychiatry* **60**, 709–717.

Kolvin, I. (1971) Studies in childhood psychoses. I. Diagnostic criteria and classification. *British Journal of Psychiatry* **118**, 381–384.

Kolvin, I., Ounsted, C. Humphrey, M., & NcNay, A. (1971) Studies in childhood psychoses. II. The phenomenology of childhood psychoses. *British Journal of Psychiatry* **118**, 385–395.

Krystal, J.H., Perry, E.B., Gueorguieva, R. *et al.* (2006) Comparative and interactive human psychopharmacologic effects of ketamine and amphetamine: implications for glutamatergic and dopaminergic model psychoses and cognitive function. *Archives of General Psychiatry* **62**, 985–995.

Kumra, S., Frazier, J.A., Jacobsen, L.K. *et al.* (1996) Childhood-onset schizophrenia: A double blind clozapine–haloperidol comparison. *Archives of General Psychiatry* **53**, 1090–1097.

Kumra, S., Jacobsen, L.K., Lenane, M. *et al.* (1998a) Childhood-onset schizophrenia: an open-label study of olanzapine in adolescents. *Journal of the American Academy of Child and Adolescent Psychiatry* **37**, 360–363.

Kumra, S., Jacobsen, L.K., Lenane, M. *et al.* (1998b) Case series: spectrum of neuroleptic-induced movement disorders and extrapyramidal side-effects in childhood-onset schizophrenia. *Journal of the American Academy of Child and Adolescent Psychiatry* **37**, 221–227.

Kumra, S., Jacobsen, L.K., Lenane, M. *et al.* (1998c) "Multidimensionally impaired disorder": is it a variant of very early-onset schizophrenia? *Journal of the American Academy of Child and Adolescent Psychiatry* **37**, 91–99.

Kumra, S., Sporn A., Hommer, D.W. *et al.* (2001) Smooth pursuit eye-tracking impairment in childhood-onset psychotic disorders. *American Journal of Psychiatry* **158**, 1291–1298.

Lam, D.H. (1991) Psychosocial family intervention in schizophrenia: a review of empirical studies. *Psychological Medicine* **21**, 423–441.

Lay, B., Blanz, B., Hartmann, M. & Schmidt, M.H. (2000) The psychosocial outcome of adolescent-onset schizophrenia: a 12-year follow-up. *Schizophrenia Bulletin* **26**, 801–816.

Leff, J. & Vaughn, C. (1985) *Expressed Emotion in Families: Its Significance for Mental Illness.* London: Guilford Press.

Lewis, S.W. & Murray, R.M. (1987) Obstetric complications, neurodevelopmental deviance and risk of schizophrenia. *Journal of Psychiatric Research* **21**, 414–421.

Lieberman, J.A., Stroup, T.S., McEvoy, J.P. *et al.* (2005) Effectiveness of antipsychotic drugs in patients with chronic schizophrenia. *New England Journal of Medicine* **353**, 1209–1223.

Lindsay, J., Ounsted, C., & Richards, P. (1979) Long-term outcome of children with temporal lobe seizures. II. Marriage, parenthood and sexual indifference. *Developmental Medicine and Child Neurology* **21**, 433–440.

Loebel, A.D., Lieberman, J.A., Alvir, J.M.N. *et al.* (1992) Duration of psychosis and outcome in first episode schizophrenia. *American Journal of Psychiatry* **149**, 1183–1188.

Marquardt, R.K., Levitt, J.G., Blanton, R.E. *et al.* (2005) Abnormal development in the anterior cingulated in childhood-onset schizophrenia: a preliminary quantitative MRI study. *Psychiatry Research* **138**, 221–233.

Matsumoto, H., Takei, N., Saito, H., Kachi, K. & Mori, N. (1999) Childhood-onset schizophrenia and obstetric complications: a case-control study. *Schizophrenia Research* **38**, 93–99.

Matsumoto, H., Takei, N., Saito, H., Kachi, K. & Mori, N. (2001) The association between obstetric complications and childhood-onset schizophrenia: a replication study. *Psychological Medicine* **31**, 907–914.

McGlashen, T.H. & Hoffman, R.E. (2000). Schizophrenia as a disorder of developmentally reduced synaptic connectivity. *Archives of General Psychiatry* **57**, 637–648.

McGorry, P.D., Yung, A.R., Philips, L.J. *et al.* (2002) Randomised controlled trial of interventions designed to reduce the risk of progression to first-episode psychosis in a clinical sample with subthreshold symptoms. *Archives of General Psychiatry* **59**, 921–928.

McGrath, J. & Murray, R. (1995) Risk factors for schizophrenia: from conception to birth. In: Hirsch, S.R. & Weinberger, D.R., eds. *Schizophrenia.* Oxford: Blackwell Science, pp. 187–205.

Morgan, C., Fisher, H. & Fearon, P. (2006) Child abuse and psychosis [comment]. *Acta Psychiatrica Scandinavica* **113**, 238; author reply 238–239.

National Institute for Clinical Excellence (2002) Guidance on the use of newer (atypical) antipsychotic drugs for the treatment of schizophrenia. *NICE Technology Appraisal Guidance No. 43.* London: NICE.

Nicholson, R.M., Giedd, J.N., Lenane, M. *et al.* (1999) Clinical and neurobiological correlates of cytogenetic abnormalities in childhood-onset schizophrenia. *American Journal of Psychiatry* **156**, 1575–1579.

Nopoulos, P.C., Giedd, J.N., Andreasen, N.C. & Rapoport, J.L. (1998) Frequency and severity of enlarged septi pellucidi in childhood-onset schizophrenia. *American Journal of Psychiatry* **155**, 1074–1079.

O'Driscoll, G.A., Benkelfat, C., Florencio, P.S. *et al.* (1999) Neural correlates of eye tracking deficits in first-degree relatives of schizophrenic patients. A positron emission tomography study. *Archives of General Psychiatry* **56**, 1127–1134.

Pantelis, C., Velakoulis, D., McGorry, P.D. *et al.* (2003) Neuroanatomical abnormalities before and after onset of psychosis: a cross sectional and longitudinal MRI comparison. *Lancet* **361**, 281–288.

Park, S., Holzman, P.S. & Goldman-Rakic, P.S. (1995) Spatial working memory deficits in the relatives of schizophrenic patients. *Archives of General Psychiatry* **52**, 821–828.

Pennington, B.F. (1997) Dimensions of executive functions in normal and abnormal development. In: Krasnegor, N., Lyon, G.R. & Goldman-Rakic, P.S., eds. *Prefrontal Cortex: Evolution, Development, and Behavioral Neuroscience.* Baltimore: Brooke Publishing, pp. 265–281.

Pettegrew, J.W., Keshavan, M.S., Panchalingam, K. *et al.* (1991) Alterations in brain high energy phosphate and membrane phospholipid metabolism in first episode, drug naive schizophrenics. A pilot study of the dorsal prefrontal cortex by *in vivo* phosphorous 31 nuclear magnetic resonance spectroscopy. *Archives of General Psychiatry* **48**, 563–568.

Pistis, M., Perra, S., Pillolla, G., Melia, M., Muntoni A.L. & Gessa, G.L. (2004) Adolescent exposure to cannabinoids induces long-lasting changes in the response to drugs of abuse of rat midbrain dopamine neurons. *Biological Psychiatry* **56**, 86–94.

Pool, D., Bloom, W., Miekle, D.H., Roniger, J.J. & Gallant, D.M. (1976) A controlled trial of loxapine in 75 adolescent schizophrenic patients. *Current Therapeutic Research* **19**, 99–104.

Poole, R. & Brabbins, C. (1996) Drug induced psychosis. *British Journal of Psychiatry* **168**, 135–138.

Poulton, R., Caspi, A., Moffitt, T.E., Cannon, M., Murray, R. & Harrington, H. (2000) Children's self-reported psychotic symptoms and adult schizophreniform disorder: a 15-year longitudinal study. *Archives of General Psychiatry* **57**, 1053–1058.

Purves, D.L. & Lichtmen, J.W. (1980) Elimination of synapses in the developing nervous system. *Science* **210**, 153–157.

Rapoport, J. & Gogtay, N. (2007) Brain neuroplasticity in healthy, hyperactive and psychotic children: Insights from neuroimaging. *Neuropsychopharmacology Reviews* **33**, 181–197.

Rapoport, J.L., Conners, C., & Reatig, N. (1985) Rating scales and assessment instruments for use in paediatric psychopharmacology research. *Psychological Bulletin* **21**, 713–1111.

Rapoport, J.L., Giedd, J., Blumenthal, J. *et al.* (1999) Progressive cortical change during adolescence in childhood-onset schizophrenia. A longitudinal magnetic resonance imaging study. *Archives of General Psychiatry* **56**, 649–654.

Rapoport, J.L., Addington, A.M. & Frangou, S. (2005) The neurodevelopmental model of schizophrenia: update 2005. *Molecular Psychiatry* **10**, 434–449.

Rapoport, J., Chavez, A., Greenstein, D., Addington, A. & Gogtay, N. (2009). Autism spectrum disorders and childhood-onset schizophrenia: Clinical and biological contributions to a relation revisited. *Journal of the American Academy of Child and Adolescent Psychiatry* **48**, 10–18.

Ratzoni, G., Gothelf, D., Brand-Gothelf, A. *et al.* (2002) Weight gain associated with olanzapine and risperidone in adolescent patients: a comparative prospective study. *Journal of the American Academy of Child and Adolescent Psychiatry* **41**, 337–343.

Read J., van Os J., Morrison A.P. & Ross C.A. (2005) Childhood trauma, psychosis and schizophrenia: a literature review with theoretical implications. *Acta Psychiatrica Scandinavica* **112**, 330–350.

Reich, W. (2000) Diagnostic Interview for Children and Adolescents (DICA). *Journal of the American Academy of Child and Adolescent Psychiatry* **39**, 59–66.

Reichenberg, A., Weiser, M., Rapp, M.A. *et al.* (2005) Elaboration on premorbid intellectual performance in schizophrenia: Premorbid intellectual decline and risk for schizophrenia. *Archives of General Psychiatry* **62**, 1297–1304.

Remschmidt, H., Schultz, E. & Martin, M. (1994). An open trial of clozapine with thirty-six adolescents with schizophrenia. *Journal of Child and Adolescent Psychopharmacology* **4**, 31–41.

Roberts, G.W., Colter, N., Lofthouse, R., Bogerts, B., Zech, M. & Crow, T.J. (1986) Gliosis in schizophrenia: a survey. *Biological Psychiatry* **21**, 1043–1050.

Robinson, D., Woerner, M.G., Alvir, J.M. *et al.* (1999) Predictors of relapse following a first episode of schizophrenia or schizoaffective disorder. *Archives of General Psychiatry* **56**, 241–247.

Rossi, A., Mancini, F., Stratta, P. *et al.* (1997) Risperidone, negative symptoms and cognitive deficit in schizophrenia: an open study. *Acta Psychiatrica Scandinavica* **95**, 40–43.

Russell, A.T., Bott, L. & Sammons, C. (1989) The phenomena of schizophrenia occurring in childhood. *Journal of the American Academy of Child and Adolescent Psychiatry* **28**, 399–407.

Rutter, M., & Plomin, R. (1997) Opportunities for psychiatry from genetic findings. *British Journal of Psychiatry* **171**, 209–219.

Sachdev, P. (1998). Schizophrenia-like psychosis and epilepsy: the status of the association. *American Journal of Psychiatry* **155**, 325–336.

Saykin, A.J., Shtasel, D.L., Gur, R.E. *et al.* (1994). Neuropsychological deficits in neuroleptic-naive patients with first episode schizophrenia. *Archives of General Psychiatry* **512**, 124–131.

Schaeffer, J.L. & Ross, R.G. (2002) Childhood-onset schizophrenia: premorbid and prodromal diagnostic and treatment histories. *Journal of the American Academy of Child & Adolescent Psychiatry* **41**, 538–545.

Schmidt, M., Blanz, B., Dippe, A., Koppe, T. & Lay, B. (1995) Course of patients diagnosed as having schizophrenia during first episode occurring under age 18 years. *European Archives of Psychiatry and Clinical Neuroscience* **245**, 93–100.

Shaffer, D., Gould M.S., Brasic, J. *et al.* (1983) A children's global assessment scale (CGAS). *Archives of General Psychiatry* **40**, 1228–1231.

Sikich, L., Frazier J.A., McLellen J. *et al.* (2008) Antipsychotics in early-onset schizophrenia and schizoaffective disorder: Findings from the early-onset schizophrenia spectrum disorders (TEOSS) study. *American Journal of Psychiatry* **165**, 1420–1431.

Simpson, G., & Angus, J.S.W. (1970) A rating scale for extrapyramidal side effects. *Acta Psychiatrica Scandinavica* **212** (Suppl.), 9–11.

Slaveska. K., Hollis. C.P. & Bramble, D. (1998) The use of antipsychotics by the child and adolescent psychiatrists of Trent region. *Psychiatric Bulletin* **22**, 685–687.

Spencer, E.K. & Campbell, M. (1994) Children with schizophrenia: Diagnosis, phenomenology and pharmacotherapy. *Schizophrenia Bulletin* **20**, 713–725.

Sporn, A.L., Greenstein, D., Gogtay, N. *et al.* (2003) Progressive brain volume loss during adolescence in childhood-onset schizophrenia. *American Journal of Psychiatry* **160**, 1281–1289.

Sporn, A.L., Addington, A.M. & Gogtay, N. *et al.* (2004a) Pervasive developmental disorder and childhood-onset schizophrenia: co-morbid disorder or phenotypic variant of a very early onset illness? *Biological Psychiatry* **55**, 989–994.

Sporn, A.L., Addington, A.M., Reiss, A.L. *et al.* (2004b) 22q11 deletion syndrome in childhood-onset schizophrenia: an update. *Molecular Psychiatry* **9**, 225–226.

Sporn, A.L., Greenstein, D., Gogtay, N. *et al.* (2005) Childhood-onset schizophrenia: smooth pursuit eye-tracking dysfunction in family members. *Schizophrenia Research* **73**, 243–252.

St Clair D., Xu M., Wang P. *et al.* (2005) Rates of adult schizophrenia following prenatal exposure to the Chinese famine of 1959–1961. *JAMA* **294**, 557–562.

Stayer, C., Sporn, A., Gogtay, N. *et al.* (2005) Multidimensionally impaired: the good news. *Journal of Child & Adolescent Psychopharmacology* **15**, 510–519.

Strandburg, R.J., Marsh, J.T., Brown. W.S. *et al.* (1999) Continuous–processing ERPs in adult schizophrenia: continuity with childhood-onset schizophrenia. *Biological Psychiatry* **45**, 1356–1369.

Susser E. & Lin S.P. (1992) Schizophrenia after prenatal exposure to the Dutch Hunger Winter of 1944–1945. *Archives of General Psychiatry* **49**, 983–988.

Tarrier, N., Beckett, R., Harwood, S., Baker, A., Yusupoff, L. & Ugartebura, I. (1993) A trial of two cognitive behavioural methods of treating drug resistant residual symptoms in schizophrenic patients: I. Outcome. *British Journal of Psychiatry* **162**, 524–532.

Thomas, M.A., Ke, Y., Levitt, J. *et al.* (1998) Preliminary study of frontal lobe ^{1}H MR spectroscopy in childhood-onset schizophrenia. *Journal of Magnetic Resonance Imaging* **8**, 841–846.

Theisen, F.M., Linden, A., Geller, F. *et al.* (2001) Prevalence of obesity in adolescent and young adult patients with and without schizophrenia and in relationship to antipsychotic medication. *Journal of Psychiatric Research* **35**, 339–345.

Toren, P., Ratner, S., Laor, N. & Weizman, A. (2004) Benefit–risk assessment of atypical antipsychotics in the treatment of schizophrenia and comorbid disorders in children and adolescents. *Drug Safety* **27**, 1135–1156.

Towbin, K.R., Dykens, E.M., Pearson, G.S. & Cohen, D.J. (1993) Conceptualising "borderline syndrome of childhood" and "childhood schizophrenia" as a developmental disorder. *Journal of the American Academy of Child and Adolescent Psychiatry* **32**, 775–782.

Tsuang, M.T., Simpson, J.C. & Kronfold, Z. (1982) Subtypes of drug abuse with psychosis. *Archives of General Psychiatry* **39**, 141–147.

Turkington, D. & Kingdon, D. (2000) Cognitive-behavioural techniques for general psychiatrists in the management of patients with psychoses. *British Journal of Psychiatry* **177**, 101–106.

Volkmar, F.R. & Cohen, D.J. (1991) Comorbid association of autism and schizophrenia. *American Journal of Psychiatry* **148**, 1705–1707.

Walsh, T., J.M. McClellan, J.M., McCarthy, S.E. *et al.* (2008) Rare structural variants disrupt multiple genes in neurodevelopmental pathways in schizophrenia. *Science* **320**, 539–543.

Weinberger, D.R. (1987) Implications of normal brain development for the pathogenesis of schizophrenia. *Archives of General Psychiatry* **44**, 660–669.

Werry, J.S., McClellan, J.M. & Chard, L. (1991) Childhood and adolescent schizophrenia, bipolar and schizoaffective disorders: A clinical and outcome study. *Journal of the American Academy of Child and Adolescent Psychiatry* **30**, 457–465.

Werry, J.S., McClellan, J.M., Andrews, L. & Ham, M. (1994). Clinical features and outcome of child and adolescent schizophrenia. *Schizophrenia Bulletin* **20**, 619–630.

White, T., Andreasen, N.C., Nopoulos, P. & Magnotta, V. (2003) Gyrifation abnormalities in childhood-onset schizophrenia. *Biological Psychiatry* **54**, 418–426.

Woods, B.T. (1998) Is schizophrenia a progressive neurodevelopmental disorder? Toward a unitary pathogeneic mechanism. *American Journal of Psychiatry* **155**, 1661–1670.

Wyatt, R.J. (1995) Early intervention in schizophrenia: can the course be altered? *Biological Psychiatry* **38**, 1–3.

Wykes, T., Reeder, C., Williams, C., Corner, J., Rice, C. & Everitt, B. (2000) Cognitive remediation—predictors of success and durability of improvements (abstract). *Schizophrenia Research* **41**, 221.

Yung, A.R., Philips, L.J., Yuen, H.P. *et al.* (2003) Psychosis prediction: 12-month follow up of a high risk ("prodromal") group. *Schizophrenia Research* **60**, 21–32.

Zahn, T.P., Jacobson, L.K., Gordon, C.T., McKenna, K., Frazier, K. & Rapoport, J.L. (1997) Autonomic nervous system markers of pathophysiology in childhood-onset schizophrenia. *Archives of General Psychiatry* **54**, 904–912.

Zahn, T.P., Jacobson, L.K., Gordon, C.T., McKenna, K., Frazier, K. & Rapoport, J.L. (1998) Attention deficits in childhood-onset schizophrenia: reaction time studies. *Journal of Abnormal Psychology* **107**, 97–108.

4

Late-onset schizophrenia

Robert Howard[1] and Dilip Jeste[2]

[1]Department of Old Age Psychiatry, Institute of Psychiatry, King's College London, London, UK
[2]Sam and Rose Stein Institute for Research on Aging, University of California, San Diego, CA, USA

Historical background and approaches to classification

Late-onset schizophrenia has historically been a contentious area from clinical and research viewpoints. For more than a century, schizophrenia has usually been thought of as a disorder with onset in adolescence or early adulthood. Yet, a distinct minority of patients with largely similar signs, symptoms, course, and treatment response, with some phenotypic differences from "typical" cases, has been known to have onset of illness in middle age and later life. There has been resistance in some quarters, especially in the US, to consider this late-onset illness as a form of schizophrenia. Today most clinicians accept the notion that there may not be a fixed and arbitrary cut-off for age of onset of schizophrenia. Controversy continues, however, about terminology. This probably illustrates the persistent conceptualization of schizophrenia as dementia praecox despite the abandonment of this term decades ago. Below

Schizophrenia, 3rd edition. Edited by Daniel R. Weinberger and Paul J Harrison © 2011 Blackwell Publishing Ltd.

we briefly review the evolution of thinking about late-onset schizophrenia since the early part of the last century.

Can schizophrenia manifest de novo in late adult life?

Both Kraepelin (1913) and Eugen Bleuler (1911) observed that there was a relatively small group of patients with schizophrenia who had an illness onset in late middle or old age and who, on clinical grounds, closely resembled those who had an onset in early adult life. Utilizing a very narrow conception of dementia praecox and specifically excluding cases of paraphrenia, Kraepelin (1913) reported that only 5.6% of 1054 patients had an onset after the age of 40 years. If the age of onset was set at 60 years or greater, only 0.2% of patients could be included.

Manfred Bleuler (1943) carried out the first specific and systematic examination of late-onset patients and defined late schizophrenia as follows:

1. onset after the age of 40;

2. symptomatology that does not differ from that of schizophrenia occurring earlier in life (or if it does differ, it should not do so in a clear or radical way); and

3. it should not be possible to attribute the illness to a neuropathological disorder because of the presence of an amnestic syndrome or associated signs of organic brain disease.

Bleuler found that between 15% and 17% of two large series of patients with schizophrenia had an onset after the age of 40. Of such late-onset cases, only 4% had become ill for the first time after the age of 60. Subsequent authors confirmed that while onset of schizophrenia after the age of 40 was unusual, onset after 60 should be considered even rarer. Of 264 elderly patients with schizophrenia admitted in Edinburgh in 1957, only seven had an illness that had begun after the age of 60 (Fish, 1958). Using very broad criteria for the diagnosis of schizophrenia (including schizoaffective, paraphrenia, and other non-organic non-affective psychoses) and studying 470 first contacts with the Camberwell Register in London, Howard *et al.* (1993) found 29% of cases to have been aged over 44 years at onset.

Kraepelin and E. Bleuler both considered late-onset cases to have much in common with more typically early-onset schizophrenia and this view was supported by M. Bleuler's report (1943) of only very mild phenomenological variance from early-onset cases. His 126 late-onset cases were, however, symptomatically milder, had less affective flattening and were less likely to have formal thought disorder than patients with a younger age at onset. Fish (1960) reported that the clinical picture presented by 23 onset-after-40 patients did not differ importantly from patients who were younger at onset, but he believed that with increasing age at onset schizophrenia took on a more "paraphrenic" form.

European use of "late paraphrenia"

The notion of paraphrenia as a distinct diagnostic entity had been discredited by Mayer's (1921) follow-up of Kraepelin's 78 original cases. At least 40% of these patients had developed clear signs of dementia praecox within a few years and only 36% could still be classified as paraphrenic. Many of the paraphrenia patients had positive family histories of schizophrenia and the presenting clinical picture of those patients who remained "true" paraphrenics did not differ from those who were later to develop signs of schizophrenia. Roth and Morrisey (1952) resurrected both the terminology and the controversy with their choice of the term "late paraphrenia" to describe patients who they believed had schizophrenia, but with an onset delayed until after the age of 55 or 60 years. The term was intended to be descriptive, to distinguish the illness from the patients with chronic schizophrenia seen in psychiatric institutions at the time, and to emphasize the clinical similarities with the illness described by Kraepelin. Choice of the term was perhaps unfortunate because two

particular points of misconception often seem to arise in relation to it and it is vital to set these straight: late paraphrenia was never intended to mean the same thing as paraphrenia, and Kraepelin certainly did not emphasize late age of onset as a feature of the illness. Kay and Roth (1961) studied a group of 39 female and three male patients diagnosed as having late paraphrenia in Graylingwell Hospital in southern England between 1951 and 1955. All but six of these cases were followed-up for 5 years. The case records of 48 female and nine male patients with late paraphrenia admitted to a hospital in Stockholm between 1931 and 1940 were also collected and these cases were followed-up until death or until 1956. Over 40% of the Graylingwell patients with late paraphrenia were living alone, compared with 12% of patients with affective disorder and 16% of those with organic psychoses who were of comparable ages. Patients with late paraphrenia were also socially isolated. Although the frequency of visual impairment at presentation (15%) was no higher than that in comparison groups with other diagnoses, some impairment of hearing was present in 40% of patients with late paraphrenia and this was considered severe in 15%. Deafness was only present in 7% of patients with affective disorder. Focal cerebral disease was identified in only 8% of patients with late paraphrenia at presentation. Primary delusions, feelings of mental or physical influence, and hallucinations were all prominent and the prognosis for recovery was judged to be poor. From a detailed analysis of 1250 first admissions to a hospital in Gothenburg, Sweden, Sjoegren (1964) identified 202 elderly individuals who conformed to the French concept of paraphrenia (Magnan, 1893): well-organized and persistent paranoid delusions with hallucinations occurring in clear consciousness. Sjoegren argued cogently that together with constitutional factors, aging itself produced effects (feelings of isolation and loneliness, social and economic insecurity, and heightened vulnerability), which contributed to the development of paranoid reactions.

Post (1966) collected a sample of 93 patients to whom he gave the non-controversial and self-explanatory label "persistent persecutory states" and made a point of including cases regardless of coexisting organic brain change. Within this broad category he recognised three clinical subtypes: a schizophrenic syndrome (34 of 93 patients), a schizophreniform syndrome (37 patients), and a paranoid hallucinosis group (22 patients). Post regarded those patients with the schizophrenic syndrome as having a delayed form of the illness with only partial expression. Post's patients were treated with phenothiazines and he was able to demonstrate that the condition was responsive to antipsychotic medication. Success or failure of treatment was related to the adequacy of phenothiazine treatment and its long-term maintenance. From a series of 45 female and two male patients with late paraphrenia (identified using the same criteria as Kay and Roth), admitted to St Francis' Hospital in Sussex, England, between 1958 and 1964, Herbert and Jacobson (1967) confirmed many of Kay and Roth's (1961) observations. In addition, these investigators found an unexpectedly high prevalence of schizophrenia among the mothers (4.4%) and siblings (13.3%) of the patients.

Based on a literature review, Harris and Jeste (1988) noted that 23% of all inpatients with schizophrenia reportedly had onset of their illness after age 40. There seemed to be a progressive decrease in the proportions of patients with onset in later years—13% in the fifth decade, 7% in the sixth decade, and only 3% after age 60.

Current diagnosis in ICD-10 and DSM-IV-TR

Diagnostic guidelines published by authoritative organizations such as the World Health Organization (WHO) or the American Psychiatric Association (APA) reflect the views of many contemporary clinicians who were consulted at the draft and field trial stages. Inclusion or exclusion of a particular diagnosis in published diagnostic schemes thus reflects the current credence given to the nosological validity of that diagnosis plus an indication of its general usefulness in clinical practice.

Late paraphrenia was included within ICD-9 (World Health Organization, 1978), but did not survive as a separate codeable diagnosis in ICD-10 (World Health Organization, 1991). There are three possible diagnostic categories available for the accommodation of patients previously diagnosed as having late paraphrenia: schizophrenia, delusional disorder, and other persistent delusional disorders. It seems likely that most cases would be coded under Schizophrenia (F20.–) (Quintal et al., 1991; Howard et al., 1994a), although the category of Delusional disorder (F22.0) is suggested as a replacement for "paraphrenia (late)" in the diagnostic guidelines. Distinction between cases of schizophrenia and delusional disorder within ICD-10 is mainly dependent on the quality of auditory hallucinations experienced by patients and is subject to some unhelpful ageism. The guidelines for delusional disorder in ICD-10 state that, "Clear and persistent auditory hallucinations (voices) … are incompatible with this diagnosis". Rather confusingly, the guidelines then suggest, however, that, "Occasional or transitory auditory hallucinations, particularly in elderly patients, do not rule out this diagnosis, provided that they are not typically schizophrenic and form only a small part of the overall clinical picture". To add further to the diagnostic dilemma, the guidelines also state that, "Disorders in which delusions are accompanied by persistent hallucinatory voices or by schizophrenic symptoms that are insufficient to meet criteria for schizophrenia" should be coded under the category Other persistent delusional disorders (F22.8). Since the majority of patients with late paraphrenia who hear distinct hallucinatory voices also have a rich variety of schizophrenic core symptoms, very few will be diagnosed as having other persistent delusional disorders.

The inclusion within DSM-IIIR (American Psychiatric Association, 1987) of a separate category of late-onset schizophrenia for cases with an illness onset after the age of 44 years seems largely to have been a reaction to the unsatisfactory and arbitrary upper age limit for onset that had been included for DSM-III (American Psychiatric Association, 1980) for a diagnosis of schizophrenia. DSM-IV (American Psychiatric Association, 1994) contains no separate category for late-onset schizophrenia and this presumably reflects the current general North American view that there is a direct continuity between cases of schizophrenia whatever their age at onset. DSM-IV-TR (American Psychiatric Association, 2000) did not change the diagnostic criteria given in DSM-IV.

Terminology and classification for the future

The important questions now are: have ICD-10 and DSM-IV-TR been fair to abandon any facility for coding a late-onset subtype within schizophrenia, and do we need diagnostic categories that distinguish the functional psychoses with onset in later life from schizophrenia? These questions provided the spur to establish an international consensus on diagnosis and terminology (Howard et al., 2000), which may form the basis for consideration of these patients within future revisions of DSM and ICD, i.e., DSM-V and ICD-11, which are expected to be completed around 2013 and 2015 respectively. When the Late-Onset Schizophrenia International Consensus Group met in 1998, we agreed that the available evidence from the areas of epidemiology, phenomenology, and pathophysiology supported heterogeneity within schizophrenia with increasing age at onset up to the age of 60 years. Schizophrenia-like psychosis with onset after the age of 60 years (i.e., what some of the psychiatrists used to call late paraphrenia) was considered to be distinct from schizophrenia. The consensus group recommended that schizophrenia with onset between 40 and 59 years be termed late-onset schizophrenia and that chronic psychosis with onset after 60 years be called very late-onset schizophrenia-like psychosis (VLOSLP). The latter term is long-winded and unmemorable but at least is unambiguous and had the unprecedented support of bothEuropean and North American old-age psychiatrists as well as those from several parts of the world. There was no consensus regarding the exact age cut-offs of 40 and 60 years, and these were considered provisional until further research established evidence-based cut-points. From this point in this chapter the term late paraphrenia will be used only for patients already described as such in the literature.

Clinical features

Psychotic symptoms

Although M. Bleuler (1943) believed that it was not possible to separate early- and late-onset patients on clinical grounds, he acknowledged that a later onset was accompanied by less affective flattening and a more benign course. Formal thought disorder is seen in only about 5% of cases of DSM-III-R late-onset schizophrenia (Pearlson *et al.*, 1989) and could not be elicited from any of 101 patients with late paraphrenia (Howard *et al.*, 1994a). First-rank symptoms of Schneider are seen, but may be somewhat less prevalent in later-onset cases. Thought-insertion, block, and withdrawal seem to be particularly uncommon (Grahame, 1984; Pearlson *et al.*, 1989; Howard *et al.*, 1994b) and negative symptoms are less severe (Almeida *et al.*, 1995a).

Delusions

Persecutory delusions usually dominate the presentation, although in a series of 101 patients with late paraphrenia, delusions of reference (76%), control (25%), grandiose ability (12%), and of a hypochondriacal nature (11%) were also present (Howard *et al.*, 1994a). Partition delusions are found in about two-thirds of cases and refer to the belief that people, animals, materials or radiation can pass through a structure that would normally constitute a barrier to such passage. This barrier is generally the door, ceiling, walls or floor of a patient's home and the source of intrusion is frequently a neighboring residence (Herbert & Jacobson, 1967; Howard & Levy, 1992; Pearlson *et al.*, 1989).

In a multicenter study of late-onset schizophrenia, Jeste *et al.* (1988) found that delusions, particularly of persecution, and auditory hallucinations were prominent in patients with late-onset schizophrenia. The authors observed that late-onset schizophrenia typically resembled the paranoid subtype of early-onset schizophrenia. Other subtypes of schizophrenia, including catatonic and disorganized types, were very rare in old age. Jeste *et al.* (1995b) reported that there was no difference between late-onset schizophrenia, "early-onset schizophrenia-young", and "early-onset schizophrenia-old", in terms of the severity of global psychopathology and of positive symptoms. On the severity of negative symptoms, however, there was a significant difference: patients with late-onset schizophrenia had less severe negative symptoms than the two early-onset schizophrenia groups.

Affective symptoms

The coexistence of affective features in late-onset schizophrenia is well recognized clinically but there have been no controlled studies comparing such features between early- and late-onset cases. Atypical, schizoaffective, and cycloid psychoses are all characterized by affective features, tend to arise later in life, and affect women more than men (Cutting *et al.*, 1978; Kendell, 1988; Levitt & Tsuang, 1988). Among patients with late paraphrenia, Post (1966) reported depressive admixtures in 60% of cases, while Holden (1987) considered that 10 of his 24 "functional" patients with late paraphrenia had affective or schizoaffective disorders. These patients also had a better outcome in terms both of institutionalization and 10-year survival compared with patients who were paranoid. Such observations have led to the suggestion that some patients with late-onset schizophrenia or late paraphrenia may have variants of primary affective disorder (Murray *et al.*, 1992).

Cognitive deficits

Attempts to identify and characterize the patterns of cognitive impairment associated with these conditions began with Hopkins and Roth (1953) who administered the vocabulary subtest from the Wechsler–Bellevue Scale, a shortened form of the Raven's Progressive Matrices, and a general test of orientation and information, to patients with a variety of diagnoses. Twelve patients with late paraphrenia performed as well as a group of elderly patients who were depressive and better than patients with dementia on all three tests.

Naguib and Levy (1987) evaluated 43 patients with late paraphrenia (having already excluded subjects with a diagnosable dementia) with the Mental Test Score, Digit Copying Test, and Digit Symbol Substitution Test. Patients performed less well than age-matched controls on the latter two tasks.

Miller *et al.* (1991) published neuropsychological data on patients with what they termed "late life psychosis". These patients performed less well than age-matched controls on the Mini Mental State Examination, the Wechsler Adult Intelligence Scale – Revised, the Wisconsin Card Sorting Test, Logical Memory and Visual Reproduction subtests from the Wechsler Memory Scale, a test of verbal fluency, and the Warrington Recognition Memory Test. Patients were, however, not well matched with controls for educational attainment and premorbid intelligence and some clearly had affective psychoses and dementia syndromes (Miller *et al.*, 1992) so that it is probably not fair to equate them with patients with late paraphrenia or late-onset schizophrenia.

Almeida *et al.* (1995b) carried out a detailed neuropsychological examination of 40 patients with late paraphrenia in south London. Using cluster analysis of the results, he identified two groups of patients. The first was a "functional" group characterized by impairment restricted to executive functions, in particular a computerized test assessing extra- and intra-dimensional attention set shift ability and a test of planning. Such patients had a high prevalence and severity of positive psychotic symptoms and lower scores on a scale of neurological abnormalities. A second "organic" group of patients with late paraphrenia showed widespread impairment of cognitive functions together with a lower frequency of positive psychotic symptoms and a high prevalence of abnormalities on neurological examination.

Paulsen et al. (1996) examined the integrity of semantic memory in both patients with late- and early-onset schizophrenia and found a striking dissimilarity. The organization of semantic memory was almost normal in the patients with late-onset schizophrenia, whereas it was significantly impaired in the patients with early-onset schizophrenia. A follow-up of these patients over a period of 2 years or longer showed no deterioration in neuropsychological functioning (Gladsjo et al., 1996), suggesting that late-onset schizophrenia is primarily a non-dementing disorder.

In a multiple group comparison study, Heaton et al. (1993) evaluated neuropsychological performance in 38 normal comparison subjects, 83 currently younger patients with early-onset schizophrenia ("early-onset schizophrenia-young"), 22 subjects with late-onset schizophrenia, 35 currently older patients with early-onset schizophrenia ("early-onset schizophrenia-old"), and 42 patients with Alzheimer disease. All subjects received an expanded Halstead–Reitan neuropsychological test battery. Raw scores on the neuropsychological tests were converted to age-, education-, and gender-corrected deficit scores for eight cognitive ability areas. All the schizophrenia groups were worse than the normal comparison group on deficit scores for all the ability areas except for memory. The late-onset schizophrenia, early-onset schizophrenia-old, and early-onset schizophrenia-young groups were similar to one another in all of the cognitive ability areas. Age of onset and duration of schizophrenia did not have a major impact on the neuropsychological impairment. Furthermore, the patterns of deficits were different when comparing patients with schizophrenia and Alzheimer disease. Patients with schizophrenia were impaired in their ability to learn new information but were normal with respect to recalling such information after a delay, whereas the patients with Alzheimer disease performed worse than the normal subjects on all the deficit scores including memory, and had greater learning and memory impairments than the schizophrenia groups. According to the neurodevelopmental model (Weinberger, 1987; see Chapter 19), the brain lesion(s) putatively related to the pathogenesis of schizophrenia are of developmental origin and are not progressive or degenerative in nature. Furthermore, long-term treatment with antipsychotics and other environmental factors are not major contributors to cognitive deficits and brain abnormalities associated with schizophrenia. The study of Heaton et al. suggests that the neurodevelopmen-

tal model applies to late-onset schizophrenia too. Consistent with this notion, Lohr et al. (1997) found that patients with late-onset schizophrenia, similar to patients with early-onset schizophrenia, had an elevated number of minor physical anomalies compared to normal comparison subjects and patients with Alzheimer disease. Differences in severity and specific locations or nature of the "lesions" may account for the delayed onset of schizophrenia in late-onset cases. Additionally, the peak in dopaminergic activity related to the schizophrenic breakdown, as per the neurodevelopmental theory (Weinberger, 1987), might be delayed until later in life in the patients with late-onset schizophrenia. Consideration of a neurodevelopmental basis to late-onset schizophrenia may need to take sex differences into account (Castle & Murray, 1991; see below).

Etiology

Genetic factors

Reviewing the literature on family history in schizophrenia, Gottesman and Shields (1982) reported that the overall risk of schizophrenia in the relatives of an affected proband was about 10% compared with a risk of around 1% for the general population (see Chapter 13). Kendler et al. (1987) concluded that there was no consistent relationship between age at onset and familial risk for schizophrenia, but data from patients with an onset in old age were not included in this analysis. The literature on familiality in late-onset schizophrenia and related psychoses of late life is sparse and inconclusive, partly due to variations in illness definition and age at onset, but principally because of the difficulties inherent in conducting family studies in patients who often have only a small number of surviving first-degree relatives. The results of the few studies specifically of late-onset psychoses, reviewed by Castle and Howard (1992), suggest a trend for increasing age at onset of psychosis to be associated with reduced risk of schizophrenia in first-degree relatives. Thus, studies involving subjects with illness onset after the age of 40 or 45 years have reported rates of schizophrenia in relatives of between 4.4% and 19.4% (Bleuler, 1943; Huber et al., 1975; Pearlson et al., 1989), while those with onsets delayed to 50 or 60 years have yielded rates of between 1.0% and 7.3% (Funding, 1961; Post, 1966; Herbert & Jacobson, 1967). More recently, studies of patients with psychosis onset after the age of 50 (Brodaty et al., 1999) and after 60 years (Howard et al., 1997) reported no increase in the prevalence of schizophrenia among relatives of patients compared to those of healthy comparison subjects. The findings of Howard et al. (1997) emerged from a controlled family study of data from 269 first-degree relatives of patients who had an onset after 60 years, and 272 relatives of healthy elderly subjects. The estimated lifetime risk for schizophrenia (with an onset range of 15–90 years) was 2.3% for the relatives of cases and 2.2% for the relatives of controls.

Brain abnormalities seen with imaging

Exclusion from computerized tomography (CT) studies of patients with obvious neurological signs or a history of stroke, alcohol abuse or dementia, has shown that structural abnormalities other than large ventricles in patients with late paraphrenia are probably no more common than in healthy aged controls. Despite adhering to such exclusions, however, Flint *et al.* (1991) found unsuspected cerebral infarction on the scans of five of 16 of their patients with late paraphrenia. Most of these infarcts were subcortical or frontal and they were more likely to occur in patients who had delusions but no hallucinations. The results of this study need to be interpreted with some caution, since only 16 of a collected sample of patients had actually undergone CT scanning and it is of course possible that these represented the more "organic" cases, or at least those who were thought most likely to have some underlying structural abnormality.

The superiority of magnetic resonance imaging (MRI) over CT, both in terms of gray/white matter resolution and visualization of deep white matter is established. The results of MRI studies of changes in periventricular and deep white matter in patients with late-onset schizophrenia and related disorders must, however, be viewed with some caution since few have assessed abnormalities in the white matter in any kind of standardized manner, and appropriate control populations, matched for cerebrovascular risk factors, are rarely used. In a series of studies, Miller *et al.* (1989, 1991, 1992) reported the results of structural MRI investigations in patients with what they termed "late life psychosis". They found that 42% of patients who were not demented with an onset of psychosis after the age of 45 (mean age at scanning 60 years) had white matter abnormalities on MRI, compared to only 8% of a healthy age-matched control group. The appearance of large patchy white matter lesions (WMLs) was six times more likely in the temporal lobe, and four times more common in the frontal lobes, of patients than controls (Miller *et al.*, 1991). These authors hypothesized that, although insufficient to give rise to focal neurological signs, WMLs might produce dysfunction in the overlying frontal and temporal cortex and that this could contribute to psychotic symptomatology. They acknowledged that since WMLs in the occipital lobes could also be implicated, it might not be possible to pinpoint an isolated anatomical WML that predisposed to psychosis. When comparisons were made between the patients who had structural brain abnormalities on MRI (10) with those who did not (7), there were no significant differences on age, educational level, IQ or performance on a wide battery of neuropsychological tests. Measurements

of ventricle–brain ratio (VBR) indicated a non-significant increase in patients (10.6%) compared to controls (8.8%). The DSM-III-R diagnoses of the 24 patients at entry to this study were schizophrenic disorder (late-onset type) (10), delusional disorder (7), schizophreniform psychosis (2), and psychosis not otherwise specified (5), but at least 12 were shown to have organic cerebral conditions.

Howard *et al.* (1995) studied WMLs among patients with very late-onset schizophrenia-like psychosis from whom the authors tried to exclude organic cases, and found they may be no more common in such patients than in healthy community-living elderly controls. Examination of individual white matter tracts in fine anatomical detail using diffusion tensor imaging has also failed to demonstrate differences between patients and healthy aged controls (Jones *et al.*, 2005).

Pearlson *et al.* (1993) reported a volumetric MRI study of patients with late-onset schizophrenia based on a sample of 11 individuals with an illness onset after the age of 55 years. Third ventricle volume was significantly greater in patients with late-onset schizophrenia than in an age-matched control group. VBR estimations were greater among the patients with late-onset schizophrenia (mean 9.0) than controls (mean 7.1), but this difference did not reach statistical significance.

Howard *et al.* (1994b) carried out volumetric MRI scans on 47 patients with late paraphrenia, 31 of whom satisfied ICD-10 criteria for a diagnosis of schizophrenia and 16 for delusional disorder. While total brain volume was not reduced in the patients compared with 35 elderly community-living controls, lateral and third ventricle volumes were increased. Measurements of the frontal lobes, hippocampus, parahippocampus, thalamus, and basal ganglia structures failed to further demonstrate differences between patient and control subjects.

Symonds *et al.* (1997) found no significant differences among the age-comparable late-onset schizophrenia, early-onset schizophrenia-old, and normal comparison groups in terms of clinically relevant structural brain abnormalities such as strokes, tumors, cysts, or other lesions that were apparent to a clinical neuroradiologist reporting on the MRI.

Corey-Bloom *et al.* (1995) compared MRI brain scans of 16 patients with late-onset and 14 with early-onset schizophrenia and 28 normal elderly controls. All subjects were over the age of 45 years. Patients with late-onset schizophrenia had significantly larger lateral ventricles than normal comparison subjects and significantly larger thalamic volumes than the patients with early-onset schizophrenia.

Gender

The female preponderance of individuals who have an onset of schizophrenia or a schizophrenia-like psychosis in middle or old age is a consistent finding. Among patients with late-onset schizophrenia (onset after 40–50 years), females have been reported to constitute 66% (Bleuler, 1943), 72% (Klages, 1961), 82% (Gabriel, 1978), 85% (Marneros & Deister, 1984) or 87% (Pearlson *et al.*, 1989) of patients. In those with an illness onset at 60 years or older, the female preponderance appears even greater: 75% (Sternberg, 1972), 86% (Howard *et al.*, 1994a), 88% (Kay & Roth, 1961) or 91% (Herbert & Jacobson, 1967).

Two recent reports have indicated the presence of a subgroup of female patients with schizophrenia with later illness onset who typically do not have a positive family history of schizophrenia (Gorwood *et al.*, 1995; Shimizu & Kurachi, 1989). Later illness onset, particularly in females, is typically associated with a milder symptom profile and better outcome, better premorbid social adjustment, and a lower prevalence of structural brain abnormalities than in (mostly male) patients with early illness onset. This has led to the suggestion that sex differences in schizophrenia may reflect different psychiatric disorders. Castle and Murray (1991) have suggested that early-onset, typically male, schizophrenia is essentially a heritable neurodevelopmental disorder, while late-onset schizophrenia in females may have etiologically more in common with affective psychosis than with the illness seen in males.

Lewine (1981) proposed two competing theories to account for age of onset and gender differences—the timing model and the subtype model. According to the timing model, men and women have the same form of schizophrenia but the age at onset of illness is different. There may be an earlier onset for men or a delayed onset for women because of biological and/or psychosocial gender differences. In this model, the age of onset should account for most of the gender differences. In the subtype model, men are differentially susceptible to a "typical" subtype of the illness, which includes early onset, while women are more susceptible to the "atypical" subtype of schizophrenia, more frequently characterized by a later onset. According to the subtype model, there are two distinct forms of schizophrenia—"male" schizophrenia and "female" schizophrenia (Lindamer *et al.*, 2000). It has been consistently demonstrated that women with schizophrenia have a milder clinical presentation and course, which could be explained by Lewine's timing model. In other words, the less severe symptoms and course of schizophrenia that is seen in women might be explained by the delayed onset of illness. Given the lack of consistent evidence for important psychosocial factors in the age at onset differential, biological factors gain more credence as possible mediators of the timing effect. As a potential way of explaining gender differences in the distribution of age at onset in this "timing" model, numerous investigators have speculated that sex hormones may play a role (Seeman, 1981; Lindamer *et al.*, 1997, 1999). Little convincing evidence exists to suggest

that androgens serve as a "trigger" in promoting schizophrenia in men (Castle, 1999). On the other hand, several lines of evidence suggest that estrogen could act as one important neuroendocrine mediator to delay and/or protect against the illness. Seeman (1981, 1999; Seeman & Lang, 1990) has long proposed an important role for sex hormones, especially estrogen, in the development of schizophrenia. It is hypothesized that women with a genetic predisposition to schizophrenia are afforded protection between puberty and menopause due to estrogen, therefore delaying the onset of the illness (Riecher-Rossler *et al.*, 1994; Lindamer *et al.*, 2000). However, there is so far no direct evidence to confirm this theory.

Sensory deficits

Deafness has been experimentally and clinically associated with the development of paranoid symptoms. Deficits of moderate to severe degree affect 40% of patients with late paraphrenia (Kay & Roth, 1961; Herbert & Jacobson, 1967) and are more prevalent than in elderly depressed patients or normal controls (Post, 1966; Naguib and Levy, 1987). Deafness associated with late-life psychosis is more usually conductive than degenerative (Cooper *et al.*, 1974) and generally of early onset, long duration, bilateral, and profound (Cooper, 1976; Cooper & Curry, 1976). Corbin and Eastwood (1986) suggested that deafness may reinforce a pre-existing tendency to social isolation, withdrawal, and suspiciousness. Further, auditory hallucinations are the psychopathological phenomenon most consistently associated with deafness (Keshavan *et al.*, 1992). There are several reports of improvement in psychotic symptoms after the fitting of a hearing aid (Eastwood *et al.*, 1981; Khan *et al.*, 1988; Almeida *et al.*, 1993), although it has to be said that clinical experience suggests that this is not usually the case. Visual impairment, most commonly a consequence of cataract or macular degeneration, is also commoner in elderly patients with paranoid psychosis than in those with affective disorder, and there is a higher coincidence of visual and hearing impairment in patients who are paranoid than in those who are affective (Cooper & Curry, 1976). An association between visual impairment and the presence of visual hallucinations (Howard *et al.*, 1994a) echoes Keshavan's findings with deafness.

Prager and Jeste (1993) reached a different conclusion about the nature of the association between sensory deficits and late-onset schizophrenia. These authors reviewed the literature and found 27 studies of sensory (visual or auditory) impairment in patients who were psychotic, published over the past 40 years. Twenty-two of the studies assessed sensory loss among patients with late-life psychosis, and five examined psychopathology in subjects with sensory impairment. The authors then conducted a case–control study involving a comparison of patients with schizophrenia (early-onset and late-onset cases) with patients with mood disorder and normal control subjects in terms of visual and auditory impairment. The results showed that all the psychiatric groups were similar to normal controls on uncorrected vision or hearing, but were significantly more impaired on corrected (i.e., with eyeglasses or hearing aids) sensory function. From this study, Prager and Jeste (1993) suggested that the association between sensory impairment and late-life psychosis may be, at least in part, a result of insufficient correction of sensory deficits in older patients with schizophrenia as compared to normal controls. This could reflect a difficulty for these patients to access optimal healthcare, especially for the treatment of sensory impairment.

Premorbid personality

Premorbid personality in patients with late and mid-life paranoid psychoses and the quality of premorbid relationships within families and with friends were assessed retrospectively by Kay et al. (1976). This study is an important one because, through use of structured patient and informant interviews, it represented a first effort to overcome some of the problems inherent in any retrospective attempt at defining premorbid personality. From a consecutive series of first admissions to a psychiatric hospital, the authors selected 54 cases of paranoid and 57 of affective psychosis over the age of 50. Patients and close relatives or friends were independently given a semi-structured clinical interview, designed to cover a wide range of paranoid traits. The patients who were paranoid were rated more highly, both by themselves and informants, on items that suggested that they had greater difficulty in establishing and maintaining satisfactory relationships premorbidly. They had also been significantly moreshy, reserved, touchy, and suspicious, and less able to display sympathy or emotion. Through principal components analysis of the results, the authors derived a "prepsychotic schizoid personality factor"; consisting of unsociability, reticence, suspiciousness, and hostility.

Retterstol (1966) argued that since personality deviations in patients who are paranoid are recognizable at a very early age, factors in the childhood and adolescence of patients are important in determining a predisposition to paranoid psychosis later in life. Key experiences in the later development of paranoid psychoses are proposed to be those which provoke feelings of insecurity or which damage the self-image of an individual whose personality is already overtly sensitive. Gurian et al. (1992) also provided evidence for the importance of childhood experiences in the development of late-onset psychosis. Among nine Israeli patients with delusional disorder, these authors found a high prevalence of "war refugees". These were individuals who had survived the Armenian or Nazi holo-causts or been forced to leave their native country. The authors proposed an association between the presence of extremely life-threatening experiences in childhood, a failure to produce progeny, and the development of paranoid delusional symptoms in late life in response to a stressful situation such as widowhood. Just how early the threatening experience needs to be is not clear. Cervantes et al. (1989) found the risk of developing a paranoid psychosis to be doubled in immigrants to the US from Mexico and Central America who were escaping war or political unrest compared with those who had moved for economic reasons. Thus, the period during which a personality may be rendered sensitive to the later development of paranoid psychosis by exposure to trauma is presumably not limited to early childhood. African- and Caribbean-born elders in the UK are at higher risk of developing non-affective non-organic psychosis after the age of 60 than indigenous elders (Reeves et al., 2001) and patients from such migrant groups have a less marked female preponderance and a younger age of onset of psychosis (Mitter et al., 2005).

Young adults with schizophrenia with persecutory delusions make explicit mentalizing errors when determining the intentions of others (Corcoran et al., 1995), jump to conclusions on the basis of insufficient evidence when reasoning under conditions of uncertainty (Garety et al., 1991), and are more likely than normal subjects to attribute the cause of negative events to other people (Kaney & Bentall, 1989). Patients with very late-onset schizophrenia-like psychosis perform as well as healthy controls on tasks involving probabilistic reasoning and making attributions, but are impaired on deception mentalizing tasks (Moore et al., 2006). Mentalizing errors may contribute to the development of persecutory delusions in patients with very late-onset schizophrenia-like psychosis who do not seem to have the wider range of cognitive biases described in younger patients with schizophrenia.

Management

Establishing a therapeutic relationship

Although patients with late-onset schizophrenia are often described as hostile, and their relationships with neighbors, primary care physicians, and the local police may be affected by their psychotic symptoms by the time psychiatric referral is considered, the authors' experience is that they are often extremely lonely. Without entering into any kind of collusion, it is always possible to take the time to listen to the patient's account of their persecution, and not difficult to express sympathy for the distress they are experiencing. Sometimes a brief admission to hospital or the establishment of regular community psychiatric nurse (CPN) visits can be rendered acceptable as an attempt to "get to the bottom" of whatever is going on. Once a relationship of trust and support has been established, patients will often accept medication and visits from members of the psychiatric team. Use of compulsory admission powers should be reserved until all else has failed. Relatives and friends should be advised to encourage the patient to reserve discussion of such complaints to the time that the CPN visits, if this is possible. Of course, there is no single strategy which is best for all patients. For most patients, interventions delivered to their own homes (CPN or volunteer visits, home helps, and meals on wheels) seem to be most acceptable and, although some will respond well to the activities and company provided by a day hospital or center, some may decline to attend. The potential role of psychological treatments in the management of psychotic symptoms in younger patients is becoming clearer (see Chapter 32), and it is unfortunate and unfair that older patients who are psychotic are not routinely considered for these (Aguera-Ortiz & Reneses-Prieto, 1999).

Rehousing

Since some patients may have highly restricted and encapsulated delusional systems, their complaints about neighbors or the home environment are sometimes taken at face value by staff in Social Services or other agencies. Hence, by the time of first psychiatric referral, a patient might have been rehoused at least once in the preceding months. As a general rule, even if it results in a brief reduction of complaints from the sufferer, provision of new accommodation is followed within a few weeks by a re-emergence of symptoms. The obvious distress this causes is sufficient reason to always advise patients and social workers against such moves unless they are being considered for non-delusional reasons or following successful treatment of psychosis.

Psychosocial and behavioral treatments

In recent years there has been development and testing of novel psychosocial interventions for older adults with schizophrenia (a proportion of whom had onset of illness after age 40). Granholm et al. (2005) conducted a randomized, controlled trial in 76 middle-aged and older stable outpatients with schizophrenia and schizoaffective disorder to examine the effects of cognitive–behavioral social skills training (CBSST) in patients on (mostly atypical) antipsychotics. The CBSST manualized group therapy was aimed at teaching cognitive and behavioral coping techniques, social functioning skills, problem solving, and compensatory aids for neurocognitive impairments. The investigators found that CBSST led to significantly increased frequency of social functioning activities, greater cognitive insight (more objectivity in reappraising psychotic symptoms), and greater skill mastery than did treatment as usual. CBSST had no significant effect on symptoms

in these patients who had already been on stable dosages of antipsychotic medications. At 12-month follow-up, the CBSST group had maintained the greater skill acquisition and performance of everyday living skills. However, the greater cognitive insight seen with CBSST at the end of the treatment was not maintained at 12-month follow-up, possibly indicating a need for booster sessions (Granholm et al., 2007).

Patterson et al. (2006) conducted a randomized controlled trial of a behavioral group intervention called Functional Adaptation Skills Training (FAST) in 240 middle-aged and older adults with schizophrenia or schizoaffective disorder. FAST was a manualized intervention which sought to improve everyday living skills such as medication management, social skills, communication, organization and planning, transportation, and financial management. Compared to the control group, the FAST-treated patients had a significant improvement in daily living skills and social skills, but not medication management. The FAST intervention has also been culturally adapted and pilot tested in Spanish-speaking Mexican–American patients with schizophrenia. The latter therapy, called "Programa de Entrenamiento para el Desarrollo de Aptitudes para Latinos" (PEDAL), was compared in a randomized controlled pilot study of 29 patients to a time-equivalent friendly support group (Patterson et al., 2005). The results showed a significant improvement in everyday living skills with PEDAL that was maintained at 12-month follow-up.

A randomized controlled trial of two methods of work rehabilitation among middle-aged and older adults with schizophrenia by Twamley et al. (2005) found that a program which placed the patients in a job chosen with a vocational counselor and then offered individualized on-site support ("place-then-train") was more successful than the one that employed a train-then-place approach. The rates of volunteer or paid work with these two programs were 81% and 44%, respectively.

Antipsychotic medication

Although management of late-onset schizophrenia is an important area of study, there is limited published research addressing its pharmacological treatment. Moreover, the available studies are often characterized by small sample sizes and are most often case reports or case series rather than well-controlled double-blind studies. As the number of reports in late-onset schizophrenia is limited, we will also include studies related to other psychotic disorders (e.g., early-onset schizophrenia, delusional disorder/paranoid psychosis) in late life. Studies related to these other disorders may be applicable to the population of older patients with late-onset schizophrenia.

In general, antipsychotic medications are the most effective symptomatic treatment for both early- and late-onset chronic schizophrenia as they improve both the acute symptoms and prevent relapses (Jeste *et al.*, 1993). Alterations in pharmacokinetics and pharmacodynamics, however, complicate pharmacotherapy in older patients; an exaggerated or otherwise altered response to medications may be seen. In comparison to younger patients, geriatric patients show an increased variability of response and an increased sensitivity to medications (Salzman, 1990).

Conventional or typical antipsychotics

The older studies of these drugs reported low response rates in patients with late-onset schizophrenia. For example, Rabins *et al.* (1984) found little or only partial response in 43% of patients with schizophrenia with an onset at age older than 44 years, while Pearlson *et al.* (1989) reported that 54% of their patients fell into this category. In reports of patients with late paraphrenia, the comparable rates range from 49% (Post, 1966) to 75% (Kay & Roth 1961). The general conclusion from such studies was that while drugs relieved some target symptoms, the overall treatment response to medication was modest. Pearlson *et al.* (1989) found poor response to antipsychotics to be associated with the presence of thought disorder and with schizoid premorbid personality traits. The presence of first-rank symptoms, family history of schizophrenia, and gender had no effect on treatment response. In a late paraphrenia patient group, Holden (1987) found auditory hallucinations and affective features to predict a favorable response. This may, of course, simply reflect a better natural history in such patients. In a group of 64 patients with late paraphrenia prescribed antipsychotic medication for at least 3 months, 42% showed no response, 31% a partial response, and 27% a full response to treatment (Howard & Levy, 1992). Adherence to medication, receiving depot rather than oral medication, and use of a CPN if the patient was an outpatient all had a positive effect on treatment response. Patients prescribed depot medication received on average a lower daily dose in chlorpromazine equivalents than those prescribed oral medication.

Rockwell *et al.* (1994) studied 10 patients with late-onset psychosis, with a mean age of 63, who had somatic delusions. These patients were compared to two groups who were similar in age and education (10 normal comparison patients and nine patients with late-onset psychosis without somatic delusions). The patients who were delusional showed the worst adherence to psychiatric treatment recommendations and rarely benefited from short-term psychopharmacological (mainly antipsychotic) intervention.

In four North American clinical centers, the mean daily dose prescribed to patients with late-onset schizophrenia, whose mean age was 61 years, was 192 mg chlorpromazine equivalents (mg CPZE) compared to 1437 mg CPZE in a group of young patients with schizophrenia (Jeste & Zisook, 1988). Jeste and McClure (1997) found that the

mean daily dose of antipsychotics used in patients with late-onset schizophrenia was significantly smaller than that prescribed to age-comparable patients with early-onset schizophrenia.

As well as dosage differences, the occurrence of adverse effects of typical antipsychotics may differ in late-onset from early-onset schizophrenia, notably tardive dyskinesia (TD; see Chapter 27). In one study of elderly patients, ranging in age from 55 to 99 years, the incidence of TD was 31% after 43 weeks of cumulative antipsychotic treatment (Saltz *et al.*, 1991). Jeste *et al.* (1999) reported the cumulative incidence of dyskinetic movements in elderly patients to be 29% following 12 months of typical antipsychotic use. This cumulative annual incidence of TD in older adults is five to six times that reported in younger adults. Higher dosage and longer duration of antipsychotic treatment as well as other factors, including alcohol dependence and subtle movement disorder at baseline, were found to increase the risk of TD in the older patient population (Jeste *et al.*, 1995a).

Atypical antipsychotics

Double-blind controlled data on atypical antipsychotics in patients with late-onset schizophrenia are very limited. Risperidone, olanzapine, quetiapine, and aripiprazole have been studied more extensively in elderly patients, mainly those with psychosis or agitation associated with dementia. Clozapine has been investigated in patients with Parkinson disease with psychosis.

The only large-scale randomized, double-blind controlled trial comparing two atypical antipsychotics in elderly patients with schizophrenia (many of whom probably had onset of illness before age 40) was a multisite international study of risperidone and olanzapine (Jeste *et al.*, 2003). One hundred and seventy-five patients with schizophrenia or schizoaffective disorder aged 60 years or older were randomly assigned to receive risperidone (1–3 mg/day, median dose 2 mg/day) or olanzapine (5–20 mg/day, median dose 10 mg/day). Both groups had significant improvement in symptoms and reduction in extrapyramidal symptoms. The overall therapeutic and adverse effects of the two drugs were similar except that clinically relevant weight gain was more common with olanzapine than with risperidone.

Of all the atypical agents, clinical experience with risperidone in older patients with psychotic disorders has been most extensive. Risperidone has efficacy in the treatment of hallucinations and delusions in such patients at relatively low doses. It should be prescribed in patients with late-onset schizophrenia at considerably lower doses than those recommended for younger adults. The initial doses of risperidone should be between 0.25 and 0.5 mg/day, with increases not to exceed 0.5 mg/day. Maximum doses in patients with schizophrenia should remain at 3 mg/day or less. Olanzapine has a somewhat similar receptor binding profile as clozapine but does not appear to cause the severe anticholinergic problems seen with clozapine. For olanzapine, a starting dose of 2.5–5 mg/day is generally well tolerated and can be increased to 10 mg/day if no adverse events appear. The starting dose of quetiapine in elderly patients should be 25–50 mg/day. The optimal target dose is suggested to be between 100 and 200 mg/day. Ziprasidone and aripiprazole have been studied in older adults with schizophrenia in open-label or retrospective studies only.

In the elderly, atypical antipsychotics have been shown to have a lower risk of extrapyramidal symptoms and TD compared to typical antipsychotics, but do carry a risk of various other side effects. Jeste et al. (1999) compared the 9-month cumulative incidence of TD with risperidone to that with haloperidol in 122 older patients. The two groups were matched on age, diagnosis, and length of pre-enrollment antipsychotic intake, and the median daily dose of each medication was 1 mg. Over the 9-month period, risperidone was associated with a significantly lower cumulative incidence of TD than haloperidol. A subsequent study comparing conventional (mainly haloperidol) and atypical (risperidone, olanzapine, and quetiapine) agents confirmed the lower risk of TD with atypical than with typical antipsychotics in a high-risk group of older patients who had borderline dyskinesia at baseline (Dolder et al., 2004). There were no significant differences among the three atypicals in the incidence of TD (Jones et al., 2006). Clozapine is difficult to use in elderly persons due to the risk of agranulocytosis as well as orthostasis, sedation, and anticholinergic effects. The necessity of regular blood tests also poses a problem for older patients. Risperidone, olanzapine, and aripiprazole in higher doses carry a greater risk of extrapyramidal side effects. Other possible side effects of all the atypical agents, especially clozapine and quetiapine, include orthostatic hypotension and sedation.

Atypical antipsychotics, especially clozapine and olanzapine (followed by risperidone and aripiprazole), have a high risk of side effects related to metabolic function (see Chapter 28). Common metabolic side effects include excessive weight gain, glucose intolerance, new-onset Type 2 diabetes mellitus, diabetic ketoacidosis, and dyslipidemia (Wirshing et al., 1998; Allison et al., 1999; Jin et al., 2002, 2004). The American Diabetic Association/American Psychiatric Association monitoring recommendations for metabolic effects (American Diabetes Association, American Psychiatric Association, American Association of Clinical Endocrinologists, and North American Center for the Study of Obesity, 2004) are applicable. As elderly patients tend to be at higher risk for cardiovascular disease, closer monitoring may be necessary for older than for younger adults.

Given the data on the increased risk of strokes and mortality in elderly patients with dementia treated with atypi-cal antipsychotics and the consequent Food and Drug Administration black box warnings (Jeste et al., 2008), clinicians should exercise caution, clinical judgment, and shared decision-making when using these drugs in all older patients, although there are no data to support or refute the applicability of these findings to people with schizophrenia.

Guidelines for prescribing

There is no evidence that any particular antipsychotic is more effective than others in this group of patients. The choice of antipsychotic drug for each individual patient should thus be based on considerations of concomitant physical illness and other treatments received together with the specific side effect profile of the drug. Treatment should usually be commenced at a low dose of an oral preparation and it is easy to argue that this should be one of the atypical agents because of the reduced risk of early and delayed emergent motor side effects. Patients who do not respond to oral treatment (whether due to poor adherence or genuine treatment resistance) may be treated with depot medications, although there are limited published data on their use in older patients. Successful treatment of elderly patients with depot can often be at very modest doses. For example, the mean dose of prescribed depot in Howard and Levy's (1992) study was 14.4 mg of flupenthixol decanoate or 9 mg of fluphenazine decanoate every fortnight. In those patients who continue to experience psychotic symptoms after receiving depot for several weeks, the dose can be increased by 10% every 2–3 weeks until a response is seen or side effects emerge. Trials of depot risperidone are in progress at the time of writing. If these trials prove successful, this may represent a useful way of delivering antipsychotic treatment to at least some of these patients.

Alexopoulos et al.'s (2005) expert consensus survey of 48 American experts on treatment of older adults reported that the experts' first-line recommendation for late-life schizophrenia was risperidone (1.25–3.5 mg/day) followed by quetiapine (100–300 mg/day), olanzapine (7.5–15 mg/day), and aripiprazole (15–30 mg/day). There was limited support for the use of clozapine, ziprasidone, and high-potency conventional antipsychotics.

Conclusions

The history of schizophrenia and schizophrenia-like psychoses that have onset in later life is a long one, but it is only in the last three decades that any real attempts have been made to study patients with these conditions and understand how they might relate to psychoses which arise earlier in the life cycle. The etiological roles of premorbid personality functioning, degenerative and genetic factors are still not elucidated fully, although most recent brain imaging studies indicate that gross degenerative changes are not present. Although late-onset schizophrenia is less common than early-onset schizophrenia, the many similarities between patients whose schizophrenia onset is in early adulthood and those whose onset occurred at middle age suggests that true schizophrenia can manifest in midlife. The differences between patients with early- and late-onset schizophrenia suggest that the latter condition may be a neurobiologically distinct subtype. If adherence with antipsychotic medication at optimal doses can be maintained and appropriate psychosocial therapies provided, the prognosis for functional improvement can be good.

Acknowledgement

This work was supported, in part, by the National Institute of Mental Health grant P30 MH66248 and by the Department of Veterans Affairs.

References

Aguera-Ortiz, L. & Reneses-Prieto, B. (1999) The place of non-biological treatments. In: Howard, R., Rabins, P.V., Castle, D.J., eds. *Late-Onset Schizophrenia*. Petersfield: Wrightson Biomedical.

Alexopoulos, G.S., Jeste, D.V., Chung, H. *et al.* (2005) Treatment of dementia and its behavioural disturbance. *Postgraduate Medicine Supplement* 3–110.

Allison, D.B., Mentore, J.L., Heo, M. *et al.* (1999) Antipsychotic-induced weight gain: A comprehensive research synthesis. *American Journal of Psychiatry* **156**, 1686–1696.

Almeida, O., Forstl, H., Howard, R. & David, A.S. (1993) Unilateral auditory hallucinations. *British Journal of Psychiatry* **162**, 262–264.

Almeida, O.P., Howard, R.J., Levy, R. & David, A.S. (1995a) Psychotic states arising in late life (late paraphrenia): Psychopathology and nosolgy. *British Journal of Psychiatry* **165**, 205–214.

Almeida, O.P., Howard, R.J., Levy, R. *et al.* (1995b) Clinical and cognitive diversity of psychotic states arising in late life (late paraphrenia). *Psychological Medicine* **25**, 699–714.

American Diabetes Association, American Psychiatric Association, American Association of Clinical Endocrinologists, North American Center for the Study of Obesity (2004) Consensus Development Conference on Antipsychotic Drugs and Obesity and Diabetes. *Journal of Clinical Psychiatry* **65**, 267–272.

American Psychiatric Association (1980) *Diagnostic and Statistical Manual of Mental Disorders, Third Edition*. Washington, DC: American Psychiatric Press.

American Psychiatric Association (1987) *Diagnostic and Statistical Manual of Mental Disorders, Third Edition-Revised*. Washington, DC: American Psychiatric Press.

American Psychiatric Association (1994) *Diagnostic and Statistical Manual of Mental Disorders, Fourth Edition*. Washington, DC American Psychiatric Press.

American Psychiatric Association (2000) *Diagnostic and Statistical Manual of Mental Disorders, Fourth Edition, Text Revision*. Washington, DC: American Psychiatric Press.

Bleuler, E.P. (1911) *Dementia Praecox or the Group of Schizophrenias*. Leipzig: Deuticke.

Bleuler, M. (1943) Die spatschizophrenen krankheitsbilder. *Fortschritte der Neurologie Psychiatrie* **15**, 259–290.

Brodaty, H., Sachdev, P., Rose, N. *et al.* (1999) Schizophrenia with onset after age 50 years. 1. Phenomenology and risk factors. *British Journal of Psychiatry* **175**, 410–415.

Castle, D.J. (1999) Gender and age at onset in schizophrenia. In: Howard, R., Rabins, P.V., Castle, D.J., eds. *Late Onset Schizophrenia*. Philadelphia: Wrightson Biomedical Publishing, Ltd.

Castle, D.J. & Howard, R. (1992) What do we know about the aetiology of late-onset schizophrenia. *European Psychiatry* **7**, 99–108.

Castle, D.J. & Murray, R.M. (1991) The neurodevelopmental basis of sex differences in schizophrenia. *Psychological Medicine* **21**, 565–575.

Cervantes, R.C., Salgado-Snyder, V.N. & Padilla, A.M. (1989) Post-traumatic stress in immigrants from Central American and Mexico. *Hospital and Community Psychiatry* **40**, 615–619.

Cooper, A.F. (1976) Deafness and psychiatric illness. *British Journal of Psychiatry* **129**, 216–226.

Cooper, A.F. & Curry, A.R. (1976) The pathology of deafness in the paranoid and affective psychoses of later life. *Journal of Psychosomatic Research* **20**, 97–105.

Cooper, A.F., Curry, A.R., Kay, D.W.K. *et al.* (1974) Hearing loss in paranoid and affective psychoses of the elderly. *Lancet* **2**, 851–854.

Corbin, S.L. & Eastwood, M.R. (1986) Sensory deficits and mental disorders of old age: Causal or coincidental associations? *Psychological Medicine* **16**, 251–256.

Corcoran, R., Frith, C.D. & Mercer, G. (1995) Schizophrenia, symptomatology and social inference: investigating theory of mind in people with schizophrenia. *Schizophrenia Research* **17**, 5–13.

Corey-Bloom, J., Jernigan, T., Archibald, S. *et al.* (1995) Quantitative magnetic resonance imaging of the brain in late-life schizophrenia. *American Journal of Psychiatry* **152**, 447–449.

Cutting, J.C., Clare, A.W. & Mann, A.H. (1978) Cycloid psychosis: Investigation of the diagnostic concept. *Psychological Medicine* **8**, 637–648.

Dolder, C.R., Lacro, J.P. & Jeste, D.V. (2004) Antipsychotic in late life depression. In Roose, S.P. & Sackeim, H.A., eds. *Late Life Depression Textbook*. Oxford: Oxford University Press.

Eastwood, R., Corbin, S. & Reed, M. (1981) Hearing impairment and paraphrenia. *Journal of Otolaryngology* **10**, 306–308.

Fish, F. (1958) A clinical investigation of chronic schizophrenia. *British Journal of Psychiatry* **104**, 34–54.

Fish, F. (1960) Senile schizophrenia. *Journal of Mental Science* **106**, 938–946.

Flint, A.J., Rifat, S.I. & Eastwood, M.R. (1991) Late-onset paranoia: Distinct from paraphrenia? *International Journal of Geriatric Psychiatry* **6**, 103–109.

Funding, T. (1961) Genetics of paranoid psychosis of later life. *Acta Psychiatrica Scandanavica* **37**, 267–282.

Gabriel, E. (1978) *Die Langfristige Entwicklung der Spatschizophrenien*. Basel: Karger.

Garety, P., Phil, M., Hemsley, D.R. & Wessely, S. (1991) Reasoning in deluded schizophrenic and paranoid patients. *Journal of Nervous and Mental Disease* **179**, 194–201.

Gladsjo, J.A., Heaton, R.K., Paulsen, J.S. & Jeste, D.V. (1996) Relationship of neuropsychological functioning and psychiatric symptoms in schizophrenia: a one-year follow-up. *Journal of the International Neuropsychological Society* **2**, 55.

Gorwood, P., Leboyer, M., Jay, M. *et al.* (1995) Gender and age at onset in schizophrenia: impact of family history. *American Journal of Psychiatry* **152**, 208–212.

Gottesman, I.I. & Shields, J. (1982) *Schizophrenia: The Epigenetic Puzzle*. Cambridge: Cambridge University Press.

Grahame, P.S. (1984) Schizophrenia in old age (late paraphrenia). *British Journal of Psychiatry* **145**, 493–495.

Granholm, E., McQuaid, J.R., McClure, F.S. *et al.* (2005) A randomized, controlled trial of cognitive behavioral social skills training for middle-aged and older outpatients with chronic schizophrenia. *American Journal of Psychiatry* **162**, 520–529.

Granholm, E., McQuaid, J.R., McClure, F.S. *et al.* (2007) Randomized controlled trial of cognitive behavioral social skills training for older people with schizophrenia: 12-month follow-up. *Journal of Clinical Psychiatry* **68**, 730–737.

Gurian, B.S., Wexler, D. & Baker, E.H. (1992) Late-life paranoia: Possible association with early trauma and infertility. *International Journal of Geriatric Psychiatry* **7**, 277–284.

Harris, M.J. & Jeste, D.V. (1988) Late-onset schizophrenia: an overview. *Schizophrenia Bulletin* **14**, 39–55.

Heaton, R., Paulsen, J., McAdams, L.A. *et al.* (1993) Neurospsychological deficits in schizophrenia: relationship to age, chronicity and dementia. *Archives of General Psychiatry* **51**, 469–476.

Herbert, M.E. & Jacobson, S. (1967) Late paraphrenia. *British Journal of Psychiatry* **113**, 461–469.

Holden, N.L. (1987) Late paraphrenia or the paraphrenias: A descriptive study with a 10-year follow-up. *British Journal of Psychiatry* **150**, 635–639.

Hopkins, B. & Roth, M. (1953) Psychological test performance in patients over sixty: II. Paraphrenia, arteriosclerotic psychosis and acute confusion. *Journal of Mental Science* **99**, 451–463.

Howard, R. & Levy, R. (1992) Which factors affect treatment response in late paraphrenia? *International Journal of Geriatric Psychiatry* **7**, 667–672.

Howard, R., Castle, D., Wessely, S. & Murray, R.M. (1993) A comparative study of 470 cases of early and late-onset schizophrenia. *British Journal of Psychiatry* **163**, 352–357.

Howard, R., Almeida, O. & Levy, R. (1994a) Phenomenology, demography and diagnosis in late paraphrenia. *Psychological Medicine* **24**, 397–410.

Howard, R.J., Almeida, O., Levy, R. *et al.* (1994b) Quantitative magnetic resonance imaging volumetry distinguishes delusional disorder from late-onset schizophrenia. *British Journal of Psychiatry* **165**, 474–480.

Howard, R., Cox, T., Almeida, O. *et al.* (1995) White matter signal hyperintensities in the brains of patients with late paraphrenia and the normal community-living elderly. *Biological Psychiatry* **38**, 86–91.

Howard, R., Graham, C., Sham, P. *et al.* (1997) A controlled family study of late-onset non-affective psychosis (late paraphrenia). *British Journal of Psychiatry* **170**, 511–514.

Howard, R., Rabins, P.V., Seeman, M.V. *et al.* (2000) Late-onset schizophrenia and very-late-onset schizophrenia-like psychois: An international consensus. *American Journal Psychiatry* **157**, 172–178.

Huber, G., Gross, G. & Schuttler, R. (1975) Spat schizophrenie. *Archives of Psychiatrie Nervenkrankheiten* **22**, 53–66.

Jeste, D.V. & McClure, F.S. (1997) Psychoses: diagnosis and treatment in the elderly. In: Schneider, L, ed. *Updates in Geriatric Psychiatry, New Directions for Mental Health Services.* San Francisco: Jossey-Bass, pp. 53–70.

Jeste, D.V. & Zisook, S. (1988) Preface to psychosis and depression in the elderly. *Psychiatric Clinics of North America* **11**, xiii–xv.

Jeste, D.V., Harris, M.J., Pearlson, G.D. *et al.* (1988) Late-onset schizophrenia: Studying clinical validity. *Psychiatric Clinics of North America* **11**, 1–14.

Jeste, D.V., Lacro, J.P., Gilbert, P.L. *et al.* (1993) Treatment of late-life schizophrenia with neuroleptics. *Schizophrenia Bulletin* **19**, 817–830.

Jeste, D.V., Caligiuri, M.P., Paulsen, J.S. *et al.* (1995a) Risk of tardive dyskinesia in older patients: A prospective longitudinal study of 266 outpatients. *Archives of General Psychiatry* **52**, 756–765.

Jeste, D.V., Paulsen, J. & Harris, M.J. (1995b) Late-onset schizophrenia and other related psychoses. In: Bloom, F.L. & Kupfer, D.J., eds. *Psychopharmacology: The Fourth Generation of Progress.* New York: Raven Press, pp. 1437–1446.

Jeste, D.V., Lacro, J.P., Palmer, B.W. *et al.* (1999) Incidence of tardive dyskinesia in early stages of low-dose treatment with typical neuroleptics in older patients. *American Journal of Psychiatry* **156**, 309–311.

Jeste, D.V., Barak, Y., Madhusoodanan, S. *et al.* (2003) An international multisite double-blind trial of the atypical antipsychotic risperidone and olanzapine in 175 elderly patients with chronic schizophrenia. *American Journal of Geriatric Psychiatry* **11**, 638–647.

Jeste, D.V., Blazer, D., Casey, D.E. *et al.* (2008) ACNP White Paper: update on the use of antipsychotic drugs in elderly persons with dementia. *Neuropsychopharmacology* **33**, 957–970.

Jin, H., Meyer, J.M. & Jeste, D.V. (2002) Phenomenology of and risk factors for new-onset diabetes mellitus and diabetic ketoacidosis associated with atypical antipsychotics: An analysis of 45 published cases. *Annals of Clinical Psychiatry* **14**, 59–64.

Jin, H., Meyer, J.M. & Jeste, D.V. (2004) Atypical antipsychotics and glucose dysregulation: a systematic review. *Schizophrenia Research* **71**, 195–212.

Jones, D.K., Catani, M., Pierpaoli, C. *et al.* (2005) A diffusion tensor magnetic resonance imaging study of frontal cortex connections in very-late-onset schizophrenia-like psychosis. *American Journal of Geriatric Psychiatry* **13**, 1092–1099.

Jones, P.B., Barnes, T.R., Davies, L. *et al.* (2006) Randomized controlled trial of the effect on quality of life of second- vs first-generation antipsychotic drugs in schizophrenia: Cost Utility of the Latest Antipsychotic Drugs in Schizophrenia Study (CUtLASS 1). *Archives of General Psychiatry* **63**, 1079–1087.

Kaney, S. & Bentall, R.P. (1989) Persecutory delusions and attributional style. *British Journal of Medical Psychology* **62**, 191–198.

Kay, D.W.K. & Roth, M. (1961) Environmental and hereditary factors in the schizophrenias of old age ("late paraphrenia") and their bearing on the general problem of causation in schizophrenia. *Journal of Mental Science* **107**, 649–686.

Kay, D.W.K., Cooper, A.F., Garside, R.F. & Roth, M. (1976) The differentiation of paranoid from affective psychoses by patients' premorbid characteristics. *British Journal of Psychiatry* **129**, 207–215.

Kendell, R.E. (1988) Other functional psychoses. In: Kendell, R.E. & Zealley, A.K., eds. *Companion to Psychiatric Studies.* Edinburgh: Churchill Livingstone.

Kendler, K.S., Tsuang, M.T. & Hays, P. (1987) Age at onset in schizophrenia: A familial perspective. *Archives of General Psychiatry* **44**, 881–890.

Keshavan, M.S., David, A.S., Steingard, S. & Lishman, W.A. (1992) Musical hallucinations: A review and synthesis. *Neuropsychology, Neuropsychiatry, and Behavioral Neurology* **5**, 211–223.

Khan, A.M., Clark, T. & Oyebode, F. (1988) Unilateral auditory hallucinations. *British Journal of Psychiatry* **152**, 297–298.

Klages, W. (1961) *Die Spatschizophrenie.* Stuttgart: Enke.

Kraepelin, E. (1913) *Psychiatrie*, 8th edn, Vol. 3, Part 2. Translated by Barclay, R.M. as *Dementia Praecox and Paraphrenia.* Edinburgh: ES Livingstone.

Levitt, J.J. & Tsuang, M.T. (1988) The heterogeneity of schizoaffective disorder: Implications for treatment. *American Journal of Psychiatry* **145**, 926–936.

Lewine, R. (1981) Sex differences in schizophrenia: Timing or subtype? *Psychological Bulletin* **90**, 432–444.

Lindamer, L.A., Lohr, J.B., Harris, M.J. & Jeste, D.V. (1997) Gender, estrogen, and schizophrenia. *Psychopharmacology Bulletin* **33**, 221–228.

Lindamer, L.A., Lohr, J.B., Harris, M.J. *et al.* (1999) Gender-related clinical differences in older patients with schizophrenia. *Journal of Clinical Psychiatry* **60**, 61–67.

Lindamer, L.A., Harris, M.J., Gladsjo, J.A. *et al.* (2000) Gender and schizophrenia. In: Morrison, M., ed. *Sex Hormones, Aging, and Mental Disorders.* Washington, DC: National Institute of Mental Health, pp. 223–239.

Lohr, J.B., Alder, M., Flynn, K. *et al.* (1997) Minor physical anomalies in older patients with late-onset schizophrenia, early-onset schizophrenia, depression, and Alzheimer's disease. *American Journal of Geriatric Psychiatry* **5**, 318–323.

Magnan, V. (1893) *Lecons cliniques sur les maladies mentales.* Paris: Bureaux de Progres Medical.

Marneros, A. & Deister, A. (1984) The psychopathology of "late schizophrenia". *Psychopathology* **17**, 264–174.

Mayer, W. (1921) Uber paraphrene psychosen. *Zeitschrift fur die Gesamte Neurologie und Psychiatrie* **71**, 187–206.

Miller, B.L., Lesser, I.M., Boone, K. *et al.* (1989) Brain white-matter lesions and psychosis. *British Journal of Psychiatry* **155**, 73–78.

Miller, B.L., Lesser, I.M., Boone, K.B. *et al.* (1991) Brain lesions and cognitive function in late-life psychosis. *British Journal of Psychiatry* **158**, 76–82.

Miller, B.L., Lesser, I.M., Mena, I. *et al.* (1992) Regional cerebral blood flow in late-life-onset psychosis. *Neuropsychology, Neuropsychiatry, and Behavioral Neurology* **5**, 132–137.

Mitter, P., Reeves, S., Romero-Rubiales, F. *et al.* (2005) Migrant status, age, gender and social isolation in very late-onset schizophrenia-like psychosis. *International Journal of Geriatric Psychiatry* **20**, 1046–1051.

Moore, R., Blackwood, N., Corcoran, R. *et al.* (2006) Misunderstanding the intentions of others: an exploratory study of the cognitive etiology of persecutory delusions in very late-onset schizophrenia-like psychosis. *American Journal of Geriatric Psychiatry* **14**, 410–418.

Murray, R.M., O'Callaghan, E., Castle, D.J. & Lewis, S.W. (1992) A neurodevelopmental approach to the classification of schizophrenia. *Schizophrenia Bulletin* **18**, 319–332.

Naguib, M.& Levy, R. (1987) Late paraphrenia: neuropsychological impairment and structural brain abnormalities on computed tomography. *International Journal of Geriatric Psychiatry* **2**, 83–90.

Patterson, T.L., Bucardo, J., McKibbin, C.L. *et al.* (2005) Development and pilot testing of a new psychosocial intervention for older Latinos with chronic psychosis. *Schizophrenia Bulletin* **31**, 922–930.

Patterson, T.L., McKibbin, C., Mausbach, B.T. *et al.* (2006) Functional Adaptation Skills Training (FAST): a randomized trial of a psychosocial intervention for middle-aged and older patients with chronic psychotic disorders. *Schizophrenia Research* **86**, 291–299.

Paulsen, J.S., Romero, R., Chan, A. *et al.* (1996) Impairment of the semantic network in schizophrenia. *Psychiatry Research* **63**, 109–121.

Pearlson, G.D., Kreger, L., Rabins, R.V. *et al.* (1989) A chart review study of late-onset and early-onset schizophrenia. *American Journal of Psychiatry* **146**, 1568–1574.

Pearlson, G.D., Tune, L.E., Wong, D.F. *et al.* (1993) Quantitative D₂ dopamine receptor PET and structural MRI changes in late onset schizophrenia. *Schizophrenia Bulletin* **19**, 783–795.

Post, F. (1966) *Persistent Persecutory States of the Elderly.* London: Pergamon Press.

Prager, S. & Jeste, D.V. (1993) Sensory impairment in late-life schizophrenia. *Schizophrenia Bulletin* **19**, 755–772.

Quintal, M., Day-Cody, D. & Levy, R. (1991) Late paraphrenia and ICD-10. *International Journal of Geriatric Psychiatry* **6**, 111–116.

Rabins, P.V., Pauker, S. & Thomas, J. (1984) Can schizophrenia begin after age 44? *Comprehensive Psychiatry* **25**, 290–293.

Reeves, S., Sauer, J., Stewart, R. *et al.* (2001) Increased first contact rates for very late onset schizophrenia like psychosis in African- and Caribbean-born elders. *British Journal of Psychiatry* **179**, 172–174.

Retterstol, N. (1966) *Paranoid and Paranoiac Psychoses. A Personal Follow-Up Investigation with Special Reference to Aetiological, Clinical and Prognostic Aspects.* Springfield: Oslo Universitetsforlaget.

Riecher-Rossler, A., Hafner, H., Stumbalum, M. *et al.* (1994) Can estradiol modulate schizophrenic symptomatology? *Schizophrenia Bulletin* **20**, 203–213.

Rockwell, E., Krull, A.J., Dimsdale, J. & Jeste, D.V. (1994) Late-onset psychosis with somatic delusions. *Psychosomatics* **35**, 66–72.

Roth, M. & Morrisey, J.D. (1952) Problems in the diagnosis and classification of mental disorders in old age. *Journal of Mental Science* **98**, 68–80.

Saltz, B.L., Woerner, M.G., Kane, J.M. *et al.* (1991) Prospective study of tardive dyskinesia incidence in the elderly. *JAMA* **266**, 2402–2406.

Salzman, C. (1990) Principles of psychopharmacology. In: Bienenfeld, D., ed. *Verwoerdt's Clinical Geropsychiatry.* Baltimore, MD: Williams and Wilkins, pp. 235–249.

Seeman, M.V. (1981) Gender and the onset of schizophrenia: neurohumoral influences. *Psychiatric Journal of the University of Ottawa* **6**, 136–138.

Seeman, M.V. (1999) Oestrogens and psychosis. In: Howard, R., Rabins, P.V. & Castle, D.J., eds. *Late Onset Schizophrenia.* Philadelphia: Wrightson Biomedical Publishing Ltd.

Seeman, M.V. & Lang, M. (1990) The role of estrogens in schizophrenia gender differences. *Schizophrenia Bulletin* **16**, 185–194.

Shimizu, A & Kurachi, M. (1989) Do women without a family history of schizophrenia have a later onset of schizophrenia? *Japanese Journal of Psychiatry and Neurology* **43**, 133–136.

Sjoegren, H. (1964) Paraphrenic, melancholic and psychoneurotic states in the pre-senile and senile periods of life. *Acta Psychiatrica Scandanavica* **176** (Suppl.).

Sternberg, E. (1972) Neuere forschungsergebnisse bei spatschizophrenen psychosen. *Fortschritte der Neurologie Psychiatrie* **40**, 631–646.

Symonds, L.L., Olichney, J.M., Jernigan, T.L. *et al.* (1997) Lack of clinically significant structural abnormalities in MRIs of older patients with schizophrenia and related psychoses. *Journal of Neuropsychiatry and Clinical Neurosciences* **9**, 251–258.

Twamley, E.W., Padin, D.S., Bayne, K.S. *et al.* (2005) Work rehabilitation for middle-aged and older people with schizophrenia: a comparison of three approaches. *Journal of Nervous and Mental Diseases* **193**, 596–601.

Weinberger, D.R. (1987) Implications of normal brain development for the pathogenesis of schizophrenia. *Archives of General Psychiatry* **44**, 660–669.

Wirshing, D.A., Spellberg, B.J., Erhart, S.M. *et al.* (1998) Novel antipsychotics and new onset diabetes. *Biological Psychiatry* **44**, 778–783.

World Health Organization (1978) *Mental Disorders: Glossary and Guide to Their Classification in Accordance with the Ninth Revision of the International Classification of Diseases.* Geneva: World Health Organization.

World Health Organization (1991) *ICD-10. The International Statistical Classification of Diseases and Related Health Problems. Vol. 1, 2.* American Psychiatric Press.

CHAPTER 5

The schizophrenia spectrum personality disorders

Eran Chemerinski and Larry J. Siever

Mount Sinai School of Medicine, New York, NY and James J. Peters Veterans Affairs Medical Center, Bronx NY, USA

Introduction

Classical phenomenological studies by Kraepelin (1919/1971) and Bleuler (1950) initially reported that schizophrenia is present in a continuum. Thus, the assessment of this disorder has increasingly encompassed candidate genes, imaging, and cognitive science strategies that employ populations other than those with schizophrenia itself (Siever et al., 2002). These include relatives of patients with schizophrenia who might exhibit mild psychotic-like symptoms, and subjects in prodromal stages of schizophrenia and schizophrenia-related personality disorders. A strategy recently employed in schizophrenia research is the examination of similarities and differences between schizophrenia spectrum disorders and chronic schizophrenia. This strategy recognizes the naturalistic variability of schizophrenia. More importantly, it permits the discrimination of the pathophysiological mechanisms associated with the core cognitive and social impairments of the schizophrenia spectrum from those associated with psychosis and extreme cognitive and social deficits of chronic schizophrenia.

Schizotypal personality disorder (SPD) is the prototypic schizophrenia-related personality disorder. Patients with this disorder share common genetic, biological, phenomenological, prognosis, and treatment response characteris-

Schizophrenia, 3rd edition. Edited by Daniel R. Weinberger and Paul J Harrison © 2011 Blackwell Publishing Ltd.

Table 5.1 DSM-IV diagnostic criteria for schizotypal personality disorder (American Psychiatric Association, 1994).

A A pervasive pattern of social and interpersonal deficits marked by acute discomfort with, and reduced capacity for, close relationships as well as by cognitive or perceptual distortions and eccentricities of behavior, beginning by early adulthood and present in a variety of contexts, as indicated by five (or more) of the following:
  1. Ideas of reference (excluding delusions of reference)
  2. Odd beliefs or magical thinking that influences behavior and is inconsistent with subcultural norms (e.g., superstitiousness, belief in clairvoyance, telepathy or "sixth sense"; in children or adolescents, bizarre fantasies or preoccupations)
  3. Unusual perceptual experiences, including bodily illusions
  4. Odd thinking and speech (e.g., vague, circumstantial, metaphorical, overelaborate, or stereotyped)
  5. Suspiciousness or paranoid ideation
  6. Inappropriate or constricted affect
  7. Behavior or appearance that is odd, eccentric or peculiar
  8. Lack of close fiends or confidants other than first-degree relatives
  9. Excessive social anxiety that does not diminish with familiarity and tends to be associated with paranoid fears rather than negative judgements about self

B Does not occur exclusively during the course of Schizophrenia, a Mood Disorder With Psychotic Features, another Psychotic Disorder, or a Pervasive Developmental Disorder

Note: If criteria are met prior to the onset of schizophrenia, add "premorbid", e.g., "schizotypal personality disorder (premorbid)".

tics with the more severely ill patients with chronic schizophrenia. The diagnosis of SPD derives from the clinical features of "borderline schizophrenia" or "latent schizophrenia" identified by Kety *et al.* (1975) in relatives of probands with schizophrenia. Since its first inclusion in the DSM-III (Table 5.1; American Psychiatric Association, 1980), SPD has been a part of the "odd" cluster of the personality disorders. SPD shares with chronic schizophrenia analogous symptom dimensions, such as ideas of reference, magical thinking, and suspiciousness (i.e., psychotic-like symptoms), and deficit-like symptoms, discriminated by factor analyses in the independent dimensions of social deficit and either cognitive disorganization or paranoid symptoms (Raine *et al.*, 1994; Bergman *et al.*, 1996). The pervasive asociality and cognitive impairments observed in patients with SPD are usually milder and more circumscribed than those of schizophrenia. Furthermore, in contrast to patients with schizophrenia, patients with SPD do not suffer from the consequences of chronic psychosis, such as prolonged functional impairment, multiple hospitalizations, and long-term and ongoing exposure to psy-

chotropic medication. Thus, the study of SPD provides an exceptional prospect to examine a population with analogous cognitive and social deficit observed in schizophrenia but devoid of the potential confounding artifacts resulting from the effects of chronic psychosis. Additionally, the recognition of factors that spare patients with SPD from psychosis and severe cognitive and functional deterioration might be translated in the formulation of treatments that successfully reduce the morbidity of psychotic exacerbations in schizophrenia. Since the publication of our chapter in the previous edition of this book (O'Flynn *et al.*, 2002) there have been numerous studies on the pathophysiology of SPD.

Phenomenology

Individuals with SPD suffer from attenuated psychotic-like symptoms, such as ideas of reference and cognitive-perceptual distortions as well as deficit-like symptoms of constricted affect, social isolation, and peculiar appearance and speech (Table 5.1). The ideas of reference of SPD are not held with the same certainty as in schizophrenia, but are nevertheless pervasive and disturbing to the patient. Individuals with SPD contemplate odd and idiosyncratic beliefs that are not part of the social norms of their culture. An example of this is the belief that the mind is able to change the physical world or "magical thinking". The idiosyncratic beliefs and manners of this population frequently extend to their speech and appearance. Patients with SPD also experience perceptual distortions such as illusions during periods of decreased awareness. The social deficits exhibited by these patients in their relatedness to others range from poor and inappropriate rapport to social isolation resulting from significant suspiciousness of the intentions of other people.

Individuals with schizoid personality disorder share with subjects with SPD the lack of close friends or confidants. However, individuals with schizoid personality disorder might not experience the cognitive–perceptual distortions that are criteria for SPD. Asociality is a core trait of schizoid personality disorder. However, in contrast to SPD, it is not secondary to distrust from others, but to a frank desire to be alone due to lack of pleasure from casual or intimate relationships. Furthermore, individuals who are schizoid remain indifferent to criticism and praise from others. In paranoid personality disorder, the diagnostic criteria lay emphasis on these individuals' suspiciousness and mistrust. The perceived hidden threatening meanings that justify their preconceptions result in an expectation of malicious intent from others and volatile responses to perceived slights. Paranoid personality disorder individuals are also reluctant to confide in others since they question the loyalty and are fearful of the ill-will of even close friends.

The study of SPD has begun to provide new opportunities to disentangle the genetics and pathophysiology of schizophrenia. By contrasting and comparing schizotypal, schizophrenic, and healthy volunteer subjects, commonalities and distinctions between SPD and schizophrenia are being mapped using neurochemical, imaging, and pharmacological tools. As arrays of candidate genes begin to be identified in relation to schizophrenia disorders, the genes that are associated with both schizotypal and schizophrenia disorders and those that are unique to schizophrenia and psychosis may be identified. Clusters of schizotypal traits and/or cognitive dysfunctions may be used to provide intermediate phenotypes to more finely hone our understanding of the character of genetic or phenomenological relationships in the spectrum. Furthermore, individuals with SPD also afford a unique opportunity to pilot pharmacological interventions that might serve to enhance cognitive function or improve negative symptoms because they have more reversible cognitive and social deficits than patients with chronic schizophrenia and are less vulnerable to potential worsening of psychosis.

A valid question drawn from the observation of the significant overlap of clinical samples of patients with SPD, schizoid and paranoid disorders (Kalus et al., 1996) is whether these disorders are discrete disorders or actually gradations of severity along the schizophrenia spectrum. The overlap in these disorders could be a result of similarity in criteria and/or comorbidity. The reported frequency of these disorders in the community varies with the type of population being assessed. For example, schizoid personality is least commonly reported in clinical settings, perhaps because these individuals do not experience the dysphoria and disruption of relationships and work activities that normally lead to the seeking of clinical treatment. In contrast, studies of mood disturbances in personality disorders reported that a significant number of individuals with SPD and paranoid disorder had experienced episodes of major depression (Bernstein et al. 1996; Siever et al. 1996). A study by Kavoussi and Siever (1992) found that the overlap initially observed between schizophrenia spectrum personality disorders and borderline personality disorder is reduced when the psychotic-like symptoms of borderline personality disorder are viewed as transient and dissociative, in contrast to the ones observed in SPD, which are more relentless and accompanied by affective instability. Individuals with avoidant personality disorder may appear socially distant and exhibit similar cognitive impairments to those observed in the schizophrenia spectrum disorders (Cohen et al., 1996). However, the criteria for this disorder emphasize that the social isolation of these individuals results, not from lack of desire for relatedness, but from their substantial anxiety and need for reassurance that they will not be rejected when attempting to interact with others.

Relationship of schizotypal personality disorder to schizophrenia

As previously mentioned, shared underlying genetic diathesis interacting with environmental insults are hypothesized to cause neurodevelopmentally-based cortical pathology (e.g., temporal pathology and prefrontal cortical hypodopaminergia; Siever & Davis, 2004) that ultimately results in the cognitive impairment observed in patients with chronic schizophrenia and schizophrenia spectrum disorders (Siever et al., 2002). SPD, the prototypic disorder of this spectrum, shares with schizophrenia similar phenomenological features, such as asociality and cognitive impairment, presumably emerging from common spectrum-related risk factors (Siever et al., 2002). However, the observation that the cognitive deficits and social deterioration in SPD are more circumscribed and of lesser degree than in chronic schizophrenia suggests that, irrespective of the DSM-IV (American Psychiatric Association, 1994) categorical point of view, schizophrenia spectrum disorders would be better conceptualized as continuous or dimensional in nature (Fossati et al., 2005). In this context, subjects with schizophrenia spectrum disorders are believed to share a common underlying liability (Battaglia et al., 1997; Holzman et al., 1988; Meehl, 1962, 1990; Lenzenweger & Korfine, 1995; Faraone et al., 2001) identified by some authors as "schizotaxia" (Meehl, 1962, 1990; Lenzenweger & Korfine, 1995; Faraone et al., 2001). This term was coined by Meehl (1962) to describe a set of signs and symptoms present in individuals genetically predisposed for schizophrenia who, while lacking the clinical manifestations of schizophrenia, usually display some evidence of deviant psychological functioning or "schizotypy". On the other hand, patients with chronic schizophrenia, who normally exhibit severe and generalized deterioration across a variety of domains, are placed in the "end-stage" of the schizophrenia continuum. The more profound level of cognitive deterioration in chronic schizophrenia compared to SPD could be explained by the capacity of individuals with SPD to recruit other related brain regions to compensate for dysfunctional areas during cognitive demands. Furthermore, while the temporal lobe and hippocampus display a reduction in volume across the schizophrenia spectrum disorders, the frontal lobe volume is generally reduced in patients with schizophrenia but either normal or increased in individuals with SPD (Buchsbaum et al., 2002). Greater frontal reserves may protect individuals with SPD from the severe cognitive deterioration and social deficits associated with chronic schizophrenia. Additionally, in contrast to chronic schizophrenia, patients with SPD are significantly less vulnerable to psychosis and thus, spared from multiple hospitalizations and long-term and ongoing exposure to psychotropic medication. Psychosis is hypothesized to result from increased levels of subcortical presynaptic dopamine (DA) release as well as elevated DA receptor sensitivity. While the frontal lobe is usually spared from any structural or functional dysfunction in subjects with SPD, prefrontal cortical (PFC) DA system lesions and PFC–striatum disconnection observed in chronic schizophrenia lead to up-regulation of subcortical DA activity (Pycock *et al.*, 1980; Lipska & Weinberger, D., 2000). Subcortical DA activity elevation, when propagated to fronto-temporal regions, normally gives rise to psychosis exacerbation (Siever & Davis, 2004). Thus, the characterization of factors that mitigate the emergence of psychosis and serious cognitive deterioration in ndividuals with SPD might improve the likelihood of utilizing strategies and agents that will successfully prevent or ameliorate social and cognitive dysfunction in schizophrenia without triggering psychotic exacerbations. For example, the administration of the DA-releasing agent amphetamine results in cognitive function improvement in both chronic schizophrenia and populations with SPD. However, in contrast to patients with chronic schizophrenia, amphetamine administration to subjects with SPD does not lead to an emergence of psychotic symptoms (Siegel *et al.*, 1996; Kirrane *et al.*, 2000) due to increased DA release (Laruelle *et al.*, 2002).

Psychometric assessment

The interaction of numerous genetic and psychosocial factors gives rise to individuals who have neurodevelopmental vulnerabilities for the development of schizophrenia spectrum disorders (Murray & Lewis, 1987; Weinberger, 1987; Keshavan, 1997; Andreasen, 1999). The term schizotypy, first coined by Rado (1956), was utilized by Meehl (1962) to refer to the personality organization that represents the expression of these vulnerabilities. The majority of schizotypy individuals, however, will never decompensate into clinical psychosis (Kwapil *et al.*, 2008). Thus, confounding consequences of clinical psychosis, such as long-term psychotropic therapy and hospitalization, are not present in studies of these individuals. On the other hand, due to presumably shared neurodevelopmental pathways with patients with schizophrenia, schizotypy subjects usually exhibit similar, although often less severe, deficits in cognitive and psychophysiological functioning (Raine & Lencz, 1995). Following the appearance of the original measure of schizotypy (Chapman *et al.*, 1976, 1978), many instruments have been developed to measure psychosis proneness in these non-clinical populations (Eckblad & Chapman, 1983; Claridge & Broks, 1984; Venables *et al.*, 1990; Raine, 1991; Mason *et al.*, 1995; Linscott, 2007; Cornblatt *et al.*, 2007). These instruments, however, vary in a wide range of techniques and conceptual frameworks. Additionally, there have been only a few studies examining the factor structure underlying them. Despite these limitations, these scales are non-invasive and inexpensive tools that permit the assessment of schizotypy in

individuals at risk for schizophrenia (Compton *et al.*, 2007), as well as in large numbers of individuals from the general population, such as in the New York High-Risk Project (Erlenmeyer-Kimling *et al.*, 1993). Data gathered with the use of these instruments have provided findings, such as the factor structure underlying schizotypy, that are relevant to the elucidation of the pathophysiology of schizophrenia spectrum disorders. One example of this is the elevated risk for psychological and physiological deficits similar to those seen in schizophrenia in non-psychotic individuals with markedly elevated scores on questionnaires designed to measure dimensions reported to characterize patients prone to schizophrenia, such as magical ideation, perceptual aberration, as well as physical and social anhedonia (Chapman *et al.*, 1995). In schizotypy individuals, social anhedonia was found to be an effective predictor for the development of a schizophrenia-spectrum illness (Kwapil, 1998).

Schizotypy has been described as a multidimensional construct consisting of a "positive" (i.e., psychotic-like cognitive and perceptual experiences; Muntaner *et al.*, 1988; Bentall *et al.*, 1989; Hewitt & Claridge, 1989; Raine & Allbutt, 1989; Venables *et al.*, 1990; Kendler & Hewitt, 1992; Gruzelier, 1996) and a "negative" schizotypy factor (i.e., interpersonal or deficit-like characteristics; Muntaner *et al.*, 1988; Bentall *et al.*, 1989; Kendler & Hewitt, 1992). Less consistently replicated factors include "cognitive disorganization" (Bentall *et al.*, 1989) and "non-conformity" (Muntaner *et al.*, 1988; Bentall *et al.*, 1989; Raine & Allbutt, 1989; Kendler & Hewitt, 1992), as well as a combination of these features and activation (Gruzelier, 1996; Gruzelier & Doig, 1996). The dimensional formulation in schizotypy, while not unanimously accepted, provides candidate factors consistent with those hypothesized to comprise schizophrenia (Raine, 2006; Arndt *et al.*, 1991; Bilder *et al.*, 1985; Liddle, 1987, Peralta *et al.*, 1992), supporting the view that a neurodevelopmental vulnerability for schizophrenia is present across the continuum of schizotypy. Furthermore, the characterization in schizotypy individuals of these distinct dimensions may assist in the elucidation of the pathophysiolagal pathways leading to negative and positive symptoms of schizophrenia, hypothesized to be distinct (Siever, 1991). Finally, findings from a study by Kendler and Hewitt (1992) suggest that genetic factors play an important role in schizotypy by contributing to the development of the "positive", "non-conformity", and "social" schizotypy dimension.

Spectrum personality disorders in premorbid clinical profiles of patients with schizophrenia

During the last decade, there has been increased research activity in the field of early intervention in putative prodromal stages of schizophrenia (Olsen & Rosenbaum,

2006). However, behavioral disturbances in subjects before the onset of psychosis were reported by Kraepelin as early as 1919. The study of premorbid personality features in schizophrenia could also assist in characterizing the relationship between schizophrenia and schizophrenia spectrum personality disorders, presently viewed as milder schizophrenia-related disorders. For example, in some patients with schizophrenia, SPD is a developmental precursor of psychosis (Trotman et al., 2006). During adolescence and early adulthood, these patients manifest a gradual decline in functioning that involves the development of SPD symptoms (Walker & Lewine, 1990; Walker & Walder, 2003). Miller et al. (2002) and Yung et al. (2003) estimated that between 40% and 50% of those who meet SPD criteria in young adulthood, and show gradual functional decline, eventually develop an Axis I psychotic disorder. However, different features of the schizophrenia prodrome could show significant inconsistencies among patients. For example, Schultze-Lutter et al. (2007) found in a large retrospective population-based study that the initial schizophrenia prodrome varied greatly in duration between weeks and decades, with men showing the first signs of mental disturbance on average at the age of 22.5 and women at 25.4 years. Therefore, these differences in the schizophrenia prodromal stage time course and symptom patterns (Yung & McGorry, 1996) merit questioning whether a unitary model should be employed for the characterization of this stage or whether there are several prodromal subgroups with different duration and symptom patterns. A retrospective analysis from a birth cohort study by Crow et al. (1995), found that children developing schizophrenia as adults exhibited consistent symptom features, such as anxiety, depression, social withdrawal, aversive behavior, poor motor control, and cognitive underachievements, particularly in verbal abilities.

Studies that prospectively followed children with increased genetic risk for developing schizophrenia as adults have found significant behavioral differences from normal controls, such as poor affective control, cognitive disturbance, social withdrawal, irritability, and maladaptive behavior (Glish et al., 1982; Parnas et al., 1982; Olin & Mednick, 1996). Furthermore, attentional deficits potentiated by anhedonia were found in the New York High-Risk study (Freedman et al., 1998). Additionally, a recent study by Ho (2007) suggests that in genetically high-risk adolescent or young adult relatives of individuals with schizophrenia, premorbid magnetic resonance imaging (MRI) brain abnormalities, including decreased whole brain, frontal, temporal, and parietal gray matter, and increased white matter, specifically in the parietal lobe, may be of predictive value for the early identification of schizophrenia. Conversely, findings from a recent study by Shioiri et al. (2007) supported the view that the disorders frequently present for some years before the onset of schizo-

phrenia are non-specific. The authors reported that, before the onset of schizophrenia, approximately 24% of 219 inpatients with schizophrenia met criteria for distinct Axis I disorders, including mood, anxiety, obsessive-compulsive, adjustment, and eating disorder. Furthermore, the premorbid features of high-risk subjects who later develop predominantly negative-symptom schizophrenia are hypothesized to be different from those present in subjects who later develop predominantly positive-symptom schizophrenia (Cannon et al., 1990). Finally, Squires-Wheeler et al. (1989, 1992) reported that, in the New York High-Risk Project, rates of schizotypal personality traits did not differ between the offspring of parents with schizophrenia and those of parents with affective disorder. Taken together, these results provide evidence that the prodromal stage of schizophrenia is characterized by a lack of specific symptom dimensions. Despite this lack of symptom specificity, it has been consistently recognized that a significant fraction of adults with schizophrenia exhibit deviant characteristics, including schizoid and schizotypal traits, before the onset of illness (Fish, 1986; Hogg et al., 1990; Foerster et al., 1991; Peralta et al., 1991). Thus, the study of the schizophrenia spectrum personality disorders in a variety of populations, such as premorbid personalities of patients with schizophrenia, non-affected relatives of patients with schizophrenia, and clinically referred patients with personality disorder, could provide key explanations of the role of early personality disturbances in the development of schizophrenia.

Genetics

Genes play an important role in the etiology of schizophrenia (Sanders & Gill, 2007; Tsuang et al., 1991; McGuffin et al., 1995; see also Chapters 12 and 13.). However, this genetic liability is not specific to schizophrenia alone but to several related disorders (Siever, 2005; Appels et al., 2004). For example, paranoid (Baron et al., 1985; Kendler et al., 1993a; Tsuang et al., 1999), schizoid (Kendler et al., 1993a), and SPD (Siever, 2005; Baron et al., 1983, 1985; Kendler & Gruenberg, 1984; Kendler et al., 1993a, 1995a,b; Battaglia et al., 1991, 1995; Cadenhead & Braff, 2002) are associated with the genetic risk for schizophrenia. Among these disorders, the symptom traits present in SPD show the strongest familial relationship to traits observed in schizophrenia (Kendler et al., 1993a, Vollema & Hoijtink, 2000; Webb & Levinson, 1993; Ingraham & Kety, 2000). The genetic relationship between schizophrenia and SPD has also been suggested by several family and adoption studies (Tienari et al., 2003; Kendler et al., 1981, 1993b, 1994; Frangos et al., 1985; Kendler, 1985, 1988; Gershon et al., 1988; Lichtermann et al., 2000) and, more recently, by the use of linkage methods (Fanous et al., 2007). Among the relatives of probands with schizophrenia, family studies reported a significantly higher incidence of SPD compared with relatives of healthy controls (Kendler *et al.*, 1981, 1993b; Baron *et al.*, 1982; Gunderson *et al.*, 1983). On the other hand, compared with relatives of healthy controls, there is a higher incidence of schizophrenia (Tienari *et al.*, 2003; Schulz *et al.*, 1986; Battaglia *et al.*, 1995) and schizophrenia-related disorders (Tienari *et al.*, 2003; Siever *et al.*, 1990b) in families of probands with SPD. Additional support for a common genetic substrate for the two disorders is the fact that probands with SPD and with schizophrenia have similar likelihood of having a relative with schizophrenia (6.9% *vs.* 6.5%; Kendler *et al.*, 1993b). However, since schizophrenic symptom factors probably occur on an etiological continuum with their personality-based counterparts, continuous rather than categorical measures of psychopathology may provide greater statistical power to detect susceptibility loci for schizophrenia.

There is emerging evidence that the psychotic-like and deficit-like symptoms might have independent heritability in subjects with schizophrenia spectrum disorders. In an assessment of the Roscommon Family Study, Fanous *et al.* (2001) reported that positive and negative symptoms in probands with schizophrenia predicted different symptom dimensions of schizotypy in their first-degree non-psychotic relatives. A twin study by Kendler *et al.* (1991) also found that positive and negative symptoms associated with SPD represent two relatively independent, strongly heritable dimensions. These data are consistent with partially independent transmission of one set of genetic factors common to the spectrum that are largely manifest in social and cognitive deficits ("spectrum phenotype") and another set of distinct genetic factors related to psychosis ("psychotic phenotype") (Siever & Davis, 2004). Furthermore, when compared to positive psychotic-like SPD traits, the deficit-like SPD symptom dimensions, such as social and cognitive deficits, appear to better characterize the relatives of proband with schizophrenia (Gunderson *et al.*, 1983; Kendler, 1985; Torgersen *et al.*, 1993; Webb & Levinson, 1993; Ingraham & Kety, 2000).

Genetic studies of cognition in the schizophrenia spectrum

Catechol-O-methyltransferase (*COMT*) is an excellent candidate gene for modulation of PFC-mediated cognitive task performance (Tunbridge *et al.*, 2004). *COMT* is an essential component in the regulation of PFC DA levels by its catabolic action on this neurotransmitter (Karoum *et al.*, 1994). *COMT* variations translate into variable neural strategies for working memory (Tan *et al.*, 2007). An evolutionarily recent mutation of the *COMT* gene that translates into a substitution of methionine (Met) for valine (Val) at codon 108/158 results in PFC DA increased activity. This is explained because the enzyme containing Met exerts one-

quarter of the DA-catabolizing activity of the enzyme containing Val (Lotta *et al.*, 1995; Lachman *et al.*, 1996). On the contrary, the DA transmission is reduced due to greater catabolism of DA in the PFC when the Val in this gene is substituted for Met (Weinberger *et al.*, 2001). A large number of studies (Bilder *et al.*, 2002; Joober *et al.*, 2002; Malhotra *et al.*, 2002; Mattay *et al.*, 2003) have replicated initial findings by Egan *et al.* (2001) of greater efficiency of working memory tasks by subjects carrying the Met allele as measured by functional MRI (fMRI). Specifically, the extent of cortical recruitment visualized by the blood-oxygen-level-dependent (BOLD) signal with increasing working memory load was attenuated in these subjects in association with better performance than subjects carrying the Val allele. These findings were replicated in other disorders associated with DA abnormalities, such as Parkinson disease (Foltynie *et al.*, 2004) and attention-deficit/hyperactivity disorder (Bellgrove *et al.*, 2005). In schizophrenia, however, genetic studies examining the correlation between risk of schizophrenia and Val allele increased load have provided ambiguous results. While Glatt *et al.* (2003) reported the existence of this correlation, more recent studies did not confirm this finding (Sanders *et al.*, 2008; Tsai *et al.*, 2006; Munafò *et al.*, 2005). Results from a study by Smyrnis *et al.* (2007a) reported that increasing Val loading in patients with SPD resulted in a dose-dependent increase in the factor loading for the relation between negative schizotypy and cognitive performance accuracy. On the other hand, a study by our group of *COMT* genotype variation in patients with SPD and healthy controls (Minzenberg *et al.*, 2006) found that the Val/Val genotype was significantly associated with worse performance on executive functioning and PFC-dependent memory tasks, regardless of diagnosis. These findings suggest that *COMT* genotype variation exerts effects on cognition independent of clinical status.

Neurochemistry

Dopaminergic systems in the brain

Working memory, motor/sensorimotor coordination, reward, and attention are some functions consistently recognized to be mediated by the dopaminergic system. Dopaminergic projections to the striatum can be divided into three systems: nigrostriatal, mesolimbic, and mesocortical (Lindvall & Bjorklund, 1983). The nigrostriatal system is mainly involved in initiation of movement and sensorimotor coordination. The role of DA in motor function is well known. However, recent evidence suggested that this neurotransmitter also plays an important role in modulating learning and motivation (Wise, 2004). Structures included in the mesocortical system are important anatomical substrates not only for drug-related reward but for natural rewards, such as food, sex, and social interactions (Nestler & Carlezon, 2006). The mesocortical system includes structures involved in complex functions, such as working memory, attention, affective behavior, language, and motor control (Viggiano et al., 2003).

Dopamine and cognitive performance

The DA system has been consistently identified as a modulator of those cognitive processes believed to be subserved by the frontal cortex, striatum, and associative structures (Cropley et al., 2006). Evidence of a role for the DA pathway at D_1 receptors in human cognitive processes has been provided by animal, genetic, imaging, and pharmacological challenge studies. Furthermore, the essential role of DA in working memory processes was first identified by Brozowski et al. (1979). In their study the authors reported that 6-hydroxdopamine lesions of the dorso-lateral prefrontal cortex (DLPFC) in non-human primates lead to delay-dependent impairments in working memory similar to those observed with PFC ablation.

The positive correlation between PFC D_1 receptor alteration and cognitive impairments was initially reported in *animal studies*. Funahashi et al. (1993) demonstrated that discrete microinjection of a D_1, but not a D_2, antagonist leads to mnemonic scotomas that resemble those resulting from PFC microlesions. Consistent with these findings, enhancement of working memory in aged monkeys is observed after D_1 agonist treatment (Castner & Goldman-Rakic, 2004). Furthermore, pharmacological modulation of working memory impairment by use of a D_1 agonist in monkeys treated with antipsychotics demonstrated lasting benefit 1 year later (Castner et al., 2000). These findings support the use of an agent with specific activity at D_1 receptors to enhance working memory performance in situations where PFC DA activity is reduced.

In *humans*, positive correlations were reported between a decline in DA activity with age and alterations of cognitive function (El-Ghundi et al., 2007). DA has also been implicated in the cognitive dysfunction observed in a variety of neuropsychiatric disorders, such as Parkinson disease (Owen & Robbins, 1998; Rinne et al., 2000), Huntington disease, traumatic brain injury, and stroke (Lange et al., 1992; McDowell, 1996), attention deficit hyperactivity disorder (ADHD; Dinn et al., 2001; Shallice et al., 2002), and schizophrenia spectrum disorder (Trestman et al., 1995; Roitman et al., 2000).

In schizophrenia, working memory is the best predictor of social reintegration and propensity for relapse (Bowie & Harvey, 2005). Its malfunction in these patients has been associated with impaired goal-oriented behavior, disorganized cognitive function, and diminished self-monitoring (Reichenberg & Harvey, 2007). A study by Meyer-Lindenberg et al. (2001) found that patients with schizo-phrenia who showed poor performance on cognitive tests exhibited less DLPFC activation and greater activation of the hippocampus in contrast to patients whose performance was near to that of normal controls, who showed greater activation of the left DLPFC. However, recent findings suggest that, besides DLPFC DA, subcortical DA integrity contributes to performance in spatial working memory tasks (Collins et al., 2000; Pillon et al., 2003).

Dopamine function in the schizophrenia spectrum

Evidence from imaging, postmortem, and metabolite studies suggests the existence of DA abnormalities in the schizophrenia spectrum (Davis et al., 1991; see Chapter 20). The "classical" DA hypothesis of schizophrenia postulates that DA hyperactivity in the striatum leads to the psychotic symptoms present in this disorder (Carlsson & Lindqvist, 1963). Studies that used the activity of dopa-decarboxylase, an enzyme involved in DA synthesis, as a measure of dopamine release, found the presence of subcortical hyper-dopaminergia in patients with schizophrenia who were experiencing psychotic symptoms (Hietala et al., 1999; Lindstrom et al., 1999). Similarly, concentration levels of the DA metabolite homovanillic acid (HVA) were found to be higher in medication-free patients with schizophrenia who were experiencing more severe psychosis. Contrary to this, patients who experienced clinical improvement after treatment with psychotropic medication were found to have lower plasma levels of this metabolite (Pickar et al., 1984; Davis et al., 1991). Further support of this hypothesis is provided by reports of a correlation between clinical doses of the DA D_2 receptor antagonists and their antipsychotic effect (Creese et al., 1976). The "revised" DA hypothesis of schizophrenia (Weinberger, 1987; Davis et al., 1991) is a more recent view of the relationship between DA dysfunction and schizophrenia. This hypothesis proposes the existence of a more generalized dysregulation of DA transmission in this disorder. This hypothesis not only states that in patients with schizophrenia positive symptoms result from subcortical hyperdopaminergia secondary to hyperactivity of mesolimbic DA projections, but also correlates the deficit symptoms and cognitive impairment experienced by these patients with decreased dopaminergic activity in frontal cortical regions (frontal hypodopaminergia) caused by hypoactivity of mesocortical DA projections to the PFC. This concept is supported by reports of similar cognitive impairments (e.g., working memory deficit) to the ones observed in schizophrenia in non-human primates with reduced stimulation of D_1 receptors in the PFC (Goldman-Rakic et al., 2000).

Schizophrenia spectrum disorders are hypothesized to share a common neurodevelopmentally-based cortical temporal (Nestor et al., 1993) and prefrontal pathology

(Siever *et al.*, 1993a; Haber *et al.*, 2000), accounting for their common cognitive, social, and attentional deficits. However, subjects with SPD do not exhibit the frontal volume reductions observed in patients with schizophrenia. Furthermore, the capacity in subjects with SPD to recruit other related regions to compensate for dysfunctional areas accounts for their milder cognitive and social deterioration compared to patients with schizophrenia. Subjects with SPD also have reduced vulnerability to psychosis (Siever *et al.*, 1993a). This protection might be provided by factors that "buffer" these subjects against DA hyperactivity. These factors include reduced vulnerability to subcortical DA, up-regulation secondary to frontal cortical DA deficit, and reduced propagation of dysfunctions to frontal and cortical regions (Kirrane & Siever, 2000). However, the relationship between DA and SPD has not yet been fully elucidated. Early studies of the DA system in SPD found that plasma and cerebral spinal fluid (CSF) concentrations of HVA, a DA metabolite, were positively correlated (Siever & Davis, 2004). CSF and plasma concentrations of this metabolite were also found to be significantly increased in subjects with SPD compared with other personality disorder patients or controls. Furthermore, increased levels of this metabolite were found to be associated in subjects with SPD with severity of psychotic-like symptoms. However, when data analysis included these symptoms as a covariate, the difference between the groups was no longer apparent (Siever *et al.*, 1991, 1993b). In contrast to previous findings, reduced plasma HVA levels were found in patients with SPD who exhibit poor performance on cognitive testing (Siever *et al.*, 1993b), as well as in those patients with SPD with deficit-like symptoms (Amin *et al.*, 1997).

More recent studies of the DA system in SPD, instead of relying on metabolites such as HVA, evaluate DA synaptic output by taking advantage of the fact that synaptic DA competes with some positron emission tomography (PET) and single photon emission computed tomography (SPECT) D_2 receptor radiotracers such as [^{11}C] raclopride and [^{123}I] IBZM (i.e., measuring the reduction of binding of a radioligand bound to the D_2 receptor). The use of these radiotracers has made it possible to measure the DA synaptic output following administration of amphetamine. An example of this is the assessment of the potential action of amphetamine in ameliorating the cognitive impairments of patients with schizophrenia by increasing DA activity in the frontal cortex. Unfortunately, in these patients, the magnitude of DA release induced by the amphetamine challenge was also found to be correlated with the degree of worsening of psychotic symptoms. Thus, in schizophrenia, psychosis can be induced by agents that increase DA activity such as amphetamine or cocaine. This phenomenon is dependent on the dose, the duration of administration, and the susceptibility of the subjects. Additionally,

larger amphetamine-induced DA release was observed in patients with schizophrenia during periods of illness exacerbation compared to during remission periods (Laruelle *et al.*, 1996; Breier *et al.*, 1997; Abi-Dargham *et al.*, 1998). Thus, the DA transmission disorder observed in these patients is associated with positive symptoms and fluctuates with the phases of illness.

In subjects with SPD, findings of plasma response to physiological stressors (α2-deoxyglucose infusion) (Mitropoulou *et al.*, 2004) and of subcortical DA release following amphetamine infusions suggest that patients with SPD have subcortical DA that is decreased compared to patients with schizophrenia and more like that of normal controls (Siever *et al.*, 2002). The administration of amphetamine in a placebo-controlled study resulted in significant performance improvement on the Wisconsin Card Sort Test (WCST) in subjects with SPD (Siegel *et al.*, 1996). Also, in this study the subjects with SPD with the lowest scores on placebo showed the most post-amphetamine improvement. Further studies also showed improved performance on tests of visuospatial working memory and attentional capacity [the DOT test and Continuous Performance Test (CPT), respectively] in patients with SPD compared to those with other personality disorders (Kirrane *et al.*, 2000). However, in contrast to patients with schizophrenia, amphetamine improved cognitive function in subjects with SPD without causing or worsening psychotic-like symptoms, supporting the notion that these subjects are protected against increases in subcortical DA activity associated with psychosis (Abi-Dargham *et al.*, 1998; Kirrane *et al.*, 2000; Siever *et al.*, 2002). A recent [^{123}I] IBZM SPECT study by Abi-Dargham *et al.* (2004) found that the degree of striatal amphetamine-induced DA release was significantly lower in SPD and remitted patients with schizophrenia than that observed in patients with schizophrenia during illness exacerbation. Since the degree of subcortical DA release following amphetamine administration is associated with worsening of psychotic symptoms in schizophrenia, the above results are consistent with the hypothesis that patients with SPD are protected from overt psychotic symptoms of schizophrenia by reduced subcortical DA activity. However, when compared to normal controls, patients with SPD showed significantly higher levels of amphetamine-induced DA release in the striatum, which suggests that patients with SPD exhibit dysregulation of DA transmission in this area. These findings support the notion that DA dysregulation in schizophrenia spectrum disorders has a trait component, present in remitted patients with schizophrenia and in patients with SPD, as well as a state component, associated with psychotic exacerbations but not SPD. It is worth mentioning that amphetamine studies, while offering a more direct assessment of DA activity compared to HVA studies, do not provide measures of baseline synaptic DA. Instead, these studies only evaluate synaptic DA transmission changes resulting from non-physiological challenges (Abi-Dargham & Laruelle, 2005).

Norepinephrine

The norepinephrine (NE) system has been implicated in cognitive functions such as attention (Lange *et al.*, 1992; Aston-Jones *et al.*, 1999) and memory consolidation (McDowell, 1996). The dorsal NE bundle, comprised of axons of the locus ceruleus' noradrenergic cell bodies, innervates the PFC (Aoki *et al.*, 1994). This structure has a high density of α_{2a}-adrenergic subtype receptors. Animal studies have shown that NE depletion of the PFC, by means of surgical ablation, toxin exposure, or aging, leads to spatial working memory deficits (Brozowski *et al.*, 1979; Cai & Arnsten, 1997), which are reversed after the administration of clonidine, an α_2-adrenergic agonist (Arnsten & Goldman-Rakic, 1985). Furthermore, working memory performance has been shown to improve in animal models (Arnsten & Goldman-Rakic, 1985; Marjamaki *et al.*, 1993; Uhlén *et al.*, 1995) and healthy subjects (Jäkälä *et al.*, 1999) by enhancing post-synaptic α_2-adrenergic receptor signals with guanfacine. Further support for targeting α_2-adrenergic receptors to enhance cognition in psychiatric disorders comes from preliminary findings from our ongoing studies. These show that subjects with SPD experience significant improvements in cognitive processing tests (i.e., PASAT, Letter-Number Sequence, and Trail Making Test B) after 4 weeks of guanfacine administration. Similarly, atomoxetine, an NE reuptake inhibitor that indirectly increases DA concentration in PFC is presently being tested as a potential therapy for the cognitive deficits of schizophrenia (Friedman *et al.*, 2004). However, it has been proposed that while moderate levels of NE enhance PFC functions through actions at postsynaptic α_2-adrenoreceptors, the release of high levels of NE activates α_1-adrenoceptors lead to cognitive dysfunction (Arnsten *et al.*, 1999; Birnbaum *et al.*, 1999; Mao *et al.*, 1999).

Cognitive impairment in the schizophrenia spectrum

Findings from meta-analytical studies (Green, 1996; Green *et al.*, 2000) support the early recognized notion of cognitive dysfunction as being a core feature of schizophrenia (Kraepelin, 1919; Bleuler, 1911). In patients with this disorder, cognitive impairments have been shown to precede the onset of psychosis (Cornblatt Erlenmeyer-Kimling, 1985; Davidson *et al.*, 1999), remain stable through much of the course of the disorder (Heaton *et al.*, 2001; Friedman *et al.*, 2001), and persist even after other symptoms have been effectively treated (Heinrichs, 2005). In schizophrenia, these impairments are not "global" as they were initially thought to be, but mild to moderate in most cognitive domains (such as attention and language skills) and severe on episodic memory and executive functions (Bilder *et al.*, 2000; Saykin *et al.*, 1991; see Chapter 8). Moreover, significant resources have been placed in understanding and treating these deficits since they have been recognized to be associated in patients with schizophrenia with worse functional outcome (Heaton & Pendleton, 1981; Bowie *et al.*, 2008).

The elucidation of differences in cognitive impairment profiles between schizophrenia spectrum personality disorders and schizophrenia might provide the key to recognizing areas of cognitive dysfunction associated with psychosis. Among the schizophrenia spectrum personality disorders, SPD has the most similar neuropsychological profile to that of schizophrenia, with comparable deficits in working memory, context processing, verbal episodic learning, and memory (Siever & Davis, 2004). However, the stability of these findings in SPD is not as well understood as in schizophrenia. Furthermore, few studies have examined the true functional ability level of subjects with SPD. One study reported that subjects with SPD considered themselves to be occupationally disabled and, compared to patients with major depression disorder, had fewer years of education (Skodol *et al.*, 2002).

Attention

Attention is an executive function that encompasses the identification and sustained focus on relevant information while ignoring competing irrelevant stimuli. Attention deficits are hypothesized to underlie dysfunctions in other cognitive domains of the schizophrenia spectrum. For example, poor performance on frontal lobe tests, such as the WCST, Trail Making, and verbal fluency tests, have been reported to occur when, in patients with schizophrenia, attention deficits were present along with perceptual distortion and social anhedonia (Obiols *et al.*, 1999). Attentional deficits, as assessed by the negative priming paradigm, have been found to be significantly more prevalent in acutely psychotic patients with schizophrenia with elevated positive symptoms than in medicated patients with schizophrenia with low positive symptoms (Park *et al.*, 2002). The CPT is a measure of attention that involves the random brief rapid visual presentation of letters or digits. The task, consisting of pressing a key to target stimuli, can be made more difficult by increasing the load on working memory or decreasing the load on perceptual processing. Using this task, several authors demonstrated that patients with schizophrenia, including those in remission, suffer from moderate attentional deficits. Furthermore, these deficits were also shown to be present in children with a schizophrenic parent and other first-degree relatives and in patients with SPD (Cornblatt & Keilp, 1994; Franke *et al.*, 1994; Roitman *et al.*, 1997; Laurent *et al.*, 2000, Minas

& Park, 2007, Cosway *et al.*, 2002). The attentional deficits, in subjects with SPD, while less severe, became similar to those exhibited by patients with schizophrenia as task demands increased (Harvey *et al.*, 2000; Moriarty *et al.*, 2003).

Context processing

Context processing is the ability to maintain information to be used to mediate later task- appropriate responses against interference such as competing processes. Subjects with schizophrenia and those with SPD exhibit context processing impairments. Furthermore, Barch *et al.* (2004) reported that the further along the schizophrenia spectrum, the more profound the level of impairment in maintaining context representations.

Our group assessed the performance of subjects with SPD in four different context processing tasks (Barch *et al.*, 2004). One of these tasks was a classical N-back working memory test, while the other three were variants of the AX-CPT. Compared to healthy volunteers, subjects with SPD exhibited context processing abnormalities (i.e., poorer maintenance of strong contextual representations) in all four tests. The level of reduced performance of subjects with SPD in these tests was substantial, reaching levels of severity similar to those for patients with schizophrenia. On the other hand, a recent study by our group (McClure *et al.*, 2007a) found that people with other personality disorders without schizotypal features are indistinguishable from health controls on context processing tests.

Working memory

Impairment in working memory is one of the most replicated cognitive dysfunctions in schizophrenia and the schizophrenia spectrum. The Paced Auditory Serial Addition Task (PASAT; Stuss *et al.*, 1988) is a measure of verbal working memory. In it, the subject is asked to add adjacent numbers that are orally presented. Working memory is needed in this task to continually "update" the material in order to perform simple calculations. A study by Heinrichs and Zakzanis (1998) found that, compared with healthy volunteers, the mean effect size for impaired performance on PASAT in patients with schizophrenia was about 1.5. The performance on the PASAT of subjects with SPD has been described to be in the moderate to severe range, a level similar to that observed in patients with schizophrenia (Mojtabai *et al.*, 2000). Furthermore, a study by our group (Mitropoulou *et al.*, 2002) showed that subjects with SPD presented similar effect sizes (d = 1.49) as patients with schizophrenia when compared to healthy volunteers. Levels of performance for subjects with other personality disorders reached levels that were significantly better than for patients with SPD and similar to healthy volunteers. Taken together, these findings suggest that

verbal working memory impairment represents a core feature and a potential endophenotype of the schizophrenia spectrum (Eastvold *et al.*, 2007; Simone *et al.*, 2007). However, results from a recent study by Wang *et al.* (2008) suggest that compared to subjects with SPD, patients with schizophrenia exhibit working memory deficits that are more severe and generalized. More recent work from our group has found that among all neuropsychological variables, the PASAT is the only test that accounts for all of the variance between SPD and other personality disorders (OPDs) (Mitropoulou *et al.*, 2005). More specifically, when the PASAT score was used as a covariate in a MANOVA comparing subjects with SPD, subjects with OPD, and healthy controls on all cognitive measures, it abolished the statistically significant group differences across the other 10 neuropsychological tests for the three groups. In fact, the profile of performance of patients with SPD looked remarkably normal after impairment on the PASAT was controlled for statistically.

The DOT test provides an index of visuo-spatial working memory. This test requires the subject to remember the spatial location of a stimulus on a piece of paper while a different material acting as an "interference stimuli" is verbally presented to the subject. Studies from our group (Keefe *et al.*, 1995) demonstrated that, when compared to healthy volunteers, the performance of subjects with SPD on this test is impaired (Lees-Reitman *et al.*,1997) with levels of impairment similar to those observed in patients with schizophrenia (Heinrichs & Zakzanis, 1998).

Episodic memory

Impairments in verbal episodic learning and memory are also among the most widely replicated and pronounced in schizophrenia (Saykin *et al*, 1991; Mitropoulou *et al.*, 2002). These processes are typically assessed with a list learning task, in which the subject listens to and then recalls a list of words or the content of stories. Subjects with SPD have been shown to recall fewer words than comparison groups at both the initial learning trial (Dickey *et al.*, 2005) and following a long delay (McClure *et al.*, 2007a). However, even with the use of the same instruments, verbal learning and memory impairments has not been consistently replicated in all studies (Mitropoulou *et al.*, 2002).

Executive functioning

Impairment in set changing and perseveration in the WCST are associated with deficits in frontal lobe executive functions, and have been reported to be present in subjects with schizophrenia and their first-degree relatives, as well as SPD and schizotypes in the normal population (Raine *et al.*, 1992; Battaglia *et al.*, 1994; Trestman *et al.*, 1995; Voglmaier *et al.*, 1997; Matsui *et al.*, 2007; Klemm *et al.*, 2006). However, while patients with schizophrenia show moderate to severe impairments across all executive function tasks, the impairment in subjects with SPD is mild and confined to distinct tasks. For example, a study by Trestman *et al.* (1995) found that impairments in subjects with SPD were confined to concept formation and cognitive flexibility as measured by the WCST and the Trail Making Test. These subjects did not show deficits on disinhibition, as measured by the Stroop Color–Word interference score. Evidence pointing to which cognitive aspects of the spectrum constitute risk factor for developing schizophrenia might be provided by the analysis of impairments in distinct executive functions.

Language skills

Language ability is typically assessed with verbal fluency tests. In patients with schizophrenia, impairments in language skills tend to be moderate to severe (Bowie *et al.*, 2004). Contrary to this, the impairment in subjects with SPD only reaches very mild levels (Voglmaier *et al.*, 1997; Trestman *et al.*, 1995).

Furthermore, a recent study by Maher *et al.* (2005) showed that patients with schizophrenia produce an elevated rate of normative thought associations in verbal utterances. This abnormality was also present in schizotypic subjects with no prior history of psychosis (Lenzenweger *et al.*, 2007), supporting the presence of hyperassociative processes in those deemed to be at elevated risk for schizophrenia. Furthermore, schizotypal characteristics in a non-clinical population were associated with impairments in the ability to correctly identify emotions as expressed in facial, paralinguistic, and postural cues (Shean *et al.*, 2007).

Neuroimaging

Structural imaging

Most neuroimaging studies of the schizophrenia spectrum have focused on cortical (i.e., frontal and temporal) and subcortical (i.e., thalamus and striatum) regions. Early findings of increased CSF volume associated with cortical atrophy in patients with schizophrenia have been consistently replicated and, more recently, observed to be present in subjects with SPD (Buchsbaum *et al.*, 1997; Koo *et al.*, 2006a; Silverman *et al.*, 1998). Dickey *et al.* (2000) reported that, compared to healthy volunteers, men with SPD showed a significantly larger CSF volume not attributable to ventricular volume (e.g., sulcal CSF) and a trend-level smaller cortical gray matter volume. In a recent study, Koo *et al.* (2006a) found that, compared to female controls, women with SPD exhibited smaller left and right neocortical gray matter relative volumes. In these patients, the cor-

tical abnormalities were associated with the presence of larger left and right sulcal CSF relative volumes. Additionally, voxel-based morphometry applied to determine global and regional volume deficits showed that the neocortical deficits in SPD were especially prominent in the left superior and middle temporal gyri, left inferior parietal region with postcentral gyrus, and right superior frontal and inferior parietal gyri. Furthermore, in the SPD group, larger lateral ventricle volumes correlated with more severe symptoms on the Structured Interview for Schizotypy and the Schizotypal Personality Questionnaire–Brief Version.

While in subjects with SPD, frontal lobe volume was reported to inversely correlate with deficit-like symptoms and poor performance in tests of executive function, temporal lobe volume is hypothesized to be inversely associated with disorganized symptoms as well as poor performance on verbal learning tasks (McCarley *et al.*, 1996).

A recent study by our group (Hazlett *et al.*, 2008) examined cortical gray/white matter volumes in a large sample of unmedicated patients with schizophrenia spectrum disorders (n = 79 SPD; n = 57 schizophrenia) and 148 healthy controls. Patients with schizophrenia had reduced gray matter volume widely across the cortex but more marked in frontal and temporal lobes. The gray matter volume reductions in patients with SPD, while present in the same regions, were only about half of those observed in schizophrenia. Furthermore, in patients with SPD, key prefrontal regions such as Brodmann area (BA) 10 were spared. In schizophrenia, greater fronto-temporal volume loss was associated with greater negative symptom severity and in SPD, greater interpersonal and cognitive impairment. Overall, our findings suggest that increased prefrontal volume in BA10 and sparing of volume loss in the temporal cortex (BAs 22 and 20) may be a protective factor in SPD, which reduces vulnerability to psychosis.

Volume reductions in frontal cortical areas have been associated with cognitive impairments and deficit symptoms of patients with schizophrenia (McCarley *et al.*, 1996). While SPD and patients with schizophrenia appear to show some common cortical abnormalities, patients with SPD do not appear to show volumetric decreases in frontal cortex to the same extent as schizophrenia (Kawasaki *et al.*, 2004; Siever *et al.*, 1990b, 2002; Siever & Davis, 2004; Suzuki *et al.*, 2005). In idividuals with SPD, frontal cortical volume does not differ from that in healthy controls (Siever, 2000; Buchsbaum, 2002). Subjects with SPD who exhibit lower frontal volumes displayed traits associated with schizophrenia-related psychopathology (Downhill *et al.*, 2001; Siever *et al.*, 1993b; Raine, 2006; Diwadkar *et al.*, 2006).

Temporal volume reduction is believed to be present across the schizophrenia spectrum. This abnormality has been consistently reported in schizophrenia (Wright *et al.*, 2000; Davidson & Heinrichs, 2003; Shenton, 2001; Downhill *et al.*, 2001; Gur *et al.*, 2000; Hirayasu *et al.*, 2000) and more recently, in subjects with SPD (Takahashi *et al.*, 2007). Recent MRI studies have found that patients with SPD, like patients with schizophrenia, have decreased gray matter volume in the superior temporal gyrus (Dickey *et al.*, 1999; Kawasaki, 2008) and Heschl's gyrus (Dickey *et al.*, 2002), as well as in the inferior and middle temporal gyri (Downhill *et al.*, 2001). However, in contrast to schizophrenia, the volumes of middle temporal regions, such as the amygdala and hippocampal complex, have not been consistently observed to be reduced in SPD (Gur *et al.*, 2000; Seidman *et al.*, 2003; Takahashi *et al.*, 2006).

The thalamus is a subcortical area of interest and has been shown to be reduced in size in patients with schizophrenia (Andreasen *et al.*, 1998; Crespo Facorro *et al.*, 2007). This structure is a nodal relay station for incoming sensory information to the cortex, as well as an essential contributor to cortical activation. MRI studies have demonstrated differences in the thalamus volume reduction of SPD compared to schizophrenia. Within the thalamus, the pulvinar has close connections with temporal lobe structures. This nucleus is reduced in both cohorts in relation to normal comparison subjects (Byne *et al.*, 2001). However, in contrast to patients with schizophrenia, the volume of the medial dorsal nucleus, associated with the PFC, is no different in schizotypal patients in relation to normal comparison subjects (Byne *et al.*, 2001). These findings suggest that in SPD, the reductions in thalamic nuclei parallel the reductions in associated cortical regions (i.e., temporal but not frontal volume reductions).

The striatum and its connections to the cortex are targets for the D_2 antagonist action of antipsychotic medications due to their high dopamine concentration. Preliminary findings suggest that in the schizophrenia spectrum, changes in striatal volumes may partially reflect DA activity. For example, striatal volumes in subjects with SPD and never-medicated patients with schizophrenia may be normal or even slightly reduced. On the other hand, in long-term neuroleptic medicated patients with schizophrenia, these volumes have been consistently reported to be increased (Staal *et al.*, 2000; Shihabuddin, 2001; Chakos *et al.*, 1994). Striatal volume increase in these patients is believed to result from compensatory increases in DA dendrites or mitochondria after long-term neuroleptic administration (Chakos *et al.*, 1994). Thus, the reduced striatal volume in patients with SPD might be compatible with reduced DA activity in these patients compared to patients with schizophrenia. In SPD, striatal volumes reported to be decreased include the caudate (Levitt *et al.*, 2002, 2004; Koo *et al.*, 2006b) and the putamen (Shihabuddin *et al.*, 2001).

There has been little attention given to whether parietal lobe structural deficits are present in patients with schizophrenia and related personality disorders. A recent study by Zhou *et al.* (2007) examined parietal volume alterations in SPD, schizophrenia and healthy control subjects. The authors reported that, compared to healthy controls, gray matter volumes in patients with schizophrenia were reduced in all parietal subregions. White matter volumes in the superior parietal gyrus (SuPG) and postcentral gyrus (PoCG) were also reduced. In contrast, subjects with SPD had gray matter reductions only in the PoCG, while other regions were not affected. In addition, patients with schizophrenia exhibited a lack of normal significant leftward asymmetry in the supramarginal gyrus (SMG). These findings suggest that volume reductions in the somatosensory cortices are a common morphological characteristic in the schizophrenia spectrum disorders. Furthermore, the additional volume alterations in schizophrenia may support the notion that a deficit in the posterior parietal region is critical for the manifestation of overt psychotic symptoms.

Functional imaging

Cognitive function in the schizophrenia spectrum has been consistently reported to be impaired. However, this impairment appears to be less severe in SPD than in schizophrenia. Functional imaging studies have been carried out in SPD to assess if these subjects counteract dysfunctions in primary regions associated with a specific cognitive function by recruiting brain regions not normally associated with this function. As noted earlier, working memory appears to be a core cognitive deficit within the schizophrenia spectrum. In healthy volunteers, working memory task performance leads to increased activation in specific brain regions. These regions, identified by functional imaging studies, include the ventral PFC, the supplementary motor area, the premotor area, the DLPFC, as well as several parietal areas (Barch & Csernansky, 2007; Koenigsberg *et al.*, 2005). During working memory tasks, subjects with SPD appear to exhibit different patterns of activation from healthy volunteers. Subjects with SPD show decreased left/increased right prefrontal activation during the WCST (Buchsbaum *et al.*, 1997). A more recent PET study by Buchsbaum *et al.* (2002) showed that Patients with SPD exhibited less activity in the precentral gyrus compared to healthy volunteers. The opposite is true for the middle frontal gyrus, with subjects with SPD showing increased activity compared to healthy volunteers. This might suggest that individuals with SPD recruit different PFC areas as compensatory mechanism while performing cognitive tasks (Siever & Davis, 2004). It is worth noting that within the PFC, the D_1 receptor system is presumed to constitute the cellular basis for working memory by selectively modulating neurons that exhibit "memory fields" (Funahashi *et al.*, 1993). PFC dysfunction was correlated with poor WCST performance in medication-naïve patients with schizophrenia (Abi-Dargham *et al.*, 2002).

Functional imaging studies performed by our group have also focused on striatal structures (Shihabuddin et al., 2001). Compared to patients with schizophrenia and healthy volunteers, subjects with SPD show increased metabolic activity in the ventral putamen. Subjects with SPD with greater activation in this area exhibited less psychotic-like symptoms than those with reduced activation. Thus, the lack of psychosis in SPD compared to schizophrenia is hypothesized to result from DA-mediated inhibition of the putamen by the ventral putamen, an area rich in D_2 receptors. In schizophrenia, subcortical D_2 receptor hyperactivity has been associated with the emergence of psychotic symptoms. Thus, the differences in increased ventral putamen activation between subjects with SPD and subjects with schizophrenia are not believed to result from an artifact of different medication histories since they were also seen in never-medicated patients with SPD compared to never-medicated patients with schizophrenia. Findings for the cingulate cortex are currently mixed, with one study observing normal anterior functioning (Mohanty et al., 2005) and another observing increased posterior activation during a working memory task (Haznedar et al., 2004).

Neurochemical imaging

A recent SPECT study using [^{123}I] iodobenzamide (IBZM) (Abi-Dargham et al., 1998) reported that, compared to healthy subjects, amphetamine induces greater release of DA in patients with schizophrenia. Following the administration of a single dose of amphetamine, radiolabeled IBZM is displaced from D_2 receptors. This phenomenon can be used as a measure of amphetamine-stimulated striatal DA release. In a related study (Abi-Dargham et al., 2004) these authors reported that the degree of striatal amphetamine-induced DA release was significantly lower in SPD than that observed in patients with schizophrenia during illness exacerbation. The degree of subcortical DA release following amphetamine administration is associated with worsening of psychotic symptoms in schizophrenia. Thus, the above results are consistent with the hypothesis that patients with SPD are protected from overt psychotic symptoms of schizophrenia by reduced subcortical DA activity. However, when compared to normal controls, patients with SPD showed significantly higher levels of amphetamine-induced DA release in the striatum. This suggests that patients with SPD exhibit dysregulation of DA transmission in this area.

PET measurement studies of D_1 receptors with [^{11}C] NNC 112 reported that patients with schizophrenia tended to show significantly higher DLPFC [^{11}C] NNC 112 BP compared to controls (Abi-Dargham et al., 2002). Findings from this study also suggest that [^{11}C] NNC 112 in vivo binding might be up-regulated selectively in the DLPFC in drug-free patients with schizophrenia, and that this up-regulation is predictive of poorer working memory performance as measured by the N-back test. In medication-free and medication-naïve patients with schizophrenia down-regulation of D_1 binding in DLPFC also correlated with impaired performance on the WCST (Okubo et al., 1997), a test of central executive function.

Preliminary findings from an ongoing PET study from our group measuring D_1 receptors with [^{11}C] NNC 112 in patients with SPD suggested that there is increased NNC 112 binding, more in subcortical areas, with decreased D_1 receptor availability associated with the presence of anhedonia in these patients. These findings are consistent with increased D_1 binding in SPD compared to controls, but relative decreases associated with anhedonia. These findings are also consistent with the well-known pleasure-reinforcement action of DA and the hypothesis that subjects who fail to up-regulate DA receptors exhibit anhedonia. However, these are preliminary findings that need to be clarified in larger samples (Siever, unpublished data).

Psychophysiology

Prepulse inhibition

The human startle reflex is a simple physiological phenomena with sensitivity to different stimulus intensities, habituation, and fear potentiation (Davis et al., 1999). This reflex is modifiable by external events. One such event is a prepulse, which is a non-startling stimulus preceding the startling stimulus (Graham, 1975). The phenomenon of reflex reduction or inhibition by pairing a startling and non-startling stimulus is known as prepulse inhibition (PPI) (Ison & Hammond, 1971). PPI is thought to represent the ability of the higher brain centers to "gate" or filter sensory information (Graham, 1975; Davis et al., 1982; Geyer & Braff, 1987; Braff & Geyer, 1990; Dawson et al., 1997). Numerous authors have reported that patients with schizophrenia have sensory information processing or "filtering" deficits of exteroceptive and interoceptive stimuli that lead to diminished PPI (Braff et al., 1991; Braff & Light, 2005; Grillon et al., 1992; Bolino et al., 1994; Ludewig et al., 2003). Sensory gating and information processing dysfunction have been associated with clinical features, such as impaired inhibition of internal stimuli with an increased awareness of "preconscious" material, leading to hallucinations and delusions (Frith, 1979). Additionally, PPI has been shown to be associated with attention deficits (Dawson et al., 1993, 2000; Hazlett et al., 1998), resulting in poor performance on cognitive tasks (Cornblatt et al., 1989; Butler et al., 1991; Karper et al., 1996). A study by Mackeprang et al. (2002) failed to find any influence of treatment with antipsychotic drugs on sensorimotor gating deficits in patients with schizophrenia, suggesting that PPI impairment is a stable vulnerability indicator of this disorder. To address this, several studies examined subjects psychometrically similar to patients with schizophrenia but free of symptoms and medications. Reduced PPI was found to be present in asymptomatic first-degree relatives of patients with schizophrenia and in subjects with SPD (Cadenhead *et al.*, 1993, 2000a,b, 2002; Kumari *et al.*, 2005; Evans *et al.*, 2005). However, these results have been inconsistent. Some studies failed to show diminished PPI in schizophrenia (Dawson *et al.*, 1993) and in both positive and negative dimensions of schizotypy measured with the Chapman scales of perceptual aberration/magical ideation and anhedonia (Cadenhead *et al.*, 1996). On the other hand, more subtle individual differences than simple positive–negative syndromes may assist with syndrome correlates. Swerdlow *et al.* (1995) reported an association of PPI with low Minnesota Multiphasic Personality Inventory (MMPI) hysteria scores, i.e., low scores on somatic anxiety, lassitude, social naivety, and inhibited aggression. Thus, PPI is believed not to vary with a specific component of schizotypy, but is associated with a general schizotypy score, reflecting a general "proneness to psychosis" or vulnerability (Abel *et al.*, 2004).

Eye movements

Classical studies have reported that patients with schizophrenia exhibit impaired smooth pursuit eye movements (Diefendorf & Dodge, 1908). More recent reports suggest that this impairment results from intrusive and anticipatory saccadic eye movements (Grove *et al.* 1991; Clementz *et al.*, 1994; Ross *et al.*, 1996, 1998). Additionally, patients with schizophrenia have been shown to perform less accurately in antisaccade (i.e., failure to inhibit reflexive saccades following instruction) and motion detection tasks (Holzman, 2000; Clementz *et al.*, 1994; Katsanis *et al.*, 1997; McDowell & Clementz 1997). These abnormalities have been shown to correlate with the social deficits and interpersonal isolation exhibited by patients with schizophrenia (Siever *et al.*, 1982). Smooth-pursuit eye movements are mediated by the frontal and temporal cortex and the brainstem, while motion detection is mediated by the inferior temporal cortex (Chen *et al.*, 1999). Several studies have reported that relatives of patients with schizophrenia exhibit significantly poorer performances on ocular pursuit paradigms than controls (Clementz *et al.*, 1994; Crawford *et al.*, 1998; Curtis *et al.*, 2001; Holzman *et al.*, 1974; Karoumi *et al.*, 2001; Lee & Williams, 2000). Thus, eye-tracking impairments could be used as genetic vulnerability markers for schizophrenia (Boudet *et al.*, 2005). Eye-tracking impairments were found to be present in SPD but not other personality disorders (Siever *et al.* 1989, 1990a). Additionally, in non-clinical populations, such as adult healthy volunteers (Lenzenweger & O'Driscoll, 2006), college students (Siever *et al.*, 1984), and military conscripts aged 18–25

(Smyrnis *et al.*, 2007b), these impairments have been associated with schizotypy. The presence of significant differences in pursuit performance only for predefined high schizotypy groups favors the hypothesis that individuals with high schizotypy might present one or more high-risk groups, distinct from the general population, that are prone to eye tracking dysfunction, as observed in schizophrenia.

Evidence of a functional basis to the deficit follows demonstration in recent-onset schizophrenia of improvement by attentional manipulations, suggesting an association with diminished voluntary attention in keeping with frontal involvement in smooth pursuit (White & Yee, 1997). Smooth pursuit impairment has been also correlated with clinical symptoms such as physical (Simons & Katkin, 1985) and social anhedonia (Clementz *et al.*, 1992) and deficit-like symptoms (Siever, 1991; Siever *et al.*, 1993a). On the other hand, perceptual aberrations were found to be associated with both antisaccade and smooth pursuit deficits (O'Driscoll *et al.*, 1998). A recent study that evaluated the presence of eye-tracking disorders in schizotypy subjects and healthy volunteers (Holahan & O'Driscoll, 2005) found that a significantly larger percentage of schizotypy individuals with positive-like symptoms than controls showed elevated antisaccade error rates on standard antisaccade tasks. On the other hand, the percentage of schizotypy participants with negative-like symptoms that exhibited elevated antisaccade error rates did not differ from that of control subjects.

Event-related potentials

Event-related potentials (ERPs) are electroencephalographic changes to external stimuli that provide objective measurement of information processing in the human brain (Korostenskaja *et al.*, 2005). Auditory ERPs such as P300 can be used for studying different aspects of the neural bases of cognitive dysfunction. P300 is a potential occurring at an approximate latency of 300 ms that is evoked by the presentation of a novel behaviorally relevant target stimulus. This potential is embedded among irrelevant stimuli while the subject is actively reacting (pressing a button or mentally counting) on the presence of the target stimuli (McCarley *et al.*, 1991, 1993). P300 is interpreted as the electrophysiological correlate of updating of working memory (Donchin & Coles, 1988) because its latency corresponds to cognitive processing speed, activation of immediate memory, and attention allocation (Kok, 1997; Polich & Kok, 1995). Amplitude reduction of the P300 is often found in schizophrenia (McCarley *et al.*, 1993, Muir *et al.*, 1991, Hirayasu *et al.*, 1998; Jeon & Polich, 2001) and is also hypothesized to be a vulnerability marker for the disorder due to its lack of association with antipsychotic effects (Ford *et al.*, 1994; Laurent *et al.*, 1999) and clinical improvement (Gallinat *et al.*, 2001; Frodl *et al.*, 2002). Furthermore, the existence of auditory ERP abnormalities in individuals at high genetic risk for schizophrenia, such as relatives of patients with this disorder (Schreiber *et al.*, 1992, Frangou *et al.*, 1997; Karoumi *et al.*, 2000, Winterer *et al.*, 2003) suggests that similar impairments might be found in individuals with SPD. A recent study by Gassab *et al.* (2006) in a non-clinical population from the community found that those participants with higher scores on the Schizotypal Personality Questionnaire (SPQ) also exhibited auditory ERP abnormalities, such as smaller P300 amplitudes and delayed P300 latencies. In SPD, P300 amplitude reduction has been reported by a number of groups (Trestman *et al.*, 1996, Klein *et al.*, 1999, Kimble *et al.*, 2000; Mannan *et al.*, 2001, Niznikiewicz *et al.*, 2000). However, the findings concerning delayed P300 latency have been less consistent (Kutcher *et al.*, 1989, Trestman *et al.*, 1996, Nuchpongsai *et al.*, 1999; Mannan *et al.*, 2001), perhaps due to psychometric instruments and selection criteria discrepancies. Furthermore, studies of patients with schizophrenia (Gruzelier, 1999) or SPD (Siever, 1991) were not able to characterize an association between P300 abnormalities and specific symptoms of these disorders. However, a recent study by Renoult *et al.* (2007) found that in schizophrenia, P300 asymmetry was correlated with severity of positive symptoms and worse global functioning (GAF), a good predictor of poor outcome.

P50 suppression

The P50 ERP test is a measure of sensory gating involving a two-stimulus (S1, S2) evoked potential paradigm in which the amplitude of the P50 wave is measured in response to each of two auditory clicks (conditioning and test) (Adler *et al.*, 1982; White & Yee, 2006). In normal subjects the second P50 wave is suppressed, or "gated", because of the inhibitory effects of the first click. On the other hand, gating deficit at short interstimulus intervals is measured by a reduced ratio or difference between the two positive-going response amplitudes (P50s) at around 50 ms. Since the P50 ERP objectively assesses attention and information processing (Cadenhead *et al.*, 2000a), impaired suppression of the P50 wave has been identified as a vulnerability marker for the sensory gating deficits observed in patients with schizophrenia and their first-degree relatives, as well as subjects with SPD (Siegel *et al.*, 1984; Waldo *et al.*, 1991, 2000; Clementz *et al.*, 1998; Cadenhead *et al.*, 2000a, 2002; Patterson *et al.*, 2008). Furthermore, Croft *et al.* (2001) found that healthy volunteers with higher schizotypal characteristics exhibited poorer P50 suppression. Reports from animal studies suggest that P50 gating abnormalities result form α7 nicotinic receptor desensitization (Griffith *et al.*, 1998), which is modulated at the CA3 hippocampal level (Flach *et al.*, 1996).

Treatment

Psychotropic medication studies

In contrast to patients with schizophrenia, most subjects with SPD never receive psychotropic medication. The use of these medications in the treatment of psychotic-like symptoms and social anxiety in SPD is justified by the biological and clinical similarities between this disorder and schizophrenia. Initial studies employed low doses of typical antipsychotic medication. A study by Goldberg *et al.* (1986) reported that social isolation, illusions, and ideas of reference significantly decreased in 13 patients with SPD with low doses of thiothixene compared to placebo. Similarly, low doses of haloperidol were significantly effective in reducing psychotic-like symptoms in patients with SPD (Hymowitz *et al.*, 1986) and in a mixed SPD and borderline personality disorder (BPD) inpatient population (Soloff *et al.*, 1986, 1989). On the other hand, an open-label study of amoxapine (a medication with antipsychotic and antidepressant action) reported beneficial effects of this drug in subjects with SPD but not BPD (Jensen & Andersen, 1989). Despite the fact that atypical antipsychotics are becoming the first line of treatment for psychotic disorders, few studies have investigated these medications in the treatment of SPD. A recent, 26-week, open-label study with a flexible dose of olanzapine in 11 patients with SPD reported significant improvements in ratings of psychosis, depression, and overall functioning (Keshavan *et al.*, 2004). Another recent placebo-controlled study by our group (Koenigsberg *et al.*, 2003) reported Positive and Negative Syndrome Scale (PANSS) general, positive and negative symptom scores improvement in an patient population with SPD with the use of low doses of risperidone. In subjects with SPD, it is important to consider that lack of effectiveness of antipsychotics could result from poor adherence due to side effects overwhelming treatment benefits. A recent review of psychotropic medication treatment of patients with SPD failed to find reliable evidence for the efficacy of antidepressants in the treatment of schizotypal symptoms (Herpertz *et al.*, 2007).

Cognitive enhancement studies

Multiple studies have attempted to improve cognitive performance and overall functioning of patients with SPD with the use of pharmacological interventions. DA agonists have been the agents of choice in these interventions due to reports from non-human primate studies that the dopaminergic circuit is critical for cognitive performance (Goldman-Rakic *et al.*, 2000). In these studies, working memory in non-human primates was improved after the administration of DA agonists (Williams & Goldman-Rakic 1995) and worsened after the administration of DA antagonists (Sawaguchi & Goldman-Rakic, 1991). Additionally, while some patients with SPD may exhibit the cognitive impairments found in schizophrenia, they do not manifest psychosis. Thus, dopamine agonists may improve cognition in these patients without inducing psychosis.

Amphetamine, a non-selective DA agonist that releases DA and blocks its re-uptake, was found to have beneficial effects on working memory. Dopaminergic agents may enhance cognition in patients with schizophrenia spectrum disorders. In patients with schizophrenia, cognitive enhancement studies using amphetamine reported amelioration of working memory (Carter et al., 1998; Stevens et al., 1998) and selective attention impairment (Carter et al., 1997), as well as increase in PFC blood flow (Daniel et al., 1991).

In a double-blind placebo controlled study by our group, subjects with schizophrenia spectrum disorder (n = 30) who demonstrated impairment at baseline (measured as >1 standard deviation of the healthy control mean for any of the cognitive measures) experienced improvement in visuo-spatial working memory (DOT test: $F[1,29] = 6.8$; $p < 0.02$) and auditory working memory (Paced Auditory Serial Addition Test; $F[1,15] = 5.4$; $p < 0.04$) after the oral administration of 30 mg of a single dose of D-amphetamine (Mitropoulou et al., 2004). Those patients with schizophrenia spectrum disorders with poorer baseline working memory were more likely to experience an improvement in their performance during cognitive enhancement compared to patients with less impaired performance at baseline. Also, no secondary worsening of psychotic-like symptoms accompanied this improvement, suggesting that, despite their common cortical hypodopaminergia, patients with SPD are not susceptible to the subcortical hyperdopaminergia present in patients with schizophrenia (Siever et al., 1993a). Amphetamine acts largely through D_1 receptors in the frontal cortex, which are known to modulate visuo-spatial working memory performance in primates (Williams & Goldman-Rakic, 1995). However, the relationship between DA and cognitive deficit is complex. Mattay et al. (2000) have demonstrated that amphetamine improves performance on working memory tasks in those individuals who were relatively poor baseline performers, but impairs performance in individuals with good baseline performance. Furthermore, a study by Kirrane et al. (2000) reported that an equal dose of amphetamine resulted in reduction in errors on working memory and verbal learning test in patients with SPD but not in other personality-disordered patients.

Bromocriptine and pergolide

Studies that employed bromocriptine, a D_2 agonist agent, have reported improvements in cognitive tasks, more so at lower doses than at higher doses (Luciana et al., 1992, 1998;

Mehta et al., 2001), perhaps because at higher doses this agent is more likely to cause adverse effects. While a number of cognitive enhancement studies have used bromocriptine as the agent of choice, the non-human primate literature has focused much more on the role that D_1 receptors play in working memory.

The administration of the D_1/D_2 agonist pergolide, which has a preferential activity at D_1 receptors (Fici et al., 1997), improved tests of frontal function and memory in patients with Parkinson disease (Kulisevsky et al., 2000), as well as visual memory and attention in sleep disorders and ADHD (Walters et al., 2000). Additionally, pergolide, but not the D_2 agonist bromocriptine, improved visuo-spatial working memory in healthy individuals (Muller et al., 1998), pointing to a preferential role of D_1 receptors in the modulation of working memory. This fact also supported the utility of an evaluation of the effects of pergolide on working memory and attention in the schizophrenic spectrum disorders. Recent cognitive enhancement studies by our group demonstrated cognitive improvement in patients with SPD tested after a 2-week administration of escalating doses of pergolide. Specifically, compared to placebo, pergolide improved working memory performance as demonstrated by increased accuracy on the n-back task. Moreover, pergolide improved performance on the PASAT in all subjects compared to the baseline testing day, which supports the notion that pergolide improves working memory performance. Word list learning and reaction times on the flanker test also improved in several of the subjects with SPD, while clinical symptoms remained either unchanged or slightly improved. While there is enough data to support the assessment of pergolide on cognitive performance in the schizophrenia spectrum, reports from studies by Zanettini et al. (2007) and Schade et al. (2007) raised concerns about the possibility of increased valvular heart disease in patients treated with ergot-derived dopamine agonists such as pergolide.

Guanfacine

The role of the noradrenergic system in cognitive functions has been systematically evaluated in numerous studies. Acting on the PFC, post-synaptic α_{2a} adrenoceptors, moderate levels of norepinephrine (NE) increase "signal-to-noise" ratio in the processing of sensory stimuli, enhance long-term memory consolidation in the amygdala and hippocampus, and has a significant role in the regulation of working memory and attention functions of the PFC (Ramos & Arnsten, 2007). NE has also been found to modulate cognitive flexibility for insight-based problem solving (Choi et al., 2006). Guanfacine is an α_{2a} post-synaptic agonist noradrenergic agent. Its action in the PFC provides a promising possibility for the treatment of cognitive deficits in schizophrenia and the schizophrenia spectrum disorders

(Friedman *et al.*, 2004). In a 4-week, placebo-controlled, double-blind study of guanfacine on a wide range of cognitive tasks (McClure *et al.*, 2007b), we found that in contrast to participants with other personality disorders (OPD), subjects with SPD displayed improved context processing following treatment with this agent. However, guanfacine did not appear to affect the performance of either participants with SPD or with OPD on verbal and visuo-spatial episodic memory tasks. Thus, the specificity of guanfacine to tasks involving context processing and to individuals with SPD lends further evidence to the hypothesis that deficits in the working memory system may in fact underlie the range of cognitive deficits within the spectrum.

Dihydrexidine

There is a need to identify pharmacological compounds with a high ratio of D_1/D_2 activity to enhance cognitive functions in subjects with schizophrenia spectrum disorders. One such compound, dihydrexidine, has been extensively studied in animals and in patients with Parkinson disease (Blanchet *et al.*, 1998). A recent study (George *et al.*, 2007) reported that the administration of this drug to patients with schizophrenia did not result in improvement in their cognitive deficits. However, this cognitive enhancement may be detected more sensitively in subjects with SPD since this population appears to have cognitive deficits that are somewhat less severe and more readily reversible than those of patients with schizophrenia.

Outcome

A study by Mehlum *et al.* (1991) that compared the outcome of individuals with personality disorders found that those with SPD exhibited the poorest ratings on social adjustment and global functioning. More recently, a study by Ullrich *et al.* (2007) that compared life-success in the community in individuals with different personality disorders reported that subjects with SPD exhibited low scores in factors representing "status and wealth" and "successful intimate relationships". Additionally, the outcome of patients with SPD has been found to be similar (McGlashan, 1986), but somewhat more variable, to that of patients with chronic schizophrenia. Thus, an important caveat to consider when analyzing reports of SPD outcome is that patients with this disorder suffering from social and cognitive disturbances as profound as those with chronic schizophrenia are, perhaps, more frequently assessed in clinical settings than higher functioning individuals with SPD. It is also important to recognize that a number of subjects meeting criteria for SPD in cross-sectional studies might in fact be in the prodromal stage of schizophrenia (Seeber & Cadenhead, 2005). A study by Schulz and Soloff (1987) found that up to 25% of young adults with SPD went on to develop schizophrenia. Reported predictors of the later onset of schizophrenia in patients with SPD include paranoid ideation, magical thinking, and social isolation (Fenton & McGlashan 1989).

Conclusions

The study of populations with SPD has proven to be a fruitful approach in the attempt to unravel the pathophysiological factors that give rise to schizophrenia. Differences and similarities between SPD and schizophrenia are being examined with genetic, neurochemical, imaging, and pharmacological instruments. For example, an array of candidate genes, associated with all the disorders included in the schizophrenia spectrum, is being identified and contrasted with those unique to schizophrenia and psychosis. A strategy employed for the elucidation of the genetic and phenomenological relationships in the spectrum involves the characterization of intermediate phenotypes comprised of clusters of cognitive disturbances as well as SPD traits. Additionally, subjects with SPD constitute an ideal population to employ in pharmacological cognitive enhancement studies due to their more readily cognitive and social deficit improvement after the use of cognitive enhancement agents and their decreased vulnerability to psychotic exacerbations. Our review of various neurocognitive and neurophysiological studies supports the notion that schizotypy may not be distinguished from psychosis by preservation of one particular class of correlates. Thus, while deficits in schizophrenia may be more severe than in SPD, all features of these two disorders overlap. This overlap precludes the use of any particular vulnerability indicator as a diagnostically reliable tool to distinguish schizotypy from psychosis.

References

Abel, K., Jolley, S., Hemsley, D. *et al.* (2004) The influence of schizotypy traits on prepulse inhibition in young healthy controls. *Journal of Psychopharmacology* **18**, 181–188.

Abi-Dargham, A., Gil, R., Krystal, J. *et al.* (1998) Increased striatal dopamine transmission in schizophrenia: confirmation in a second cohort. *American Journal of Psychiatry* **155**, 761–767.

Abi-Dargham, A., Mawlawi, O. & Lombardo, I. (2002) Prefrontal dopamine D1 receptors and working memory in schizophrenia. *Journal of Neuroscience* **22**, 3708–3719.

Abi-Dargham, A., Kegeles, L., Zea-Ponce, Y. *et al.* (2004) Striatal amphetamine-induced dopamine release in patients with schizotypal personality disorder studied with single photon emission computed tomography and [123I] iodobenzamide. *Biological Psychiatry* **55**, 1001–1006.

Abi-Dargham, A. & Laruelle, M. (2005) Mechanisms of action of second generation antipsychotic drugs in schizophrenia: insights from brain imaging studies. *European Psychiatry* **20**, 15–27.

Adler, L., Pachtman, E., Franks, R. *et al.* (1982) Neurophysiological evidence for a defect in neuronal mechanisms involved in sensory gating in schizophrenia. *Biological Psychiatry* **17**, 639–654.

American Psychiatric Association (1980) *Diagnostic and Statistical Manual of Mental Disorders*, 3rd edn. Washington, DC: American Psychiatric Association.

American Psychiatric Association (1994) *Diagnostic and Statistical Manual of Mental Disorders*, 4th edn. Washington, DC: American Psychiatric Association.

Amin, F., Davidson, M., Kahn, R. *et al.* (1997) Assessment of the central dopaminergic index of plasma HVA in schizophrenia. *Schizophrenia Bulletin* **21**, 53–66.

Andreasen, N. (1999) A unitary model of schizophrenia: Bleuler's "fragmented phrene" as schizencephaly. *Archives of General Psychiatry* **56**, 781–793.

Andreasen, N., Paradiso, S. & O'Leary, D. (1998) "Cognitive dysmetria" as an integrative theory of schizophrenia: a dysfunction in cortical-subcortical-cerebullar circuitry? *Schizophrenia Bulletin* **24**, 203–218.

Aoki, C., Go, C., Venkatesan, C. & Kurose H. (1994) Perikaryal and synaptic localization of alpha 2A-adrenergic receptor-like immunoreactivity. *Brain Research* **650**, 181–204.

Appels, M., Sitskoorn, M., Vollema, M. & Kahn, R. (2004) Elevated levels of schizotypal features in parents of patients with a family history of schizophrenia spectrum disorders. *Schizophrenia Bulletin* **30**, 781–790.

Arndt, S., Alliger, R.J. & Andreasen, N.C. (1991) The distinction of positive and negative symptoms. The failure of a two-dimensional model. *British Journal of Psychiatry* **158**, 317–322.

Arnsten, A. & Goldman-Rakic, P. (1985) Alpha-2 adrenergic mechanisms in prefrontal cortex associated with cognitive decline in aged non human primates. *Science* **230**, 1273–1276.

Arnsten, A., Mathew, R., Ubriani, R. *et al.* (1999) Alpha-1 noradrenergic receptor stimulation impairs prefrontal cortical cognitive function. *Biological Psychiatry* **45**, 26–31.

Aston-Jones, G., Rajkowski, J. & Cohen, J. (1999) Role of locus coeruleus in attention and behavioral flexibility. *Biological Psychiatry* **46**, 1309–1320.

Barch, D. & Csernansky, J. (2007) Abnormal parietal cortex activation during working memory in schizophrenia: verbal phonological coding disturbances versus domain-general executive dysfunction. *American Journal of Psychiatry* **164**, 1090–1098.

Barch, D., Mitropoulou, V., Harvey, P. *et al.* (2004) Context-processing deficits in schizotypal personality disorder. *Journal of Abnormal Psychology* **113**, 556–568.

Baron, M., Gruen, R., Rainer, J. *et al.* (1982) Schizoaffective illness, schizophrenia, and affective disorders: morbidity risk and genetic transmission. *Acta Psychiatrica Scandinavica* **65**, 253–262.

Baron, M., Gruen, R., Asnis, L., Kane, J. (1983) Familial relatedness of schizophrenia and schizotypal states. *American Journal of Psychiatry* **140**, 1437–1442.

Baron, M., Gruen, R., Asnis, L. & Lord, S. (1985) Familial transmission of schizotypal and borderline personality disorders. *American Journal of Psychiatry* **142**, 927–934.

Battaglia, M., Gasperini, M., Sciuto, G. *et al.* (1991) Psychiatric disorders in the families of schizotypal subjects. *Schizophrenia Bulletin* **17**, 659–668.

Battaglia, M., Abbruzzese, M., Ferri, S. *et al.* (1994) An assessment of the Wisconsin Card Sorting Test as an indicator of liability to schizophrenia. *Schizophrenia Research* **14**, 39–45.

Battaglia, M., Bernardeschi, L., Franchini, L. *et al.* (1995) A family study of schizotypal disorder. *Schizophrenia Bulletin* **21**, 33–46.

Battaglia, M., Cavallini, M.C., Macciardi, F. & Bellodi, L. (1997) The structure of DSM-IIIR schizotypal personality disorder diagnosed by direct interview. *Schizophrenia Bulletin* **23**, 83–92.

Bellgrove, M., Domschke, K. & Hawi, Z. (2005) The methionine allele of the COMT polymorphism impairs prefrontal cognition in children and adolescents with ADHD. *Experimental Brain Research* **163**, 352–360.

Bentall, R., Claridge, G. & Slade, P. (1989) The multidimensional nature of schizotypal traits: a factor analytic study with normal subjects. *British Journal of Clinical Psychology* **28**, 363–375.

Bergman, A., Harvey, P., Mitropoulou, V. *et al.* (1996) The factor structure of schizotypal symptoms in a clinical population. *Schizophrenia Bulletin* **22**, 501–509.

Bernstein, D., Useda, D. & Siever, L. (1996) Paranoid personality disorder. In: Widiger, T.A., Frances, A.J., Pincus, H.A., Ross, R., First, M.B. & Davis, W.W., eds. *DSM-IV Sourcebook, Vol. 2.* Washington, DC: American Psychiatric Association, pp. 665–674.

Bilder, R., Mukherjee, S., Rieder, R. & Pandurangi, A. (1985) Symptomatic and neuropsychological components of defect states. *Schizophrenia Bulletin* **11**, 409–419.

Bilder, R., Goldman, R., Robinson, D. *et al.* (2000) Neuropsychology of first-episode schizophrenia: initial characterization and clinical correlates. *American Journal of Psychiatry* **157**, 549–559.

Bilder, R., Volavka, J., Czobor, P. *et al.* (2002) Neurocognitive correlates of the COMT Val (158) Met polymorphism in chronic schizophrenia. *Biological Psychiatry* **52**, 701–707.

Birnbaum, S., Gobeske, K., Auerbach, J. *et al.* (1999) A role for norepinephrine in stress-induced cognitive deficits: alpha-1-adrenoceptor mediation in the prefrontal cortex. *Biological Psychiatry* **46**, 1266–1274.

Blanchet, P., Fang, J., Gillespie, M. *et al.* (1998) Effects of the full dopamine D1 receptor agonist dihydrexine in Parkinson's disease. *Clinical Neuropharmacology* **21**, 339–343.

Bleuler, E. (1911/1950) *Dementia Praecox or the Group of Schizophrenias.* New York: International Universities Press.

Bolino, F., Di Michele, V., DiCicco, L. *et al.* (1994) Sensorimotor gating and habituation evoked by electro-cutaneous stimulation in schizophrenia. *Biological Psychiatry* **36**, 670–679.

Boudet, C., Bocca, M. & Chabot, B. (2005) Are eye movement abnormalities indicators of genetic vulnerability to schizophrenia? *European Psychiatry* **20**, 339–345.

Bowie, C. & Harvey, P. (2005) Cognition in schizophrenia: impairments, determinants, and functional importance. *Psychiatric Clinics of North America* **28**, 613–633.

Bowie, C., Harvey, P., Moriarty, P. *et al.* (2004) A comprehensive analysis of verbal fluency deficit in geriatric schizophrenia. *Archives of Clinical Neuropsychology* **19**, 289–303.

Bowie, C.R., Leung, W.W., Reichenberg, A. *et al.* (2008) Predicting schizophrenia patients' real-world behavior with specific neuropsychological and functional capacity measures. *Biological Psychiatry* **63**, 505–511.

Braff, D. & Geyer, M. (1990) Sensorimotor gating and schizophrenia: human and animal studies. *Archives of General Psychiatry* **47**, 181–188.

Braff, D. & Light, G. (2005) The use of neurophysiological endophenotypes to understand the genetic basis of schizophrenia. *Dialogues in Clinical Neuroscience* **7**, 125–135.

Braff, D., Saccucco, D. & Geyer M. (1991) Information processing dysfunctions in schizophrenia: studies of visual backward masking, sensorimotor gating, and habituation. In: Steinhauser, S.R., Gruzelier, J.H. & Zubin, J., eds. *Handbook of Schizophrenia, Vol. 5 Neuropsychology, Psychophysiology and Information Processing*. Amsterdam: Elsevier, pp. 303–334.

Breier, A., Su, T. & Saunders, R (1997) Schizophrenia is associated with elevated amphetamine-induced synaptic dopamine concentrations: evidence from a novel positron emission tomography method. *Proceedings of the National Academy of Sciences USA* **94**, 2569–2574.

Brozowski, T., Brown, R., Rosvold, H. & Goldman, P. (1979) Cognitive deficit caused by regional depletion of dopamine in prefrontal cortex of rhesus monkey. *Science* **205**, 929–932.

Buchsbaum, M., Yang, S., Hazlett, E. *et al.* (1997) Ventricular volume and asymmetry in schizotypal personality disorder and schizophrenia assessed with magnetic resonance imaging. *Schizophrenia Research* **27**, 45–53.

Buchsbaum, M., Nenadic, I., Hazlett, E. *et al.* (2002) Differential metabolic rates in prefrontal and temporal Brodman areas in schizophrenia and schizotypal personality disorder. *Schizophrenia Research* **54**, 141–150.

Butler, R., Jenkins, M., Geyer, M. & Braff, D. (1991) Wisconsin card sorting deficits and diminished sensorimotor gating in a discrete subgroup of schizophrenic patients. In: Tamminga, C.A. & Schulz, S.C., eds. *Advances in Neuropsychiatry and Psychopharmacology, Vol. I: Schizophrenia Research*. New York: Raven Press.

Byne, W., Buchsbaum, M., Kemether, E. *et al.* (2001) MRI assessment of medial and dorsal pulvinar nuclei of the thalamus in schizophrenia and schizotypal personality disorder. *Archives of General Psychiatry* **58**, 133–140.

Cadenhead, K. & Braff, D. (2002) Endophenotyping schizotypy: a prelude to genetic studies within the schizophrenia spectrum. *Schizophrenia Research* **54**, 47–57.

Cadenhead, K., Geyer, M. & Braff, D. (1993) Impaired startle prepulse inhibition and habituation in patients with schizotypal personality disorder. *American Journal of Psychiatry* **150**, 1862–1867.

Cadenhead, K., Perry, W., Braff, D. (1996) The relationship of information-processing deficits and clinical symptoms in schizotypal personality disorder. *Biological Psychiatry* **40**, 853–858.

Cadenhead, K., Light, G., Geyer, M. & Braff, D. (2000a) Sensory gating deficits assessed by the P50 event-related potential in subjects with schizotypal personality disorder. *American Journal of Psychiatry* **157**, 55–59.

Cadenhead K., Swerdlow, N., Shafer, K. *et al.* (2000b) Modulation of startle response and startle laterality in relatives of schizo-phrenic patients and in subjects with schizotypal personality disorder: evidence of inhibitory deficits. *American Journal of Psychiatry* **157**, 1660–1668.

Cadenhead K., Light G., Geyer M. *et al.* (2002) Neurobiological measures of schizotypal personality disorder: defining an inhibitory endophenotype? *American Journal of Psychiatry* **159**, 869–871.

Cai, J. & Arnsten, A. (1997) Dose-dependent effects of the dopamine D1 receptor agonists A77636 or SKF81297 on spatial working memory in aged monkeys. *Journal of Pharmacology and Experimental Therapeutics* **283**, 183–189.

Cannon, T., Mednick, S. & Parnas, J. (1990) Antecedents of predominantly negative- and predominantly positive-symptom schizophrenia in a high risk population. *Archives of General Psychiatry* **47**, 622–632.

Carlsson, A. & Lindqvist, M. (1963) Effect of chlorpromazine or haloperidol on formation of 3-methoxytyramine and normetanephrine in mouse brain. *Acta Pharmacologica Toxicologica* **20**, 140–144.

Carter, C., Mintun, M., Nichols, T. & Cohen, J. (1997) Anterior cingulate gyrus dysfunction and selective attention deficits in schizophrenia: [15O] H2O PET study during single-trial Stroop task performance. *American Journal of Psychiatry* **154**, 1670–1675.

Carter, C., Perlstein, W. & Ganguli, R. (1998) Functional hypofrontality and working memory dysfunction in schizophrenia. *American Journal of Psychiatry* **155**, 1285–1287.

Castner, S. & Goldman-Rakic, P. (2004) Enhancement of working memory in aged monkeys by a sensitizing regimen of dopamine D1 receptor stimulation. *Journal of Neuroscience* **24**, 1446–1450.

Castner, S., Williams, G. & Goldman-Rakic P. (2000) Reversal of anitpsychotic-induced working memory deficts by short-term dopamine D1 receptor stimulation. *Science* **287**, 2020–2022.

Chakos, M., Lieberman, J., Bilder, R. *et al.* (1994) Increase in caudate nuclei volumes of first-episode schizophrenic patients taking antipsychotic drugs. *American Journal of Psychiatry* **151**, 1430–1436.

Chapman J., Chapman L. & Kwapil T. (1995) Scales for the measurement of schizotypy. In: Raine, A., Lencz, T., Mednick, S., eds. *Schizotypal Personality Disorder*. Cambridge: Cambridge University Press, pp. 79–106.

Chapman, L., Chapman, J. & Raulin, M. (1976) Scales for physical and social anhedonia. *Journal of Abnormal Psychology* **85**, 374–382.

Chapman, L., Chapman, J. & Raulin, M. (1978) Body-image aberration in schizophrenia. *Journal of Abnormal Psychology* **87**, 399–407.

Chen, Y., Nakayama, K., Levy, D. *et al.* (1999) Psychophysical isolation of a motion-processing deficit in schizophrenia and their relatives and its association with impaired smooth pursuit. *Proceedings of the National Academy of Sciences USA* **96**, 4724–4729.

Choi, Y., Novak, J., Hillier, A. *et al.* (2006) The effect of alpha-2 adrenergic agonists on memory and cognitive flexibility. *Cognitive and Behavioral Neurology* **19**, 204–207.

Claridge, G. & Broks, P. (1984) Schizotypy and hemisphere function I. Theoretical considerations and the measurement of schizotypy. *Personality and Individual Differences* **5**, 633–648.

Clementz, B., McDowell, J. & Zisook, S. (1994) Saccadic system functioning among schizophrenia patients and their first-degree biological relatives. *Journal of Abnormal Psychology* **103**, 277–287.

Clementz, B., Geyer, M. & Braff, D. (1998) Poor P50 suppression among schizophrenia patients and their first-degree biological relatives. *American Journal of Psychiatry* **155**, 1691–1694.

Clementz, B., Grove, W., Iacono, W. & Sweeney, J. (1992) Smooth pursuit eye movement dysfunction and liability for schizophrenia: implications for genetic modeling. *Journal of Abnormal Psychology* **101**, 117–129.

Cohen, L., Hollander, E., DeCaria, C. *et al.* (1996) Specificity of neuropsychological impairment in obsessive–compulsive disorder: a comparison with social phobic and normal control subjects. *Journal of Neuropsychiatry and Clinical Neurosciences* **8**, 82–85.

Collins, P., Wilkinson, L. & Everitt, B. (2000) The effect of dopamine depletion from the caudate nucleus of the common marmoset (Callithrix jacchus) on tests of prefrontal cognitive function. *Behavioral Neuroscience* **114**, 3–17.

Compton, M., Chien, V. & Bollini, A. (2007) Psychometric properties of the Brief Version of the Schizotypal Personality Questionnaire in relatives of patients with schizophrenia-spectrum disorders and non-psychiatric controls. *Schizophrenia Research* **91**, 122–131.

Cornblatt, B. & Erlenmeyer-Kimling, L. (1985) Global attentional deviance as a marker of risk for schizophrenia: specificity and predictive validity. *Journal of Abnormal Psychology* **94**, 470–486.

Cornblatt, B. & Keilp, J. (1994) Impaired attention, genetics and the pathophysiology of schizophrenia. *Schizophrenia Bulletin* **20**, 31–46.

Cornblatt, B., Lenzenweger, M., Erlenmeyer-Kimling, L. (1989) The Continuous Performance Test, Identical Pairs version: II. Contrasting attentional profiles in schizophrenic and depressed patients. *Psychiatry Research* **29**, 65–86.

Cornblatt, B., Auther, A., Niendam, T. *et al.* (2007) Preliminary findings for two new measures of social and role functioning in the prodromal phase of schizophrenia. *Schizophrenia Bulletin* **33**, 688–702.

Cosway, R., Byrne, M. & Clafferty, R. (2002) Sustained attention in young people at high risk for schizophrenia. *Psychological Medicine* **32**, 277–286.

Crawford, T., Sharma, T. & Puri, B., (1998) Saccadic eye movements in families multiply affected with schizophrenia: the Maudsley family study. *American Journal of Psychiatry* **155**, 1703–1710.

Creese, I., Burt, D. & Snyder, S. (1976) Dopamine receptor binding predicts clinical and pharmacological potencies of antischizophrenic drugs. *Science* **19**, 481–483.

Crespo-Facorro, B., Roiz-Santiáñez, R., Pelayo-Terán J. *et al.* (2007) Reduced thalamic volume in first-episode non-affective psychosis: correlations with clinical variables, symptomatology and cognitive functioning. *Neuroimage* **35**, 1613–1623.

Croft, R., Lee, A., Bertolot, J. & Gruzelier, J. (2001) Associations of P50 suppression and desensitization with perceptual and cognitive features of "unreality" in schizotypy. *Biological Psychiatry* **50**, 441–446.

Cropley, V., Fujita, M. & Innis, R. (2006) Molecular imaging of the dopaminergic system and its association with human cognitive function. *Biological Psychiatry* **59**, 898–907.

Crow, T., Done, D. & Sacker, A. (1995) Birth cohort study of the antecedents of psychosis: ontogeny as witness to phylogenetic origins. In: Haefner, H. & Gattaz, W.F., eds. *Search for the Causes of Schizophrenia*, Vol. **3**. Berlin: Springer, pp. 3–20.

Curtis, C., Calkins, M. & Iacono, W. (2001) Saccadic disinhibition in schizophrenia patients and their first-degree biological relatives. A parametric study of the effects of increasing inhibitory load. *Experimental Brain Research* **137**, 228–236.

Daniel, E., Weinberger, D. & Goldberg, T. (1991) The effect of amphetamine on regional cerebral blood flow during cognitive activation in schizophrenia. *Journalof Neuroscie nce* **11**, 1907–1917.

Davidson, L. & Heinrichs, R. (2003) Quantification of frontal and temporal lobe brain-imaging findings in schizophrenia: a meta-analysis. *Psychiatry Research* **122**, 69–87.

Davidson, M., Reichenberg, A. & Rabinowitz, J. (1999) Behavioral and intellectual markers for schizophrenia in apparently healthy male adolescents. *American Journal of Psychiatry* **156**, 1328–1335.

Davis, M., Gendelman, D., Tischler, M. & Gendelman, P. (1982) A primary acoustic startle circuit: lesion and stimulation studies. *Journal of Neuroscience* **2**, 791–805.

Davis, K., Kahn, R., Ko, G. & Davidson, M. (1991) Dopamine and schizophrenia: a reconceptualisation. *American Journal of Psychiatry* **148**, 1474–1486.

Davis M., Walker D.L. & Lee Y. (1999) Neurophysiology and neuropharmacology of startle and its affective modification. In: Dawson, M.E., Schell, A.M. *et al.*, eds. *Startle Modification: Implications for Neuroscience, Cognitive Science, and Clinical Science*. New York: Cambridge University Press, pp. 114–133.

Dawson, M., Hazlett, A., Filion, D. *et al.* (1993) Attention and schizophrenia: impaired modulation of the startle reflex. *Journal of Abnormal Psychology* **102**, 633–641.

Dawson M., Schell A., Swerdlow N. & Filion, D. (1997) Cognitive, clinical and neuropsychological implications of startle modification. In: Lang, P.J., Simons, R.F. & Balaban M.T., eds. *Attention and Orienting: Sensory and Motivational Processes*. Hillsdale, NJ: Erlbaum.

Dawson, M., Schell, A. & Hazlett, E. (2000) On the clinical and cognitive meaning of impaired sensorimotor gating in schizophrenia. *Psychiatry Research* **96**, 187–197.

Dickey, C., McCarley, R., Volgmaier, M. *et al.* (1999) Schizotypal personality disorder and MRI abnormalities of temporal lobe grey matter. *Biological Psychiatry* **45**, 1393–1402.

Dickey, C., Shenton, M., Hirayasu, Y. *et al.* (2000) Large CSF volume not attributable to ventricular volume in schizotypal personality disorder. *American Journal of Psychiatry* **157**, 48–54.

Dickey, C., McCarley, R. & Voglmaier, M. (2002) Smaller left Heschl's gyrus volume in patients with schizotypal personality disorder. *American Journal of Psychiatry* **159**, 1521–1527.

Dickey, C., McCarley R., Niznikiewicz, M. *et al.* (2005) Clinical, cognitive, and social characteristics of a sample of neuroleptic-naive persons with schizotypal personality disorder. *Schizophrenia Research* **78**, 297–308.

Diefendorf, A. & Dodge, R. (1908) An experimental study of ocular reactions of the insane from photographic records. *Brain* **31**, 451–489.

Dinn, W., Robbins, N. & Harris, C. (2001) Adult attention-deficit/hyperactivity disorder: neuropsychological correlates and clinical presentation. *Brain and Cognition* **46**, 114–121.

Diwadkar, V., Montrose, D., Dworakowski, D. (2006) Genetically predisposed offspring with schizotypal features: an ultra high-risk group for schizophrenia? *Progress in Neuro-Psychopharmacol and Biological Psychiatry* **30**, 230–238.

Donchin, E. & Coles, G. (1988) Is the P300 manifestation of context updating? *Behavioral and Brain Sciences* **11**, 357–374.

Downhill, J., Buchsbaum, M. & Hazlett, E. (2001) Temporal lobe volume determined by magnetic resonance imaging in schizotypal personality disorder and schizophrenia. *Schizophrenia Research* **48**, 187–199.

Eastvold, A., Heaton, R. & Cadenhead, K. (2007) Neurocognitive deficits in the (putative) prodrome and first episode of psychosis. *Schizophrenia Research* **93**, 266–277.

Eckblad, M. & Chapman, L. (1983) Magical ideation as an indicator of schizotypy. *Journal of Consulting and Clinical Psychology* **51**, 215–225.

Egan, M., Goldberg, T. & Kolachana, B. (2001) Effect of COMT Val108/158 Met genotype on frontal lobe function and risk for schizophrenia. *Proceedings of the National Academy of Sciences USA* **98**, 6917–6922.

El-Ghundi, M., O'Dowd, B. & George S. (2007) Insights into the role of dopamine receptor systems in learning and memory. *Annual Review of Neuroscience* **18**, 37–66.

Erlenmeyer-Kimling, L., Cornblatt, B.A., Rock, D. *et al.* (1993) The New York High-Risk Project: anhedonia, attentional deviance, and psychopathology. *Schizophrenia Bulletin* **19**, 141–153.

Evans, L., Gray, N. & Snowden, R. (2005) Prepulse inhibition of startle and its moderation by schizotypy and smoking. *Psychophysiology* **42**, 223–231.

Fanous, A., Gardner, C., Walsh, D. & Kendler, K. (2001) Relationship between positive and negative symptoms of schizophrenia and schizotypal symptoms in nonpsychotic relatives. *Archives of General Psychiatry* **58**, 669–673.

Fanous, A., Neale, M., Gardner, C. *et al.* (2007) Significant correlation in linkage signals from genome-wide scans of schizophrenia and schizotypy. *Molecular Psychiatry* **12**, 958–965.

Faraone, S., Green, A., Seidman, L. & Tsuang M. (2001) Schizotaxia: clinical implications and new directions for research. *Schizophrenia Bulletin* **27**, 1–18.

Fenton, T. & McGlashan, T. (1989) Risk of schizophrenia in character disordered patients. *American Journal of Psychiatry* **146**, 1280–1284.

Fici, G., Wu, H., VonVoigtlander, P. & Sethy, V. (1997) D1 dopamine receptor activity of anti-parkisonian drugs. *Life Science* **60**, 1597–1603.

Fish, B. (1986) Antecedents of an acute schizophrenic break. *Journal of the American Academy of Child Psychiatry* **25**, 595–600.

Flach, K., Adler, L., Gerhardt, G. *et al.* (1996) Sensory gating in a computer model of the CA3 neural network of the hippocampus. *Biological Psychiatry* **40**, 1230–1245.

Foerster, A., Lewis, S., Owen, M. & Murray, R. (1991) Low birth weight and a family history of schizophrenia predict poor premorbid functioning in psychosis. *Schizophrenia Research* **5**, 13–20.

Foltynie, T., Goldberg, T. & Lewis, S. (2004) Planning ability in Parkinson's disease is influenced by the COMT val158met polymorphism. *Movement Disorders* **19**, 885–891.

Ford, J., White, W., Csernansky, J. *et al.* (1994) ERPs in schizophrenia: effects of antipsychotic medication. *Biological Psychiatry* **36**, 153–170.

Fossati, A., Citterio, A., Grazioli, F. *et al.* (2005) Taxonic structure of schizotypal personality disorder: A multiple-instrument, multi-sample study based on mixture models. *Psychiatry Research* **137**, 71–85.

Frangos, E., Athanassenas, G., Tsitourides, S. *et al.* (1985) Prevalence of DSM III schizophrenia among the first-degree relatives of schizophrenic probands. *Acta Psychiatrica Scandinavica* **72**, 382–386.

Frangou, S., Sharma, T. & Alarcon, G. (1997) The Maudsley Family Study. II. Endogenous event-related potentials in familial schizophrenia. *Schizophrenia Research* **23**, 45–53.

Franke, P., Maier, W., Hardt, J. *et al.* (1994) Attentional abilities and measures of schizotypy: their variation and covariation in schizophrenic patients, their siblings, and normal control subjects. *Psychiatry Research* **54**, 259–272.

Freedman, L., Rock, D., Roberts, S. *et al.* (1998) The New York High-Risk Project: attention, anhedonia and social outcome. *Schizophrenia Research* **30**, 1–9.

Friedman, J., Harvey, P., Coleman, T. *et al.* (2001) Six-year follow-up study of cognitive and functional status across the lifespan in schizophrenia: a comparison with Alzheimer's disease and normal aging. *American Journal of Psychiatry* **158**, 1441–1448.

Friedman, J., Stewart, D. & Gorman, J. (2004) Potential noradrenergic targets for cognitive enhancement in schizophrenia. *CNS Spectrum* **9**, 350–355.

Frith, C. (1979) Consciousness, information processing and schizophrenia. *British Journal of Psychiatry* **134**, 225–235.

Frodl, T., Meisenzahl, E. & Müller, D. (2002) P300 subcomponents and clinical symptoms in schizophrenia. *International Journal of Psychophysiology* **43**, 237–246.

Funahashi, S., Bruce, C. & Goldman-Rakic, P. (1993) Dorsolateral prefrontal lesions and oculomotor delayed-response performance: evidence for mnemonic "scotomas". *Journal of Neurosciences* **13**, 1479–1497.

Gallinat, J., Riedel, M., Juckel, G. *et al.* (2001) P300 and symptom improvement in schizophrenia. *Psychopharmacology* **158**, 55–65.

Gassab, L., Mechri, A., Dogui, M. *et al.* (2006) Abnormalities of auditory event-related potentials in students with high scores on the Schizotypal Personality Questionnaire. *Psychiatry Research* **144**, 117–122.

George, M., Molnar, C., Grenesko, E. *et al.* (2007) A single 20mg dose of dihydrexidine (DAR-0100), a full dopamine D1 agonist, is safe and tolerated in patients with schizophrenia. *Schizophrenia Research* **93**, 42–50.

Gershon, E., DeLisi, L., Hamovit, J. *et al.* (1988) A controlled family study of chronic psychoses. *Archives of General Psychiatry* **45**, 328–336.

Geyer, M. & Braff, D. (1987) Startle habituation and sensorimotor gating in schizophrenia and related animal models. *Schizophrenia Bulletin* **13**, 643–668.

Glatt, S., Faraone, S. & Tsuang, M. (2003) Association between a functional catechol O-methyltransferase gene polymorphism and schizophrenia: meta-analysis of case-control and family-based studies. *American Journal of Psychiatry* **160**, 469–476.

Glish, M.A., Erlenmeyer-Kimling, L. & Watt, N.F. (1982) Parental assessment of the social and emotional adaptation of children at high risk for schizophrenia. In: Lahey, B. & Kazdin, A., eds. *Advances in Child Clinical Psychology*. New York: Wiley.

Goldberg, S., Schulz, C., Schulz, M. et al. (1986) Borderline and schizotypal personality disorders treated with low dose thioxene vs. placebo. *Archives of General Psychiatry* **43**, 680–686.

Goldman-Rakic, P., Muly, E. & Williams, G. (2000) D1 receptors in prefrontal cells and circuits. *Brain Research Reviews* **31**, 295–301.

Graham, F. (1975) The more or less startling effects of weak prestimulation. *Psychophysiology* **12**, 238–248.

Green, M. (1996) What are the functional consequences of neurocognitive deficits in schizophrenia? *American Journal of Psychiatry* **153**, 321–330.

Green, M., Kern, R., Braff, D. & Mintz, J. (2000) Neurocognitive deficits and functional outcome in schizophrenia: Are we measuring the "right stuff"? *Schizophrenia Bulletin* **26**, 119–136.

Griffith, J., O'Neill, J., Petty, F. et al. (1998) Nicotinic receptor desensitization and sensory gating deficits in schizophrenia. *Biological Psychiatry* **44**, 98–106.

Grillon, C., Ameli, R., Charney, D., Krystal, J. & Braff, D. (1992) Startle gating deficits occur across prepulse intensities in schizophrenic patients. *Biological Psychiatry* **32**, 939–943.

Grove, W., Lebow, B., Clementz, B. et al. (1991) Familial prevalence and coaggregation of schizotypy indicators: a multitrait family study. *Journal of Abnormal Psychology* **100**, 115–121.

Gruzelier, J. (1996) The factorial structure of schizotypy. I. Affinities and contrasts with syndromes of schizophrenia. *Schizophrenia Bulletin* **22**, 611–620.

Gruzelier, J. (1999) Functional neuro-psychophysiological asymmetry in schizophrenia: a review and reorientation. *Schizophrenia Bulletin* **25**, 91–120.

Gruzelier, J. & Doig, A. (1996) The factorial structure of schizotypy. II. Patterns of cognitive asymmetry, arousal, handedness and gender. *Schizophrenia Bulletin* **22**, 621–634.

Gunderson, J., Siever, L. & Spaulding, E. (1983) The search for the schizotype: crossing the border again. *Archives of General Psychiatry* **40**, 15–22.

Gur, R., Turetsky, B., Cowell, P. et al. (2000) Temporolimbic volume reductions in schizophrenia. *Archives of General Psychiatry* **57**, 769–775.

Haber, S., Fudge, J. & McFarland, N. (2000) Striatonigrostriatal pathways in primates form an ascending spiral from the shell to the dorsolateral striatum. *Journal of Neuroscience* **20**, 2369–2382.

Harvey, P., Moriarty, P., Serper, M. et al. (2000) Practice-related improvement in information processing with novel antipsychotic treatment. *Schizophrenia Research* **46**, 139–148.

Hazlett, E., Buchsbaum, M., Haznedar, M. et al. (1998) Prefrontal cortex glucose metabolism and startle eye blink modification abnormalities in unmediated schizophrenia patients. *Psychophysiology* **35**, 186–198.

Hazlett, E., Buchsbaum, M., Haznedar, M. et al. (2008) Cortical gray and white matter volume in unmedicated schizotypal and schizophrenia patients. *Schizophrenia Research* **101**, 111–123.

Haznedar, M., Buchsbaum, M., Hazlett, E., Shihabuddin L., New, A. & Siever, L. (2004) Cingulate gyrus volume and metabolism in the schizophrenia spectrum. *Schizophrenia Research* **71**, 249–262.

Heaton, R. & Pendleton, M. (1981) Use of neuropsychological tests to predict patients everyday functioning. *Journal of Consulting and Clinical Psychology* **49**, 807–821.

Heaton, R., Gladsome, J., Palmer, B. et al. (2001) Stability and course of neuropsychological deficits in schizophrenia. *Archives of General Psychiatry* **58**, 24–32.

Heinrichs, R. (2005) The primacy of cognition in schizophrenia. *American Psychologist* **60**, 229–242.

Heinrichs, R. & Zakzanis, K. (1998) Neurocognitive deficit in schizophrenia: a quantitative review of the evidence. *Neuropsychology* **12**, 426–445.

Herpertz S., Zanarini, M., Schulz, C., Siever, L., Lieb, K., Möller, H.; WFSBP Task Force on Personality Disorders; World Federation of Societies of Biological Psychiatry (WFSBP) (2007) World Federation of Societies of Biological Psychiatry (WFSBP) guidelines for biological treatment of personality disorders. *World Journal of Biological Psychiatry* **8**, 212–244.

Hewitt, J. & Claridge, G. (1989) The factor structure of schizotypy in a normal population. *Personality and Individual Differences* **10**, 323–329.

Hietala, J., Syvalahti, E., Vilkman, H. et al. (1999) Depressive symptoms and presynaptic dopamine functions in neuroleptic-naïve schizophrenia. *Schizophrenia Research* **35**, 41–50.

Hirayasu, Y., Asato, N., Ohta, H. et al. (1998) Abnormalities of auditory event related potentials in schizophrenia prior to treatment. *Biological Psychiatry* **43**, 244–253.

Hirayasu, Y., McCarley, R., Salisbury, D. et al. (2000) Planum temporale and Heschl gyrus volume reduction in schizophrenia: a magnetic resonance imaging study of first-episode patients. *Archives of General Psychiatry* **57**, 692–699.

Ho, B. (2007) MRI brain volume abnormalities in young, nonpsychotic relatives of schizophrenia probands are associated with subsequent prodromal symptoms. *Schizophrenia Research* **96**, 1–13.

Hogg, B., Jackson, H.J, Rudd, R.P. & Edwards, J. (1990) Diagnosing personality disorders in recent-onset schizophrenia. *Journal of Nervous and Mental Disease* **178**, 194–199.

Holahan, A. & O'Driscoll, G. (2005) Antisaccade and smooth pursuit performance in positive- and negative-symptom schizotypy. *Schizophrenia Research* **76**, 43–54.

Holzman, P. (2000) Eye movements and the search for the essence of schizophrenia. *Brain Research* **31**, 350–356.

Holzman, P., Proctor, L. & Levy, D. (1974) Eye-tracking dysfunctions in schizophrenic patients and their relatives. *Archives of General Psychiatry* **31**, 143–151.

Holzman, P., Kringlen, E. & Matthysse, S. (1988) A single dominant gene can account for eye tracking dysfunctions and schizophrenia in offsprings of discordant twins. *Archives of General Psychiatry* **45**, 641–647.

Hymowitz, P., Francis, A., Jacobsberg, L. *et al.* (1986) Neuroleptic treatment of schizotypal personality disorders. *Comprehensive Psychiatry* **27**, 267–271.

Ingraham, L. & Kety, S. (2000) Adoption studies of schizophrenia. *American Journal of Medical Genetics* **97**, 18–22.

Ison, J. & Hammond, G. (1971) Modification of the startle reflex in the rat by changes in auditory and visual environments. *Journal of Comparative Physiology* **75**, 435–452.

Jäkälä, P., Riekkinen, M. & Sirviö, J. (1999) Guanfacine, but not clonidine, improves planning and working memory performance in humans. *Neuropsychopharmacology* **20**, 460–470.

Jensen, H. & Andersen, J. (1989) An open, noncomparative study of amoxapine in borderline disorders. *Acta Psychiatrica Scandinavica* **79**, 89–93.

Jeon, Y. & Polich, J. (2001) P300 asymmetry in schizophrenia: a meta-analysis. *Psychiatry Research* **104**, 61–74.

Joober, R., Gauthier, J. & Lal, S. (2002) Catechol-O-methyltransferase Val-108/158-Met gene variants associated with performance on the Wisconsin Card Sorting Test. *Archives of General Psychiatry* **59**, 662–663.

Kalus, O., Bernstein, D. & Siever, L. (1996) Schizoid personality disorder. In: Widiger, T.A., Frances, A.J., Pincus, H.A., Ross, R., First, M.B. & Davis, W.W., eds. *DSM-IV Sourcebook, Vol. 2*. Washington, DC: American Psychiatric Association, pp. 675–684.

Karoum, F., Chrapusta, S. & Egan, M. (1994) 3-Methoxytyramine is the major metabolite of released dopamine in the rat frontal cortex: reassessment of the effects of antipsychotics on the dynamics of dopamine release and metabolism in the frontal cortex, nucleus accumbens, and striatum by a simple two pool model. *Journal of Neurochemistry* **63**, 972–979.

Karoumi, B., Laurent, A., Rosenfeld, F. *et al.* (2000) Alteration of event related potentials in siblings discordant for schizophrenia. *Schizophrenia Research* **41**, 325–334.

Karoumi, B., Saoud, M., d'Amato, T. *et al.* (2001) Poor performance in smooth pursuit and antisaccadic eye-movement tasks in healthy siblings of patients with schizophrenia, *Psychiatry Research* **101**, 209–219.

Karper, L., Freeman, G., Grillon, C. *et al.* (1996) Preliminary evidence of an association between sensorimotor gating and distractibility in psychosis. *Journal of Neuropsychiatry and Clinical Neurosciences* **8**, 60–66.

Katsanis, J., Kortenkamp, S., Iacono, W.G. & Grove, W.M. (1997) Antisaccade performance in patients with schizophrenia and affective disorder. *Journal of Abnormal Psychology* **106**, 468–472.

Kavoussi, R. & Siever, L. (1992) Overlap between borderline and schizotypal personality disorders. *Comprehensive Psychiatry* **33**, 7–12.

Kawasaki, Y., Suzuki, M., Nohara, S. *et al.* (2004) Structural brain differences in patients with schizophrenia and schizotypal disorder demonstrated by voxel-based morphometry. *European Archives of Psychiatry and Clinical Neuroscience* **254**, 406–414.

Kawasaki, Y., Suzuki, M., Takahashi, T. *et al.* (2008) Anomalous cerebral Asymmetry in patients with schizophrenia demonstrated by voxel-based morphometry. *Biological Psychiatry* **63**, 793–800.

Keefe, R., Roitman, S., Harvey, P. *et al.* (1995) A pen and paper human analogue of a monkey prefrontal cortex activation task: Spatial working memory in patients with schizophrenia. *Schizophrenia Research* **17**, 25–33.

Kendler, K. (1985) Diagnostic approaches to schizotypal personality disorder: a historical perspective. *Schizophrenia Bulletin* **11**, 538–553.

Kendler, K. (1988) Familial aggregation of schizophrenia and schizophrenia spectrum disorders: evaluation of conflicting results. *Archives of General Psychiatry* **45**, 377–383.

Kendler, K. & Gruenberg, A. (1984) An independent analysis of the Danish Adoption Study of Schizophrenia. VI. The relationship between psychiatric disorders as defined by DSM-III in the relatives and adoptees. *Archives of General Psychiatry* **41**, 555–564.

Kendler, K. & Hewitt, J. (1992) The structure of self-report schizotypy in twins. *Journal of Personality Disorders* **6**, 1–17.

Kendler, K., Gruenberg, A. & Strauss, J. (1981) An independent analysis of the Copenhagen sample of the Danish adoption study of schizophrenia. II. The relationship between schizotypal personality disorder and schizophrenia. *Archives of General Psychiatry* **38**, 982–987.

Kendler, K.S., Ochs, A.L., Gorman, A.M. *et al.* (1991) The structure of schizotypy: a multitrait twin study. *Psychiatry Research* **36**, 19–36.

Kendler, K.S., McGuire, M., Gruenberg, A.M. *et al.* (1993a) The Roscommon Family Study. III. Schizophrenia-related personality disorders in relatives. *Archives of General Psychiatry* **50**, 781–788.

Kendler, K., McGuire, M., Gruenberg, A.M. *et al.* (1993b) The Roscommon Family Study. I. Methods, diagnosis of probands and risk of schizophrenia in relatives. *Archives of General Psychiatry* **50**, 527–540.

Kendler, K., Gruenberg, A. & Kinney, D. (1994) Independent diagnosis of adoptees and relatives as defined by DSM-III in the provincial and national samples of the Danish adoption study of schizophrenia. *Archives of General Psychiatry* **51**, 456–468.

Kendler, K., Neale, M. & Walsh, D. (1995a) Evaluating the spectrum concept of schizophrenia in the Roscommon Family Study. *American Journal of Psychiatry* **152**, 749–754.

Kendler, K., McGuire, M., Gruenberg, A. & Walsh, D. (1995b) Schizotypal symptoms and signs in the Roscommon Family Study. Their factor structure and familial relationship with psychotic and affective disorders. *Archives of General Psychiatry* **52**, 296–303.

Keshavan, M. (1997) Neurodevelopment and schizophrenia: quo vadis? In: Keshavan, M.S. & Murray, R.M., eds. *Neurodevelopment and Adult Psychopathology*. Cambridge: Cambridge University Press, pp. 267–277.

Keshavan, M., Shad, M., Soloff, P. & Schooler, N. (2004) Efficacy and tolerability of olanzapine in the treatment of schizotypal personality disorder. *Schizophrenia Research* **71**, 97–101.

Kety, S., Rosenthal, D., Wender, P. *et al.* (1975) Mental illness in the biological and adoptive families of adopted individuals who have become schizophrenic: preliminary report based o psychiatric interviews. In: Fieve, R.R., Rosenthal, D. & Brill, H., eds. *Genetic Research in Psychiatry.* Baltimore: Johns Hopkins University Press, pp. 147–165.

Kimble, M., Lyons, M. & O'Donnell, B. (2000) The effect of family status and schizotypy on electrophysiologic measures of attention and semantic processing. *Biological Psychiatry* **47**, 402–412.

Kirrane, R. & Siever, L. (2000) New perspectives on schizotypal personality disorder. *Current Psychiatry Reports* **2**, 62–66.

Kirrane, M., Mitropoulou, V., Nunn, M. *et al.* (2000) Effects of amphetamine on visuospatial working memory in schizophrenia spectrum personality disorder. *Neuropsychopharmacology* **22**, 14–18.

Klein, C., Berg, P., Rockstroh, B. & Andresen, B. (1999) Topography of the auditory P300 in schizotypal personality. *Biological Psychiatry* **45**, 1612–1621.

Klemm, S., Schmidt, B., Knappe, S. & Blanz, B. (2006) Impaired working speed and executive functions as frontal lobe dysfunctions in young first-degree relatives of schizophrenic patients. *European Child and Adolescent Psychiatry* **15**, 400–408.

Koenigsberg, H., Reynolds, D., Goodman, M. *et al.* (2003) Risperidone in the treatment of schizotypeal personality disorder. *Journal of Clinical Psychiatry* **64**, 628–634.

Koenigsberg, H., Buchsbaum, M. & Buchsbaum, B. (2005) Functional MRI of visuospatial working memory in schizotypal personality disorder: a region-of-interest analysis. *Psychological Medicine* **35**, 1019–1030.

Kok, A. (1997) Event-related potentials (ERP) reflections of mental resources: a review and synthesis. *Biological Psychology* **45**, 19–56.

Koo, M., Dickey, C., Park, H. *et al.* (2006a) Smaller neocortical gray matter and larger sulcal cerebrospinal fluid volumes in neuroleptic-naive women with schizotypal personality disorder. *Archives of General Psychiatry* **63l**, 1090–1100.

Koo, M., Levitt, J. & McCarley, R. (2006b) Reduction of caudate nucleus volumes in neuroleptic-naive female subjects with schizotypal personality disorder. *Biological Psychiatry* **60**, 40–48.

Korostenskaja, M., Dapsys, K. & Siurkute, A. (2005) Effects of olanzapine on auditory P300 and mismatch negativity (MMN) in schizophrenia spectrum disorders. *Progress in Neuropsychopharmacoly and Biological Psychiatry* **29**, 543–548.

Kraepelin, E. (1919/1971) *Manic-Depressive Insanity and Paranoia.* Translated by Barclay, R.M. Edinburgh: E. & S. Livingstone.

Kulisevsky, J., Garcia-Sanchez, C., Berthier, M. *et al.* (2000) Chronic effects of dopaminergic replacement on cognitive function in Parkinson's disease: a two-follow-up study of previously untreated patients. *Movement Disorders* **15**, 613–636.

Kumari, V., Das, M., Zachariah, E. *et al.* (2005) Reduced prepulse inhibition in unaffected siblings of schizophrenia patients. *Psychophysiology* **42**, 588–594.

Kutcher, S., Blackwood, D., Gaskell, D. *et al.* (1989) Auditory P300 does not differentiate borderline personality disorder from schizotypal personality disorder. *Biological Psychiatry* **26**, 766–774.

Kwapil, T. (1998) Social anhedonia as a predictor of the development of schizophrenia-spectrum disorders. *Journal of Abnormal Psychology* **107**, 558–565.

Kwapil, T., Barrantes-Vidal N. & Silvia P. (2008) The dimensional structure of the Wisconsin schizotypy scales: Factor identification and construct validity. *Schizophrenia Bulletin* **34**, 444–457.

Lachman, H., Papolos, D., Saito, T. *et al.* (1996) Human catechol-O-methyltransferase pharmacogenetics: description of a functional polymorphism and its potential application to neuropsychiatric disorders. *Pharmacogenetics* **6**, 243–250.

Lange, K., Robbins, T., Marsden, C. *et al.* (1992) L-dopa withdrawal in Parkinson's disease selectively impairs cognitive performance in tests sensitive to frontal lobe dysfunction. *Psychophamocology* **107**, 394–404.

Laruelle, M., Abi-Dargham, A. & van Dyke, C. (1996) Single photon emission computerized tomography imaging of amphetamine-induced dopamine release in drug-free schizophrenic patients. *Proceedings of the National Academy of Sciences USA* **93**, 9235–9240.

Laruelle, M., Kegeles, L. & Zea-Ponce, Y. (2002) Amphetamine-induced dopamine release in patients with schizotypal personality disorders studies by SPECT and [123] IBZM. *Neuroimage* **16**, S61.

Laurent, A., Garcia-Larrea, L., d'Amato, T. *et al.* (1999) Auditory event-related potentials and clinical scores in unmedicated schizophrenic patients. *Psychiatry Research* **86**, 229–238.

Laurent, A., Biloa-Tang, M., Bougerol, T. *et al.* (2000) Executive/attentional performance and measures of schizotypy in patients with schizophrenia and in their nonpsychotic first-degree relatives. *Schizophrenia Research* **46**, 269–283.

Lee, L. & Williams, L. (2000) Eye movement dysfunction as a biological marker of risk for schizophrenia. *Australian and New Zealand Journal of Psychiatry* **34**, S91–S100.

Lees-Reitman, S., Cornblatt, B., Bergman, A. *et al.* (1997) Attentional functioning in schizotypal personality disorder. *American Journal of Psychiatry* **154**, 655–660.

Lenzenweger, M. & O'Driscoll, G. (2006) Smooth pursuit eye movement and schizotypy in the community. *Journal of Abnormal Psychology* **115**, 779–786.

Lenzenweger, M. & Korfine, L. (1995) Tracking the taxon: on the latent structure and base rate of schizotypy. In: Raine, A., Lencz, T. & Mednick, S.A., eds. *Schizotypal Personality.* New York: Cambridge University Press, pp. 135–167.

Lenzenweger, M., Miller, A., Maher, B. & Manschreck, T. (2007) Schizotypy and individual differences in the frequency of normal associations in verbal utterances. *Schizophrenia Research* **95**, 96–102.

Levitt, J., McCarley, R. & Dickey, C. (2002) MRI study of caudate nucleus volume and its cognitive correlates in neuroleptic-naive patients with schizotypal personality disorder. *American Journal of Psychiatry* **159**, 1190–1197.

Levitt, J., Westin, C., Nestor, P. *et al.* (2004) Shape of caudate nucleus and its cognitive correlates in neuroleptic-naive schizotypal personality disorder. *Biological Psychiatry* **55**, 177–184.

Lichtermann, D., Karbe, E. & Maier, W. (2000) The genetic epidemiology of schizophrenia and of schizophrenia spectrum disorders. *European Archives of Psychiatry and Clinical Neuroscience* **250**, 304–310.

Liddle, P. (1987) The symptoms of chronic schizophrenia: a re-examination of the positive-negative dichotomy. *British Journal of Psychiatry* **151**, 145–151.

Lindstrom, L., Gefvert, O., Hagberg, G. *et al.* (1999) Increased dopamine synthesis rate in medial prefrontal cortex and striatum in schizophrenia indicated by L-(Beta-11C) Dopa and PET. *Biological Psychiatry* **46**, 681–688.

Lindvall, O. & Bjorklund, A. (1983) *Chemical Neuroanatomy*. New York: Raven Press, pp. 229–255.

Linscott, R. (2007) The latent structure and coincidence of hypohedonia and schizotypy and their validity as indices of psychometric risk for schizophrenia. *Journal of Personality Disorders* **21**, 225–242.

Lipska, B. & Weinberger, D. (2000) To model a psychiatric disorder in animals: schizophrenia as a reality test. *Neuropsychopharmacology* **23**, 223–239.

Lotta, T., Vidgren, J. & Tilgmann, C. (1995) Kinetics of human soluble and membrane-bound catechol O-methyltransferase: a revised mechanism and description of the thermolabile variant of the enzyme. *Biochemistry* **34**, 4202–4210.

Luciana, M., Depue, R., Arbisi, P. & Leon, A. (1992) Facilitation of working memory in humans by a D2 dopamine receptor agonist. *Journal of Cognitive Neuroscience* **4**, 58–68.

Luciana, M., Collins, P. & Depue, R. (1998) Opposing roles for dopamine and serotonin in the modulation of human spatial working memory functions. *Cerebral Cortex* **8**, 218–226.

Ludewig, K., Geyer, M. & Vollenweider, F. (2003) Deficits in prepulse inhibition and habituation in never-medicated, first-episode schizophrenia. *Biological Psychiatry* **54**, 121–128.

Mackeprang, T., Kristiansen, K. & Glenthoj, B. (2002) Effects of antipsychotics on prepulse inhibition of the startle response in drug-naïve schizophrenic patients. *Biological Psychiatry* **52**, 863–873.

Maher, B., Manschreck, T., Linnert, J. & Candela, S., (2005) Quantitative assessment of the frequency of normal associations in the utterances of schizophrenia patients and healthy controls. *Schizophrenia Research* **78**, 219–224.

Malhotra, A., Kestler L. & Mazzanti, C. (2002) A functional polymorphism in the COMT gene and performance on a test of prefrontal cognition. *American Journal of Psychiatry* **159**, 652–654.

Mannan, M., Hiramatsu, K., Hokama, H. & Ohta, H. (2001) Abnormalities of auditory event-related potentials in students with schizotypal personality disorder. *Psychiatry and Clinical Neurosciences* **55**, 451–457.

Mao, Z., Arnsten, A. & Li, B. (1999) Local infusion of an alpha-1 adrenergic agonist into the prefrontal cortex impairs spatial working memory performance in monkeys. *Biological Psychiatry* **46**, 1259–1265.

Marjamaki, A., Luomala, K., Ala-Uotila, S. & Scheinin, M. (1993) Use of recombinant human alpha 2-adrenoceptors to characterize subtype selectively of antagonist binding. *European Journal of Pharmacology* **246**, 219–226.

Mason, O., Claridge, G. & Jackson, M. (1995) New scales for the assessment of schizotypy. *Personality and Individual Differences* **18**, 7–13.

Matsui, M., Yuuki, H., Kato, K. *et al.* (2007) Schizotypal disorder and schizophrenia: a profile analysis of neuropsychological functioning in Japanese patients. *Journal of the International Neuropsychological Society* **13**, 672–682.

Mattay, V., Callicott, J., Bertolino, A. *et al.* (2000) Effects of dextroamphetamine on cognitive performance and cortical activation. *Neuroimage* **12**, 268–275.

Mattay, V., Goldberg, T., Fera, F. *et al.* (2003) Catechol O-methyltransferase val158-met genotype and individual variation in the brain response to amphetamine. *Proceedings of the National Academy of Sciences USA* **100**, 6186–6191.

McCarley, R., Faux, S., Shenton, M. *et al.* (1991) Event-related potentials in schizophrenia: their biological and clinical correlates and a new model of schizophrenic pathophysiology. *Schizophrenia Research* **4**, 209–231.

McCarley, R., Shenton, M., O'Donnell, B. *et al.* (1993) Auditory P300 abnormalities and left posterior superior temporal gyrus volume reduction in schizophrenia. *Archives of General Psychiatry* **50**, 190–197.

McCarley, R., Hsiao, J. & Freedman, R. (1996) Neuroimaging and the cognitive neuroscience of schizophrenia. *Schizophrenia Bulletin* **22**, 703–725.

McClure, M., Romero, M., Bowie, C. *et al.* (2007a) Visual-spatial learning and memory in schizotypal personality disorder: continued evidence for the importance of working memory in the schizophrenia spectrum. *Archives of Clinical Neuropsychological* **22**, 109–116.

McClure, M., Barch, D., Romero, M. *et al.* (2007b) The effects of guanfacine on context processing abnormalities in schizotypal personality disorder. *Biological Psychiatry* **61**, 1157–1160.

McDowell SK (1996) A role for dopamine in executive function deficits. *Journal of Head Trauma Rehabilitation* **11**, 89–92.

McDowell, J. & Clementz, B. (1997) The effect of fixation condition manipulations on antisaccade performance in schizophrenia: studies of diagnostic specificity. *Experimental Brain Research* **115**, 333–344.

McGlashan, T. (1986) Schizotypal personality disorder, Chestnut Lodge follow-up study. VI. Long-term follow-up perspective. *Archives of General Psychiatry* **43**, 329–334.

McGuffin, P., Owen, M. & Farmer, A. (1995) Genetic basis of schizophrenia. *Lancet* **346**, 678–682.

Meehl, P.E. (1962) Schizotaxia, schizotypy, schizophrenia. *American Psychologist* **17**, 827–839.

Meehl, P. (1990) Toward an integrated theory of schizotaxia, schizotypy, and schizophrenia. *Journal of Personality Disorders* **4**, 1–99.

Mehlum, L., Friis, S., Irion, T. *et al.* (1991) Personality disorders 2–5 years after treatment: a prospective follow-up study. *Acta Psychiatrica Scandinavica* **84**, 72–77.

Mehta, M., Swainson, R., Ogilvie, A. *et al.* (2001) Improved short-term spatial memory but impaired reversal learning following the dopamine D(2) agonist bromocriptine in human volunteers. *Psychopharmacology* **159**, 10–20.

Meyer-Lindenberg, A., Poline, J., Kohn, P. *et al.* (2001) Evidence for abnormal cortical functional connectivity during working memory in schizophrenia. *American Journal of Psychiatry* **158**, 1809–1817.

Miller, T., McGlashan, T., Rosen, J. *et al.* (2002) Prospective diagnosis of the initial prodrome for schizophrenia based on the structured interview for prodromal syndromes: preliminary evidence of interrater reliability and predictive validity. *American Journal of Psychiatry* **159**, 863–865.

Minas, R. & Park, S. (2007) Attentional window in schizophrenia and schizotypal personality: Insight from negative priming studies. *Applied and Preventive Psychology* **12**, 140–148.

Minzenberg, M., Xu, K. & Mitropoulou, V. (2006) Catechol-O-methyltransferase Val158Met genotype variation is associated with prefrontal-dependent task performance in schizotypal personality disorder patients and comparison groups. *Psychiatric Genetics* **16**, 117–124.

Mitropoulou, V., Harvey, P., Maldari, L. *et al.* (2002) Neuropsychological performance in schizotypal personality disorder: evidence regarding diagnostic specificity. *Biological Psychiatry* **52**, 1175–1182.

Mitropoulou, V., Goodman, M., Sevy, S. *et al.* (2004) Effects of acute metabolic stress on the dopaminergic and pituitary-adrenal axis activity in patients with schizotypal personality disorder. *Schizophrenia Research* **70**, 27–31.

Mitropoulou, V., Harvey, P., Zegarelli, G. *et al.* (2005) Neuropsychological performance in schizotypal personality disorder: importance of working memory. *American Journal of Psychiatry* **162**, 1896–1903.

Mohanty, A., Herrington, J.D., Koven, N.S. *et al.* (2005) Neural mechanisms of affective interference in schizotypy. *Journal of Abnormal Psychology* **114**, 16–27.

Mojtabai, R., Bromet, E., Harvey, P. *et al.* (2000) Neuropsychological differences between first-admission schizophrenia and psychotic affective disorders. *American Journal of Psychiatry* **157**, 1453–1460.

Moriarty, P., Harvey, P., Mitropoulou, V. *et al.* (2003) Reduced processing resource availability in schizotypal personality disorder: evidence from a dual-task CPT study. *Journal of Clinical and Experimental Neuropsychology* **25**, 335–347.

Muir, W., St Clair, D. & Blackwood, D. (1991) Long latency auditory event related potentials in schizophrenia and in bipolar and unipolar affective disorder. *Psychological Medicine* **21**, 867–879.

Muller, U., von Cramon, D. & Pollman, S. (1998) D1- versus D2-receptor modulation of visuospatial working memory in humans. *Journal of Neuroscience* **18**, 2720–2728.

Munafò, M., Bowes, L., Clark, T. & Flint, J. (2005) Lack of association of the COMT (Val158/108 Met) gene and schizophrenia: a meta-analysis of case-control studies. *Molecular Psychiatry* **10**, 765–770.

Muntaner, C., Garcia-Sevilla, L., Alberto, A., Torrubia, R. (1988) Personality dimensions, schizotypal and borderline personality traits and psychosis proneness. *Personality and Individual Differences* **9**, 257–268.

Murray, R.M. & Lewis, S.W. (1987) Is schizophrenia a neurodevelopmental disorder? *British Medical Journal* **295**, 681–682.

Nestler, E. & Carlezon, W., Jr. (2006) The mesolimbic dopamine reward circuit in depression. *Biological Psychiatry* **59**, 1151–1159.

Nestor, P., Shenton, M. & McCarley, R. (1993) Neuropsychological correlates of MRI temporal lobe abnormalities in schizophrenia. *American Journal of Psychiatry* **150**, 1849–1855.

Niznikiewicz, M., Voglmaier, M., Shenton, M. *et al.* (2000) Lateralized P3 deficit in schizotypal personality disorder. *Biological Psychiatry* **48**, 702–705.

Nuchpongsai, P., Arkaki, H., Langman, P. & Ogura, C. (1999) N2 and P3b components of the event-related potential in students at risk for psychosis. *Psychiatry Research* **88**, 131–141.

Obiols, J.E., Serrano, F., Caparros, B., Subira, S. & Barrantes, N. (1999) Neurological soft signs in adolescents with poor performance on the continuous performance test: markers of liability for schizophrenia spectrum disorders? *Psychiatry Research* **86**, 217–228.

O'Driscoll, G., Lenzenweger, M. & Holzman, P. (1998) Antisaccades and smooth pursuit eye tracking and schizotypy. *Archives of General Psychiatry* **55**, 837–843.

O'Flynn, K., Gruzelier, J., Bergman, A. & Siever, L. (2002) The schizophrenia spectrum personality disorder. In: Hirsch, S. & Weinberger, D., eds. *Schizophrenia*, 2nd edn. Wiley, John & Sons, Inc., pp. 80–101.

Okubo, Y., Suhara, T., Suzuki, K. *et al.* (1997) Decreased prefrontal dopamine D1 receptors in schizophrenia revealed by PET. *Nature* **385**, 634–636.

Olin, S. & Mednick, S. (1996). Risk factors of psychosis: Identifying vulnerable populations premorbidly. *Schizophrenia Bulletin* **22**, 223–240.

Olsen, K. & Rosenbaum, B. (2006) Prospective investigations of the prodromal state of schizophrenia: review of studies. *Acta Psychiatrica Scandinavica* **113**, 247–272.

Owen, A. & Robbins, T. (1998) Attention and working memory in movement disorders. In: Jahanashi, M. & Brown, R., eds. *Neuropsychology of Movement Disorders*. Amsterdam: North-Holland.

Park, S., Puschel, J., Sauter, B. *et al.* (2002) Spatial selective attention and inhibition in schizophrenia patients during acute psychosis and at 4-month follow-up. *Biological Psychiatry* **51**, 498–506.

Parnas, J., Schulsinger, F., Schulsinger, H., Mednick, S. & Teasdale, T. (1982) Behavioral precursors of schizophrenia spectrum. *Archives of General Psychiatry* **39**, 658–664.

Patterson, J., Hetrick, W., Boutros, N. *et al.* (2008) P50 sensory gating ratios in schizophrenics and controls: A review and data analysis. *Psychiatry Research* **158**, 226–247.

Peralta, V., Cuesta, M.J. & de Leon, J. (1991) Premorbid personality and positive and negative symptoms in schizophrenia. *Acta Psychiatrica Scandinavica* **84**, 336–339.

Peralta, V., Cuesta, M. & de Leon J. (1992) Positive versus negative schizophrenia and basic symptoms. *Comprehensive Psychiatry* **33**, 202–206.

Pickar, D., Labarac, R., Linnoila, M. *et al.* (1984) Neuroleptic-induced decrease in plasma homovanillic acid and antipsychotic activity in schizophrenic patients. *Science* **225**, 954–956.

Pillon, B., Czernecki, V. & Dubois, B. (2003) Dopamine and cognitive function. *Current Opinion in Neurology* **16**, S17–22.

Polich, J. & Kok, A. (1995) Cognitive and biological determinants of P300: an integrative review. *Biological Psychology* **41**, 103–146.

Pycock, C., Kerwin, R. & Carter, C (1980) Effects of lesions of cortical dopamine terminals on subcortical dopamine receptors in rats. *Nature* **286**, 74–77.

Rado, S. (1956) *Psychoanalysis of Behavior*. New York: Grune & Stratton.

Raine, A. (1991) The SPQ: a scale for the assessment of schizotypal personality based on DSM-IIIR criteria. *Schizophrenia Bulletin* **17**, 555–564.

Raine, A. (2006) Schizotypal personality: neurodevelopmental and psychosocial trajectories. *Annual Review of Clinical Psychology* **2**, 291–326.

Raine, A. & Allbutt, J. (1989) Factors of schizoid personality. *British Journal of Clinical Psychology* **28**, 31–40.

Raine, A. & Lencz, T. (1995) Conceptual; and theoretical issues in schizotypal personality disorder research. In: Raine, A., Lencz, T. & Mednick, S., eds. *Schizotypal Personality*. Cambridge: Cambridge University Press, pp. 3–15.

Raine, A., Lencz, T. & Reynolds, G. (1992) An evaluation of structural and functional prefrontal deficits in schizophrenia: MRI and neuropsychological measures. *Psychiatry Research* **45**, 123–137.

Raine, A., Reynolds, C., Lencz, T. & Scerbo, A. (1994) Cognitive-perceptual, interpersonal, and disorganized features of schizotypal personality. *Schizophrenia Bulletin* **20**, 191–201.

Ramos, B. & Arnsten, A. (2007) Adrenergic pharmacology and cognition: focus on the prefrontal cortex. *Pharmacology and Therapeutics* **113**, 523–536.

Reichenberg, A. & Harvey, P. (2007) Neuropsychological impairments in schizophrenia: Integration of performance-based and brain imaging findings. *Psychological Bulletin* **133**, 833–858.

Renoult, L., Prévost, M., Brodeur, M. *et al.* (2007) P300 asymmetry and positive symptom severity: a study in the early stage of a first episode of psychosis. *Schizophrenia Research* **93**, 366–373.

Rinne, J., Portin, R., Ruottinen, H. *et al.* (2000) Cognitive impairment and the brain dopaminergic system in Parkinson disease: [18F] fluorodopa positron emission tomographic study. *Archives of Neurology* **57**, 470–475.

Roitman, S.E., Cornblatt, B.A., Bergman, A. *et al.* (1997) Attentional functioning in schizotypal personality disorder. *American Journal of Psychiatry* **154**, 655–660.

Roitman, S.E., Mitropoulou, V., Keefe, R.S. *et al.* (2000) Visuospatial working memory in schizotypal personality disorder patients. *Schizophrenia Research* **41**, 447–455.

Ross, R.G., Hommer, D., Radant, A., Roath, M. & Freedman, R. (1996) Early expression of smooth-pursuit eye movement abnormalities in children of schizophrenic parents. *Journal of the American Academy of Child and Adolescent Psychiatry* **35**, 941–949.

Ross, R.G., Olincy, A., Harris, J.G. *et al.* (1998) Anticipatory saccades during smooth pursuit eye movements and familial transmission of schizophrenia. *Biological Psychiatry* **44**, 690–697.

Sanders, J. & Gill, M. (2007) Unravelling the genome: a review of molecular genetic research in schizophrenia. *Irish Journal of Medical Science* **176**, 5–9.

Sanders, A., Duan, J., Levinson, D. *et al.* (2008) No significant association of 14 candidate genes with schizophrenia in a large European ancestry sample: Implications for psychiatric genetics. *American Journal of Psychiatry* **165**, 497–506; erratum 165, 1359.

Sawaguchi, T. & Goldman-Rakic, P. (1991) D1 dopamine receptors in prefrontal cortex involvement in working memory. *Science* **251**, 947–950.

Saykin, A., Gur, R.C., Gur, R.E. *et al.* (1991) Neuropsychological function in schizophrenia. Selective impairment in memory and learning. *Archives of General Psychiatry* **48**, 618–624.

Schade, R., Andersohn, F. & Suissa, S. (2007) Dopamine agonists and the risk of cardiac-valve regurgitation. *New England Journal of Medicine* **356**, 29–38.

Schreiber, H., Stolz-Born, G., Kornhuber, H. & Born, J. (1992) Event-related potential correlates of impaired selective attention in children at high risk for schizophrenia. *Biological Psychiatry* **32**, 634–651.

Schultze-Lutter, F., Ruhrmann, S. & Hoyer, C. (2007) The initial prodrome of schizophrenia: different duration, different underlying deficits? *Comprehensive Psychiatry* **48**, 479–488.

Schulz, P.M. & Soloff, P.H. (1987) Still borderline after all these years. 140th Annual Meeting of the American Psychiatric Association, Chicago, IL.

Schulz, P.M., Schulz, S.C., Goldberg, S.C. *et al.* (1986) Diagnoses of the relatives of schizotypal outpatients. *Journal of Nervous and Mental Disorders* **174**, 457–463.

Seeber, K. & Cadenhead, K. (2005) How does studying schizotypal personality disorder inform us about the prodrome of schizophrenia? *Current Psychiatry Reports* **7**, 41–50.

Seidman, L., Pantelis, C. & Keshavan, M. (2003) A review and new report of medial temporal lobe dysfunction as a vulnerability indicator for schizophrenia: a magnetic resonance imaging morphometric family study of the parahippocampal gyrus. *Schizophrenia Bulletin* **29**, 803–830.

Shallice, T., Marzocchi, G.M. & Coser, S. (2002) Executive function profile of children with attention deficit hyperactivity disorder. *Developmental Neuropsychology* **21**, 43–71.

Shean, G., Bell, E. & Cameron, C. (2007) Recognition of nonverbal affect and schizotypy. *Journal of Psychology* **141**, 281–291.

Shenton, M., Dickey, C., Frumin, M. & McCarley, R (2001) A review of MRI findings in schizophrenia. *Schizophrenia Research* **49**, 1–52.

Shihabuddin, L., Buchsbaum, M.S., Hazlett, E. *et al.* (2001) Striatal size and relative glucose metabolic rate in schizotypal personality disorder and schizophrenia. *Archives of General Psychiatry* **58**, 877–884.

Shioiri, T., Shinada, K., Kuwabara, H. & Someya, T. (2007) Early prodromal symptoms and diagnoses before first psychotic episode in 219 inpatients with schizophrenia. *Psychiatry and Clinical Neurosciences* **61**, 348–354.

Siegel, C., Waldo, M., Mizner, G., Adler, L.E. & Freedman, R. (1984) Deficits in sensory gating in schizophrenic patients and their relatives: evidence obtained with auditory evoked responses. *Archives of General Psychiatry* **41**, 607–612.

Siegel, B.V., Trestman, R.L., O'Flaithbheartaigh, S. *et al.* (1996) D-amphetamine challenge effects on Wisconsin Card Sort test: performance in schizotypal personality disorder. *Schizophrenia Research* **20**, 29–32.

Siever, L.J. (1991) The biology of the boundaries of schizophrenia. In: Tamminga, C.A. & Schulz, S.C., eds. *Advances in Neuropsychiatry and Psychopharmacology, Vol. 1, Schizophrenia Research*. New York: Raven Press, pp. 181–191.

Siever, L.J. (2000) Genetics and neurobiology of personality disorders. *European Psychiatry* **15**, 54–57.

Siever, L. (2005) Endophenotypes in the personality disorders. *Dialogues in Clinical Neuroscience* **7**, 139–151.

Siever, L.J. & Davis, K.L. (2004) The pathophysiology of the schizophrenic disorders: Perspective from the spectrum. *American Journal of Psychiatry* **161**, 398–413.

Siever, L., Haier, R. & Coursey, R. (1982) Smooth pursuit eye movements in non-psychiatric populations: relationship to other "markers" for schizophrenia and psychological correlates. *Archives of General Psychiatry* **39**, 1001–1005.

Siever, L.J., Coursey, R.D., Alterman, I.S., Buchsbaum, M.S. & Murphy, D.L. (1984) Impaired smooth-pursuit eye movement: vulnerability marker for schizotypal personality disorder in a normal volunteer population. *American Journal of Psychiatry* **141**, 1560–1566.

Siever, L.J., Coursey, R.D., Alterman, I.S. *et al.* (1989) Clinical, psychophysiologic, and neurologic characteristics of volunteers with impaired smooth pursuit eye movements. *Biological Psychiatry* **26**, 35–51.

Siever, L.J., Keefe, R., Bernstein, D.P. *et al.* (1990a) Eye tracking impairment in clinically identified schizotypal personality disorder patients. *American Journal of Psychiatry* **147**, 740–745.

Siever, L.J., Silverman, J.M., Horvath, T.B. *et al.* (1990b) Increased morbid risk for schizophrenia-related disorders in relatives of schizotypal personality disordered patients. *Archives of General Psychiatry* **47**, 634–640.

Siever, L.J., Amin, F., Coccaro, E.F. *et al.* (1991) Plasma homovanillic acid in schizotypal personality disorder patients and controls. *American Journal of Psychiatry* **148**, 1246–1248.

Siever, L.J., Kalus, O. & Keefe, R. (1993a) The boundaries of schizophrenia. *Psychiatry Clinics of North America* **16**, 217–244.

Siever, L.J., Amin, F., Coccaro, E.F. *et al.* (1993b) CSF homovanillic acid in schizotypal personality disorder. *American Journal of Psychiatry* **150**, 149–151.

Siever, L.J., Bernstein, D.P. & Silverman, J.M. (1996) Schizotypal personality disorder. In: Widiger, T.A., Frances, A.J., Pincus, H.A. *et al.*, eds. *DSM-IV Sourcebook*, Vol. **2** Washington: American Psychiatric Association, pp. 685–701.

Siever, L.J., Koenigsberg, H.W. & Harvey, P. (2002) Cognitive and brain function in schizotypal personality disorder. *Schizophrenia Research* **54**, 157–167.

Silverman, J.M., Smith, C.J., Guo, S.L. *et al.* (1998) Lateral ventricular enlargement in schizophrenic probands and their siblings with schizophrenia-related disorders. *Biological Psychiatry* **43**, 97–106.

Simone, A., Cattapan-Ludewig, K., Zmilacher, S. *et al.* (2007) Cognitive functioning in the schizophrenia prodrome. *Schizophrenia Bulletin* **33**, 761–771.

Simons, R. & Katkin, W. (1985) Smooth pursuit eye movements in subjects reporting physical anhedonia and perceptual aberrations. *Psychiatry Research* **14**, 275–289.

Skodol, A., Gunderson, J., McGlashan, T. *et al.* (2002) Functional impairment in patients with schizotypal, borderline, avoidant, or obsessive-compulsive personality disorder. *American Journal of Psychiatry* **159**, 276–283.

Smyrnis, N., Avramopoulos, D., Evdokimidis, I. *et al.* (2007a) Effect of schizotypy on cognitive performance and its tuning by COMT val158 met genotype variations in a large population of young men. *Biological Psychiatry* **61**, 845–853.

Smyrnis, N., Evdokimidis, I., Mantas, A. *et al.* (2007b) Smooth pursuit eye movements in 1,087 men: effects of schizotypy, anxiety, and depression. *Experimental Brain Research* **179**, 397–408.

Soloff, P., George, A. & Nathan, S. (1986) Amitriptyline and haloperidol in unstable and schizotypal borderline disorders. *Psychopharmacology Bulletin* **22**, 177–182.

Soloff, P., George, A. & Nathan, S. (1989) Amitriptyline versus haloperidol in borderlines: final outcomes and predictors of response. *Journal of Clinical Psychopharmacology* **9**, 238–246.

Squires-Wheeler, E., Skodol, A.E., Bassett, A. & Erlenmeyer-Kimling, L. (1989) DSM-IIIR schizotypal personality traits in offspring of schizophrenic disorder, affective disorder, and normal control parents. *Journal of Psychiatric Research* **23**, 229–239.

Squires-Wheeler, E., Skodol, A.E. & Erlenmeyer-Kimling, L. (1992) The assessment of schizotypal features over two points in time. *Schizophrenia Research* **6**, 75–85.

Staal, W.G., Hulshoff Pol, H.E. & Schnack, H.G. (2000) Structural brain abnormalities in patients with schizophrenia and their healthy siblings. *American Journal of Psychiatry* **157**, 416–421.

Stevens, A.A., Goldman-Rakic P.S. & Gore J.C. (1998) Cortical dysfunction in schizophrenia during auditory word and tone working memory demonstrated by functional magnetic imaging. *Archives of General Psychiatry* **55**, 1097–1103.

Stuss, D., Stethem, L., Pelchat, G. (1998) Three tests of attention and rapid information processing: An extension. *Clinical Neuropsychology* **2**, 246–250.

Suzuki, M., Zhou, S., Takahashi, T. *et al.* (2005) Differential contributions of prefrontal and temporolimbic pathology to mechanisms of psychosis. *Brain* **128**, 2109–2122.

Swerdlow, N.R., Filion, D., Geyer, M.A. & Braff, D.L. (1995) Normal personality correlates of sensorimotor, cognitive and visuospatial gating. *Biological Psychiatry* **37**, 286–299.

Takahashi, T., Suzuki, M. & Zhou, S. (2006) Temporal lobe gray matter in schizophrenia spectrum: a volumetric MRI study of the fusiform gyrus, parahippocampal gyrus, and middle and inferior temporal gyri. *Schizophrenia Research* **87**, 116–126.

Takahashi, T., Suzuki, M., Hagino, H. *et al.* (2007) Prevalence of large cavum septi pellucidi and its relation to the medial temporal lobe structures in schizophrenia spectrum. *Progress in Neuropsychopharmacology and Biological Psychiatry* **31**, 1235–1241.

Tan, H., Callicott, J., Weinberger, D. (2007) Dysfunctional and compensatory prefrontal cortical systems, genes and the pathogenesis of schizophrenia. *Cerebral Cortex* **17** (Suppl. 1), i171–181.

Tienari, P., Wynne, L. & Läksy, K., (2003) Genetic boundaries of the schizophrenia spectrum: evidence from the Finnish Adoptive Family Study of Schizophrenia. *American Journal of Psychiatry* **160**, 1587–1594.

Torgersen, S., Onstad, S., Skre, I., Edvardsen, J. & Kringlen, E. (1993) "True" schizotypal personality disorder: a study of co-twins and relatives of schizophrenic probands. *American Journal of Psychiatry* **150**, 1661–1667.

Trestman, R.L., Keefe, R.S.E., Mitropoulou, V. *et al.* (1995) Cognitive function and biological correlates of cognitive performance in schizotypal personality disorder. *Psychiatry Research* **59**, 127–136.

Trestman, R.L., Horvath, T., Kalus, O. *et al.* (1996) Event-related potentials in schizotypal personality disorder. *Journal of Neuropsychiatry and Clinical Neuroscience* **8**, 33–40.

Trotman, H., McMillan, A. & Walker, E. (2006) Cognitive function and symptoms in adolescents with schizotypal personality disorder. *Schizophrenia Bulletin* **32**, 489–497.

Tsai, S., Hong, C., Hou, S. & Yen, F. (2006) Lack of association of catechol-O-methyltransferase gene Val108/158Met polymorphism with schizophrenia: a family-based association study in a Chinese population. *Molecular Psychiatry* **11**, 2–3.

Tsuang, M., Gilbertson, M. & Faraone, S. (1991) The genetics of schizophrenia. Current knowledge and future directions. *Schizophrenia Research* **4**, 157–171.

Tsuang, M., Stone, W. & Faraone, S. (1999) Schizophrenia: a review of genetic studies. *Harvard Review of Psychiatry* **7**, 185–207.

Tunbridge, E., Bannerman, D., Sharp, T. & Harrison, P. (2004) Catechol-o-methyltransferase inhibition improves set-shifting performance and elevates stimulated dopamine release in the rat prefrontal cortex. *Journal of Neuroscience* **24**, 5331–5335.

Uhlén, S., Muceniece, R., Rangel, N. *et al.* (1995) Comparison of the binding activities of some drugs on alpha 2A, alpha 2B and alpha 2C-adrenoceptors and non-adrenergic imidazoline sites in the guinea pig. *Pharmacology and Toxicology* **76**, 353–364.

Ullrich, S., Farrington, D. & Coid, J. (2007) Dimensions of DSM-IV personality disorders and life-success. *Journal of Personality Disorders* **21**, 657–663.

Venables, P., Wilkins, S., Mitchell, D. *et al.* (1990) A scale for the measurement of schzotypy. *Personality and Individual Differences* **11**, 481–495.

Viggiano, D., Vallone, D., Ruocco, L. & Sadile, A. (2003) Behavioural, pharmacological, morpho-functional molecular studies reveal a hyperfunctioning mesocortical dopamine system in an animal model of attention deficit and hyperactivity disorder. *Neuroscience and Biobehavioral Reviews* **27**, 683–689.

Voglmaier, M.M., Seidman, L.J., Salisbury, D. & McCarley, R.W. (1997) Neuropsychological dysfunction in schizotypal personality disorder: a profile analysis. *Biological Psychiatry* **41**, 530–540.

Vollema, M. & Hoijtink, H. (2000) The multidimensionality of self-report schizotypy in a psychiatric population: an analysis using multidimensional Rasch models. *Schizophrenia Bulletin* **26**, 565–575.

Waldo, M., Carey, G., Myles-Worsley, M. *et al.* (1991) Codistribution of a sensory gating deficit and schizophrenia in multi-affected families. *Psychiatry Research* **39**, 257–268.

Waldo, M., Adler, L., Leonard, S. *et al.* (2000) Familial transmission of risk factors in the first-degree relatives of schizophrenic people. *Biological Psychiatry* **47**, 231–239.

Walker, E. & Lewine, R. (1990) Prediction of adult-onset schizophrenia from childhood home movies of the patients. *American Journal of Psychiatry* **147**, 1052–1056.

Walker, E. & Walder, D. (2003) Neurohormonal aspects of the development of psychotic disorders. In Cicchetti, D. & Walker, E., eds. *Neurodevelopmental Mechanisms in Psychopathology.* New York: Cambridge University Press, pp. 526–543.

Walters, A., Mandelbaum, D. & Lewin, D. (2000) Dopaminergic therapy in children with restless legs/periodic limb movements in sleep and ADHD: Dopaminergic therapy study group. *Pediatric Neurology* **22**, 182–186.

Wang, Y., Chan, R., Xin, Yu. *et al.* (2008) Prospective memory deficits in subjects with schizophrenia spectrum disorders: A comparison study with schizophrenic subjects, psychometrically defined schizotypal subjects, and healthy controls. *Schizophrenia Research* **105**, 114–124.

Webb, C.T. & Levinson, D.F. (1993) Schizotypal and paranoid personality disorder in the relatives of patients with schizophrenia and affective disorders: a review. *Schizophrenia Research* **11**, 81–92.

Weinberger, D.R. (1987) Implications of normal brain development for the pathogenesis of schizophrenia. *Archives of General Psychiatry* **44**, 660–669.

Weinberger, D.R., Egan, M.F. & Bertolino, A. (2001) Prefrontal neurons and the genetics of schizophrenia. *Biological Psychiatry* **50**, 825–844.

White, P.M. & Yee, C.M. (1997) Effects of attentional and stressor manipulations on the P50 gating response. *Psychophysiology* **34**, 703–711.

White P. & Yee C. (2006) P50 sensitivity to physical and psychological state influences, *Psychophysiology* **43**, 320–328.

Williams, G.V. & Goldman-Rakic, P.S. (1995) Modulation of memory fields by dopamine D1 receptors in prefrontal cortex. *Nature* **376**, 572–575.

Winterer, G., Egan, M., Raedler, T. *et al.* (2003) P300 and genetic risk for schizophrenia. *Archives of General Psychiatry* **60**, 1158–1167.

Wise, R.A. (2004) Dopamine, learning and motivation. *Nature Reviews Neuroscience* **5**, 483–494.

Wright, I., Rabe-Hesketh, S., Woodruff, P. *et al.* (2000) Meta-analysis of regional brain volumes in schizophrenia. *American Journal of Psychiatry* **157**, 16–25.

Yung, R. & McGorry, P. (1996) The prodromal phase of first-episode psychosis: past and current conceptualizations. *Schizophrenia Bulletin* **22**, 353–370.

Yung, A., Phillips, L., Yuen, H. *et al.* (2003) Psychosis prediction: 12-month follow-up of a high-risk ("prodromal") group. *Schizophrenia Research* **60**, 21–32.

Zanettini, R., Antonini, A. & Gatto, G. (2007) Valvular heart disease and the use of dopamine agonists for Parkinson's disease. *New England Journal of Medicine* **356**, 39–46.

Zhou, S., Suzuki, M., Takahashi, T. *et al.* (2007) Parietal lobe volume deficits in schizophrenia spectrum disorders. *Schizophrenia Research* **89**, 35–48.

CHAPTER 6

The prodrome of schizophrenia

Jean Addington[1] and Shôn W. Lewis[2]

[1]Department of Psychiatry, University of Calgary, Canada
[2]Department of Psychiatry, University of Manchester, UK

Introduction

One important current concept is that detection and intervention very early in the course of the illness offers what could be the field's best practical hope for realizing substantive improvements in the outcome of schizophrenia or schizophrenia spectrum disorders. McGlashan *et al.* (2003) suggest that psychosis is "brewing" long before its manifestation as a diagnosable illness and that there are identifiable signs and symptoms that precede the development of frank psychotic symptoms. Typically, early psychosis work targets those who are presenting with a first episode of psychosis. Over the last decade there has been a worldwide movement to develop comprehensive early intervention programs for schizophrenia (Addington, 2008).

Might it be possible to intervene before the onset of the full disorder? Pre-onset studies are more controversial because the development of a disorder is only a probability. These studies deal with the future risk of schizophrenia. Premorbidly, the predictive power of the genetic risk for the disorder is prohibitively small (Cornblatt & Obuchowski, 1997), but it is possible to identify an "at-risk mental state" in which individuals have an ultra-high risk,

i.e., 15–30% chance of developing a full-blown psychotic illness in the medium term. These are individuals who are seeking help for their presenting concerns as well as interventions to delay or prevent the onset of the psychotic illness. In this putatively prodromal phase, the formation of symptoms and disability has already begun, and may provide enough predictive power for the disorder to be tested as a new diagnostic threshold (McGlashan *et al.*, 2003). Many individuals experiencing prodromal symptoms are help-seeking since their symptoms, although attenuated or subthreshold for psychosis, are already debilitating. This raises the importance of intervention in the prodromal stage using preventive approaches, so-called "indicated prevention". Reducing the duration of untreated psychosis (DUP) in the first episode may prevent or limit the future severity of symptoms, chronicity of the disorder, or resultant collateral damage. Goals of treatment in the prodromal phase include all of the above aims plus ameliorating, delaying or even preventing the onset of the disorder. Rapid intervention for individuals experiencing their first episode of psychosis has a high likelihood of resulting in remission of psychotic symptoms. However, it is common for remitted first-episode patients to experience persisting difficulties in everyday functioning. A large percentage of such individuals have difficulty working, and find themselves disabled and unable to support themselves (Addington *et al.*, 2003a,b). It is believed that this disability

Schizophrenia, 3rd edition. Edited by Daniel R. Weinberger and
Paul J Harrison © 2011 Blackwell Publishing Ltd.

develops in the years preceding the onset of psychotic symptoms, the prodromal period, in which social withdrawal and the evolution of negative symptoms form the foundation on which psychotic symptoms develop (Häfner et al., 1999).

What is the prodrome?

The term prodrome describes a retrospective concept because until there is an established psychotic illness such as schizophrenia it cannot be defined (Yung et al., 1996). For those who have a psychotic illness, the prodrome refers to the time period characterized by mental state features which represent a change from a person's premorbid functioning up until the onset of frank psychotic features (Yung et al., 1996). Approximately 80–90% of patients with schizophrenia report a variety of symptoms, including changes in perception, beliefs, cognition, mood, affect, and behavior that preceded psychosis, although approximately 10–20% develop psychotic symptoms precipitously without any apparent significant prodromal period (Yung & McGorry, 1996a). The typical pattern is that the non-specific symptoms and negative symptoms develop first, followed by attenuated, or mild, positive symptoms, together with distress and decreased functioning (Häfner et al., 1998). Although most individuals with schizophrenia have probably experienced a prodromal period, it is less clear how many of those who experience prodromal symptoms will subsequently develop a psychotic illness. Thus, a precondition for early intervention is the accurate detection of prodromal states, i.e. knowing who may be at risk of conversion to psychosis.

Terminology of high-risk syndromes can be confusing. Table 6.1 summarizes their characteristics. Schizotypy is a trait which is genetically related to schizophrenia and appears to confer some increased risk. Isolated psychotic symptoms represent another risk state which has been identified in epidemiological community surveys. Such symptoms are usually self-limiting and not accompanied by distress. "Early" prodromal symptoms are a collection of trait-like perceptual abnormalities (described below), which confer long-term increased psychosis risk. "Late" prodromal symptoms, or clinical high risk, are the focus of this chapter.

Prodromal criteria

If we are interested in practical and useful prepsychotic intervention, we need to address this in those whose risk of converting to psychosis is much higher than the 10% risk that we see in those with high genetic risk, in terms of an affected first-degree relative. One strategy has been the detection of attenuated or subthreshold psychotic symptoms suggestive of imminent psychosis to define a group who appear to be at clinical high risk for psychosis, since this risk is based on detection of these attenuated or subthreshold symptoms. Yung et al. (1996) in Melbourne, Australia developed a specialized clinical setting, the Personal Assistance and Crisis Evaluation Clinic (PACE) to study and treat individuals who present for help and are concerned about symptoms that appear to be psychotic in nature. These individuals have subclinical or attenuated positive symptoms and were considered to be at "ultra-high risk", which is the term adopted by the Melbourne group as a technically correct alternative to "prodromal". Other terms have been introduced such as clinical high risk. In this chapter, for consistency, the term clinical high risk (CHR) will be used to describe those who meet the criteria for a putative prodromal state.

Yung and McGorry (1996a,b) defined criteria for three syndromes that they proposed reflect a CHR for developing a psychotic disorder in the near future (PACE criteria) (Table 6.2). The criteria include the recent onset of a functional decline plus genetic risk (as implied by the presence of pre-existing schizotypal disorder, or a first-degree family history of psychosis), or recent onset of either subthreshold or brief, self-limiting psychotic symptoms which are of insufficient severity or duration to meet diagnostic criteria for an Axis 1 psychotic disorder, such as schizophreniform disorder. Using these new criteria, the risk of converting to

Table 6.1 Terminology and characteristics of at-risk syndromes.

Construct	Alternative names	Increased risk of psychosis	Presence of psychotic symptomatology	Distress	Help seeking	Treatment indicated
Schizotypy	Psychosis proneness	Yes	No	No	No	No
Isolated psychotic symptoms	Psychosis-like symptoms	Yes	Yes	No	No	No
Early prodromal	Basic symptoms	Yes	Yes	Yes	Sometimes	No
Late prodromal	Clinical high risk At-risk mental state Ultra-high risk	Yes	Yes	Yes	Yes	Probably
First-episode psychosis		Yes	Yes	Yes	Usually	Yes

Table 6.2 Melbourne criteria for ultra-high-risk mental state based on Comprehensive Assessment of "At-Risk Mental State" (CAARMS).

1. Vulnerability group
   1.1 First-degree relative with psychosis *or* patient with schizotypal personality disorder
   1.2 30% drop in Global Assessment of Function (GAF) score from premorbid level, sustained for 1 month
   1.3 Change in functioning occurred in the last year

2. Attenuated symptom group
   2.1 Specified severity rating on at least one or more attenuated positive symptoms*
   2.2 Specified frequency rating over a given time period*
   2.3 Symptoms present in past year and for not longer than 5 years

3. Brief Limited Intermittent Psychotic Symtpoms (BLIPS) group
   3.1 Specified severity rating of brief psychotic symptoms*
   3.2 Specified frequency rating over a given time period*
   3.3 Each episode of symptoms is present for <1 week and spontaneously remit on every occasion
   3.4 Symptoms present in past year and for not longer than 5 years

*Range of possible severity and frequency ratings are given in the CAARMS manual.

psychosis increases from approximately 10% in the genetic high-risk group to approximately 30–50% as reported in several studies (Yung *et al.*, 1998a,b). Reliability of this diagnosis has been shown to be excellent, and studies using these criteria support the view that putatively prodromal persons are symptomatic and at high and imminent risk for psychosis (Schaffner & McGorry, 2001). Almost identical criteria, the Criteria for Prodromal Syndrome (COPS), have been developed by McGlashan at Yale University (Miller *et al.*, 2002).

A second approach to operationally identifying these CHR individuals involves examining so-called "basic" symptoms. The basic symptom concept originated in the observation of deficits that were perceived by individuals with schizophrenia often years before the first manifestation of psychotic symptoms. These mild, often subclinical but troublesome, self-experiences of drive and affect, thought, speech, perception, motor action, and vegetative symptoms were called Basic Symptoms. Starting in the late 1960s with Huber in Germany (Gross, 1989), the Bonn Scale for the Assessment of Basic Symptoms (BSABS) was developed and later elaborated on by Klosterkötter *et al.* (1997, 2001). The BSABS assesses self-perceived neuropsychological, perceptual, and mood disturbances, offers detailed psychopathological description of early symptoms, and has demonstrated the ability to predict conversion to schizophrenia over a relatively long time-scale (Klosterkötter *et al.*, 2001). The Cologne Early Recognition Study (CER)

prospectively studied patients in a possible prodromal phase prior to a first episode. In this study of 160 subjects, 49.4% had developed schizophrenia during the 10-year follow-up period. This demonstrates that the presence of certain basic symptoms predicted schizophrenia with a probability of 70% (Klosterkötter *et al.*, 2001), although it has been noted that the original sampling frame comprising patients referred for assessment of psychotic symptoms may have acted to boost this predictive power.

Klosterkötter's group uses both BSABS and COPS in the German Early Recognition Centre where they focus on identifying and treating persons at risk of schizophrenia. What is notable is that BSABS identifies subjects at an earlier stage than does COPS. This allows possible identification of those who may be in the early pre-onset stage of a psychotic illness as well as those in the late pre-onset stage for whom psychosis is potentially more imminent. The terms "early prodromal" and "late prodromal" have been used to define these two at-risk groups.

Studies with CHR cohorts have shown that individuals who meet prodromal criteria experience an extremely diverse array of symptoms and behaviors. These experiences extend beyond the subthreshold psychotic symptoms that form the basis of the criteria, with depression, anxiety, substance use problems, and personality disorder traits commonly reported (Meyer *et al.*, 2005; Svirkis *et al.*, 2005). Although these symptoms do not always reach diagnostic thresholds, 22% of young people who meet prodromal criteria also meet criteria for more than one DSM-IV non-psychotic diagnosis when they are first assessed (Yung *et al.*, 2004). How do we identify these young people? They are distressed; they are functioning poorly and have significant disability. They are help-seeking and are, or at least their parents are, willing to accept professional help. They are different from a subgroup who report isolated psychotic symptoms in the apparent absence of distress, disability or progressive change, and who do not desire assistance.

Assessment and clinical rating scales for the prodrome

There is, therefore, the need for operational instruments to characterize, quantify, and track putatively prodromal symptoms and "at-risk mental states" for clinical and research purposes. In order to promote accurate and valid assessment of CHR individuals, three specific scales have been developed that will only be briefly described here (Addington, 2004).

Comprehensive Assessment of "At Risk Mental State" (CAARMS)

The CAARMS was specifically designed to prospectively measure the psychopathology of the "at-risk mental state"

(ARMS), which is the CHR mental state that may represent the prodrome or precursor state to a first psychotic episode (Yung *et al.*, 1996, 2000; Yung & McGorry, 1996a). Developed in 1994, the CAARMS incorporates seven dimensions of psychopathology, operationally defines the ultra-high-risk criteria for transition, as well as the threshold for established psychosis, and has demonstrated good reliability and predictive validity (Yung, *et al.*, 1996, 2003). A revised version, the CAARMS II, was constructed in 2000. The first aim of the CAARMS is to determine if an individual meets the criteria for an ARMS, i.e., the Melbourne criteria, and to rule out or confirm criteria for acute psychosis. The second purpose is to describe a range of psychopathology and functioning factors over time in these individuals. The CAARMS was designed to be a dimensional instrument capable of quantifying severity and includes more than just the positive symptoms used to define criteria for ARMS. There are seven dimensions with a total of 27 symptoms (Table 6.3). The CAARMS manual (Yung *et al.*, 2000) provides detailed anchor points, definitions, and questions for each symptom, allowing the assessment to be conducted in a semi-structured interview. The positive items are rated on a 0–6 scale with 0 = absent/never and 6 = psychotic and severe. These seven-point scales cover severity variance in the subpsychotic or attenuated range. The other dimensions include items that may be salient during the prodromal phase of psychotic illness, such as negative symptoms, deterioration of role functioning, sleep disturbance, and impaired tolerance to normal stress.

Scale of Prodromal Symptoms (SOPS) and Structured Interview of Prodromal Symptoms (SIPS)

Using the Australian criteria, the Yale group lead by McGlashan developed the Scale of Prodromal Symptoms (SOPS) embedded within a structured interview (Structured Interview of Prodromal Symptoms; SIPS) (Miller *et al.*, 2002, 2003a; McGlashan, 2001). Since the definition of prodromal states also includes the family history, Global Assessment of Function (GAF), and schizotypal personality disorder, these and the SOPS are incorporated in the SIPS. The interview includes 29 questions to probe for each positive symptom item in the SOPS. The SIPS can then be used to determine the presence or absence of a psychotic state, of a prodromal (CHR) state, and of which prodromal state, as well as the severity of the latter once diagnosed. Based on the groups described by Yung *et al.* (1998a) as presented in Table 6.2, McGlashan *et al.* operationalized these groups in the Criteria of Prodromal Syndromes (COPS) (McGlashan *et al.*, 2003; Miller *et al.*, 2002). The COPS criteria are presented in Table 6.4.

The goal of the SIPS and SOPS was to identify operationally the presence of these prodromal symptoms and to measure their severity over time, as well as their ability to predict conversion to actual psychosis. The SOPS, like the

Table 6.3 Comprehensive Assessment of "At-Risk Mental State" (CAARMS).

1. Positive
   1.1. Disorders of thought content
   1.2. Perceptual abnormalities
   1.3. Disorganized speech

2. Cognitive change/attention concentration
   2.1. Subjective experience
   2.2. Observed cognitive change

3. Emotional disturbance
   3.1. Subjective emotional disturbance
   3.2. Observed blunted affect
   3.3. Observed inappropriate affect

4. Negative
   4.1. Alogia
   4.2. Avolition/apathy
   4.3. Anhedonia

5. Behavioral change
   5.1. Social isolation
   5.2. Impaired role functioning
   5.3. Disorganizing/odd stigmatizing behaviors
   5.4. Aggression/dangerous behaviors

6. Motor/physical changes
   6.1. Subjective complaints of impaired motor function
   6.2. Informant reported or observed changes in motor functioning
   6.3. Subjective complaints of impaired bodily sensation
   6.4. Subjective complaints of autonomic functioning

7. General psychopathology
   7.1. Mania
   7.2. Depression
   7.3. Suicidality and self-harm
   7.4. Mood swings/lability
   7.5. Anxiety
   7.6. Obsessive-compulsive disorder (OCD) symptoms
   7.7. Dissociative symptoms
   7.8. Impaired tolerance to normal stress

DSM-IV, defines psychosis as the presence of at least one positive symptom at psychotic intensity for sufficient length of time. In the SOPS, psychosis threshold is defined as the presence of at least one of the five attenuated positive symptoms at a psychotic level of intensity and at sufficient frequency, duration or urgency. Frequency/duration is operationalized as at least 1 hour a day at an average frequency of 4 days per week over 1 month, i.e., definite presence for more than half the days over 1 month. Urgency is any positive psychotic symptom that is seriously disorganizing or dangerous no matter what the duration.

The SOPS was designed as a dimensional instrument with the potential of quantifying severity. In addition to the five attenuated positive symptoms, the SOPS includes

Table 6.4 Criteria of prodromal symptoms (COPS).

1. Genetic risk and deterioration syndrome (GRD)
    1.1 First-degree relative with psychosis *or* relative or patient with schizotypal personality disorder
    1.2 30% drop in Global Assessment of Function (GAF) score from premorbid level, sustained for 1 month
    1.3 Change in functioning occurred in the last year

2. Attenuated positive symptom syndrome (APSS)
    2.1 Rating of 3, 4 or 5 on any one of the five positive symptoms in Scale of Prodromal Symptoms (SOPS)
    2.2 Symptom occurs at above severity level at an average frequency of at least once per week in the past month
    2.3 Symptom must have begun in the past year or currently rate at least one scale point higher than rated 12 months previously

3. Brief intermittent psychotic syndrome (BIPS)
    3.1 Rating of 6 (psychotic intensity) on any one of the five positive symptoms in the SOPS
    3.2 Present at least several minutes per day at a frequency of at least once per month
    3.3 Symptom must have begun in the past 3 months
    3.4 Symptom not seriously disorganizing or dangerous, does not last for > 1 hour a day at an average frequency of 4 days per week over 1 month

Table 6.5 Scale of Prodromal Symptoms (SOPS).

1. Positive
    1.1. Unusual thought content
    1.2. Suspiciousness
    1.3. Grandiosity
    1.4. Perceptual abnormalities
    1.5. Conceptual disorganization

2. Negative
    2.1. Social isolation or withdrawal
    2.2. Avolition
    2.3. Decreased expression of emotion
    2.4. Decreased experience of emotion
    2.5. Decreased ideational richness
    2.6. Deterioration in role functioning

3. Disorganization
    3.1. Odd behavior or appearance
    3.2. Bizarre thinking
    3.3. Trouble with focus and attention
    3.4. Impairment in personal hygiene

4. General symptoms
    4.1. Sleep disturbance
    4.2. Dysphoric mood
    4.3. Motor disturbances
    4.4. Impaired tolerance to stress

negative, disorganized, and general psychopathology scales. The four subscales and symptoms are presented in Table 6.5. Using the SIPS, outpatients were identified who met symptomatic syndromal criteria for the prodrome with excellent interrater reliability. Kappa coefficients of interrater agreement were computed with a mean kappa of 0.81 (Miller *et al.*, 2002). Within the same study, interrater agreement was within the excellent range ($r \geq 0.95$) for the total score of the SOPS and for 17 of the 19 individual items. Values of 0.70 and 0.72 were obtained for the remaining items (Miller *et al.*, 2002). The predictive value of the SIPS was examined in the same sample of 29. These results give a positive predictive value (PPV) of 54%, a psychotic/non-psychotic sensitivity of 1.0, and a specificity of 0.73 (Miller *et al.*, 2002). These results support the validity of the criteria for defining prodromal states that mark high imminent risk for the psychosis-6 scale, but with the difference that the level 6 stands for a psychotic level of severity.

Schizophrenia Prediction Instrument for Adults (SPI-A)

Unlike the CAARMS and SOPS, the SPI-A is aimed at identifying early rather than late prodromal symptoms (see Table 6.1). The SPI-A was developed from work on Basic Symptoms (described above). The BSABS assesses self-perceived neuropsychological disturbances, offers detailed psychopathological description of early symptoms, and

has demonstrated excellent ability to predict conversion to schizophrenia (Klosterkötter *et al.*, 2001).

The Cologne Early Recognition Study (CER) prospectively studied patients in a possible prodromal phase prior to a first episode (Klosterkötter *et al.*, 2001). Following this study, additional work was done on the Bonn Scale. Based first on a hierarchical cluster analysis of the CER data, followed by a confirmatory approach for construct validation (Weineke *et al.*, 2002) with a large inpatient sample, the SPI-A was developed from the total BSABS (Weineke *et al.*, 2002). This instrument has six dimensions with 32 items (Table 6.6).

In a newly published English-language manual (Schultze-Lutter *et al.*, 2007), the SPI-A provides operational definitions for these pre-psychotic deviations, along with typical statements of patients and examples of questions which allow the assessment to be conducted in a semi-structured interview. Besides specific questions, there are general guiding questions for symptoms. Only symptoms that are subjectively experienced by the person and are not present in what the person considers their premorbid stage are assessed as a definite basic symptom (BS).

Transition to psychosis

The above criteria reliably identify young people who are at CHR of psychosis, or who are in the early stages of the

Table 6.6 Schizophrenia Prediction Instrument for Adults (SPI-A).

A. Affective-dynamic disturbances
  A1 Impaired tolerance to certain stressors
    A1.1 Impaired tolerance to unusual, unexpected or specific novel demands
    A1.2 Impaired tolerance to certain social everyday situations
    A1.3 Impaired tolerance to working under pressure of time or rapidly changing different demands
  A2 Change in mood and emotional responsiveness
  A3 Decrease in positive emotional responsiveness towards others

B. Cognitive-attentional impediments
  B1 Inability to divide attention
  B2 Feeling overly distracted by stimuli
  B3 Difficulties concentrating
  B4 Difficulties holding things in mind for less than half an hour
  B5 Slowed-down thinking
  B6 Lack of "thought energy", purposive thoughts

C. Cognitive disturbances
  C1 Increased indecisiveness with regard to insignificant choices between equal alternatives
  C2 Thought interference
  C3 Thought blockages
  C4 Disturbance of receptive speech
  C5 Disturbance of expressive speech
  C6 Disturbance of immediate recall

D. Disturbances in experiencing self and surrounding
  D1 Decreased capacity to discriminate between different kinds of emotions
  D2 Increased emotional reactivity in response to routine social interactions
  D3 Thought pressure
  D4 Unstable ideas of reference
  D5 Changed perception of the face or body of others

E. Body perception disturbances
  E1 Bodily sensations of numbness and stiffness
  E2 Bodily sensations of pain in a distinct area
  E3 Bodily sensations migrating through the body
  E4 Bodily sensations of being electrified
  E5 Bodily sensations of movement or pressure
  E6 Bodily sensations of body/body parts changing size

F. Perception disturbances
  F1 Hypersensitivity to light/optic stimuli
  F2 Photopsia
  F3 Micropsia, macropsia
  F4 Hypersensitivity to sounds/noise
  F5 Changed intensity/quality of acoustic stimuli
  F6 Somatopsychic bodily depersonalization

onset of illness. The 12-month transition rate to full-blown psychosis of young people who meet the ARMS, or late prodromal, criteria approached 40% in earlier follow-up studies despite the provision of supportive psychotherapy and, where appropriate, antidepressant or anxiolytic medication (Cadenhead, 2002; Mason *et al.*, 2004; Miller *et al.*, 2003b; Morrison *et al.*, 2004; Yung *et al.*, 2003). This rate of progression to illness is much higher than the incidence rate in the general population of between 0.2 and 0.5 new cases per 1000 population per year (Jablensky *et al.*, 1992) and the 10–12% statistical risk a child of a parent with schizophrenia has of developing the illness later in life (see Chapter 10).

Two large-scale, multisite studies, one from North America and one from Europe, have aimed to better quantify the level of risk, and also to identify particular predictors of transition to psychosis. In the first, a consortium of investigators from the USA and Canada pooled data from individual prodromal studies using similar or identical CHR criteria, conducted at eight sites. The research centers comprising the North American Prodrome Longitudinal Study (NAPLS) ascertained CHR individuals and followed them at regular intervals for a period of up to 2.5 years (Addington *et al.*, 2007). Although originally developed as independent studies, the sites employed similar ascertainment and longitudinal assessment methods, making it possible to form a standardized protocol for mapping acquired data into a new scheme representing the common components across sites (Addington *et al.*, 2007), yielding the largest database of longitudinally followed CHR cases worldwide. Of the 370 subjects enrolled in the study, 291 (79%) had at least one follow-up assessment. Approximately 35% of these 291 subjects converted to psychosis over the 2.5-year follow-up period (Cannon *et al.*, 2008). Five features assessed at baseline contributed uniquely to the prediction of psychosis: a genetic risk for schizophrenia with recent deterioration in functioning, higher levels of unusual thought content, higher levels of suspicion/paranoia, greater social impairment, and history of substance abuse. Algorithms combining two or three of these variables resulted in dramatic increases in positive predictive power (i.e., to 68–80%) compared with the prodromal criteria alone (Cannon *et al.*, 2008), although this method reduces sensitivity, leading to a higher rate of false negatives. By comparing the transition rates in this sample with the incidence rates for psychosis in the general population over the same time period, it was possible to quantify the relative risk of psychosis at 405.

The European Prediction of Psychosis Study (EPOS; Ruhrman *et al.*, 2010) is a prospective, multicentre European study led from Cologne and including sites in the Netherlands, the UK, Spain, and Norway. Inclusion criteria were the CHR criteria as used in NAPLS, plus the cognitive symptom cluster from SPI-A in help-seeking people aged 16–35. The aims of the study were to assess the rate of transition to psychosis over an 18-month follow-up, plus to identify baseline variables predictive of transition. From the total sample of 245 enrolled, 90% met CHR criteria on the SIPS. Of the 183 who were followed up over 18 months, transition rates of 14% at 12 months and 19% over 18 months' follow-up were seen. DSM-IV diagnosis following transition were schizophrenia in 62%, mood disorder with psychotic features in 16%, and the rest mainly divided between schizoaffective and schizophreniform disorder. Multiple regression analysis, controlling for confounds, identified six baseline variables that independently predicted transition: SIPS positive score (the severity of positive symptoms); bizarre thinking; sleep disturbance; schizotypal personality; low functioning in past year on the GAF scale; and years of education. Combining these into a four-class "prognostic index", as is done with cancer staging for instance, proved useful in refining predictive power. Relating the transition rate data to known incidence rates in the reference population showed a relative risk over 18 months of psychosis in this group to be 365, similar to that of 405 shown in the NAPLS.

Predictors of transition

Several cohort studies and trials have reported on demographic, clinical, and other predictors of transition in samples of people seeking help who meet CHR criteria. There is incomplete overlap between findings, partly because different studies have collected different variables. The best replicated is baseline positive symptom severity, whether this is measured by Positive and Negative Syndrome Scale (PANSS), CAARMS, or SIPS. This was shown in the NAPLS, EPOS, and Melbourne PACE cohort (Yung *et al*, 2003), as well as treatment trials such as the EDIE (Morrison *et al.*, 2004). It seems to predict both transition and time to transition. In the PACE cohort, duration of symptoms also predicted transition. In terms of individual psychotic symptoms, both the NAPLS and EPOS reported that unusual thought content, suspicion/paranoia, and bizarre thinking (a disorganization syndrome feature) predicted transition. The PACE and NAPLS reported negative symptoms also to be predictive, although not as strongly as positive symptoms. Both the NAPLS and EPOS reported low functioning as measured by GAF over the previous year to predict transition. From first principles, it might seem that street drug use, especially cannabis and amphetamines, would predict transition. In the NAPLS, however, a history of any substance use, including alcohol, was a weak predictor.

Cognitive deficits

Over the past 5 years, at least 10 research groups around the world have published results of cognitive functioning during the prodrome to psychosis (Brewer *et al.*, 2006). Findings from cross-sectional studies have consistently documented the presence of widespread cognitive deficits

intermediate between healthy control (HC) and first-episode psychosis (FEP) samples (Hawkins *et al.*, 2004; Keefe *et al.*, 2006) and that cognitive functioning is related to course of illness (Keefe *et al.*, 2006; see also Chapter 8). A number of deficits have been noted in the prodrome, most reliably in spatial working memory (Smith *et al.*, 2006; Wood *et al.*, 2003), verbal declarative learning and memory (Brewer *et al.*, 2005; Hawkins *et al.*, 2004; Lencz *et al.*, 2006), and attention (Francey *et al.*, 2005; Hawkins *et al.*, 2004; Niendam *et al.*, 2006). Executive functions such as verbal fluency and set-shifting have also been implicated but less consistently (Hawkins *et al.*, 2004; Lencz *et al.*, 2006). Some deficits such as sustained attention may represent stable vulnerability markers (Wood *et al.*, 2003; Brewer *et al.*, 2005) while others, such as verbal declarative memory, may be more predictive of conversion to psychosis (Smith *et al.*, 2006; Brewer *et al.*, 2005).

Social functioning

Poor social functioning is a hallmark of schizophrenia. An association between low or deteriorated functioning and onset of psychosis has been reported (Mason *et al.*, 2004; Yung *et al.*, 2003, 2004). For example, Yung *et al.* (2003) reported that a GAF score of 50 or below at baseline was associated with psychosis at 12-month follow-up. In a small sample, Pinkham *et al.* (2007) demonstrated that CHR subjects had significantly impaired social skills relative to normal controls and did not differ from those in the early stages of a psychotic illness. One study examined subjective experience of functioning (particularly in school and work settings) and demonstrated that young CHR individuals were similar to first-episode adolescents in terms of their impairment relative to normal controls (Ballon *et al.*, 2007). In a recent study with a large sample (Addington *et al.*, 2008a), the CHR group did not differ significantly from first- and multi-episode patients on measures of social functioning and work adjustment, and all three groups were impaired relative to a sample of non-psychiatric controls. This study demonstrates that even at the prepsychotic phase of the illness, these young people are demonstrating significant deficits in social functioning. This implies that social deficits are present long before the onset of psychotic symptoms.

In schizophrenia research, an interest in social cognition has recently emerged partly due to its association with poor social functioning. Facial affect recognition is one component of social cognition and it has been well established in the literature that individuals with schizophrenia generally show deficits in both identification and discrimination of facial affect at all stages of the illness. These are stable deficits that appear to be unrelated to symptoms (Addington *et al.*, 2006; Kee *et al.*, 2003). We had already demonstrated that social deficits precede the onset of full-blown symptoms, but also found in this sample of CHR subjects that deficits in facial affect recognition appear to be present before the onset of psychosis and are possibly a vulnerability marker (Addington *et al.*, 2008b).

Imaging findings

Structural brain imaging

In a classical structural magnetic resonance imaging (MRI) experiment, Pantelis *et al.* (2003) tested the hypotheses that measurable structural abnormalities were seen in people with CHR of psychosis, and that progressive changes accompanied that transition. For 75 people with CHR who underwent MRI scans, the 31% who developed psychosis were compared using MR at baseline and follow-up with the 69% who had not. Baseline and 1-year follow-up MRI data from these two subgroups were compared. In the between-group comparison at baseline, the subjects who did develop the disorder had less gray matter in the right medial temporal, lateral temporal, and inferior frontal cortex, and in the cingulate cortex bilaterally, than those who did not make the transition. Furthermore, when re-scanned, individuals who had developed psychosis showed a reduction in gray matter in the left parahippocampal, orbito-frontal, and cerebellar cortices, and the cingulate gyri. This suggests that these changes were progressive and occurred in association with transition to psychosis. The nature of these changes has been further investigated by Sun *et al.* (2009) who used advanced image analysis techniques to show that the changes were particularly seen as surface contraction in the right prefrontal cortex. Overall, these studies suggest that transition to psychosis is accompanied by a patterned loss of gray matter which may well continue during the first years of active illness (see Chapter 16).

Functional brain imaging

Functional MRI (fMRI) studies, like neuropsychological studies, tend to show results in ARMS subjects which are intermediate between subjects with schizophrenia and healthy volunteers. In a study where performance was matched between CHR subjects, first-episode patients and normal controls, fMRI activation deficits were qualitatively the same in CHR as in psychosis. Compared to controls, reduced prefrontal and parietal cortex activation was observed during a verbal working memory task (the n-back task), while verbal fluency performance was associated with reductions in prefrontal and anterior cingulate activation.

Molecular imaging has been helpful in clarifying the neurotransmitter abnormality in ARMS and, by doing this, confirming a pathophysiological continuity with the full psychosis phenotype. Using positron emission (PET) and single photon emission tomography (SPECT) in drug-free patients with acute psychosis, it has been shown in a series of experiments that, although resting dopamine release is not greatly different from that in healthy subjects, a single dose administration of D-amphetamine will lead to a surge in striatal dopamine which is much higher in patients than controls. These experiments constituted the first direct evidence in support of the dopamine hypothesis, initially proposed over 30 years earlier (see Chapter 20). Moreover, the magnitude of this pharmacologically-induced surge in dopamine release was shown to predict acute clinical response to subsequent antipsychotic drug treatment. Further experiments have used related PET imaging techniques such as radiolabeled L-DOPA (6-[^{18}F]fluoro-L-DOPA) uptake to show increased levels of presynaptic dopamine uptake in the striatum in schizophrenia. Howes *et al.* (2009) applied this technique to study striatal dopamine in 24 people with CHR compared to 12 matched healthy volunteers. The results showed that striatal dopamine uptake was significantly elevated in the CHR cases compared to controls. The elevation was confined to the associative subdivision of the striatum, rather than the limbic or sensorimotor subdivisions. Also, there was a significant correlation between dopamine uptake and both CAARMS and PANSS scores in the CHR group ($r = 0.5$), as well as an inverse correlation with semantic verbal fluency. The authors noted that the associative striatum serves to regulate information flow to the prefrontal cortex, which mediates verbal fluency. Whether those CHR cases with the highest levels of presynaptic dopamine uptake will prove to be those most at risk of transition to psychosis remains to be seen.

The work of Howes and colleagues suggests that, at the level of pathophysiology, there is a continuity between the attenuated psychotic symptoms seen in individuals with CHR and those with full psychosis. It still leaves open the question of what factors dictate the transition over the threshold of psychosis and whether there is something inherent in this transition which makes psychosis, and specifically schizophrenia, a more persistent and even progressive disorder.

Intervention in the prodrome

Ideally, providing effective treatment for young people at ultra-high risk of developing a psychotic disorder could potentially stop or at least delay the later conversion to psychosis. Even if it were not possible to completely prevent the development of a psychotic episode, early intervention might minimize the impact that the episode has on functioning, as the development of disability during the prodromal phase of illness creates a ceiling for eventual recovery (Häfner *et al.*, 1995).

The first study to address intervention at this stage was carried out by McGorry *et al.* (2002) in Melbourne, Australia. They randomized 59 CHR subjects to 6 months of active treatment (risperidone 1–3 mg/day plus a modified cognitive-behavioral therapy; CBT) or needs-based intervention. By the end of treatment significantly fewer individuals in the active treatment group had progressed to a first episode of psychosis (9.7% *vs.* 36%). Six months after treatment ended the differences were no longer significant as more of the active treatment group converted to psychosis (19% *vs.* 36%). Adherence to medication suggested a sustained effect as participants in the active treatment group who were compliant with antipsychotic medication were less likely to develop psychosis than those who were less compliant. These results suggest that a combination of antipsychotic medication and CBT may delay but not necessarily prevent the onset of psychosis in symptomatic CHR subjects. Furthermore, McGorry *et al.* (2002) reported that high-risk individuals who did not progress to psychosis showed improvement in a range of symptoms and functioning when they received the combination of risperidone and CBT. This was a landmark study in considering the possibility of delaying or even preventing psychosis. However, as with many early studies, there were some methodological limitations which should be acknowledged. First, there was no blinding of subjects or raters to group assignment. Second, combining pharmacological and psychological treatments in the active treatment group does not allow us to determine the relative contribution of medication or CBT. Third, it was difficult to control for adherence to medication.

A second trial with a more rigorous design was initiated in 1999 by McGlashan *et al.* (2003) at Yale University and included additional sites at Calgary, Toronto and North Carolina. The PRIME (Prevention through Risk Identification Management & Education) study is a randomized double-blind parallel study of 60 CHR subjects comparing the efficacy of a low-dose antipsychotic (olanzapine) *versus* placebo in preventing or delaying the onset of psychosis. Subjects were randomized to medication or placebo for 1 year and then in the second year did not receive any medications. Efficacy measures included the conversion-to-psychosis rate and the SOPS scores. At initial presentation, these subjects were help-seeking and symptomatic with a broad range of attenuated positive and negative symptoms. On average they were rated at study entry as "Moderately Ill" on the Clinical Global Impression (CGI) scale with significant impairment in functioning as indicated by a mean rating of 42 on the GAF scale (Miller *et al.*, 2003b). Short-term analyses at 8 weeks suggested that olanzapine is associated with significantly greater symptomatic improvement in prodromal symptoms than placebo (Woods *et al.*, 2003). At 1-year follow-up, 16% of olanzapine-treated subjects converted to psychosis compared to 35%

of placebo-treated subjects. Furthermore, the hazard of conversion to psychosis among placebo-treated patients was about 2.5 times that among olanzapine-treated patients, a trend level difference (McGlashan *et al.*, 2006). Interpretation of these findings is likely limited by the small sample size. In year two, the conversion-to-psychosis rate did not differ significantly between groups. Of the former olanzapine subjects, three converted (33%), and of the former placebo subjects two (25%) converted. Ruhrmann *et al.* (2007) reported preliminary data from a randomized trial of needs-focused support with or without amisulpride, which showed greater improvements in psychotic symptoms and functioning in the drug treatment group at 12 weeks.

Further, a recently reported naturalistic study indicates that antidepressants may also offer benefits for clinical high-risk youths (Cornblatt *et al.*, 2007). The researchers examined naturalistically prescribed antidepressants (n = 20) and second-generation antipsychotics (n = 28). The two groups did not differ in baseline symptom profiles, with the exception of disorganized thinking, which was more severe in those on second-generation antipsychotic medication. Improvement in three of five positive symptoms over time was significant and similar for both medications. Disorganized thought, however, did not improve with either medication. Twelve of the 48 adolescents developed a psychotic disorder, with all converters having been on antipsychotics, and none on antidepressants. However, treatment outcome was confounded with medication adherence, in that 11 of the 12 converters were non-adherent, and participants were more likely to be non-adherent to second-generation antipsychotics than to antidepressants.

These preliminary reports of trials attempting to prevent or delay onset, with one exception, have involved medications, mainly antipsychotics. Medication seems to alleviate the early symptoms in those who may be prodromal for schizophrenia, and to delay onset. Subjects entering medication trials (McGorry *et al.*, 2002; Miller *et al.*, 2003b) are usually in the late pre-onset period as reflected by their high rate of attenuated psychotic symptoms, poor level of functioning, and high rates of conversion to psychosis. It may be that individuals who are not yet disabled and are less symptomatic may have the potential to benefit from non-medical interventions.

Concerns about early treatment

In the absence of infallible markers of vulnerability or risk of illness, the feasibility, safety, and ethics of early intervention research needs to be seriously considered. Clinical trials using medication with putatively prodromal subjects has generated a great deal of controversy and debate (Bentall & Morrison, 2002). Despite offering some advantages over the first-generation medications (see Chapter 25), there are medical risks associated with the newer antipsychotics, such as weight gain and diabetes (see Chapters 27 and 28). This is of particular concern for false-positive cases. Adherence is also a problem in this group (McGorry *et al.*, 2002) and the use of medications for prevention inevitably leads to the difficult question of how long they should be prescribed.

There is, however, another essential concern. The potential merit in preventing, delaying or attenuating the onset of acute psychotic illness is undeniable from individual, family, and societal perspectives. Yet the majority of these young people choose not to participate in trials and it is therefore likely that results in this field may have been affected by biases in subject selection. For example, data from the Calgary PRIME clinic demonstrated that only 14% of all eligible individuals who met criteria for CHR chose to be in the trial (Addington & Addington, 2005). Forty-seven percent of the eligible subjects were concerned, bothered, and debilitated by their symptoms but did not feel they required medication. Second, those who opted for the medication trial had increased symptoms compared to those who refused the trial. The majority of eligible subjects who had less marked symptoms chose to be involved in a range of interventions that included psychoeducation about risk, management of stress and symptoms, and ongoing monitoring of the symptoms with immediate access to a physician if necessary. This is supported by the 95% rate of participation in the EDIE trial (described below).

Psychological treatment approaches

These issues have led to a logical case for considering the application of psychological treatment approaches for psychotic symptoms in the emergent phase of psychotic disorders. Bentall and Morrison (2002) suggest that the evaluation of psychological treatment approaches in this early phase of psychotic disorders would be a more acceptable and safer first step in the development of preventive interventions, which might in itself reduce or avoid the need for drug treatment. Furthermore, since these subjects are help-seeking, they may benefit from a psychological intervention even if they are false positives (i.e., not at risk of psychosis).

There is one published trial of psychological intervention alone, which was completed in Manchester, UK. The Early Detection and Intervention Evaluation (EDIE) was a single-blind randomized controlled trial of cognitive therapy (CT) with individuals at clinical high risk of psychosis (Morrison *et al.*, 2004). In this study 58 individuals were randomized to either CT or monitoring. CT was provided for the first 6 months and all patients were monitored on a monthly basis for 12 months. CT was found to significantly reduce the

likelihood of progression to psychosis as defined on the PANSS over 12 months (6% *vs.* 22%), of being prescribed antipsychotic medication (6% *vs.* 30%), and of meeting criteria for a DSM-IV diagnosis of a psychotic disorder (6% *vs.* 26%). CT also improved positive symptoms in the sample. It is of note that 95% of eligible subjects consented to participate and that drop-out rates were considerably lower than in the PACE and PRIME trials. A 3-year follow-up study (Morrison *et al.*, 2007) showed that the effects of therapy disappeared, although follow-up rates were only 50%.

The CT utilized in this trial was based on an empirically validated cognitive model of psychosis (Morrison, 2001). The therapy adhered to the structure and principles of CT (Beck, 1976), being time-limited (up to a maximum of 26 sessions over 6 months; average number of sessions was 12), problem-orientated, collaborative, and involving the use of homework tasks and guided discovery. Initial stages of therapy included a cognitive-behavioral assessment, the development of a shared list of problems and goals, and the generation of a case formulation based on the cognitive model. Common techniques, which were collaboratively selected on the basis of a shared case formulation, included the examination of advantages and disadvantages associated with particular ways of thinking and behaving, consideration of evidence, generations of alternative explanations, and the use of behavioral experiments to evaluate beliefs. A comprehensive description is provided in the treatment manual utilized in the trial (French & Morrison, 2004).

There are several arguments to support why CBT may be a beneficial psychological intervention for the CHR group. First, CBT is likely to help with both the attenuated and brief intermittent psychotic symptoms. CBT has demonstrated effectiveness for those with schizophrenia to cope with psychotic symptoms, and to reduce associated distress (Lewis *et al.*, 2002; Pilling *et al.*, 2002; Sensky *et al.*, 2000; Tarrier *et al.*, 1998) and risk of relapse (Birchwood *et al.*, 1989; Gumley *et al.*, 2003). Second, a CBT approach is a valuable intervention for the non-specific emotional problems that are often observed during the at-risk mental state. CBT is an effective treatment for both depression and anxiety, which are common in schizophrenia and in its prodromal stage (Yung *et al.*, 2003). McGorry *et al.* (2002) reported that 37% of those who did not develop a psychotic illness met criteria for either a mood or anxiety disorder. Increased problems with meta-cognition and self-schemas, which are psychological processes typically targeted during CBT, have been observed in those at ultra-high risk (Morrison *et al.*, 2002). CBT approaches have also been useful in addressing substance use, which is believed to be a common and important contributing factor in the development of psychosis in those at risk (van Os *et al.*, 2002). Third, CBT interventions fit very well in a stress–

vulnerability model and may be an invaluable therapy to teach the types of coping strategies that may offer protection against environmental stresses that contribute to conversion (Roberts, 1991). Thus, CBT is the model of psychological intervention that holds the greatest promise for being effective in (1) addressing the range of symptoms and concerns present in the ultra-high-risk period and (2) teaching potentially effective strategies to protect against the impact of environmental stressors that may contribute to the emergence of psychosis. Furthermore, work is beginning in other areas to explore the usefulness of other psychological interventions at this early phase, such as cognitive remediation, group and family work, and a focus on substance use (Addington et al., 2006). See also Chapter 32 for a discussion of CBT in established schizophrenia.

Conclusions

Overall, we believe that there are different phases to the prodromal period of schizophrenic psychosis and that different treatments, including *both* pharmacotherapy and psychological interventions, may be appropriate and effective at different times during this period. Indeed, supporters of the medication trials report that those being randomized for treatment are highly symptomatic and in these trials several individuals convert in the first several weeks, indicating that they were already very close to developing a full-blown psychotic illness. Antipsychotics might be expected to be important in the later phases of the prodrome when attenuated psychotic symptoms are clearly evident and the individual is potentially on the cusp of a conversion. Psychological interventions might be expected to be most promising at earlier and less symptomatic stages of the prodrome. In fact, in the early stages of the prodromal period, the presenting symptoms are not only less severe but also less specific. These individuals present with a wider constellation of concerns. They need and want to understand their perceptual difficulties, to manage the stress, depression, anxiety, sleep disturbance, and decline in functioning, and to be supported through this difficult period (Yung et al., 2003). These symptoms and concerns may be more modifiable with a psychological intervention than with medication.

References

Addington, J. (2004) The diagnosis and assessment of individuals prodromal for schizophrenic psychosis. *CNS Spectrums* **9**, 588–594.

Addington, J. (2008) The promise of early intervention. *Early Intervention in Psychiatry* **1**, 294–307.

Addington, J. & Addington, D. (2005) Clinical trials during the prodromal stage of schizophrenia. *American Journal of Psychiatry* **162**, 1387.

Addington, J., Leriger, E. & Addington, D. (2003a) Symptom outcome one year after admission to an early psychosis program. *Canadian Journal of Psychiatry* **48**, 204–207.

Addington, J., Young, J. & Addington, D. (2003b) Social outcome in early psychosis. *Psychological Medicine* **33**, 1119–1124.

Addington, J., Francey, S. M. & Morrison, A.P. (2006) *Working With People at High Risk of Developing Psychosis: A Treatment Handbook*. Chichester: John Wiley & Sons.

Addington, J., Cadenhead, K.S., Cannon, T.D. et al. (2007) North American Prodrome Longitudinal Study (NAPLS): A collaborative multi-site approach to prodromal schizophrenia research. *Schizophrenia Bulletin* **33**, 665–672.

Addington, J., Penn, D.L., Woods, S.W., Addington, D. & Perkins, D.O. (2008a) Social functioning in individuals at clinical high risk for psychosis. *Schizophrenia Research* **99**, 119–124.

Addington, J., Penn, D.L., Woods, S.W., Addington, D. & Perkins, D.O. (2008b) Facial affect recognition in individuals at clinical high risk for psychosis. *British Journal of Psychiatry* **192**, 67–68.

Ballon, J.S., Kaur, T., Marks, I.I. & Cadenhead, K.S. (2007) Social functioning in young people at risk for schizophrenia. *Psychiatry Research* **151**, 29–35.

Beck, A.T. (1976) *Cognitive Therapy and the Emotional Disorders*. New York: International Universities Press.

Bentall, R.P. & Morrison, A.P. (2002) More harm than good: The case against using antipsychotic drugs to prevent severe mental illness. *Journal of Mental Health* **11**, 351–356.

Birchwood, M., Smith, J., MacMillan, F. et al. (1989) Predicting relapse in schizophrenia: The development and implementation of an early signs monitoring system using patients and families as observers, a preliminary investigation. *Psychological Medicine* **19**, 649–656.

Brewer, W.J., Francey, S.M., Wood, S.J. et al. (2005) Memory impairments identified in people at ultra-high risk for psychosis who later develop first-episode psychosis. *American Journal of Psychiatry* **162**, 71–78.

Brewer, W.J., Wood S.J., Phillips L.J. et al. (2006) Generalized and specific cognitive performance in clinical high-risk cohorts: A review highlighting potential vulnerability markers for psychosis. *Schizophrenia Bulletin* **32**, 538–555.

Cadenhead, K. (2002) Vulnerability markers in the schizophrenia spectrum: Implications for phenomenology, genetics and the identification of the schizophrenia prodrome. *Psychiatric Clinics of North America* **25**, 837–853.

Cannon, T.D., Cadenhead, K., Cornblatt, C. et al. (2008) Prediction of psychosis in ultra high risk youth: A multi-site longitudinal study in North America. *Archives of General Psychiatry* **65**, 28–37.

Cornblatt, B. & Obuchowski, M. (1997) Update of high-risk research: 1987–1997. *International Review of Psychiatry* **9**, 447.

Cornblatt, B.A., Lencz, T., Smith, C.W. et al. (2007) Can antidepressants be used to treat the schizophrenia prodrome? Results of a prospective, naturalistic treatment study of adolescents. *Journal of Clinical Psychiatry* **68**, 546–557.

Francey, S.M., Jackson, H.J., Phillips, L.J., Wood, S.J., Yung, A.R. & McGorry, P.D. (2005) Sustained attention in young people at high risk of psychosis does not predict transition to psychosis. *Schizophrenia Research* **79**, 127–136.

French, P. & Morrison, A.P. (2004) *Early Detection and Cognitive Therapy for People at High Risk of Developing Psychosis: A Treatment Approach.* Chichester: John Wiley & Sons.

Gross, G. (1989) The "basic" symptoms of schizophrenia. *British Journal of Psychiatry* **155**, 21–25.

Gumley, A.I., O'Grady, M., McNay, L., Reilly, J., Power, K.G. & Norrie, J. (2003) Early Intervention for relapse in schizophrenia: results of a 12 month randomized controlled trial of cognitive-behavior therapy. *Psychological Medicine* **33**, 419–431.

Häfner, H., Hambrecht, M., Loffler, W., Munk-Jorgensen, P. & Riecher-Rossler, A. (1998) Is schizophrenia a disorder of all ages? A comparison of first episodes and early course across the life-cycle. *Psychological Medicine* **28**, 351–365.

Häfner, H., Nowotny, B., Löffler, W., an der Heiden, W. & Maurer, K. (1995) When and how does schizophrenia produce social deficits? *European Archives of Psychiatry and Clinical Neuroscience* **246**, 17–28.

Häfner, H., Loffler, W., Maurer, K., Hambrecht, M. & an der Heiden, W. (1999) Depression, negative symptoms, social stagnation and social decline in the early course of schizophrenia. *Acta Psychiatrica Scandinavcia* **100**, 105–118.

Hawkins, K.A., Addington, J., Keefe, R.S.E. *et al.* (2004) Neuropsychological status of subjects at high risk for a first episode of psychosis. *Schizophrenia Research* **67**, 115–122.

Howes, O.D., Montgomery, A.J., Asselin, M.C. *et al.* (2009) Elevated striatal dopamine function linked to prodromal signs of schizophrenia. *Archives of General Psychiatry* **66**, 13–20.

Jablensky, A., Sartorius, N., Ernberg, G. *et al.* (1992) Schizophrenia: manifestations, incidence and course in different cultures. A World Health Organization ten-country study. *Psychological Medicine—Monograph Supplement* **20**, 1–97.

Kee, K.S., Green, M.F., Mintz, J. & Brekke, J.S. (2003) Is emotion processing a predictor of functional outcome in schizophrenia? *Schizophrenia Bulletin* **29**, 487–497

Keefe, R.S.E., Perkins, D.O., Gu, H., Zipursky, R.B., Christensen, B.K. & Lieberman, J.A. (2006) A longitudinal study of neurocognitive function in individuals at-risk for psychosis. *Schizophrenia Research* **88**, 26–35.

Klosterkötter, J., Gross, G., Huber, G., Wieneke, A., Steinmeyer, E. M. & Schultze-Lutter, F. (1997) Evaluation of the "Bonn Scale for the Assessment of Basic Symptoms—BSABS" as an instrument for the assessment of schizophrenia proneness: A review of recent findings. *Neurology, Psychiatry and Brain Research* **5**, 137–150.

Klosterkötter, J., Hellmich, M., Steinmeyer, E.M. & Schultze-Lutter, F. (2001) Diagnosing schizophrenia in the initial prodromal phase. *Archives of General Psychiatry* **58**, 158–164.

Lencz, T., Smith, C.W., Mclaughlin, D. *et al.* (2006) Generalized and specific neurocognitive deficits in prodromal schizophrenia. *Biological Psychiatry* **59**, 863–871.

Lewis, S., Tarrier, N., Haddock, G. *et al.* (2002) Randomised controlled trial of cognitive-behavioral therapy in early schizophrenia: acute-phase outcomes. *British Journal of Psychiatry* **181**, s91–s97.

Mason, O., Startup, M., Halpin, S., Schall, U., Conrad, A. & Carr, V. (2004) Risk factors for transition to first episode psychosis among individuals with "at-risk mental states". *Schizophrenia Research* **71**, 227–237.

McGlashan, T.H. (2001) Psychosis treatment prior to psychosis onset: Ethical issues. *Schizophrenia Research* **51**, 47–54.

McGlashan, T.H., Zipursky, R., Perkins, D.O. *et al.* (2003) A randomized double blind clinical trial of olanzapine vs placebo in patients at risk for being prodromally symptomatic for psychosis: I Study rationale and design. *Schizophrenia Research* **61**, 7–18.

McGlashan, T.H., Zipursky, R.B., Perkins, D. *et al.* (2006) Randomized, double-blind trial of olanzapine versus placebo in patients prodromally symptomatic for psychosis. *American Journal of Psychiatry* **163**, 790–799.

McGorry, P.D., Yung, A.R., Phillips, L.J. *et al.* (2002) Randomized controlled trial of interventions designed to reduce the risk of progression to first-episode psychosis in a clinical sample with subthreshold symptoms. *Archives of General Psychiatry* **59**, 921–928.

Meyer, S.E., Bearden, C.E., Lux, S.R. *et al.* (2005) The psychosis prodrome in adolescent patients viewed through the lens of DSM-IV. *Journal of Child and Adolescent Psychopharmacology* **15**, 434–451.

Miller, T.J., McGlashan, T.H., Rosen, J.L. *et al.* (2002) Prospective diagnosis of the initial prodrome for schizophrenia based on the structured interview for prodromal syndromes: Preliminary evidence of interrater reliability and predictive validity. *American Journal of Psychiatry* **159**, 863–865.

Miller, T.J., McGlashan, T.H., Rosen, J.L. *et al.* (2003a) Prodromal assessment with the Structured Interview for Prodromal Syndromes and the Scale of Prodromal Symptoms: Predictive validity, interrater reliability, and training to reliability. *Schizophrenia Bulletin* **29**, 703–715.

Miller, T.J., Zipursky, R., Perkins, D.O. *et al.* (2003b) A randomized double blind clinical trial of olanzapine vs placebo in patients at risk for being prodromally symptomatic for psychosis: II Recruitment and baseline characteristics of the "prodromal" sample. *Schizophrenia Research* **61**, 19–30.

Morrison, A.P. (2001) The interpretation of intrusions in psychosis: An integrative cognitive approach to hallucinations and delusions. *Behavioural and Cognitive Psychotherapy* **29**, 257–276.

Morrison, A.P., Bentall, R., French, P. *et al.* (2002) Randomised controlled trial of early detection and cognitive therapy for preventing transition to psychosis in high-risk individuals. *British Journal of Psychiatry* **181**, s78–s84.

Morrison, A.P., French, P., Walford, L. *et al.* (2004) Cognitive therapy for the prevention of psychosis in people at ultra-high risk. *British Journal of Psychiatry* **185**, 291–297.

Morrison, A.P., French, P., Parker, S. *et al.* (2007) Three year follow-up of a randomised controlled trial of cognitive therapy for the prevention of psychosis in people at ultra high-risk. *Schizophrenia Bulletin* **33**, 682–687.

Niendam, T.A., Bearden, C.E., Johnson, J.K. *et al.* (2006) Neurocognitive performance and functional disability in the psychosis prodrome. *Schizophrenia Research* **84**, 100–111.

Pantelis, C., Velakoulis, D., McGorry, P. *et al.* (2003) Neuroanatomical abnormalities before and after onset of psychosis: a cross sectional and longitudinal MRI comparison. *Lancet* **361**, 281–287.

Pilling, S., Bebbington, P., Kuipers, E. *et al.* (2002) Psychological treatments in schizophrenia: I Meta-analyses of family intervention and cognitive behavior therapy. *Psychological Medicine* **32**, 763–782.

Pinkham, A.E., Penn, D.L., Perkins, D.O., Graham, K. & Siegal, M. (2007) Emotion perception and social skill over the course of psychosis: a comparison of individuals "at risk" for psychosis and individuals with early and chronic schizophrenia spectrum illness. *Cognitive Neuropsychiatry* **12**, 198–212.

Roberts, G. (1991) Delusional belief system and meaning in life: a preferred reality. *British Journal of Psychiatry* **158**, 19–28.

Ruhrmann, S., Bechdolf, A., Kuhn, K.U. *et al.* (2007) Acute effects of treatment for people putatively in a late initial prodromal phase of psychosis. *British Journal Psychiatry* **51** (Suppl.), 88–95.

Ruhrmann, S., Schultze-Lutter, F., Salokangas, R.K. *et al.* (2010) Prediction of psychosis in adolescents and young adults at high risk: results from the prospective European prediction of psychosis study. *Archives of General Psychiatry* **67**, 241–251

Schaffner, K.F. & McGorry, P.D. (2001) Preventing severe mental illnesses—new prospects and ethical challenges. *Schizophrenia Research* **51**, 3–15.

Schultze-Lutter, F., Addington, J., Ruhrmann, S., Klosterkotter, J. & Giovanni Fioriti Editore (2007) *Schizophrenia Proneness Instrument, Adult Version (SPI-A).* Rome, Italy.

Sensky, T., Turkington, D., Kingdon, D. *et al.* (2000) A randomized controlled trial of cognitive-behavioral therapy for persistent symptoms in schizophrenia resistant to medication. *Archives of General Psychiatry* **57**, 165–172.

Smith, C.W., Park, S. & Cornblatt, B. (2006) Spatial working memory deficits in adolescents at clinical high risk for schizophrenia. *Schizophrenia Research* **81**, 211–215.

Sun, D., Stewart, G.W., Jenkinson, M. *et al.* (2009) Brain surface contraction mapped in first episode schizophrenia: a longitudinal magnetic resonance imaging study. *Molecular Psychiatry* **14**, 976–986.

Svirkis, T., Korkeila, J., Heinimaa, M. *et al.* (2005) Axis I disorders and vulnerability to psychosis. *Schizophrenia Research* **75**, 439–446.

Tarrier, N., Yusopoff, L., Kinney, C. *et al.* (1998) Randomized controlled trial of intensive cognitive behavior therapy for patients with chronic schizophrenia. *British Medical Journal* **317**, 303–307.

van Os, J., Bak, M., Hanssen, M., Bijl, R.V., de Graaf, R. & Verdoux, H. (2002) Cannabis use and psychosis: a longitudinal population-based study. *American Journal of Epidemiology* **156**, 319–327.

Weineke, A., Schultze-Lutter, F., Picker, H., Steinmeyer, E.M., & Klosterkotter, J. (2002) The Schizophrenia Prediction Instrument (SPI-A): first preliminary results of the evaluation study. *Schizophrenia Research* **53**, S37.

Wood, S.J., Pantelis, C., Proffitt, T. *et al.* (2003) Spatial working memory ability is a marker of risk-for-psychosis. *Psychological Medicine* **33**, 1239–1247.

Woods, S.W., Breier, A., Zipursky, R.B. *et al.* (2003) Randomized trial of olanzapine versus placebo in the symptomatic acute treatment of the schizophrenic prodrome. *Society of Biological Psychiatry* **54**, 453–464.

Yung, A.R. & McGorry, P.D. (1996a) The initial prodrome in psychosis: Descriptive and qualitative aspects. *Australian and New Zealand Journal of Psychiatry* **30**, 587–599.

Yung, A.R. & McGorry, P.D. (1996b) The prodromal phase of first-episode psychosis: Past and current conceptualizations. *Schizophrenia Bulletin* **22**, 353–370.

Yung, A.R., McGorry, P.D., McFarlane, C.A., Jackson, H.J., Patton, G.C. & Rakkar, A. (1996) Monitoring and care of young people at incipient risk of psychosis. *Schizophrenia Bulletin* **22**, 283–303.

Yung, A.R., Phillips, L.J. & McGorry, P.D. (2004) *Treating Schizophrenia in the Prodromal Phase.* London: Taylor & Francis.

Yung, A.R., Phillips, L.J., McGorry, P. *et al.* (1998a) Can we predict the onset of first-episode psychosis in a high-risk group? *International Clinical Psychopharmacology* **13**, S23–S30.

Yung, A.R., Phillips, L.J., McGorry, P. *et al.* (1998b) Prediction of psychosis: A step towards indicated prevention of schizophrenia. *British Journal of Psychiatry* **172**, 14–20.

Yung, A.R., Phillips, L.J., McGorry, P.D., Ward, J.L. & Thompson, K. (2000) *The comprehensive assessment of at-risk mental states (CAARMS).* Melbourne: University of Melbourne.

Yung, A.R., Phillips, L.J., Yuen, H. *et al.* (2003) Psychosis prediction: a 12-month follow-up of a high-risk ("prodromal") group. *Schizophrenia Research* **60**, 21–32.

CHAPTER 7

Course and outcome

Wolfram an der Heiden[1] and Heinz Häfner[2]

[1]Central Institute of Mental Health, Mannheim, Germany
[2]University of Heidelberg, Heidelberg, Germany

Introduction

Studies on the natural history of schizophrenia aim at shedding light on the variance in the natural course and outcome, on the spectrum of consequences, as well as on the factors influencing the disorder. Kraepelin (1893), preoccupied with the course of dementia praecox throughout his professional life, believed he had found the basis for this "disease entity" in the combination of symptomatology and course. In the end, his belief was shaken when he came to realize the great variety of courses (Kraepelin, 1920).

Most recent longitudinal studies have, of necessity, examined the treated rather than the natural course of schizophrenia. The only exceptions have been retrospec-

tive investigations limited to periods before first professional contact or studies following up placebo controls, but these are limited because of ethical problems with studying highly selected patient groups over short periods to assess the efficacy of therapeutic interventions.

Time trends

Since the turn of the 19th century, the length of hospital stay after first admission has decreased progressively, as consistently shown by several authors (Brown, 1960; Häfner & an der Heiden, 1982). Ødegård (1964) demonstrated this on successive cohorts of patients from the national Norwegian case register discharged in the periods 1936–1942, 1945–1952, and 1955–1959.

Time trends in the frequency and length of hospital stay fail to provide valid indicators of the course of the illness,

Schizophrenia, 3rd edition. Edited by Daniel R. Weinberger and
Paul J Harrison © 2011 Blackwell Publishing Ltd.

because they are influenced by disease-independent factors (Burns, 2007). an der Heiden *et al.* (1995) demonstrated in a long-term (15.6-year) first-episode study of schizophrenia a widening gap between fairly stable mean symptom scores for 10 cross-sectional assessments, and a continued decrease in hospital days per year. Simultaneously, outpatient contacts increased, reflecting the change in the system of mental-healthcare, while the treatment prevalence and the illness course have remained more or less unchanged.

Equally difficult to assess are time trends in the impact of therapy on the long-term course of schizophrenia. Shepherd *et al.* (1989) reviewed selected 20th-century outcome studies of schizophrenia and found a substantial increase in recovery rates since the 1950s. In contrast, Warner (1985), in his more comprehensive, but still selective, review, concluded that the recovery rate had scarcely improved since the early years of the 20th century.

A meta-analysis (Hegarty *et al.*, 1994) of 320 longitudinal studies that fulfilled minimum methodological standards found a recovery rate of 35% for the period 1895–1955 and a rate of 49% for 1956–1985, possibly indicating a favorable effect of neuroleptics. In the following period characterized by second-generation neuroleptics, 1986–1992, however, the rate fell back to 36%. The authors stress the difficulties in interpreting these results, e.g., the changes between these time periods in the diagnostic criteria used (Loranger, 1990; Stoll *et al.*, 1993). Furthermore, Hegarty *et al.* (1994) pointed out that not a single study they reviewed was based on a truly representative cohort.

Bleuler (1968) reported the impression that the number of "catastrophic" and severe chronic cases had decreased since the beginning of the 20th century. This sounds plausible considering the fact that acute and severe psychotic symptoms can be cured or alleviated by antipsychotic drugs, as Häfner and Kasper (1982) showed with the gradual disappearance of life-threatening catatonia in Germany. Secondary impairment (Wing & Brown, 1970) caused by social deprivation in old mental hospitals is outdated. However, the remedies currently available reduce neither predisposition to the illness nor chronic courses. Since the 1970s and 1980s the system of care provided for people with schizophrenia in most developed countries and, as a result, the social biographies of persons affected have undergone marked changes, as early recognition and intervention, outpatient treatment, and complementary care have become more and more widespread.

Methodological aspects of course and outcome research

Systematic studies into the medium- and especially the long-term course of schizophrenia require considerable effort. This explains the small number of pertinent studies and the even fewer number that meet the time-consuming methodological requirements (Castle, 2000; Gaebel & Frommann, 2000; Jablensky, 1995; Ram *et al.*, 1992). The limited standardization of study methodology leads to a considerable variation in results. For example, the proportion of recovered patients ranges from 7% (Marneros *et al.*, 1991) to 58% (Bland *et al.*, 1976). To obtain comparable results, a minimum standard of general study characteristics is required (Castle, 2000; Castle & Morgan, 2008):

- Definition of the study population;
- Research design;
- Selection of life domains (social performance, etc.) and illness domains (syndromes, etc.) for the assessment of course and outcome.

Study population

The *inclusion criteria*—diagnosis being the most important—may produce very different study sample compositions. For example, diagnostic criterion C1—persistence of symptoms for at least 6 months—for a DSM-IV diagnosis of schizophrenia (American Psychiatric Association, 1994) excludes more acute cases of schizophrenia with a good prognosis than criterion G1 in ICD-10 does, which requires persistence of symptoms for only at least 4 weeks. Only if the cohort at entry into a longitudinal study is representative of all cases diagnosed with schizophrenia in a given population or of a precisely defined subgroup, e.g. late- or early-onset schizophrenia, will the results be valid for the disorder or for the subgroup in question.

An optimal solution is a population-based prospective assessment of real-onset cases. However, due to an annual incidence rate as low as 1–2 cases per 10 000 population, including a high percentage of uncharacteristic onsets (Häfner, 1995), it is impractical to search for real-onset cases by door-to-door surveys. For this reason, first episodes are usually recruited from among first contacts with treatment services by excluding multiple episodes. It remains a controversial question whether a treated incidence calculated from inpatient data is a valid estimate of the true incidence. According to the few comparative studies addressing this question, the "lifetime" risk—its definition is variable—for persons with schizophrenia of coming into contact with inpatient services ranges from 50% to 100% (Engelhardt *et al.*, 1982; Geddes & Kendell, 1995; Goldacre *et al.*, 1994; Link & Dohrenwend, 1980; Thornicroft & Johnson, 1996; von Korff *et al.*, 1985). As the proportion of cases in inpatient care decreases with the extension of outpatient care, case recruitment should be extended to outpatient services as well. In countries with a hospital-centered system of mental healthcare, a practical alternative is to recruit first admissions for schizophrenia over a long period from all the mental hospitals serving a defined population or from case registers.

A major problem, especially with studies covering long periods, is the question whether the patient samples assessed at follow-up are representative of the initial samples (Riecher-Rössler & Rössler, 1998).

Another reason for distorted results of longitudinal studies is the considerable variation in the individual follow-up periods. An ideal solution, but one which is difficult to comply with, would be identical lengths of illness course for all individuals included in a study. For the same reason, entering subjects at different stages of illness progression should be avoided (Castle, 2000; Jablensky, 1995). In the earlier generation of long-term follow-up studies, the samples included were invariably recruited from among hospitalized cases who differed considerably in the duration of pretreatment illness (Clarke & O'Callaghan, 2003; Häfner, 2003b).

For the reasons stated, the first hospital admission is usually chosen to mark the beginning of the study. First admission, which is usually triggered by psychotic episodes, takes place at illness stages with maximum symptom presentation (Häfner *et al.*, 1995). When an initial assessment taken at around the time of hospital admission is compared with a later follow-up, the result will show an artifact of improvement, because at any cross-sectional assessment after recovery from the first episode only about 20% of the patients will be experiencing a psychotic episode (Häfner & an der Heiden, 1986; Wiersma *et al.*, 1996).

Research design

Robins (1979) distinguished three types of designs for longitudinal studies. In "follow-back" studies, case identification takes place at follow-up, e.g., by including only hospitalized patients with a duration of illness of 10 years or more. Illness onset and history are traced retrospectively from the patient's memory and/or clinical records. This design misses favorable outcomes not fulfilling the inclusion criteria.

In "real-time" prospective studies, inclusion in the study and assessments start at illness onset/first admission. Ideally, all assessments are conducted on the same cohort by the same investigators using the same instruments. This is an ideal design. Several researchers have used data from "real-time" short-term prospective studies to carry out an additional long-term follow-up assessment (e.g., an der Heiden *et al.*, 1995; Carpenter & Strauss, 1991; Harrison *et al.*, 2001; Mason *et al.*, 1996; Wiersma *et al.*, 1998). The most recent example is the WHO Coordinated Multicenter Study on the Course and Outcome of Schizophrenia (ISoS; Hopper *et al.*, 2007).

The third design, "retrospective" or "historical" cohort study (Rothman, 2002), represents a kind of compromise between "follow-back" and "real-time" prospective studies. Case identification takes place retrospectively at the beginning of the chosen follow-up period. Samples are recruited from admission or discharge records and thus inclusion is based on available data, which tend to differ in quality.

Hospital admission or discharge records alone (e.g. Eaton *et al.*, 1992a,b; Engelhardt *et al.*, 1982; Maurer, 1995) do not provide a sufficiently valid picture of illness course. Instead, they are suited to describing treatment careers or for monitoring patients' need for treatment. Local or national analyses based on case-register data provide information for planning and monitoring services, but not for a detailed analysis of the course of schizophrenia.

Longitudinal studies limited to an initial assessment and one follow-up retrospectively reconstruct the illness course over a long interval: Ciompi & Müller (1976), median period 36.9 years, age range less than 10–65 years; Huber *et al.* (1979), mean age 22.4 years, range 9–59 years; the Northwick Park Study (Johnstone, 1991), range 3–13 years; the Chestnut Lodge Study (McGlashan, 1984a,b), mean 15 years, range 2–32 years; the Vermont Longitudinal Study (Harding *et al.*, 1987a), follow-up at 5–10 years and 20–25 years, range 2–32 years. In the review by an der Heiden (1996), 34 of 50 studies spanning 10 years or more relied on a single follow-up assessment.

Some of the latest generation of long-term studies have included several waves of assessment before the final follow-up. In the Washington International Pilot Study of Schizophrenia (IPSS) (Carpenter & Strauss, 1991) patients were re-assessed 2, 5, and 11 years after first assessment. In their first-episode study over 15 years, Harrow and Jobe (2007) carried out five follow-up assessments. In the ABC (Age, Beginning, Course) first-episode study a population-based subsample was followed up at 6 months, 1, 2, 3, 5, and 12 years after first admission (Häfner *et al.*, 2008). In the Mannheim first-episode cohort of the WHO Collaborative Study on Impairments and Disabilities Associated with Schizophrenic Disorders (Jablensky *et al.*, 1980) probands were examined at 10 cross-sections over a period of 15.5 years (an der Heiden *et al.*, 1996). In this way illness course can be reconstructed on the basis of a greater number of assessments and shorter intervals. A small number of short- or medium-term studies (e.g., Ventura *et al.*, 2004) assessed illness course at very short intervals of, for example, 14 days, by quick-to-use instruments (e.g., the Brief Psychiatric Rating Scale; BPRS; Overall & Gorham, 1962).

Most instruments used for assessing the course of schizophrenia are cross-sectional in nature. They aim to provide data on the current state, usually focusing on periods 2–4 weeks preceding the interview. For measuring symptoms retrospectively over longer periods (1) information on reliability is scattered (e.g., Andreasen *et al.*, 1981; Keller *et al.*, 1987; McGuffin *et al.*, 1986, Zimmerman *et al.*, 1988) and (2) information on validity is almost non-existent (an der Heiden & Krumm, 1991).

A number of longitudinal studies focus on outcome. When analyzing changes in illness course over time, and over long periods of time in particular, it is necessary to distinguish between the comparison of initial and final follow-up—outcome research—and the analysis of the occurrence and/or persistence of changes in symptoms, functional impairment and their consequences in the interval between these follow-ups, including the construction of transphenomenal patterns of illness or trajectories. Such patterns or trajectories offer a possibility to describe the main psychopathological phenomena over time and they can serve as diagnostic criteria and as a basis for predicting future illness course in clinical practice.

Outcome studies provide information on changes in patients' illness status and life situation after a lengthy duration of illness. For studies of this type, there are approved and reliable instruments available. However, this approach, too, does not produce comparable results automatically. In Harding et al.'s (1987a,b) follow-up study of 168 inpatients with schizophrenia over a period of 32 years, 68% had a good global outcome, as operationalized by a Global Assessment Scale (GAS) score greater than 61 (Endicott et al. 1976). In comparison, Breier et al.'s (1991) study of 58 chronic patients with schizophrenia over 13 years on average, using the same instrument and measure (GAS score > 61), yielded a good outcome in only 3%.

The concepts for describing the course and outcome depend on the issues looked at. When the aim is to evaluate treatment measures, standardized, illness course-related indicators of the effectiveness and side effects of therapies are chosen. In studies on the course of schizophrenia, standards, which would allow direct comparisons of the results, are more or less lacking. One reason for this is that none of the designs can really do without using retrospective data from varying periods of time (see above).

Indicators for describing course and outcome

For the purposes of clinical and rehabilitative practice, there is a growing demand for indicators that in addition to measuring global outcome allow a differential assessment of certain domains of outcome and effects of treatment.

Today the main criteria for describing the course of schizophrenia are symptoms, cognitive and social functioning, impairment, and disability (closely associated with the illness), as well as personality-related and environmental characteristics, less closely or not associated with the illness, such as demographic and socioeconomic status, illness behavior, and quality of life. Strauss and Carpenter (1972, 1974) distinguished four domains in schizophrenic illness—without implying a causal association with the illness or other factors, which, according to the authors, are only loosely connected with one another ("open-linked systems") or with external characteristics of the illness course: social relations, occupational status, and treatment. Carpenter (2007) recommended dividing schizophrenia into (psycho-)pathologocical domains and studying their course. An important question in this context is what are the clearly distinguishable domains that make up the disease construct of schizophrenia and what are the associated psychological phenomena, e.g., coping with illness, quality of life, etc., and the environmental factors involved. Of particular interest are the symptom dimensions and the functional deficits accompanying the disorder, and the question of their interdependence versus independence. Several authors have tested these hypotheses (Breier et al., 1991; Kirkpatrick & Galderisi, 2008; Stephens et al., 1980). They reported pronounced associations between symptom measures, negative symptoms on the one hand and domains of functioning on the other. Many authors, however, did not find any correlation between changes on different symptom-related or functional dimensions and the course of schizophrenia (Gupta et al., 1997; Loebel et al., 1992; Tohen et al., 1992). An important reason for this might lie in the differences of the trajectories of these domains: for example, positive symptoms have an episodic course, negative symptoms show a higher degree of stability, and neuropsychological impairment, occupational, and marital status undergo the smallest degree of change. As a result, cross-sectional analyses and, hence, outcome at follow-up are bound to yield low correlations (an der Heiden et al., 1996; Breier et al., 1991).

Course types of schizophrenia

Without an identifiable etiology and with a distinct underlying pathophysiology still rather obscure, the disease construct of schizophrenia is currently based on tradition, clinical experience, and conventional definitions of the diagnosis. The sets of operational criteria on which the diagnosis of schizophrenia is based produce a rather heterogeneous spectrum of illness courses. For this reason the search for subtypes that help to explain this heterogeneity has been on for a long time.

Kraepelin was among the first to describe subtypes of schizophrenia on the basis of the symptoms presenting: a paranoid-hallucinatory, a hebephrenic, and a simple type. Dementia simplex, a frequent diagnosis in those days, is now rarely made, probably because modern diagnostic techniques permit most such cases to be attributed to other causes, such as neurodegenerative disorder. Whether the hebephrenic subtype, characterized by social and cognitive impairment, is explained by a progressive, malign illness course or by environmental risk factors, such as social deprivation, is yet to be clarified. Systematic analyses of Kraepelin's syndromal subtypes with regard to their courses have not yet yielded any clear-cut results except for the probability of the persistence (negative symptoms, deficits) or recurrence (psychotic episodes) of existing syndromes.

The subtypes given in the ICD-10 classification (World Health Organization, 1993) follow the Kraepelinian tradition, whereas those included in the DSM-IV (American Psychiatric Association, 1994) take some account of symptom dimensions generated by statistical analysis. Later attempts to validate these clinical subtypes on their types of course (e.g., Deister & Marneros, 1993; Fenton & McGlashan, 1991a; World Health Organization, 1979) have also failed to produce conclusive results. More recent attempts aim to distinguish biologically homogeneous subtypes. These are based on distinct symptom dimensions, e.g. primary negative (Blanchard *et al.*, 2005; Carpenter *et al.*, 1988; Dollfus *et al.*, 1996; Hwu *et al.*, 2002; Roy *et al.*, 2001; Stahl & Buckley, 2007), anhedonia (Schürhoff *et al.*, 2003), age at onset (Palmer *et al.*, 2001; Sato *et al.*, 2004; Schürhoff *et al.*, 2004; Welham *et al.*, 2000), biological indices [e.g., electrodermal activities and electroencephalogram (EEG); Sponheim *et al.*, 2001], intellectual functioning (Heinrichs *et al.*, 1997; Maccabe *et al.*, 2002) or neuropsychological deficits (Holthausen *et al.*, 2002; Seaton *et al.*, 2001). These characteristic features of the disorder can demonstrate the typical course of the domain in question. Differences in the courses of these domains indicate that schizophrenia is not a unitary disease process.

Of lasting value have been Kraepelin's attempts to reduce the great variety of course types of schizophrenia to a few simple *trajectories*. The efforts undertaken in his wake on the basis of categories such as stable, progressing and remittent, or psychosis *versus* disability, have produced course typologies whose number range from a mere four (Watt *et al.*, 1983) to as many as 79 (Huber *et al.*, 1979) (for further course types, see also Bleuler, 1972; Leon, 1989; Thara *et al.*, 1994). Ciompi (1980) added to Kraepelin's course types—simple and undulating—two further stages at the beginning and the end: onset (acute, chronic) and end state (recovery or mild, moderate or severe residua). Attempts to classify the patients of five long-term studies (Burghölzli study: Bleuler, 1972; Lausanne study: Ciompi & Müller, 1976; Vermont study: Harding *et al.*, 1987b; ISoS study: Harrison *et al.*, 2001; Chicago study: Marengo *et al.*, 1991) according to the Ciompi scheme have largely failed to show agreement (Häfner & an der Heiden, 2003).

The categories of "florid" (Kraepelin, 1893) or "acute" *versus* "chronic" (primarily negative, unproductive) symptoms are presumed to arise from different neurobiological processes (Andreasen & Olsen, 1982; Crow, 1980a,c). While the diagnosis is mainly based on symptoms—the aim being diagnostic exclusiveness—the psychological impairments (e.g., of attention, cognition, affect, speech) are less specific (Heaton *et al.*, 2001; Heinrichs & Zakzanis, 1998), because they are also encountered in other disorders, e.g., in severe

major depressive disorder. Like symptoms, the behavioral anomalies are classified as disease-inherent factors, i.e., factors associated with the disorder and its course (Schubart *et al.*, 1986).

The subdivision into a deficit and non-deficit type of schizophrenia (Carpenter *et al.*, 1988; for a review, see Kirkpatrick & Galderisi, 2008) and the distinction of Kraepelinian schizophrenia by the intensity of cognitive impairment (Keefe *et al.*, 1996) represent a further attempt to label patients according to outcome/severity with prognostic consequences for the illness course. Empirical analyses of symptoms (Bralet *et al.*, 2002; Keefe *et al.*, 1987; Kilzieh *et al.*, 2003) and magnetic resonance imaging (MRI) research (Buchsbaum *et al.*, 2002, 2003; Mitelman *et al.*, 2005) seem to delineate Kraepelinian schizophrenia, but they actually only reflect limited sections from the total schizophrenia spectrum. The hypothesis postulating autonomous psychopathological processes is still awaiting validation.

Positive and negative symptom dimensions

The terms "negative" and "positive" stem from Reynolds (1858). The underlying concept was later substantiated by Jackson's (1887) hierarchical model, according to which deficit symptoms are classified as primary or lower-level nervous dysfunctions, and secondary symptoms, such as psychosis, as reflecting responses from a higher level of the central nervous system. This clear distinction of two categories of schizophrenic symptoms is clinically useful. It gives the complex psychopathology a simple order and seems justified by different course types, outcomes, and therapy responses.

Based primarily on a distinction between positive and negative symptom dimensions, Crow (1985) proposed a dichotomous biological model: Type I schizophrenia with psychotic symptoms and good prognosis without cognitive impairment; caused by dopaminergic dysfunction, it should respond well to antidopaminergic treatment; Type II schizophrenia with a clinical poverty syndrome (Wing & Brown, 1970) and a poor prognosis, and caused by brain lesions *in utero* or perinatally. Type II was explained by stable neurodevelopmental deficits.

According to Crow, Type I and II schizophrenia were expressions of coexisting, but independent, pathophysiological processes, but he did not specify how they were related to one another. Actually, neither cross-sectionally nor over the course of the disorder have these two types been shown to be mutually exclusive (Addington & Addington, 1991; Eaton *et al.*, 1995; Marneros *et al.*, 1995; Maurer & Häfner, 1991; Peralta *et al.*, 1992).

Another attempt to categorize the symptomatology of schizophrenia and distinguish types of illness course by the positive–negative dichotomy was undertaken by Andreasen and Olsen (1982). After failing to validate their own study by means of factor analysis, the authors tried to analyze the symptoms and course of schizophrenia based on one single dimension. At one extreme were cases characterized by brain anomalies, negative symptoms, and poor prognosis; at the other extreme were cases with positive symptoms, good outcome, and no cognitive impairment. The results of their follow-up study of first episodes of schizophrenia over 4 years lead the authors finally to abandon the model (Andreasen, 1990).

Negative symptoms are a frequent and fairly persistent characteristic of a poor prognosis. First emerging at the prodromal stage, mostly in conjunction with depression and long before the first psychotic episode (Gourzis et al., 2002; Häfner et al., 1995), they cannot be just a residuum of a florid or psychotic episode, as postulated by Kraepelin (1893). Carpenter et al. (1988) distinguished between primary and secondary negative symptoms. The primary negative or deficit syndromes (anhedonia, flattening and narrowing of affect, poverty of speech, avolition, and reduced social activity), the authors believed, precede psychosis onset and frequently persist over the entire course of the disorder. These syndromes neither respond to antipsychotic treatment nor vary with depressive symptoms, anxiety or dosage of medication [Schedule for Deficit Syndrome (SDS); Kirkpatrick et al., 1989; Kirkpatrick & Galderisi, 2008].

In Jablensky's (2000) opinion, it is more plausible to presume a continuum of negative symptomatology with two extremes differing in their prognosis: a severe deficit syndrome at one end and a mild negative syndrome at the other.

Primary negative symptoms, by definition, are traits. They should be stable over time and largely independent of environmental factors (Carpenter & Kirkpatrick, 1988). In contrast, the amount and course of secondary negative symptoms, such as psychomotor poverty/slowness, anergia, social withdrawal, and lack of perseverence, are presumed to fluctuate with psychotic episodes, depression, side effects of medication, and physical morbidity (Carpenter et al., 1991; Kirkpatrick & Galderisi, 2008; Whiteford & Peabody, 1989).

An attempt to test the validity of this hypothesis showed that the course of the secondary or "non-deficit syndrome" did not depend on extrinsic factors, as originally expected. In contrast, the more severely ill subgroup with "primary" negative symptoms showed significant correlations with these factors, whereas the group with secondary negative symptoms did less so (Maurer & Häfner, 1991). The authors interpreted this result according to Jablensky's (2000) model: patients with a deficit syndrome, who are more severely ill than patients presenting "milder" non-deficit negative symptoms, are also more sensitive to adversity.

Functional and cognitive impairment

A growing body of evidence has emerged indicating that negative symptoms might have a pathophysiological basis distinct from that of positive symptoms. In this context, their association especially with cognitive impairment and brain dysfunctions has been explored (Addington & Addington,1991; Arndt et al., 1995; Bell & Mishara, 2006; Lieberman et al., 2001b; Stahl & Buckley, 2007; Tamminga et al., 1998).

Persons with schizophrenia—compared with healthy controls—are, on average, impaired in several neuropsychological tests (e.g., visual and auditory attention, working and episodic memory, executive functions and language, to the degree of 0–2 SDs; Eastvold et al., 2007; Goldberg et al., 2003; Heinrichs & Zakzanis, 1998; Kane & Lencz, 2008; Kurtz, 2005). The amount and profile of cognitive and functional impairment vary between individuals, ranging from absence of any impairment to presence of severe cognitive deficits. The most frequent type is the impairment of working memory and other executive functions, which indicate dysfunction in the prefrontal areas (Pantelis et al., 1999; Perlstein et al., 2001; Weinberger & Berman, 1996). Keefe (2008) called for adding cognitive impairment to DSM-V as a diagnostic criterion for schizophrenia. Some authors supported the idea, but Kane and Lencz (2008) contradicted him, rightly pointing out that while the standard deviatons in schizophrenia were profound (maximum 2 SD) the small differences between schizophrenia and depression (around 0.5 SD) demonstrate only limited specificity.

With regard to the course of cognitive deficits, Saykin et al. (1994) demonstrated that the onset and profiles of cognitive impairment in 37 new, untreated cases of schizophrenia hardly differed from those of unmedicated, formerly treated patients with long histories of illness, as also subsequently demonstrated by Albus et al. (1996) in a large number of cases. Sobizack et al. (1999), too, found no differences in memory functions, speech, and cognitive flexibility/abstraction between 66 first-episode patients and 49 chronic cases of schizophrenia. However, both patient groups differed highly significantly from 40 healthy controls.

A review based on 15 studies with follow-up periods of 1 year or more (Rund, 1998) also showed that the mean values for deficits in verbal skills, memory, and attentional span are fairly stable over time. Profiles of cognitive impairment at early and later stages of schizophrenia, including in patients receiving antipsychotic treatment, indicate fairly reliably that, as long as we lack the means of treating them effectively, cognitive and functional deficits are bound to persist almost unchanged in the course of the disorder (Bilder et al., 2000; Buchanan et al., 2005; Goldberg et al., 1993). Hence, from the first episode on, a stable pattern of the neuropsychological deficits exists in most patients and persists for a lifetime. Only a small group of patients shows gradual progression of these deficits over the course of schizophrenia. Harvey *et al.* (1998, 1999) reported that a certain proportion of patients with long illness courses experience mostly slow, but serious decline in cognitive and functional abilities in old age, i.e., beyond age 65 years. The authors stress that this form of "schizophrenia dementia" is free of the pathology encountered in Alzheimer disease (Harvey *et al.*, 1999). The causes of these late and rare, presumably neurodegenerative, processes are still obscure.

Clear-cut and stable deficits can be interpreted as indicating structural brain changes. Goldberg *et al.* (1993) explain them as a "static" encephalopathy, other authors as stable vulnerability factors (Nopoulos *et al.*, 1994; Nuechterlein & Dawson, 1984; Rund *et al.*, 1997). They correspond to the neurodevelopmental model of schizophrenia (Murray & Lewis, 1987; Weinberger, 1995). The question of their onset is not easy to answer: the latest analyses based on genetically defined high-risk cases of the Edinburgh study (Johnstone *et al.*, 2002, 2005) and descriptively defined ultra-high-risk cases of the Melbourne study (Yung *et al.*, 2003) show that prior to psychosis onset there is a clear increase in cognitive deficits and in pre-existing brain anomalies (also see Fuller *et al.*, 2002; Ho *et al.*, 2003a; Keshavan *et al.*, 2005). Hence, it is reasonable to presume that cognitive impairment occurring premorbidly or accumulating in the prodromal period represents an exacerbation of a neurodevelopmental disorder (Jarskog *et al.*, 2004; Wood *et al.*, 2004). After the early illness stage, the majority of patients, however, show no progression of the neuropsychological parameters, of the cognitive one in particular, in the medium and long term.

Functional and cognitive impairment and symptoms

While in some studies an association between positive symptoms and cognitive functioning has not been demonstrated (Goldberg *et al.*, 1993; Hoff *et al.*, 1999; Weickert *et al.*, 2000), weak to medium-sized positive correlations have been found between negative symptoms and cognitive deficits (Addington & Addington, 2000; Bilder *et al.*, 1985; Carlsson *et al.*, 2006; McGurk & Mueser, 2003; Milev *et al.*, 2005; Paulsen *et al.*, 1995; Putnam & Harvey, 2000).

In most of these studies, the association between negative symptoms and cognitive impairment was analyzed based on comparisons between first-episode samples and samples with long histories of illness. Attempts to analyze the relation between both domains longitudinally, e.g., by determining whether change in neuropsychological functioning is accompanied by change in negative symptoms, have not revealed any clear correlations. Hughes *et al.*

(2002) assessed 62 patients with chronic DSM-IV schizophrenia and found no evidence of a relationship between changes in negative symptoms and cognitive function (IQ, verbal fluency, verbal memory) over time. However, both dimensions showed only little change, and cross-sectionally, cognitive impairments were strongly correlated with seven negative symptoms from the Positive and Negative Syndrome Scale (PANSS) (Kay *et al.*, 1987). Bell and Mishara (2006), too, did not find an association between change in negative symptoms and neurocognition in a larger group of 267 patients with schizophrenia.

In contrast, Gold *et al.* (1999) found that changes in verbal and full-scale IQ were significantly related to changes in negative but not positive or disorganized symptoms. A few studies have reported positive correlations between negative symptoms and cognitive impairment in the course of schizophrenia (e.g., Censits *et al.* 1997), but not on the basis of associated changes in the two variables. Tandon *et al.* (2000) found that in 60 drug-free patients with DSM-IIIR schizophrenia enduring negative symptoms, which the authors distinguished from phasic symptoms, these were significantly associated with lower scores in a few neuropsychological tests (IQ, reaction time, and verbal fluency), while negative symptoms of the phasic type were not. Low cognitive performance at admission was a predictor of negative symptoms at year 1, but not at year 3, in a study of 120 first-episode patients with a DSM-IV psychotic disorder, including affective psychosis (Carlsson *et al.* 2006).

Thus, results for the association of negative symptoms and cognitive impairment over the course of schizophrenia are not fully consistent. While in most cross-sectional studies the two dimensions show low to medium-size correlation coefficients, they exhibit either no or weak positive correlations for changes over the course of the illness. The lack of consistency is probably accounted for by the small degree of change these dimensions undergo.

Cognitive impairment and brain anomalies

Except at the early stages of illness and in a few deteriorating cases, negative symptoms and neuropsychological deficits do not generally seem to progress. Does this also hold good for the morphological and functional brain anomalies involved? Like cognitive deficits, they are already measurable in the first illness episode (Fannon *et al.*, 2000; Ho *et al.*, 2003b; Lawrie, 2004; Weinberger, 1995). Based on their review of 34 studies of various designs, Antonova *et al.* (2004) reported the well-known correlation between brain volume and general intelligence, and a number of correlations between specific alterations in brain structure and mostly non-specific cognitive deficiencies in schizophrenia. In a review of 65 studies of patients with schizophrenia who had never been treated with antipsychotic medications, Torrey (2002) found significant abnormalities in brain structure and function. In many studies, however, the degree of morphological changes shows no correlation with the duration of illness (Harrison *et al.*, 2003; Johnstone, 1999; Lawrie & Abukmeil, 1998; Lewis, 1990; Nair *et al.*, 1997).

In an MRI study comparing 34 recent-onset patients with schizophrenia with a chronically ill group (n = 22) and normal controls (n = 14), Chakos *et al.* (2005) found that hippocampal volumes were smaller in older/chronic patients than in younger patients, as compared with age-matched controls. Similar results were reported by Lieberman *et al.* (2001a), Hulshoff Pol *et al.* (2002), Velakoulis *et al.* (2002), and Woods *et al.* (2005). Patients at a high genetic risk for schizophrenia (Lawrie *et al.*, 1999; Schreiber *et al.*, 1999) already frequently show signs of volume reduction in the hippocampus and adjoining temporal gyri in premorbid examinations. In cases with transition to psychosis, the atrophy tends to increase (Lawrie, 2004; Pantelis *et al.*, 2003).

Mildly progressing morphological brain changes associated with cognitive and/or functional impairment can be found not only in the most active early course in high-risk individuals (Lawrie, 2004; Nair *et al.*, 1997), but also in the long-term course (Cahn *et al.*, 2002; Falkai *et al.*, 2004; Rapoport *et al.*, 1999). In a prospective 5-year follow-up study, DeLisi *et al.* (1997) compared 50 first-admission patients with a DSM-IIIR diagnosis of schizophrenia with 20 age-, sex- and IQ-matched controls by means of automated MRI analysis. They found a significant reduction in brain volume and gray matter in the period studied, but no regional or white matter reduction in subjects with schizophrenia. The widespread cognitive deficits, already present at first admission, remained stable in the course of the disorder and showed no correlation with morphological brain changes. Only the verbal memory deficit increased in parallel with brain atrophy. In severe and mainly deteriorating cases of childhood-onset schizophrenia, Jacobsen *et al.* (1998) found progressive reduction in temporal lobe volume and Keller *et al.* (2003) progressive loss of cerebellar volume.

In males with schizophrenia, Mathalon *et al.* (2001) found mild, progressive volume reduction associated with clinical deterioration. The progression in brain volume reduction was associated with pronounced neurocognitive changes present at inclusion, which did not remit in the 5 years studied. Gender-specific associations were also reported by Antonova *et al.* (2004) who reviewed 35 MRI studies carried out since 1990: the overall brain volume tended to correlate both with general intelligence and detailed cognitive functions in female, but not in male, patients with schizophrenia.

Ho *et al.* (2003b) found small, but ongoing, morphological changes in the brains of 73 patients with recent-onset DSM-IV schizophrenia over the 3 years following initial assessment and despite continued antipsychotic drug treatment. These progressive changes appeared to concentrate around the frontal lobes and to correlate with functional impairment. Woods (1998), too, reported slight increases in morphological brain changes subsequent to the first illness episode in comparison with healthy controls.

With reference to the considerable methodological problems of such long-term studies, which require sophisticated, time-consuming, and expensive assessment methods, the current state of knowledge on progressive brain changes in the course of schizophrenia can be summarized as follows: childhood-onset and severe cases with a high genetic load appear to be associated with mild progressive brain changes located primarily in the prefrontal cortex and the hippocampus. In less severe, adult-onset cases of schizophrenia, progressive changes exceeding normal age-related phenomena are rare. It has not yet been possible to demonstrate a causal association between these changes and specific symptoms. Moreover, it has been noted in several studies that antipsychotic drug treatment also correlates with progressive changes on MRI scanning, raising the possibility that these changes may not be fundamental characteristics of the pathological course of the illness.

Course of empirical symptom dimensions

Following the early attempts to reduce the diversity of schizophrenic symptoms to a few latent variables (Bilder *et al.*, 1985; Lorr *et al.*, 1963; World Health Organization, 1973), the factor-analytical studies by Liddle (1987a,b) and Liddle and Barnes (1990) have attracted widespread attention. In their three-factor model, negative symptoms (affective non-response, apathy, anhedonia) loaded on a single factor, called psychomotor poverty. Delusions, hallucinations, and psychotic thought disorders loaded on a more restricted psychotic factor (reality distortion). The authors called a third factor, including speech and thought disorders, a disorganization syndrome. Liddle (1994) presumed that psychomotor poverty and disorganization are located in two different regions of the frontal lobe. The factor "reality distortion" was associated with fewer deficits.

From studies which include social parameters, a social-dysfunction factor was added to the three-factor model (Peralta *et al.*, 1994; Toomey *et al.*, 1997). A five-factor solution with additional depressive and manic dimensions is found when measures of affective symptoms are not excluded (Lindenmayer *et al.*, 2004).

The number of factors required to explain an optimum degree of the variance depends on the type and number of symptoms fed into the model and on the patient sample studied (Jablensky, 2000). Samples of chronic patients deliver fewer positive and depressive symptoms

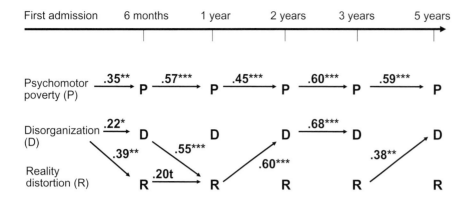

Pearson correlations: t: p < 0.1; *:p < 0.05; **:p <0.01; ***: p <0.001

Fig. 7.1 Correlations within and between syndrome ratings at six points in time over 5 years. The factors were tested by explorative orthogonal factor analysis at each of the five follow-ups. ABC subsample of 115 first episodes (from Löffler & Häfner, 1999b with permission from Elsevier).

than patients in psychotic episodes. Instruments yielding data on most of the affective symptoms also produce a depression factor, particularly in first-admission samples (Arora *et al.*, 1997; Davidson & McGlashan, 1997; Kay & Sevy, 1990; Salokangas, 1997; White *et al.*, 1997), or an overall neuroticism factor (Rey *et al.*, 1994), which more or less encompasses the depression factor.

It appears that the latent symptom factors generated from established cases of psychosis provide reasonably replicable solutions in diagnostic groups over time, but the factor structure may be less stable around the time of first presentation (Drake *et al.*, 2003; Löffler & Häfner, 1999a).

The stability and change over time in the symptom dimensions of schizophrenia have not been much studied yet. Arndt *et al.* (1995) showed the validity of Liddle's three-factor model over 2 years and Salokangas (1997) over 5 years, both in samples of first-episode patients. The three factors varied independently of each other. In both studies the negative and the delusion factor remained stable until follow-up.

Löffler and Häfner (1999a,b) assessed 115 patients with first illness episodes of schizophrenia from the ABC sample at six cross-sections from illness onset to 5 years after first hospital admission. They compared four models: the severity-liability model (Gottesman *et al.*, 1987), Andreasen and Olsen's (1982) bipolar symptom model, Crow's (1980b,c) two-factor model, and Liddle and Barnes' (1990) three-factor model—by means of confirmatory factor analysis. Only Liddle and Barnes' three-factor model produced results that were in satisfactory agreement with the data. As expected, all symptoms showed significant positive loadings on the three factors, but the associations with risk factors and clinical variables did not have much power in discriminating between the three dimensions. The only exceptions were disorganization, associated with a higher degree of familial loading, and the negative factor, which showed significant correlations with pre- and peri-natal complications, although the coefficients were low throughout the measurements.

Figure 7.1 illustrates the stability of and the transitions occurring between the three factors tested at each of the five follow-up assessments. The factor "negative symptoms" remained stable and independent of the other factors over the whole period of observation, showing significant or highly significant coefficients with each new follow-up. The factors "disorganization" and "positive symptoms" showed inconsistent and low correlations at the follow-ups. Contrary to the two other factors, which showed no prognostic power with respect to social outcome, the presence of negative symptoms at 6 months after first admission, mostly after the remission of the acute episode, was a highly significant predictor of the patients' social status up until 3-year follow-up (Löffler & Häfner, 1999b).

The dimensions "positive symptoms" and "disorganization" appear not to be separable as two independent and stable factors in the medium-term course. Negative symptoms, stable over time, associated with overall functional impairment, and of prognostic power, constitute the only factor so far that might reflect independent brain dysfunction persisting after the first illness episode.

Cechnicki and Walczewski (1999) in a controlled prospective study with follow-ups at 1, 3, and 7 years, and Biehl *et al.* (1986) in a study of a sample of patients at first-admission with schizophrenia (ICD-8/9: 295) followed up at seven cross-sections over 5 years applied a clinical approach and obtained different results: small to medium-sized correlations between positive and negative symptom sum scores. Lenzenweger *et al.* (1991) and Löffler and Häfner (1999a) have suggested a plausible explanation: the two modes of operationalizing positive and negative symptom scores differ in subsuming disorganization symptoms under the positive and negative clusters or treating them as a separate category. The correlations sometimes found between positive and negative symptoms can be explained by their covariation with disorganization symptoms (Fenton & McGlashan, 1991b). These findings once more underscore that both the clinical symptom clusters and the latent symptom dimensions are merely heuristic representations of specific patterns of dysfunction and impairment—not free from overlap—and their underlying brain anomalies.

Since categorical diagnoses are usually of limited prognostic power and the inclusion criteria frequently comprise characteristics of illness course, van Os et al. (1996, 1999), Ratakonda et al. (1998), Peralta et al. (2002), Rosenman et al. (2003), Murray et al. (2005), and Dikeos et al. (2006) studied the question of whether the prediction of course and outcome could be improved by focusing on symptom dimensions. Categorical diagnoses, such as that of schizophrenia according to DSM-IV with its 6-month criterion, have been shown to better predict duration of illness (Peralta et al., 2002), use of support services, and a deteriorating course (Rosenman et al., 2003). However, understandably, it is not possible to reliably predict single outcome domains, such as level of impairment during episodes, deterioration in functioning or response to antipsychotic treatment either by categorical or dimensional models (Dikeos et al., 2006). For this reason van Os et al. (1996) and Allardyce et al. (2007) suggest applying a combination of categorical and dimensional representations of psychosis in patients with psychotic disorder, because this is considerably better than either representation alone. In other words, with regard to our still limited knowledge of the disease construct of schizophrenia and its neurobiological components, for practical purposes, expressing patients' functioning, disabilities, and symptoms both dimensionally and categorically may be more useful in predicting outcome than either one alone.

Prepsychotic prodromal stage and early psychotic stage

As mentioned, the study of the transformation from health to the prodromal stage of schizophrenia in prospective population studies is faced with the problems of the low incidence rate, the poor predictive power of developmental antecedents (Jones, 1999; Malmberg et al., 1998), and the frequent onset of schizophrenia with non-specific signs (Häfner & Maurer, 2003).

One of the difficulties in generating biological indicators of the onset of the disorder lies in the fact that current knowledge of the underlying neurobiological disease process is still limited. Most of the biological changes are trait factors that are associated with lifetime risk, but not causally involved in onset (Cornblatt et al., 1998; Isohanni et al., 1999).

For these reasons, psychosis onset can currently be depicted only retrospectively with self-experienced symptoms and observable behavior. Nonetheless, the monitoring of these signs of the disorder and of accompanying neuropsychological and neurophysiological changes from the earliest possible timepoint on is a highly promising approach to modeling the early course of schizophrenia and to early preventive action (see Chapter 6).

Prodromal symptoms and behaviors include mood symptoms (e.g., depressive mood, anxiety, dysphoria, and irritability), cognitive symptoms (e.g., distractibility and difficulty concentrating), social withdrawal, obsessive behaviors and—mostly after a prepsychotic stage—also brief (<1 week) attenuated positive symptoms (e.g., illusions, ideas of reference, and magical thinking), to name but a few (Davidson & McGlashan, 1997; Häfner et al., 2003b; Yung & McGorry, 1996). The most frequent prepsychotic symptoms belong to two dimensions: depressive (most frequent) and negative (second in frequency). Among the latter are indicators of cognitive impairment, such as difficulty with thinking and concentration, and loss of energy, pointing to early consequences of the disorder.

On the basis of IRAOS data collected in the ABC cohort of 232 first episodes of schizophrenia, Häfner et al. (1999b) found that prodromal symptoms, such as social impairment, depressed mood along with loss of self-confidence, and feelings of guilt, tended to occur an average of 4.8 years (median: 2.3 years) before psychosis onset with odds ratios ranging from 3 to 5 compared with healthy controls. Positive symptoms appeared 1.3 years (median: 0.8 years) before first admission. At the prepsychotic prodromal stage most of the depressive and negative symptoms appeared. After the appearance of the first psychotic symptom—mainly in the last year preceding the climax of the first episode—all three symptom categories accumulated rapidly.

All the milestones of the early illness course—first symptom, first negative and positive symptom, climax of the episode (=maximum of symptoms)—have shown a widely reported significant age difference of 3–4 years between the sexes (e.g., Leung & Chue, 2000; Thorup et al., 2007), which is crucial for the social course of the illness.

The distribution of the durations of early illness course is markedly skewed: 33% of cases with schizophrenia spectrum disorder took less than 1 year to develop; 18% had an acute type of onset of 4 weeks or less, and 68% a chronic type of onset of 1 year or more. Only 6.5% started with positive symptoms exclusively, 20.5% presented with both positive and negative symptoms within the same month, and 73% with depressive, negative or non-specific symptoms, thus experiencing a prepsychotic prodromal stage.

Besides the type of onset, the duration of pretreatment illness appears to be determined also by patients' help-seeking behavior, social isolation, availability of care, and premorbid functioning (Drake *et al.*, 2000; Larsen *et al.*, 2004; Morgan *et al.*, 2006; Norman *et al.*, 2007; Skeate *et al.*, 2002; Verdoux *et al.*, 2001).

Risk factors or prodromal signs?

The identification in the population at risk of prodromal symptoms that could potentially predict the onset of psychotic illness would offer a good chance for early intervention. To date, the majority of studies have concentrated on subclinical, attenuated or brief (≤1 week) positive symptoms. Epidemiological study results from the US, France, the Netherlands, New Zealand, the UK, and Germany suggest that the lifetime prevalence of subclinical psychotic experiences is high (Eaton *et al.*, 1991; Kendler *et al.*, 1996; Poulton *et al.*, 2000; Spauwen *et al.*, 2003; van Os *et al.*, 2000; Verdoux *et al.*, 1998; Wittchen *et al.*, 2004), fluctuating around 5–20% depending on the type of psychotic-like experiences (e.g., single *vs.* multiple hallucinations, one-time *vs.* frequent occurrence) and the age of the population studied. The identification of such subclinical psychotic experiences and their predictive power for the transition to full-blown psychosis are of great interest for early intervention.

Prepsychotic prodromal signs and symptoms are non-specific in nature. They may occur without a temporal association with a first psychotic episode. Prodromal stages, too, can remit. From a clinical point of view, non-specific subclinical psychotic symptoms, especially if they have manifested themselves in childhood, should not be classified as part of the illness course. They are attracting a keen interest today in the context of etiological hypotheses and preventive prospects.

Chapman *et al.* (1994) found elevated rates of transition to psychotic disorders in individuals who had rated high on magical ideation and perceptual aberration on their Chapman Scales (Chapman *et al.*, 1976) 10 years previously. In the Dunedin birth-cohort study (Silva & Stanton, 1996), children who had reported hallucinations at age 11 years showed a 16-fold risk (25%) for schizophreniform disorder at age 26 years compared with children without psychotic experiences (Poulton *et al.*, 2000).

The Swedish conscript study (Malmberg *et al.*, 1998) among 50054 young men aged 18–20 years showed that deficits in socializing are a crucial prognostic indicator: the four items "having fewer than two friends", "preference for socializing in small groups", "feeling more sensitive than others", and "not having a steady girlfriend" were associated with a high relative risk (OR 30.7) for being hospitalized with a diagnosis of schizophrenia in a period of 15 years after first assessment. However, in the total sample, a positive response to all four items predicted psychosis only in 3%, because of the high prevalence of these features in the male population of that age.

Davidson *et al.* (1999) and Rabinowitz *et al.* (2000) studied 16–17-year-old male conscripts born during a 7-year period in Israel. Using the National Hospitalisation Psychiatric Case Register, the authors identified 692 individuals who had been hospitalized for schizophrenia for the first time in an average period of 9 years following the initial testing. The results for these subjects, who were compared with the entire conscript population and matched controls, pointed in the same direction as the results of the Swedish study. With effect sizes ranging from 0.40 to 0.58, the young males later hospitalized for schizophrenia faired significantly worse in cognitive and behavioral functioning than did controls. As in the Swedish study, the main indicator of risk for psychosis was poor social functioning with an effect size difference of 1.25.

Hanssen *et al.* (2005) followed-up a representative population-based sample of 7076 individuals aged 16–65 years from the Dutch NEMESIS study for 2 years. Cases with psychotic experiences showed a 2-year transition rate to psychotic disorder of 8%, representing a greater than 60-fold increase in risk compared to those without incident psychotic experiences. The risk for developing psychosis in need of treatment was about 3% for those experiencing one psychotic symptom, 14% for those with two, 20% for those with three, and 50% for those with four. These results reveal a dose–response relationship, as did those of a prospective population German study (Wittchen *et al.*, 2004).

Persons who at inclusion in the same Dutch study reported having had hallucinations showed an elevated risk (16%) of developing psychosis if they had also experienced depression in the first year of the follow-up period (Krabbendam *et al.*, 2005).

When short follow-up periods of up to 3 years are being studied, a higher proportion of prodromal stages of already evolving cases will be included among the symptom carriers compared with longer or lifetime follow-up periods. This fact should be kept in mind when looking at the high rates of transitions to psychosis in these studies in comparison with long-term follow-up studies.

In terms of its functional relevance, a robust result was yielded by the controlled 3–5-year follow-up of a carefully assessed young population cohort aged 14–24 years at inclusion in Germany (Wittchen *et al.*, 2004). The authors demonstrated a continuous distribution of Composite International Diagnostic Interview (CIDI)-based psychotic symptoms in the population. An increase in depressive symptoms during the follow-up period led to an elevated risk for schizophrenia spectrum disorder (odds ratio 2.92), and the odds ratio for developing schizophrenia increased to 1.92 if anxiety was present. When depressive symptoms decreased in that period, the odds ratio for developing psychosis fell to 0.69 and to 0.61 when anxiety decreased. These findings suggest that prepsychotic prodromal symptoms may represent psychopathological expressions of the underlying neurobiological process, which may evolve into a psychotic stage, remain unchanged or remit.

Related questions are (1) How many individuals have subclinical psychotic experiences that *remain* subclinical and (2) How many of these symptoms *disappear* over time. In the above-mentioned Dutch epidemiological study, Hanssen *et al.* (2005) found that 8% of people who had had any incident subclinical symptoms at baseline (comprising 17 core psychosis items on delusions and hallucinations) also had persistence of the psychotic experiences 2 years later, and that an additional 8% made the transition to clinical disorder. Thus, the overwhelming majority (84%—who were false positives!) no longer described subclinical psychotic experiences. A study in a British population using a slightly different screen for prevalent psychotic experiences (at least one of four key items on thought insertion, paranoia, strange experiences, and hallucinations) at baseline and a shorter follow-up (18 months) yielded a higher persistence rate of 30% (Wiles *et al.*, 2006). Here, too, the great majority of psychotic experiences (70% at 1½-year follow-up) did not persist.

An important observation is that the generally good outcome of subclinical psychotic experiences can be modified to poorer outcomes if subjects are exposed to additional environmental risk factors. A notable example is cannabis misuse, especially in adolescence (see below; (Kristensen & Cadenhead, 2007; Murray *et al.*, 2003) and possibly trauma.

Predicting illness course from the duration of untreated psychosis

In the last two decades, several instruments for an early recognition of psychosis risk were developed and their validity was tested. They permit us to assess prepsychotic signs and psychotic prodromal symptoms, and to predict transition to psychosis with different probabilities (for reviews, see Häfner & Maurer, 2006; Miller *et al.*, 1999; Yung, 2006).

The availability of detailed information on the lengthy course of schizophrenia preceding the first treatment contact has prompted the question whether the duration of untreated psychosis (DUP) or untreated illness (DUI) is a predictor of a poor illness course. Results from studies on associations with various indicators of a poor course—symptoms, cognitive deficits, social decline and frequency of relapses—are not fully consistent. The reason lies in the lack of standardized study group composition, and definition and measurement of the onset of DUP and DUI. [For a discussion of some of the methodological pitfalls, see Friis *et al.* (2003).] Various speculative explanations have been proposed. Wyatt (1991) and in his wake Loebel *et al.* (1992), Lieberman *et al.* (2001b), and Jarskog *et al.*

(2004) regarded untreated psychosis as an "active morbid process" "toxic" to the brain. McGlashan and Johannessen (1996) and McGlashan (2006) presumed that deficits may result from an attenuated synaptic plasticity of the brain. If the underlying disease process of psychosis is not treated with antipsychotic medications, it might become chronic. The authors believed that antipsychotic therapy might have a benign effect on the underlying pathological process or help to preserve the plasticity of the brain.

Most of the studies have examined the association between DUP, mostly defined by the first manifestation of persistent psychotic symptoms, and indicators of the course of the first episode or 1-year outcome using primarily clinical interviews. The main results were significantly positive correlations of prolonged DUP with a slower remission of psychotic episodes and level of positive and negative symptoms (Drake *et al.*, 2000; Emsley *et al.*, 2007; Harrigan *et al.*, 2003; Loebel *et al.*, 1992; Simonsen *et al.*, 2007), and partly also with global functioning, quality of life, and frequency of readmissions. It seems plausible to presume that a delayed treatment of the first psychotic episode delays the remission of the episode. However, it should be kept in mind that a lengthy prodromal stage is associated with a longer duration of the first episode compared with acute psychotic episodes not preceded by a prodrome.

Outcome studies covering 1 year or more have confirmed the results from short-term follow-up studies concerning a positive association between DUP and increased positive symptoms (Addington *et al.*, 2004; Löffler & Häfner, 1999a). In contrast, de Haan *et al.* (2003) found a significant correlation only with negative symptoms over 6 years and Bottlender *et al.* (2003) with both positive and negative symptoms over a 15-year period. In a naturalistic study with 318 first-episode patients followed up for 8 years after initial treatment, Harris *et al.* (2005) found a moderate positive correlation between DUP and severity of positive symptoms, and reduced social and occupational functioning, but no association between DUP and negative symptoms.

Only a few studies have tested the predictive power of DUI following the first sign of illness. Using the IRAOS, a semi-structured interview (Häfner *et al.*, 2003a), which produces reliable data on both DUI and DUP, Löffler and Häfner (1999a) assessed a population-based sample of 115 first-episode cases of schizophrenia spectrum disorder at five cross-sections over 5 years following first admission. The result confirmed the significant association between a longer DUP and elevated positive and neurotic symptom scores, and between a longer DUI and elevated scores for negative (avolition, apathy, asociality) and depressive (depression, anxiety, disturbed sleep, etc.) symptoms at 5-year follow-up. An explanation for this is provided by the fact that the preponderances of prepsychotic prodromal symptoms in DUI and of positive symptoms in DUP correspond to the long-term courses of these symptom dimensions (see above, Course types of schizophrenia), which means that the symptoms of each category are predictive only of the same symptom dimension.

Studies on predicting neuromotor and neurocognitive functioning by DUP have so far not yielded clear-cut results. Emsley et al. (2005) found no association between DUP and neurological abnormalities as measured by the Neurological Evaluation Scale (NES; Buchanan & Heinrichs, 1989) in 66 medication-naïve patients from an early-psychosis unit. Available studies of patients treated with neuroleptic medications or without treatment information are not informative.

The association between DUP and neuropsychological test results are negative according to most, but not all, studies. A reason for this might be that cognitive impairment runs a stable course more or less independent of the symptom dimensions and, in addition, is not defined consistently across the studies. Lappin et al. (2007) found a positive correlation between DUP and reduced verbal IQ, verbal learning, and verbal working memory, but no information on treatment was given. No association was found by Robinson et al. (1999a,b), Craig et al. (2000)—over 24 months after first assessment, Ho et al. (2000), Hoff et al. (2000), Barnes et al. (2000), Norman et al. (2001), and Rund et al. (2007).

Due to the divergence of the study results, especially those concerning the outcome parameters, reviews and meta-analyses can be seen as merely indicating a tendency of consistency. Perkins et al. (2005) in their meta-analysis, based on 43 publications up to l 2004, concluded that a short DUP is negatively associated with global psychopathology, positive and negative symptoms and functional outcome, that this association seems to be independent of the effects of other variables, and that DUP does not appear to be associated with the rather stable symptom dimension of neurocognitive functioning. The authors also reported that there is no relationship with abnormities of brain morphology, but evidence for this conclusion is still thin.

Marshall et al. (2005), more cautiously reviewing 26 studies published up to 2004, found no correlation between DUP and initial clinical evaluation of psychopathology and social functioning. Almost all associations, however, attained significance with a lengthening follow-up period (6, 12, and 24 months). In 12 studies, the effect of DUP seemed robust even after controlling for premorbid adjustment, and this was confirmed by Singh (2007). In a critical review of 10 studies published between 1992 and 2000, Norman and Malla (2001) stated that although there seems some evidence for a relationship between DUP and initial response to treatment, the robustness of these findings and their independence from confounding variables are yet to be established.

As the associations between DUP and outcome might be confounded or moderated by third factors, many of the above studies have attempted to control for these possible influences. As control in observational studies cannot be introduced in the same way as in experimental designs, it must be substituted mainly by adjusting design variables through statistical methods. Again, results are far from unambiguous (e.g., de Haan et al., 2003; Harris et al., 2005; Selten et al., 2007; Verdoux et al., 2001).

A significant indication that moderating influences might be at work is provided by the correlation reported between an extended (pre-)psychotic prodromal stage and negative symptoms (Binder et al., 1998; Bottlender et al., 2000; de Haan et al., 2000; Haas et al., 1998; Häfner et al., 2002; Harrigan et al., 2003; Scully et al., 1997; Waddington et al., 1995). A long prodromal stage associated with negative symptoms and an insidious illness onset is—regardless of treatment—a predictor of a poor illness course (Ciompi & Müller, 1976; Müller et al., 1986; Sartorius et al., 1986). An acute onset of psychosis is a predictor of a favorable illness course, as shown by studies conducted before neuroleptic medications became available (Sartorius et al., 1977).

The clinically crucial question is whether shortening DUP by early intervention is capable of warding off unfavorable consequences of the disorder. Controlled intervention trials in early illness and with sufficiently long follow-up periods are required to establish whether it is the duration of the active disease process before the beginning of an efficacious treatment or an unfavorable type of the disorder, indicated by an insidious onset, that actually determines a poor prognosis.

A few controlled studies of cognitive–behavioral and/or low-dose neuroleptic treatment of early positive symptoms in patients with prodromal symptoms and at increased or ultra-high psychosis risk of different definitions have consistently reported weak, but significantly favorable, treatment effects on symptoms and a reduction in transitions to psychosis (French et al., 2007; Lewis et al., 2002; McGorry et al., 2002). Effects on the long-term illness course are not yet known. In summary, for the time being these studies can be seen as merely indicating that early intervention administered in the first episode can have benign effects.

The pretreatment illness course of several years' duration has implications for the interpretation of the results from studies that have used first admission as the definition of illness onset. This is the case, for example, with the reports of a significant excess of incidence rates for schizophrenia from the lowest social class and their interpretation along the lines of the social-causation hypothesis (Eaton, 1999; Faris & Dunham, 1939; Kohn, 1969), because these factors might also influence patients' help-seeking behavior.

Social course of schizophrenia

Indicators of the social course of schizophrenia are social competence and functioning on the one hand, social impairment and social disability (e.g., low socioeconomic status, poor integration in the labor market) on the other. The latter factors are to some extent codetermined by the sociocultural environment. Therefore, in studies into the social course of schizophrenia, comparisons with age- and sex-matched controls from the population of the study area—instead of national statistics—are necessary.

Significant social impairment in people with schizophrenia can already be seen between illness onset and the end of the early illness stage (Addington et al., 2008; Ballon et al., 2007; Gourzis et al., 2002; Häfner & Nowotny, 1995; McGorry et al., 1996). In a comparison of the level of social functioning of 86 clinical high-risk (CHR) individuals with three control groups (first-episode patients, multiepisode patients, non-psychiatric individuals), CHR patients did not differ in social deficits from the other clinical groups, but were significantly worse than normal controls (Addington et al., 2008). While at the first sign of the disorder, patients from the ABC study fulfilling six major social roles (e.g., completed school education, occupational training, employment, own income, own accommodation, marriage or stable partnership) did not differ from age- and sex-matched "healthy" controls (Häfner et al., 1999a), some 6 years later, at first admission, persons with schizophrenia already showed significant differences from controls and a considerable degree of social impairment. Most severely affected were marriages and partnerships: 52% of the women and 28% of the men were married or lived in a stable partnership at illness onset, but by the first admission the corresponding figures were 33% for women, compared to 78% for healthy controls, and 17% for men, compared to 60% for controls. Studies of the early course of schizophrenia conducted by McGorry et al. (1995), Yung et al. (1998), and McGlashan (1998) confirmed what the analyses of symptoms and functional impairment indicated, namely that the prodromal stage and the first psychotic episode are the pathologically most active phases in schizophrenia.

In most cases of schizophrenia social disability becomes manifest with accumulating negative symptoms and increasing cognitive impairment long before the first psychiatric contact (Bilder, 1998; Gourzis et al., 2002). According to prospective epidemiological studies on the course of schizophrenia extending over several years after first admission (an der Heiden et al., 1995; Jablensky et al., 1992; Leff et al., 1992; Shepherd et al., 1989; Vazquez-Barquero et al., 1995), the scores and profiles of social disability remain more or less stable after remission of the first episode, as do negative symptoms and cognitive impairment. The studies are also consistent in showing significantly poorer social outcomes for men than women, particularly in the medium-term course, whereas the symptom-related outcomes show no difference between the sexes (Häfner et al., 1998; Simonsen et al., 2007; Usall et al., 2002).

Social disadvantage in the course of schizophrenia is not a consequence of the disorder alone. In almost all studies, poor premorbid social functioning is the most powerful predictor of social course and outcome in schizophrenia. Nevertheless, it is contaminated with the prodromal illness stage (Addington et al., 2003; Haas & Sweeney, 1992; Häfner & Nowotny, 1995; Maziade et al., 1996; Rakfeldt & McGlashan, 1996). Using the IRAOS and applying a regression model, Häfner et al. (2003b) assessed social course up to 5 years after first admission in a subsample of 170 patients from the ABC cohort who had experienced a prepsychotic prodromal stage characterized by non-specific (including depressive) and negative symptoms. The only significant predictors of a poor 5-year social outcome were impaired social development at psychosis onset and the socially adverse illness behavior of young men. The influence of the traditional predictors, age, gender, type of onset (chronic, acute), and symptomatology, was mediated by these two variables assessed at the end of the prepsychotic prodromal stage.

The individual's level of social development at illness onset is the baseline against which social course is measured. At young age, illness onset occurs at a low level of social development and presumably of cognitive development as well. The disorder impairs further social development and leads to social and possibly also cognitive stagnation. In contrast, a later illness onset at a high level of social development may result in social decline. In cultures that offer equal education and employment opportunities, women, in whom illness onset is on average 4 years older than in men, attain a higher level of social development and a larger proportion of marriages than men do before falling ill with schizophrenia. In the rare very late-onset cases of psychosis, e.g., at retirement age, socioeconomic conditions and partnership relations tend to be so stable that the disorder hardly has any impact on them. This explains the good social prognosis of late-onset schizophrenia.

Population studies have consistently shown that adolescent and young adult males show a significantly higher frequency of socially adverse behavior (e.g., alcohol and drug abuse, self-neglect, aggressive behavior, and poor sociocultural integration, etc.) than their female counterparts (Choquet & Ledoux, 1994; Döpfner et al.,1997; Häfner et al., 1998; Maccoby & Jacklin, 1980). As a result, women with schizophrenia show significantly better social adaptation at the early illness stage than do males (Häfner, 2003a). This difference in illness behavior leads to a reduced compliance with treatment and poor social adjustment in young male patients in the course of the disorder.

Consequently, the significantly poorer medium-term social course of schizophrenia in young males may result from their socially adverse illness behavior and their lower level of social development at the earlier onset of their illness.

As the protective effect of estrogens in women disappears after the menopause and socially adverse male behavior becomes less frequent with age, women show poorer illness courses in later age, while men have milder symptoms and a significantly more favorable social course of illness (Häfner *et al.*, 2001b; Opjordsmoen, 1998).

Purely illness-related prognostic indicators of the social course are previous illness course or poor premorbid functioning, negative symptoms, and cognitive impairment (Milev *et al.*, 2005). They directly influence social functioning and, hence, the outcome of psychosocial rehabilitation as well as community outcome in general (Green, 1996). Such patient-related outcome criteria are not the only factors determining community outcome. It also depends on the patients' acceptance in the community, e.g., on the prevalence of stigma and discrimination, on the availability of suitable employment and good-quality care, and on the patients' acceptance by their families (Giron & Gomez-Beneyto, 2004).

Medium- and long-term course of schizophrenia

According to first-episode studies, the proportion of patients who improve and have no relapses over a 5-year period varies from 21% (Bland & Orn, 1978) to 25% (Biehl *et al.*, 1986) to 30% (The Scottish Schizophrenia Research Group, 1992), but in these studies, the definition of a relapse varied. In the World Health Organization (WHO) cohort of the IPSS (Leff *et al.*, 1992), 22% of the patients, including both first and multiple episodes of schizophrenia (ICD-9), had experienced no psychotic relapses.

The proportion of differently defined unfavorable outcomes of illness parameters, e.g., non-remitting negative or frequently recurring psychotic symptoms, shows more marked variation, ranging from 22% in the WHO cohort to 60% in an der Heiden *et al.'s* (1996) study.

Course of symptom dimensions

In order to gain a better understanding of the heterogeneous course, probably accounted for by several neurobiological processes, of the disease construct of schizophrenia, both the course of transphenomenal factors (see above, Course of empirical symptom dimensions) and descriptive symptom dimensions (see above, Positive and negative symptom dimensions) have been studied. Considering the subdiagnostic presence of the symptom dimensions in the

Table 7.1 Number of months (raw data) spent with at least one symptom of the main clinical categories in the 134-month (11.2-year) follow-up period.

Symptom	Mean	SD
Depressive	76.9	56.2
Manic	9.0	24.8
Negative	45.1	54.5
Positive	26.7	42.6
Disorganization	6.3	19.2

general population, it is reasonable to study them also as components of the disorder.

First steps towards an analytical deconstruction of the "disease entity" of schizophrenia were undertaken with the isolation of positive and negative symptoms and the study of their course in the population-based ABC study. To study the four sufficiently frequent and psychopathologically discrete symptom dimensions: positive, negative, depressive, and manic, the average follow-up period of 12.3 years was homogenized on the basis of IRAOS data to 11.2 years or 134 monthly intervals by the shortest course included (an der Heiden et al., unpublished observations). The relative frequency of the four roughly defined, clinically relevant syndromes was measured by the number of months in which these syndromes were present. Table 7.1 shows that the depressive syndrome was by far the most prevalent, as was the case at the prodromal stage of the disorder. Exclusion of overlapping symptoms (e.g., between negative and depressive symptoms such as lack of initiative, slowness, etc., and between positive and manic symptoms) yielded core syndromes, each consisting of four to five most frequent (>1%), non-overlapping symptoms. The complex negative syndrome, including domains such as lack of initiative, social dysfunctioning, emotional and cognitive impairment, could not be reduced to a core syndrome and, hence, was entered in the analysis as comprising the 19 single IRAOS symptoms. Again, the most frequent depressive core symptom, present for 30.4 months, was predominant compared with the most frequent positive symptom, verbal hallucinations, present for 4.8 months (Table 7.2).

Figure 7.2 shows the percentage of patients with depressive, manic, and psychotic core syndromes in 134 monthly assessments. After remission of the first episode and all the symptoms, all three dimensions showed a plateau-like course. The hierarchy of the syndromes, too, remained unchanged with depression predominating. The illness-related syndromes, positive and depressive, showed no sex difference. This finding lends support to the conclusion drawn from the early illness course that the disorder as such does not differ between men and women, except for the sex difference in age of onset and in "normal" social behavior.

In this study, the mean values neither for the symptom dimensions, nor for the social course, subject to influence by external factors, showed a discernible trend: both at first admission and at 11.2-year follow-up, some 30% of the patients were in regular employment, whereas the figure for "healthy" controls was 70%.

Table 7.2 Mean duration (in months) of depressive, manic and psychotic core symptoms in the long-term (11.2-year) course of schizophrenia.

	Months with symptoms
Depressive symptoms	
Depressed mood (≥14 days)	30.4
Loss of self-confidence	27.9
Feelings of guilt	8.2
Suicidal thoughts/attempt	4.2
Manic symptoms	
Elated mood	5.8
Reduced need for sleep	3.8
Pressure of speech	3.6
Hyperactivity	0.8
Flight of ideas	0.7
Psychotic symptoms	
Verbal hallucination	4.8
Thought insertion	2.4
Thought withdrawal	1.7
Thought echo	1.2

Unlike the other symptom dimensions, negative symptoms, which were assessed based on the 19 single symptoms, remit at a different pace in men and women and, overall, more slowly than the other syndromes after the first episode. Some 5 years after the climax of the first episode, negative symptoms, too, show a stable, plateau-like course in both men and women. The factors explaining the slower remission of negative symptoms in men in the medium-term course are not yet known. However, they probably relate to the differences in the normal behavioral dispositions of men and women, as seen with the early illness course.

Frequency of relapse episodes

The frequency of relapses in the short- and medium-term course was discussed in the previous section. The proportion of patients free of relapses in the medium-term course was 20%.

In the ABC study 107 first-episode patients experienced a total of 333 psychotic relapses (defined as persistence of or increase in positive symptoms over a period of at least 2 weeks after and before a 4-week period of absence of symptoms or of declining symptoms; range: 0–29) in the 11.2-year follow-up period (an der Heiden *et al.*, 2005); 17% suffered neither relapses nor persisting symptoms or cognitive and functional impairment in the long-term course. For 44.2% of the time patients spent in psychotic relapse episodes they also suffered from depressive symptoms, whereas, at 34.5%, the corresponding figure for psychosis-free intervals was considerably lower. Most of the patients studied received neuroleptic medication. Seventy-three episodes (18%) were free of psychotic symptoms and purely depressive in type. A consistent finding has been

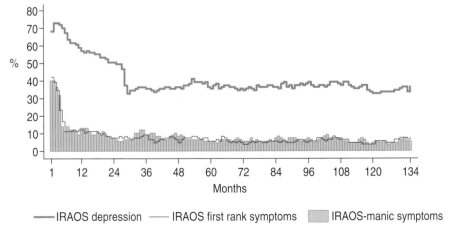

—IRAOS depression ——— IRAOS first rank symptoms ▨ IRAOS-manic symptoms

Fig. 7.2 Long-term course of three symptom dimensions in schizophrenia based on a homogenized duration of illness.

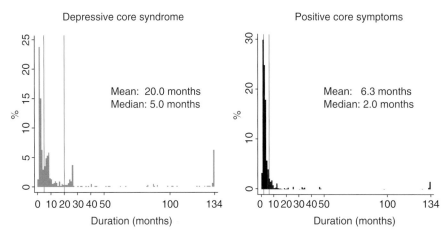

Fig. 7.3 Duration of spells with depressive and positive symptoms.

reported from a 2-year follow-up in the WHO Ten-Country Study (n = 543; Jablensky, 2003): a prevalence of 16% for affective episodes. Bressan *et al.* (2003) followed up 80 clinically stable outpatients with schizophrenia (first episodes) for 1½ years; 16.3% of the relapse episodes were major depressive episodes according to DSM-IV, a proportion close to that found in the long-term course.

To explore whether the symptom dimensions of schizophrenia run monotonous courses, some of them only rarely interrupted by episodes, or show frequent exacerbations and, if they do, to study the temporal pattern of these exacerbations, the individual data had to be assessed without an operationalized definition of their duration. Only a very small proportion (1%) of cases showed permanently persisting positive symptoms indicative of a chronic psychosis (Fig. 7.3), the figure for depressive symptoms being 6% and for negative symptoms 7%. In the majority of cases, the three dimensions studied showed exacerbations and intervals that were very different in length. However, the differences between means and medians and the histogram depicted in Figure 7.3 indicate that short spells of exacerbation predominate. The mean duration of an episode was 6.3 months for positive symptoms (median: 2.0), 20.0 months for depressive symptoms (median: 5.0), and 23.3 months for negative symptoms (median: 5.0). The asynchronous courses are an indication of the independence of the symptom dimensions. The only aspect running somewhat counter to this impression is the moderate increase in depressive symptoms within psychotic episodes. To date analyses on how these individual types of course of the symptom dimensions influence the overall course of schizophrenia have produced fairly stable mean values and a plateau-like course. However, they have also revealed a high degree of interindividual variability, hidden behind the mean values depicting the course of the complex disease construct.

Prognostic indicators

Prognostic indicators are studied for two reasons: first, to obtain good prognostic tools for clinical practice. Such indicators are predominantly characteristics that reflect the disease process, because, as a rule, it is possible to predict the further course of a disease from its earlier stages. The second reason is to find risk factors that are independent of the disease process itself but help elucidate the underlying etiology. The prognostic power of early factors contributing to the risk of illness tends to decrease with increasing duration of illness (Carpenter & Strauss, 1991; Möller *et al.*, 1986).

The prognostic value of a wide range of clinical variables has been examined, including risk factors such as family history of psychotic disorder, sociodemographic background, and prognostic indicators such as premorbid personality, the symptom profiles and diagnoses given at presentation, cognitive functioning, and treatment response. Recent studies have examined the predictive validity of the DSM-IV and ICD-10 categorical diagnoses and have found that the predictive power of the diagnostic categories is improved when used in conjunction with a dimensional symptom score (Dikeos *et al.*, 2006).

Long-lasting poor premorbid social and occupational functioning prior to first contact, frequently associated with a prolonged prodromal stage, have been shown to be a powerful predictor of an unfavorable course of schizophrenia and also of other chronic diseases and disease-independent biographies. Insidious onset, young age at onset, male gender, and not being married have consistently been related to a poor prognosis of overall outcome (Harrison *et al.*, 1996; Malmberg *et al.*, 1998; Wiersma *et al.*, 2000). Hence, irrespective of their association with the disease process, these factors can be regarded as robust indicators of the medium-term (under

5-year) clinical outcome, although their effects are very different.

The current evidence on most of the prognostic variables is inconclusive. The explanatory power of any prognostic indicator in psychosis varies with the study setting and patient sample. To date, most predictor studies have only been able to explain around a third of the total variance seen in outcome, and no single clinical characteristic or background variable has been found to have a strong association with long-term clinical outcome.

The prediction of single domains or symptom dimensions of the disorder by precisely defined factors is slightly more promising. At certain stages in life, age and sex are predictive of social outcome due to the influence they have on the level of social and cognitive development at onset and sex-specific social behavior (Häfner et al., 1999a). Childhood onset may be associated with severe developmental deficits, disorganizational syndromes, and cognitive impairment, and involves an elevated risk of a poor symptom-related and social course, whereas a very late onset is associated with paranoid symptomatology and less or no social decline in the medium- and long-term course (Häfner et al., 2001a; Howard & Jeste, 2003).

Negative and positive symptoms, for the most part, predict only these same symptom dimensions (Löffler & Häfner, 1999a; Möller et al., 1982, 2002; Pietzcker & Gaebel 1983; Strauss & Carpenter, 1977). The negative symptom domain is usually more stable over time and is more strongly associated with neurocognitive impairments, brain abnormalities, and social and employment disability (Davidson & McGlashan, 1997) (see above, Functional and cognitive impairment). The positive symptom domain is of poor predictive power for the clinical course, except for the probability of psychotic relapses.

Ventura et al. (2004) reported a slightly improved mutual prognostic power of positive and negative syndromes by solving the problem of different trajectories. They defined six periods in relation to psychotic exacerbation. The authors rated 46 recent-onset cases of schizophrenia spectrum disorder on the Brief Psychiatric Rating Scale (BPRS) every 2 weeks over a mean period of 3 years. Studying the exacerbations of positive (in 77%) and negative symptoms (in 42%), they found a significant, slightly increased correlation of exacerbations and intervals between these syndromes. The authors presumed that there is a weak functional association between the two syndromes.

The traditional subtypes are generally of limited prognostic value. However, evidence of differential outcome has been demonstrated between the hebephrenic and the schizoaffective type (Jablensky, 2000). In a prospective follow-up study conducted after remission of acute symptoms (6 months after first admission), Ohta et al. (1990) attempted to improve the prognosis by focusing on empirical subtypes. They identified three clusters of patients on the basis of PANSS data: (1) 31% with negative symptoms, (2) 32% with persisting delusions and hallucinations, and (3) 37% in full remission. As expected, the two symptom-related clusters allowed a fairly reliable prognosis of an elevated relapse rate, higher symptom scores, and impaired attention 2 years later.

Prognostic scales have been developed which attempt to increase the predictive power of the known indicators. However, such complex predictor patterns are difficult to use in practice.

Möller and von Zerssen (1995) compared six prognostic scales with outcome criteria in their own and in a replication sample at 5-year follow-up. The highest degree of variance was explained by the Stephens scale and the Strauss–Carpenter scale (Möller et al., 1982, 1984).

Jablensky (2000) has given an overview of the clinically practical, sufficiently validated prognostic indicators, which we have supplemented and adapted to the results of recent predictor studies:

1. Sociodemographic characteristics (gender, age or level of social and cognitive development at psychosis onset);
2. Level of social and occupational functioning prior to illness onset;
3. Past psychotic episodes and successful treatments (rapid remission vs. persisting symptoms);
4. Type of illness onset (acute vs. chronic) and duration of untreated illness;
5. Severe negative symptoms, cognitive and social impairment at the initial illness stage and in the first episode);
6. Illness behavior (socially adverse behaviour, poor compliance);
7. Cortical atrophy at first admission (Gattaz et al., 1995; Vita et al., 1991);
8. Alcohol and drug abuse, pre- and co-morbidly.

Transnational differences in the course of schizophrenia

Acute and transient psychoses, which according to Wig & Parhee (1989) show rapid remissions in developing countries (Craig et al., 1997; Varma et al., 1996), have also a favorable short- and medium-term prognosis regarding symptomatology, cognitive impairment, and social course. That acute, transient psychosis with a good prognosis also occurs in developed countries has been shown by Marneros et al. (1991) in a controlled prospective study. However, an 18-year follow-up of recent-onset schizophrenia among Afro-Caribbeans in England showed significantly higher recovery rates compared with British persons (Takei et al., 1998). McKenzie et al. (1995) have reported a similar finding. The main difference seems to be that these transient acute-onset psychoses have a considerably lower incidence in the developed world. In developed countries psychotic symptoms are relevant for the social prognosis only in special cases, e.g., when psychotic episodes are extremely frequent or the persisting psychotic symptoms are particularly severe (Carpenter & Kirkpatrick, 1988; McGlashan, 1998).

The high rates of compulsory admissions or admissions involving the police among Afro-Caribbeans in Great Britain raised the question of whether or not these minorities are affected by a delay in treatment or a longer DUP. The ÆSOP study (Morgan *et al.*, 2006), however, showed that this minority group did not have a longer DUP than persons of British origin with schizophrenia. In both groups, DUP was strongly associated with other predictors of a poor illness course, in particular an insidious onset.

Attempts to compare the medium- and long-term course of schizophrenia in the transnational samples of the IPSS (World Health Organization, 1979), the Ten-Country Study (Jablensky *et al.*, 1992), and the pooled data from the International Study of Schizophrenia (ISoS study; Hopper *et al.*, 2007) have yielded different results. Nevertheless, it can be concluded that schizophrenia in some developing countries has a better prognosis than in developed countries (Jablensky *et al.*, 1992; Leff *et al.*, 1992; Murphy & Raman, 1971).

Long-term clinical course and outcome of schizophrenia

In the last decades textbooks discussing the long-term course and outcome of schizophrenia, with few exceptions, have cited the same studies in spite of their generally poor designs: three large-scale studies by Ciompi and Müller (1976; Lausanne study), the Bonn Study (Huber *et al.*, 1979), and the Burghölzli Study (Bleuler, 1972) from German-speaking countries in the 1970s, and three long-term studies of schizophrenia in the US: the Chestnut Lodge Follow-up Study (McGlashan 1984a,b), the Vermont Longitudinal Study (Harding *et al.*, 1987a,b), and the Washington IPSS cohort study (Carpenter & Strauss, 1991).

In a review, an der Heiden (1996) analyzed 59 long-term studies of schizophrenia—including those cited above—that covered follow-up periods of 10 years or more and were published in the years 1932–1996. The overarching finding did not support the general impression of consistency in the results. On the contrary, results on course and outcome are very heterogeneous. Given the differences in the study designs, patient samples, course and outcome criteria, and lengths of follow-up periods, it is, contrary to the widespread opinion in the textbooks, nearly impossible to draw any valid conclusions from these results.

Since 1990, the WHO has coordinated a long-term follow-up of former WHO studies of schizophrenia [International Study of Schizophrenia (ISoS); Hopper *et al.*, 2007; Sartorius *et al.*, 1996]. Fifteen- and 25-year follow-ups have been conducted on the cohorts of the former IPSS (World Health Organization, 1979), the WHO Collaborative Study on the Assessment and Reduction of Social Disability (RAPyD; Jablensky *et al.*, 1980), and the Determinants of Outcome of Severe Mental Disorders Study (Ten-Country Study, DOSMeD; Sartorius *et al.*, 1986). Eighteen research centers in 13 countries participated (n = 1043). The results from these studies, too, confirm the heterogeneity of course and outcome. The means show no early trend to deterioration after first admission. The same was true for the medium-term course of schizophrenia. The clinical status of more than half of the subjects was rated as "recovered".

From the Sofia cohort of the WHO Disability Study (n = 55 at follow-up 16 years after index admission), Ganev (2000) has reported a predominantly favorable long-term outcome of psychotic symptoms: 55% of the patients improved in the first 10 years after first admission and only 20% deteriorated. Mason *et al.* (1996) from Nottingham (13-year follow-up) and Wiersma *et al.* (1998) from Groningen found no indication of a late recovery. The Groningen study rather showed that chronicity (continued positive or persisting negative symptoms) increased slightly on average and the length of episodes increased with each episode.

During the last decade several efforts have been undertaken (e.g., an der Heiden *et al.*, 1996; Andreasen *et al.*, 2005; Bebbington *et al.*, 2006; Liberman *et al.*, 2002; Nuechterlein *et al.*, 2006) to tackle the problem of differing definitions of remission, relapse, and outcome status, a major reason why comparability is problematic. All these approaches have in common (1) a better standardization and operationalization of outcome criteria; and (2) instead of relying on single cross-sectional assessments for measuring outcome data, an assessment period between 6 months and 2 years to take into account the undulating character of schizophrenic syndromes.

The criteria for defining recovery proposed by the Remission in Schizophrenia Working Group (Andreasen *et al.*, 2005) consist of two components: (1) diagnostically relevant schizophrenia core syndromes (psychoticism, disorganization, negative symptoms) operationalized by approved diagnostic instruments, developed primarily by the authors: Scale for the Assessment of Positive Symptoms (SAPS; Andreasen, 1984); Scale for the Assessment of Negative Symptoms (SANS; Andreasen, 1989); PANSS (Kay *et al.*, 1987); and BPRS (Overall & Gorham, 1962); and (2) a mild or reduced rating of all symptoms during a 6-month period. An alternative concept proposed by Liberman *et al.* (2002; Liberman & Kopelowicz, 2005) includes: (1) symptom criteria: operationalized by a BPRS score of 4 or less on all positive and negative psychosis items; and (2) social criteria: at least half-time work or school, independent living without supervision, no full dependence on financial support from disability insurance, and at least once weekly contact with peers; each of the criteria should last for at least 2 consecutive years.

The system of Nuechterlein et al. (2006) differs from the others in so far as it gives additional criteria for relapse and exacerbation. Based on the rating in three symptoms (unusual thought content, hallucinations, and conceptual disorganization) from the expanded version of the BPRS (Lukoff et al., 1986), during a period of 9–12 months the authors define nine types of "episodic" outcome, e.g., continuous remission, remission followed by relapse, and stable persisting symptoms.

In an earlier attempt to evaluate long-term outcome, an der Heiden et al. (1996) argued that besides the recording of the schizophrenic core syndromes as measured by approved instruments (SANS, PSE, BPRS), criteria for improved outcome must be supplemented by treatment criteria. In this way, remission—or recovered outcome—is defined by only mild core symptoms, no neuroleptic in- or out-patient treatment, and this state must be stable for a period of 9 months.

While in the majority of recent long-term studies data are collected through personal interviews, Bebbington et al. (2006) used routine clinical notes from in- and out-patient treatment to extract information at monthly intervals to evaluate remission and relapse. Based on the assessment of positive symptoms, the authors defined states of full, partial or non-remission, as well as relapse/non-relapse according to clinical ratings of consecutive periods.

Recently, several studies have been undertaken to evaluate the various remission criteria in different settings. Wunderink et al. (2007) explored the Andreasen criteria, as did de Hert et al. (2007), Emsley et al. (2007), Helldin et al. (2007), and van Os et al. (2006a,b). To summarize, the Andreasen criteria possess concurrent and predictive validity, and change in remission status correlates with changes in relevant domains, such as unmet needs, global functioning, satisfaction with services, and quality of life.

Others have attempted to evaluate the Liberman remission criteria (Kopelowicz et al., 2005) or to compare the Andreasen remission criteria with a criterion set proposed by Lieberman et al. (Dunayevich et al., 2006). [The Lieberman approach differs from Andreasen's definition of remission in two main characteristics: (1) change score; remission requires a 50% reduction in total BPRS score from baseline with no score greater than "mild" on five psychosis items (unusual thought content, suspiciousness, hallucinations, conceptual disorganization, mannerisms, posturing); and (2) no use of a time criterion.]

According to the Mannheim criteria, 60.7% of patients from the Mannheim cohort of the former WHO Collaborative Study on Impairments and Disabilities Associated with Schizophrenic Disorders (Jablensky et al., 1980) were symptomatic 14 years after first hospital admission, 12.5% were symptom-free while treated with neuroleptics, and 26.8%

were remitted (an der Heiden et al., 1996). Remitted patients had significantly fewer hospital readmissions during the follow-up period, had lower psychotic symptom scores at seven cross-sectional assessments until 14-year follow-up, and were less socially disabled. In a second analysis, the defined remission criteria were used to analyze outcome in the ABC study (see above) on average 12.3 years after first hospital admission. Symptoms and treatment data in a 9-month period before long-term follow-up were assessed retrospectively with the IRAOS (Häfner et al., 1992). Of the ABC cohort, 29.9% seemed to have recovered—they neither showed any of the clinical symptoms nor were they treated with neuroleptics during the 9-month period; 7.5% were free of symptoms while treated with neuroleptics; and 62.6% showed significant positive and/or negative symptoms. The similarity with the results from the Mannheim Long-Term Study of Schizophrenia cohort (former "Disability" cohort) is obvious. The breakdown of the ABC cohort into three outcome groups is also mirrored by occupational and treatment data, considering the total period of observation: belonging to the remitted outcome group correlates with more time in regular employment, less time in sheltered working conditions, and a lower share of early retirement. These patients also show a lower number of readmissions to hospital and they spend in total fewer days in hospital.

The application of three different remission criteria (Andreasen, Liberman, Mannheim) in patients from the ABC cohort (possible because the IRAOS symptom list was conceptualized on the basis of approved instruments, e.g. SANS, SAPS, BPRS, PANSS, and symptoms, treatment, and biographical data were assessed on a longitudinal basis) showed that 20.6% of the patients complied with the Liberman criteria, 31.8% with the Andreasen criteria, and 29.9% with the Mannheim criteria. Pairwise agreement was highest between Andreasen and Mannheim (88.8%; kappa = 0.74), and almost identical but lower between Andreasen and Liberman (79.4%; kappa = 0.48), and Mannheim and Liberman (79.4%; kappa = 0.46). Only 15 patients (14%) equally fulfilled the remission criteria of all three sets. This result is an impressive illustration of the crucial importance that uniform criteria for defining the key design variables has in studying and describing the course of schizophrenia.

Comorbidity with substance abuse as a predictor of course

The abuse of alcohol and illicit drugs is very common in schizophrenia (Cantor-Graae et al., 2001; Chen & Murray, 2004; Larsen et al., 2006; Soyka et al., 1993), and the most often misused substances are alcohol and cannabis (Margolese et al., 2004). As it is estimated that roughly one-quarter of patients with schizophrenia spectrum disorders currently use or misuse cannabis (Green *et al.*, 2005)—though great local variation occurs, this substance has gained special interest as a possible factor in the etiology of the disorder. Verdoux *et al.* (2002) found an association between the frequency of cannabis use and the intensity of psychotic-like experiences in a non-clinical population of 571 female students. Ferdinand *et al.* (2005) carried out a 14-year follow-up of 1580 initially 4–16-year-old children and found that cannabis use predicted psychotic symptoms in adulthood independently of other putative predictors. From a review of five general population cohort studies (Swedish Conscript Study: Andreasson *et al.*, 1987; Dunedin Study: Arseneault *et al.*, 2002; Caspi *et al.*, 2005; Christchurch Study: Fergusson *et al.*, 2005; EDSP Study: Henquet *et al.*, 2005; NEMESIS Study: van Os *et al.*, 2002). Fergusson *et al.* (2006) concluded that epidemiological research has produced suggestive evidence of a causal link between the use of cannabis and the development of psychosis or psychotic symptoms (also see Arseneault *et al.*, 2004).

Looking from the opposite direction, prodromal patients show a higher rate of current and lifetime diagnoses of cannabis abuse and dependence (Rosen *et al.*, 2006), and the use of cannabis results in an earlier age at onset as well as at different milestones (first social/occupational dysfunction, first negative symptom, first psychotic episode) in the development of schizophrenia (Barnes *et al.*, 2006; Bühler *et al.*, 2002; Veen *et al.*, 2004).

Further evidence for a causal relationship is suggested from looking at the temporal relationship between substance use and the development of schizophrenia. In the ABC study, drug misuse preceded non-specific signs of the onset of schizophrenia in 27.5% of cases, began in the same month in 34.6%, and followed in 37.9% of cases (Hambrecht & Häfner, 1996).

In the medium- and long-term course of schizophrenia, cannabis increases the risk for relapse and hospital readmission (Wade *et al.*, 2006). Persistent substance users (drugs and/or alcohol) have significantly more severe positive symptoms and greater overall severity of symptoms, but not of depressive symptoms (Harrison *et al.*, 2008; Hides *et al.*, 2006; Margolese *et al.*, 2006). With respect to the influence of cannabis on the negative syndrome, Talamo *et al.* (2006) in a meta-analysis of eight cross-sectional surveys found that comorbid patients had significantly lower PANSS negative scores (also see Dubertret *et al.*, 2006). In contrast, Boydell *et al.* (2006) found no evidence of fewer negative symptoms amongst cannabis users in 757 cases of first-onset schizophrenia. As the dose of cannabis is unknown, both results may be correct. In a follow-up of a Dutch incidence cohort of 181 patients—125 with a DSM-IV diagnosis of schizophrenic disorder, Selten *et al.* (2007) found that 30 months after first contact, poor course was best predicted by male sex, long duration of dysfunctioning before psychosis onset, and heavy cannabis use during the follow-up period. (However, after adjusting for sex in a multivariate analysis, the association was no longer significant, at least not in males.) A controlled first-episode study of schizophrenia over 11.2 years, too, showed that cannabis use was associated with an increase in positive and negative symptoms, but not in depression (Häfner, 2008).

Earlier studies frequently reported that cannabis does not have a negative impact on cognitive functioning. With reference to the dopaminergic effect of tetrahydrocannabinol (THC), some studies even reported better test performances in cannabis users compared with controls (McCleery *et al.*, 2006; Stirling *et al.*, 2005).

Meanwhile a few robust studies have appeared showing cannabis use to be associated with weak or even considerable impairment of cognitive functioning in patients with schizophrenia, and also in some healthy individuals (D'Souza *et al.*, 2009). The development of morphological brain changes has been demonstrated in some cases. However, it is not yet clear why only some at-risk persons develop neurobiological abnormalities.

Substance users are more likely to be young, male, and have lower levels of education (Kavanagh *et al.*, 2004; Larsen *et al.*, 2006; Salyers & Mueser, 2001). Because of an overrepresentation of men among comorbid patients, alcohol and drug abuse has a compounding effect on the sex difference in the social course of schizophrenia. In the long term, substance misuse is associated with an increased social risk: for divorce, unemployment, and crime (Addington & Addington, 1998; Brennan *et al.*, 2000; Salyers & Mueser, 2001). Substance abuse also leads to reduced compliance with care measures (rehabilitation) and antipsychotic drug treatment (Margolese *et al.*, 2004).

Suicide in the course of schizophrenia

Schizophrenia is associated with an enhanced risk for both natural and unnatural deaths, and most of the unnatural deaths are due to suicide (Brown, 1997; see also Chapters 28 and 31). Basically, there are three parameters indicating excess mortality in schizophrenia: crude mortality rates (CMR: number of deaths in a population during a specified period), standardized mortality ratio (SMR: number of observed deaths divided by the number of expected deaths, usually defined by population rates), and number/percentage of patients dying during a defined period of observation. While CMR and number/percentage gain additional significance by comparing numbers or rates between different groups, the comparison is already included in the SMR. The suicide rates for patients with schizophrenia are determined by those for the respective general populations.

Sartorius *et al.* (1987) found at the 5-year follow-up of the WHO Determinants of Outcome Study that nearly 4% of patients with a diagnosis of schizophrenia had committed suicide. Wilkinson (1982) reported a rate of 8% for suicide from a retrospective case-register-based analysis covering 10–15 years. Among the patients of the Chestnut Lodge Study, 6.4% committed suicide over a mean period of 19 years (Fenton *et al.*, 1997). Krausz *et al.* (1995) reported a rate of 13.1% among adolescents with schizophrenia after a minimum of 11 years and Häfner (2008) of 6.5% over a follow-up period of 12.3 years in a population-based first-episode sample aged 12–59 years at first admission. In a study of lifetime suicide rates, five of the 133 (3.8%) North-West Wales first-admission cohort from 1984–1988 committed suicide during a 5-year follow-up period (Healy *et al.*, 2006).

Long-term studies of first episodes of schizophrenia in Europe covering 14–16 years of illness have found rates ranging from 3% to 4% (Ganev, 2000; Mason *et al.*, 1995) up to 10% (an der Heiden *et al.*, 1995; Ganev, 2000; Wiersma *et al.*, 1998).

Based on his meta-analysis of 18 publications, Brown (1997) calculated an aggregate CMR of 189 deaths per 10 000 population a year, an aggregate SMR of 151 (Brown multiplies the SMR by 100), and a 10-year survival rate of 81%. According to his estimates, 28% of the excess mortality is accounted for by suicide and 12% by accidents. The remaining 60% is attributable to the same causes as in the general population.

In the above meta-analysis, the SMR for suicide was 838, was significantly higher for men than women, and showed a tendency to decrease with age (also see Krausz *et al.*, 1995). Osby *et al.* (2000) have also reported moderate gender differences from a linkage study based on the inpatient register and the national cause-of-death register of Stockholm County/Sweden. SMRs, calculated by 5-year age classes and 5-year calendar periods, were at their highest for suicide as a single cause of death. In this study, though, the rates for women at 19.7 were slightly higher than those for men at 15.7. Baxter and Appleby (1999), combining data from the Salford Psychiatric Case Registers and the NHS Central Registers in Great Britain, found an excess rate for suicide risk or undetermined external cause of 11.4 for men and of 13.7 for women. In a more recent 10-year follow-up study of 3470 patients with schizophrenia (4.1% of whom died from suicide) from 122 French public departments for adult psychiatry, Limosin *et al.* (2007) reported an SMR of 15.8 for schizophrenic men and 17.7 for schizophrenic women.

It is an established fact that there is an increased risk for suicide in schizophrenia, although the rates vary between studies depending on the frequency of follow-ups, ethnicity, age, and sex.

Risk factors for suicide

In a meta-analysis of 29 case–control and cohort studies, Hawton *et al.* (2005) found that risk of suicide in people with schizophrenia was strongly associated with depression, previous suicide attempts, drug misuse, agitation or motor restlessness, fear of mental disintegration, poor adherence to treatment, and recent loss. On the other hand, reduced risk was associated with hallucinations. In contrast, Kaplan and Harrow (1996) in a comparison of 70 patients with schizophrenia and 97 depressed patients reported that psychotic symptoms in patients with schizophrenia, such as delusions and hallucinations, were correlated with a later attempt of suicide. However, concomitant depression, usually increased in psychotic episodes, was not controlled for in that study. In a study by Grunebaum *et al.* (2001) in a diagnostically mixed population (schizophrenia, major depression, bipolar disorder) of 429 patients, reported no evidence for a correlation between the presence of delusions and a history of suicide attempts in the schizophrenic subgroup (n = 147).

Fenton *et al.* (1997; Kaplan & Harrow, 1996), studying patients from the Chestnut Lodge Study (McGlashan, 1984a,b), a highly selected sample, demonstrated a significant association between a low score for negative symptoms at index admission and death from suicide. Conversely, being classified as belonging to the paranoid schizophrenia subtype was associated with an excess risk of 12% for suicide. Presence of depressive symptoms, as well as fewer negative symptoms, were also identified as risk factors in a case—control study by McGirr *et al.* (2006) of 45 subjects with schizophrenia with completed suicide and 36 matched controls.

Depression alone accounted for over 80% of the explained variance in suicidal behavior in two independent studies of outpatients with schizophrenia by Bartels *et al.* (1992). The importance of depression as a risk factor for suicide was also emphasized in two other reviews (Caldwell & Gottesman, 1990; Miles, 1977). Thus, depression, the most frequent syndrome in the overall course of schizophrenia (Häfner *et al.*, 2005), but not adequately recorded in all pertinent studies, plays an important role as a risk factor for suicide.

Age and duration of illness were also linked to risk for suicide in the studies of Heilä *et al.* (2005), Clarke *et al.* (2006), Barak *et al.* (2004) and de Hert *et al.* (2001).

The risk for suicide seems to be highest for patients with the best chances for a good outcome and preserved insight (Fenton, 2000). Life events appear to enhance the risk for suicide (Heilä *et al.*, 1999a), whereas appropriate antipsychotic medication reduces it (Heilä *et al.*, 1999b).

Quality of life

Besides the classical indicators, constructs such as quality of life (QOL) or life satisfaction have attained special importance in the outcome assessment of schizophrenia and the evaluation of treatment measures (Becker *et al.*, 1998; Dunayevich *et al.*, 2006; Lehman, 1996; Lehman *et al.*, 2003; World Health Organization, 1998).

QOL depends not only on the disorder, but also on the individual person in question, as well as on several domains of life, e.g., economic and sociocultural conditions that the patient lives in. Hence, its assessment requires comparisons with controls from the general population, with people with other illnesses, more rarely also with the patients' goals, expectations, and coping resources (Michaelos, 1980) or their baseline in the social context (Campbell et al., 1976).

Subjective QOL also determines to a high degree how patients rate their experience of their symptoms. Comparable studies have been conducted by von Zerssen and Hecht (1987), who studied the associations between mental health, happiness, and life satisfaction, by Huber et al. (1988), who compared QOL between persons with psychiatric illness and healthy individuals; and by Malm et al. (1981), Oliver & Mohamad (1992), Mechanic et al. (1994), and Priebe et al. (2000).

Weber (1997) analyzed patients' individual aspirations and their judgments of achieving or missing these aspirations. The study was based on patients from the Mannheim Long-Term Study of Schizophrenia cohort assessed at 15.5 years after first admission. Weber assessed the patients' global life satisfaction and their aspirations and achievements in different domains of life. The age- and gender-matched controls from the general population had better starting conditions than patients for attaining their aspirations, they were more confident that the conditions would continue to be favorable in the future, and that they would be able to influence the achievement of their goals. In the context of the generally negative cognition of people with schizophrenia, it should be kept in mind that depression is the most frequent symptom in schizophrenia. Two studies (Huppert et al., 2001; Wetherell et al., 2003) found that the influence of anxiety on subjective QOL was even stronger than that of depressive symptoms. [For a review, also comprising determinants of QOL, see Malla and Payne (2005).] Aspirations were equally important to patients and controls, but after long histories of illness patients—women more frequently than men—reduced their aspirations and in this way preserved a certain degree of life satisfaction.

In summary, there is evidence that the QOL of people with schizophrenia is impaired, on both subjective and objective criteria, including their work and financial situation (Bengtsson-Tops & Hansson, 1999). Their quality of life is already reduced by the time of first contact with professional services (Browne et al., 2000), but the later outcome depends on their symptoms and the adjustment of their aspirations.

Becker et al. (1998) studied how the size of social network influences QOL and found that a medium number of social contacts were associated with the highest degree of QOL.

Rudnick and Kravetz (2001) found that social-support seeking may influence outcome favorably, but does not correlate with QOL. Caron et al. (2005) and Malla et al. (2004) identified a full range of sociodemographic characteristics having differential associations with different aspects of QOL. However, Ho et al.'s (2000) study failed to confirm most of these findings.

The role of medication—mostly first-generation neuroleptics—was assessed in a survey of 565 patients with schizophrenia in Germany (Angermeyer & Matschinger, 2000). The authors concluded that side effects of medications such as extrapyramidal motor symptoms affect patients' QOL. These results to some extent coincide with those of Sullivan et al. (1992) that QOL varies with depressive symptoms, family interaction, and side effects of medications. In many countries, the now almost complete transition to antipsychotic drugs that have significantly reduced extrapyramidal side effects has more or less eradicated this source of erosion to the QOL of people with schizophrenia.

Conclusions

The last few years of research into the course and outcome of schizophrenia have led us to bid farewell to the traditional long-term studies and their heterogeneous results. Progress in research methods, including precisely defined inclusion criteria (diagnosis without selective course criteria), epidemiological first-episode samples, more or less comparable follow-up periods, standardized assessment procedures and prospective, in part controlled, study designs have yielded increasingly consistent data on various course and outcome patterns and the trajectories of the course of schizophrenia. The average course of the disorder shows neither progressive deterioration, as described by Kraepelin for dementia praecox, nor pronounced improvement in symptoms and impairments at later stages of the illness. After the remission of the first episode, mean scores for neurocognitive impairments and the leading symptom dimensions of schizophrenia—depressive, negative, positive, and manic—exhibit a plateau-like trajectory and a surprising degree of intraindividual stability, although negative and depressive symptoms tend to unfold in longer waves.

In contrast with the traditional view, schizophrenia now has a lifelong perspective. The underlying neurobiological dysfunctions seem to appear first as risk factors mostly manifesting themselves as a subtle retardation of development from early childhood on, but the majority of these risk factors do not result in psychosis. Risk factors in late childhood and adolescence are mild cognitive, social, and emotional anomalies, and impaired socioeconomic development. These factors, too, only rarely lead to transit to the disorder. An indicator of increased susceptibility is the occurrence of rare psychotic symptoms in mentally healthy individuals or of mild psychopathological states. Rarely occurring or mild symptoms are associated with a low risk for developing psychosis, but that risk increases considerably with an increasing frequency of those symptoms. Age at illness onset, too, is a good indicator of risk: the lower that age, the higher the severity of symptoms and consequences of the disorder and, *vice versa*, the higher the age at onset, the milder the consequences. The most active part of the disease process is the period from illness onset until the climax of the first psychotic episode, marked by the accumulation of symptoms and of cognitive and social impairment. Even today, treatment usually begins only after most of the social consequences have become reality.

The course of schizophrenia shows a high degree of interindividual variability. There are cases with prodromal stages of several years' duration, increasingly severe negative symptoms, functional impairment, and subsequently persisting disability. A small group shows gradual progression over time. Other cases begin with an acute psychotic episode without any negative symptoms, followed by a sustained remission.

The different components of the disease construct of schizophrenia—positive, negative, depressive, and manic syndromes and cognitive impairment—differ in their frequencies. Depression is the most frequent symptom of schizophrenia. It occurs from the initial stages on and persists throughout a lifetime, being particularly pronounced in psychotic episodes and depressive relapses. The course of the negative syndrome differs most from those of the other domains. All the symptom dimensions—except neuropsychological deficits—evolve in asynchronous waves of exacerbations and symptom-free intervals, which differ in their durations and show a high degree of interindividual variability. These waves are shortest for positive symptoms and longest for depressive and negative symptoms. After remission of the first episode of schizophrenia, on average, there is usually no trend of either improvement or deterioration. Nevertheless, it does not have the stability of a neurodevelopmental brain defect. Schizophrenia can be understood as dynamic processes involving selective temporary dysfunction and plastic restitution. The factors precipitating these dysfunctions and waves of symptom exacerbation are not yet known. Credit for the advances in course and outcome research in the past two decades goes to a few controlled prospective first-admission studies, which have produced data on symptomatology, neuropsychological functioning, and morphological changes visible in magnetic resonance tomography. The first recent-onset studies, in which psychopathological and social data were correlated with morphological MRI data, revealed associations of cognitive and symptom-related phenomena with morphological changes, which may progress. The causal mechanisms of these processes, though perhaps not yet sufficiently clarified, are described in the chapters that follow.

Acknowledgments

We thank Professor Andreas Meyer-Lindenberg for taking the time to carefully read the manuscript. His critical comments and numerous suggestions have been invaluable. We also thank Dr Judith Allardyce, who, invited by Professor Jim van Os, provided suggestions to supplement or revise the passages on "The course of empirical symptom dimensions", "Risk factors or prodromal signs?", and "Prognostic indicators". Most of these suggestions have been adopted unchanged or in a slightly modified form.

References

Addington, J. & Addington, D. (1991) Positive and negative symptoms of schizophrenia. Their course and relationship over time. *Schizophrenia Research* **5**, 51–59.

Addington, J. & Addington, D. (1998) Effect of substance misuse in early psychosis. *British Journal of Psychiatry* **172** (Suppl. 33), 134–136.

Addington, J. & Addington, D. (2000) Neurocognitive and social functioning in schizophrenia: a 2.5 year follow-up study. *Schizophrenia Research* **44**, 47–56.

Addington, J., Young, J. & Addington, D. (2003) Social outcome in early psychosis. *Psychological Medicine* **33**, 1119–1124.

Addington J., Van Mastrigt S., Addington D. (2004) Duration of untreated psychosis: impact on 2-year outcome. *Psychological Medicine* **34**, 277–284.

Addington, J., Penn, D.L., Woods, S.W. *et al.* (2008) Social functioning in individuals at clinical high risk for psychosis. *Schizophrenia Research* **99**, 119–124.

Albus, M., Hubmann, W., Ehrenberg, C. *et al.* (1996) Neuropsychological impairment in first-episode and chronic schizophrenic patients. *European Archives of Psychiatry and Clinical Neuroscience* **246**, 249–255.

Allardyce, J., McGreadie, R.G., Morrison, G. & van Os, J. (2007) Do symptom dimensions or categorial diagnosis best discriminate between known risk factors for psychosis? *Social Psychiatry and Psychiatric Epidemiology* **42**, 429–437.

American Psychiatric Association (1994) *DSM-IV: Diagnostic and Statistical Manual of Mental Disorders*, 4th edn. Washington, DC: American Psychiatric Association.

an der Heiden, W. (1996) Der Langzeitverlauf der schizophrenen Psychosen—eine Literaturübersicht. *Zeitschrift für Medizinische Psychologie* **5**, 8–21.

an der Heiden, W. & Krumm, B. (1991) The course of schizophrenia—some remarks on a yet unsolved problem of data collection. *European Archives of Psychiatry and Clinical Neuroscience* **240**, 303–306.

an der Heiden, W., Krumm, B., Müller, S. *et al.* (1995) Mannheimer Langzeitstudie der Schizophrenie: Erste Ergebnisse zum Verlauf der Erkrankung über 14 Jahre nach stationärer Erstbehandlung. *Nervenarzt* **66**, 820–827.

an der Heiden, W., Krumm, B., Müller, S. *et al.* (1996) Eine prospektive Studie zum Langzeitverlauf schizophrener Psychosen: Ergebnisse der 14-Jahres-Katamnese. *Zeitschrift für Medizinische Psychologie* **5**, 66–75.

an der Heiden, W., Könnecke, R., Maurer, K. *et al.* (2005) Depression in the long-term course of schizophrenia. *European Archives of Psychiatry and Clinical Neuroscience* **255**, 174–184.

Andreasen, N.C. (1984) *The Scale for the Assessment of Positive Symptoms (SAPS).* Iowa City, IA: University of Iowa.

Andreasen, N.C. (1989) The Scale for the Assessment of Negative Symptoms (SANS). *British Journal of Psychiatry* **155** (Suppl. 7), 53–58.

Andreasen, N.C. (1990) Positive and negative symptoms: historical and conceptual aspects. In: Andreasen, N.C., ed. *Schizophrenia: Positive and Negative Symptoms and Syndromes* Basel: Karger, pp. 1–42.

Andreasen, N.C. & Olsen, S.A. (1982) Negative vs. positive schizophrenia: definition and validation. *Archives of General Psychiatry* **39**, 789–794.

Andreasen, N.C., Grove, W.M., Shapiro, R.W. *et al.* (1981) Reliability of lifetime diagnosis. *Archives of General Psychiatry* **38**, 400–405.

Andreasson, S., Allebeck, P., Engstrom, A. & Rydberg U. (1987) Cannabis and schizophrenia: A longitudinal study of Swedish conscripts. *Lancet* **ii**, 1483–1485.

Andreasen, N.C., Carpenter, W.T., Kane, J.M. *et al.* (2005) Remission in schizophrenia: proposed criteria and rationale for consensus. *American Journal of Psychiatry* **162**, 441–449.

Angermeyer, M.C. & Matschinger, H. (2000) Neuroleptika und Lebensqualität. Ergebnisse einer Patientenbefragung. *Psychiatrische Praxis* **27**, 64–68.

Antonova, E., Sharma, T., Morris, R. & Kumari, V. (2004) The relationship between brain structure and neurocognition in schizophrenia: a selective review. *Schizophrenia Research* **70**, 117–145.

Arndt, S., Andreasen, N.C., Flaum, M. *et al.* (1995) A longitudinal study of symptom dimensions in schizophrenia—Prediction and patterns of change. *Archives of General Psychiatry* **52**, 352–360.

Arseneault, L., Cannon, M., Poulton, R., Murray, R., Caspi, A. & Moffitt, T.E. (2002) Cannabis use in adolescence and risk for adult psychosis: longitudinal prospective study. *British Medical Journal* **325**, 1212–1213.

Arseneault, L., Cannon, M., Witton, J. & Murray, R.M. (2004) Causal association between cannabis and psychosis: examination of the evidence. *British Journal of Psychiatry* **184**, 110–117.

Arora, A., Avasthi, A. & Kulhara, P. (1997) Subsyndromes of chronic schizophrenia: a phenomenological study. *Acta Psychiatrica Scandinavica* **96**, 225–229.

Ballon, J.S., Kaur, T., Marks, I.I. & Cadenhead, K.S. (2007) Social functioning in young people at risk for schizophrenia. *Psychiatry Research* **151**, 29–35.

Barak, Y., Knobler, C.Y. & Aizenberg, D. (2004) Suicide attempts among elderly schizophrenic patients: a 10-year case-control study. *Schizophrenia Research* **71**, 77–81.

Barnes, T.R.E., Hutton, S.B., Chapman, M.J. *et al.* (2000) West London first-episode study of schizophrenia. Clinical correlates of duration of untreated psychosis. *British Journal of Psychiatry* **177**, 207–211.

Barnes, T.R.E., Mutsatsa, S.H., Hutton, S.B., Watt, H.C. & Joyce, E.M. (2006) Comorbid substance use and age at onset of schizophrenia. *British Journal of Psychiatry* **188**, 237–242.

Bartels, S.J., Drake, R.E. & McHugo, G.J. (1992) Alcohol abuse, depression, and suicidal behavior in schizophrenia. *American Journal of Psychiatry* **149**, 394–395.

Baxter, D. & Appleby, L. (1999) Case register study of suicide risk in mental disorders. *British Journal of Psychiatry* **175**, 322–326.

Bebbington, P.E., Craig, T., Garety, P. *et al.* (2006) Remission and relapse in psychosis: operational definitions based on case-note data. *Psychological Medicine* **36**, 1551–1562.

Becker, T., Leese, M., Clarkson, P. *et al.* (1998) Links between social network and quality of life: an epidemiologically representative study of psychotic patients in south London. *Social Psychiatry and Psychiatric Epidemiology* **33**, 229–304.

Bell, M.D. & Mishara, A.L. (2006) Does negative symptom change relate to neurocognitive change in schizophrenia? *Schizophrenia Research* **81**, 17–27.

Bengtsson-Tops, A. & Hansson, L. (1999) Subjective quality of life in schizophrenic patients living in the community. Relationship to clinical and social characteristics. *European Psychiatry* **14**, 256–263.

Biehl, H., Maurer, K., Schubart, C. *et al.* (1986) Prediction of outcome and utilization of medical services in a prospective study of first onset schizophrenics. *European Archives of Psychiatry and Neurological Sciences* **236**, 139–147.

Bilder, R.M. (1998) The neuropsychology of schizophrenia: what, when, where, how? In: Fleischhacker, V.W., Hinterhuber, H. & Meise, U., eds. *Schizophrenie Störrungen: State of the Art II.* Innsbruck: Vrelag Integrative Psychiatrie, pp. 155–171.

Bilder, R.M., Goldman, R.S., Robinson, D. *et al.* (2000) Neuropsychology of first-episode schizophrenia: initial characterization and clinical correlates. *American Journal of Psychiatry* **157**, 549–559.

Bilder, R.M., Mukherjee, S., Rieder, R.O. & Pandurangi, A.K. (1985) Symptomatic and neuropsychological components of defect status. *Schizophrenia Bulletin* **11**, 409–419.

Binder, J., Albus, M., Hubmann, W. *et al.* (1998) Neuropsychological impairment and psychopathology in first-episode schizophrenic patients related to the early cousre of the illness. *European Archives of Psychiatry and Clinical Neuroscience* **248**, 70–77.

Blanchard, J.J., Horan, W.P. & Collins, L.M. (2005) Examining the latent structure of negative symptoms: is there a distinct subtype of negative symptom schizophrenia? *Schizophrenia Research* **77**, 151–165.

Bland, R.C. & Orn, H. (1978) Fourteen-years outcome in early schizophrenia. *Psychological Medicine* **4**, 244–254.

Bland, R.C., Parker, J.H. & Orn, H. (1976) Prognosis in schizophrenia. A ten-year follow-up of first admissions. *Archives of General Psychiatry* **33**, 949–954.

Bleuler, M. (1968) A 23-year longitudinal study of 208 schizophrenics and impressions in regard to the nature of schizophenia. In: Rosenthal, D. & Kety, S.S., eds. *The Transmission of Schizophrenia.* Oxford: Pergamon Press, pp. 3–12.

Bleuler, M. (1972) *Die schizophrenen Geistesstörungen im Lichte langjähriger Kranken- und Familiengeschichten.* Stuttgart: Thieme.

Bottlender, R., Strauss, A. & Möller, H.-J. (2000) Impact of duration of symptoms prior to first hospilization on acute outcome in 998 schizophrenic patients. *Schizophrenic Research* **44**, 145–150.

Bottlender, R., Sato, T., Jager, M. *et al.* (2003) The impact of the duration of untreated psychosis prior to first psychiatric admission on the 15-year outcome in schizophrenia. *Schizophrenia Research* **62**, 37–44.

Boydell, J., van Os, J., Caspi, A. *et al.* (2006) Trends in cannabis use prior to first presentation with schizophrenia, in South-East London between 1965 and 1999. *British Journal of Psychiatry* **36**, 1441–1446.

Bralet, M.C., Loas, G., Yon, V. & Maréchal, V. (2002) Clinical characteristics and risk factors for Kraepelinian subtype of schizophrenia: replication of previous findings and relation to summer birth. *Psychiatry Research* **111**, 147–154.

Breier, A., Schreiber, J.L., Dyer, J. & Pickar, D. (1991) National Institute of Mental Health longitudinal study of chronic schizophrenia: prognosis and predictors of outcome. *Archives of General Psychiatry* **48**, 239–246.

Brennan, P.A., Mednick, S.A. & Hodgins, S. (2000) Major mental disorders and criminal violence in a Danish birth cohort. *Archives of General Psychiatry* **57**, 494–500.

Bressan, R.A., Chaves, A.C., Pilowsky, L.S. *et al.* (2003) Depressive episodes in stable schizophrenia: critical evaluation of the DSM-IV and ICD-10 diagnostic criteria. *Psychiatry Research* **117**, 47–56.

Brown, G.W. (1960) Length of hospital stay and schizophrenia: a review of statistical studies. *Acta Psychiatrica et Neurologica Scandinavica* **35**, 414–430.

Brown, S. (1997) Excess mortality of schizophrenia. A meta-analysis. *British Journal of Psychiatry* **171**, 502–508.

Browne, S., Clarke, M., Gervin, M. *et al.* (2000) Determinants of quality of life at first presentation with schizophrenia. *British Journal of Psychiatry* **176**, 173–176.

Buchanan, R.W. & Heinrichs, D.W. (1989) The Neurological Evaluation Scale (NES): a structured instrument for the evaluation of neurological signs in schizophrenia. *Psychiatry Research* **27**, 335–350.

Buchanan R.W., Ball M.P., Weiner E. *et al.* (2005) Olanzapine treatment of residual positive and negative symptoms. *American Journal of Psychiatry* **162**, 124–129.

Buchsbaum, M.S., Shihabuddin, L., Hazlett, E.A. *et al.* (2002) Kraepelinian and non-Kraepelinian schizophrenia subgroup differences in cerebral metabolic rate. *Schizophrenia Research* **55**, 25–40.

Buchsbaum, M.S., Shihabuddin, L., Brickman, A.M. *et al.* (2003) Caudate and putamen volumes in good and poor outcome patients with schizophrenia. *Schizophrenia Research* **64**, 53–62.

Bühler, B., Hambrecht, M., Löffler, W., an der Heiden, W. & Häfner, H. (2002) Precipitation and determination of the onset and course of schizophrenia by substance abuse: a retrospective and prospective study of 232 population-based first illness episodes. *Schizophrenia Research* **54**, 243–251.

Burns, T. (2007) Hospitalisation as an outcome measure in schizophrenia. *British Journal of Psychiatry* **191** (Suppl. 50), s37–s41.

Cahn, W., Hulshoff Pol, H.E., Bongers, M. *et al.* (2002) Brain morphology in antipsychotic-naïve schizophrenia: a study of multiple brain structures. *British Journal of Psychiatry* **43** (Suppl.), s66–72.

Caldwell, C.B. & Gottesman, I.I. (1990) Schizophrenics kill themselves too: a review of risk factors of suicide. *Schizophrenia Bulletin* **16**, 571–589.

Campbell, A., Converse, R.E. & Rodgers, W.L. (1976) *The Quality of American Life: Perception, Evaluations, and Satisfactions*. New York: Russell Sage Foundation.

Cantor-Graae, E., Nordström, L.G. & McNeil, T.F. (2001) Substance abuse in schizophrenia: a review of the literature and a study of correlates in Sweden. *Schizophrenia Research* **48**, 69–82.

Carlsson, R., Nyman, H., Ganse, G. & Cullberg, J. (2006) Neuropsychological functions predict 1- and 3-year outcome in first-episode psychosis. *Acta Psychiatrica Scandinavica* **113**, 102–111.

Caron, J., Mercier, C., Diaz, P. & Martin, A. (2005) Socio-demographic and clinical predictors of quality of life in patients with schizophrenia or schizo-affective disorder. *Psychiatry Research* **137**, 203–213.

Carpenter, W.T. (2007) Commentary: Deconstructing and reconstructing illness syndromes associated with psychosis. *World Psychiatry* **6**, 28–29.

Carpenter, W.T. & Kirkpatrick, B. (1988) The heterogeneity of the long-term course of schizophrenia. *Schizophrenia Bulletin* **14**, 645–652.

Carpenter, W.T. & Strauss, J.S. (1991) The prediction of outcome in schizophrenia. IV: Eleven-year follow-up of the Washington IPSS cohort. *Journal of Nervous and Mental Disease* **179**, 517–525.

Carpenter, W.T., Heinrichs, D.W. & Wagman, A.M.I. (1988) Deficit and nondeficit forms of schizophrenia: the concept. *American Journal of Psychiatry* **145**, 578–583.

Carpenter, W.T., Buchanan, R.W., Kirkpatrick, B., Thaker, G. & Tamminga, C. (1991) Negative symptoms: a critique of current approaches. In: Marneros, N.C., Andreasen, N.C. & Tsuang, M.T., eds. *Negative Versus Positive Schizophrenia*. Berlin: Springer, pp. 126–133.

Caspi, A., Moffitt, T.E., Cannon, M. *et al.* (2005) Moderation of the effect of adolescent-onset cannabis use on adult psychosis by a functional polymorphism in the catechol-O-methyltransferase gene: longitudinal evidence of a gene X environment interaction. *Biolological Psychiatry* **57**, 1117–1127.

Castle, D. (2000) Women and schizophrenia. In: Castle, D., McGrath, J. & Kulkarni, J., eds. *Women and Schizophrenia*. Cambridge: Cambridge University Press, pp. 19–33.

Castle, D.J. & Morgan, V. (2008) Epidemiology. In: Mueser, K.T. & Jeste, D.V., eds. *Clinical Handbook of Schizophrenia*. New York: Guilford Press, pp. 14–24.

Cechnicki, A. & Walczewski, K. (1999) Dynamic of positive and negative syndrome in schizophrenia—prospective study. In: López-Ibor, J., Sartorius, N., Gaebel, W. *et al.*, eds. *Psychiatry on New Thresholds. Abstracts of the XI World Congress of Psychiatry, Hamburg, August 6–11, 1999*.

Censits, D.M., Ragland, J.D., Gur, R.C. & Gur, R.E. (1997) Neuropsychological evidence supporting a neurodevelopmental model of schizophrenia: a longitudinal study. *Schizophrenia Research* **24**, 289–298.

Chakos, M., Schobel, S.A., Gu, H. *et al.* (2005) Duration of illness and treatment effects on hippocampal volume in male patients with schizophrenia. *British Journal of Psychiatry* **186**, 26–31.

Chapman, L.J., Chapman, J.P. & Roulin, M.L. (1976) Scales for physical and social anhedonia. *Journal of Abnormal Psychology* **87**, 374–407.

Chapman, L.J., Chapman, J.P., Kwapil, T.R. *et al.* (1994) Putatively psychosis-prone subjects 10 years later. *Journal of Abnormal Psychology* **103**, 171–183.

Chen, C.-K. & Murray, R.M. (2004) How does drug abuse interact with familial and developmental factors in the etiology of schizophrenia? In: Keshavan, M.S., Kennedy, J. & Murray, R.M., eds. *Neurodevelopment and Schizophrenia*. Cambridge: Cambridge University Press, pp. 248–269.

Choquet, M. & Ledoux, S. (1994) Epidémiologie et adolescence. *Confrontations psychiatriques* **27**, 287–309.

Ciompi, L. (1980) Catamnestic long-term study on the course of life and aging of schizophrenics. *Schizophrenia Bulletin* **6**, 606–618.

Ciompi, L. & Müller, C. (1976) *Lebensweg und Alter der Schizophrenen*. Berlin: Springer.

Clarke, M. & O'Callaghan, E. (2003) The value of first-episodes studies in schizophrenia. In: Murray, R.M., Cannon, M., Jones, P. *et al.*, eds. *The Epidemiology of Schizophrenia*. New York: Cambridge University Press, pp. 148–166.

Clarke, M., Whitty, P., Browne, S. *et al.* (2006) Suicidality in first episode psychosis. *Schizophrenia Research* **86**, 221–225.

Cornblatt, B., Obuchowski, M., Schnur, D.B. & O'Biran, J. (1998) Hillside study of risk and early detection in schizophrenia. *British Journal of Psychiatry* **172** (Suppl. 3), 26–32.

Craig, T.J. Sigel, C., Hopper, K., Lin, S. & Sartorius, N. (1997) Outcome in schizophrenia and related disorders compared between developing and developed countries: a recursive partitioning re-analysis of the WHO DOSMeD data. *British Journal of Psychiatry* **170**, 229–233.

Craig, T.J., Bromet, E.J., Fennig, S. *et al.* (2000) Is there an association between duration of untreated psychosis and 24-month clinical outcome in a first-admission series? *American Journal of Psychiatry* **157**, 60–66.

Crow, T.J. (1980a) Discussion: positive and negative schizophrenic symptoms and the role of dopamine. *British Journal of Psychiatry* **137**, 383–386.

Crow, T.J. (1980b) Molecular pathology of schizophrenia: more than one disease process. *British Medical Journal* **260**, 66–68.

Crow, T.J. (1980c) Positive and negative schizophrenic symptoms and the role of dopamine. *British Journal of Psychiatry* **137**, 383–386.

Crow, T.J. (1985) The two-syndrome concept: Origins and current status. *Schizophrenia Bulletin* **11**, 471–486.

Davidson, L. & McGlashan, T.H. (1997) The varied outcomes of schizophrenia. *Canadian Journal of Psychiatry* **42**, 34–43.

Davidson, M., Reichenberg, A., Rabinowitz, J. *et al.* (1999) Behavioral and intellectual markers for schizophrenia in apparently healthy male adolescents. *American Journal of Psychiatry* **156**, 1328–1335.

de Haan, L., van Der Gaag, M. & Wolthaus, J. (2000) Duration of untreated psychosis and the long-term course of schizophrenia. *European Psychiatry* **15**, 264–267.

de Haan, L., Linszen, D.H., Lenior, M.E. *et al.* (2003) Duration of untreated psychosis and outcome of schizophrenia: delay in intensive psychosocial treatment versus delay in treatment with antipsychotic medication. *Schizophrenia Bulletin* **29**, 341–348.

de Hert, M., McKenzie, K. & Peuskens, J. (2001) Risk factors for suicide in young people suffering from schizophrenia: a long-term follow-up study. *Schizophrenia Research* **47**, 127–134.

de Hert, M., van Winkel, R., Wampers, M. *et al.* (2007) Remission criteria for schizophrenia: evaluation in a large naturalistic cohort. *Schizophrenia Research* **92**, 68–73.

Deister, A. & Marneros, A. (1993) Long-term stability of subtypes in schizophrenic disorders: a comparison of four diagnostic systems. *European Archives of Psychiatry and Clinical Neuroscience* **242**, 184–190.

DeLisi, L.E., Sakuma, M., Tew, W. *et al.* (1997) Schizophrenia as a chronic active brain process: a study of progressive brain structural change subsequent to the onset of schizophrenia. *Psychiatry Research* **74**, 129–140.

Dikeos, D.G., Wickham, H., McDonald, C.D. *et al.* (2006) Distribution of symptom dimensions across Kraepelinian divisions. *British Journal of Psychiatry* **189**, 346–353.

Dollfus, S., Everitt, B., Ribeyre, J.M. *et al.* (1996) Identifying subtypes of schizophrenia by cluster analyses. *Schizophrenia Bulletin* **22**, 545–555.

Döpfner, M., Plück, J., Berner, W. *et al.* (1997) [Mental disturbances in children and adolescents in Germany. Results of a representative study:age,gender and rater effects, in German] *Z Kinder Jugendpsychiatr Psychother* **25**, 218–233.

Drake, R.J., Haley, C.J., Akhtar, S. & Lewis S.W. (2000) Causes and consequences of duration of untreated psychosis in schizophrenia. *British Journal of Psychiatry* **177**, 511–515.

Drake, R.J., Dunn, G., Tarrier, N., Haddock, G., Haley, C. & Lewis, S. (2003) The evolution of symptoms in the early course of non-affective psychosis. *Schizophrenia Research* **63**, 171–179.

Dubertret, C., Bidard, I., Adès, J. & Gorwood, P. (2006) Lifetime positive symptoms in patients with schizophrenia and cannabis abuse are partially explaines by co-morbid addiction. *Schizophrenia Research* **86**, 284–290.

Dunayevich, E., Sethuraman, G., Enerson, M., Taylor, C.C. & Lin, D. (2006) Characteristics of two alternative schizophrenia remission definitions: Relationship to clinical and quality of life outcomes. *Schizophrenia Research* **86**, 300–308.

D'Souza, D.C., Sewell, R.A. & Ranganathan, M. (2009) Cannabis and psychosis/schizophrenia: human studies. *European Archives of Psychiatry and Clinical Neuroscience* **259**, 413–431.

Eastvold, A.D., Heaton, R.K. & Cadenhead, K.S. (2007) Neurocognitive deficits in the (putative) prodrome and first episode of psychosis. *Schizophrenia Research* **93**, 266–277.

Eaton, W.W. (1999) Evidence for universitality and uniformity of schizophrenia around the world: assessment and implications. In: Gattaz, W.F. & Häfner, H., eds. *Search for the Causes of Schizophrenia, Vol. IV. Balance of the Century*. Darmstadt: Steinkopff Verlag, pp. 21–33.

Eaton, W.W., Romanoski, A., Anthony, J.C. & Nestadt, G. (1991) Screening for psychosis in the general population with a self-report interview. *Journal of Nervous and Mental Disease* **179**, 689–693.

Eaton, W.W., Mortensen, P.B., Herman, H. *et al.* (1992a) Long-term ciyrse if hospitalization for schizophrenia. I. Risk for rehospitalization. *Schizophrenia Bulletin* **18**, 217–227.

Eaton, W.W., Bukjerm W., Haro, J.M. *et al.* (1992b) Long-term course of hospitalization for schizophrenia. II. Change with passage of time. *Schizophrenia Bulletin* **18**, 229–241.

Eaton, W.W., Thara, R., Federman, B., Melton, B. & Liang, K.Y. (1995) Structure and course of positive and negative symptoms in schizophrenia. *Archives of General Psychiatry* **52**, 217–134.

Emsley, R., Turner, H.J., Oosthuizen, P.P. & Carr, J. (2005) Neurological abnormalities in first-episode schizophrenia: temporal stability and clinical and outcome correlates. *Schizophrenia Research* **75**, 35–44.

Emsley, R., Rabinowitz, J., Medori, R. & Early Psychosis Global Working Group (2007) Remission in early psychosis: rates, predictors, and clinical and functional outcome correlates. *Schizophrenia Research* **89**, 129–139.

Endicott, J., Spitzer, R.L., Fleiss, J.L. & Cohen, J. (1976) The Global Assessment Scale. A procedure for measurement overall severity of psychiatric disturbance. *Archives of General Psychiatry* **33**, 766–771.

Engelhardt, D.M., Rosen, B., Feldman, J. *et al.* (1982) A 15-year followup of 646 schizophrenic outpatients. *Schizophrenia Bulletin* **8**, 493–503.

Falkai, P., Tepest, R., Honer, W.G. *et al.* (2004) Shape changes in prefrontal, but not parieto-occipital regions: brains of schizophrenic patients come closer to a circle in coronal and sagittal view. *Psychiatry Research* **132**, 261–271.

Fannon, D., Chitnis, X. & Doku, V. (2000) Features of structural brain abnormality detected in first-episode psychosis. *American Journal of Psychiatry* **157**, 1829–1834.

Faris, R.E.L. & Dunham, H.W. (1939) *Mental Disorders in Urban Areas: An Ecological Study of Schizophrenia and Other Psychosis.* Chicago: University or Chicago Press.

Fenton, W.S. (2000) Depression, suicide, and suicide prevention in schizophrenia. *Suicide & Life Threatening Behavior* **30**, 34–49.

Fenton, W.S. & McGlashan, T.H. (1991a) Natural history of schizophrenia subtypes. I. Longitudinal study of paranoid, hebephrenic, and undifferentiated schizophrenia. *Archives of General Psychiatry* **48**, 969–977.

Fenton, W.S. & McGlashan, T.H. (1991b) Natural history of schizophrenia subtypes. II. Positive and negative symptoms and long-term course. *Archives of General Psychiatry* **48**, 978–986.

Fenton, W.S., McGlashan, T., Victor, B.J. & Blyler, C.R. (1997) Symptoms, subtype, and suicidality in patients with schizophrenia spectrum disorders. *American Journal of Psychiatry* **154**, 199–204.

Ferdinand, R.F., van der Ende, J., Bongers, I. *et al.* (2005) Cannabis—psychosis pathway independent of other types of psychopathology. *Schizophrenia Research* **79**, 289–295.

Fergusson, D.M., Horwood, L.J. & Ridder, E.M. (2005) Tests of causal linkages between cannabis use and psychotic symptoms. *Addiction* **100**, 354–366.

Fergusson, D.M., Poulton, R., Smith, P.F. & Boden, J.M. (2006) Cannabis and psychosis. *British Medical Journal* **332**, 172–176.

French, P., Shryane, N., Bentall, R.P., Lewis, S.W. & Morrison, A.P. (2007) Effects of cognitive therapy on the longitudinal development of psychotic experiences in people at high risk of developing psychosis. *British Journal of Psychiatry* **51** (Suppl), s82–87.

Friis, S., Larsen, T.K., Melle, I. *et al.* (2003) Methodological pitfalls in early detection studies—the NAPE lecture 2002. *Acta Psychiatrica Scandinavica* **107**, 3–9.

Fuller, R., Nopoulos, P., Arndt, S. *et al.* (2002) Longitudinal assessment of premorbid cognitive functioning in patients with schizophrenia through examination of standardized scholastic test performance. *American Journal of Psychiatry* **159**, 1183–1189.

Gaebel, W. & Frommann, N. (2000) Long-term course in schizophrenia: concepts, methods and research strategies. *Acta Psychiatrica Scandinavica* **102** (Suppl. 407), 49–53.

Ganev, K. (2000) Long-term trends of symptoms and disability in schizophrenia and related disorders. *Social Psychiatry and Psychiatric Epidemiology* **35**, 389–395.

Gattaz, W.F., Brunner, J., Schmidt, A. & Maras, A. (1995) Increased breakdown of membrane phospholipids in schizophrenia: implications for the hypofrontality hypothesis. In: Häfner, H. & Gattaz, W.F., eds. *Search for the Causes of Schizphrenia*, **Vol. III**. Berlin: Springer, pp. 215–226.

Geddes, J.R. & Kendell, R.E. (1995) Schizophrenic subjects with no history of admission to hospital. *Psychological Medicine* **25**, 859–868.

Giron, M. & Gomez-Beneyto, M. (2004) Relationship between family attitudes and social functioning in schizophrenia: a nine-month follow-up prospective study in Spain. *Journal of Nervous and Mental Disease* **192**, 414–420.

Gold, A., Arndt, S., Nopoulos, P. *et al.* (1999) Longitudinal study of cognitive function in first-episode and recent-onset schizophrenia. *American Journal of Psychiatry* **156**, 1342–1348.

Goldacre, M., Shiwach, R. & Yeates, D. (1994) Estimating incidence and prevalence of treated psychiatric disorders from routine statistics: the example of schizophrenia in Oxfordshire. *Journal of Epidemiology and Community Health* **48**, 318–322.

Goldberg, T.E., Hyde, T.M., Kleinman, J.E. & Weinberger, D.R. (1993) Course of schizophrenia: neuropsychological evidence for a static encephalopathy. *Schizophrenia Bulletin* **19**, 797–804.

Goldberg, T.E., David, A. & Gold J.M. (2003) Neurocognitive deficits in schizophrenia. In: Hirsch, S.R. & Weinberger, D.W., eds. *Schizophrenia*, 2nd edn. Oxford: Blackwell Publishing, pp. 168–184.

Gourzis, P., Katrivanou, A. & Beratis, S. (2002) Symptomatology of the initial prodromal phase in schizophrenia. *Schizophrenia Bulletin* **28**, 415–429.

Gottesman, I.I., McGuffin, P. & Farmer, A.E. (1987) Clinical genetics as clue to the "real" genetics of schizophrenia (a decade of modest gains while playing for a time). *Schizophrenia Bulletin* **13**, 23–47.

Green, M.F. (1996) What are the functional consequences of neurocognitive deficits in schizophrenia. *American Journal of Psychiatry* **153**, 321–330.

Green, B., Young, R. & Kavanagh, D. (2005) Cannabis use and misuse prevalence among people with psychosis. *British Journal of Psychiatry* **187**, 306–313.

Grunebaum, M.F., Oquendo, M.A., Harkavy-Friedman, J.M. et al. (2001) Delusions and suicidality. *American Journal of Psychiatry* **158**, 742–747.

Gupta, S., Andreasen, N.C., Arndt, S. et al. (1997) The Iowa Longitudinal Study of Recent Onset Psychosis: one-year follow-up of first episode patients. *Schizophrenia Research* **23**, 1–13.

Haas, G.L. & Sweeney, J.A. (1992) Premorbid and onset features of first-episode schizophrenia. *Schizophrenia Bulletin* **18**, 373–386.

Haas, G., Gattatt, L.S. & Sweeney, J.A. (1998) Delay to first antipsychotic medication in schizophrenia: impact on symptomatology and clinical course of illness. *Journal of Psychiatric Research* **32**, 151–159.

Häfner, H. (1995) Epidemiology of schizophrenia. The disease model of schizophrenia in the light of current epidemiological knowledge. *European Psychiatry* **10**, 228–236.

Häfner, H. (2003a) Gender differences in schizophrenia. *Psychoneuroendocrinology* **28**, 17–54.

Häfner, H. (2003b) Prodrome, onset and early course of schizophrenia. In: Murray, R.M., Cannon, M., Jones, P. et al., eds. *The Epidemiology of Schizophrenia*. New York: Cambridge University Press, pp. 124–147.

Häfner, H. (2008) *Cannabis und Schizophrenie*. Speech at the 26. Psychiatrietage Königslutter. Nov 20–21, 2008. Königslutter.

Häfner, H. & an der Heiden, W. (1982) Evaluation gemeindenaher Versorgung psychisch Kranker. *Archiv für Psychiatrie und Nervenkrankheiten* **232**, 71–95.

Häfner, H. & an der Heiden, W. (1986) The contribution of European case registers to research on schizophrenia. *Schizophrenia Bulletin* **12**, 26–51.

Häfner, H. & an der Heiden, W. (2003) Course and outcome of schizophrenia. In: Hirsch, S.R. & Weinberger, D.R., eds. *Schizophrenia*, 2nd edn. Oxford: Blackwell Publishing, pp. 101–141.

Häfner, H. & Kasper, S. (1982) Akute lebensbedrohliche Katatonie. Epidemiologische und klinische Befunde. *Nervenarzt* **53**, 385–394.

Häfner, H. & Maurer, K. (2003) The prodromal phase of psychosis. In: Miller, T., ed. *Early Intervention in Psychotic Disorder*. Amsterdam: Kluwer Academic Publishers, pp. 71–100.

Häfner, H. & Maurer, K. (2006) Early Detection of Schizophrenia: current evidence and future perspectives. *World Psychiatry* **5**, 130–138.

Häfner, H. & Nowotny, B. (1995) Epidemiology of early-onset schizophrenia. *European Archives of Psychiatry and Clinical Neuroscience* **245**, 80–92.

Häfner, H., Riecher-Rössler, A., Hambrecht, M. et al. (1992) IRAOS: an instrument for the assessment of onset and early course of schizophrenia. *Schizophrenia Research* **6**, 209–223.

Häfner, H., Maurer, K., Löffler, W. et al. (1995) Onset and early course of schizophrenia. In: Häfner, H. & Gattaz, W.F., eds. *Search for the Causes of Schizophrenia. Vol. III*. Berlin: Springer, pp. 43–66.

Häfner, H., and der Heiden, W., Behrens, S. et al. (1998) Causes and consequences of the gender difference in age at onset of schizophrenia. *Schizophrenia Bulletin* **24**, 99–113.

Häfner, H., Löffler, W., Maurer, K. et al. (1999a) Depression, negative symptoms, social stagnation and social decline in the early course of schizophrenia. *Acta Psychiatrica Scandinavica* **100**, 105–118.

Häfner, H., Maurer, K., Löffler, W. et al. (1999b) Onset and prodromal phase as determinants of the course. In: Gattaz, W.F. & Häfner, H., eds. *Search for the Causes of Schizophrenia, Vol. IV: Balance of the Century*. Darmstadt: Steinkopff, pp. 35–58.

Häfner, H., Löffler, W., Riecher-Rössler, A. & Häfner-Ranabauer, W. (2001a) Schizophrenie und Wahn im höheren und hohen Lebensalter. Epidemiologie und ätiologische Hypothesen. *Nervenarzt* **72**, 347–357.

Häfner, H., Maurer, K., Löffler, W. et al. (2001b) Onset and early course of schizophrenia—a challenge for early intervention. *Psychiatrica Fennica* **32** (Suppl. 2), 81–108.

Häfner, H., Maurer, K., Löffler, W., an der Heiden, W., Könnecke, R. & Hambrecht, M. (2002) The early course of schizophrenia. In: Häfner, H., ed. *Risk and protective factors in schizophrenia*. Darmstadt: Steinkopff, pp. 207–228.

Häfner, H., Löffler, W., Maurer, K. et al. (2003a) *IRAOS Interview for the Retrospective Assessment of the Onset and Course of Schizophrenia and Other Psychoses*. Göttingen: Hogrefe & Huber Publishers.

Häfner, H., Maurer, K., Löffler, W. et al. (2003b) Modeling the early course of schizophrenia. *Schizophrenia Bulletin* **29**, 325–340.

Häfner, H., Maurer, K., Trendler, G. et al. (2005) The early course of schizophrenia and depression. *European Archives of Psychiatry and Clinical Neuroscience* **255**, 167–173.

Häfner, H., an der Heiden, W. & Maurer, K. (2008) Evidence for separate diseases? Stages of one disease or different combinations of symptom dimensions? *European Archives of Psychiatry and Clinical Neuroscience* **258** (Suppl. 2), 85–96.

Hambrecht, M. & Häfner, H. (1996) Substance abuse and the onset of schizophrenia. *Biological Psychiatry* **40**, 1155–1163.

Hanssen, M., Bak, M., Bijl, R.V. et al. (2005) The incidence and outcome of subclinical psychotic experiences in the general population. *British Journal of Clinical Psychology* **44**, 181–191.

Harding, C.M., Brooks, G.W., Ashikaga, T. et al. (1987a) The Vermont longitudinal study of persons with severe mental illness. I: Methodology, study sample, and overal status 32 years later. *American Journal of Psychiatry* **144**, 718–726.

Harding, C.M., Brooks, G.W., Ashikaga, T. et al. (1987b) The Vermont longitudinal study of persons with severe mental illness. II: Long-term outcome of subjects who retrospectively met DSM-III criteria for schizophrenia. *American Journal of Psychiatry* **144**, 727–735.

Harrigan, S.M., McGorry, P.D. & Krstev, H. (2003) Does treatment delay in first-episode psychosis really matter? *Psychological Medicine* **33**, 97–110.

Harris, M.G., Henry, L.P., Harrigan, S.M. et al. (2005) The relationship between duration of untreated psychosis and outcome: An eight-year prospective study. *Schizophrenia Research* **79**, 85–93.

Harrison, G., Croudace, T., Mason, P., Glazebrook, C. & Medley, I. (1996) Predicting the long-term outcome of schizophrenia. *Psyclogical Medicine* **26**, 697–705.

Harrison, G., Hopper, K., Craig, T. *et al.* (2001) Recovery from psychotic illness: A 15 and 25 year international follow-up study. *British Journal of Psychiatry* **178**, 506–517.

Harrison, P.J., Freemantle, N. & Geddes, J.R. (2003) Meta-analysis of brain weight in schizophrenia. *Schizophrenia Research* **64**, 25–34.

Harrison, I., Joyce, E.M., Mutsatsa, S. *et al.* (2008) Naturalistic follow-up of co-morbid substance use in schizophrenia: The West London first episode study. *Psychological Medicine* **38**, 79–88.

Harrow, M. & Jobe, T.H. (2007) Factors involved in outcome and recovery in schizophrenic patients not on antipsychotic medications: a 15-year multifollow-up study. *Journal of Nervous and Mental Disease* **195**, 406–414.

Harvey, P.D., Howanitz, E., Parrella, M., White, L. & Davidson, M. (1998) Symptoms, cognitive functioning, and adaptive skills in geriatric patients with lifelong schizophrenia: a comparison across treatment sites. *American Journal of Psychiatry* **155**, 1080–1086.

Harvey, P.D., Parrella, M., White, L. *et al.* (1999) Convergence of cognitive and adaptive decline in late-life schizophrenia. *Schizophrenia Research* **35**, 77–84.

Hawton, K., Sutton, L., Haw, C. *et al.* (2005) Schizophrenia and suicide: systematic review of risk factors. *British Journal of Psychiatry* **187**, 9–20.

Healy, D., Harris, M., Tranter, R. *et al.* (2006) Lifetime suicide rates in treated schizophrenia: 1875–1924 and 1994–1998 cohorts compared. *British Journal of Psychiatry* **188**, 223–228.

Heaton, R.K., Gladsjo, J.A., Palmer, B.W. *et al.* (2001) Stability and course of neuropsychological deficits in schizophrenia. *Archives of General Psychiatry* **58**, 24–32.

Hegarty, J.D., Baldessarini, R.J., Tohen, M. *et al.* (1994) One hundred years of schizophrenia: a meta-analysis of the outcome literature. *American Journal of Psychiatry* **151**, 1409–1416.

Heilä, H., Heikkinen, M.E., Isometsä, E.T. *et al.* (1999a) Life events and completed suicide in schizophrenia: a comparison of suicide victims with and without schizophrenia. *Schizophrenia Bulletin* **25**, 519–531.

Heilä, H., Henriksson, M.M., Heikkinen, M.E. & Marttunen, M.J. (1999b) Suicide victims with schizophrenia in different treatment phases and adequacy of antipsychotic medication. *Journal of Clinical Psychiatry* **60**, 200–208.

Heilä, H., Haukka, J., Suvisaari, J. & Lönnqvist, J. (2005) Mortality among patients with schizophrenia and reduced psychiatric hospital care. *Psychological Medicine* **35**, 725–732.

Heinrichs, R.W. & Zakzanis, K.K. (1998) Neurocognitive deficit in schizophrenia: a quantitative review of the evidence. *Neuropsychology* **12**, 426–445.

Heinrichs, R.W., Ruttan, L., Zakzanis, K.K. & Case, D. (1997) Parsing schizophrenia with neurocognitive tests: evidence of stability and validity. *Brain and Cognition* **35**, 207–224.

Helldin, L., Kane, J.M., Karilampi, U. *et al.* (2007) Remission in prognosis of functional outcome: a new dimension in the treatment of patients with psychotic disorders. *Schizophrenia Research* **93**, 160–168.

Henquet, C., Krabbendam, L., Spauwen, J. *et al.* (2005) Prospective cohort study of cannabis use, predisposition for psychosis, and psychotic symptoms in young people. *BMJ* **330**, 11.

Hides, L., Dawe, S., Kavanagh, D.J. & Young, R.M. (2006) Psychotic symptom and cannabis relapse in recent-onset psychosis. Prospective study. *British Journal of Psychiatry* **189**, 137–143.

Ho, B.-C., Andreasen, N.C., Flaum, M. *et al.* (2000) Untreated initial psychosis: its relation to quality of life and symptom remission in first-episode schizophrenia. *American Journal of Psychiatry* **157**, 808–815.

Ho, B.-C., Alicata, D., Ward, J. *et al.* (2003a) Untreated initial psychosis: relation to cognitive deficits and brain morphology in first-episode schizophrenia. *American Journal of Psychiatry* **160**, 142–148.

Ho, B.-C., Andreasen, N.C., Nopoulos, P. *et al.* (2003b) Progressive structural brain abnormalities and their relationship to clinical outcome: a longitudinal magnetic resonance imaging study early in schizophrenia. *Archives of General Psychiatry* **60**, 585–594.

Hoff, A.L., Sakuma, M., Wieneke, M. *et al.* (1999) Longitudinal neuropsychological follow-up study of patients with first-episode schizophrenia. *American Journal of Psychiatry* **156**, 1336–1341.

Hoff, A.L., Sakuma, M., Razi, K. *et al.* (2000) Lack of association between duration of untreated illness and severity of cognitive and structural brain deficits at the first episode of schizophrenia. *American Journal of Psychiatry* **157**, 1824–1828.

Holthausen, E.A., Wiersma, D., Sitskoorn, M.M. *et al.* (2002) Schizophrenic patients without neuropsychological deficits: subgroup, disease severity or cognitive compensation? *Psychiatry Research* **112**, 1–11.

Hopper, K., Harrison, G., Janca, A., & Sartorius, N. (2007) *Recovery from Schizophrenia—An International Perspective. A Report from the WHO Collaborative Project, the International Study of Schizophrenia.* Oxford: Oxford University Press.

Howard, R. & Jeste, D.V. (2003) Late-onset schizophrenia. In: Hirsch, S.R. & Weinberger, D.R., eds. *Schizophrenia*, 2nd edn. Oxford: Blackwell Publishing, pp. 68–79.

Huber, G., Gross, G. & Schüttler, R. (1979) *Schizophrenie. Eine verlaufs- und sozialpsychiatrische Langzeitstudie.* Berlin: Springer.

Huber, D., Henrich, G. & Herschbach, P. (1988) Measuring the quality of life: a comparison between physically and mentally chronically ill patients and healthy persons. *Pharmacopsychiatria* **21**, 453–455.

Hughes, C., Kumari, V., Soni, W. *et al.* (2002) Longitudinal study of symptoms and cognitive function in chronic schizophrenia. *Schizophrenia Research* **59**, 137–146.

Hulshoff Pol, H.E., Schnack, H.G., Bertens, M.G.B.C. *et al.* (2002) Volume changes in gray matter in patients with schizophrenia. *American Journal of Psychiatry* **159**, 244–250.

Huppert, J.D., Weiss, K.A., Lim, R., Pratt, S. & Smith, T.E. (2001) Quality of life in schizophrenia: contributions of anxiety and depression. *Schizophrenia Research* **51**, 171–180.

Hwu, H.G., Chen, C.H., Hwang, T.J. *et al.* (2002) Symptom patterns and subgrouping of schizophrenic patients: significance of negative symptoms assessed on admission. *Schizophrenia Research* **56**, 105–119.

Isohanni, M., Isohanni, I., Järvelin, M.R. *et al.* (1999) Childhood and adolescent predictors of schizophrenia. In: López-Ibor, J., Sartorius, N, Gaebel, W. & Haasen, C., eds. *Psychiatry on New*

Thresholds. Abstracts of the XI World Congress of Psychiatry, Hamburg, August 6–11, 1999.

Jablensky, A. (1995) Schizophrenia: the epidemiological horizon. In: Hirsch, S.R. & Weinberger, D.R., eds. *Schizophrenia.* Oxford: Blackwell Science, Ltd., pp. 206–252.

Jablensky, A. (2000) Symptome schizophrener Störungen. In: Helmchen, H., Henn, F., Lauter, H. *et al. Psychiatrie der Gegenwart. Vol. 5,* 4th edn. Berlin: Springer, pp. 3–51.

Jablensky, A. (2003) The epidemiological horizon. In: Hirsch, S.R. & Weinberger, D.R., eds. *Schizophrenia,* 2nd edn. Oxford: Blackwell Publishing, pp. 203–231.

Jablensky, A., Schwarz, R. & Tomov, T. (1980) WHO collaborative study on impairments and disabilities associated with schizophrenic disorders. A preliminary communication: objectives and methods. *Acta Psychiatrica Scandinavica* (Suppl. 285), 152–163.

Jablensky, A., Sartorius, N., Ernberg, G. *et al.* (1992) Schizophrenia: manifestations, incidence and course in different cultures. A World Health Organization Ten-Country Study. *Psychological Medicine* (Suppl. 20).

Jackson, J.H. (1887) Remarks on the evolution and dissolution of the nervous system. *Journal of Mental Science* **33**, 25–48.

Jacobsen, L.K., Giedd, J.N., Castellanos, X. *et al.* (1998) Progressive reduction of temporal lobe structures in childhood-onset schizophrenia. *American Journal of Psychiatry* **155**, 678–685.

Jarskog, F., Gilmore, J.H., & Lieberman, J.A. (2004) Neurodegenerative models of schizophrenia. In: Keshavan, M., Kennedy, J. & Murray, R., eds. *Neurodevelopment and Schizophrenia.* Cambridge: Cambridge University Press, pp. 373–389.

Johnstone, E.C. (1991) Disabilities and circumstances of schizophrenic patients—a follow-up study. *British Journal of Psychiatry* **159** (Suppl.13).

Johnstone, E.C. (1999) Brain imaging and function: the balance of the century. In: Gattaz, W.F. & Häfner, H., eds. *Search for the Causes of Schizophrenia,* Vol. **IV**. Balance of the Century. Darmstadt: Steinkopff, pp. 293–305.

Johnstone, E.C., Lawrie, S.M. & Cosway, R. (2002) What does the Edinburgh high-risk study tell us about schizophrenia? *American Journal of Medical Genetics (Neuropsychiatric Genetics)* **114**, 906–912.

Johnstone E.C., Ebmeier, K.P., Miller, P., Owens, D.G. & Lawrie, S.M. (2005) Predicting schizophrenia: findings from the Edinburgh High-Risk Study. *British Journal of Psychiatry* **186**, 18–25.

Jones, P.B. (1999) Longitudinal approaches to the search of the cause of schizophrenia: past, present and future. In: Gattaz, W.F. & Häfner, H., eds. *Search for the Causes of Schizophrenia, Vol. IV. Balance of the Century.* Darmstadt: Steinkopff Verlag, pp. 91–119.

Kane, J.M. & Lencz, T. (2008) Cognitive deficits in schizophrenia: short-term and long-term. *World Psychiatry* **7**, 29–30.

Kaplan, K.J. & Harrow, M. (1996) Positive and negative symptoms as risk factors for later suicidal activity in schizophrenics. *Suicide & Life Threatening Behavior* **26**, 105–121.

Kavanagh, D.J., Waghorn, G., Jenner, L. *et al.* (2004) Demographic and clinical correlates of comorbid substance use disorders in psychosis: multivariate analyses from an epidemiological sample. *Schizophrenia Research* **66**, 115–124.

Kay, S.R. & Sevy, S. (1990) Pyramidical model of schizophrenia. *Schizophrenia Bulletin* **16**, 537–545.

Kay, S.R., Fiszbein, A. & Opler, L.A. (1987) The Positive and Negative Syndrome Scale (PANSS) for schizophrenia. *Schizophrenia Bulletin* **13**, 261–276.

Keefe, R.S.E. (2008) Should cognitive impairment be included in the diagnostic criteria for schizophrenia? *World Psychiatry* **7**, 22–28.

Keefe, R.S., Mohs, R.C., Losonczy, M.F. *et al.* (1987) Characteristics of very poor outcome schizophrenia. *American Journal of Psychiatry* **144**, 889–895.

Keefe, R.S., Frescka, E., Apter, S.H. *et al.* (1996) Clinical characteristics of Kraepelinian schizophrenia: replication and extension of previous findings. *American Journal of Psychiatry* **153**, 806–811.

Keller, M.B., Lavori, P.W., Friedman, B. *et al.* (1987) The longitudinal interval follow-up evaluation. A comprehensive method for assessing outcome in prospective longitudinal studies. *Archives of General Psychiatry* **44**, 540–548.

Keller, A., Castellanos, X., Vaituzis, C. *et al.* (2003) Progressive loss of cerebellar volume in childhood-onset schizophrenia. *American Journal of Psychiatry* **160**, 128–133.

Kendler, K.S., Gallagher, T.J., Abelson, J.M. & Kessler, R.C. (1996) Lifetime prevalence, demographic risk factors, and diagnostic validity of nonaffective psychosis as assessed in a US community sample. The National Comorbidity Survey. *Archives of General Psychiatry* **53**, 1022–1031.

Keshavan, M.S., Diwadkar, V.A., Montrose, D.M. *et al.* (2005) Premorbid indicators and risk for schizophrenia: a selective review and update. *Schizophrenia Research* **79**, 57.

Kilzieh, N., Wood, A.E., Erdmann, J., Raskind, M. & Tapp, A. (2003) Depression in Kraepelinian schizophrenia. *Comprehensive Psychiatry* **44**, 1–6.

Kirkpatrick, B. & Galderisi, S. (2008) Deficit schizophrenia: an update. *World Psychiatry* **7**, 143–147.

Kirkpatrick, B., Buchanan, R.W., McKenney, P.D., Alphs, L.D. & Carpenter, W.T. (1989) The Schedule for the Deficit Syndrome: an instrument for research in schizophrenia. *Psychiatry Research* **30**, 119–123.

Kohn, M. (1969) *Class and Conformity: A Study of Values.* Homewood, IL: Dorsey Press.

Kopelowicz, A., Liberman, R.P., Ventura, J. *et al.* (2005) Neurocognitive correlates of recovery from schizophrenia. *Psychological Medicine* **35**, 1165–1173.

Krabbendam, L., Myin-Germeys, I., Hanssen, M. *et al.* (2005) Development of depressed mood predicts onset of psychotic disorder in individuals who report hallucinatory experiences. *British Journal of Clinical Psychology* **44**, 113–125.

Kraepelin, E. (1893) *Psychiatrie. Ein Lehrbuch für Studierende und Ärzte,* 4 edn. Leipzig: Barth.

Kraepelin, E. (1920) Die Erscheinungsformen des Irreseins. *Zeitschrift für die gesamte Neurologie und Psychiatrie* **62**, 1–29.

Krausz, M., Müller-Thomsen, T. & Haasen, C. (1995) Suicide among schizophrenic adolescents in the long-term course of illness. *Psychopathology* **28**, 95–103.

Kristensen, K. & Cadenhead, K.S. (2007) Cannabis abuse and risk for psychosis in a prodromal sample. *Psychiatry Research* **151**, 151–154.

Kurtz, M.M. (2005) Neurocognitive impairment across the lifespan in schizophrenia: an update. *Schizophrenia Research* **74**, 15–26.

Lappin, J.M., Morgan, K.D., Morgan, C. *et al.* (2007) Duration of untreated psychosis and neuropsychological function in first episode psychosis. *Schizophrenia Research* **95**, 103–110.

Larsen, T.K., Friis, S., Haahr, U. *et al.* (2004) Premorbid adjustment in first-episode non-affective psychosis: distinct patterns of pre-onset course. *British Journal of Psychiatry* **185**, 108–115.

Larsen, T.K., Melle, I., Auestad, B. *et al.* (2006) Substance abuse in first-episode non-affective psychosis. *Schizophrenia Research* **88**, 55–62.

Lawrie, S.M. (2004) Premorbid structural abnormalities in schizophrenia. In: Keshavan, M., Kennedy, J. & Murray, R., eds. *Neurodevelopment and Schizophrenia*. Cambridge: Cambridge University Press, pp. 347–372.

Lawrie, S.M. & Abukmeil, S.S. (1998) Brain abnormality in schizophrenia: a systematic and quantitative review of volumetric magnetic resonance imaging studies. *British Journal of Psychiatry* **172**, 110–120.

Lawrie, S.M., Whalley, H. & Kestelman, J.N. (1999) Magnetic resonance imaging of brain in people at high risk of developing schizophrenia. *Lancet* **353**, 30–33.

Leff, J.P., Sartorius, N., Jablensky, A. *et al.* (1992) The International Pilot Study of Schizophrenia: five-year follow-up findings. *Psychological Medicine* **22**, 131–145.

Lehman, A.F. (1996) Evaluating outcomes of treatments for persons with psychotic disorders. *Journal of Clinical Psychiatry* **57** (Suppl. 11), 61–67.

Lehman, A.F., Fischer, E.P., Postrado, L. *et al.* (2003) The Schizophrenia Care and Assessment Program Health Questionnaire (SCAP-HQ): an instrument to assess outcomes of schizophrenia care. *Schizophrenia Bulletin* **29**, 247–256.

Lenzenweger, M.F., Dworkin, R.H. & Wethington, E. (1991) Examining the underlying structure of schizophrenic phenomenology: evidence for a three-process model. *Schizophrenia Bulletin* **17**, 515–524.

Leon, C.A. (1989) Clinical course and outcome of schizophrenia in Cali, Colombia: a 10-year follow-up study. *Journal of Nervous and Mental Disease* **177**, 593–606.

Leung, A. & Chue, P. (2000) Sex differences in schizophrenia, a review of the literature. *Acta Psychiatrica Scandinavica* **401**, 3–38.

Lewis, S.W. (1990) Computerised tomography in schizophrenia 15 years on. *British Journal of Psychiatry* **157** (Suppl. 9), 16–24.

Lewis, S., Tarrier, N., Haddock, G. *et al.* (2002) Randomized, controlled trial of cognitive-behaviour therapy in early schizophrenia: acute phase outcomes. *British Journal of Psychiatry* **181**, 91–97.

Liddle, P.F. (1987a) Schizophrenic syndromes, cognitive performance and neurological dysfunction. *Psychological Medicine* **17**, 49–57.

Liddle, P.F. (1987b) The symptoms of chronic schizophrenia: a re-examination of the positive–negative dichotomy. *British Journal of Psychiatry* **151**, 145–151.

Liddle, P.F. (1994) Volition and schizophrenia in psychological medicine. In: David, A.S. & Cutting, J.C., eds. *The Neuropsychology of Schizophrenia*. Hove: Lawrence Erlbaum, pp. 39–49.

Liddle, P.F. & Barnes, T.R.E. (1990) Syndromes of chronic schizophrenia. *British Journal of Psychiatry* **157**, 558–561.

Liberman, R.P. & Kopelowicz, A. (2005) Recovery from schizophrenia: a concept in search of research. *Psychiatric Services* **56**, 735–742.

Liberman, R.P., Kopelowicz, A., Ventura, J. & Gutkind, D. (2002) Operational criteria and factors related to recovery from schizophrenia. *International Review of Psychiatry* **14**, 256–272.

Lieberman, J.A., Chakos, M., Wu, H. *et al.* (2001a) Longitudinal study of brain morphology in first episode schizophrenia. *Biological Psychiatry* **49**, 487–499.

Lieberman, J.A., Perkins, D., Belger, A. *et al.* (2001b) The early stages of schizophrenia: speculations on pathogenesis, pathophysiology, and therapeutic approaches. *Biological Psychiatry* **50**, 884–897.

Limosin, F., Loze, J.-Y., Philippe, A. *et al.* (2007) Ten-year prospective follow-up study of the mortality by suicide in schizophrenic patients. *Schizophrenia Research* **94**, 23–28.

Lindenmayer, J.P., Brown, E., Baker, R.W. *et al.* (2004) An excitement subscale of the Positive and Negative Syndrome Scale. *Schizophrenia Research* **68**, 331–337.

Link, B.G. & Dohrenwend, B.P. (1980) Formulation of hypotheses about the ratio of untreated to treated cases in the true prevalence studies of functional psychiatric disorders in adults in the United States. In: Dohrenwend, B.P., Dohrenwend, B.S., Schwartz, G.M. *et al.*, eds. *Mental Illness in the United States. Epidemiological Estimates*. New York, Praeger, pp. 133–149.

Loebel, A.D., Lieberman, J.A., Alvir, J.M.J. *et al.* (1992) Duration of psychosis and outcome in first-episode schizophrenia. *American Journal of Psychiatry* **149**, 1183–1188.

Löffler, W. & Häfner, H. (1999a) Dimensionen der schizophrenen Symptomatik—Vergleichende Modellprüfung an einem Erstepisodensample. *Nervenarzt* **70**, 416–429.

Löffler, W. & Häfner, H. (1999b) Ecological pattern of first admitted schizophrenics in two German cities over 25 years. *Social Science & Medicine* **49**, 93–108.

Loranger, A.W. (1990) The impact of DSM-III on diagnostic practice in a university hospital: a comparison of DSM-II and DSM-III in 10914 patients. *Archives of General Psychiatry* **47**, 672–675.

Lorr, M., Klett, C.J. & McNair, D.M. (1963) *Syndromes in Psychosis*. New York: Pergamon Press.

Lukoff, D., Nuechterlein, K.H. & Ventura, J. (1986) Manual for Expanded Brief Psychiatric Rating Scale (BPRS). *Schizophrenia Bulletin* **12**, 594–602.

Maccabe, J.H., Aldouri, E., Fahy, T.A. *et al.* (2002) Do schizophrenic patients who managed to get to university have a non-developmental form of illness? *Psychological Medicine* **32**, 535–544.

Maccoby, E.E. & Jacklin, C.N. (1980) Sex differences in aggression: a rejoinder and reprise. *Child Development* **51**, 964–980.

Malla, A.K., Norman, R.M.G., McLean, T.S. *et al.* (2004) Determinants of quality of life in first-episode psychosis. *Acta Psychiatrica Scandinavica* **109**, 46–54.

Malla, A.K. & Payne, J. (2005) First-episode psychosis: psychopathology, quality of life, and functional outcome. *Schizophrenia Bulletin* **31**, 650–671.

Malm, U., May, P.R.A. & Dencker, S.J. (1981) Evaluation of the quality of life of the schizophrenic outpatient: a checklist. *Schizophrenia Bulletin* **7**, 477–487.

Malmberg, A., Lewis, G., David, A. & Allebeck, P. (1998) Premorbid adjustment and personality in people with schizophrenia. *British Journal of Psychiatry* **172**, 308–313.

Marengo, J.T., Harrow, M., Sands, J. & Galloway, C. (1991) European versus U.S. data on the course on schizophrenia. *American Journal of Psychiatry* **148**, 606–611.

Margolese, H.C., Malchy, L., Negrete, J.C. *et al.* (2004) Drug and alcohol use among patients with schizophrenia and related psychoses: levels and consequences. *Schizophrenia Research* **67**, 157–166.

Margolese, H.C., Carlos Negrete, J., Tempier, R. & Gill, K. (2006) A 12-month prospective follow-up study of patients with schizophrenia-spectrum disorders and substance abuse: changes in psychiatric symptoms and substance use. *Schizophrenia Research* **83**, 65–75.

Marneros, A., Deister, A., & Rohde, A. (1991) *Affektive, schizoaffektive und schizophrene Psychosen. Eine vergleichende Langzeitstudie*. Berlin: Springer.

Marneros, A., Rohde, A. & Deister, A. (1995) Psychotic continuum under longitudinal considerations. In: Marneros, A., Andreasen, N.C. & Tsuang, M.T., eds. *Psychotic Continuum*. Berlin: Springer, pp. 17–30.

Marshall, M., Lewis, S., Lockwood, A. *et al.* (2005) Association between duration of untreated psychosis and outcome in cohorts of first-episode patients. *Archives of General Psychiatry* **62**, 975–983.

Mason, P., Harrison, G., Glazebrook, C., Medley, I., Dalkin, T. & Croudace, T. (1995) Characteristics of outcome in schizophrenia at 13 years. *British Journal of Psychiatry* **167**, 596–603.

Mason, P., Harrison, G., Glazebrook, C. *et al.* (1996) The course of schizophrenia over 13 years. A report from the International Study on Schizophrenia (ISoS) coordinated by the World Health Organization. *British Journal of Psychiatry* **169**, 580–586.

Mathalon, D.H., Sullivan, E.V., Lim, K.O. & Pfefferbaum, A. (2001) Progressive brain volume changes and the clinical course of schizophrenia in men: a longitudinal magnetic resonance imaging study. *Archives of General Psychiatry* **58**, 148–157.

Maurer, K. (1995) *Der geschlechtsspezifische Verlauf der Schizophrenie über 10 Jahre*. Hamburg: Dr Kovac.

Maurer, K. & Häfner, H. (1991) Dependence, independence or interdependence of positive and negative symptoms. In: Marneros, A., Andreasen, N.C. & Tsuang, M.T., eds. *Negative Versus Positive Schizophrenia*. Berllin: Springer, pp. 160–182.

Maziade, M., Bouchard, S., Gingras, N. *et al.* (1996) Long-term stability of diagnosis and symptom dimensions in a systematic sample of patients with onset of schizophrenia in childhood and early adolescence. II. Positive–negative distinction and childhood predictors of adult outcome. *British Journal of Psychiatry* **169**, 371–378.

McCleery, A., Addington, J. & Addington, D. (2006) Substance misuse and cognitive functioning in early psychosis: a 2 year follow-up. *Schizophrenia Research* **88**, 187–191.

McGirr, A., Tousignant, M., Routhier, D. *et al.* (2006) Risk factors for completed suicide in schizophrenia and other chronic psychotic disorders: a case-control study. *Schizophrenia Research* **84**, 132–143.

McGlashan, T.H. (1984a) The Chestnut Lodge follow-up study. I. Follow-up methodology and study sample. *Archives of General Psychiatry* **41**, 573–585.

McGlashan, T.H. (1984b) The Chestnut Lodge follow-up study, II. LOng-term outcome of schizophrenia and the affective disorders. *Archives of General Psychiatry* **41**, 586–601.

McGlashan, T.H. (1998) Early detection and intervention of schizophrenia: rationale and research. *British Journal of Psychiatry* **172** (Suppl. 33), 3–6.

McGlashan, T.H. (2006) Is active psychosis neurotoxic? *Schizophrenia Bulletin* **32**, 609–613.

McGlashan, T.H. & Johannessen, J.O. (1996) Early detection and intervention with schizophrenia: rationale. *Schizophrenia Bulletin* **22**, 201–222.

McGorry, P.D., McFarlane, C., Patton, G.C. *et al.* (1995) The prevalence of prodromal symptoms of schizophrenia in adolescence: a preliminary survey. *Acta Psychiatrica Scandinavica* **92**, 241–249.

McGorry, P.D., Edwards, J., Mihalopoulos, C., Harrigan, S.M. & Jackson, H.J. (1996) EPPIC: An evolving system of early detection and optimal management. *Schizophrenia Bulletin* **22**, 305–326.

McGorry, P.D., Yung, A.R., Phillips, L.J. *et al.* (2002) Randomized controlled trial of interventions designed to reduce the risk of progression to first episode psychosis in a clinical sample with subthreshold symptoms. *Archives of General Psychiatry* **59**, 921–928.

McGuffin, P., Katz, R. & Aldrich, J. (1986) Past and Present State Examination: the assessment of lifetime ever psychopatholgy. *Psychological Medicine* **16**, 461–465.

McGurk, S.R. & Mueser, K.T. (2003) Cognitive functioning and employment in severe mental illness. *Journal of Nervous and Mental Diseases* **191**, 789–798.

McKenzie, K., van Os, J., Fahy, T. *et al.* (1995) Psychosis with good prognosis in Afro-Caribbean people now living in the United KOngdom. *British Medical Journal* **311**, 1325–1327.

Mechanic, D., McAlpine, D., Rosenfield, S. & Davis, D. (1994) Effects of illness attribution and depression on the quality of life among persons with serious mental illness. *Social Science & Medicine* **39**, 155–164.

Michaelos, A.L. (1980) Satisfaction and happiness. *Social Indicators Research* **8**, 385–422.

Miles, C.P. (1977) Conditions predisposing to suicide: a review. *Journal of Nervous and Mental Disease* **164**, 231–246.

Milev, P., Ho, B.-C., Arndt, S. & Andreasen, N.C. (2005) Predictive values of neurocognition and negative symptoms on functional outcome in schizophrenia: a longitudinal first-episode study with 7-Year follow-up. *American Journal of Psychiatry* **162**, 495–506.

Miller, T.J., McGlashan, T.H. Woods, S.W. *et al.* (1999) Symptoms assessment in schizophrenic prodromal states. *Psychiatric Quarterly* **70**, 273–287.

Mitelman, S.A., Shihabuddin, L., Brickman, A.M., Hazlett, E.A. & Buchsbaum, M.S. (2005) Volume of the cingulate and outcome in schizophrenia. *Schizophrenia Research* **72**, 91–108.

Möller, H.-J. & von Zerssen, D. (1995) Course and outcome of schizophrenia. In: Hirsch, S.R. & Weinberger, D.R., eds. *Schizophrenia*. Oxford: Blackwell Science, Ltd., pp. 106–127.

Möller, H.-J., Schmid-Bode, W. & von Zerssen, D. (1986) Prediction of long-term outcome in schizophrenia by prognostic scales. *Schizophrenia Bulletin* **12**, 225–235.

Möller, H.-J., von Zerssen, D., Werner-Eilert, K. & Wüschner-Stockheim, M. (1982) Outcome in schizophrenia and simlar paranoid psychosis. *Schizophrenia Bulletin* **8**, 99–108.

Möller, H.-J., Scharl, W. & von Zerssen, D. (1984) Strauss-Carpenter-Skala: Überprüfung ihres prognostischen Wertes für das 5-Jahres-'Outcome' schizophrener Patienten. *European Archives of Psychiatry and Neurological Science* **234**, 112–117.

Möller, H.J., Bottlender, R., Grob, A. *et al.* (2002) The Kraepelinian dichotomy: preliminary results of a 15-year follow-up study on functional psychoses: focus on negative symptoms. *Schizophrenia Research* **56**, 87–94.

Morgan, C., Dazzan, P., Morgan, K. *et al.* (2006) First episode psychosis and ethnicity: initial findings from the AESOP study. *World Psychiatry* **5**, 40–46

Müller, P., Guenther, U. & Lohmeyer, J. (1986) Behandlung und Verlauf schizophrener Psychosen über ein Jahrzehnt. *Nevenarzt* **57**, 332–341.

Murphy, H.B. & Raman, A.C. (1971) The chronicity of schizophrenia in indigenous tropical peoples. Results of a twelve-year follow-up survey in Mauritius. *British Journal of Psychiatry* **118**, 489–497.

Murray, R.M. & Lewis, S.W. (1987) Is schizophrenia a neurodevelopmental disorder? *British Medical Journal* **295**, 681–682.

Murray, R.M., Grech, A., Phillips, P. & Johnson, S. (2003) What is the relationship between substance abuse and schizophrenia? In: Murray, R.M., Jones, P.B., Susser, E. *et al.*, eds. *The Epidemiology of Schizophrenia*. Cambridge: Cambridge University Press, pp. 317–342.

Murray, V., McKee, I., Miller, P.M. *et al.* (2005) Dimensions and classes of psychosis in a population cohort: a four-class, four-dimension model of schizophrenia and affective psychoses. *Psychological Medicine* **35**, 499–510.

Nair, T.R., Christensen, J.D., Kingsbury, S.J. *et al.* (1997) Progression of cerebrovascular enlargement and the subtyping of schizophrenia. *Psychiatry Research* **74**, 141–150.

Nopoulos, P., Flashman, L., Flaum, M. *et al.* (1994) Stability of cognitive functioning early in the course of schizophrenia. *Schizophrenia Research* **14**, 29–37.

Norman, R.M.G. & Malla, A.K. (2001) Duration of untreated psychosis: a critical examination of the concept and its importance. *Psychological Medicine* **31**, 381–400.

Norman, R.M.G., Townsend, L.A. & Malla, A.K. (2001) Duration of untreated psychosis and cognitive functioning in first-episode patients. *British Journal of Psychiatry* **179**, 340–345.

Norman R.M., Malla, A.K. & Manchanda, R. (2007) Early premorbid adjustment as a moderator of the impact of duration of untreated psychosis. *Schizophrenia Research* **95**, 111–114.

Nuechterlein, K.H. & Dawson, M.E. (1984) A heuristic vulnerability/stress model of schizophrenic episodes. *Schizophrenia Bulletin* **10**, 300–312.

Nuechterlein, K.H., Miklowitz, D.J., Ventura, J. *et al.* (2006) Classifying episodes in schizophrenia and bipolar disorder: criteria for relapse and remission applied to recent-onset samples. *Psychiatry Research* **144**, 153–166.

Ødegård, Ø. (1964) Patterns of discharge from Norwegian psychiatric hospitals before and after the introduction of psychotropic drugs. *American Journal of Psychiatry* **120**, 772–778.

Ohta, Y., Nagata, K., Yoshitake, K. *et al.* (1990) Changes in negative symptoms of schizophrenic patients two years later. *Japanese Journal of Psychiatry and Neurology* **44**, 521–529.

Oliver, J.P. & Mohamad, H. (1992) The quality of life of the chronically mentally ill: a comparison of public, private and voluntary residential provisions. *British Journal of Social Work* **22**, 391–404.

Opjordsmoen, S. (1998) Delusional disorders. I. Comparative long-term outcome. *Acta Psychiatrica Scandinavica* **80**, 603–612.

Osby, U., Correia, N., Brandt, L. *et al.* (2000) Mortality and causes of death in schizophrenia in Stockholm county, Sweden. *Schizophrenia Research* **45**, 21–28.

Overall, J.E. & Gorham, D.R. (1962) The Brief Psychiatric Rating Scale. *Psychological Reports* **10**, 799–812.

Palmer, B.W., McClure, F.S. & Jeste, D.V. (2001) Schizophrenia in late life: findings challenge traditional concepts. *Harvard Review of Psychiatry* **9**, 51–58.

Pantelis, C., Barber, F.Z., Barnes, T.R., Nelson, H.E., Owen, A.M. & Robbins T.W. (1999) Comparison of set-shifting ability in patients with chronic schizophrenia and frontal lobe damage. *Schizophrenia Research* **37**, 251–270.

Pantelis, C., Velakoulis, D., McGorry, P.D. *et al.* (2003) Neuroanatomical abnormalities befor and after onset of psychosis: a cross-sectional and longitudinal MRI comparison. *Lancet* **361**, 281–288.

Paulsen, J.S., Heaton, R.K., Sadek, J.R. *et al.* (1995) The nature of learning and memory impairments in schizophrenia. *Journal of the International Neuropsychological Society* **1**, 88–99.

Peralta, V., de Leon, J. & Cuesta, M.J. (1992) Are there more than two syndromes in schizophrenia? A critique of the positive–negative dichotomy. *British Journal of Psychiatry* **161**, 335–343.

Peralta, V., Cuesta, M.J. & de Leon, J. (1994) An empirical analysis of latent structures underlying schizophrenic symptoms. *Biological Psychiatry* **36**, 726–736.

Peralta, V., Cuesta, M.J., Giraldo, C. *et al.* (2002) Classifying psychotic disorders: issues regarding categorial vs. dimensional approaches and time frame to assess symptoms. *European Archives of Psychiatry and Clinical Neuroscience* **252**, 12–18.

Perkins, D.O., Gu, H., Boteva, K. & Lieberman, J.A. (2005) Relationship between duration of untreated psychosis and outcome in first-episode schizophrenia: a critical review and meta-analysis. *American Journal of Psychiatry* **162**, 1785–1804.

Perlstein, W.M., Carter, C.S., Noll, D.C. & Cohen, J.D. (2001) Relation of prefrontal cortex dysfunction to working memory and symptoms in schizophrenia. *American Journal of Psychiatry* **158**, 1105–1113.

Pietzcker, A. & Gaebel, W. (1983) Prediction of "natural" course, relapse and prophylactic response in schizophrenic patients. *Pharmaco-psychiatria* **16**, 206–211.

Poulton, R., Caspi, A., Moffitt, T.E. *et al.* (2000) Children's self-reported psychotic symptoms and adult schizophreniform disorder: a 15-year longitudinal study. *Archives of General Psychiatry* **57**, 1053–1058.

Priebe, S., Roeder-Wanner, U.U. & Kaiser, W. (2000) Quality of life in first admitted schizophrenic patients: a follow-up study. *Psychological Medicine* **30**, 225–230.

Putnam, K.M. & Harvey, P.D. (2000) Cognitive impairment and enduring negative symptoms: a comparative study of geriatric and nongeriatric schizophrenia patients. *Schizophrenia Bulletin* **26**, 867–878.

Rabinowitz, J., Reichenberg, A., Weiser, M. *et al.* (2000) Cognitive and behavioural functioning in men with schizophrenia both before and shortly after first admission to hospital. Cross-sectional analysis. *British Journal of Psychiatry* **177**, 26–32.

Rakfeldt, J. & McGlashan, T.H. (1996) Onset, course, and outcome of schizophrenia. *Current Opinion in Psychiatry* **9**, 73–76.

Ram, R., Bromet, E.J., Eaton, W.W., Pato, C. & Schwartz, J.E. (1992) The natural course of schizophrenia: a review of first-admission studies. *Schizophrenia Bulletin* **18**, 185–207.

Rapoport, J.L., Giedd, J.N., Blumenthal, J. *et al.* (1999) Progressive cortical change during adolescence in childhood-onset schizophrenia. A longitudinal magnetic resonance imaging study. *Archives of General Psychiatry* **56**, 649–654.

Ratakonda, S., Gorman, J.M., Yale, S.A. & Amador, X.F. (1998) Characterization of psychotic conditions. Use of the domains of psychopathology model. *Archives of General Psychiatry* **55**, 75–81.

Rey, E.-R., Bailer, J., Bräuer, W. *et al.* (1994) Empirische Analysen zur Gültigkeit des Anhedonie-Konstruktes bei ersthospitalisierten Schizophrenen. *Zeitschrift für Klinische Psychologie* **23**, 93–104.

Reynolds, J.R. (1858) On the pathology of convulsions, with special reference to those of children. *Liverpool Medical and Chirurgical Journal* **2**, 1–14.

Riecher-Rössler, A. & Rössler, W. (1998) The course of schizophrenic psychoses: what do we really know ? A selective review from an epidemiological perspective. *European Archives of Psychiatry and Clinical Neuroscience* **248**, 189–202.

Robins, L.N. (1979) Longitudinal methods in the study of normal and pathological development. In: Kisker, K.P., Meyer, J.-E., Müller, C. *et al.*, eds. *Psychiatrie der Gegenwart. Forschung und Praxis. Grundlagen und Methoden der Psychiatrie, Bd.I.* Berlin: Springer, pp. 627–684.

Robinson, D.G., Woerner, M.G., Alvir, J.M. *et al.* (1999a) Predictors of relapse following response from a first episode of schizophrenia or schizoaffective disorder. *Archives of General Psychiatry* **156**, 241–247.

Robinson, D.G., Woerner, M.G., Alvir, J.M. *et al.* (1999a) Predictors of treatment response from a first episode of schizophrenia or schizoaffective disorder. *Archives of General Psychiatry* **156**, 544–549.

Rosen, J.L., Miller, T.J., D'Andrea, J.T. *et al.* (2006) Comorbid diagnoses in patients meeting criteria for the schizophrenia prodrome. *Schizophrenia Research* **85**, 124–131.

Rosenman, S., Korten, A., Medway, J. & Evans, M. (2003) Dimensional vs. categorical diagnosis in psychosis. *Acta Psychiatrica Scandinavica* **107**, 378–384.

Rothman, K.J. (2002) *Epidemiology*. Oxford: Oxford University Press.

Roy, M.-A., Merette, C. & Maziade, M. (2001) Subtyping schizophrenia according to outcome or severity: a search for homogeneous subgroups. *Schizophrenia Bulletin* **27**, 115–138.

Rudnick, A. & Kravetz, S. (2001) The relation of social support-seeking to quality of life in schizophrenia. *Journal of Nervous and Mental Disease* **189**, 258–262.

Rund, B.R. (1998) A review of longitudinal studies of cognitive functions in schizophrenia patients. *Schizophrenia Bulletin* **24**, 425–435.

Rund, B.R., Landro, N.I. & Orbeck, A.L. (1997) Stability in cognitive dysfunctions in schizophrenic patients. *Psychiatry Research* **69**, 131–141.

Rund, B.R., Melle, I., Friis, S. *et al.* (2007) The course of neurocognitive functioning in first-episode psychosis and its relation to premorbid adjustment, duration of untreated psychosis, and relapse. *Schizophrenia Research* **91**, 132–140.

Salokangas, R.K.R. (1997) Structure of schizophrenic symptomatology and its changes over time: prospective factor-analytical study. *Acta Psychiatrica Scandinavica* **95**, 32–39.

Salyers, M.P. & Mueser, K.T. (2001) Social functioning, psychopathology, and medication side effects in relation to substance use and abuse in schizophrenia. *Schizophrenia Research* **48**, 109–123.

Sartorius, N., Jablensky, A. & Shapiro, R.W. (1977) Two-year follow-up of the patients included in the WHO International Pilot Study of Schizophrenia. *Psychological Medicine* **7**, 529–541.

Sartorius, N., Jablensky, A., Korten, A. *et al.* (1986) Early manifestation and first-contact incidence of schizophrenia in different cultures. A preliminary report on the initial evaluation phase of the WHO Collaborative Study on determinants of outcome of severe mental disorders. *Psychological Medicine* **16**, 909–928.

Sartorius, N., Jablensky, A., Ernberg, G. *et al.* (1987) Course of schizophrenia in different countries: some results of a WHO international comparative 5-year follow-up study. In: Häfner, H., Gattaz, W.F. & Janzarik, W., eds. *Search for the causes of schizophrenia, Vol. I* Berlin: Springer, pp. 107–113.

Sartorius, N., Gulbinat, W.H., Harrison, G., Laska, E. & Siegel, C. (1996) Long-term follow-up of schizophrenia in 16 countries: a description of the International Study of Schizophrenia conducted by the World Health Organization. *Social Psychiatry and Psychiatric Epidemiology* **31**, 249–258.

Sato, T., Bottlender, R., Schröder, A. & Möller, H.-J. (2004) Psychopathology of early-onset versus late-onset schizophrenia revisited: an observation of 473 neuroleptic-naive patients before and after first-admission treatments. *Schizophrenia Research* **67**, 175–183.

Saykin, A.J., Shtasel, D.L., Gur, R.E. *et al.* (1994) Neuropsychological deficits in neuroleptic naive patients with first-episode schizophrenia. *Archives of General Psychiatry* **51**, 124–131.

Schreiber, H., Baur-Seack, K. & Kornhuber, H.H. (1999) Brain morphology in adolescents at genetic risk for schizophrenia assessed by qualitative and quantitative magnetic resonance imaging. *Schizophrenia Research* **40**, 81–84.

Schubart, C., Schwarz, R., Krumm, B., & Biehl, H. (1986) *Schizophrenie und soziale Anpassung*. Berlin: Springer.

Schürhoff, F., Szöke, A., Bellivier, F. *et al.* (2003) Anhedonia in schizophrenia: a distinct familial subtype? *Schizophrenia Research* **61**, 59–66.

Schürhoff, F., Golmard, J.-L., Szöke, A. *et al.* (2004) Admixture analysis of age at onset in schizophrenia. *Schizophrenia Research* **71**, 35–41.

Scully, P.J., Coakley, G., Kinsella, A. & Waddington, J.L. (1997) Executive (frontal) dysfunction and negative symptoms in schizophrenia: apparent gender differences in "static" v. "progressive" profiles. *British Journal of Psychiatry* **171**, 154–158.

Seaton, B.E., Goldstein, G. & Allen, D.N. (2001) Sources of heterogeneity in schizophrenia: the role of neuropsychological functioning. *Neuropsychology Reviews* **11**, 45–67.

Selten, J.-P., Veen, N.D., Hoek, H.W. *et al.* (2007) Early course of schizophrenia in a representative Dutch incidence cohort. *Schizophrenia Research* **97**, 79–87.

Shepherd, M., Watt, D., Falloon, I.R.H. & Smeeton, N. (1989) The natural history of schizophrenia: a five-year follow-up study of outcome and prediction in a representative sample of schizophrenics. *Psychological Medicine* (Suppl.15).

Silva, P.A. & Stanton, W.R. (1996) *From Child to Adult: The Dunedin Multidisciplinary Health and Development Study.* Auckland: Oxford University Press.

Simonsen, E., Friis, S., Haahr, U. *et al.* (2007) Clinical epidemiologic first-episode psychosis: 1-year outcome and predictors. *Acta Psychiatrica Scandinavica* **116**, 54–61.

Singh, S.P. (2007) Outcome measures in early psychosis. Relevance of duration of untreated psychosis. *British Journal of Psychiatry* **191** (Suppl. 50), s58–s63.

Skeate, A., Jackson, C., Birchwood, M. & Jones, C. (2002) Duration of untreated psychosis and pathways to care in first-episode psychosis. Investigation of help-seeking behaviour in primary care. *British Journal of Psychiatry* **43** (Suppl.), s73–77.

Sobizack, N., Albus, M., Hubmann, W. *et al.* (1999) Neuropsychologische Defizite bei ersterkrankten schizophrenen Patienten. *Nervenarzt* **70**, 408–415.

Soyka, M., Albus, M., Kathmann, N. *et al.* (1993) Prevalence of alcohol and drug abuse in schizophrenic inpatients. *European Archives of Psychiatry and Clinical Neuroscience* **242**, 362–372.

Spauwen, J., Krabbendam, L., Lieb, R., Wittchen, H.U. & van Os, J. (2003) Sex differences in psychosis: normal or pathological? *Schizophrenia Research* **62**, 45–49.

Sponheim, S.R., Iacono, W.G., Thuras, P.D. & Beiser, M. (2001) Using biological indices to classify schizophrenia and other psychotic patients. *Schizophrenia Research* **50**, 139–150.

Stahl, S.M. & Buckley, P.F. (2007) Negative symptoms and schizophrenia: a problem that will not go away. *Acta Psychiatrica Scandinavica* **115**, 4–11.

Stephens, J.H., Ota, K.Y. & Carpenter, W.T. (1980) Diagnostic criteria for schizophrenia: Prognostic implications and diagnostic overlap. *Psychiatry Research* **2**, 1–12.

Stirling, J., Lewis, S., Hopkins, R. & White, C. (2005) Cannabis use prior to first onset psychosis predicts spared neurocognition at 10-year follow-up. *Schizophrenia Research* **75**, 135–137.

Stoll, A.L. Hohen, M. Baldessarini, R.J. *et al.* (1993) Shifts in diagnositc frequencies of schizophrenia and major affective disorders at six North American psychiatric hospitals, 1972–88. *Americal Journal of Psychiatry* **150**, 1668–1673.

Strauss, J.S. & Carpenter, W.T. (1972) The prediction of outcome in schizophrenia. I. Characteristics of outcome. *Archives of General Psychiatry* **27**, 739–746.

Strauss, J.S. & Carpenter, W.T. (1974) Characteristic symptoms and outcome in schizophrenia. *Archives of General Psychiatry* **30**, 429–434.

Strauss, J.S. & Carpenter, W.T. (1977) The prediction of outcome in schizophrenia. II. Five-year outcome and its predictors. *Archives of General Psychiatry* **34**, 159–163.

Sullivan, G., Wells, K.B. & Leake, B. (1992) Clinical factors associated with better quality of life in a seriously mentally ill population. *Hospital and Community Psychiatry* **43**, 794–798.

Takei, N., Persaud, R., Woodruff, P. *et al.* (1998) First episodes of psychosis in Afro-Caribbean and White people. An 18-year follow-up population-based study. *British Journal of Psychiatry* **172**, 147–153.

Talamo, A., Centorrino, F., Tondo, L. *et al.* (2006) Comorbid substance-use in schizophrenia: relation to positive and negative symptoms. *Schizophrenia Research* **86**, 251–255.

Tamminga, C.A., Buchanan, R.W. & Gold, J.M. (1998) The role of negative symptoms and cognitive dysfunction in schizophrenia outcome. *International Clinical Psychopharmacology* **13** (Suppl.), 21–26.

Tandon, R., DeQuardo, J.R., Taylor, S.F. *et al.* (2000) Phasic and enduring negative symptoms in schizophrenia: biological markers and relationship to outcome. *Schizophrenia Research* **45**, 191–201.

Thara, R., Henrietta, M., Joseph, A. *et al.* (1994) Ten-year course of schizophrenia—the Madras longitudinal study. *Acta Psychiatrica Scandinavica* **90**, 329–336.

The Scottish Schizophrenia Research Group (1992) The Scottish first episode schizophrenia study. VIII. Five-year follow-up: clinical and psychosocial findings. The Scottish Schizophrenia Research Group. *British Journal of Psychiatry* **161**, 496–500.

Thornicroft, G. & Johnson, S. (1996) True versus treated prevalence of psychosis—The Prism Case Identification Study. *European Psychiatry* **11** (Suppl. 4), 185.

Thorup, A., Petersen, L., Jeppesen, P. *et al.* (2007) Gender differences in young adults with first-episode schizophrenia spectrum disorders at baseline in the Danish OPUS study. *Journal of Nervous and Mental Disease* **195**, 396–405.

Tohen, M., Stoll, A.L., Strakowski, S.M. *et al.* (1992) The McLean First-Episode Psychosis Project: six-month recovery and recurrence outcome. *Schizophrenia Bulletin* **18**, 273–282.

Torrey, E.F. (2002) Studies of individuals with schizophrenia never treated with antipsychotic medications: a review. *Schizophrenia Research* **58**, 101–115.

Toomey, R., Kremen, W.S., Simpson, J.C. *et al.* (1997) Revisiting the factor structure for positive and negative symptoms: evidence from a large heterogeneous group of psychiatric patients. *American Journal of Psychiatry* **154**, 371–377.

Usall, J., Haro, J.M., Ochoa, S., Márquez, M. & Araya, S.; Needs of Patients with Schizophrenia group. (2002) Influence of gender on social outcome in schizophrenia. *Acta Psychiatrica Scandinavica* **106**, 337–342.

van Os, J., Fahy, T.A., Jones, P. *et al.* (1996) Psychopathological syndromes in the functional psychoses: associations with course and outcome. *Psychological Medicine* **26**, 161–176.

van Os, J., Gilvarry, C., Bale, R. *et al.* (1999) A comparison of the utility of dimensional and categorical representations of psychosis. UK700 Group. *Psychological Medicine* **29**, 595–606.

van Os, J., Hanssen, M., Bijl, R.V. & Ravelli, A. (2000) Strauss (1969) revisited: a psychosis continuum in the general population? *Schizophrenia Research* **45**, 11–20.

van Os, J., Bak, M., Hanssen, M., Bijl, R.V., de Graaf, R. & Verdoux, H. (2002) Cannabis use and psychosis: a longitudinal population-based study. *American Journal of Epidemiology* **156**, 319–327.

van Os, J., Drukker, M., À Campo, J., Meijer, J., Bak, M. & Delespaul, P. (2006a) Validation of remission criteria for schizophrenia. *American Journal of Psychiatry* **163**, 2000–2002.

van Os , J., Burns, T., Cavallaro, R. *et al.* (2006b) Standardized remission criteria in schizophrenia. *Acta Psychiatrica Scandinavica* **113**, 91–95.

Varma, V.K., Malhotra, S. & Yao, E.S. (1996) Course and outcome of acute non-organic psychotic states. *Indian Psychiatric Quarterly* **67**, 195–207.

Vazquez-Barquero, J.L., Cuesta-Nunez, M.J., de la Varga, M. *et al.* (1995) The Cantabria first episode schizophrenia study: a summary of general findings. *Acta Psychiatrica Scandinavica* **91**, 156–162.

Veen, N.D., Selten, J.P., van der Tweel, I., Feller, W.G., Hoek, H.W. & Kahn, R.S. (2004) Cannabis use and age at onset of schizophrenia. *American Journal of Psychiatry* **161**, 501–506.

Velakoulis, D., Wood, S.J., Smith, D.J. *et al.* (2002) Increased duration of illness is associated with increased volume in right medial temporal/anterior cingulate grey matter in patients with chronic schizophrenia. *Schizophrenia Research* **57**, 43–49.

Ventura, J., Nuechterlein, K.H., Green, M.F. *et al.* (2004) The timing of negative symptom exacerbation in relationship to positive symptom exacerbation in the early course of schjizophrenia. *Schizophrenia Research* **69**, 333–342.

Verdoux, H., Maurice-Tison, S., Gay, B., van Os, J., Salamon, R. & Bourgeois, M.L. (1998) A survey of delusional ideation in primary-care patients. *Psychological Medicine* **28**, 127–134.

Verdoux, H., Liraud, F., Bergey, C., Assens, F., Abalan, F. & van Os, J. (2001) Is the association between duration of untreated psychosis and outcome confounded? A two year follow-up study of first-admitted patients. *Schizophrenia Research* **49**, 231–241.

Verdoux, H., Sorbara, F., Gindre, C. *et al.* (2002) Cannabis use and dimensions of psychosis in a nonclinical population of female subjects. *Schizophrenia Research* **59**, 77–84.

Vita, A., Dieci, M., Giobbio, G.M. *et al.* (1991) CT scan abnormalities and outcome of chronic schizophrenia. *American Journal of Psychiatry* **148**, 1577–1579.

von Korff, M., Nestadt, G., Romanoski, A. *et al.* (1985) Prevalence of treated and untreated DSM-III schizophrenia. Results of a two-stage community survey. *Journal of Nervous and Mental Disease* **173**, 577–581.

von Zerssen, D. & Hecht, H. (1987) Gesundheit, Glück, Zufriedenheit im Lichte einer katamnestischen Erhebung an psychiatrischen Patienten und gesunden Probanden. *Psychotherapie und Medizinische Psychologie* **37**, 83–96.

Wade, D., Harrigan, S., Edwards, J. *et al.* (2006) Course of substance misuse and daily tobacco use in first-episode psychosis. *Schizophrenia Research* **81**, 145–150.

Waddington, J.L., Youssef, H.A. & Kinsella, A. (1995) Sequential cross-sectional and 10-year prospective study of severe negative symptoms in relation to duration of initially untreated psychosis in chronic schizophrenia. *Psychological Medicine* **25**, 849–857.

Warner, R. (1985) *Recovery from schizophrenia. Psychiatry and Political Economy.* London: Routledge & Kegan Paul.

Watt, D.C., Katz, K. & Shepherd, M. (1983) The natural history of schizophrenia: a 5-year prospective follow-up of a representative sample of schizophrenics by means of a standardized clinical and social assessment. *Psychological Medicine* **13**, 663–670.

Weber, I. (1997) *Die Lebenszufriedenheit einer Kohorte Schizophrener 15,5 Jahre nach stationärer Erstaufnahme.* Doctoral dissertation, Fakultät für Klinische Medizin Mannheim der Ruprecht-Karls-Universität Heidelberg.

Weickert, T.W., Goldberg, T.E., Gold, J.M., Bigelow, L.B., Egan, M.F. & Weinberger D.R. (2000) Cognitive impairments in patients with schizophrenia displaying preserved and compromised intellect. *Archives of General Psychiatry* **57**, 907–913. Erratum in: 57, 1122.

Weinberger, D.R. (1995) Schizophrenia as a neurodevelopmental disorder. In: Hirsch, S.R. & Weinberger, D.R., eds. *Schizophrenia.* Oxford: Blackwell, pp. 293–323.

Weinberger, D.R. & Berman, K.F. (1996) Prefrontal function in schizophrenia: confounds and controversies. *Philosophical Transactions of the Royal Society London B Biological Science* **351**, 1495–503.

Welham, J., McLachlan, G., Davies, G. & McGrath, J. (2000) Heterogeneity in schizophrenia; mixture modelling of age-at-first-admission, gender and diagnosis. *Acta Psychiatrica Scandinavica* **101**, 312–317.

Wetherell, J.L., Palmer, B.W., Thorp, S.R., Patterson, T.L., Golshan, S. & Jeste, D.V. (2003) Quality of life in schizophrenia: contributions of anxiety and depression. *Journal of Clinical Psychiatry* **64**, 1476–1482.

White, L., Harvey, P.D., Opler, L. & Lindenmayer, J.P. (1997) Empirical assessment of the factorial structure of clinical symptoms in schizophrenia: a multisite, multimodel evaluation of the factorial structure of the Positive and Negative Syndrome Scale. The PANSS Study Group. *Psychopathology* **30**, 263–274.

Whiteford, H.A. & Peabody, C.A. (1989) The differential diagnosis of negative symptoms in chronic schizophrenia. *Australian and New Zealand Journal of Psychiatry* **23**, 491–496.

Wing, J.K. & Brown, G.W. (1970) *Institutionalism and Schizophrenia: A Comparative Study of THree Mental Hospitals 1960–1968.* Cambridge: Cambridge University Press.

Wiersma, D., Giel, R., de Jong, A. *et al.* (1996) Assessment of the need for care 15 years after onset of a Dutch cohort of patients with schizophrenia, and an international comparison. *Social Psychiatry and Psychiatric Epidemiology* **31**, 114–121.

Wiersma, D., Nienhuis, F.J., Slooff, C.J. & Giel, R. (1998) Natural course of schizophrenic disorders: a 15-year followup of a Dutch incidence cohort. *Schizophrenia Bulletin* **24**, 75–85.

Wiersma, D., Wideerling, J., Dragonmirecka, E. et al. (2000) Social disability in schizophrenia: its development and prediction over 15 years in incidence cohorts in six European centres. *Psychological Medicine* **30**, 1155–1167.

Wig, N.N. & Parhee, R. (1989) Acute and transient psychoses: a view from the developing countries. In: Mezzich, J.E. & Cranach, M., eds. *International Classification in Psychiaty: Unity and Diversity*. Cambridge: Cambridge University Press, pp. 115–121.

Wiles, N.J., Zammit, S., Bebbington, P. *et al.* (2006) Self-reported psychotic symptoms in the general population. *British Journal of Psychiatry* **188**, 519–526.

Wilkinson, D.G. (1982) The suicide rate in schizophrenia. *British Journal of Psychiatry* **140**, 138–141.

Wing, J.K. & Brown, G.W. (1970) *Institutionalism and Schizophrenia. A Comparative Study of Three Mental Hospitals 1960–1968*. Cambridge: Cambridge University Press.

Wittchen, H.U., Höfler, M., Lieb, R. *et al.* (2004) Depressive und psychotische Symptome in der Bevölkerung—eine prospektiv-longitudinale Studie (EDSP) an 2.500 Jugendlichen und jungen Erwachsenen (Abstract). Paper presented at the DGPPN Congress, Berlin, Nov. 24–27, 2004. *Nervenarzt* **75** (Suppl. 2), 87.

Wood, S.J., De Luca, C.R., Anderson, V., & Pantelis, C. (2004) Cognitive development in adolescence: cerebral underpinnings, neural trajectories, and the impact of abberations. In: Keshavan, M., Kennedy, J. & Murray, R., eds. *Neurodevelopment and Schizophrenia* Cambridge: Cambridge University Press, pp. 69–88.

Woods, B.T. (1998) Is schizophrenia a progressive neurodevelopmental disorder? Toward a unitary pathogenetic mechanism. *American Journal of Psychiatry* **155**, 1661–1670.

Woods, B.T., Ward, K.E. & Johnson, E.H. (2005) Meta-analysis of the time-course of brain volume reduction in schizophrenia: implications for pathogenesis and early treatment. *Schizophrenia Research* **73**, 221–228.

World Health Organization (1973) *The International Pilot Study of Schizophrenia*, Vol. **1**. Geneva, WHO.

World Health Organization (1979) *Schizophrenia. An International Follow-Up Study*. New York: Wiley.

World Health Organization (1993) *The ICD-10 classification of mental and behavioural disorders: diagnostic criteria for research*. Geneva: WHO.

World Health Organization (1998) The World Health Organization Quality of Life Assessment (WHOQOL): development and general psychometric properties. *Social Science and Medicine* **46**, 1569–1585.

Wunderink, L., Nienhuis, F.J., Sytema, S. & Wiersma, D. (2007) Predictive validity of proposed remission criteria in first-episode schizophrenic patients responding to antipsychotics. *Schizophrenia Bulletin* **33**, 792–796.

Wyatt, R.J. (1991) Neuroleptics and the natural course of schizophrenia. *Schizophrenia Bulletin* **17**, 325–351.

Yung, A.R. (2006) Identification of the population. In: Addington, J., Francey, S.M. & Morrison A.P. eds. *Working with people at high risk of developing psychosis: a treatment handbook*. Chichester-New York: John Wiley & Sons, pp. 7–24.

Yung, A.R. & McGorry, P.D. (1996) The prodromal phase of first-episode psychosis: past and current conceptualizations. *Schizophrenia Bulletin* **22**, 353–370.

Yung, A.R., Phillips, L.J., McGorry, P.D. *et al.* (1998) Prediction of psychosis. A step towards indicated prevention of schizophrenia. *British Journal of Psychiatry* **172** (Suppl. 33), 14–20.

Yung, A.R., Phillips, L.J., Yuen, H.P. *et al.* (2003) Psychosis prediction: 12-month follow up of a high-risk ("prodromal") group. *Schizophrenia Research* **60**, 21–32.

Zimmerman, M., Coryell, W., Pfohl, B. & Stangl, D. (1988) The reliability of the Family History Method for psychiatric diagnosis. *Archives of General Psychiatry* **45**, 320–322.

CHAPTER 8

Neurocognitive impairments in schizophrenia: their character and role in symptom formation

Terry E. Goldberg[1], Anthony David[2], and James. M. Gold[3]

[1]Albert Einstein College of Medicine, Zucker Hillside Hospital/Litwin Zucker Alzheimer's Disease Research Center, Feinstein Institute Manhasset, NY USA
[2]Institute of Psychiatry, London, UK
[3]Maryland Psychiatric Research Center, Crownsville, MD, USA

Introduction

Abnormalities in attentional, associative, and volitional cognitive processes have been considered central features of schizophrenia since the original clinical descriptions of Kraepelin (1919) and Bleuler (1911, 1950). The application of formal psychological assessment techniques in hundreds of studies in dozens of independent laboratories over the past 70 years has more than amply documented that such abnormalities are common occurrences in patients with the disorder. For example, about 60 years ago, Rappaport *et al.* (1945/1946) published *Diagnostic Psychological Testing*, an influential work reporting findings from the application of a broad test battery to a wide variety of psychiatric patients. In describing patients with deteriorated chronic schizophrenia, they noted that such patients had their greatest impairments in "judgment, attention, concentration, planning ability and anticipation". They

further commented on the memory difficulties, inadequate concept formation, and general intellectual inefficiency of patients with schizophrenia. Although interpreted within a psychodynamic framework and prior to the narrowing of the diagnostic conceptualization of schizophrenia and introduction of modern pharmacotherapy, the empirical observations made in the early 1940s are remarkably consistent with current findings. Indeed, we would suggest that the vast body of data on cognitive functioning in schizophrenia has been remarkably uniform over many years. What has changed is the significance attributed to these results.

In recent years, the routine use of clinical neuropsychological assessment and experimental neuropsychological paradigms has offered a new perspective to the understanding of schizophrenia and has thrown light on several of the more problematic facets of the disorder. In particular, they have made important contributions to understanding the course of cognitive impairment, the specificity of profiles of cognitive impairment to schizophrenia, and the prognostic importance of deficits. More recently still, the putative importance of cognitive impairment in

Schizophrenia, 3rd edition. Edited by Daniel R. Weinberger and Paul J Harrison © 2011 Blackwell Publishing Ltd.

understanding a cardinal symptom of schizophrenia (thought disorder) and the genetics of schizophrenia is coming to be appreciated. In this chapter we will attempt to address some of the classical issues inherent in neuro-cognitive approaches to schizophrenia and present newer componential accounts of impairments in attention, working memory, and episodic memory. Additionally, we will review novel applications of neurocognition in schizophrenia, relating specific types of cognitive processing to symptoms.

Course of cognitive impairment

Accumulating evidence from the prospective study of large birth cohorts has indicated that individuals later diagnosed as having schizophrenia have relatively subtle develop-mental delays in a variety of milestones, including stand-ing, toileting, and speech. The magnitude of the delays usually falls within the normal range, i.e., does not form a distinct distribution (Jones & Cannon, 1998). The data are consistent with views that schizophrenia is a neurodevel-opmental disorder in which pathological processes interact with normal developmental processes and societal demands to form a distinct symptom constellation at each stage (see Chapter 19).

Surrogate measures for cognition in individuals prior to the clinical onset of the illness, involving use of school grades or academic achievement in childhood and adoles-cence, have yielded somewhat inconsistent findings. For instance, Bilder et al. (2006) used a variety of achievement-based scores and observed an increasing gap between con-trols and patients through elementary and high school. Fuller et al. (2002) found that some, but not all, measures from the Iowa Achievement Tests were impaired at specific phases of adolescent development. A novel approach to this issue was developed by Weickert et al. (2000) and helps to integrate these findings. They used a surrogate measure of premorbid IQ based on reading ability and current ("morbid") IQ to define three subgroups. One, consisting of attenuations in both premorbid and current IQ and global neurocognitive test impairments appeared to reflect obvious neurodevelopmental compromise. A second group (modal in that 50% of patients demonstrated the pattern) had intact premorbid IQ but reduced current IQ, suggesting a decline during the early stages of the disorder and a more circumscribed pattern of cognitive impair-ments in which executive function, attention, and episodic memory were impaired. A third group had current and premorbid IQs within the normal range, but demonstrated subtle impairments in executive function. These results have been observed by Mockler et al. (1997) and Reichenberg et al. (2002, 2005). Consistent evidence for cognitive attenu-ation in the schizophrenia prodrome has come from population-based studies of male conscripts. In a compel-ling set of investigations, patients with schizophrenia were shown to have had lower cognitive test scores than control peers in late adolescence while being evaluated for entry into the Israeli Defense Force (Reichenberg et al., 2002, 2005). Moreover, declines in general cognitive function using a surrogate measure of premorbid ability predicted schizophrenia outcomes. In a Scandinavian cohort (David et al., 1997), found that lower cognitive scores were associ-ated with a later diagnosis of schizophrenia.

Evidence for cognitive stability in the middle part of the course of the illness comes from several cross-sectional and longitudinal studies. Crucially, deterioration does not appear to occur during the early chronic phase of the illness, which thus appears to be self-arresting. For instance, over intervals of 8 years, the performance of patients did not decline on tests such as the Wechsler Adult Intelligence Scale (WAIS) and Halstead–Reitan measures when assessed longitudinally (Klonoff et al., 1970; Rund, 1998; Smith, 1964). In several large cross-sectional studies using tests known to be sensitive to progressive dementias, using IQ, or using variants of the Halstead–Reitan Battery, no differ-ences were found between patients with longer durations of illness and those with shorter durations above and beyond aging (Mockler et al., 1997 Goldstein & Zubin, 1990; Heaton et al., 1994; Hyde et al., 1994). Several correlational studies have not shown cognitive deterioration with increasing chronicity. In perhaps the best of these, Gold et al. (1999b) found in a large and well-characterized sample that associations between duration of illness and cognitive level were weak and non-significant (but see Cuesta et al., 1998).

In later life the clinical picture becomes more dynamic again. In a large series of studies, Bowie and colleagues determined that a significant minority of patients show marked cognitive decline and meet criteria for dementia using such instruments as the Mini Mental State and Clinical Dementia Rating Scale (Bowie et al., 2006). Such patients when followed longitudinally demonstrate cog-nitive declines that are much steeper than those seen in healthy controls. Moreover, their pattern of memory impairment changes from one suggestive of fronto-striatal dysfunction to one suggestive of cortical/medial temporal dysfunction. Friedman et al. (2002) found that both baseline cognitive impairment and magnitude of cognitive decline over 18 months predicted subsequent decline in perform-ance of everyday living skills in institutionalized patients. Nevertheless, it should be appreciated that these individu-als do not have Alzheimer disease, either in terms of cogni-tive profile or neuropathology (see Chapter 18). Note also that this pattern of decline reported by Harvey and others was seen in patients who were chronically institutionalized and/or were discharged to nursing homes and were over the age of 65 years, and likely does not apply to ambulatory patients living in the community.

While we have highlighted results which support the notion that schizophrenia is a static encephalopathy, and that are consistent with the observation of Kraepelin (1919), "As a rule, if no essential improvement intervenes in at most two or three years after the appearance of the more striking morbid phenomena, a state of weak mindedness will be developed, which usually changes only slowly and insignificantly", several lines of evidence suggest that cognitive function may be more dynamic than previously thought. Taken in sum, types of evidence from imaging (which demonstrates volumetric decline around the time of the emergence of clinical symptoms), relative neurocognitive stability, and symptomatic improvement (with treatment) remain remarkably unaligned.

Tradition of clinical neuropyschological studies of schizophrenia

The original observations of Kraepelin (1919) and Bleuler (1911) suggesting that impairments of cognition were central to the disorder has been supported by a rich tradition of empirical research, including the pioneering work of Goldstein (1959), Shakow (1972), and many others. This body of experimental and psychological assessment research took on new significance when, and was reinvigorated by, findings from the initial neuroimaging studies showed that schizophrenia involved structural brain abnormalities. In essence, the evidence that the illness compromised brain structure naturally led to the question of whether the observed impairments in brain function could be directly and causally related to structural brain abnormalities. To investigate this question, clinical neuropsychological methods rapidly became commonplace in the mainstream schizophrenia literature in the late 1970s and 1980s.

The importation of assessment methods from clinical neuropsychology brought with it an interpretive framework that had been shaped by the study of previously healthy adults who had suffered discrete lesions. Thus, the validity of assessment methods was primarily established by the demonstration of sensitivity to "brain damage" in general and, more importantly, as sensitivity to specific, localized lesions. Given this framework, performance on specific tests was sometimes proposed to measure the function of specific brain areas. Following from this, much of the schizophrenia neuropsychology literature of the 1970s and 1980s focused on the extent to which patients demonstrated the severity and/or pattern of impairment commonly observed in patients with verified brain injuries using broad neuropsychological batteries such as the Halstead–Reitan Battery or a variety of briefer screening tests (Chelune *et al.*, 1979; Goldstein, 1978; Heaton *et al.*, 1979). In addition, much of the literature focused on patient performance on a small number of tests [such as the Wisconsin Card Sorting Test (WCST)] as a means of assessing the role of frontal lobe dysfunction (Braff *et al.*, 1991; Goldstein *et al.*, 1996). By the mid–late1980s the common neuropsychological understanding of the illness was that a substantial number of patients demonstrated easily detectable levels of impairment, with most research attention focused on aspects of executive function and episodic memory performance, thought to correspond to the abnormalities of the frontal and temporal lobes that had been documented in the imaging literature (see Chapter 16). To a large degree, this remains the modal understanding of the disorder.

However, the weight of accumulated evidence has begun to shift this modal understanding. Heinrichs and Zakzanis (1998) published an influential meta-analysis that documented substantial impairment on every task examined, with effect sizes varying from a low of 0.46 on Block Design to a high of 1.41 on verbal memory, with an overall effect size of 0.92. That is, across tests, patients with schizophrenia tended to score approximately one standard deviation below that observed in healthy controls. The most frequently documented island of relatively preserved function in the literature involved tests of crystallized verbal knowledge, such as word reading and vocabulary. Performance on such tests is typically thought to reflect "premorbid" intellectual capacity, with poorer performance in other cognitive domains thought to reflect illness-onset associated loss of efficiency. While there was variability in the precise level of impairment across tests and cognitive domains in the Heinrichs and Zakzanis review, this documentation of an impressive level of general impairment presented a challenge to localizationist views for several reasons. First, the level of impairment observed on measures of memory and executive function was not clearly larger than that seen on many other measures. Second, patients demonstrated reliable impairment on measures that were not thought to be critically dependent upon the integrity of the frontal or temporal lobes. Thus, differential impairment, if present at all, was a matter of degree, not of kind. Further, this accumulation of evidence of impairment on tasks thought to measure the outputs of different neural systems poses substantial interpretive problems. In essence, the literature is consistent with either a wide variety of different, putatively independent deficits, or more parsimoniously, the impact of a smaller number of deficits that have wide ramifications. In either case, the fact of general impairment rises to the foreground.

The recent meta-analysis by Dickinson *et al.* (2007b) provides even more impressive evidence of a general deficit that had been underappreciated. Specifically, the Digit Symbol subtest from the WAIS, a brief measure of processing speed that is thought to have little localizing value, was shown to have the largest effect size ($g = -1.57$) reported in

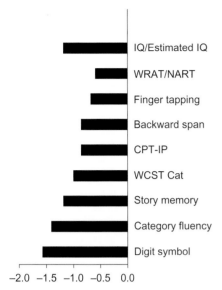

Fig. 8.1 Meta-analytical results from Dickinson *et al.* (2007b). WRAT, Wide Range Achievement Test; NART, National Adult Reading Test; CPT-IP, Continuous Performance Test, Identical Pairs version, WCST, Wisconsin Card Sort Test.

the schizophrenia clinical neuropsychology literature. As seen in Figure 8.1, the level of impairment on digit symbol was substantially higher (often significantly so) than observed in some of the domains that are the major focus of schizophrenia cognition research, such as working memory, executive functioning, and verbal memory. Of note, the next largest effect size was documented on the category fluency, another measure thought to assess processing speed. Also remarkable is the fact that the IQ effect size is substantial, and larger than observed on many other measures. It appears likely that the implicit localizationist framework that has informed the field led to a failure to appreciate what appears to be the most reliable and robust deficit that has been documented in this research tradition. In essence the field had largely ignored the largest deficit, a deficit documented in dozens of studies over many years, perhaps because a deficit in processing speed was difficult to conceptualize in terms of localized dysfunction.

Several other lines of evidence are consistent with the idea that there is a generalized cognitive impairment. Patient performance across tasks thought to measure independent abilities tends to be moderately to highly intercorrelated (Dickinson *et al.*, 2007b). That is, performance on one task (thought to reflect the output of a discrete brain area) tends to be highly predictive of performance on tasks thought to reflect the output of different, discrete brain areas. Similarly, multiple factor analytic studies have documented a very robust first factor with loadings from nearly all measures (Dickinson *et al.*, 2006, Gladsjo *et al.*, 2004;

Keefe *et al.*, 2006). Thus, even when datasets provide evidence of separable factors after the imposition of various rotations, such factors tend to explain very little variance, whereas the general, or common factor, tends to explain a substantial amount of the total variance. Further, through the use of single common factor analysis, Dickinson *et al.* (2004) have shown that most of the between-group variance observed across the Wechsler Intelligence and Memory scales was shared. This suggested that the extent to which patients and healthy controls differ across different cognitive domains (with demonstrated factor analytic validity) can be understood largely in terms of an underlying difference on a single common factor. While there was some evidence that impairment on a few measures (notably processing speed and memory) exceeded that predicted by the single common factor, these specific deficits accounted for very little variance compared to the variance explained by impairment of a single common "deficit" factor. Note, this literature does not rule out the existence of substantial specific and differential deficits. It does, however, suggest that commonly used methods borrowed from the clinical neuropsychological literature are unlikely to be capable of producing such evidence given the weight of accumulated findings.

If neuropsychological batteries primarily provide variegated assessments of a single underlying dimension of impairment, it should be possible to achieve reliable estimates of this general level of impairment using a much smaller number of tasks. Indeed, there are now several published demonstrations that very brief assessment approaches provide for reliable measures of the general impairment level documented on extensive test batteries and provide a useful means of tracking clinical change as might occur in the context of a treatment trial (Gold *et al.*, 1999a; Keefe *et al.*, 2004; Velligan *et al.*, 2004). Thus, there are important practical assessment implications of the recognition that clinical neuropsychological measures are primarily assessing a general dimension of cognitive performance.

Experimental approaches to the study of specific cognitive functions in schizophrenia

In addition to the clinical neuropsychological literature, there is a rich history of experimental studies focused on specific cognitive functions that are thought to be either differentially impaired, might be responsible for more general impairment, or which may provide particularly compelling evidence of dysfunction in specific neural substrates. Three cognitive functions have attracted a great deal of research interest: episodic memory, working memory, and attention, and will be briefly reviewed here. In addition, we will briefly discuss recent evidence that more elementary perceptual operations may also be impaired in the illness.

Episodic memory

Interest in episodic memory has been driven by several observations, including evidence of anatomical abnormalities in the hippocampus, a structure known to play a critical role in normal memory function; evidence from several influential clinical neuropsychological battery studies suggesting that memory was the most impaired aspect of the cognitive profile, and evidence that performance on memory measures is among the most robust correlates of several different aspects of functional outcome (Green, 1996; Nelson *et al.*, 1998; Saykin *et al.*, 1991, 1994). These psychometric and biological findings are consistent with clinical observations: patients frequently complain of poor memory. Thus, there is converging evidence that memory function may be a critical core feature of the illness, pointing towards both biology and important clinical features.

Both meta-analytic and experimental studies provide important evidence about the nature of memory impairment in schizophrenia. First, the impairment is not modality specific, with reliable deficits noted with both verbal and visual materials (Aleman *et al.*, 1999). Second, impairment is maximally evident using free recall methods, with somewhat reduced, but still reliable evidence of impairment when subjects are tested using recognition memory methods (i.e., Did I show you this face before?; Pelletier *et al.*, 2005). Third, and perhaps most surprisingly, the extent of patient impairment does not appear to be reliably amplified by increasing the delay interval between initial learning and later test (Aleman *et al.*, 1999; Dickinson *et al.*, 2007b; Gold *et al.*, 2000). Thus, the deficit is better described as a problem in learning, in the acquisition of information, rather than as a deficit in memory *per se*.

There is growing evidence that failures in the initial encoding of to-be-remembered material may underlie the learning impairment. That is, patients fail to initially process material in a fashion that allows for later efficient retrieval. For example, when presented with lists of words that are semantically related, healthy subjects tend to recall related items together, whereas patients with schizophrenia are less apt to do so (Paulsen *et al.*, 1995). If these semantic relationships are highlighted at the time of initial presentation, patients are much more likely to use this information to boost their recall (Gold *et al.*, 1992a). It appears that patients fail to fully process and spontaneously integrate the different features of, or relationships among, to-be-remembered information (Gold *et al.*, 2004). Such "information-poor" representations are harder to retrieve, as recollection of one aspect of a scene or of a recent experience will not serve as a powerful cue to

retrieve a more complete representation. Thus, some failures in encoding may result from failures to engage in a number of strategic, organizational, and control processes that are typically thought to be mediated by non-medial temporal lobe structures (Barch *et al.*, 2002; Barch, 2005; cf. the computational approach described below). However, deficits in these other systems provide critical constraints on memory performance. While initial interest in the study of memory was largely motivated by the idea that it provided a specific behavioral assay for hippocampal dysfunction, more recent evidence, from both behavioral and functional neuroimaging studies, implicate a wider network, including the prefrontal cortex (Barch, 2005). Parsing the contributions of different aspects of the network to the easily observed behavioral deficit remains an active area of investigation.

A novel approach to understanding episodic memory impairments in schizophrenia involved computational modeling, in a study which yielded results surprisingly consistent with some aspects of the view outlined above (Talamini *et al.*, 2005). In this model, the medial temporal lobe binds memories and their instance-specific context, and then stores their code for later retrieval. The model described here is based on studies showing that the bulk of hippocampal cortical input is segregated over two pathways. One of these may convey spatio-temporal information about context; the other conveys information regarding items and objects. The two streams are interconnected at various levels within the entorhinal cortex, which likely contributes to the integration of cortical inputs into a representation of their co-occurrence. The hippocampus proper may quickly associate a small code to the conjunction of cortical inputs, such that similar entorhinal patterns come to be separated via their associated hippocampal patterns. These hippocampal patterns are thus not directly associated with individual features, but serve to separate the large number of overlapping entorhinal patterns. The representational overlap in entorhinal cortex, combined with the pattern separation system in the hippocampus proper, enormously increases the capacity of the memory store with respect to any single layer system, and allows recall of episodic memories. The model was first shown to learn and retrieve in a manner consistent with known behavior in learning and memory. Next, various in silico lesions were made in the model, including sharp reductions in connectivity between various levels or modules, the addition of noise, and reduction of elements (i.e., "neurons"). Connectivity reductions appeared to recapitulate schizophrenia memory impairments most closely. At the network level, this reduced connectivity led to compromised cross-association of episodic features (i.e., item and context) and a superimposed, mild reduction of pattern separation in the system. This preferentially affected tasks with a large retrieval demand, such as free recall. Thus, what appeared to be disproportionate failures in retrieval were due to compromised encoding.

Working memory

Working memory, the ability to maintain representations in an activated, easily retrieved state in the service of ongoing behavior and cognitive processing, has been one of the central concerns of cognitive schizophrenia research in the last two decades. Several factors likely account for this focus. First, the elegant evidence of sustained firing of primate prefrontal neurons during the delay period of working memory tasks, by Patricia Goldman-Rakic among others, suggested that it might be possible to build a highly detailed translational model of human working memory (Castner et al., 2004) and inspired dozens of human functional imaging studies that demonstrate activation of the prefrontal cortex during performance of working memory tasks (D'Esposito, 2007). In light of earlier evidence that patients with schizophrenia demonstrated both behavioral and neurophysiological evidence of prefrontal dysfunction during the performance of more cognitively complex tasks (such as the WCST), the idea that relatively elementary aspects of working memory might also be evidence of prefrontal dysfunction in schizophrenia was highly attractive (Weinberger & Berman, 1988). This interest was bolstered by the burgeoning literature demonstrating that working memory was a critical resource required by many different cognitive operations, such as reasoning, language comprehension, and mental arithmetic (Baddeley, 1986). Thus, impairment in working memory would be expected to cause widespread impairments—a plausible single deficit that might account for the general deficit. When one adds to this the evidence that abnormalities of dopamine function may impair working memory performance, it is easy to understand why the study of working memory in schizophrenia became, and remains, a vigorous enterprise (Goldman-Rakic et al., 2004).

Several reliable conclusions emerge from the experimental literature (Lee & Park, 2005). First, working memory deficits are observed across multiple modalities. Second, deficits have been found with loads as low as a single target item or location with deficits amplified at higher loads. Thus, the deficit involves the use (or precision) both of available capacity as well as capacity limits. Third, impairments are consistently found at short delay intervals, suggesting that there is a deficit in the formation of working memory representations (Lee & Park, 2005; Fuller et al., 2005). Fourth, there is conflicting evidence about whether the extent of impairment in schizophrenia is amplified with increasing retention intervals, suggesting that working memory decay results are strongly influenced by the methods employed (Javitt et al., 1999; Lencz et al., 2003; Tek et al., 2002); the meta-analysis of Lee and Park (2005)

suggests that the extent of impairment is not reliably magnified by increasing retention intervals. As predicted from the normal cognitive literature, there is evidence that working memory impairments in schizophrenia are indeed related to higher-order reasoning and problem-solving deficits, suggesting that the deficits may play a substantial role in the generalized deficit observed in schizophrenia (Gold et al., 1997; Glahn et al., 2000). These behavioral findings are richly corroborated by the functional neuroimaging literature where abnormalities of prefrontal physiology have been reliably documented during the performance of working memory tasks (Glahn et al., 2005).

Two issues emerge from this impressive body of work that require comment. First, while the idea that working memory impairment may be implicated in the generalized deficit of schizophrenia has obvious conceptual appeal, the working memory effect sizes are not among the largest in the overall cognitive literature. Lee and Park (2005) found an overall working memory effect size of 0.45, which is substantially smaller than the global mean effect size (0.92 in Heinrichs & Zakzanis, 1998, and 0.98 in Dickinson et al., 2007a). It is difficult to understand how a relatively small deficit on a measure thought to be a relatively pure measure of working memory would lead to a substantially larger deficit on tasks that involve multiple component processes hypothesized to be less impaired than working memory. That is, even if working memory is a critical "resource" for multiple cognitive processes, in order for working memory deficits to explain other impairments, one would have to posit that the working memory deficit is somehow substantially amplified when in the context of other processes. Second, much of the interest in working memory was based on the idea that this was a critical resource for the ongoing adaptive control of behavior. That is, it is thought that working memory is the basis of executive control: task goals and rules must be held in an activated state in order to influence the selection and direction of other cognitive operations. While this is a critical form of working memory, it is not clear that much of the experimental work on the precision and capacity of working memory offers important traction in understanding higher-order working memory processes that mediate executive control. For example, the temporal frame of the typical working memory capacity measure is of the order of seconds, whereas tasks that are thought to involve executive uses of working memory can span many minutes. It is unlikely that the same precise architecture mediates these different types of performance, or that findings from one domain may be simply translated to the other. Thus, it remains for further work to delineate the contribution of elementary forms of working memory for the executive control functions that are typically seen as being mediated by the prefrontal cortex (Cohen et al., 1999).

While episodic and working memory are generally thought of as distinct cognitive systems, the similarities of the patient impairment in both systems is striking and unlikely to be coincidental. In both systems the impairments are amodal, are not robustly amplified by delay, and appear to implicate abnormalities in the formation of representations that are precise, durable in the face of interference, and easily retrieved. While speculative, it is difficult to dismiss the notion that the impairments of both systems are due to a more general mechanism that compromises the formation of distributed representations.

Attention

Attention has been the most "elastic" concept in the schizophrenia literature, the term being used to refer to a wide array of clinical observations, and performance on numerous different tasks. At the level of clinical phenomenology, patients often appear preoccupied or distracted by their own thoughts and perceptions, and have difficulty sustaining expected engagement with the external environment. In the experimental literature, particularly research motivated by the information processing theories or broader clinical neuropsychological models, deficits in attention, or in attentional "resources" were often proposed as explanations for poor performance on tasks ranging from measures of short-term memory, vigilance, grapho-motor speed, and problem solving (Mirsky *et al.*, 1995; Nuechterlein & Dawson 1984). The lack of clarity about how to define and measure attention has led to considerable confusion in the literature and a lack of clear cumulative progress despite extensive study.

Some of this confusion can be easily understood in light of recent cognitive neuroscience research where attention is seen as serving a modulatory role across cognitive systems, facilitating performance in the face of information overload (Luck & Vecera, 2002). Attention serves to focus perceptual systems when they are taxed by multiple inputs, guides working memory encoding to optimize the use of limited storage capacity, and guides response selection processes when they are confronted by competing response alternatives. As such, attention indirectly influences behavior by modulating the operation of other cognitive systems, and it can be difficult to isolate impairments of attention *per se*. Thus, there can be no such thing as an "attention test"; it is a function that can only be studied in terms of how it influences the operation of other systems. Therefore, the nature of attentional mechanisms differs in different cognitive systems.

One useful distinction is to separate the control of attention *versus* the implementation of selection (Gold *et al.*, 2007). This distinction may be grasped with the metaphor of a flashlight. The control of attention has to do with whether the light is pointed at the most advantageous location to meet task demands. In contrast, the implementation of selection corresponds to the brightness of the beam—does it provide sufficient light to enhance task performance? There is surprising evidence that the implementation of selection may be relatively intact in schizophrenia. For example, patients are able to use both central/endogenous and peripheral/exogenous cues to guide spatial attention, with normal levels of attentional orienting observed in a large majority of studies using the Posner cuing method (Bustillo *et al.*, 1997; Gold *et al.*, 1992b; Maruff *et al.*, 1995; Oie *et al.*, 1998; Posner *et al.*, 1988; Strauss *et al.*, 1992). Gold *et al.* (2006) recently demonstrated that patients are able to selectively store information in working memory when to-be-remembered items differed from to-be-ignored items on the basis of color or shape, or where peripheral cue boxes or central arrows were used to indicate the relevant items. In all conditions, patients and controls selectively stored the relevant items and excluded the irrelevant items from memory. Further evidence for intact implementation of selection was documented by Luck *et al.* (2006) using event-related potentials recorded during a visual search task. In this experiment subjects needed to make a perceptual discrimination on a salient color target. The shift of attention to the target was indexed by the N2pc, a well-established correlate of visual attention (Luck *et al.*, 1997; Luck & Hillyard 1994). In this study, the onset and magnitude of the N2pc was highly similar in patients and controls. Thus, there is now ample evidence that specific aspects of attention are surprisingly functional in schizophrenia when selection can be achieved on the basis of salient perceptual features.

There is, however, abundant evidence of failures in the control of attention. For example, patients have difficulty resisting orienting attention to highly salient stimuli when it is maladaptive to do so, as seen in experiments requiring subjects to make eye movements or shift attention away from a peripheral stimulus or cue (e.g., Maruff *et al.*, 1996, 1998; Sereno & Holzman, 1996). Thus, patients fail to use the task rule ("shift attention away from the stimulus") to guide their responses when confronted by a salient, but task-irrelevant stimulus. Moreover, there is consistent evidence that patients have difficulty using task instructions to overcome pre-potent response tendencies, as seen in studies of the Stroop and in "context" versions of the Continuous Performance Test (CPT; e.g., Barch *et al.*, 1999, 2003; Cohen *et al.*, 1999). In the latter task, subjects are asked to respond to a target sequence of the letter A followed by an X that occurs on 70% of trials. On 10% of trials, subjects see a B followed by an X, and patients typically make inappropriate target responses in this condition. Such errors suggest failures to use the task rule (only respond to X following an A) to bias response selection systems to inhibit the experimentally-induced tendency to respond to X stimuli. Thus, attentional control breaks down when task goals are challenged by competition from stimuli or responses that are highly salient. When task goals face little competition, or where salient stimuli and responses are consistent with task success, patients performance may be relatively intact as such situations do not require a significant input from control systems. Thus, the attention deficits in schizophrenia appear in the face of specific task demands that tax control systems. It appears likely a deficit in the ability to maintain goals, i.e., maintain the appropriate task set, may be critically implicated in the types of behavioral failures that are typically attributed to deficits in attention.

Perceptual processes

While much of the research literature has focused on higher-level cognitive processes, there is a growing body of evidence that the illness also may impact more basic sensory perceptual processes. For example, there is replicated electrophysiological and behavioral evidence suggesting that patients have reduced ability to detect changes in simple auditory features such as frequency and duration (Javitt et al., 1998). There is similar evidence that visual perceptual processes may be compromised, including contrast sensitivity and the early organizational processes that integrate individual features and the context in which they appear in order to perceive integrated objects (Butler et al., 2005; Uhlhaas & Silverstein, 2005). Such failures in integrative processing can provide paradoxical performance advantages to patients. For example, patients may be less susceptible than controls to certain visual illusions that are created by the normal tendency to group and organize visual input (Uhlhaas & Silverstein, 2005). While less frequently studied than higher-order cognitive processes, impairments of perceptual processing appear to be associated with illness chronicity and functional disability (Swerdlow et al., 2006, Uhlhaas & Silverstein, 2005); e.g., impairments in mismatch negativity may progress over the course of the illness (Salisbury et al., 2007; Umbricht et al., 2006). It remains unclear the extent to which impairments in basic perceptual processes are a correlate or a cause of higher-order impairments. If a correlate, then one might consider the impairment of perceptual processing, to the extent that it is not protypical of the illness, to be a marker of unusually severe global impairment. On the other hand, degradation of perceptual representations could be seen as causally related to higher-order deficits as the function of these latter processes is compromised by having to operate on imprecise inputs (Haenschel et al., 2007). These questions have yet to be resolved.

How many deficits? Many, few, none?

The fact that patients with schizophrenia demonstrate a widespread deficit on numerous cognitive measures is now a well established and accepted fact. However, the implications of this empirical observation are not so clear cut. There is broad recognition that many conventional cognitive tasks have limited localizing value. Thus, the comparison of performance levels across tasks provides only a very rough guide to the neural systems that are maximally and minimally impacted by the illness. Is it plausible that a much smaller number of "core" impairments might account for the broad impairment pattern documented in the meta-analytic literature? Certainly one could argue that impairments of attention and/or working memory could account for such a pattern. While an attractive argument, there are reasons to think this will not prove to be the case. For example, Gold et al. (2006) recently documented that patients demonstrated the intact operation of selective attention mechanisms in the context of working memory encoding. This was accompanied by a reliable reduction in working memory capacity in these same patients who showed intact selection. Thus, the working memory impairment cannot be explained on the basis of poor selective attention. While this result does not rule out a role for impairments in other aspects of attention that may impact working memory, it does suggest that a straightforward account based on poor selection of to-be-remembered items cannot account for visual object working memory. Recall that the effect sizes documented in experimental studies of working memory are not among the largest seen in the literature. Thus, it appears unlikely that the two most widely studied and theoretically attractive candidate mechanisms (attention and working memory) will provide an adequate account of the breadth and depth of the impairments documented in the literature. Might a deficit in the ability to maintain task goals provide a more parsimonious and plausible explanation? This attractive hypothesis has yet to be rigorously studied.

A further puzzle is how should one expect the findings of generalized impairment in the clinical neuropsychology literature to map onto the more precise methods developed in the recent cognitive neuroscience literature? Is it reasonable to expect that all functions are impaired, and that more precise measurement approaches might yield even larger effect sizes? There are already some surprises documented in the literature. For example, as noted, Dickinson et al. (2007a) reported that the largest effect size in the clinical neuropsychology literature is seen on the Digit Symbol subtest of the WAIS, a measure of processing speed. However, Luck et al. (2006) recently reported that the speed of attentional shifting appears to be normal in schizophrenia, and there is no question that performance of the Digit Symbol task requires repeated shifts of visual attention. Other examples can be cited of nearly normal/fully normal performance by patients with schizophrenia, including in aspects of selective attention, retention in episodic memory, and in aspects of skill learning, among others (Gold et al.,

2000, 2006; Goldberg *et al.*, 1993; Michel *et al.*, 1998). Thus, it is already clear that the generalized deficit documented in the neuropsychological literature is not fully "generalizable" to more precise experimental approaches. Indeed, it is our view that demonstrating areas of relatively intact performance among patients with schizophrenia may prove to be among the most useful data that could be introduced into the field and would serve to constrain thinking about how the illness impacts brain function.

It is possible that contradictory evidence emerging from experimental *versus* clinical assessment methods may be understood by considering how these methods typically differ. The best cognitive experimental paradigms are designed to isolate the role of a specific cognitive process, and minimize the contribution of other processes. Thus, the Posner visual orienting paradigm uses easily perceived stimuli, requires minimal response selection, and uses the pattern or observed reaction times (not just the overall reaction time) to highlight the role of spatial attention (Posner *et al.*, 1988). In contrast, clinical neuropsychological measures that are thought to require attention, such as Digit Symbol, involve visual search, memory, and precise response selection. Thus, the clinical test is likely to be more sensitive to a variety of impairments, but it is not possible to determine which process is deficient based on a single overall performance measure by itself. Further, clinical tasks typically require the coordinated and sequential operation of several different cognitive processes, whereas most experimental paradigms attempt to minimize this complexity. If schizophrenia involves a deficit in the ability to mobilize and coordinate distributed networks, many clinical tests are much more likely to be sensitive to patient impairment than more refined experimental measures. Thus, impairments on clinical tests may be more likely than on experimental tests for a number of potentially interesting theoretical reasons that may provide for new approaches to understanding the nature of impairment in schizophrenia.

Cognition, functional outcome, and the cognitive effects of antipsychotics

In two influential reviews, Green (1996; Green *et al.*, 2000) documented that cognitive performance was an important correlate of various aspects of outcome in schizophrenia, ranging from ratings of ability to function in the community, to laboratory measures of social skill, and the ability to acquire psychosocial skills. While the degree of correlation varied across cognitive constructs, generally favoring verbal memory, there was a clear main effect: better cognitive performance was associated with better outcome. The overall effect sizes varied from the small to large range, with composite cognitive measures explaining more than half the variance in functional outcome in some studies. In some of the reviewed studies, cognitive measures demonstrated a much more robust relationship to functional outcome than did conventional clinical ratings of symptom severity, suggesting that the cognitive signal was not simply a proxy for overall illness severity and that the path to disability reduction in schizophrenia likely passed through cognitive function.

Nevertheless, as the cognition–outcome literature has grown, the evidence has become less clear that specific aspects of cognitive performance are consistently related to different dimensions of outcome (such as social functioning, instrumental functioning, etc.). In part, this results from the fact that studies use a wide variety of cognitive assessment methods as well as outcome assessment methods, making it difficult to carefully compare studies. Across studies, it appears that broader cognitive measures have a more robust relationship to outcome, although contradictory evidence for specificity can certainly be found (Bowie *et al.*, 2006; Dickinson *et al.*, 2007b; McGurk *et al.*, 2004). However, the fact that arguments for specificity have been advanced for so many different cognitive functions (memory, processing speed, executive function, etc.) diminishes confidence that there is a robust function-specific outcome relationship that will emerge over time.

In part, this view is influenced by the broader literature on intellectual performance. It is important to recognize that the cognition–outcome relationship is in no way unique to schizophrenia. The birth of intellectual assessment came in the context of evaluating school children in order to determine appropriate class placement—the ability to function in school is clearly a critical "outcome" for children. There is substantial evidence in healthy adult subjects that measures of general intellectual ability correlate at approximately 0.50 with occupational outcome (job complexity), supervisor ratings, and performance in vocational training (Schmidt & Hunter, 2004). Measures of general mental ability appear to have a marked advantage over more specific ability measures in the prediction of occupational performance in healthy populations. Thus, to a very large degree, the findings in the schizophrenia literature are completely consistent with the larger literature on the role of intellectual ability in adaptive functioning. This does not make cognitive impairment any less interesting as a therapeutic target in schizophrenia, but it does suggest that it may be wise to consider a variety of pharmacological strategies, including mechanisms that may not be specific to schizophrenia.

Specificity: a necessary digression

The identification of a characteristic neurocognitive profile of schizophrenia relative to other disorders would provide useful information concerning the fundamental validity of the accumulated findings. Differences in overall global impairment may have important implications for everyday functioning, whereas differences in the profile of impairment may help sharpen the discussion of anatomical implications of deficits, and identify useful measures for intermediate phenotypes in genetic linkage or association studies. Furthermore, differential deficits derived from comparative studies could provide targets for rehabilitative and pharmacological treatment efforts. However, the assumptions that underlie this view have recently been challenged.

One interesting way to approach issues of specificity in neurocognition in schizophrenia comes from recent studies that have examined the distinctiveness of profiles in schizophrenia and bipolar disorder. Until about a decade ago, there were several reasons to consider the two disorders as distinct diagnostic entities, including the attenuated number of individuals with high levels of expertise and achievement in schizophrenia, the use of different medications, and seemingly different neurocognitive profiles. This view has begun to change. First, second-generation antipsychotics have demonstrated efficacy in the treatment of manic episodes and in the reduction of mood episodes. Second, from a genetics standpoint, striking evidence has emerged that schizophrenia and bipolar disorder (both highly heritable) share linkage regions and susceptibility genes (see Chapters 12 and 13). It is unclear whether the gene products are most relevant to psychotic symptoms, mood instability or cognition; nevertheless, the work implies that notions about specificity itself lose relevance as etiological mechanisms become known. Third, structural neuroimaging studies have found volumetric reductions in both disorders. Finally, and critically, large-scale cognitive studies undertaken when patients with bipolar disorder were euthymic indicated the presence of rather widespread cognitive impairments in a profile similar to that observed in schizophrenia, albeit somewhat less severe (e.g., 0.5 z score units as opposed to 1.0 z score units) (Schretlen *et al.*, 2007; Martínez-Arán *et al.*, 2004). Together this work suggests that dimensional approaches to classification in psychotic disorders may be more fruitful than categorical approaches (see Chapter 1).

Antipsychotic medications

Clearly, any antipsychotic drug that had differential efficacy for cognition would have a substantial advantage over other available medications. Thus, cognitive measures were used in many of the large-scale clinical trials of the second-generation antipsychotics. Unfortunately, the interpretation about cognitive advantages of second-generation drugs as a class, or for particular compounds, has recently been questioned

Numerous recent studies have suggested that second-generation antipsychotic medications significantly enhance

cognition in schizophrenia. However, none included healthy controls undergoing repeated testing to assess the possibility that "improvements" actually reflect simple practice effects. In a study of 104 first-episode patients (Goldberg *et al.*, 2007), we were able to address several sources of bias or problematic methodologies which made interpretation of earlier results complex:

1. We directly compared two of the most widely prescribed second-generation drugs in the US, olanzapine and risperidone, in a randomized, blinded trial on key measures of neurocognition (increasing the generalizability of the result);

2. The study was federally sponsored;

3. The large majority of patients were drug naïve at baseline (thus changes over the following weeks could not be attributed to a switch in medication, or withdrawal from prior medication; and, *pari passu*, patients did not have long and/or complex histories of antipsychotic treatment that might play a role in drug response that cannot easily studied, not less quantified);

4. Perhaps most critically, a healthy control group (n = 84) was assessed over repeated visits to measure practice effects.

Fifty-one first-episode patients were randomized to olanzapine (modal dose 12.7 mg) and 53 to risperidone (modal dose 3.7 mg). Assessments occurred at baseline, 6 weeks later, and 16 weeks later; tests included multiple measures of working memory and attention, speed of processing, episodic memory, and executive function. No differential drug effects were observed. Of 16 cognitive measures, nine demonstrated improvement over time. Of these, only two (visual memory for designs, trail-making speed) demonstrated greater rates of change than those observed in the control group undergoing repeated assessment. The composite effect size in the control group was 0.33; in the patients, 0.36. Results suggest that cognitive change was consistent in magnitude to practice effects and thus does not reflect cognitive enhancement *per se*. These findings have important implications for drug discovery and the design of registration trials that attempt to show cognitive enhancement, demonstrating that serial assessments of cognition may confound cognitive improvement and practice effects, and raising the possibility that cognitive enhancement may be an artifact of repeated assessment (Goldberg *et al.*, 2007). Data collected in a large clinical trial in which patients with chronic schizophrenia remained on a second-generation antipsychotic over a 12-week period, during which they were cognitively assessed three times, supports these findings (Keefe *et al.*, 2007). Large improvements upon repeated testing were observed on an extensive neuropsychological test battery; the effect size was 0.45. Interestingly, practice effects were found even on tests in which alternate forms were used (e.g., verbal list learning). This study demonstrates that practice effects are not restricted to a "rarified" first-episode group, but are also present in middle-aged, chronic patients.

At face value, practice effects may be clinically advantageous, since optimal performance of activities in daily life is dependent on practice or repetition. However, there is little evidence that improvements in practiced tasks generalize to other tasks, since a practice effect is either paradigm specific (e.g., familiarity with testing instructions and demands) or item specific (e.g., words on a list). As a result, practice effects may not reflect changes in the compromised neurobiology that are necessary for improvement in broad domains of cognition. Furthermore, practice effects will not compensate for baseline differences between patients with schizophrenia and healthy subjects who also practice. Possible ways of minimizing practice effects in research include utilizing cross-over study designs, incorporating a healthy control group for assessment of practice effects in cognition, and using tests that are not prone to practice effects.

Parenthetically, the conclusion that second-generation antipsychotics have not been shown to enhance cognition is in keeping with the emerging evidence that (in contrast to earlier views) they do not have a distinct advantage in antipsychotic efficacy, or a unifying or distinctive pharmacology, compared to first-generation drugs (see Chapters 23 and 25); it is also consistent with the fact that D_2 receptor blockade, the property shared by all antipsychotics, is not clearly beneficial for cognitive processes in healthy human subjects or in animals, and may be impairing (Artaloytia et al., 2006; McCartan et al., 2001; Morrens et al., 2007).

Summary

To summarize, over the last decade, neurocognitive deficits have emerged as a critical focus of schizophrenia research, and are seen as a core feature of the disorder (Goldberg & Green, 2002). In particular, the role of neurocognitive abnormalities in mediating both acute treatment response and long-term patient outcome has been identified as key priorities for National Institute of Mental Health (NIMH) USA. Cognitive impairment is now considered a legitimate therapeutic target in schizophrenia, hopefully stimulating the development of innovative therapeutic strategies. Because of its potential critical importance to the design of future cognitive studies, the NIMH has recently launched a consensus-driven initiative to provide a standardized neurocognitive test battery for intervention studies in schizophrenia (MATRICS, Nuechterlein et al., 2008). The measures have recently undergone extensive testing to establish reliability, and other psychometric and practical characteristics for use in intervention research. The MATRICS battery itself takes approximately 60–90 min to administer and is comprised of the following tests: fluency

(for the category animals), symbol coding, trail making, Continuous Performance Test, Identical Pairs Version (CPT-IP), letter-number span, spatial span, Hopkins verbal learning, Brief Visuospatial Memory test, Mazes, and Managing Emotions. The battery is able to capture broadband cognitive impairment. Moreover, the MATRICS tests were selected to tap each of seven dissociable cognitive factors that have been replicably identified in the schizophrenia literature (Nuechterlein et al., 2004).

Neuropsychological investigations of psychotic symptoms

Is there any relationship between cognitive deficits and symptoms or syndromes within the schizophrenic group of disorders? Liddle (1987a) examined the relationships between symptoms rated on a symptomatic assessment scale in 40 patients with chronic schizophrenia, and demonstrated that symptoms segregated into three syndromes: *psychomotor poverty* (reduced speech, lack of spontaneous movement, and blunting of affect); *disorganization* (inappropriate affect, poverty of content of speech, and disturbances in the form of thought); and *reality distortion* (delusions and hallucinations). Examination of the correlations between syndrome severity and performance on a range of well-standardized clinical neuropsychological tests revealed that each of the syndromes was associated with a specific pattern of neuropsychological impairment (Liddle, 1987b). Whereas the psychomotor poverty syndrome was associated with poor performance in tests of conceptual thinking, object naming, and long-term memory, the two syndromes linked with the presence of positive symptoms were associated with a different pattern of cognitive dysfunction. The disorganization syndrome was associated with poor performance in tests of concentration, immediate recall, and word learning, and the reality distortion syndrome was associated with poor figure-ground perception. A similar approach using factor analysis was undertaken by Basso et al. (1998) with 62 patients with schizophrenia on whom a wide variety of clinical, demographic, and neuropsychological measures were available. Negative symptoms were associated with a range of abnormalities such as impaired global IQ, executive function, motor skill, vigilance, attention and memory indices, while disorganization correlated with a subset of these (IQ, attention, and motor tasks). Psychotic symptoms did not correlate with the standard tests.

Other research has focused on specific symptoms to understand their neuropsychological basis. This endeavor involves a shift away from the search for "deficits" and requires a wider conception of cognitive processes, including excesses as well as deficits, dysfunctions, and abnormal interactions (see Halligan & David, 2001) in order to generate mechanistic accounts of symptoms.

Hallucinations

There have been no convincing studies to suggest that auditory verbal hallucinations (AVHs) correlate with deficits on standard neuropsychological tests, unlike, for example, negative symptoms (see above, and David, 1994a).

Hemisphere dysfunction in auditory hallucinations has been examined utilizing the technique of dichotic listening. This entails competition between the right and left hemispheres in the identification of auditory stimuli presented simultaneously, one to each ear. When the stimuli are words or consonant–vowel syllables, input to the left hemisphere predominates, especially in right handers. This right ear/left hemisphere advantage appears to be attenuated in patients who are hallucination-prone (Bruder *et al.*, 1995; Green *et al.*, 1994) and correlates with symptom severity (Levitan *et al.*, 1999). This pattern could be interpreted as a left hemisphere abnormality with or without overactivity of the right hemisphere. Studies using functional magnetic resonance imaging (fMRI) have shown that the right hemisphere shows more activity relative to the left in response to external speech (Woodruff *et al.*, 1997). More recently, however, Hoffman *et al.* (2007) have been able to identify possible sources of AVH in left-hemisphere language circuits which, when targeted for temporary disruption by repetitive transcranial magnetic stimulation, lead to reduced experience of the hallucination.

Language and hallucinations

Schizophrenic auditory hallucinations, the characteristic "voices" talking to or about the subject, have a precise content which is often highly personalized to the voice-hearer (Nayani & David, 1996). It has been suggested that consistency of semantic content of AVHs leads the voice-hearer to personify the experience (Hoffman *et al.*, 1994). Often a complex relationship develops between the patient and "the voices"—usually that of the powerless and the powerful, respectively (Chadwick & Birchwood, 1994). This is in contradistinction to the idea that hallucinations are the random productions of a disordered neocortex (David, 1994a).

The observation that the universal experience of inner speech resembles some AVHs continues to stimulate neurocognitive research. A single case study of a woman with continuous hallucinations showed that inner speech, or more specifically short-term maintenance of phonological representations, can coexist with AVHs (David & Lucas, 1993). This implies that AVHs are not synonymous with inner speech in any simple sense. A battery of short-term memory tests requiring an intact phonological store was used in a group comparison of schizophrenic patients who had recently reported hallucinations *versus* patients who had not (Haddock *et al.*, 1995). The authors tested the general hypothesis that any abnormality could affect monitoring of inner speech, leading to an increased vulnerability to AVHs. All patients performed less well than controls but there was no significant interaction with the presence or absence of hallucinations. Similarly, the verbal transformation effect (the sensation that when a word like "life" is repeated over and over, it turns into "fly") has been used in this context and most recent findings suggest that hallucinators are no more prone to the effect than controls. However, Haddock *et al.* (1995) demonstrated that this effect is vulnerable to motivational factors (i.e., suggestion). In contrast, a separate case study suggested that thought insertion (a pathological experience akin to hearing voices) does appear to be incompatible with effective short-term or working memory (David, 1994b).

Evans *et al.* (2000) carried out an in-depth study of seven patients with no history of AVH and 12 with a strong history of AVH using auditory imagery paradigms which tapped into the functioning of the "inner ear", the "inner voice", and the "inner ear–inner voice" partnership (Smith *et al.*, 1995). These included: parsing meaningful letter strings, pitch judgments, verbal transformations, and a range of tasks requiring phonological judgments. The results showed a wide range of abilities and deficits in both groups, but no clear pattern, and hence do not support an abnormality in inner speech and phonological processing in patients vulnerable to AVHs. However, problems in attribution of inner speech, for example, or theories of hallucinations based on lower level perceptual or physiological processes are not ruled out (see below).

Reality or source monitoring

The problem of deciding whether one imagined hearing a voice, heard someone else speaking, and if the latter, deciding who it was, falls under the rubric of source (or reality) monitoring (Johnson *et al.*, 1988). Hallucinations and delusions of control can therefore be conceived of as failures of source monitoring—either due to a general failure and hence source confusion or a systematic failure or bias so that imagined voices (planned utterances) tend to be remembered as "heard". The first empirical test of this was by Bentall *et al.* (1991), and the results were somewhat equivocal, with hallucinators being no more prone to monitoring errors than other groups. Morrison and Haddock (1997) introduced an innovation to this paradigm by examining source monitoring for words with emotional content. They found that such words tended to disrupt source monitoring but only in terms of immediate ratings of subjective ownership. Seal *et al.* (1997) manipulated several task parameters, including emotional content, and found trends toward more self-to-other misattributions in hallucinators *versus* non-hallucinators. Other research using similar methodology has shown that patients with schizophrenia may well be prone to making source monitoring errors, but the relationship to hallucinations has not emerged (Vinogradov *et al.*, 1997). Indeed a confounding effect of low IQ (Vinogradov *et al.*, 1997) and poor verbal memory (Seal *et al.*, 1997) has been problematic. In perhaps the most complete study, Keefe *et al.* (1999) used a systematic multinomial model to dissect memory level and source, and found that patients not only had difficulty remembering both internal and external sources, but showed a bias in reporting that stimuli came from external sources. Unfortunately, only weak relations with various positive symptoms were discerned. Finally, Brébion *et al.* (2005, 2007) have used increasingly refined episodic memory paradigms to explore the link between memory for context and content in relation to hallucinations and other symptoms in schizophrenia. They found poor source discrimination—assigning words from one list to another—was linked with auditory hallucinations, as were intrusions (the erroneous recall of words that were not presented in a target list). This suggests a combination of lack of inhibition or response bias plus source memory deficits.

Frith's model (1987, 1992) proposes that source monitoring is achieved by a corollary discharge-like mechanism, whereby ownership of a speech act is signaled at the intention stage. The hypothesized failure of this mechanism in AVHs was tested by Cahill *et al.* (1996) using distorted auditory feedback. The aim was to produce a dissonance between external and "internal" monitoring. Reliance solely on the external route would lead to the attribution of an alien source to the heard speech. By lowering or raising the pitch of the patients' speech, the authors did indeed induce hallucination-like experiences. However, this tendency correlated more strongly with the presence of delusions than hallucinations. Johns and McGuire (1999) repeated the experiment using 10 patients with schizophrenia with hallucinations (and delusions) and eight with delusions alone plus normal volunteers. The results showed that, while uncertainty as to the source of the speech was a feature of both schizophrenia groups, external attribution was more common in the hallucinators, a tendency more evident when derogatory material was heard. Goldberg *et al.* (1997) used delayed auditory feedback on the assumption that the dysfluency this usually causes is due to the mismatch between planned and perceived speech output. The authors argued that if the speech production is not anticipated (due to a disconnection between intentions and the monitored output), then this adverse effect on speech should be *less* in those with hallucinations compared to those without. The results showed the opposite, that is, speech output was even more affected in the hallucinators and patients with delusions of control. However, the role of attention in this paradigm has been questioned, though it is unclear why this effect would specifically impact hallucinations.

Indirect psychological evidence for a failure in self-monitoring comes from examining speech repairs, especially when these occur rapidly, often within a word, before external acoustic feedback can have come into play. Leudar *et al.* (1994) found that internal error detection occurred much less commonly in patients with schizophrenia compared with normal controls. However, there was no difference between patients with and without AVHs.

Summary

In summary, inner speech itself appears not to be differentially impaired in hallucinators while data on auditory feedback is contradictory. There is some inconsistent support for reality monitoring errors. An attempt to integrate all these approaches within a single cognitive neuropsychiatric model has been made (David, 2004) with suggestions for future studies.

Delusions

There have been several cognitive models proposed to explain delusion formation. One explanation is that they result from the natural interpretations of abnormal experiences (Maher, 1974). Delusions can occur, however, in the absence of abnormal perceptions and *vice versa*, and different delusional beliefs can be present in various subjects with abnormal perceptions (Chapman & Chapman, 1989). Other theories of delusion formation have therefore emphasized abnormalities in attentional bias, such as increased attention to threatening stimuli in patients with persecutory delusions. Evidence for this includes the significantly longer time that patients with persecutory delusions require to name the print colors of threatening compared with depressive and neutral words in an emotional Stroop test (Kaney & Bentall, 1989), and demonstrations of preferential recall of threat-related propositions in a story recall task (Kaney *et al.*, 1992).

It has also been proposed that patients with persecutory delusions have abnormal attributional processes. Such accounts hold that delusions arise out of habitual tendencies to attribute the causes to events or outside forces (externalizing; Kaney & Bentall, 1989) or people (personalizing) rather than oneself (internalizing), especially where accepting blame would be unpalatable or threatening to self-esteem (self-serving bias) (see Beck & Proctor, 2002, for review).

Reasoning

More recent studies have examined the nature of reasoning biases in patients with delusions about non-persecutory themes. Leafhead *et al.* (1996) employed the emotional Stroop paradigm to investigate the attentional bias in a patient with the Cotard delusion, the belief that one is dead. The patient was found to have increased attention to death-related words. Rossell *et al.* (1998) administered a sentence verification task to patients with delusions. When asked to judge whether statements were real (true), e.g., "fish swim in rivers"; unlikely, e.g., "passengers have sex on trains"; nonsense (untrue), e.g., "the bible is a car catalog", deluded subjects, whose overall performance matched that of controls, made significantly more incorrect responses to sentences that had an emotional content congruent with their delusional beliefs, especially in the intermediate unlikely category. These findings suggest that reasoning abnormalities in deluded patients become particularly evident with tasks related to the theme of the delusional belief, and also indicate the presence of disturbed higher-order semantic processes in these patients. However, it is unclear if delusions cause misinterpretations, or misinterpretations cause delusions, or if delusional subjects are relatively preoccupied with certain emotional themes.

Early work suggested that delusions were the consequence of faulty syllogistic reasoning (von Domarus, 1944), i.e., *I am a man, Napoleon is a man, I am Napoleon.* An investigation of logical reasoning ability, including conditional (Byrne, 1989) and syllogistic (Evans *et al.*, 1993) reasoning tasks, has demonstrated that such reasoning is not impaired in relatively high functioning deluded patients—at least no more than in non-deluded patients (Kemp *et al.*, 1997). Relatively difficult problems were given, such as:

No religious people are criminals
Some priests are criminals
then:
Some religious people are not priests (true/false)
or:
Some priests are not religious people (true/false).

All subjects tended to be swayed by their common-sense understanding rather than working through the problems logically.

Further studies have emphasized abnormalities in hypothesis-testing in deluded patients, with patients with persecutory delusions requiring less information before reaching a conclusion than non-deluded controls—based on judgments of probability of occurrence (Huq *et al.*, 1988; Garety *et al.*, 1991). Tasks have involved being presented with a bead of one of two colors and judging from which of two jars the bead was most likely to have come, given the known proportion of each colored bead in the two jars (e.g. 85:15 in one and 15:85 in the other). Deluded patients tended to reach a judgment after a single bead had been presented while controls tend to wait for more beads before deciding. More naturalistic versions of the task have also been devised and the results are comparable (Dudley *et al.*, 1997). These and similar tasks have also shown that patients are more inclined to stick to their hypotheses even in the presence of negative feedback (Young & Bentall, 1995; Freeman, 2007; Bell *et al.*, 2006). A few conclusions can now

be drawn. First, the "jumping to conclusions" pattern of responding is perhaps best viewed as a data gathering bias, i.e., the tendency to accept an outcome with minimal supporting evidence and failing to seek or wait for further, possibly disconfirming, evidence. This formulation more accurately describes the data (rather than Bayesian norms) and is heuristically valuable. Second, the bias is a rather reliable finding in schizophrenia. However, its close—and presumed causal—association with delusions is not so certain. There have been, for example, reports of a lack of correlation between delusions within a group of patients with schizophrenia (Mortimer *et al.*, 1996) and intriguing emerging findings suggesting a similar "jumping to conclusions" bias in relatives of patients and those identified as psychosis-prone (Freeman, 2007) while some longitudinal studies suggest a state-like association with delusions. It would be of interest to explore how the "beads task" relates to other executive functions, such as impulse control, set shifting, resistance to interference, etc., and which brain systems are involved.

These perceptual and reasoning biases would appear to provide a better explanation for the predisposition to and formation of persecutory delusions rather than their maintenance once formed. Freeman (2007) argues that in paranoia, it is the anxiety, depression, and general distress caused by the beliefs that maintain them by leading to vicious cycles of biased information processing.

The difficulty in distinguishing between the effects of beliefs on current perception and reasoning, and the effects of the latter on belief formation, has been highlighted in the investigation of delusional misidentification, in which it has been argued that abnormal beliefs distort current perceptual experiences in a top-down fashion (Fleminger, 1994). Delusional misidentification (as in the Capgras delusion), is however more commonly seen in patients' neurological syndromes, such as stroke or dementia, than "functional" psychoses. Interest in cognitive neuropsychiatric phenomenology has revived debates as to whether delusions are compatible with normal reasoning (see Maher, 1974) in the presence of abnormal perceptions of the sort that might be expected following cortical damage, or whether additional reasoning deficits are also required (Bell *et al.*, 2006).

Theory of mind

Chris Frith (1992) was the first person to suggest that a theory of mind (ToM)—the ability to infer another's mental state, their beliefs, desires, and intentions—might plausibly be related to delusions. Interest in ToM reasoning arose from developmental psychology and was given a boost following demonstrations that a profound deficit in ToM might underlie autism. Frith speculated that rather than ToM ability failing to develop, as in autism, a later acquired abnormality might lead to inaccurate or inappropriate inferences. This has provoked an explosion of cognitive research, with a variety of stimuli and paradigms being applied to various groups and subgroups of patients with schizophrenia. It was quickly demonstrated that ToM tasks were generally performed less well by people with schizophrenia than healthy controls; a necessary first step but hardly earth shattering. Next came the usual impetus to relate such deficits to particular symptoms or subsyndromes (and the allied state *vs.* trait issue) and to show that the deficits were "specific" and not due to a lower level impairment (say in attention or memory). These studies have been extensively reviewed (Harrington *et al.*, 2005; Brüne, 2005) and subjected to meta-analysis (Sprong *et al.*, 2007). The overall association between ToM deficits and schizophrenia yields a large standardized effect size (Cohen's d = 0 1.26), the strongest being with disorganization, but positive (paranoid) and negative symptoms are related too. Negative symptoms might be considered more "developmental" so, by analogy with autism, they might be expected to lead to more pervasive problems even where so-called first-order ToM tasks are used (e.g., he thinks that …). The more demanding second-order deficits (he thinks that she thinks. …) are more likely to uncover deficits in positive-symptom patients. Patients in remission still show a strong effect (d = 0.69), supporting trait-like properties for ToM deficits, although other evidence supports state-like effects too (Pousa *et al.*, 2008).

ToM research has extended into neurological patients and has been linked to amygdala and frontal lesions, especially where the amygdala lesions are long-standing (Fine *et al.*, 2001; Shaw *et al.*, 2004). Functional imaging has been used to locate the neural networks involved; medial frontal systems come up time and again (Lee *et al.*, 2004; Frith & Frith, 1999).

ToM deficits do not explain why particular types of faulty inferences are made regarding others' intentions—most commonly that they are malign. This is precisely the object of attributional accounts of delusions and is amenable to experimental manipulation using materials borrowed from the social psychology laboratory (see above). Hence, ToM deficits combined with attributional biases may be the necessary components of a paranoid belief.

Other approaches to delusions

David and Howard (1994) employed a type of reality monitoring methodology to study cognitively intact patients with delusional memories. The phenomenal characteristics of each person's delusional memory were contrasted with a real memorable event and a fantasy. It was found that delusional memories were more vivid and tangible even than real events (although delusions tended to be "rehearsed" more mentally) and this vividness could lead to reality confusion. However, a detailed case-study approach revealed coincident reasoning aberrations as well on, for example, the cognitive estimates task.

Other psychophysiological methods have been employed to aid the understanding of delusions. Monitoring directed attention in subjects in real time—an "on-line" measurement of attention—has the advantage over off-line measures in that it allows the presence of "abnormal" information processing strategies. The measurement of visual scan paths is one method which has potential as a monitor of real-time visual information processing. The visual scan path is, literally, a map which traces the direction and extent of gaze when an individual comprehends a complex scene (Norton & Stark, 1971), i.e., a psychophysiological "marker" of sensory input and directional attention on viewing a stimulus. A small number of studies have investigated visual scan paths in schizophrenia (see Phillips & David, 1994). A relationship between symptomatology and viewing strategy has been demonstrated, with positive symptoms being associated with increased scanning and negative symptoms with increased staring (Gaebel *et al.*, 1987; Streit *et al.*, 1997). Other studies have aimed to investigate specific abnormalities in the visual scan paths, i.e., specific attentional deficits, in deluded patients with schizophrenia compared with non-deluded patients with schizophrenia (Phillips & David, 1994, 1997, 1998). They have demonstrated that deluded patients with schizophrenia employ abnormal strategies when viewing salient visual stimuli, human faces—viewing non-feature areas to a significantly greater extent than both well-matched, non-deluded patients with schizophrenia and normal controls. Such strategies "normalize" with recovery. One interpretation is that deluded patients with schizophrenia rely on less salient visual information when appraising complex stimuli compared with controls.

Insight

Insight in psychosis may be defined as the awareness that one has a mental disorder, combined with the ability to label unusual mental events as pathological and the acknowledgement that these require treatment. Lack of insight is a hallmark of schizophrenia and has been considered to be relevant to cognition. Reasons for this include the analogy with neurological syndromes such as anosognosia, but also the intuition that cognitive processes, such as self-awareness and self-reflection, and judgments about the self are components of insight. Interest in the cognitive underpinnings of insight has generated a large body of research which has been subject to systematic review and meta-analysis (Morgan & David, 2004; Aleman *et al.*, 2006). An association with general intellectual function (e.g., IQ) is frequently observed, as is a small but consistent association with executive functioning. Here the correlation coefficients are small–moderate (around 0.2–0.3). Thus it is clear that self-processing may rely, in part, on information processing efficiency or may be considered as an executive function, but a considerable proportion of the insight construct is not explained by cognition and instead is related to psychopathology (inversely: more psychopathology, worse insight), mood (lower mood, better insight) (Mintz *et al.*, 2003), and probably social, cultural, and personality factors.

Summary

The negative symptoms of schizophrenia seem by their very nature to be eminently reducible to cognitive deficits (although there is a danger of circularity, e.g., reduced verbal fluency correlating with poverty of speech). However, linking cognitive abnormalities with positive symptoms has proven to be a challenge. It appears that standard neuropsychological tests lack the specificity and sensitivity to shed light on the cognitive basis of such phenomena as hallucinations and delusions. More successes have been claimed when individual symptoms or symptom complexes or awareness of these have been the focus of investigation, coupled with the use of experimental tasks with a sound theoretical basis. Novel approaches influenced by theories from cognitive development (ToM) have proved fruitful. Contrasting individual cases with clear-cut phenomenology and relatively few intellectual impairments is a strategy worth employing. Within-subject designs with and without the symptoms of interest is another potentially powerful approach. Finally, the remit of neuropsychology needs to expand into social psychology and take account of concepts such as attribution and bias, and perhaps into cognitive and computation neuroscience (e.g., Kapur, 2003) to incorporate models of dopamine function on human behavior.

Conclusions

This chapter has attempted to demonstrate that cognitive paradigms can be utilized to constrain thinking about schizophrenia (for instance, the nature of episodic memory impairments), make important observations about what is "wrong" with patients (in the sense of the identification of core impairments), and be used in novel ways to provide novel mechanistic accounts of symptoms. The modal pattern of the developmental trajectory of cognitive impairment reflects deterioration from some higher level of functioning and then stabilization, but at the illnesses onset and in late life there may be more fluctuation in cognitive performance. Working memory and episodic memory dysfunctions are prominent, but may reflect a more general intellectual deficit. Speed of processing has been underappreciated as an important impairment that monitors the general deficit and predicts outcome. Because these deficits

may account for some of the social and vocational morbidity associated with schizophrenia, they probably should be considered targets for various remediation modalities. These should ultimately include novel cognitive enhancing medications, provided confounders such as practice effects can be controlled in clinical trials.

References

Aleman, A., Hijman, R., de Haan, E.H. & Kahn, R.S. (1999) Memory impairment in schizophrenia: a meta-analysis. *American Journal of Psychiatry* **156**, 1358–1366.

Aleman, A., Agrawal, N., Morgan, K. & David, A.S. (2006) Insight in psychosis and neuropsychological function: meta-analysis. *British Journal of Psychiatry* **189**, 204–212.

Artaloytia, J.F., Arango, C., Lahti, A. *et al.* (2006) Negative signs and symptoms secondary to antipsychotics: a double-blind, randomized trial of a single dose of placebo, haloperidol, and risperidone in healthy volunteers. *American Journal of Psychiatry* **163**, 488–493.

Baddeley, A.D. (1986) *Working Memory*. Oxford: Clarendon.

Barch, D.M. (2005) The cognitive neuroscience of schizophrenia. *Annual Review of Clinical Psychology* **1**, 321–353.

Barch, D.M., Carter, C.S., Hachten, P.C., Usher, M. & Cohen, J.D. (1999) The "benefits" of distractibility: mechanisms underlying increased Stroop effects in schizophrenia. *Schizophrenia Bulletin* **25**, 749–762.

Barch, D.M., Csernansky, J.G., Conturo, T. & Snyder, A.Z. (2002) Working and long-term memory deficits in schizophrenia: is there a common prefrontal mechanism? *Journal of Abnormal Psychology* **111**, 478–494.

Barch, D.M., Carter, C.S., MacDonald, A.W. 3rd, Braver, T.S. & Cohen, J.D. (2003) Context-processing deficits in schizophrenia: diagnostic specificity, 4-week course, and relationships to clinical symptoms. *Journal of Abnormal Psychology* **112**, 132–143.

Basso, M.R., Nasrallah, H.A., Olson, S.C. & Bornstein, R.A. (1998) Neuropsychological correlates of negative, disorganized and psychotic symptoms in schizophrenia. *Schizophrenia Research* **31**, 99–111.

Beck, A.T. & Proctor, N.A. (2002) Delusions: A cognitive perspective. *Journal of Cognitive Psychotherapy* **16**, 455–468.

Bell, V., Halligan, P.W. & Ellis, H.D. (2006) Explaining delusions: a cognitive perspective. *Trends in Cognitive Sciences* **10**, 219–226.

Bentall, R., Baker, G. & Havers, S. (1991) Reality monitoring and psychotic hallucinations. *British Journal of Clinical Psychology* **30**, 213–222.

Bilder, R.M., Reiter, G., Bates, J. *et al.* (2006) Cognitive development in schizophrenia: follow-back from the first episode. *Journal of Clinical and Experimental Neuropsychology* **28**, 270–282.

Bleuler, E. (1911) *Dementia Praecox or the Group of Schizophrenias*. New York: International Universities Press.

Bleuler, E. (1950) *Dementia Praecox or the Group of Schizophrenia*. New York: International Universities Press.

Bowie, C.R., Reichenberg, A., Patterson, T.L., Heaton, R.K. & Harvey, P.D. (2006) Determinants of real-world functional performance in schizophrenia subjects: correlations with cognition, functional capacity, and symptoms. *American Journal of Psychiatry* **163**, 418–425.

Braff, D.L., Heaton, R., Kuck, J. *et al.* (1991) The generalized pattern of neuropsychological deficits in outpatients with chronic schizophrenia with heterogeneous Wisconsin Card Sorting Test results. *Archives of General Psychiatry* **48**, 891–898.

Brébion, G., David, A.S., Jones, H.M. & Pilowsky, L.S. (2005) Hallucinations, negative symptoms, and response bias in a verbal recognition task in schizophrenia. *Neuropsychology* **19**, 612–617.

Brébion, G., David, A.S., Jones, H.M., Ohlsen, R. & Pilowsky, L.S. (2007) Temporal context discrimination in patients with schizophrenia: Associations with auditory hallucinations and negative symptoms. *Neuropsychology* **45**, 817–823.

Bruder, G., Rabinowicz, E., Towey, J. *et al.* (1995) Smaller right ear (left hemisphere) advantage for dichotic fused words in patients with schizophrenia. *American Journal of Psychiatry* **152**, 932–935.

Brüne, M. (2005) "The theory of mind" in schizophrenia: A review of the literature. *Schizophrenia Bulletin* **31**, 21–42.

Bustillo J.R., Thaker G., Buchanan R.W., Moran M., Kirkpatrack B. & Carpenter W.T. (1997) Visual information-processing impairments in deficit and nondeficit schizophrenia. *American Journal of Psychiatry* **154**, 647–654.

Butler, P.D., Zemon, V., Schechter, I. *et al.* (2005) Early-stage visual processing and cortical amplification deficits in schizophrenia. *Archives of General Psychiatry* **62**, 495–504.

Byrne, R. (1989) Suppressing valid inferences with conditionals. *Cognition* **31**, 61–83.

Cahill, C., Silbersweig, D. & Frith, C. (1996) Psychotic experiences induced in deluded patients using distorted auditory feedback. *Cognitive Neuropsychiatry* **1**, 201–211.

Castner, S.A., Goldman-Rakic, P.S. & Williams, G.V. (2004) Animal models of working memory: insights for targeting cognitive dysfunction in schizophrenia. *Psychopharmacology (Berlin)* **174**, 111–125.

Chadwick, P. & Birchwood, M. (1994) The omnipotence of voices: a cognitive approach to auditory hallucinations. *British Journal of Psychiatry* **164**, 190–201.

Chapman, L.J. & Chapman, J.P. (1989) Strategies for resolving the heterogeneity of schizophrenics and their relatives using cognitive measures. *Journal of Abnormal Psychology* **98**, 357–366.

Chelune, G.J., Heaton, R.K., Lehman, R.A. & Robinson, A. (1979) Level versus pattern of neuropsychological performance among schizophrenic and diffusely brain-damaged patients. *Journal of Consulting and Clinical Psychology* **47**, 155–163.

Cohen, J.D., Barch, D.M., Carter, C. & Servan-Schreiber, D. (1999) Context-processing deficits in schizophrenia: Converging evidence from three theoretically motivated cognitive tasks. *Journal of Abnormal Psychology* **108**, 120–133.

Cuesta, M.J., Peralta, V. & Zarzuela, A. (1998) Illness duration and neuropsychological impairments in schizophrenia. *Schizophrenia Research* **33**, 141–150.

D'Esposito, M. (2007) From cognitive to neural models of working memory. *Philosophical Transactions of the Royal Society of London. Series B Biological Sciences* **362**, 761–772.

David, A.S. (1994a) The neuropsychology of auditory-verbal hallucinations. In: David, A. & Cutting, J., eds. *The Neuropsychology of Schizophrenia*. Hove: Lawrence Erlbaum Associates, pp. 269–312.

David, A.S. (1994b) Thought echo reflects the activity of the phonological loop. *British Journal of Clinical Psychology* **33**, 81–europsychiatry of auditory verbal hallucinations: an overview. *Cognitive Neuropsychiatry* **9**, 107–123.

David, A.S. (2004) The cognitive neuropsychiatry of auditory verbal hallucinations: an overview. *Cognitive Neuropsychiatry* **9**, 107–123.

David, A.S. & Howard, R. (1994) An experimental phenomenological approach to delusional memory in schizophrenia and late paraphrenia. *Psychological Medicine* **24**, 515–524.

David, A.S. & Lucas, P. (1993) Auditory–verbal hallucinations and the phonological loop: a cognitive neuropsychological study. *British Journal of Clinical Psychology* **32**, 431–441.

David, A.S., Malmberg, A., Brandt, L., Allebeck, P. & Lewis, G. (1997) IQ and risk for schizophrenia: a population-based cohort study. *Psychological Medicine* **27**, 1311–1323.

Dickinson, D., Iannone, V.N., Wilk, C.M. & Gold, J.M. (2004) General and specific cognitive deficits in schizophrenia. *Biological Psychiatry* **55**, 826–833.

Dickinson, D., Ragland, J.D., Calkins, M.E., Gold, J.M. & Gur, R.C. (2006) A comparison of cognitive structure in schizophrenia patients and healthy controls using confirmatory factor analysis. *Schizophrenia Research* **85**, 20–29.

Dickinson, D., Bellack, A.S. & Gold, J.M. (2007a) Social/communication skills, cognition, and vocational functioning in schizophrenia. *Schizophrenia Bulletin* **33**, 1213–1220.

Dickinson, D., Ramsey, M.E. & Gold, J.M. (2007b) Overlooking the obvious: a meta-analytic comparison of digit symbol coding tasks and other cognitive measures in schizophrenia. *Archives of General Psychiatry* **64**, 532–542.

Dudley, R.E.J., John, C.H., Young, A.W. & Over, D.E. (1997) Normal and abnormal reasoning in people with delusions. *British Journal of Clinical Psychology* **36**, 243–258.

Evans, J. St. B.T., Newstead, S.E. & Byrne, R.M.J. (1993) *Human Reasoning*. Hove: Erlbaum.

Evans, C., McGuire, P. & David, A.S. (2000). Is auditory imagery defective in patients with auditory hallucinations? *Psychological Medicine* **30**, 137–148.

Fine, C., Lumsden, J. & Blair, R.J.R. (2001) Dissociation between "theory of mind" and executive functions in a patient with early left amygdala damage. *Brain* **124**, 287–298.

Fleminger, S. (1994) Top-down processing and delusional misidentification. In: David, A.S. & Cutting, J.C., eds. *The Neuropsychology of Schizophrenia*. Hove: Lawrence Erlbaum Associates, Ltd.

Freeman, D. (2007) Suspicious minds: the psychology of persecutory delusions. *Clinical Psychology Review* **27**, 425–457.

Friedman, J.I., Harvey, P.D., McGurk, S.R. *et al.* (2002) Correlates of change in functional status of institutionalized geriatric schizophrenic patients: focus on medical comorbidity. *American Journal of Psychiatry* **159**, 1388–1394.

Frith, C.D. (1987) The positive and negative symptoms of schizophrenia reflect impairments in the perception and initiation of action. *Psychological Medicine* **17**, 631–648.

Frith, C. (1992) *Cognitive Neuropsychology of Schizophrenia*. Hove: Erlbaum.

Frith, C.D. & Frith, U. (1999) Interacting minds—a biological basis. *Science* **286**, 1692–1695.

Fuller, R.L., Nopoulos, P., Arndt, S., O'Leary, D., Ho, B.C. & Andreasen, N.C. (2002) Longitudinal assessment of premorbid cognitive functioning in patients with schizophrenia through examination of standardized scholastic test performance. *American Journal of Psychiatry* **159**, 1183–1189.

Fuller, R.L., Luck, S.J., McMahon, R.P. & Gold, J.M. (2005) Working memory consolidation is abnormally slow in schizophrenia. *Journal of Abnormal Psychology* **114**, 279–290.

Gaebel, W., Ulrich, G. & Frick, K. (1987) Visuomotor performance of schizophrenic patients and normal controls in a picture viewing task. *Biological Psychiatry* **22**, 1227–1237.

Garety, P.A., Hemsley, D.R. & Wessely, S. (1991) Reasoning in deluded schizophrenic and paranoid patients. Biases in performance on a probabilistic inference task. *The Journal of Nervous and Mental Disease* **179**, 194–201.

Gladsjo, J.A., McAdams, L.A., Palmer, B.W., Moore, D.J., Jeste, D.V. & Heaton, R.K. (2004) A six-factor model of cognition in schizophrenia and related psychotic disorders: relationships with clinical symptoms and functional capacity. *Schizophrenia Bulletin* **30**, 739–754.

Glahn, D.C., Cannon, T.D., Gur, R.E., Ragland, J.D. & Gur, R.C. (2000) Working memory constrains abstraction in schizophrenia. *Biological Psychiatry* **47**, 34–42.

Glahn, D.C., Ragland, J.D., Abramoff, A. *et al.* (2005) Beyond hypofrontality: a quantitative meta-analysis of functional neuroimaging studies of working memory in schizophrenia. *Human Brain Mapping* **25**, 60–69.

Gold, J.M., Randolph, C., Carpenter, C.J., Goldberg, T.E. & Weinberger, D.R. (1992a) Forms of memory failure in schizophrenia. *Journal of Abnormal Psychology* **101**, 487–494.

Gold, J.M., Randolph, C., Coppola, R., Carpenter, C.J., Goldberg, T.E. & Weinberger, D.R. (1992b) Visual orienting in schizophrenia. *Schizophrenia Research* **7**, 203–209.

Gold, J.M., Carpenter, C., Randolph, C., Goldberg, T.E. & Weinberger, D.R. (1997) Auditory working memory and Wisconsin Card Sorting Test performance in schizophrenia. *Archives of General Psychiatry* **54**, 159–165.

Gold, J.M., Queern, C., Iannone, V.N. & Buchanan, R.W. (1999a) Repeatable battery for the assessment of neuropsychological status as a screening test in schizophrenia I: sensitivity, reliability, and validity. *American Journal of Psychiatry* **156**, 1944–1950.

Gold, S., Arndt, S., Nopoulos, P., O'Leary, D.S. & Andreasen, N.C. (1999b) Longitudinal study of cognitive function in first-episode and recent-onset schizophrenia. *American Journal of Psychiatry* **156**, 1342–1348.

Gold, J.M., Rehkemper, G., Binks, S.W. 3rd *et al.* (2000) Learning and forgetting in schizophrenia. *Journal of Abnormal Psychology* **109**, 534–538.

Gold, J.M., Poet, M.S., Wilk, C.M. & Buchanan, R.W. (2004) The family pictures test as a measure of impaired feature binding in schizophrenia. *Journal of Clinical and Experimental Neuropsychology* **26**, 511–520.

Gold, J.M., Fuller, R.L., Robinson, B.M., McMahon, R.P., Braun, E.L. & Luck, S.J. (2006) Intact attentional control of working memory encoding in schizophrenia. *Journal of Abnormal Psychology* **115**, 658–673.

Gold, J.M., Fuller, R.L., Robinson, B.M., Braun, E.L. & Luck, S.J. (2007) Impaired top-down control of visual search in schizophrenia. *Schizophrenia Research* **94**, 148–155.

Goldberg, T.E. & Green, M.F. (2002) Neurocognitive functioning in patients with schizophrenia: An overview. In: Davis, K.L., ed. *Psychopharmacology: The Fifth Generation of Progress*. New York: Raven Press.

Goldberg, T.E., Torrey, E.F., Gold, J.M., Ragland, J.D., Bigelow, L.B. & Weinberger, D.R. (1993) Learning and memory in monozygotic twins discordant for schizophrenia. *Psychological Medicine* **23**, 71–85.

Goldberg, T.E., Gold, J.M., Coppola, R. & Weinberger, D.R. (1997) Unnatural practices, unspeakable actions: a study of delayed auditory feedback in schizophrenia. *American Journal of Psychiatry* **154**, 858–860.

Goldberg, T.E., Goldman, R.S., Burdick, K.E. *et al.* (2007) Cognitive improvement after treatment with second-generation antipsychotic medications in first-episode schizophrenia: is it a practice effect? *Archives of General Psychiatry* **64**, 1115–1122.

Goldman-Rakic, P.S., Castner, S.A., Svensson, T.H., Siever, L.J. & Williams, G.V. (2004) Targeting the dopamine D1 receptor in schizophrenia: insights for cognitive dysfunction. *Psychopharmacology (Berlin)* **174**, 3–16.

Goldstein, K. (1959) Concerning the concreteness in schizophrenia. *Journal of Abnormal Psychology* **59**, 146–148.

Goldstein, G. (1978) Cognitive and perceptual differences between schizophrenics and organics. *Schizophrenia Bulletin* **4**, 160–185.

Goldstein, G. & Zubin, J. (1990) Neuropsychological differences between young and old schizophrenics with and without associated neurological dysfunction. *Schizophrenia Research* **3**, 117–120.

Goldstein, G., Beers, S.R., & Shemansky, W.J. (1996) Neuropsychological differences between schizophrenic patients with heterogeneous Wisconsin Card Sorting Test performance. *Schizophrenia Research* **21**, 13–18.

Green, M.F. (1996) What are the functional consequences of neurocognitive deficits in schizophrenia? *American Journal of Psychiatry* **153**, 321–330.

Green, M.F., Hugdahl, K. & Mitchell, S. (1994) Dichotic listening during auditory hallucinations in patients with schizophrenia. *American Journal of Psychiatry* **151**, 357–362.

Green, M.F., Kern, R.S., Braff, D.L. & Mintz, J. (2000) Neurocognitive deficits and functional outcome in schizophrenia: Are we measuring the "right stuff"? *Schizophrenia Bulletin* **26**, 119–136.

Haddock, G., Slade, P.D. & Bentall, R.P. (1995) Auditory hallucinations and the verbal transformation effect: the role of suggestions. *Personality and Individual Differences* **19**, 301–306.

Haenschel, C., Bittner, R.A., Haertling, F. *et al.* (2007) Contribution of impaired early-stage visual processing to working memory dysfunction in adolescents with schizophrenia: a study with event-related potentials and functional magnetic resonance imaging. *Archives of General Psychiatry* **64**, 1229–1240.

Halligan, P.W. & David, A.S. (2001) Cognitive neuropsychiatry: towards a scientific psychopathology. *Neuroscience: Nature Reviews* **2**, 209–215.

Harrington, L., Siegert, R.J. & McClure, J. (2005) Theory of mind in schizophrenia: a critical review. *Cognitive Neuropsychiatry* **10**, 249–286.

Heaton, R.K., Vogt, A.T., Hoehn, M.M., Lewis, J.A., Crowley, T.J. & Stallings, M.A. (1979) Neuropsychological impairment with schizophrenia vs. acute and chronic cerebral lesions. *Journal of Clinical Psychology* **35**, 46–53.

Heaton, R., Paulsen, J.S., McAdams, L.A. *et al.* (1994) Neuropsychological deficits in schizophrenics. Relationship to age, chronicity and dementia. *Archives of General Psychiatry* **51**, 469–476.

Heinrichs, R.W. & Zakzanis, K.K. (1998) Neurocognitive deficit in schizophrenia: a quantitative review of the evidence. *Neuropsychology* **12**, 426–445.

Hoffman, R.E., Oates, E., Hafner, J., Hustig, H.H. & McGlashan, T.H. (1994) Semantic organization of hallucinated "voices" in schizophrenia. *American Journal of Psychiatry* **151**, 1229–1230.

Hoffman, R.E., Hampson, M., Wu, K. *et al.* (2007) Probing the pathophysiology of auditory/verbal hallucinations by combining functional magnetic resonance imaging and transcranial magnetic stimulation. *Cerebral Cortex* **17**, 2733–2743.

Huq, S.F., Garety, P.A. & Hemsley, D.R. (1988) Probabilistic judgments in deluded and non-deluded subjects. *The Quarterly Journal of Experimental Psychology* **40A**, 801–812.

Hyde, T.M., Nawroz, S., Goldberg, T.E. *et al.* (1994) Is there cognitive decline in schizophrenia, A cross-sectional study. *British Journal of Psychiatry* **164**, 494–500.

Javitt, D.C., Grochowski, S., Shelley, A.M. & Ritter, W. (1998) Impaired mismatch negativity (MMN) generation in schizophrenia as a function of stimulus deviance, probability, and interstimulus/interdeviant interval. *Electroencephalography and Clinical Neurophysiology* **108**, 143–153.

Javitt, D.C., Liederman, E., Cienfuegos, A. & Shelley, A.M. (1999) Panmodal processing imprecision as a basis for dysfunction of transient memory storage systems in schizophrenia. *Schizophrenia Bulletin* **25**, 763–775.

Johns, L.C. & McGuire, P.K. (1999) Verbal self-monitoring and auditory hallucinations in schizophrenia. *Lancet* **353**, 469–470.

Johnson, M.K., Foley, M.A. & Leach, K. (1988) The consequence for memory of imagining in another person's voice. *Memory and Cognition* **16**, 337–342.

Jones, P. & Cannon, M. (1998) The new epidemiology of schizophrenia. *Psychiatric Clinics in North America* **21**, 1–25.

Kaney, S. & Bentall, R.P. (1989) Persecutory delusions and attributional style. *British Journal of Medical Psychology* **62**, 191–198.

Kaney, S., Wolfenden, M., Dewey, M.E. & Bentall, R.P. (1992) Persecutory delusions and the recall of threatening and non-threatening propositions. *British Journal of Clinical Psychology* **31**, 85–87.

Kapur, S. (2003) Psychosis as a state of aberrant salience: A framework linking biology, phenomenology, and pharmacology in schizophrenia. *American Journal of Psychiatry* **160**, 13–23.

Keefe, R.S.E., Silva, S.G., Perkins, D.O. & Lieberman, J.A. (1999) The effects of atypical antipsychotic drugs on neurocognitive impairment in schizophrenia: a review and meta-analysis. *Schizophrenia Bulletin* **25**, 201–222.

Keefe, R.S., Goldberg, T.E., Harvey, P.D., Gold, J.M., Poe, M.P. & Coughenour, L. (2004) The Brief Assessment of Cognition in Schizophrenia: reliability, sensitivity, and comparison with a standard neurocognitive battery. *Schizophrenia Research* **68**, 283–297.

Keefe, R.S., Bilder, R.M., Harvey, P.D. *et al.* (2006) Baseline neurocognitive deficits in the CATIE schizophrenia trial. *Neuropsychopharmacology* **31**, 2033–2046.

Keefe, R.S., Bilder, R.M., Davis, S.M. *et al.*; CATIE Investigators: Neurocognitive Working Group (2007) Neurocognitive effects of antispsychotic medications in patients with chronic schizophrenia in the CATIE Trial. *Archives of General Psychiatry* **64**, 633–647.

Kemp, R., Chua, S., McKenna, P. & David, A.S. (1997) Reasoning and delusions. *British Journal of Psychiatry* **170**, 398–405.

Klonoff, H., Hutton, G.H. & Fibiger, C.H. (1970) Neuropsychological patterns in chronic schizophrenia. *Journal of Nervous and Mental Disease* **150**, 291–300.

Kraepelin, E. (1919) *Dementia Praecox and Paraphrenia*, Robertson, G.M., ed. (translated by Barclay, R.M & Krieger, R.E.) (1971) Huntington, New York.

Leafhead, K.M., Young, A.W. & Szulecka, T.K. (1996) Delusions demand attention. *Cognitive Neuropsychiatry* **1**, 5–16.

Lee, J. & Park, S. (2005) Working memory impairments in schizophrenia: a meta-analysis. *Journal of Abnormal Psychology* **114**, 599–611.

Lee, K.H., Farrow, T.F.D., Spence, S.A. & Woodruff, P.W.R. (2004) Social cognition, brain networks and schizophrenia. *Psychological Medicine* **34**, 391–400.

Lencz, T., Bilder, R.M., Turkel, E. *et al.* (2003) Impairments in perceptual competency and maintenance on a visual delayed match-to-sample test in first-episode schizophrenia. *Archives of General Psychiatry* **60**, 238–243.

Leudar, I., Thomas, P. & Johnston, M. (1994) Self-monitoring in speech production: effects of verbal hallucinations and negative symptoms. *Psychological Medicine* **24**, 749–761.

Levitan, C., Ward, P.B. & Catts, S.V. (1999) Superior temporal gyral volumes and laterality correlates of auditory hallucinations in schizophrenia. *Biological Psychiatry* **46**, 955–962.

Liddle, P.F. (1987a) The symptoms of chronic schizophrenia: a re-examination of the positive–negative dichotomy. *British Journal of Psychiatry* **151**, 145–151.

Liddle, P.F. (1987b) Schizophrenic syndromes, cognitive performance and neurological dysfunction. *Psychological Medicine* **17**, 49–57.

Luck, S.J. & Hillyard, S.A. (1994) Spatial filtering during visual search: Evidence from human electrophysiology. *Journal of Experimental Psychology: Human Perception and Performance* **20**, 1000–1014.

Luck, S.J. & Vecera, S.P. (2002) Attention. In: Yantis, S., ed. *Stevens' Handbook of Experimental Psychology: Vol 1: Sensation and Perception*, 3rd edn. New York: Wiley.

Luck, S.J., Girelli, M., McDermott, M.T. & Ford, M.A. (1997) Bridging the gap between monkey neurophysiology and human perception: An ambiguity resolution theory of visual selective attention. *Cognitive Psychology* **33**, 64–67.

Luck, S.J., Fuller, R.L., Braun, E.L., Robinson, B., Summerfelt, A. & Gold, J.M. (2006) The speed of visual attention in schizophrenia: Electrophysiological and behavioral evidence. *Schizophrenia Research* **85**, 174–195.

Maher, B.A. (1974) Delusional thinking and perceptual disorder. *Journal of Individual Psychology* **30**, 85–95.

Martínez-Arán, A., Vieta, E., Reinares, M. *et al.* (2004) Cognitive function across manic or hypomanic, depressed, and euthymic states in bipolar disorder. *American Journal of Psychiatry* **161**, 262–270.

Maruff, P., Hay, D., Malone, V. & Currie, J. (1995) Asymmetries in the convert orienting of visual spatial attention in schizophrenia. *Neuropsychologia* **33**, 1205–1223.

Maruff, P., Pantelis, C., Danckert, J., Smith, D. & Currie, J. (1996) Deficits in the endogenous redirection of covert visual attention in chronic schizophrenia. *Neuropsychologia* **34**, 1079–1084.

Maruff, P., Danckert, J., Pantelis, C. & Currie, J. (1998) Saccadic and attentional abnormalities in patients with schizophrenia. *Psychological Medicine* **28**, 1091–1100.

McCartan, D., Bell, R., Green, J.F. *et al.* (2001) The differential effects of chlorpromazine and haloperidol on latent inhibition in healthy volunteers. *Journal of Psychopharmacology* **15**, 96–104.

McGurk, S.R., Coleman, T., Harvey, P.D. *et al.* (2004) Working memory performance in poor outcome schizophrenia: relationship to age and executive functioning. *Journal of Clinical and Experimental Neuropsychology* **26**, 153–160.

Michel, L., Danion, J.M., Grangé, D. & Sandner, G. (1998) Cognitive skill learning and schizophrenia: implications for cognitive remediation. *Neuropsychology* **12**, 590–599.

Mintz, A.R., Dobson, K.S. & Romney, D.M. (2003) Insight in schizophrenia: a meta-analysis. *Schizophrenia Research* **61**, 75–88.

Mirsky, A.F., Yardley, S.L., Jones, B.P., Walsh, D. & Kendler, K.S. (1995) Analysis of the attention deficit in schizophrenia: a study of patients and their relatives in Ireland. *Journal of Psychiatric Research* **29**, 23–42.

Mockler, D., Riordan, J. & Sharma, T. (1997) Memory and intellectual deficits do not decline with age in schizophrenia. *Schizophrenia Research* **26**, 1–7.

Morgan, K.D. & David, A.S. (2004) Neuropsychological studies of insight in patients with psychotic disorders. In: Amador, X.F. & David, A.S., eds. *Insight and Psychosis: Awareness of Illness in Schizophrenia and Related Disorders*, 2nd edn. Oxford: Oxford University Press, pp. 177–193.

Morrens, M., Wezenberg, E., Verkes, R.J., Hulstijn, W., Ruigt, G.S. & Sabbe, B.G. (2007) Psychomotor and memory effects of haloperidol, olanzapine, and paroxetine in healthy subjects after short-term administration. *Journal of Clinical Psychopharmacology* **27**, 15–21

Morrison, A.P. & Haddock, G. (1997) Cognitive factors in source monitoring and auditory hallucinations. *Psychological Medicine* **27**, 669–679.

Mortimer, A.M., Bentham, P., McKay, A.P. *et al.* (1996) Delusions in schizophrenia: A phenomenological and psychological exploration. *Cognitive Neuropsychiatry* **1**, 289–304.

Nayani, T.H. & David, A.S. (1996) The auditory hallucination: a phenomenological survey. *Psychological Medicine* **26**, 177–189.

Nelson, M.D., Saykin, A.J., Flashman, L.A. & Riordan, H.J. (1998) Hippocampal volume reduction in schizophrenia as assessed by magnetic resonance imaging: a meta-analytic study. *Archives of General Psychiatry* **55**, 433–440.

Norton, D. & Stark, L. (1971) Eye movements and visual perception. *Scientific American* **224**, 35–43.

Nuechterlein, K.H. & Dawson, M.E. (1984) Information processing and attentional functioning in the developmental course of schizophrenic disorders. *Schizophrenia Bulletin* **10**, 160–203.

Nuechterlein, K.H., Barch, D.M., Gold, J.M., Goldberg, T.E., Green, H.F. & Heaton, R.K. (2004) Identification of separable cognitive factors in schizophrenia. *Schizophrenia Research* **72**, 29–39.

Nuechterlein, K.H., Green, M.F., Kern, R.S. *et al.* (2008) The MATRICS Consensus Cognitive Battery, part 1: test selection, reliability, and validity. *American Journal of Psychiatry* **165**, 203–213.

Oie, M., Rund, B.R. & Sundet, K. (1998) Covert visual attention in patients with early-onset schizophrenia. *Schizophrenia Research* **34**, 195–205.

Paulsen, J.S., Heaton, R.K., Sadek, J.R. *et al.* (1995) The nature of learning and memory impairments in schizophrenia. *Journal of the International Neuropsychological Society* **1**, 88–99.

Pelletier, M., Achim, A.M., Montoya, A., Lal, S. & Lepage, M. (2005) Cognitive and clinical moderators of recognition memory in schizophrenia: a meta-analysis. *Schizophrenia Research* **74**, 233–252.

Phillips, M.L. & David, A.S. (1994) Understanding the symptoms of schizophrenia using visual scan paths. *British Journal of Psychiatry* **165**, 673–675.

Phillips, M.L. & David, A.S. (1997) Visual scan paths are abnormal in deluded schizophrenics. *Neuropsychologia* **35**, 99–105.

Phillips, M.L. & David, A.S. (1998) Abnormal visual scan paths: a psychophysiological marker of delusions in schizophrenia. *Schizophrenia Research* **29**, 235–245.

Posner, M.I., Early, T.S., Reiman, E., Pardo, P.J. & Dhawan, I.M. (1988) Asymmetries in hemispheric control of attention in schizophrenia. *Archives of General Psychiatry* **45**, 814–821.

Pousa, E., Duñó, R., Brebion, G., David, A.S., Ruiz, A.I. & Obiols, J.E. (2008) Theory of mind deficits in chronic schizophrenia: evidence for state dependence. *Psychiatry Research* **158**, 1–10.

Rappaport, D., Gill, M. & Schafer, R. (1945/1946) *Diagnostic Psychological Testing*. Chicago: Year Book Publishers.

Reichenberg, A., Weiser, M., Rabinowitz, J. *et al.* (2002) A population-based cohort study of premorbid intellectual, language, and behavioral functioning in patients with schizophrenia, schizoaffective disorder, and nonpsychotic bipolar disorder. *American Journal of Psychiatry* **159**, 2027–2035.

Reichenberg, A., Weiser, M., Rapp, M. *et al.* (2005) Elaboration on premorbid intellectual performance in schizophrenia: premorbid intellectual decline and risk for schizophrenia. *Archives of General Psychiatry* **62**, 1297–1304.

Rossell, S.L., Shapleske, J. & David, A.S. (1998) Sentence verification and delusions: a content-specific deficit. *Psychological Medicine* **28**, 1189–1198.

Rund, B.R. (1998) A review of longitudinal studies of cognitive functions in schizophrenia patients. *Schizophrenia Bulletin* **24**, 425–435.

Salisbury, D.F., Kuroki, N., Kasai, K., Shenton, M.E. & McCarley, R.W. (2007) Progressive and interrelated functional and structural evidence of post-onset brain reduction in schizophrenia. *Archives of General Psychiatry* **64**, 521–529.

Saykin, A.J., Gur, R.C., Gur, R.E. *et al.* (1991) Neuropsychological function in schizophrenia. Selective impairment in memory and learning. *Archives of General Psychiatry* **48**, 618–624.

Saykin, A.J., Shatasel, D.L., Gur, R.E. *et al.* (1994) Neuropsychological deficits in neuroleptic naïve patients with first-episode schizophrenia. *Archives of General Psychiatry* **51**, 124–131.

Schmidt, F.L. & Hunter, J. (2004) General mental ability in the world of work: occupational attainment and job performance. *Journal of Personality and Social Psychology* **86**, 162–173.

Schretlen, D.J., Cascella, N.G., Meyer, S.M. *et al.* (2007) Neuropsychological functioning in bipolar disorder and schizophrenia. *Biological Psychiatry* **62**, 179–186.

Seal, M.L., Crowe, S.F. & Cheung, P. (1997) Deficits in source monitoring in subjects with auditory hallucinations may be due to differences in verbal intelligence and verbal memory. *Cognitive Neuropsychiatry* **2**, 273–290.

Sereno, A.B. & Holzman, P.S. (1996) Spatial selective attention in schizophrenic, affective disorder, and normal subjects. *Schizophrenia Research* **20**, 33–50.

Shakow, D.J. (1972) The Worcester State Hospital Research on schizophrenia (1927–1946). *Journal of Abnormal Psychology* **80**, 67–110.

Shaw, P., Lawrence, E.J., Radbourne, C., Bramham, J., Polkey, C.E. & David, A.S. (2004) The impact of early and late damage to the human amygdala on "theory of mind" reasoning. *Brain* **127**, 1–14.

Smith, A. (1964) Mental deterioration in chronic schizophrenia. *Journal of Nervous and Mental Disease* **39**, 479–487.

Smith, J.D., Wilson, M. & Reisberg, D. (1995) The role of subvocalization in auditory imagery. *Neuropsychologia* **33**, 1433–1454.

Sprong, M., Schothorst, P., Vos, E., Hox, J. & van Engeland, H. (2007) Theory of mind in schizophrenia: meta-analysis. *British Journal of Psychiatry* **191**, 5–13.

Strauss, M.E., Alphs, L. & Boekamp, J. (1992) Disengagement of attention in chronic schizophrenia. *Psychiatry Research* **43**, 87–92.

Streit, M., Woelwer, W. & Gaebel, W. (1997) Facial-affect recognition and visual scanning behaviour in the course of schizophrenia. *Schizophrenia Research* **24**, 311–317.

Swerdlow, N.R., Light, G.A., Cadenhead, K.S., Sprock, J., Hsieh, M.H. & Braff, D.L. (2006) Startle gating deficits in a large cohort of patients with schizophrenia: relationship to medications, symptoms, neurocognition, and level of function. *Archives of General Psychiatry* **63**, 1325–1335.

Talamini, L., Mateer, M., Elvevaag, B.E., Murre, J. & Goldberg, T.E. (2005) A computational account of parahippocampal abnormalities in schizophrenia during memory processing. *Archives of General Psychiatry* **62**, 485–493.

Tek, C., Gold, J., Blaxton, T., Wilk, C., McMahon, R.P. & Buchanan, R.W. (2002) Visual perceptual and working memory impairments in schizophrenia. *Archives of General Psychiatry* **59**, 146–153.

Uhlhaas, P.J. & Silverstein, S.M. (2005) Perceptual organization in schizophrenia spectrum disorders: empirical research and theoretical implications. *Psychological Bulletin* **131**, 618–632.

Umbricht, D.S., Bates, J.A., Lieberman, J.A., Kane, J.M. & Javitt, D.C. (2006) Electrophysiological indices of automatic and controlled auditory information processing in first-episode, recent-onset and chronic schizophrenia. *Biological Psychiatry* **59**, 762–772.

Velligan, D.I., DiCocco, M., Bow-Thomas, C.C. *et al.* (2004) A brief cognitive assessment for use with schizophrenia patients in community clinics. *Schizophrenia Research* **71**, 273–283.

Vinogradov, S., Willis-Shore, J., Poole, J.H., Marten, E., Ober, B.A. & Shenaut, G.K. (1997) Clinical and neurocognitive aspects of source monitoring errors in schizophrenia. *American Journal of Psychiatry* **154**, 1530–1537.

von Domarus, E. (1944) The specific laws of logic in schizophrenia. *Language and Thought in Schizophrenia* 104–114.

Weickert, T.W., Goldberg, T.E., Gold, J.M., Bigelow, L.B., Egan, M.F. & Weinberger, D.R. (2000) Cognitive impairments in patients with schizophrenia displaying preserved and compromised intellect. *Archives of General Psychiatry* **57**, 907–913.

Weinberger, D.R. & Berman, K.F. (1988) Speculation on the meaning of cerebral metabolic hypofrontality in schizophrenia. *Schizophrenia Bulletin* **14**, 157–168.

Woodruff, P.W., Wright I.C., Bullmore, E. *et al.* (1997) Auditory hallucinations and the temporal cortical response to speech in schizophrenia: a functional magnetic resonance imaging study. *American Journal of Psychiatry* **154**, 1676–1682.

Young, H.F. & Bentall, R.P. (1995) Hypothesis testing in patients with persecutory delusions: comparison with depressed and normal subjects. *British Journal of Clinical Psychology* **34**, 353–369.

PART 2

Biological Aspects

CHAPTER 9

The secondary schizophrenias

Thomas M. Hyde[1] and Maria A. Ron[2]

[1]Lieber Institute for Brain Development, Baltimore, MD, USA
[2]Institute of Neurology, University College London, London, UK

Schizophrenia is a behavioral disorder that is a diagnosis of exclusion, despite decades of research establishing its biological underpinnings. There are no established laboratory tests, neuroimaging studies, electrophysiological paradigms or neuropsychological testing batteries that can explicitly confirm this disorder to the exclusion of phenocopies. This was explicitly recognized by Kraepelin and Bleuler, and particularly by Schneider, as a caveat in the delineation of his first-rank symptoms.

The existence of a disparate range of brain disorders that can, uncommonly, give rise to schizophrenia-like symptomatology presents psychiatry with a problem and an opportunity. On the one hand, it poses nosological dilemmas about the limits of the definition of schizophrenia; on the other, it provides insights into the biological mechanisms underlying the generation of schizophrenic symptoms.

This chapter first outlines the nosological challenges and how recent classification systems have dealt with these, distinguishing secondary schizophrenia-like psychoses

arising from defined neuropathological processes and those secondary to cerebral complications of systemic illness. Second, it attempts to estimate the prevalence of such secondary schizophrenias in relation to schizophrenia in general. Third, it examines the evidence for symptomatic differences between secondary and primary schizophrenia and discusses their clinical diagnosis. Finally, the chapter reviews broadly which specific brain diseases seem to present a particularly increased risk of schizophrenic symptoms.

Terminology and classification

In the past, mental disorders have been subdivided into "organic" and "functional" categories. Within this framework, schizophrenia was assigned to a class of disorders conventionally known as "functional psychoses" and this was the terminology that held sway in ICD-9 (World Health Organization, 1978). Although the ICD-9 had several disadvantages, most particularly the absence of clearly defined reliable operational diagnostic criteria, one potential advantage was the adherence to a descriptive pattern of phenomenological definition. Thus, the term "organic", as opposed to "functional", was not intended to

Schizophrenia, 3rd edition. Edited by Daniel R. Weinberger and Paul J Harrison © 2011 Blackwell Publishing Ltd.

imply a "physical" etiology, but specifically to describe a set of symptoms of cognitive impairment, such as disorientation, reduced level of consciousness, and impairments of memory. This allowed schizophrenia secondary to coarse brain disease (with a clearly identifiable neuropathology) to be classed under the rubric of schizophrenia, with appropriate subdiagnosis according to the pathology of the causative agent or disease. In DSM-III and DSM-IIIR, the term "organic" was redefined in an important way, so as to imply a specific pathological etiology, rather than to describe particular symptoms in the mental state. Thus, separate categories of "organic mental disorders" were introduced. Cases of psychosis without cognitive impairment, but in the presence of "evidence from the history, physical examination or laboratory tests of a specific organic factor judged to be etiologically related", were now called "organic delusional syndrome" or "organic hallucinosis", depending on the predominant symptoms. Nevertheless, in DSM-III it was acknowledged that symptoms in these "organic" mental disorders could be "essentially identical with schizophrenia". This convention put the diagnostician in the problematic position of having to rename a syndrome whenever a likely organic cause became apparent (Lewis *et al.*, 1987). The DSM-IV and DSM-IVR attempted to rectify this problem by eliminating the section delineating a separate category of "organic mental syndromes and disorders". Implicit in the classification of some forms of mental illness as "organic" was the assumption, by contrast, that some must arise purely from experience rather than physical changes in brain anatomy and function. Thankfully, this artificial dichotomization is disappearing, as the biological bases of all major mental disorders become more apparent.

In so far as all behavioral disorders have a biological component, the differentiation between *schizophrenia-like* symptoms arising from a definite cause and those with an obscure etiology is an inherently dissatisfying process. As we better define the biological basis of psychosis in schizophrenia, the etiology of these pathological processes will become apparent. As it now stands, in a sense, schizophrenia is a term reserved for those "idiopathic" cases of chronic psychosis.

Potential problems with the term "organic" are exemplified by treatment of the term in the ICD-10 (World Health Organization, 1992), particularly in the section on "Other organic mental disorders" (F06). It is worthwhile examining this in a little detail so as to advance the argument that the term organic should be abandoned as a descriptor for schizophrenias caused by coarse brain disease. The ICD-10 use of the term organic introduces a paradox that is referred to in the text thus: "use of the term organic does not imply that conditions elsewhere in this classification are nonorganic". Moreover, the criteria put forward in ICD-10 by which to identify disorders such as an organic schizophrenia-like disorder are not strictly logical. One of the two requirements to justify a diagnosis is "a temporal relationship (weeks or a few months) between the development of the underlying disease and the onset of the syndrome". In reality, this time-scale limits inclusion to what are essentially precipitating factors rather than true causes which, as will be discussed later, seem often to take several years before generating schizophrenia-like symptoms. A further problem with the notion of splitting off "organic" schizophrenias from schizophrenia in general is that our knowledge base as to the epidemiology of the first group, and of the relationship in general between the two groups, is very limited. The greatest difficulty in confidently diagnosing a case of organic schizophrenia-like disorder is in the attribution of the symptoms to a particular organic cause. This is seldom simple, particularly because there may be little time congruence between onset of the physical disorder and onset of the schizophrenic symptoms. It is this difficulty in attribution that seems to have led to the comparatively poor interrater reliability reported in recent field trials of ICD-10 for these organic categories, as compared with their "functional" counterparts (Sartorius *et al.*, 1993).

Spitzer *et al.* (1992) argued cogently for retiring the term "organic mental disorders". In this review we shall follow their lead. They asserted that the term "organic" has insoluble problems attached to it and for this reason another term should be chosen. They considered the term "symptomatic", but noted that this can be ambiguous and proposed that the term "secondary" should be used instead. Secondary disorders should be distinguished from substance-induced disorders and are recognized if they are caused by medical disorders that are classified outside the mental disorder section of the ICD. Schizophrenic symptoms can thus be categorized in any individual case to being primary, or secondary "to a non-psychiatric medical disorder", or substance-induced.

The DSM-IV (American Psychiatric Association, 2000) has adopted this approach, which harkens back to the phenomenological basis of classification in ICD-9. Sensibly, the introduction to the organizational plan in DSM-IV states that "the term organic mental disorder is no longer used in DSM-IV because it incorrectly implies that the other mental disorders in the manual do not have a biologic basis". Thus, schizophrenic symptoms secondary to a non-psychiatric medical disorder are now headed under section 293.8 "psychotic disorder due to a general medical condition".

Secondary schizophrenias can be thought of as falling into two categories:

1. Where the psychotic symptoms arise from the cerebral involvement of a systemic illness known to affect the brain. This is the category headed 293.8 in DSM-IV.

2. Where schizophrenic symptoms arise in the context of a demonstrable, often clinically unsuspected, neuropathologically defined disorder that is not part of an ongoing systemic disease process.

This latter area has become considerably more important since the advent of high-resolution neuroimaging techniques in the past 20 years. In the DSM-IV, this category is subsumed into the general class of psychotic disorders due to a general medical condition. This is paradoxical because many of these disorders are restricted to the central nervous system (CNS), such as neoplasms and cerebrovascular disease.

In reviewing the literature regarding the association between psychosis and coarse brain disease, another problem frequently arises. Over the decades, the term psychosis has been applied to a wide variety of signs and symptoms. Defined criteria for primary schizophrenia have only been commonly agreed upon in the past 30 years. Even within this period, the criteria have been significantly modified. The details of case reports must be scrutinized carefully. For example, a problem arises in differentiating disorders with prominent psychotic features from delirium. Most reserve the term delirium for an agitated confusional state, with prominent sensory illusions and misperceptions. In fact, there is significant overlap between the clinical signs and symptoms of delirium, primary schizophrenia, and the secondary schizophrenias. A relatively abrupt onset and short time course helps differentiate delirium from the other two entities when reported in the literature. Frequently, however, many so-called secondary schizophrenias are actually delirious states, such as the encephalopathy associated with sepsis in the elderly.

How common are secondary schizophrenias?

Given the disputes over definition and diagnosis, it is not surprising that little is known about the detailed epidemiology of secondary schizophrenia. One difficulty in estimating prevalence is the problem of definition: how confident can one be that the well-defined brain disease is truly responsible for the presenting schizophrenic symptoms? A second difficulty is that the closer one looks, the more likely it is that structural pathology will be revealed. The widespread availability of high-resolution brain imaging techniques has shown that unsuspected cerebral lesions occur in a small but significant number of patients with schizophrenic symptoms. Most structural brain imaging research in psychosis has concentrated rather on minor quantitative changes involving widened fluid spaces and reduced volume of particular structures in the medial temporal lobe. These minor quantitative changes would not usually be reported as abnormal by most clinical radiologists. However, there are a handful of reports in the literature of gross focal brain lesions in schizophrenia.

Two large imaging studies using X-ray-based computerized tomography (CT) enable an estimate to be made of the prevalence of such unequivocal focal lesions in schizophrenia. Owens *et al.* (1980) in their series of 136 patients with schizophrenia found "unsuspected intracranial pathology" as a focal finding on CT in 12 cases (9%), after excluding lesions resulting from leucotomy. This was a relatively elderly sample: five of these 12 cases were aged over 65. Lewis (1990) examined a series of 228 Maudsley Hospital patients who met Research Diagnostic Criteria (RDC) for schizophrenia and who had been consecutively scanned for clinical reasons. Patients with a history of epilepsy or intracranial surgery, or who were aged over 65 at the time of scan, were excluded. The original scan reports were examined and the films of those not unequivocally normal were reappraised by a neuroradiologist blind to the original report. In 41 patients the scan showed a definite intracranial abnormality. This was in the nature of enlarged fluid spaces in 28 cases, but in 13 patients (6%) there was a discrete focal lesion. These lesions varied widely in location and probable pathology, although left temporal and right parietal regions were most commonly implicated.

Given the differences in the nature of the patient samples, these two studies are in rough agreement about the prevalence of unexpected focal abnormalities on CT: between 6% and 9%. One magnetic resonance imaging (MRI) study has also examined the issue of the prevalence of focal abnormalities in schizophrenia. Given the higher resolution of MRI technology, one might predict a higher lesion detection rate than with CT. O'Callaghan *et al.* (1992) scanned 47 patients under the age of 65 meeting DSM-III criteria for schizophrenia, with 25 matched controls. Four patients (9%) were revealed to have unsuspected lesions of a neurodevelopmental type: one partial agenesis of the corpus callosum; two cases of marked asymmetric dilatation of the left lateral ventricle (one with an associated porencephalic cyst); and one cerebellar hypoplasia.

The only epidemiologically sound and well-executed study to report prevalence figures for secondary schizophrenias of the type produced by systemic physical illness is the study by Johnstone *et al.* (1987). The study examined a sample of 328 consecutive patients presenting with a first episode of schizophrenia between the age of 15 and 70 years. Patients were screened clinically, without routine diagnostic neuroimaging, for the presence of organic illnesses that the authors judged were "of definite or possible etiological significance". Thirteen patients fell into the category of substance-induced schizophrenia, including one patient who was judged to have developed schizophrenia-like symptoms secondary to treatment with steroids. Nine patients (3%) were regarded as falling into the category of schizophrenia secondary to non-psychiatric medical disorders. These comprised three cases of tertiary syphilis, two of neurosarcoidosis, one of multisystem autoimmune disease including systemic lupus erythematosus (SLE), one of carcinoma of the bronchus with a secondary right parietal and frontal brain infarction, one of cerebral cysticercosis, and one of chronic thyrotoxicosis. In these cases, neurological signs were the exception rather than the rule and a history of epilepsy was noted in only one case. Over half of the cases had migrated from developing countries and had presumably been at increased risk of untreated infections and other disorders. No case had a family history of schizophrenia. Two additional aspects of the data that were not specifically commented on by the authors were the relatively late age at onset of these nine cases (range 29–59 years) and, curiously, that all nine cases were female.

Inferring cause and effect

The establishment of a cause–effect relationship between a particular organic disease and schizophrenic symptoms in clinical practice can be very difficult. Coincidence does not prove causality. Table 9.1 gives general criteria by which observations are used in disease models to support the existence of a causal relationship. As can be seen, in the case of secondary schizophrenias, several of these criteria are difficult to fulfil. Neurodevelopmental formulations of etiology in schizophrenia generally are relatively recent, but mean that the temporality criterion can be difficult to demonstrate if the cause arises many years before the schizophrenic symptoms. Nonetheless, there are clear instances in the literature of cause being attributed where it is by no

means clear that the lesion predated the schizophrenia. For example, several old postmortem studies disclosed brain tumors in patients with schizophrenia without evidence that the tumor predated the psychiatric symptoms (Davison & Bagley, 1969). In addition to the problems noted in Table 9.1, there are other difficulties. In some instances both the physical disease and the schizophrenic symptoms may result from another cause. Epilepsy might be the best example of this, where both the symptoms of epilepsy—itself a syndrome—and schizophrenia may arise from some underlying brain disease, rather than epilepsy causing schizophrenia directly. Drug treatments of the physical disorder can also predispose to psychotic symptomatology; e.g., steroids and amphetamines (in the case of narcolepsy; Walterfang et al., 2005a). A further possible confounding factor is that some aspect of preschizophrenic personality might predispose to health-endangering behaviors, e.g., head injury. Despite all these caveats, a number of different physical disorders have, down the years, been linked to the emergence of secondary schizophrenia.

Co-occurrence of schizophrenia-like symptoms and organic brain disease

In 1969, Davison and Bagley (1969) published an extensive review of the world literature, backed with some 800 references, of the co-occurrence of schizophrenia-like symptoms and organic disease. This review remains a landmark in the field. It took as its starting point the operational criteria for

Table 9.1 General criteria to support causal relationships used in disease models.

CriterionObservation		Comments regarding schizophrenia
Temporality	Cause precedes effect	Cause may be several years earlier
		Problems with cross-sectional surveys of schizophrenic patients: temporality must be inferred
Consistency	Repeatedly observed	Many observations are anecdotal, single-case reports
Strength	Large relative risk	Relative risk difficult to establish because associations are often rare; best established for epilepsy
Dose–response	Larger exposure to cause associated with larger risk	May not hold for schizophrenia where specific subtle lesion may be important
Reversibility	Reduced exposure to cause associated with reduced effect	Not shown
Specificity	One cause leads to one effect	Several different causes with no clear common pathology; each cause can have different neuropsychiatric effects
Analogy	Similar exposure gives known effects	Closest analogy probably epilepsy; variety of causes, latent period, pleiomorphic behavioral syndrome
Biological plausibility	Makes sense	Neurodevelopmental model facilitates understanding of mechanisms; but what about non-neurodevelopmental causes?

schizophrenia of the 1957 WHO Committee, which were adapted slightly by Davison and Bagley so that their case material included cases which today would broadly be headed under the rubric of schizophrenia and paranoid psychosis. Criteria also included the absence of impaired consciousness and the absence of prominent affective symptoms. The authors concluded that the occurrence of schizophrenia-like symptoms exceeded chance expectation in many organic CNS disorders and that, where a discrete lesion was present, those in the temporal lobe and diencephalon seemed to be particularly significant.

Davison and Bagley reviewed the evidence for the association between schizophrenia and a large range of individual CNS disorders. Epilepsy was statistically associated with schizophrenia-like psychosis, particularly where a temporal lobe lesion existed. Head injury was also a risk factor for psychosis, again with a possible association with temporal lobe lesions. Severe closed head injury with diffuse cerebral damage was related to early development of psychotic symptoms. Encephalitic disorders, cerebral syphilis, Wilson disease, Huntington disease, Friedreich ataxia, vitamin B_{12} deficiency, subarachnoid hemorrhage, and cerebral tumor also seemed to be associated with an increased risk of schizophrenia-like symptoms. They found much less evidence to implicate other CNS disorders, such as multiple sclerosis, motor neurone disease, and Parkinson disease.

Not surprisingly, 40 years later, a few of Davison and Bagley's conclusions might be amended. For example, their association between narcolepsy and psychosis most likely reflects a side effect of amphetamines used in treatment, rather than the disease itself. Additionally the correlation between cerebral tumors and schizophrenia-like symptoms is weak. Many such instances could be better explained as chance association, unless the tumors were of the type whose natural history was very long-standing, such as hamartomas of the temporal lobe. Conversely, new evidence for these and other disorders being associated is now available, and is reviewed below.

Epilepsy

Estimates of the incidence of schizophrenic symptoms in temporal lobe epilepsy vary widely (reviewed in Hyde & Weinberger, 1997), and are obviously sensitive to artifacts of ascertainment. Roberts et al. (1990) reported that 25 of his consecutive autopsy series of 249 cases (10%) had a lifetime history of psychotic symptoms. Trimble (1988) estimated that patients with epilepsy were at three- to nine-fold increased risk of schizophrenia-like psychoses. More recently, 5.4% of patients with epilepsy treated at a tertiary care clinic demonstrated significant psychotic symptomatology (van der Feltz-Cornelis et al., 2008). In these patients, left frontal and temporal pathology was common.

The definitive case series of 69 patients by Slater and Beard (1963) noted that classical Schneiderian "positive" symptoms were predominant, often without negative symptoms. Additionally, psychoses frequently arose in the context of a normal premorbid personality, without a family history of schizophrenia. An association between medial temporal lobe, particularly dominant temporal lobe, epilepsy and Schneiderian symptoms does seem to exist. Flor-Henry's initial report (1969) about laterality actually contained 19 cases of left and 12 cases of right temporal lobe involvement (most cases had bilateral involvement), a similar proportion to Slater and Beard's original series (36 left, 32 right). The 10 independent series to examine the laterality issue do show a trend towards left-sided predominance, as reviewed by Trimble (1990). Nonetheless, the observation that about one-sixth of patients with schizophrenic psychoses of epilepsy had only right temporal lobe involvement detracts from the hypothesis that left temporal involvement is necessary: involvement of either side may be sufficient.

In temporal lobe epilepsy with psychosis, neurodevelopmental lesions in the temporal lobe, such as hamartomas, rather than the early acquired lesion of mesial temporal sclerosis, are over-represented. Taylor (1975) compared a series of 47 temporal lobectomy patients with hamartomas and focal dysplasias in the resected temporal lobe with 41 patients with mesial temporal sclerosis. Of the former group, 23% had histories of psychosis, compared with 5% in the latter group: psychosis was particularly common in left-handed females. Roberts et al. (1990) noted that in 16 of 249 cases, schizophrenic symptoms were present preoperatively; in a further nine they emerged postoperatively. Schizophrenic symptoms were more commonly found in those epilepsies associated with lesions originating in utero or perinatally, which were physiologically active at a relatively early age, as inferred from a comparatively early age at first seizure. The medial temporal lobe was most often involved. An unusual neurodevelopmental tumor, the ganglioglioma (also known as the dysembryoplastic neuroepithelioma, or DNET), was specially associated with heightened risk of psychosis, especially after surgical resection (Andermann et al., 1999). The reason for this association is unclear.

Postictal pyschosis is a transient phenomenon that occurs shortly after a seizure and lasts anywhere from 1 day to 3 months. It is differentiated from chronic psychosis associated with epilepsy ("interictal psychosis") in its transitory nature (Logsdail & Toone, 1988). However, the psychotic symptoms that occur during the acute phase of postictal psychosis are largely indistinguishable from primary schizophrenia. Most patients with postictal psychosis have complex partial seizures, with or without secondary generalization (Logsdail & Toone, 1988; Nishida et al., 2006). The epileptogenic focus usually is in the temporal lobe with postictal psychosis, implicating temporal lobe dysfunction in both primary and secondary schizophrenias (Nishida et al., 2006).

Two competing hypotheses attempt to explain the association between epilepsy and schizophrenic symptoms. Either both sets of symptoms arise from a common underlying cerebral pathology, usually in the temporal lobe, or, less plausibly, the schizophrenic symptoms arise out of a process of progressive facilitation of subthreshold electrical activity ("kindling"). The relationship between the timing of seizures and the emergence of schizophrenic symptoms can vary. Classically, the schizophrenic symptoms emerge as interictal phenomena, although occasionally schizophreniform symptoms are part of a postictal psychosis or even an ictal phenomenon during partial complex seizures (Mace, 1993). The scalp electroencephalogram (EEG) usually shows no change during interictal schizophrenic psychosis, which argues against the notion of kindling being an important mechanism. Stevens (1992) has advanced a third, neurodevelopmental explanation of the link between epilepsy and schizophrenia, proposing that abnormal neuronal regeneration and connectivity develop in adolescence in some individuals with epilepsy that predisposes to schizophrenic symptoms. Many cases of partial complex seizures develop in late childhood and early adolescence (Mendez et al., 1993). Importantly, most cases of schizophrenia develop slightly later, in late adolescence and early adulthood. The overlap in the timing of the appearance of seizures and psychosis is congruent with the notion of neurodevelopmental pathology. More refined electrophysiological studies, perhaps using magnetoencephalography, may be the most promising avenue to explore the anatomical and physiological links between schizophrenic symptoms and epilepsy (Mace, 1993).

Cerebral trauma

An increased frequency of schizophrenia after traumatic brain injury has been reported in a number of studies. Thus, an early study of a Finnish cohort of war veterans (Achté et al., 1969, 1991) described psychotic disorders in 7.6% of 762 subjects. Temporal lobe injury was most frequently associated with psychosis, and a delusional disorder was the most common clinical manifestation. Similarly, Gualtieri and Cox (1991) estimated that the risk of psychosis after traumatic brain injury was two to five times greater than in uninjured controls and that many years may elapse between the head injury and the emergence of psychosis. More recent studies, however, have shown that the incidence of schizophrenia is only modestly raised after head injury and suggested that a greater frequency of head trauma in schizophrenia may result from illness-related propensity towards accidents.

Indeed, David and Prince (2005) concluded that it is unlikely that head injury causes schizophrenia, whereas pre-existing psychosis predisposes to head injury. Nielsen et al. (2002) separately examined the rates of concussion and severe head injury in the 15 years preceding hospital admission for schizophrenia in 8288 subjects with schizophrenia and a similar number of controls, adjusting for the number of other fractures as a measure of altered premorbid accident proneness. A modest increase for both concussion and severe head injury was present only in males (odds ratio, 1.5). Harrison et al. (2006), in a nested case–control study within a very large Swedish cohort, identified 748 cases of schizophrenia and 1526 cases of non-affective psychosis, and compared each of these subjects with 20 age- and gender-matched randomly selected controls (from 14 960 matched controls for the patients with schizophrenia and 30 520 for those with non-affective psychoses). Similar numbers of hospital admissions for head injuries were recorded in patients with schizophrenia and controls (7.2% and 6.6%, respectively), but there was a modest increase in head injury in those with other non-affective psychoses compared with controls (8.6% and 6.3%, respectively). In this study, head injuries sustained in childhood or a family history of psychosis did not carry a higher risk of developing schizophrenia. Malaspina et al. (2001) in a large study of multiplex schizophrenia pedigrees have reported a greater risk for schizophrenia after head injury, suggesting a synergistic effect for brain trauma and genetic vulnerability to schizophrenia. Case–control studies have helped to clarify the characteristics of the head injury that are more likely to be associated with psychosis. Sachdev et al. (2001) examined a series of 45 patients with schizophrenia-like symptoms following brain injury and 45 non-psychotic controls matched for gender, current age, and age at the time of injury. The interval between head injury and psychosis was variable (2 weeks to 17 years, mean 54.7 months) and in a quarter the injury had occurred before the age of 16. Patients with psychosis had more extensive brain damage visible on neuroimaging, particularly in the left temporal and right parietal regions, and had more severe and diffuse cognitive impairment (lower IQ and worse memory and executive functions) than nonpsychotic controls, but epilepsy was equally common in the two groups. A family history of psychosis and the duration of unconsciousness were the best predictors of psychosis, suggesting an interaction between trauma and genetic vulnerability. However, it should be noted that the subtle neurological abnormalities associated with schizophrenia (Mittal & Walker, 2007) often predate the onset of illness, and may predispose patients towards closed head injury even in the premorbid period.

Space-occupying lesions

The clinical manifestations of intracranial tumors are determined by the infiltration and/or compression of normal brain structures, and by the more widely distributed effects of raised intracranial pressure. Behavioral and mood disturbances usually follow the neurological and cognitive deficits and schizophrenia-like symptoms are rare. Some patients exhibit transient and poorly formed visual hallucinations that suggest temporal lobe involvement, and fluctuations in the severity of mental abnormalities are common within the context of progressive neurological deterioration. In the series reported by Malamud (1967), schizophrenia-like symptoms were more common in tumors involving the temporal lobe and cingulate gyrus, and Lisanby et al. (1998) also found the temporal lobes to be more commonly involved. Frontal tumors have been implicated in some studies (Andy et al., 1981), but not in others (Davison & Bagley, 1969). Feinstein and Ron (1990) reported space-occupying lesions in eight of a series of 53 patients with schizophrenia-like symptoms associated with brain disease, but the localization of these lesions was variable. Intracranial neoplasms are rarely reported in imaging studies of unselected patients with schizophrenia (Owens et al., 1980), suggesting that a misdiagnosis of primary schizophrenia in patients with psychiatric manifestations of brain tumors is extremely rare.

Asymptomatic neurodevelopmental abnormalities, usually a chance finding, have also been reported in association with schizophrenia. These include aqueduct stenosis (Reveley & Reveley, 1983), arachnoid (Lanczik et al., 1989) and porencephalic cysts (O'Callaghan et al., 1992), arteriovenous malformations (Vaillant, 1965), and cavum of the septum pellucidum (Lewis & Mezey, 1985; George et al., 1989; DeGreef et al., 1992), but it remains unclear whether such neurodevelopmental lesions increase the risk of schizophrenia or whether they are markers of more relevant contemporaneous neurodevelopmental abnormalities.

Cerebrovascular disease

In acute stroke, short-lived paranoid delusional states, often accompanied by confusion, affective and behavioral disturbances, can be encountered. The frequent delusional misidentifications (reduplicative paramnesia, Capgra and Fragoli syndromes) experienced by these patients may occur as a result of disconnection between brain areas specialized in face and place recognition (e.g., fusiform and parahypocampal gyrus) and those subserving long-term memory and retrieval (e.g., right antero-medial temporal areas) (Hudson & Grace, 2000). Visual hallucinations, another frequent symptom, may reflect abnormalities in occipital neural circuits. Acute stroke should be considered in aging patients without a previous history of psychiatric illness who present with such symptoms. Thus, Miller et al. (1991) reported unsuspected cortical or subcortical white matter infarcts in a quarter of a series of 24 patients with late-life psychosis, compared to 6% in a non-psychotic control group. Temporal lobe stroke was most frequently

reported in those with late-onset psychosis. Post-stroke psychosis has been more frequently reported with right hemisphere infarction involving the thalamus and the temporo-parietal-occipital junction (Price & Mesulam, 1985). Pre-existing degenerative disease (e.g., Alzheimer disease) increases the risk of psychosis (Carota et al., 2002). All patients with either late-onset psychosis or known risk factors (e.g., atrial fibrillation) should be carefully evaluated for stroke, especially if the onset of psychosis is associated with focal neurological signs and/or symptoms.

It has been well reported that that cerebral SLE can give schizophrenia-like symptoms (MacNeil et al., 1976). Attributing causation in individual cases can be difficult: SLE is common, with variable course and symptoms, and its first-line treatment, corticosteroids, can produce psychotic symptoms. Additionally, cerebral involvement more often produces seizures and delirium rather than pure psychotic symptoms. The frequency of psychosis as a neuropsychiatric manifestation of SLE has been estimated at between 5% (Brey et al., 2002) and 15% (Mikdashi & Handwerger, 2004) in two large cohorts. Psychotic symptoms were found to correlate with greater disease activity and with the presence of other neuropsychiatric complications. The precise mechanisms underlying the neuropsychiatric symptoms of SLE are uncertain. In addition to the possible side effects of steroid administration, vascular occlusion and brain tissue damage by pathogenic antibodies are likely etiological mechanisms (Stojanovitch et al., 2007). Psychotic features have also been described in MELAS, a heritable disorder of mitochondrial dysfunction, characterized by myopathy, encephalopathy, lactic acidosis, and stroke-like episodes (Apostolova et al., 2005).

Movement disorders

Psychotic symptoms are a common feature in patients with Parkinson disease (PD). Nearly half of the patients with long-standing illness experience visual hallucinations and these are more likely to occur in the elderly and in those with cognitive impairment or coexisting depression (Fenelon et al., 2000). Hallucinations in clear consciousness are usually non-threatening, transient, and stereotyped images of people or animals and tend to occur at night, commonly during the "on" periods, and patients may retain insight. Sleep disturbances (fragmented and altered sleep rhythm and vivid dreams) often precede daytime hallucinations, and intrusion of rapid eye movement (REM) sleep imagery into wakefulness may be a relevant mechanism (Pappert et al., 1999). Delusions are less frequent—reported in about 10% of patients—but are often distressing and difficult to manage (Pacchetti et al., 2005). Themes of persecution, theft, phantom boarders, and infidelity are common. Severe psychosis is associated with progressive cognitive impairment and increased mortality. Psychotic symptoms may be more frequent in those receiving anticholinergic medications and dopamine agonists that stimulate the hypersensitive dopaminergic receptors in the nigrostriatal system, but the association with dosage or treatment duration is weak (Aarsland *et al.*, 1999). Although helpful, discontinuation of these drugs rarely leads to complete remission. The neuropathological substrate of psychosis in PD is little understood, but pathology related to Alzheimer disease (AD), including tangle, plaques and ApoE status, does not appear to play an important role (Camicioli *et al.*, 2005). The association of psychosis and cognitive impairment suggests involvement of several neurotransmitter systems.

Dementia with Lewy bodies (DLB) is a common and increasingly recognized form of dementia (15–25% of all cases). Psychotic symptoms are one of its core features and occur in half of patients, together with fluctuating cognitive impairment and classic parkinsonian motor symptoms. Psychotic symptoms are heterogeneous, and visual hallucinations of human and non-human forms have been described in 78% of patients, misidentifications and reduplications (e.g., Capgras syndrome, phantom boarders) in 56%, and delusions in 25% (Nagahama *et al.*, 2007). The presence and severity of psychotic symptoms is not correlated with the parkinsonian features (Borroni *et al.*, 2008). A large postmortem study of prospectively evaluated DLB patients (Ballard *et al.*, 2004) reported an inverse correlation between tangle counts and severity of visual hallucinations, and a positive correlation between numbers of neocortical Lewy bodies and delusions and hallucinations. This pattern is different from that described in AD, where psychotic features are associated with numbers of neocortical tangles. Cholinergic deficits are more severe in DLB than in AD despite fewer cortical tangles in DLB (Ballard *et al.*, 2000). The treatment of psychosis in PD and DLB is problematic, as antipsychotic medication tends to worsen the motor deficits. Clozapine is the more effective treatment of psychosis in PD (Frieling *et al.*, 2007). Cholinesterase inhibitors can be useful in DLB for their effect on cognition, as well as their tolerability.

The association of Huntington disease (HD) with an increased risk of schizophrenia is well established. HD, an autosomal dominant disorder with complete penetrance, localized to chromosome 4, is the first major neurological disorder with a well-characterized genetic defect (Gusella *et al.*, 1983). Schizophrenic symptoms were reported in 5–11% of patients with HD in the six series, each comprising at least 50 cases, reviewed by Hyde *et al.* (1992). The reviews by Davison (1983), Naarding *et al.* (2001), and van Duijn *et al.* (2007) quote similar prevalence figures. A study of confirmed carriers with and without psychosis (Tsuang *et al.*, 2000) showed no differences in the demographic or clinical characteristics of the two groups. The onset of psychosis is variable, although it is earlier in those with a high number of CAG repeats. Patients with psychosis tended to

have a higher number of CAG repeats and were more likely to have a first-degree relative with psychosis. The co-occurrence of psychosis and HD in certain families suggests that there may be modifying genetic factors that interact with the HD gene to increase the risk of psychosis (Tsuang *et al.*, 2000). Weinberger (1987) noted the age-related risk of psychosis in HD, suggesting that psychosis most often appears in the third decade of life, like primary schizophrenia itself. Developmental changes in the CNS immediately before or around this time of life may predispose towards the appearance of psychotic symptoms from a variety of causes, not just genetic abnormalities.

The association between psychosis and other diseases involving the lenticulostriatal system has been reviewed by Lauterbach *et al.* (1998). Included in this group, in addition to HD, are Wilson disease and Fahr disease (idiopathic calcification of the basal ganglia). In the latter two conditions, psychotic symptoms have been reported, although definitive studies to ascertain their frequency are not available.

Demyelinating diseases

Symptoms of anxiety and depression are common in multiple sclerosis (MS) and may present in half of the patients at some point in the illness. Psychotic symptoms are much less common. A very large epidemiological study (Patten *et al.*, 2005) has reported a prevalence of psychotic disorders in patients with MS (2–3%) double that in a normal population, making it clear that the association is greater than could be expected by chance for two common conditions. In this study, patients with MS between the ages of 15 and 24 had the highest prevalence of psychotic disorders.

Studies of small groups of patients with schizophrenia-like symptoms (Feinstein *et al.*, 1992) suggest that the onset of psychosis usually occurs when MS is well established and that paranoid delusions and lack of insight are common. In some patients, the onset of psychosis may coincide with a relapse. Symptoms usually attenuate in a few weeks and respond well to antipsychotic medication. There is some evidence that lesions around the temporal horns predispose to the development of psychosis. It is unclear if the psychotic symptoms in patients with MS are primary or a secondary manifestation of an affective disorder.

Schizophrenic symptoms also present in other conditions where the normal myelin development is interrupted. Included in this category are rare conditions such as metachromatic leukodystrophy, adrenoleukodystrophy, cerebrotendinous xanthomatosis, Schilder, Niemann–Pick and Pelizaeus–Merzbacher diseases, and phenylketonuria (Walterfang *et al.*, 2005b). The frequency of schizophrenic symptoms depends on the age at which these conditions become manifest and on where in the brain the disturbance in myelination is most severe. Thus, diseases with onset in childhood are characterized by severe cognitive and motor impairment, while those starting in adolescence and early adulthood are more likely to be associated with psychosis. Involvement of fronto-temporal white matter is also a predisposing factor for psychosis. This is the case in metachromatic leukodystrophy, an autosomal recessive disease in which the extent of the deficiency in arylsulfatase-A, leading to demyelination, dictates the age of onset. Hyde *et al.* (1992), in a review of 129 published cases, noted that 50% of the patients with onset in adolescence or early adulthood experienced hallucinations or delusions and that a clinical diagnosis of primary schizophrenia had been made in 35%. In this series, neurological signs appeared as demyelination extended to more posterior brain regions. Arylsulfatase-A abnormalities in the absence of neurological symptoms have occasionally been reported in patients with schizophrenia (Manowitz *et al.*, 1981).

Metabolic and autoimmune disorders

Metabolic disorders rarely induce psychotic symptoms; more commonly, such disorders are associated with depression or delirium. For example, thyroid-related psychoses are most usually affectively based (Davis, 1989). Hyperparathyroidism, usually an adenoma leading to hypercalcemia, often causes psychiatric symptoms, although again convincing schizophrenic symptoms seem to be rare (Johnson, 1975; Alarcon & Franceschini, 1984; Ebel *et al.*, 1992); organic mental states with delirium or depressive symptoms are more commonly seen (Gatewood *et al.*, 1975). There are numerous case reports of psychosis induced by excesses of both endogenous cortisol production (Cushing syndrome) and the use of prescription corticosteroids. Over 80% of patients with hypercortisolemia have psychiatric symptoms, including psychosis (Perantie & Brown, 2002). Vitamin B_{12} deficiency can present with mental changes, although psychosis is unusual. Zucker *et al.* (1981) reviewed the literature and found only 15 cases of "B_{12} psychosis" responding to B_{12} replacement: most of these were depressive disorders. B_{12} deficiency may more often be an effect, rather than a cause, of schizophrenic symptoms.

Childhood Sydenham chorea, an autoimmune-mediated complication of rheumatic fever with probable basal ganglia involvement, may predispose to later schizophrenia (Wilcox & Nasrallah, 1986). It also can be acutely associated with psychosis (Moore, 1996). Paraneoplastic encephalopathies are uncommon, poorly understood complications of non-CNS tumors, possibly mediated by cross-reactive tumor-directed antibodies. They can, rarely, cause schizophrenic symptoms, seemingly mediated by limbic inflammation (Van Sweden & Van Peteghem, 1986).

Encephalitis and other infections of the central nervous system

While usually causing delirium, infections of the CNS on occasion produce schizophrenic symptoms. Wilson (1976) reported three cases of viral encephalitis presenting as psychosis. Limbic encephalitis is most often associated with psychotic symptoms. Many viruses are known to cause limbic encephalitis (Glaser & Pincus, 1969; Damasio & Van Hoesen, 1985). In a review of 22 cases, Torrey (1986) noted reports of a variety of neurotropic viruses causing encephalitis leading to psychotic symptoms: Epstein–Barr, cytomegalovirus, rubella, herpes simplex, and measles. Nunn *et al.* (1986) reported four cases of psychosis arising in children after viral encephalitic illnesses of varying pathology: rubella, measles, varicella, and herpes simplex. Psychosis in Epstein–Barr virus infection is unusual (Leavell *et al.*, 1986) and most commonly depressive in form (Rubin, 1978; White & Lewis, 1987).

Subacute sclerosing panencephalitis (SSPE) is a rare presentation of measles infection of the CNS, secondary to an aberrant form of the virus. It presents as a progressive neurological disorder (Koehler & Jakumeit, 1976), with a clinical onset usually in early adult life or before, although often years after the initial measles infection. Two case histories are typical: symptoms of schizophrenia (Duncalf *et al.*, 1989) or delusional disorder (dysmorphophobia; Salib, 1988) presenting in young adults, with the emergence of rapidly progressive neurological signs several months later and death within a year. A report of schizophreniform psychosis more directly following measles infection (Stoler *et al.*, 1987) was criticized for failing conclusively to demonstrate brain involvement with the virus (McCune, 1987).

Sporadic reports of schizophrenia in other infective and inflammatory conditions exist. Neuroborreliosis (also known as *Borrelia* encephalitis and CNS Lyme disease) is a cause of schizophrenic symptoms that apparently responds to antibiotic therapy (Barnett *et al.*, 1991, Hess *et al.*, 1999). Neurocysticercosis results from invasion of the CNS with *Taenia solium* larvae, producing cysts, nodules, fibrosis, and hydrocephaly. Schizophrenia-like complications are apparently not uncommon, although this contention deserves more research (Tavares *et al.*, 1993; Forlenza *et al.*, 1997). Childhood encephalitis has emerged as a clear-cut but rare risk factor for adult schizophrenia, conferring a five-fold relative risk in epidemiological cohort studies.

Psychotic symptoms can arise in the context of human immunodeficiency virus (HIV) infection, usually acquired immune deficiency syndrome (AIDS) (McDaniel *et al.*, 1997). Harris *et al.* (1991) reviewed the literature, as well as the histories of a cohort of 124 HIV-infected patients followed up for 6 years, for new-onset psychosis, after excluding cases where psychotic symptoms arose out of substance abuse or delirium. Psychotic symptoms usually took the form of acute-onset delusions, hallucinations, and bizarre behavior, most often in the context of a mood disturbance, particularly mania or hypomania. Typical schizophrenic symptoms in clear consciousness were rarely described. In a follow-up report, Sewell et al. (1994) examined the characteristics of psychosis in HIV-infected individuals. In addition to hallucinations and delusions, the majority of patients had substantial mood symptoms. The psychotic patients also had high rates of previous substance abuse. The pathogenesis of psychosis in the setting of HIV infection has yet to be established. There have been no extensive studies of psychosis in the context of HIV infection since the advent of high activity antiretroviral therapy (HAART). The reduction in opportunistic infections and HIV-related dementia with the widespread use of HAART in HIV-infected individuals offers the potential for a significant reduction in the development of comorbid psychosis (Dolder et al., 2004).

Drug-related psychosis

Psychotic symptoms, usually transient, can be induced in healthy subjects by a variety of drugs, but the link between schizophrenia and drug use is more complex. Thus, patients with primary schizophrenia use drugs more often than control subjects and, in turn, drug use is associated with earlier age of onset, more severe symptoms, more frequent relapses, and less compliance with medication. Swartz et al. (2006) reported drug use in 60% of patients with schizophrenia entering a trial of antipsychotic medication, of which 37% had a concurrent diagnosis of substance use disorder, and Barnes et al. (2006) reported lifetime rates of 27% for alcohol-related problems and 68% for drug use in first-episode psychosis. Substance use to alleviate dysphoric symptoms has been put forward as an explanation for the high comorbidity, with limited empirical support (Gregg et al., 2007). Chambers et al. (2001) have suggested that in schizophrenia, pathology involving reward circuits may increase vulnerability to addictive behavior; at present it appears likely that several factors may influence this complex relationship.

In a large survey of subjects with psychosis attending an emergency department, Caton et al. (2005) diagnosed primary psychosis in 56% and drug-induced psychosis in 44%, using DSM-IV criteria. In the group with primary psychosis, 55% had used cannabis and 50% alcohol. Cannabis, alcohol, and cocaine alone or in combination were the substances most often involved in the drug-induced psychosis group. A national survey in UK prisons (Farrell et al., 2002) found a five-fold increase in psychosis for cocaine users, three-fold for amphetamine users and two-fold for cannabis users, with severe dependence conferring increased risk.

The best evidence for an association between schizophrenia and cannabis use comes from prospective cohort studies (Moore et al., 2007) that have reported odds ratios for schizophrenia in cannabis users ranging from 1.4 to 3.5 (van Os et al., 2002; Weiser et al., 2002; Ferdinand, 2005; Henquet et al., 2005). These studies also suggest a dose–response relationship (Henquet et al., 2005) and a very high risk for schizophrenia (odds ratio, 11) for those who used cannabis before the age of 15 (Arseneault et al., 2002). In practical terms, it has been suggested than in the UK, with a population of 15.5 million subjects aged between 15 and 34 years, 800 cases of schizophrenia could be prevented every year by avoiding cannabis use (Moore et al., 2007) The most likely explanation for this association is that cannabis triggers psychosis in genetically predisposed individuals, and polymorphism of the COMT gene may influence this vulnerability (Caspi et al., 2005). Dysregulation of the dopaminergic, GABAergic and glutamatergic neurons caused by cannabis is the likely mechanism of symptom production.

Experimental administration of amphetamine sulfate to healthy volunteers (Krystal et al., 2005) produces abnormalities of thought content (grandiosity, suspiciousness), thought disorder, and psychomotor activation, without perceptual disturbances or negative symptoms. A short-lived psychosis following heavy use of amphetamines was described by Connell in 1958. More persistent psychoses in methamphetamine users have also been described, even after long periods of abstinence (Akiyama, 2006). These psychoses are akin to paranoid schizophrenia and negative symptoms can be present. A large survey of regular methamphetamine users (McKetin et al., 2006) reported a prevalence of 18% for psychotic symptoms in subjects without primary schizophrenia, and metamphetamine also aggravated the symptoms of those with primary schizophrenia. The psychotic symptoms resulting from drugs such as amphetamines acting on the dopamine system are different from those caused by N-methyl-D-aspartate (NMDA) receptor antagonists such as ketamine and phencyclidine (PCP) (Krystal et al., 2005) that trigger perceptual changes, delusions, negative symptoms, and sedation by causing NMDA receptor hypofunction in the prefrontal cortex. The differential effects of these two types of drugs suggest that neural networks mediated by dopamine and glutamate neurotransmission are both implicated in schizophrenia.

Paranoid ideas and hallucinations are common in cocaine users, often accompanied by anxiety and depressive features (Serper et al., 1999). These symptoms usually last for hours or days, but chronic psychosis can also appear (Breslow et al., 1996). Floyd et al. (2006) reported paranoid symptoms in 71% of a group of cocaine-dependent users, some of whom also used alcohol and cannabis. The onset of regular cocaine use in adolescence was associated with greater symptom severity, although pre-existing vulnerability to psychosis cannot be excluded in cross-sectional studies. Disrupted myelination in limbic circuits has been considered a possible mechanism for cocaine-induced psychosis.

The link between heavy alcohol consumption and psychosis has received less attention in recent years. Alcoholic hallucinoses, acute episodes of auditory hallucinations and delusion in clear consciousness, have been well documented (Glass, 1989), but there is little evidence that alcohol abuse causes schizophrenia. On the other hand, schizophrenia and alcoholism comorbidity may have a profound effect on prefrontal gray matter volumetric loss, which in turn may result in more severe psychosis (Mathalon *et al.*, 2003).

Sex chromosome abnormalities

Limited evidence links sex chromosome abnormalities with schizophrenia-like disorders. The first report linked an XXXY genotype to schizophrenia (Money & Hirsch, 1963). Most of the reports are single case studies. For example, Turner syndrome (45,XO) has been associated with schizophrenia in about 10 cases. However, studies with large sample sizes (Nielsen & Stradiot, 1987) have not disclosed an increased incidence of schizophrenia in Turner syndrome: two cases in 968 female patients with schizophrenia (Kaplan & Cotton, 1968); or one case in 3558 (Akesson & O'Landers, 1969), with a likely incidence rate for Turner being 0.01% of live female births. The coincidence is so low that Bamrah and MacKay (1989) speculated that Turner syndrome was actually protective against schizophrenia. The issue is complicated by the heterogeneity of Turner: only half of cases are 45,XO, the rest being mosaics or having a structurally abnormal X chromosome (Fishbain, 1990). Other sex chromosome abnormalities reported with schizophrenia include an XX male (Muller & Endres, 1987) and an XO/XY mosaic with basal ganglia calcification (Deckert *et al.*, 1992). Schizophrenia has been described in Noonan syndrome (Turner phenotype with normal karyotype, Krishna *et al.*, 1977) and in 47,XYY males (Faber & Abrams, 1975; Dorus *et al.*, 1977).

Extra X chromosomes may confer an increased vulnerability to schizophrenia. Of 20 psychotic males with Klinefelter syndrome (47,XXY) described by Sorensen and Nielsen (1977), five fulfilled criteria for schizophrenia. The authors surprisingly concluded that this was insufficient evidence for genuine association. In a study cross-referencing sex chromosome aneuploidies with schizophrenia based on data in a national registry, Mors *et al.* (2001) concluded that possessing an extra X chromosome did not confer an increased risk of schizophrenia. More recently, a detailed study of 32 subjects with Klinefelter syndrome found high levels of schizophrenia-spectrum pathology (van Rijn *et al.*, 2006). XXXY associations have also been reported. DeLisi *et al.* (1994) found that the XXX

and XXY karyotypes are more common in the population with schizophrenia. In his review of this topic, Propping (1983) considered that the Klinefelter karyotype and the XXX karyotype were the two sex chromosomal abnormalities that had the strongest association with schizophrenia. From the data available, Propping estimated that for both XXY and XXX the risk of schizophrenia was increased three-fold. DeLisi *et al.* (1991) concurred with this conclusion, citing it as evidence for possible linkage of schizophrenia to the X chromosome. Ongoing genetic studies of schizophrenia will help resolve this controversy.

Associations with Mendelian disorders

Propping's (1983) review discussed possible associations between a variety of Mendelian disorders and schizophrenia. Table 9.2 summarizes his conclusions, dividing such disorders into probable and possible associations with increased risk of schizophrenia. Linkage and association studies have been undertaken at many laboratories and clinical centers around the world to identify candidate genes or chromosomal regions conferring an increased risk for schizophrenia or some of its biological components,

Table 9.2 Inherited disorders with an increased risk of schizophrenia (adapted from Propping, 1983 with permission from Springer).

Highly probable
　Acute intermittent porphyria
　Familial basal ganglia calcification
　Huntington disease
　Metachromatic leukodystrophy
　Porphyria variegata
　Velocardiofacial syndrome

Possible
　Congenital adrenal hyperplasia
　Erythropoietic porphyria
　Fabry disease
　Familial ataxia/spinocerebellar degeneration
　Gaucher disease, adult type
　G6PD deficiency
　Hemochromatosis
　Homocystinuria
　Hyperasparaginemia
　Ichthyosis vulgaris
　Kartaneger syndrome
　Kufs disease
　Laurence–Moon–Biedl syndrome
　Niemann–Pick type C disease
　Oculocutaneous albinism
　Phenylketonuria
　Sex chromosome aneuploides
　Wilson disease

G6PD, glucose-6-phosphate dehydrogenase.

such as abnormal frontal lobe function on neuropsychological testing batteries (Risch, 1990; Egan *et al.*, 2000).

Cytogenetic abnormalities appear to be more common in schizophrenia, and detailed analysis of these abnormalities may help identify target loci and candidate genes (Demirhan & Tastemir, 2003). One of the first genes discovered through this approach is *DISC1*; a high incidence of schizophrenia and other mental disorders were found in a Scottish family with a balanced chromosomal translocation [(1:11) (q42.1; q14.3)]. This translocation produces a truncated version of the DISC1 protein (Millar *et al.*, 2000). Subsequently, two groups identified single nucleotide polymorphisms and haplotypes within *DISC1* that were associated with an increased risk of schizophrenia (Hennah *et al.*, 2003; Callicott *et al.*, 2005). The phenotype of schizophrenia associated with both the translocation and the risk haplotypes conformed to DSM-based criteria for primary schizophrenia. As the genetic basis for schizophrenia becomes more clearly defined, the boundary between cytogenetic abnormalities associated with secondary schizophrenia and primary schizophrenia is becoming blurred (Kendler, 2003).

Acute intermittent porphyria is an autosomal dominant disorder of porphyrin metabolism resulting from a deficiency of the enzyme porphobilinogen deaminase. Acute intermittent porphyria may present with episodic psychiatric symptoms. Additionally, psychotropic medications may precipitate or exacerbate an acute attack. Psychiatric symptoms include psychosis, depression, anxiety, and/or delirium. Tishler *et al.* (1985) screened 3867 psychiatric inpatients for acute intermittent porphyria and found a prevalence of 0.21%, higher than the general population. Most of the patients had symptoms of agitated psychosis, apathy or depression, with neuropsychological impairment. In rare cases, acute intermittent porphyria may cause a transient schizophrenia-like state; however, most of the attacks are of relatively short duration. Unlike schizophrenia, with treatment, many individuals with porphyria are relatively normal between acute attacks. The link between the acute intermittent porphyria and psychosis has fuelled recent searches for linkage of schizophrenia to chromosome 11, home of both the D_2 receptor and porphobilinogen deaminase gene. Nevertheless, at least in one study, no linkage has been established (Moises *et al.*, 1991). This is not surprising given the rarity of acute intermittent porphyria even in the general psychiatric population.

It is likely that the alleged association between Wilson disease (hepatolenticular degeneration) and schizophrenic symptoms has been overemphasized. Wilson disease is an autosomal recessive disease of copper transport linked to chromosome 13 (Frydman *et al.*, 1985). Although Wilson's original series included two patients with schizophrenic symptoms, the 520 case reports up to 1959 included only eight convincing cases (Davison & Bagley 1969). Dening (1985) and Dening and Berrios (1989) reviewed psychiatric symptomatology in a series of 195 cases. Hallucinations occurred in only two cases, delusions in three. Personality and mood disorders are much more common.

Homocystinuria is an autosomal recessive disorder characterized by an abnormality in methionine metabolism. It is often caused by a defect in the gene for methylenetetrahydrofolate reductase, an essential enzyme in folate metabolism. The gene is located on chromosome 1p36.3 (Gaughan *et al.*, 2000). Homocystinuria is often associated with mental retardation, seizures, and an increased risk of stroke. While some have associated homocystinuria with schizophrenia, literature reviews do not substantiate this assertion, except in unusual cases (Bracken & Coll, 1985; Abbott *et al.*, 1987; Regland *et al.*, 1997). Interestingly, the increase in schizophrenia in cohorts exposed to famine in early gestation in the Dutch "hunger winter" of 1944–45 has been attributed to folate deficiency. In these cases, it is believed that folate deficiency produced subtle abnormalities of cerebral development, which did not become manifest until early adulthood (Susser *et al.*, 1996).

Niemann–Pick type C disease is an autosomal recessive disorder starting in adolescence or early adulthood. Vertical gaze abnormalities, ataxia, and extrapyramidal signs predominate. Cataplexy and seizures often appear as the disease evolves. Psychosis may be the initial manifestation of the disease in some cases, leading to the misdiagnosis of primary schizophrenia (Turpin *et al.*, 1991; Walterfang *et al.*, 2006). The diagnosis is made by bone marrow biopsy, which reveals sea-blue histiocytes.

Oculocutaneous albinism is an unusual genetic disorder. Cosegregation of schizophrenia and oculocutaneous albinism has been described repeatedly (Baron, 1976; Clarke & Buckley, 1989); interestingly, neurodevelopmental abnormalities, particularly of projections to the visual association cortex, occur in albinism (Clarke & Buckley, 1989). A common biochemical defect may underlie the pigmentary and psychiatric manifestations of this disorder. How the genetic defect in this form of albinism translates into neurodevelopmental abnormalities remains to be explained.

A variety of genetic disorders have been linked to schizophrenia in selected pedigrees. Although these may be chance associations, it is possible that the specific genetic defect may have protean manifestations. In most cases, the psychotic symptoms begin during the traditional window of vulnerability to schizophrenia, in the late second and third decades of life. Two families in which the autosomal dominant connective tissue disorder Marfan syndrome cosegregated with schizophrenia have been described (Sirota *et al.*, 1990), plus one additional case (Romano & Linares, 1987). An autosomal recessive syndrome causing progressive sensorineural deafness and blindness has been described in two relatively large pedigrees cosegregating with schizophrenia: Usher syndrome (Sharp *et al.*, 1993;

Wu & Chiu, 2006). A family with multiple instances of the X-linked Alport syndrome and psychosis has been described (Shields *et al.*, 1990). Recent interest has also focused on the risk of psychoses in families affected by Wolfram syndrome, an autosomal recessive disorder characterized by juvenile-onset diabetes mellitus and progressive bilateral optic nerve atrophy (Swift *et al.*, 1990). Tuberous sclerosis is an unusual autosomal dominant disorder characterized by the development of slow-growing hamartomatous tumors in many organs, including the brain. This disorder has been linked to genetic defects on chromosomes 9 and 16 (Jones *et al.*, 1997). Schizophrenia-like symptoms have been reported and seem to be linked with tumors affecting the medial temporal lobe (Heckert *et al.*, 1972). Bilateral calcification in the temporal lobe was probably the mediating link in a patient with psychotic symptoms in the context of a long-standing autosomal illness, lipoid proteinosis (Emsley & Paster, 1985). Better understanding of the precise genetic defect in each of these disorders, and the impact of the defect upon the development and integrity of the CNS, might offer intriguing clues into the neurobiology of schizophrenia.

Prader-Willi syndrome (PWS) is a rare neurodevelopmental disorder characterized by hyperphagia and obesity, impaired cognition, and marked behavioral abnormalities. The genetic basis of PWS is complicated; it may be due to a paternally derived deletion in chromosome 15q11–q13 (70% of cases) or maternal uniparental chromosome 15 disomy (25% of cases) (Bittel & Butler, 2005). Autistic-like symptoms are common in PWS (Dimitropoulos & Schultz, 2007). Recurrent psychotic episodes have been described in two cohorts of patients with PWS (Clarke *et al.*, 1998; Vogels *et al.*, 2004). A better understanding of the genetic basis of PWS potentially may help unravel the link between neurodevelopmental abnormalities, autism, and psychosis. An individual with psychosis, obesity, autistic spectrum disorder, low IQ, and a history of marked developmental delay might profit from a cytogenetic investigation for PWS.

Two unusual genetically-based neurodevelopmental disorders have attracted attention as being associated with a schizophrenia-like phenotype. Each involves a disturbance of neuronal migration and is potentially informative about the pathogenesis of schizophrenia. Kallmann syndrome is characterized by anosmia with hypogonadism. The anosmia is a result of a neurodevelopmental failure in the olfactory tracts. The hypogonadism is a result of low hypothalamic secretion of gonadotrophic-releasing hormone. The X-linked subtype is caused by a mutation at Xp22.3; an autosomal subtype also exists. Parallels between Kallmann syndrome and schizophrenia have been drawn in the literature (Cowen & Green, 1993), because patients with schizophrenia have relative anosmia and reduced fertility. However, O'Neill *et al.* (1999) found no mutations of the relevant gene (*KAL-X*) in nine patients with schizophre-

nia and Kallmann-type symptoms. The authors concluded that such a mutation rarely, if ever, causes schizophrenia. The parallels between the phenotype of Kallmann syndrome and schizophrenia are weak. Subjects with schizophrenia do not have obvious pathology in the olfactory tracts or hypogonadism. Their reduced reproductive rate may be more aptly ascribed to their deficits in social function, rather than gonadal dysfunction. It is not surprising that O'Neill *et al.* (1999) found no mutations in the relevant gene. The description of a single individual with Kallmann syndrome and schizophrenia is most likely serendipitous.

Velocardiofacial syndrome (VCFS) is a genetic disorder characterized by craniofacial structural abnormalities, cardiac defects and learning disabilities. In addition, children and adolescents with VCFS have smaller cerebellar, pontine, temporal lobe, and hippocampal volumes than normal controls (Eliez *et al.*, 2001a,b). VCFS is usually associated with deletion mutations of chromosome 22q11, the same region as for the gene for catechol-O-methyl transferase (*COMT*), an enzyme involved in the metabolism of dopamine. VCFS is associated with notably high rates of schizophrenia. Fluorescence *in situ* hybridization is the best technique to identify the deletion mutations and confirm the diagnosis of VCFS (Larson & Butler, 1995). The largest series examined to date was 50 cases in the UK ascertained mainly through clinical genetic services (Murphy *et al.*, 1999). Of these, 15 had a history of a psychotic disorder, and 12 of these met DSM-IV criteria for schizophrenia (24%). In samples of subjects with schizophrenia and clinical features suggestive of VCFS, raised rates of 22q11 deletions have been found (Bassett *et al.*, 1998). Interestingly, although the genetic defect and the dysmorphic changes are present from birth, psychotic symptoms do not develop until early adulthood. This illustrates the principle that psychosis only appears in an age-specific window of vulnerability, suggesting an interaction between genetic defects and the natural biology of human brain maturation. Clearly, the discovery of the exact genetic defect leading to psychosis in VCFS is paramount in understanding this syndrome. The role of COMT in the induction of psychosis in VCFS remains speculative at this time.

Phenomenology of primary *versus* secondary schizophrenia

Both brain imaging and clinical studies point to a prevalence rate of 5–8% for psychoses of likely identifiable organic etiology amongst series of relatively unselected patients. If this is the case, is it possible to distinguish the minority of organic cases on clinical grounds alone?

The short answer is no, in that there is a large overlap in presenting symptoms between functional and organic psychoses. Nevertheless, several studies have compared symptom profiles in the two groups and some general differences do emerge. In their review of the literature, Davison and Bagley (1969) compared rates of individual psychotic symptoms in 150 reported cases of various organic schizophrenia-like psychoses with a series of 475 patients with functional schizophrenia reported by other authors. Of 14 clinical features compared, seven occurred significantly less frequently in the organic group: flat or incongruous affect; passivity feelings; thought disorder; auditory hallucinations; tactile hallucinations; schizoid premorbid personality; and family history of schizophrenia.

Catatonic symptoms were reported more frequently in organic cases. Of the organic group, 64% showed Schneiderian first-rank symptoms, although this feature was not recorded in the control group. These results are intriguing, although they represent a retrospective survey of a varied collection of different case reports.

Cutting (1987) compared the Present State Examination (PSE)-rated symptomatology of 74 cases of organic psychosis with 74 cases of RDC acute schizophrenia, all prospectively interviewed. Like Davison and Bagley, he found auditory hallucinations to be less common in the organic group. Delusions were also less frequently found, although simple persecutory delusions were actually more common in the organic group. Contrary to the findings of Davison and Bagley, Schneiderian symptoms were rare in the organic group (3%). Thought disorder and visual hallucinations were more common. Cutting also noted a difference in the content of the phenomenology. Whereas delusions of the first rank were unusual in organic cases, in nearly one-half of the deluded organic patients, two delusional themes were patent: either belief of imminent misadventure to others, or bizarre occurrences in the immediate vicinity. Few patients with non-organic schizophrenia showed these features. Cutting offers possible explanations for these organic themes as being delusional elaborations of deficits of perception, or memory. In the area of perceptual disturbance, the mistaken identity of other people was another theme found more commonly in the organic group.

In the study of Johnstone et al. (1988), PSE-rated symptomatology was compared between 23 cases of so-called organic psychosis and 92 of non-organic psychoses matched for age, sex, and ethnicity conforming to DSM-III criteria for schizophrenia, mania, and psychotic depression. The authors found considerable overlap in symptoms. Comparing the organic and schizophrenic (n = 43) groups, nuclear (first-rank) schizophrenic symptoms tended to be less frequent in the organic group (50% vs. 74%, p = 0.06). Visual hallucinations were more common in the organic group only if consciousness was clouded.

In the series of RDC patients with schizophrenia under 65 referred to above, Lewis (1987) compared clinical features of those 41 patients with unequivocally abnormal CT scans to features in the 166 with a normal CT scan. Those with abnormal CT had significantly less evidence of a family history of schizophrenia in first-degree relatives, were more likely to have demonstrated formal thought disorder, and more often had EEG abnormalities. Clinical presentation also seemed more atypical in the abnormal scan group, in that these patients were significantly more likely to have received alternative prior hospital diagnoses and a longer interval had intervened before a diagnosis of schizophrenia was made.

Feinstein and Ron (1990) examined the symptomatology in a series of 53 patients with schizophrenia ascertained retrospectively, in whom psychotic symptoms arose secondary to overt brain disease. Symptom patterns were compared with normative data derived from the International Pilot Study of Schizophrenia. The only individual symptom difference was an excess of visual hallucinations in the secondary schizophrenia group. Feinstein and Ron (1990) noted a relatively old age at onset (mean of 34 years) and a family history of schizophrenia in first-degree relatives was present in three of 53 cases. A wide variety of organic disease was represented. Overall, 50% of cases had epilepsy, reflecting a referral bias compared with the more representative series of Johnstone et al. (1987).

Individual cases included frontal meningioma, cerebral lymphoma, tuberous sclerosis, multiple sclerosis, Huntington disease, encephalitis, cerebral abscess, and hyperparathyroidism. Three cases of schizophrenic symptoms arising after neurosurgical operation were also included. The authors noted the wide variability in brain regions involved with, in particular, no consistent lateralized temporal pathology.

In their series of cases of VCFS, Murphy et al. (1999) compared the clinical characteristics of those with schizophrenia to a large series of cases with schizophrenia without VCFS. The subjects with VCFS had a later age at onset and fewer negative symptoms than those with primary schizophrenia.

Excluding secondary schizophrenia in practice: physical investigations

Table 9.3 outlines first- and second-line physical investigations which should be considered in new cases of psychosis, including schizophrenia. Of the first-line investigations, some may dispute the need for syphilis serology; however, tertiary syphilis still occasionally presents as a psychosis in clinical practice.

The second-line investigations are dependent on other abnormal findings (e.g., autoantibodies if raised erythrocyte sedimentation rate, chromosome studies if developmental delays or unusual body morphology). In particular, an MRI scan, and EEG studies, are probably only warranted if there are neurological symptoms in the history

Table 9.3 Secondary schizophrenias: suggested screening procedures.

First line

Neurological history and examination
Full blood count and differential
Erythrocyte sedimentation rate
Electrolytes
Syphilis serology
Thyroid function tests
Liver function panel
Urinary drug screen

Second line

Sleep-deprived EEG, with attention to the temporal lobe
Brain MRI or CT
Serum calcium
HIV antibody titers
Autoantibody titers
Lyme antibody titers
Arylsulfatase-A levels
Copper and ceruloplasmin levels
Karyotype
Genetic testing
Cerebrospinal fluid analyses

(e.g., epilepsy), or neurological signs on examination, or other abnormal investigations. This is the position recently adopted in the UK by the National Institute for Health and Clinical Excellence (2008).

Conclusions

Clinically unsuspected, usually neurodevelopmental, brain lesions of etiological relevance occur in 5–10% of schizophrenic illness. Males seem to predominate. There is no indication that the discovery of such a lesion influences treatment in any specific way. The more classical variants of secondary schizophrenias are those psychotic disorders arising in the context of systemic physical disease. The best evidence available is that these account for about 3% of newly presenting schizophrenias. Clinically, it is important to detect this subtype, because recognition and treatment of the primary disorder are needed. The existence of secondary schizophrenias offers several potential avenues to illuminate the cause of primary schizophrenia. The observation of neurodevelopmental lesions was one of the building blocks of the neurodevelopmental model of schizophrenia. Association with Mendelian disorders is currently of interest in the search for candidate chromosomes or chromosomal regions and genes predisposing to primary schizophrenia. The disorders which remain unexplained are adult-onset physical disorders which produce secondary schizophrenic symptoms, although the notion of a developmental window may prove important in understanding their onset.

References

Aarsland, D., Larsen, J.P., Cummins, J.L., & Laake, K. (1999) Prevalence and clinical correlates of psychotic symptoms in Parkinson disease: a community-based study. *Archives of Neurology* **56**, 595–601.

Abbott, M.H., Folstein, S.E., Abbey, H. & Pyeritz, R.E. (1987) Psychiatric manifestations of homocystinuria due to cystathionine beta-synthase deficiency: prevalence, natural history, and relationship to neurologicl impairmnet and vitamin B6-reponsiveness. *American Journal of Medical Genetics* **26**, 959–969.

Achté, K.A., Hillbom, E. & Aalberg, V. (1969) Psychosis following war brain injuries. *Acta Psychiatrica Scandinavica* **45**, 1–18.

Achté, K., Jarho, L., Kyykka, T. & Vesterinen, E. (1991) Paranoid disorders following war brain damage. *Psychopathology* **24**, 309–315.

Akesson, H.O. & O'Landers, S. (1969) Frequency of negative sex chromatin among women in mental hospitals. *Human Heredity* **19**, 43–47.

Akiyama, K. (2006) Longitudinal clinical course following pharmacological treatment of methamphetamine psychosis which persists after long-term abstinence. *Annals of the New York Academy of Sciences* **1074**, 125–134.

Alarcon, R.D. & Franceschini, J.A. (1984) Hyperparathyroidism and paranoid psychosis case report and review of the literature. *British Journal of Psychiatry* **145**, 477–486.

American Psychiatric Association (2000) *Diagnostic and Statistical Manual of Mental Disorders*, 4th edn. Revised. American Psychiatric Association, Washington, DC.

Andermann, L.F., Savard, G., Meencke, H.J. *et al.* (1999) Psychosis after resection of ganglioglioma or DNET: evidence for an association. *Epilepsia* **40**, 83–87.

Andy, O.J., Webster, J.S. & Carranza, J. (1981) Frontal lobe lesions and behavior. *Southern Medical Journal* **74**, 968–972.

Apostolova, L.G., White, M., Moore, S.A., & Davis, P.H. (2005) Deep white matter pathological features in watershed regions. *Archives of Neurology* **62**, 1154–1156.

Arseneault, L., Cannon, M., Poulton, R. *et al.* (2002) Cannabis use in adolescence and risk for adult psychosis: longitudinal prospective study. *British Medical Journal* **325**, 1212–1213.

Ballard, C., Piggott, M., Johnson, M., *et al.* (2000) Delusions associated with elevated muscarinic binding in dementia with Lewy bodies. *Annals of Neurology* **48**, 868–876.

Ballard, C.G., Jacoby, R., Del, S.T. *et al.* (2004) Neuropathological substrates of psychiatric symptoms in prospectively studied patients with autopsy-confirmed dementia with lewy bodies. *American Journal of Psychiatry* **161**, 843–849.

Bamrah, J.S. & MacKay, M.E. (1989) Chronic psychosis in Turner's syndrome. *British Journal of Psychiatry* **155**, 857–859.

Barnes, M., Lawford, B.R., Burton, S.C. *et al.* (2006) Smoking and schizophrenia: is symptom profile related to smoking and which antipsychotic medication is of benefit in reducing cigarette use? *Austrialian and New Zealand Journal of Psychiatry* **40**, 575–580.

Barnett, W., Sigmund, D., Roelcke, U. & Mundt, C. (1991) Endogenous-like paranoid–hallucinatory syndrome due to borrelia encephalitis. *Nervenarzt* **45**, 445–447.

Baron, M. (1976) Albinism and schizophreniform psychosis: a pedigree study. *American Journal of Psychiatry* **133**, 1070–1073.

Bassett, A.S., Hodgkinson, K., Chow, E.W. *et al.* (1998) 22q11 Deletion syndrome in adults with schizophrenia. *American Journal of Human Genetics* **81**, 328–337.

Bittel, D.C. & Butler, M.G. (2005) Prader-Willi syndrome: clinical genetics, cytogenetics, and molecular biology. *Expert Review of Molecular Medicine* **7**, 1–20.

Borroni, B., Agosti, C., & Padovani, A. (2008) Behavioral and psychological symptoms in dementia with Lewy-bodies (DLB): Frequency and relationship with disease severity and motor impairment. *Archives of Gerontology and Geriatrics* **46**, 101–106.

Bracken, P. & Coll, P. (1985) Homocystinuria and schziophrenia: literature review and case report. *Journal of Nervous and Mental Disease* **173**, 51–55.

Breslow, R.E., Klinger, B.I., & Erickson, B.J. (1996) Acute intoxication and substance abuse among patients presenting to a psychiatric emergency service. *General Hospital Psychiatry* **18**, 183–191.

Brey, R.L., Holliday, S.L., Saklad, A.R., *et al.* (2002) Neuropsychiatric syndromes in lupus:prevalence using standardized definitions. *Neurology* **58**, 1214–1220.

Callicott, J.M., Straub, R.E., Pezawas, L. *et al.* (2005) Variations in DISC1 affects hippocampal structure and function and increased risk for schizophrenia. *Proceedings of the National Academy of Sciences USA* **102**, 8627–8632.

Camicioli, R., Rajput, A., Rajput, M. *et al.* (2005) Apolipoprotein E epsilon4 and catechol-O-methyltransferase alleles in autopsy-proven Parkinson's disease: relationship to dementia and hallucinations. *Movement Disorders* **20**, 989–994.

Carota, A., Staub, F.,& Bogousslavsky, J. (2002) Emotions, behaviours and mood changes in stroke. *Current Opinion in Neurology* **15**, 57–69.

Caspi, A., Moffitt, T.E., Cannon, M. *et al.* (2005) Moderation of the effect of adolescent-onset cannabis use on adult psychosis by a functional polymorphism in the Catechol-O-Methyltransferase gene: longitudinal evidence of a gene X environment interaction. *Biological Psychiatry* **57**, 1117–1127.

Caton, C.L., Drake, R.E., Hasin, D.S. *et al.* (2005) Differences between early-phase primary psychotic disorders with concurrent substance use and substance-induced psychoses. *Archives of General Psychiatry* **62**, 137–145.

Chambers, R.A., Krystal, J.H., & Self, D.W. (2001) A neurobiological basis for substance abuse comorbidity in schizophrenia. *Biological Psychiatry* **50**, 71–83.

Clarke, D.J. & Buckley, M. (1989) Familial association of albinism and schizophrenia. *British Journal of Psychiatry* **155**, 551–553.

Clarke, D.J., Boer, H., Webb, T. *et al.* (1998) Prader-Willi syndrome and psychotic symptoms: 1. Case descriptions and genetic studies. *Journal of Intellectual Disability Research* **42**, 440–450.

Cowen, M.A. & Green, M. (1993) The Kallmann's syndrome variant (KSV) model of the schizophrenias. *Schizophrenia Research* **9**, 1–10.

Cutting, J. (1987) The phenomenology of acute organic psychosis: comparison with acute schizophrenia. *British Journal of Psychiatry* **151**, 324–332.

Damasio, A.R. & Van Hoesen, G.W. (1985) The limbic system and the localisation of herpes simplex encephalitis. *Journal of Neurology, Neurosurgery and Psychiatry* **48**, 297–301.

David, A.S. & Prince, M. (2005) Psychosis following head injury: a critical review. *Journal of Neurology, Neurosurgery and Psychiatry* **76**, 53–60.

Davis, A.T. (1989) Psychotic states associated with disorders of thyroid function. *International Journal of Psychiatry in Medicine* **19**, 47–56.

Davison, K. (1983) Schizophrenia-like psychoses associated with organic cerebral disorders: a review. *Psychiatric Developments* **1**, 1–34.

Davison, K. & Bagley, C.R. (1969) Schizophrenia-like psychoses associated with organic disorders of the central nervous system. In: Herrington, R., ed. *Current Problems in Neuropsychiatry: Schizophrenia, Epilepsy, the Temporal Lobe.* Special Publication No. 4, London: *British Journal of Psychiatry.*

Deckert, J., Strik, W.K. & Fritze, J. (1992) Organic schizophrenic syndrome associated with symmetrical basal ganglia sclerosis and XO/XY-mosaic. *Biological Psychiatry* **31**, 401–403.

DeGreef, G., Bogerts, B., Falkai, P. *et al.* (1992) Increased prevalence of the cavum septum pellucidum in magnetic resonance scans and post-mortem brains of schizophrenic patients. *Psychiatry Research* **45**, 1–13.

DeLisi, L.E., Crow, T.J., Davies, K.E. *et al.* (1991) No genetic linkage detected for schizophrenia to Xq27–q28. *British Journal of Psychiatry* **158**, 630–634.

DeLisi, L.E., Friedrich, U., Wahlstrom, J. *et al.* (1994) Schizophrenia and sex chromosome anomalies. *Schizophrenia Bulletin* **20**, 495–505.

Demirhan, O. & Tastemir, D. (2003) Chromosome aberrations in a schizophrenic population. *Schizophrenia Research* **65**, 1–7.

Dening, T.R. (1985) Psychiatric aspects of Wilson's disease. *British Journal of Psychiatry* **147**, 677–682.

Dening, T.R. & Berrios, G.E. (1989) Wilson's disease: psychiatric symptoms in 195 cases. *Archives of General Psychiatry* **46**, 1126–1134.

Dimitropoulos, A. & Schultz, R.I. (2007) Autistic-like symptomatology of Prader-Willi syndrome: a review of recent findings. *Current Psychiatry Reports* **9**, 159–164.

Dolder, C.R., Patterson, T.L. & Jeste, D.V. (2004) HIV, psychosis, and aging: past, present, and future. *AIDS* **18**. S35–42.

Dorus, E., Dorus, W. & Telfer, M.A. (1977) Paranoid schizophrenia in a 47,XYY male. *American Journal of Psychiatry* **134**, 687–689.

Duncalf, C.M., Kent, J.N., Harbord, M. & Hicks, E.P. (1989) Subacute sclerosing panencephalitis presenting as schizophreniform psychosis. *British Journal of Psychiatry* **155**, 557–559.

Ebel, H., Schlegel, U. & Klosterkotter, J. (1992) Chronic schizophreniform psychoses in primary hyperparathyroidism. *Nervenarzt* **63**, 180–183.

Egan, M.F., Goldberg, T.E., Gscheidle, T. *et al.* (2000) Relative risk of attention deficits in siblings of patients with schizophrenia. *American Journal of Psychiatry* **157**, 1309–1316.

Eliez, S., Schmitt, J.E., White, C.D., Wellis, V.G. & Reiss, A.L. (2001a) A quantitative MRI study of posterior fossa development in velocardiofacial syndrome. *Biological Psychiatry* **49**, 540–546.

Eliez, S., Blasey, C.M., Schmitt, J.E. *et al.* (2001b) Velocardiofacial syndrome: are structural changes in the temporal and mesial temporal regions related to schizophrenia? *American Journal of Psychiatry* **158**, 447–453.

Emsley, R.A. & Paster, L. (1985) Lipoid proteinosis presenting with neuropsychiatric manifestations. *Journal of Neurology, Neurosurgery and Psychiatry* **48**, 1290–1292.

Faber, R. & Abrams, R. (1975) Schizophrenia in a 47,XYY male. *British Journal of Psychiatry* **127**, 401–403.

Farrell, M., Boys, A., Bebbington, P. *et al.* (2002) Psychosis and drug dependence: results from a national survey of prisoners. *British Journal of Psychiatry* **181**, 393–398.

Feinstein, A. & Ron, M.A. (1990) Psychosis associated with demonstrable brain disease. *Psychological Medicine* **20**, 793–803.

Feinstein, A., du Boulay, G. & Ron, M.A. (1992) Psychotic illness in multiple sclerosis: a clinical and magnetic resonance imaging study. *British Journal of Psychiatry* **161**, 680–685.

Fenelon, G., Mahieux, F., Huon, R., & Ziegler,M. (2000) Hallucinations in Parkinson's disease: prevalence, phenomenology and risk factors. *Brain* **123**, 733–745.

Ferdinand, K.C. (2005) Primary prevention trials: lessons learned about treating high-risk patients with dyslipidemia without known cardiovascular disease. *Current Medical Research and Opinion* **21**, 1091–1097.

Fishbain, D.A. (1990) Chronic psychoses in Turner's syndrome. *British Journal of Psychiatry* **156**, 745–746.

Flor-Henry, P. (1969) Psychosis and temporal lobe epilepsy. *Epilepsia* **10**, 363–395.

Floyd, A.G., Boutros, N.N., Struve, F.A. *et al.* (2006) Risk factors for experiencing psychosis during cocaine use: a preliminary report. *Journal of Psychiatric Research* **40**, 178–182.

Forlenza, O.V., Filho, A.H., Nobrega, J.P. *et al.* (1997) Psychiatric manifestations of neurocysticercosis: a study of 38 patients from a neurology clinic in Brazil. *Journal of Neurology, Neurosurgery, and Psychiatry* **62**, 612–616.

Frieling, H., Hillemacher, T., Ziegenbein, M. *et al.* (2007) Treating dopamimetic psychosis in Parkinson's disease: structured review and meta-analysis. *European Neuropsychopharmacology* **17**, 165–171.

Frydman, M., Bonne-Tamir, B., Farber, L.A. *et al.* (1985) Assignment of the gene for Wilson disease to chromosome 13: linkage to the esterase D locus. *Proceedings of the National Academy of Sciences of the USA* **82**, 1819–1821.

Gatewood, J.W., Organ, C.H. & Mead, B.T. (1975) Mental changes associated with hyperparathyroidsm. *American Journal of Psychiatry* **132**, 129–132.

Gaughan, D.J., Barbaux, S., Kluijtmans, L.A. & Whitehead, A.S. (2000) The human and mouse methylenetetrahydrofolate reductase (MTHFR) genes: genomic organization, mRNA structure and linkage to the CLCN6 gene. *Gene* **257**, 279–289.

George, M.S., Scott, T., Kellner, C.H. & Malcolm, R. (1989) Abnormalities of the septum pellucidum in schizophrenia. *Journal of Neuropsychiatry and Clinical Neurosciences* **1**, 385–390.

Glaser, G.H. & Pincus, J.H. (1969) Limbic encephalitis. *Journal of Nervous and Mental Disease* **149**, 59–67.

Glass, I.B. (1989) Alcoholic hallucinosis: a psychiatric enigma—2. Follow-up studies. *British Journal of Addiction* **84**, 151–164.

Gregg, L., Barrowclough, C., & Haddock, G. (2007) Reasons for increased substance use in psychosis. *Clinical Psychology Review* **27**, 494–510.

Gualtieri, T. & Cox, D.R. (1991) The delayed neurobehavioural sequelae of traumatic brain injury. *Brain Injury* **5**, 219–232.

Gusella, J.F., Wexler, N.S., Conneally, P.M. *et al.* (1983) A polymorphic DNA marker genetically linked to Huntington's disease. *Nature* **306**, 234–238.

Harris, M.J., Jeste, D.V., Gleghorn, A. & Sewell, D.D. (1991) New-onset psychosis in HIV-infected patients. *Journal of Clinical Psychiatry* **52**, 369–376.

Harrison, G., Whitley, E., Rasmussen, F. *et al.* (2006) Risk of schizophrenia and other non-affective psychosis among individuals exposed to head injury: case control study. *Schizophrenia Research* **88**, 119–126.

Heckert, E.E., Wald, A. & Romero, O. (1972) Tuberous sclerosis and schizophrenia. *Diseases of the Nervous System* **33**, 439–445.

Hennah, W., Varilo, T., Kestila, M. *et al.* (2003) Haplotype transmission analysis provides evidence of association for DISC1 to schizophrenia and suggests sex-dependent effects. *Human Molecular Genetics* **12**, 3151–3159.

Henquet, C., Krabbendam, L., Spauwen, J. *et al.* (2005) Prospective cohort study of cannabis use, predisposition for psychosis, and psychotic symptoms in young people. *British Medical Journal* **330**, 11.

Hess, A., Buchmann, J., Zetti, U.K. *et al.* (1999) Borrelia burgdorferi central nervous system infection presenting as an organic schizophrenialike disorder. *Biological Psychiatry* **45**, 795.

Hudson, A.J.& Grace, G.M. (2000) misidentification syndromes related to face specific area in the fusiform gyrus. *Journal of Neurology Neurosurgery and Psychiatry* **69**, 645–648.

Hyde, T.M. & Weinberger, D.R. (1997) Seizures and schizophrenia. *Schizophrenia Bulletin* **23**, 611–622.

Hyde, T.M., Ziegler, J.C. & Weinberger, D.R. (1992) Psychiatric disturbances in metachromatic leukodystrophy: insights into the neurobiology of psychosis. *Archives of Neurology* **49**, 401–406.

Johnson, J. (1975) Schizophrenia and Cushing's syndrome cured by adrenalectomy. *Psychological Medicine* **5**, 165–168.

Johnstone, E.C., Owens, D.G., Frith, C.D. & Crow, T.J. (1987) The relative stability of positive and negative features in chronic schizophrenia. *British Journal of Psychiatry* **150**, 60–64.

Johnstone, E.C., Cooling, N.J., Frith, C.D., Crow, T.J. & Owens, D.G. (1988) Phenomenology of organic and functional psychoses and the overlap between them. *British Journal of Psychiatry* **153**, 770–776.

Jones, A.C., Daniells, C.E., Snell, R.G. *et al.* (1997) Molecular genetic and phenotypic analysis reveals differences between TSC1 and TSC2 associated familial and sporadic tuberous sclerosis. *Human Molecular Genetics* **6**, 2155–2161.

Kaplan, A.R. & Cotton, J.E. (1968) Chromosomal abnormalities in female schizophrenics. *Journal of Nervous and Mental Diseases* **147**, 402–417.

Kendler, K.S. (2003) The genetics of schizophrenia: chromosomal deletions, attentional disturbance, and spectrum boundaries. *American Journal of Psychiatry* **160**, 1549–1553.

Koehler, K. & Jakumeit, U. (1976) Subacute sclerosing panencephalitis presenting as Leonhard's speech-prompt catatonia. *British Journal of Psychiatry* **129**, 29–31.

Krishna, N.R., Abrams, R., Taylor, M.A. & Behar, D. (1977) Schizophrenia in a 46,XY male with the Noonan syndrome. *British Journal of Psychiatry* **130**, 570–572.

Krystal, J.H., Perry, E.B., Jr., Gueorguieva, R. *et al.* (2005) Comparative and interactive human psychopharmacologic effects of ketamine and amphetamine: implications for glutamatergic and dopaminergic model psychoses and cognitive function. *Archives of General Psychiatry* **62**, 985–994.

Lanczik, M., Fritze, J., Classen, W., Ihl, R. & Maurer, K. (1989) Schizophrenia-like psychosis associated with an arachnoid cyst visualized by mapping of EEG and P300. *Psychiatry Research* **29**, 421–423.

Larson, R.S. & Butler, M.G. (1995) Use of fluorescence *in situ* hybridization (FISH) in the diagnosis fo DiGeorge sequence and related diseases. *Diagnostic and Molecular Pathology* **4**, 274–278.

Lauterbach, E.C., Cummings, J.L., Duffy, J. *et al.* (1998) Neuropsychiatric correlates and treatment of lenticulostriatal diseases: a review of the literature and overview of research opportunities in Huntington's, Wilson's, and Fahr's diseases. A report of the ANPA Committee on Research. American Neuropsychiatric Association. *Journal of Neuropsychiatry and Clinical Neurosciences* **10**, 249–266.

Leavell, R., Ray, C.G., Ferry, P.C. & Minnich, L.L. (1986) Unusual acute neurologic presentations with Epstein–Barr virus infection. *Archives of Neurology* **43**, 186–188.

Lewis, S.W. (1987) *Schizophrenia with and without intracranial abnormalities on CT scan*. M. Phil thesis, University of London.

Lewis, S.W. (1990) Computed tomography in schizophrenia fifteen years on. *British Journal of Psychiatry* **157** (Suppl. 9), 16–24.

Lewis, S.W. & Mezey, G.C. (1985) Clinical correlates of septum pellucidum cavities: an unusual association with psychosis. *Psychological Medicine* **15**, 43–54.

Lewis, S.W., Reveley, A.M., Reveley, M.A., Chitkara, B. & Murray, R.M. (1987) The familial–sporadic distinction in schizophrenia research. *British Journal of Psychiatry* **151**, 306–313.

Lisanby, S.H., Kohler, C., Swanson, C.L. & Gur, R.E. (1998) Psychosis secondary to brain tumor. *Seminars in Clinical Neuropsychiatry* **3**, 12–22.

Logsdail, S.J. & Toone, B.K. (1988) Post-ictal psychoses, a clinical and phenomenological description. *British Journal of Psychiatry* **152**, 246–252.

Mace, C.J. (1993) Epilepsy and schizophrenia. *British Journal of Psychiatry* **163**, 439–445.

MacNeil, A., Grennan, D.M., Ward, D. & Dick, W.C. (1976) Psychiatric problems in systemic lupus erythematosus. *British Journal of Psychiatry* **128**, 442–445.

Malamud, N. (1967) Psychiatric disorder with intracranial tumours of limbic system. *Archives of Neurology* **18**, 113–123.

Malaspina, D., Goetz, R.R., Friedman, J.H. *et al.* (2001) Traumatic brain injury and schizophrenia in members of schizophrenia and bipolar disorder pedigrees. *American Journal of Psychiatry* **158**, 440–446.

Manowitz, P., Goldstein, L. & Nora, R. (1981) An arylsulfatase-A variant in schizophrenic patients: preliminary report. *Biological Psychiatry* **16**, 1107–1113.

Mathalon, D.H., Pfefferbaum, A., Lim, K.O. *et al.* (2003) Compounded brain volume deficits in schizophrenia-alcoholism comorbidity. *Archives of General Psychiatry* **60**, 245–252.

McCune, N. (1987) Schizophreniform episode following measles infection. *British Journal of Psychiatry* **151**, 558–559.

McDaniel, J.S., Purcell, D.W. & Farber, E.W. (1997) Severe mental illness and HIV-related medical and neuropsychiatric sequelae. *Clinical Psychology Review* **17**, 311–325.

McKetin, R., McLaren, J., Lubman, D.I. & Hides, L. (2006) The prevalence of psychotic symptoms among methamphetamine users. *Addiction* **101**, 1473–1478.

Mendez, M.F., Grau, R., Doss, R.C. & Taylor, J.L. (1993) Schizophrenia in epilepsy: seizure and psychosis variables. *Neurology* **43**, 1073–1077.

Mikdashi, J. & Handwerger, B. (2004) Predictors of neuropsychiatric damage in systemic lupus erythematosus: data from the Maryland lupus cohort *Rheumatology* **43**, 1555–1560.

Millar, J.K., Wilson-Annan, J.C., Anderson, S. *et al.* (2000) Disruption of two novel genes by a translocation co-segregating with schizophrenia. *Human Molecular Genetics* **9**, 1415–1423.

Miller, B.L., Lesser, I.M., Boone, B.K. *et al.* (1991) Brain lesions and cognitive function in late-life psychosis. *British Journal of Psychiatry* **158**, 76–82.

Mittal, V.A. & Walker, E.F. (2007) Movement abnormalities predict conversion to Axis I psychosis among prodromal adolescents. *Journal of Abnormal Psychology* **116**, 796–803.

Moises, H.W., Gelernter, J., Giuffra, L.A. *et al.* (1991) No linkage between D$_2$ dopamine receptor gene region and schizophrenia. *Archives of General Psychiatry* **48**, 643–647.

Money, J. & Hirsch, S.R. (1963) Chromosome anomalies, mental deficiency and schizophrenia. *Archives of General Psychiatry* **7**, 242–251.

Moore, D.P. (1996) Neuropsychiatric aspects of Sydenham's chorea: a comprehensive review. *Journal of Clinical Psychiatry* **57**, 407–414.

Moore, T.H., Zammit, S., Lingford-Hughes, A. *et al.* (2007) Cannabis use and risk of psychotic or affective mental health outcomes: a systematic review. *Lancet* **370**, 319–328.

Mors, O., Mortensen, P.B. & Ewald, H. (2001) No evidence of increased risk for schizophrenia or bipolar affective disorder in persons with aneuploides of the sex chromosomes. *Psychological Medicine* **31**, 425–430.

Muller, N. & Endres, M. (1987) An XX male with schizophrenia: a case of personality development and illness similar to that in XXY males. *Journal of Clinical Psychiatry* **48**, 379–380.

Murphy, K.C., Jones, L.A. & Owen, M.J. (1999) High rates of schizophrenia in adults with velocardiofacial syndrome. *Archives of General Psychiatry* **56**, 940–945.

Naarding, P., Kremer, H.P.H. & Zitman, F.G. (2001) Huntington's disease: a review of the literature on prevalence and treatment of neuropsychiatric phenomena. *European Psychiatry* **16**, 439–445.

Nagahama, Y., Okina, T., Suzuki, N., *et al.* (2007) Classification of psychotic symptoms in dementia with Lewy bodies. *American Journal of Geriatric Psychiatry* **15**, 961–967.

National Institute for Health and Clinical Excellence (2008) Structural neuroimaging in first-episode psychosis. NICE technology appraisal guidance 136. National Institute for Healthy & Clinical Effectiveness. www.nice.org.uk/nicemedia/pdf/TA136Guidance.pdf

Nielsen, J. & Stradiot, M. (1987) Transcultural study of Turner's syndrome. *Clinical Genetics* **32**, 260–270.

Nielsen, A.S., Mortensen, P.B., O'Callaghan, E. *et al.* (2002) Is head injury a risk factor for schizophrenia? *Schizophrenia Research* **55**, 93–98.

Nishida, T., Kudo, T., Inoue, Y. *et al.* (2006) Postictal mania versus postictal psychosis: differences in clinical features, epileptogenic zone, and brain functional changes during postictal period. *Epilepsia* **47**, 2104–2114.

Nunn, K.P., Lask, B. & Cohen, M. (1986) Viruses, neurodevelopmental disorder and childhood psychoses. *Journal of Child Psychology and Psychiatry* **27**, 55–64.

O'Callaghan, E., Buckley, P., Redmond, O. *et al.* (1992) Abnormalities of cerebral structure on MRI: interpretation in relation to the neurodevelopmental hypothesis. *Journal of the Royal Society of Medicine* **85**, 227–231.

O'Neill, M., Brewer, W., Thornley, C. *et al.* (1999) Kallmann syndrome gene (*KAL-X*) is not mutated in schizophrenia. *American Journal of Medical Genetics* **88**, 34–37.

Owens, D.G.C., Johnstone, E.C., Bydder, G.M. *et al.* (1980) Unsuspected organic disease in chronic schizophrenia demonstrated by computed tomography. *Journal of Neurology, Neurosurgery and Psychiatry* **43**, 1065–1069.

Pacchetti, C., Manni, R., Zangaglia, R. *et al.* (2005) Relationship between hallucinations, delusions, and rapid eye movement sleep behavior disorder in Parkinson's disease. *Movement Disorders* **20**, 1439–1448.

Pappert, E.J., Goetz, C.G., Niederman, F.G. *et al.* (1999) Hallucinations, sleep fragmentation, and altered dream phenomena in Parkinson's disease. *Movement Disorders* **14**, 117–121.

Patten, S.B., Svenson, L.W. & Metz, L.M. (2005) Psychotic disorders in MS: population-based evidence of an association. *Neurology* **65**, 1123–1125.

Perantie, D.C. & Brown, E.S. (2002) Corticosteroids, immune suppression, and psychosis. *Current Psychiatry Reports* **4**, 171–176.

Price, B.H. & Mesulam, M.M. (1985) Psychiatric manifestations of right hemispheric infarctions. *Journal of Nervous and Mental Disease* **173**, 610–614.

Propping, P. (1983) Genetic disorders presenting as schizophrenia: Karl Bonhoffers early view of the psychoses in the light of medical genetics. *Human Genetics* **65**, 1–10.

Regland, B., Germgard, T., Gottfries, C.G., Grenfeldt, B. & Koch-Schmidt, A.C. (1997) Homozygous thermolabile methylenetretrahydrofolate reductase in schizophrenia-like psychosis. *Journal of Neural Transmission* **104**, 931–941.

Reveley, A.M. & Reveley, M.A. (1983) Aqueduct stenosis and schizophrenia. *Journal of Neurology, Neurosurgery and Psychiatry* **46**, 18–22.

Risch, N. (1990) Genetic linkage and complex diseases, with special reference to psychiatric disorders. *Genetics Epidemiology* **7**, 17–45.

Roberts, C.W., Dane, D.J., Bauton, C. & Crow, T.J. (1990) A "mock-up" of schizophrenia: temporal lobe epilepsy and schizophrenia-like psychosis. *Biological Psychiatry* **28**, 127–143.

Romano, J. & Linares, R.L. (1987) Marfan syndrome and schizophrenia: a case report. *Archives of General Psychiatry* **44**, 190–192.

Rubin, R.L. (1978) Adolescent infectious mononucleosis with psychosis. *Journal of Clinical Psychiatry* **39**, 773–775.

Sachdev, P., Smith, J.S., & Cathcart, S. (2001) Schizophrenia-like psychosis following traumatic brain injury: a chart-based descriptive and case-control study. *Psychological Medicine* **31**, 231–239.

Salib, E.A. (1988) SSPE presenting as a schizophrenia-like state with bizarre dysmorphophic features. *British Journal of Psychiatry* **152**, 709–710.

Sartorius, N., Kaelber, C.T., Cooper, J.E. *et al.* (1993) Progress toward achieving a common language in psychiatry: results from the field trials accompanying the clinical guidelines of mental and behaviourial disorders in ICD-10. *Archives of General Psychiatry* **50**, 115–124.

Serper, M.R., Chou, J.C., Allen, M.H. *et al.* (1999) Symptomatic overlap of cocaine intoxication and acute schizophrenia at emergency presentation. *Schizophrenia Bulletin* **25**, 387–394.

Sewell, D.D., Jeste, D.V., Atkinson, J.H. *et al.* (1994) HIV-associated pychosis: a study of 20 cases. San Diego HIV Neurobehavioral Research Center Groups. *American Journal of Psychiatry* **151**, 237–242.

Sharp, C.W., Muir, W.J., Blackwood, D.H. *et al.* (1993) Schizophrenia: a neuropsychiatric phenotype of the Usher syndrome type 3 allele. *Schizophrenia Research* **9**, 125.

Shields, G.W., Pataki, C. & DeLisi, E. (1990) A family with Alport syndrome and psychosis. *Schizophrenia Research* **3**, 235–239.

Sirota, P., Frydman, M. & Sirota, L. (1990) Schizophrenia and Marfan syndrome. *British Journal of Psychiatry* **157**, 433–436.

Slater, E. & Beard, A.W. (1963) The schizophrenia-like psychoses of epilepsy. *British Journal of Psychiatry* **109**, 95–112.

Sorensen, K. & Nielsen, J. (1977) Twenty psychotic males with Klinefelter's syndrome. *Acta Psychiatrica Scandinavica* **56**, 249–255.

Spitzer, R.H., First, M.B., Williams, J.B.W. *et al.* (1992) Now is the time to retire the term "organic mental disorders". *American Journal of Psychiatry* **149**, 240–244.

Stevens, J.R. (1992) Abnormal reinnervation as a basis for schizophrenia: a hypothesis. *Archives of General Psychiatry* **49**, 235–243.

Stojanovitch, L., Zandman-Goddard, G., Pavlovich, S., & Sikanich, N. (2007) Psychiatric manifestation in systemic lupus erithematosus. *Autoimmunity Reviews* **6**, 421–426.

Stoler, M., Meshulam, B., Zoldan, J. & Sirota, P. (1987) Schizophreniform episode following measles infection. *British Journal of Psychiatry* **150**, 861–862.

Susser, E., Neugebauer, R., Hoek, H.W. *et al.* (1996) Schizophrenia after prenatal famine. *Archives of General Psychiatry* **53**, 25–31.

Swartz, M.S., Wagner, H.R., Swanson, J.W. *et al.* (2006) Substance use in persons with schizophrenia: baseline prevalence and correlates from the NIMH CATIE study. *Journal of Nervous and Mental Disease* **194**, 164–172.

Swift, R.G., Sadler, D.B. & Swift, M. (1990) Psychiatric findings in Wolfram syndrome homozygotes. *Lancet* **336**, 667–669.

Tavares, A.R., Pinto, D.C., Lemow, A. & Nascimento, E. (1993) Lesion localization in schizophrenia-like disorder associated with neurocysticerosis. *Schizophrenia Research* **9**, 111.

Taylor, D. (1975) Factors influencing the occurrence of schizophrenia-like psychoses in temporal lobe epilepsy. *Psychological Medicine* **1**, 247–253.

Tishler, P.V., Woodward, B., O'Connor, J. *et al.* (1985) High prevalence of intermittent acute porphyria in a psychiatric patient population. *American Journal of Psychiatry* **142**, 1430–1436.

Torrey, E.F. (1986) Functional psychosis and viral encephalitis. *Integrated Psychiatry* **4**, 224–236.

Trimble, M.R. (1988) *Biological Psychiatry*. John Wiley, Chichester.

Trimble, M.R. (1990) First-rank symptoms of Schneider: a new perspective? *British Journal of Psychiatry* **156**, 195–200.

Tsuang, D., Almqvist, E.W., Lipe, H. *et al.* (2000) Familial aggregation of psychotic symptoms in Hungtington's disease. *American Journal of Psychiatry* **157**, 1955–1959.

Turpin, J.C., Masson, M. & Baumann, N. (1991) Clinical aspects of Niemann–Pick type C disease in the adult. *Developmental Neuroscience* **13**, 304–306.

Vaillant, G. (1965) Schizophrenia in a woman with temporal lobe arteriovenous malformations. *British Journal of Psychiatry* **111**, 307–308.

van der Feltz-Cornelis, C.M., Aldenkamp, A.P., Ader, H.J. *et al.* (2008) Psychosis in epilepsy patients and other chronic medically ill patients and the role of cerebral pathology in the onset of psychosis: a clinical epidemiological study. *Seizure* **17**, 446–456.

van Duijn, E., Kingma, E.M. & van der Mast, R.C. (2007) Psychopathology in verified Huntington's disease gene carriers. *Journal of Neuropsychiatry and Clinical Neurosciences* **19**, 441–448.

van Os, J., Bak, M., Hanssen, M. *et al.* (2002) Cannabis use and psychosis: a longitudinal population-based study. *American Journal of Epidemiology* **156**, 319–327.

van Rijn, S., Aleman, A., Swaab, H. & Kahn, R. (2006) Klinefelter's syndrome (karyotype 47,XXY) and schizophrenia-spectrum pathology. *British Journal of Psychiatry* **189**, 459–460.

Van Sweden, B. & Van Peteghem, P. (1986) Psychopathology in paraneoplastic encephalopathy: an electroclinical observation. *Journal of Clinical Psychiatry* **47**, 267–268.

Vogels, A., De Hert, M., Descheemaeker, M.J. *et al.* (2004) Psychotic disorders in Prader-Willi syndrome. *American Journal of Medical Genetics A* **127**, 238–243.

Walterfang, M., Upjohn, E., & Velakoulis, D. (2005a) Is schizophrenia associated with narcolepsy? *Cognitive and Behavioral Neurology* **18**, 113–118.

Walterfang, M., Wood, S.J., Velakoulis, D. *et al.* (2005b) Diseases of white matter and schizophrenia-like psychosis. *Australian and New Zealand Journal of Psychiatry* **39**, 746–756.

Walterfang, M., Fietz, M., Fahey, M. *et al.* (2006) The neuropsychiatry of Niemann-Pick type C disease in adulthood. *Journal of Neuropsychiatry and Clinical Neurosciences* **18**, 158–170.

Weinberger, D.R. (1987) Implications of normal brain development for pathogenesis of schizophrenia. *Archives of General Psychiatry* **44**, 660–669.

Weiser, M., Knobler, H.Y., Noy, S. & Kaplan, Z. (2002) Clinical characteristics of adolescents later hospitalized for schizophrenia. *American Journal of Medical Genetics* **114**, 949–955.

White, P.D. & Lewis, S.W. (1987) Delusional depression following infectious mononucleosis. *British Medical Journal* **295**, 297–298.

Wilcox, J.A. & Nasrallah, H.A. (1986) Sydenham's chorea and psychosis. *Neuropsychobiology* **15**, 13–14.

Wilson, L.G. (1976) Viral encephalopathy mimicking functional psychosis. *American Journal of Psychiatry* **133**, 165–170.

World Health Organization (1978) *The ICD-9 Classification of Mental and Behaviourial Disorders*. Geneva: WHO.

World Health Organization (1992) *The ICD-10 Classification of Mental and Behaviourial Disorders*. Geneva: WHO.

Wu, C.Y. & Chiu, C.C. (2006) Usher syndrome with psychotic symptoms: two cases in the same family. *Psychiatry and Clinical Neurosciences* **60**, 626–628.

Zucker, D.K., Livingston, R.L., Nakra, R. & Clayton, P.J. (1981) B12 deficiency and psychiatric disorders: case report and literature review. *Biological Psychiatry* **16**, 197–205.

Schizophrenia: the epidemiological horizon

Assen Jablensky[1], James B. Kirkbride[2], and Peter B. Jones[2]

[1]School of Psychiatry and Clinical Neurosciences, The University of Western Australia, Perth, WA, Australia
[2]Department of Psychiatry, University of Cambridge and Addenbrooke's Hospital, Cambridge, UK

Introduction

Establishing the epidemiological "signature" of a disease—its frequency in specified populations, geographical spread and spatial distribution, temporal variation, and associations with comorbid conditions and risk factors, is an essential step towards unraveling its causes and a prerequisite for its ultimate prevention and control. In a number of human diseases, the epidemiological mapping of a syndrome has revealed patterns suggestive of possible causation and has narrowed down the search area for subsequent clinical and laboratory research. Attempts to apply this approach to the study of schizophrenia have not met with comparable success, although epidemiological investiga-

tions into the schizophrenic disorders have been conducted for over a century. A principal source of difficulty is the nature of the disease concept of schizophrenia itself. The attributes defining schizophrenia are primarily inferential and depend critically on self-reported subjective experience; the underlying structural and functional pathology is insufficiently understood and there is no objective diagnostic test or validated biological marker that could provide a secure anchor for epidemiological field research. Recurring controversies in research into schizophrenia concern its delineation from other psychoses and bipolar affective disorder; the validity of the schizophrenia spectrum concept and the existence of non-psychotic *formes frustes*, such as schizotypal disorder; the utility of its categorical classification as compared to descriptive symptom dimensions or quantitative cognitive traits; and the lingering discordances between the ICD-10 and DSM-IV criteria for its diagnosis.

Schizophrenia, 3rd edition. Edited by Daniel R. Weinberger and
Paul J Harrison © 2011 Blackwell Publishing Ltd.

Notwithstanding the many unresolved issues, there is at present a broad acceptance of the notion that schizophrenia is a genetically *complex* disease, involving variants and mutations in multiple genes and gene networks, marked heterogeneity, and a significant non-genetic contribution to its phenotypic expression. Advancing the understanding of the neurobiology of such a complex disorder with ill-defined phenotype boundaries requires an epidemiological horizon for the planning and interpretation of genetic, neuropathological, and neurophysiological research. No less important is the demand for an epidemiological resource that would aid clinicians in making evidence-based diagnostic and treatment decisions. In reviewing the existing vast and often inconsistent epidemiological information about schizophrenia, it is therefore essential to identify findings that are replicable and likely to be valid, despite the variation in concepts and research methods that still confound the field. This chapter surveys a broad range of topics which add up to a composite epidemiological picture of a complex disease. Special attention is given to findings reported in the last few years and to the epidemiological implications of recent clinical and biological research.

Sources of variation in the epidemiology of schizophrenia related to the method of investigation

The measurement of the prevalence, incidence, and morbid risk of schizophrenia depends critically on (1) the capacity to identify in a given population all affected individuals (or the great majority of them); and (2) the availability of a diagnostic system which will select "true" cases corresponding to established clinical concepts. The first prerequisite refers to the sensitivity of the case finding and the second to the specificity of disease category allocation needed to minimize false-positive diagnoses. Several of these issues also apply to studies of the course and outcome of schizophrenia (see Chapter 7).

Case finding

The majority of case-finding designs fall into three groups:
1. Case detection in clinical populations;
2. Population surveys: door-to-door or representative samples;
3. Birth cohort studies.

Cases in treatment contact
At any given time, psychiatric hospital or outpatient populations contain substantial percentages of persons with the diagnosis of schizophrenia. This provides relatively easy access to cases for epidemiological investigation. However, the probability of being in treatment depends on the availability and accessibility of services, their location, and the rate of their utilization by population groups. Hospital samples are rarely representative of all the persons with a given disorder. The age and sex distribution, marital state, socioeconomic status, ethnicity, and severity of illness in hospital samples often differ from those characterizing the larger pool of people in the community exhibiting the disorder of interest. The extent of the selective bias affecting clinical populations may vary widely from one setting to another (e.g., in a developing country compared to a developed country) and between different points in time.

Under the rare circumstances of stable social conditions, adequate service provision, and lack of major changes in legislation, admission policies, and treatment philosophy, the presumption that the majority of people with schizophrenic disorders eventually get admitted to hospital may be justified (see Geddes & Kendell, 1995). However, such conditions hardly obtain anywhere at present. Worldwide, mental health care is moving away from the hospital and into the community (see Chapter 30). An increasing number of patients with schizophrenia are being managed on an outpatient basis without admission to hospital. Therefore, case finding for schizophrenia that is restricted to hospital admissions is liable to be methodologically flawed.

The deficiencies of case finding through hospitals can be overcome by extending the case detection network to community mental health services, general practitioners, private providers, and charity organizations. An example of such extension was provided by an Australian national prevalence survey of psychoses (Jablensky *et al.*, 2000) in which the great majority (82%) of cases were identified through non-hospital services and agencies. Another approach to case finding is by using psychiatric case registers, where such facilities exist. The cumulative nature of the data and the capacity for record linkage to other databases make registers highly effective tools for many types of epidemiological research. However, the advantages of the case registers do not offset the problem that an unknown number of persons with schizophrenia never contact psychiatric services. The proportion of people with schizophrenia who never consult has been estimated at about 17% in the US (Link & Dohrenwend, 1980). There is no evidence that persons with schizophrenia who are not in contact with the mental health services are treated by other agencies, such as general practitioners or private psychiatrists. In both Denmark (Munk-Jørgensen & Mortensen, 1992) and the UK (Bamrah *et al.*, 1991), the number of patients with schizophrenia managed solely by general practitioners was found to be negligible, though it may have increased during the last decade.

Short of a door-to-door community survey, no standard method of estimating the "hidden" schizophrenic morbidity is available. The presence of such latent morbidity needs to be taken into account in the planning of epidemiological surveys of schizophrenia. Its size is likely to be increasing due to diverse reasons, including the growing number of mentally ill people among prison populations, the existence of informal agencies or religious groups providing niches for people with unconventional beliefs, and the high proportion of individuals with psychotic disorders among the homeless in the large cities.

Door-to-door and sample surveys

Historically, the field survey method has produced some of the most robust epidemiological data on schizophrenia. An early version of the survey method was used by Brugger (1931) in his investigations of the prevalence of psychoses in Thuringia and Bavaria. The method was applied with great success by Scandinavian investigators in the 1930–1960s (Strömgren, 1938; Bøjholm & Strömgren, 1989; Sjögren, 1948; Bremer, 1951; Essen-Möller et al., 1956; Hagnell, 1966). In the majority of these studies, a single investigator, or a small group of researchers, interviewed and diagnosed nearly every member of a well-defined community, usually of a small size. Several of the Scandinavian studies were prospective and the original population was re-examined after intervals of 10 or more years. While the completeness of case finding and thoroughness of assessment probably remain unsurpassed, the representativeness of results obtained from selected small communities is problematic.

A viable substitute for the complete census of a population is the sample survey in which a probability sample is drawn and interviewed to establish point or lifetime prevalence. Examples include the National Institute of Mental Health (NIMH) Epidemiological Catchment Area (ECA) study in which some 20 000 persons at five sites in the US were interviewed (Robins & Regier, 1991); the National Comorbidity Survey (Kessler et al., 1994) based on a national probability sample of 5877 US residents; and the Australian National Mental Health Survey (Andrews et al., 2001), in which a national probability sample of 10 641 adults was interviewed. An important feature of these surveys is that all three used a common scheme of case detection and diagnosis, based on versions of the same generic diagnostic instrument (administered by lay interviewers). However, since all three aimed to assess general mental morbidity, the numbers of identified cases of schizophrenia were too small for epidemiological analysis. In the instance of the Australian survey, a separate, in-depth study of "low-prevalence" disorders, including schizophrenia and other psychoses, was conducted on a stratified sample of 980 cases drawn from a census of 3800 individuals found to be screen-positive for psychosis (Jablensky et al., 2000).

Birth cohorts

The birth cohort study can be a particularly effective method for determining incidence and morbid risk because its results produce a "natural" morbidity and mortality life table (Susser & Schwartz, 2006). The method was first applied to a study of the major psychoses in Germany by Klemperer (1933) and subsequently used with remarkable success by Scandinavian investigators. Studies in Denmark (Fremming, 1947) and Iceland (Helgason, 1964; Helgason & Magnusson, 1989) were able to trace 92–99% of the members of birth cohorts and to estimate the lifetime morbid risk for schizophrenia. More recent examples include the search for developmental precursors of adult schizophrenia using prospectively collected data from the UK 1946 birth cohort of the National Survey of Health and Development (NSHD) (n = 5362; Jones et al., 1994); the UK 1958 birth cohort of the National Child Development Study (NCDS) (n = 15 398; Done et al., 1994); and the North Finland 1966 birth cohort (n = 11 017; Jones et al., 1998; Isohanni et al., 2001). Samples from two birth cohorts in the US, the National Collaborative Perinatal Project 1959–1966 (n = 9236; Cannon et al., 2002b) and the Child Health and Development Study 1960–1967 (n = 19 044; Susser et al., 2000) have been drawn for follow-up studies focusing on prenatal, perinatal, and early childhood influences on the development of schizophrenia. Birth cohort samples of this kind are eminently suited for the testing of hypotheses about risk factors, especially if the original data collection included biological samples such as frozen blood or placenta specimens. Their main limitation stems from: (1) the long "latency" period before follow-up studies can generate schizophrenia incidence data; and (2) the relatively small yield of cases of schizophrenia (81 cases by age 43 in the NSHD; 45 cases by age 23 in the NCDS; 76 cases by age 28 in the Finnish cohort study). The latter factor restricts the range of data analyses because of limited statistical power. Despite their limitations, birth cohort studies have provided significant and convergent insights into possible developmental antecedents of schizophrenia (Welham et al., 2009).

Variants of the cohort design include follow-up studies of individuals who had undergone some kind of assessment at a specified age. Examples are a Swedish study including 50 087 men given a psychological examination as army conscripts at age 18–20 during 1969–1970 and followed up through the national psychiatric case register until 1983 (Malmberg et al., 1998); and a similar Israeli study based on a preconscription cognitive and behavioral assessment during 1985–1991 of 9724 male adolescents aged 16–17 and a follow-up through the psychiatric case register (Davidson et al., 1999). Follow-up studies of cohorts defined by a particular maternal exposure at a given time, e.g., the offspring of pregnant women exposed to acute undernutrition during the 1945 Dutch "hunger winter" (Susser & Lin, 1992); the stress of the 5-day *blitzkrieg* against the Netherlands in 1940 (van Os & Selten, 1998); radiation due to the Nagasaki A-bomb in 1945 (Imamura et al., 1999);

or prenatal rubella (Brown *et al.*, 2001), provide further examples of rich research opportunities using cohort data.

Diagnosis

Diagnostic concepts (see Chapter 1) play a critical role in the epidemiology of schizophrenia since: (1) a proportion of the variation in results of individual studies is due to variation in diagnostic concepts and practices; (2) the diagnostic classification of cases may not be comparable across studies; and (3) in any particular study the diagnosis of schizophrenia may include or exclude conditions of uncertain nosological status, such as acute schizophreniform episodes, schizoaffective disorders, or other "spectrum" disorders (see Chapter 5). In addition, the question of how and by whom the diagnosis was made is an important qualifier of the reported results.

Diagnosis-related bias is usually difficult to detect in past epidemiological research. Until the late 1960s, diagnostic rules were seldom explicitly stated and the description of assessment methods often lacked sufficient detail. As demonstrated by the US–UK diagnostic study (Cooper *et al.*, 1972), concepts of schizophrenia in two different psychiatric cultures diverged to an extent that practically invalidated the comparisons. The World Health Organization (WHO) International Pilot Study of Schizophrenia (IPSS) (World Health Organization, 1973, 1979) examined the diagnostic variation across nine countries by applying a computerized reference classification, CATEGO (Wing *et al.*, 1974), in addition to the clinical diagnoses made locally by psychiatrists. It transpired, reassuringly, that psychiatrists in the majority of settings were using similar diagnostic concepts of schizophrenia, broadly corresponding to the Kraepelin–Bleuler tradition. In most settings the core diagnostic concept of schizophrenia does not seem to have undergone major changes over time. In a re-analysis of Kraepelin's original cases from 1908, Jablensky *et al.* (1993) demonstrated that clinical data on dementia praecox and manic-depressive psychosis collected in the early 20th century could be coded and analyzed in terms of CATEGO syndromes and that the agreement between the 1908 diagnosis of dementia praecox and the CATEGO classification of the same cases was 88.6%.

Since 1980, the comparability of epidemiological data on schizophrenia over time has been affected by the adoption of operational diagnostic criteria such as the Research Diagnostic Criteria (RDC), DSM-III, DSM-IIIR, and DSM-IV. The introduction of such criteria has helped to resolve some old, and to create some new, diagnostic problems with epidemiological implications. Stephens *et al.* (1982), using nine diagnostic systems, established that only 7% of the cases were diagnosed as schizophrenic by all systems. The DSM-III requirement of 6 months' prior duration of symptoms and an upper age limit at 45 for a first diagnosis of schizophrenia excluded from the incidence estimates as many as two-thirds of the cases which met the ICD-9 glossary definition of the disorder. ICD-10, which requires only 4 weeks' symptom duration, agrees well with DSM-IIIR and DSM-IV on the classification of "core" cases of schizophrenia but the classifications may produce discrepant results in atypical or milder cases. Such differences may be relatively unimportant for clinical practice but are likely to result in serious bias in epidemiological and genetic studies. The inclusion of 6-month symptom duration criteria in the DSM classification aims to increase the homogeneity of patient samples and to minimize the false-positive diagnoses. However, this is not an unequivocal advantage for epidemiology. The application of restrictive diagnostic criteria at the case-finding stage of surveys is likely to exclude potential "true" cases which fall short of meeting the full set of criteria at the point of initial examination. As a rule, initial over-inclusion of false positives is less damaging than exclusion of false negatives in two-stage surveys since, once properly assessed at the second stage, false positives can be eliminated from data analysis. In contrast, erroneously rejected cases are unlikely ever to be retrieved. Until the etiology of schizophrenia is elucidated, or a validated biomarker is established, the decision as to what constitutes "true" schizophrenia will remain arbitrary. With regard to epidemiological studies, less restrictive criteria are preferable to strict exclusion rules since they allow for a broader spectrum of outcomes at the end-point of observation. This greater variation at end-point should help to identify outcome-based subgroups and to relate their characteristics to the initial symptoms and to various risk factors.

Investigators

Epidemiological studies of schizophrenia vary with regard to how and by whom potential cases are identified and diagnosed. Many of the earlier European studies were carried out by a single investigator (usually a psychiatrist) or by a small group of researchers. This had the advantage of diagnostic consistency, although systematic bias could not be excluded. Clinician-led studies are less common in current research, where multicenter collaborative designs, large samples, and cost considerations limit the use of such strategies. Lay interviewers or professionals other than psychiatrists are increasingly involved in case finding and interviewing, and the clinicians' role is often restricted to a diagnostic review of cases. The effects of interviewer-related variation (e.g., professional *vs.* lay interviewers) have only been studied in a limited way (Robins, 1989). However, there is an increasing concern that lay interviewers using structured diagnostic interviews in community surveys are liable to commit response errors, especially in rating symptom severity (Regier *et al.*, 1998).

Instruments

Instruments used in epidemiological research into the psychotic disorders differ with regard to purpose and scope, sources of data, output format, and user. At a basic conceptual level, the most widely used current diagnostic instruments fall into three categories.

The first category comprises tools designed for screening for psychosis as part of two-phase surveys. At present, there is no generally agreed, validated set of screening criteria that could serve as a "gold standard" in case finding for schizophrenia. Based on a re-analysis of ECA data, Eaton et al. (1991) have suggested that a combination of DSM-III criterion A and 16 items from the Diagnostic Interview Schedule (DIS) (Robins et al., 1981) might be capable of identifying two-thirds of the psychotic cases in a community survey, and that the addition of a single question about past psychiatric hospitalization could increase the "hit" rate to nearly 90%. A psychosis screening questionnaire (PSQ), developed for use by lay interviewers (Bebbington & Nayani, 1995), has been shown to perform with a satisfactory positive predictive value of 91.2% and a negative predictive value of 98.4%.

The second category includes fully structured interviews, such as the NIMH Diagnostic Interview Schedule (DIS) (Robins et al., 1981), and the related WHO–ADAMHA Composite International Diagnostic Interview (CIDI) (Robins et al., 1988). Both have been constrained to match the diagnostic criteria of DSM-IIIR, DSM-IV, and ICD-10. These instruments were designed for use by non-psychiatric interviewers and clinical judgment is not required in their administration and scoring.

The third category includes semi-structured interview schedules, such as the Present State Examination (PSE) (Wing et al., 1974) and the Schedules for Clinical Assessment in Neuropsychiatry (SCAN) (Wing et al., 1990, 1998), which cover a broad range of psychopathology and require clinical judgment for their administration and scoring. The data elicited by the SCAN can be processed by computer diagnostic algorithms providing ICD-10, DSM-IIIR, and DSM-IV diagnoses.

Each type of instrument has both advantages and disadvantages. The main advantage of the DIS/CIDI is that it can be used by lay interviewers who have received brief (2-week) training. It has been shown as capable of achieving high interrater reliability in generating standard diagnoses in a single-stage survey design. However, the range of psychopathology covered by DIS/CIDI and other similar instruments is restricted to the diagnostic system with which such instruments are interlocked. A major disadvantage is that their clinical validity, in terms of sensitivity and specificity in diagnosing schizophrenia, is questionable. The PSE–SCAN type of interview, on the other hand, allows a great amount of descriptive information to be collected and processed in alternative ways. Both the reliability and validity of the PSE are to a large extent a function of the training and skills of the interviewer. The main disadvantages of the PSE–SCAN system are that the interview is time-demanding, and that making a proper diagnosis often requires collateral information that may only be obtainable in a clinical setting. An abbreviated survey version of the SCAN, which partly overcomes these limitations, is also available (Brugha et al., 1999).

Measures of morbidity

Depending on the type of cases included in the numerator and the time period covered, different aspects of morbidity are captured by indices of prevalence, incidence, and morbid risk (disease expectancy). However, problems often arise in relation to the denominator, i.e., the population base from which the cases are recruited. Using the total population size (all age groups) as a denominator is appropriate when "burden of disease" or service needs are being estimated. The total population is not an appropriate base when the objective is to measure incidence since the probabilities of disease onsets are not evenly distributed over the lifespan. The denominator, person-years at risk, should reflect the pooled risks of developing schizophrenia within a given population and exclude age groups for which the risk equals or approximates zero. Three methods can be used to achieve this, depending on the design of the study. First, age correction can be applied, setting the lower limit for schizophrenia risk at 15 years. The upper limit is often set at age 54, but there is no reason why it could not be higher. Second, when determining cumulative incidence (morbid risk) in cohort studies, both the numerator and the denominator need to be adjusted by weighting each affected person in the numerator for average life-expectancy at the age of ascertainment (or at the age at death if the patient died prior to the survey), as well as by adjusting the denominator for persons who have died as unaffected prior to the survey. Weinberg's abridged method of estimating person-years of exposure (*Bezugsziffer*, BZ) to the risk of disease (Weinberg, 1925; Reid, 1960) is still widely used (see below). Third, to enable comparisons of rates, the denominator may need to be recalculated to a standard population by direct or indirect standardization.

Although relatively simple statistical methods are available for standardization and adjustment, they have been inconsistently applied in schizophrenia research. Lack of proper standardization of morbidity measures introduces uncontrolled variation and may compromise the validity of comparisons across different studies. In the last decades the epidemiological analysis of schizophrenia has been showing a trend towards increased use of statistical procedures that are standard in the epidemiology of other noncommunicable diseases, such as relative risk, incidence ratios, multivariate regression, proportional hazards models, survival analysis, etc. This signals a transition from descriptive to analytical or risk factor epidemiology of the disorder.

Descriptive epidemiology and demography of schizophrenia

The descriptive epidemiology of schizophrenia still contains gaps but the contours of the overall picture have been laid down and enable some tentative conclusions.

Incidence

The incidence rate of schizophrenia (annual number of emerging new cases in a defined population per 1000 individuals at risk) is of particular interest since its variation is sensitive to the effects of causal and risk factors. The estimation of incidence depends critically on the capacity to pinpoint disease onset or inception. There is no agreed definition of inception of schizophrenia, and the idea of onset being a point event raises fundamental difficulties. Precursors of schizophrenia, including developmental delays, cognitive abnormalities, and behavioral oddities, may appear very early in life but, at present, such developmental precursors are only identifiable *post hoc* and cannot serve as reference points for dating onset. Since the timing of the "true" onset of brain dysfunction that underlies schizophrenia is still hypothetical, epidemiological research has to operate with proxy events. The "social" onset (appearance of conspicuous behavioral abnormalities leading to consultation, admission or other action) rarely coincides with the onset of the earliest symptoms enabling a diagnosis of the disorder; the diagnostic symptoms are in the majority of cases preceded by a prodromal subclinical phase of varying duration that may be as long as 2–6 years (Häfner *et al.* 1993; see Chapter 6). Thus, any point on the continuum spanning the prodromal phase, the appearance of psychotic symptoms, and the "social" onset could be arbitrarily designated as the beginning of a schizophrenic illness. Since inconsistencies in the ascertainment of onset result in unreliable incidence estimates within or across studies, it is important for epidemiology to agree on a standard procedure in defining onset, e.g., as the earliest time when the disorder becomes diagnosable according to specified criteria. A convention addressing this problem has not yet been adopted in incidence studies of schizophrenia. In many studies, the first hospital admission is still being used as an index of onset. This is difficult to sustain in view of the wide variation across individuals and settings, and the time lag between first appearance of symptoms and first admission. A better approximation to the time of onset is provided by the first contact, i.e., the point at which some "helping agency" is contacted by an indi-

vidual with incipient psychotic illness. The majority of first contacts are ambulatory and may precede admission to hospital by many months; in a number of instances, hospitalization may not take place at all. A version of this method was used in the WHO Ten-Country Study (Jablensky *et al.*, 1992) in which case finding targeted, prospectively over 2 years, first contacts with a variety of services, including non-medical ones.

Table 10.1 provides an overview of selected incidence studies of schizophrenia. Six studies, published between 1946 and 1974, are designated as "historical" in the sense that they produced some of the earliest estimates of the incidence of schizophrenia, mostly based on counts of first admissions to hospital. The 16 studies published between 1980 and 2007 feature a diversity of methods and incidence estimates ranging from low (0.10–0.41 per 1000) to high (0.62–2.16 per 1000). While some of the variation across these surveys is likely to relate to the method of ascertainment or diagnostic criteria, the highest rates have been obtained in populations with special characteristics, such as genetic isolates (Haukka *et al.*, 2001) or areas with high density of migrant groups (Boydell *et al.*, 2003; Kirkbride *et al.*, 2006). For comparison, the variation of the incidence rates in the WHO Ten-Country Study (Jablensky *et al.*, 1992) is relatively unaffected by differences in case finding methods and diagnostic assessment, and are fairly close to the mean rates based on 147 studies from 33 countries in the systematic review by McGrath *et al.* (2004a).

The WHO study (Sartorius *et al.*, 1986; Jablensky *et al.*, 1992) generated directly comparable incidence data for different populations by using identical case finding and diagnostic procedures prospectively, based on first-in-lifetime contacts with "helping agencies" in the area (including traditional healers in developing countries) which were monitored over a 2-year period. Potential cases and key informants were interviewed using standardized instruments, and the onset of psychotic symptoms diagnostic of schizophrenia was ascertained for 1022 of the total 1379 patients. In 86% of these patients, the first appearance of diagnostic symptoms of schizophrenia was within a year of the first contact and therefore the first-contact rate could serve as a reasonable approximation to the onset rate. The differences between the rates for broadly (ICD-9) defined schizophrenia in the WHO study were significant (p < 0.001; two-tailed test) while those for the restrictively defined "nuclear", schizophrenia syndrome with first-rank (Schneiderian) symptoms, were not. The salient aspect of the WHO findings is not the lack of statistically significant differences in the rates of "nuclear" schizophrenia but, rather, the relatively modest range of variation (0.16–0.42 per 1000) in the incidence of schizophrenia when standard case definitions, case finding procedures, and assessment methods are used across very different populations. Independent replications of the design and methods of the

Table 10.1 Synopsis of selected incidence studies of schizophrenia.

Author	Country	Population	Method	Incidence rate per 1000 population at risk
Historical surveys (published before 1980)				
Ødegaard (1946a)	Norway	Total population	First admissions 1926–35 (n = 14231)	0.24
Helgason (1964)	Iceland	Total population	First admissions 1966–67 (n = 2388)	0.27
Häfner & Reimann (1970)	Germany	City of Mannheim (n = 330000)	Case register	0.54
Raman & Murphy (1972)	Mauritius	Total population (n = 257000)	First admissions	0.24 (Africans) 0.14 (Indian Hindus) 0.09 (Indian Moslems)
Lieberman (1974)	Russia	Moscow district (n = 248000)	Follow-back (to onset) of prevalent cases	0.20 (male) 0.19 (female)
Eaton et al. (1974)	USA	Maryland state	First admissions	0.30
Surveys published 1980–2007				
Joyce et al. (1987)	New Zealand	Total population	First admissions (1974–84)	0.18
Castle et al. (1991)	UK	London (Camberwell)	Case register	0.25 (ICD-9) 0.17 (RDC) 0.08 (DSM-III)
Nicole et al. (1992)	Canada	Area in Quebec (n = 338300)	First admissions	0.31 (ICD) 0.09 (DSM-III)
Lin et al. (1989)	Taiwan	Three communities (n = 39024)	Household survey	0.17
Rajkumar et al. (1993)	India	Area in Chennai (Madras) (n = 43097)	Door-to-door screen and informants (interview)	0.41
Hickling & Rodgers-Johnson (1995)	Jamaica	Total population (n = 2460000)	First contact (interview)	0.24 ("broad" SZ) 0.21 ("restrictive" SZ)
McNaught et al. (1997)	UK	London health district (n = 112127)	Two censuses, 5 years apart	0.21 (DSM-IIIR)
Brewin et al. (1997)	UK	Nottingham	Two cohorts of first contacts (1978–80 and 1992–94)	0.25 → 0.29 (all psychoses) 0.14 → 0.09 (ICD-10)
Mahy et al. (1999)	Barbados	Total population (n = 262000)	First contacts	0.32 ("broad" SZ) 0.28 ("restrictive" SZ)
Haukka et al. (2001)	Finland	National birth cohorts (1950–1969)	Case register data (ICD-8 and ICD-9)	0.62 (males) 0.63 (females)
Svedberg et al. (2001)	Sweden	Stockholm (three catchment areas)	First admissions (1991–92)	0.09 (DSM-IV)
Scully et al. (2002)	Ireland	Two counties (n = 104089)	First contacts 1995–2000 (interview)	0.35 (DSM-IV)
Boydell et al. (2003)	UK	South-East London (Camberwell)	First contact (records) (1965–97)	0.68 → 1.53 (DSM-IIIR)
Kirkbride et al. (2006)	UK ÆSOP study	Three cities	First contact (interview) (1997–99) DSM-IV diagnoses	2.16 (London) 0.82 (Nottingham) 0.82 (Bristol)

Continued

Table 10.1 *Continued*

Author	Country	Population	Method	Incidence rate per 1000 population at risk
Veling *et al.* (2006)	The Netherlands	The Hague (n = 518 000)	First contacts (2000–02)	0.22 (DSM-IV)
Menezes *et al.* (2007)	Brazil	Area in Sao Paulo (n = 2 315 000)	First contacts (2002–04)	0.10 (DSM-IV)
WHO Ten-Country Study (Jablensky *et al.*, 1992)				
	Denmark	Aarhus	First contacts	0.18 ("broad" SZ) 0.07 ("restrictive" SZ)
	India	Chandigarh (urban area)	First contacts	0.35 ("broad" SZ) 0.09 ("restrictive" SZ)
	India	Chandigarh (rural area)	First contacts	0.42 ("broad" SZ) 0.11("restrictive" SZ)
	Ireland	Dublin	First contacts	0.22 ("broad" SZ) 0.09 ("restrictive" SZ)
	Japan	Nagasaki	First contacts	0.21 ("broad" SZ) 0.10 ("restrictive" SZ)
	Russia	Moscow	First contacts	0.28 ("broad" SZ) 0.02 ("restrictive" SZ)
	UK	Nottingham	First contacts	0.24 ("broad" SZ) 0.14 ("restrictive" SZ)
	USA	Honolulu	First contacts	0.16 ("broad" SZ) 0.09 ("restrictive" SZ)
Systematic review (McGrath *et al.*, 2004a)				
	Data from 33 countries	147 studies	Cumulative plots of incidence rates	0.24 (mean, both sexes) 0.22 (mean, males) 0.21 (mean, females)

SZ, schizophrenia.

WHO study have subsequently been carried out, with similar results, by researchers in India (Rajkumar *et al.*, 1993), the Caribbean (Hickling & Rodgers-Johnson, 1995; Mahy *et al.*, 1999) and the UK ÆSOP study (Kirkbride *et al.*, 2006).

Prevalence and disease expectancy (morbid risk)

The prevalence of a disorder is defined as the total number of cases (per 1000 persons at risk) present in a population at a given time or over a defined period (prevalence is a *proportion*, while incidence is a *rate*). Point prevalence refers to cases which are active (i.e., symptomatic) on a given date, or within a brief interval around a census date as midpoint. Since cases in remission are likely to be missed in point prevalence surveys, the assessment of the present mental state in such studies needs to be supplemented with information about past episodes of the disorder. This should result in a *lifetime prevalence* index, or proportion of survivors affected (PSA). In disorders tending towards a continuous course, such as schizophrenia, point and lifetime prevalence estimates are similar or may even be identical. Generally, period prevalence is a less useful index of morbidity since it confounds point prevalence with incidence.

Lifetime morbid risk (LMR) or *disease expectancy* is the probability that an individual born into a particular population will develop the disease if they survive through the entire period of risk for that disease (usually 15–54 years of age in the instance of schizophrenia). If age- and sex-specific incidence rates are available, LMR can be estimated directly by summing up the rates across the age groups within the period of risk. An indirect approximation can be obtained from census data using the so-called abridged method of Weinberg (1925):

$$P = \frac{A}{B - (B_o + 1/2 B_m)}$$

where P is LMR or disease expectancy (%); A is the number of prevalent cases; B is the total population surveyed; B_0 is the number of persons who have not yet entered the risk period; and B_m is the number of persons within the risk period. A modification of this method (Bøjholm & Strömgren. 1989), weights the numerator for excess mortality among patients with schizophrenia. Whether estimated directly from age-specific incidence rates, or indirectly from prevalence data, LMR enables a more reliable comparison of the lifetime risk of schizophrenia in different populations than the prevalence or incidence rates.

An overview of selected prevalence studies of schizophrenia spanning a period of some 60 years is given in Table 10.2. The studies differ in their methodology but have in common a high intensity of case finding (many of them were census investigations). Several studies included repeat surveys in which the original population was re-examined at some later time (the resulting follow-up prevalence figures are indicated in the Table 10.2 by →).

Two recent studies based on large samples have produced reliable lifetime prevalence estimates that are surprisingly similar to those reported by earlier, pre-DSM-III, studies. In Sweden, a national population-based cohort of 7 739 202 individuals was created by record linkage across the national registration database and the hospital discharge register. Using a stringent definition of schizophrenia "caseness", Lichtenstein *et al.* (2006) estimated a lifetime prevalence of 4.07 per 1000 and a high proportion (3.81%) of affected families with multiple affected members. In a study of a nationally representative sample of 8028 adults in Finland, Perälä *et al.* (2007) used interview data, self-reports, case notes, and national psychiatric register records to assess the lifetime prevalence of all psychotic disorders (30.6 per 1000) and schizophrenia (8.7 per 1000). These are unusually high lifetime prevalence estimates, exceeding by two-fold those in the neighboring Swedish population. Since both studies utilized national register data, which are known to be comprehensive and accurate, the differences between the two populations are unlikely to be artifactual. One of the possible sources for the divergent findings is the different demographic and genetic structure of the two populations, including an internal isolate in north-eastern Finland with unusually high schizophrenia prevalence (Hovatta *et al.*, 1999).

A recent systematic review of some 180 published studies (Saha *et al.*, 2005) estimated median values of 4.6 per 1000 population at risk for point prevalence; 4.0 per 1000 for lifetime prevalence; and 7.2 per 1000 for disease expectancy (morbid risk). No significant differences in prevalence were found between males and females, or between urban and non-urban sites. The population subgroups of migrants tended to have a higher prevalence, with a risk ratio of 1.8 (0.9–6.4) (see Chapter 11). In the majority of the studies the differences between the lowest and highest quantiles of prevalence were 5–6.5-fold. Considering the many possible sources of variation, this range is relatively modest for a low-prevalence disorder. However, similar prevalence

Table 10.2 Synopsis of selected prevalence studies of schizophrenia.

Author	Country	Population (size)	Method	Prevalence per 1000 population at risk
Historical surveys (published 1930–80)				
Brugger (1931)	Germany	Area in Thuringia (n = 37 561)	Census	2.4 (point)
Strömgren (1938); Bøjholm & Strömgren (1989)	Denmark	Island population (n = 50 000)	Repeat census	3.9 → 3.3 (point)
Lemkau *et al.* (1943)	USA	Household sample	Census	2.9 (point)
Essen-Möller *et al.* (1956); Hagnell (1966)	Sweden	Community in southern Sweden	Repeat census	6.7 → 4.5 (point)
Rin & Lin (1962); Lin *et al.* (1989)	Taiwan	Population sample	Repeat census	2.1 → 1.4 (point)
Bash & Bash-Liechti (1969)	Iran	Rural area (n = 11 585)	Census	2.1 (point)
Crocetti *et al.* (1971)	Croatia	Sample of 9201 households	Census	5.9 (point)
Dube & Kumar (1972)	India	Four areas in Agra (n = 29 468)	Census	2.6 (point)
Rotstein (1977)	Russia	Population sample (n = 35 590)	Census	3.8 (lifetime)

Continued

Table 10.2 *Continued*

Author	Country	Population (size)	Method	Prevalence per 1000 population at risk
Surveys published 1981–2007				
Padmavathi *et al.* (1987)	India	Urban area (n = 101 229)	Census	2.5 (point)
Indian Council of Medical Research (1988)	India	Rural area (n = 46 380)	Census	2.2 (point)
Robins & Regier (1991)	USA	Aggregated data across five study sites	Sample survey	7.0 (point) 15.0 (lifetime)
Salan (1992)	Indonesia	Slum area in West Jakarta (n = 100 107)	Two-stage survey	1.4 (point)
Kendler & Walsh (1995)	Ireland	Roscommon County (n = 32 775)	Register-based family study	Lifetime: 5.4 (males) 4.3 (females)
Jeffreys *et al.* (1997)	UK	London health district (n = 112 127)	Census; interviews of a sample (n = 172)	5.1 (point)
Jablensky *et al.* (2000)	Australia	Four urban areas (n = 1 084 978)	Census; interviews of a sample (n = 980)	4.7 (point, SZ and NAP)
Waldo (1999)	Kosrae (Micronesia)	Island population (n = 5 500)	Key informants and interviews	6.8 (point), age 15+
Kebede & Alem (1999)	Ethiopia	District (n = 227 135) Mixed urban and rural	Two-stage survey	7.1 (point)
Scully *et al.* (2004)	Ireland	Rural area population (n = 29 542)	Census; interviews	Point: 4.0 (males) 3.8 (females)
Arajärvi *et al.* (2005)	Finland	Birth cohort including isolate population (n = 12 368)	Case register data; interviews	Lifetime: 15.0 (SZ) 19.0 (SZ spectrum)
Phillips *et al.* (2004)	China	National survey sample (n = 19 223)	Interviews	Point: 4.7 (both sexes) 3.4 (males) 6.0 (females)
Wu *et al.* (2006)	USA	~3 million insured persons	Estimation based on insurance claims	Period (12 months): 5.1
Lichtenstein *et al.* (2006)	Sweden	National cohort (n = 7 739 202)	Case register data	4.07 (lifetime)
Ayuso-Mateos *et al.* (2006)	Spain	Extrapolation to total population	Estimation based on disease modelling, region of Cantabria	Lifetime: 3.0 (males) 2.8 (females)
Perälä *et al.* (2007)	Finland	Representative national sample (n = 8 028)	Two-stage survey; case register data	8.7 (lifetime)
Systematic reviews				
Goldner *et al.* (2002)	Data from 9 countries	18 prevalence studies	Pooled best-estimate rates; heterogeneity analysis	3.4 (period, 12-month) 5.5 (lifetime)
Saha *et al.* (2005)	Data from 46 countries	188 prevalence studies	Cumulative plots of prevalence estimates	4.6 (point) 3.3 (period) 4.0 (lifetime) 7.2 (morbid risk)

SZ, schizophrenia; NAP, non-affective psychosis.

figures may mask important differences in incidence rates between populations. Crude prevalence figures are difficult to interpret in the absence of essential background demographic data, such as differential mortality, age structures of populations, and migration rates. Since such differences across populations exist, the LMR is likely to be a more reliable estimator of the "true" extent of schizophrenia risk. Most studies have produced LMR estimates in the range 0.50–1.60% (0.72% in the systematic review by Saha *et al.*, 2005). Therefore, the "rule of thumb" that the morbid risk for schizophrenia is approximately 1% is not very far off the mark.

Secular trends in the incidence and prevalence of schizophrenia

The rarity of descriptions of schizophrenia in the medical literature before the 18th century has led to speculation that the condition was rare, until the industrial revolution (Hare, 1983). The earliest references to psychotic states matching the clinical picture of schizophrenia can be found in Pinel (1803) and Haslam (1809). Nineteenth century asylum statistics suggests that "monomaniac insanity" or "delusional insanity" (the diagnostic groups likely to contain patients with schizophrenia in the pre-Kraepelinian era) comprised between 5.3% and 18.9% of all institutionalized patients (Jablensky, 1986). The records of the Munich University Psychiatric Clinic, under the direction of Kraepelin in 1908, indicate that dementia praecox accounted for less than 10% of the first admissions annually (Jablensky *et al.*, 1993). During much of the 19th century, schizophrenia was probably less conspicuous than it is today, due to the much higher prevalence of organic brain diseases such as general paresis. The number of people hospitalized with schizophrenia increased rapidly in the early decades of the 20th century. It remains unclear whether this was due to increased use of the diagnosis, social pressure to institutionalize the mentally ill, or a real rise in incidence.

The question whether long-term trends in the incidence of schizophrenia can be detected has attracted renewed interest following reports since the 1970s suggesting a 40% or more reduction in first admissions with a diagnosis of schizophrenia in Denmark, the UK, and New Zealand (Weeke & Strömgren, 1978; Eagles *et al.*, 1988). Such data have not been consistently replicated; some reports have shown increases (Castle *et al.*, 1991; Bamrah *et al.*, 1991); or no change (Harrison *et al.*, 1991). Other studies have pointed to compensatory increases in other diagnoses, such as paranoid states, reactive psychoses, or borderline personality disorder (Der *et al.*, 1990; Harrison *et al.*, 1991; Munk-Jørgensen, 1986). Although a trend of diminishing rates of schizophrenia cannot be excluded, the combined effect of several factors could explain the observed changes: variations in the definition of first admission or first contact;

changes in diagnostic practices over time; changes in the treatment modalities and settings; increases in the mortality of patients with schizophrenia; and changes in the age composition of the populations concerned. The reported size of the compensatory increase of other diagnoses on first admission is sufficient to account for the drop in schizophrenia diagnoses. In addition, the time lag in the diagnosis of schizophrenia, which in many instances amounts to years after the first service contact, may artificially depress the first admission rates for the most recent years of the observation period. The gradual "disappearance" of schizophrenia, therefore, is a rather unlikely hypothesis.

Spatial variation in the incidence and prevalence of schizophrenia

There is growing evidence to suggest that a range of population-related biological and environmental factors may be contributing to the onset of schizophrenia and to the maintenance of its incidence and prevalence in populations (see Chapter 11). Many of the environmental factors are likely to interact with genetic vulnerability at the individual level. Peaks and troughs do exist in the epidemiological landscape of schizophrenia, resulting from likely interactions between genetic variation across human groups, culture, migration and habitat, the social fabric, nutrition, and geography. These sources of variation merit the attention of epidemiologists, social anthropologists, and biological researchers alike.

Populations with high and low rates of schizophrenia: genetic isolates

Very high rates of schizophrenia (two to three times the national or regional rate) have been reported for population isolates, such as an area in northern Sweden (Böök *et al.*, 1978) and several areas in Finland (Hovatta *et al.*, 1999; Arajärvi *et al.*, 2005). Even higher rates have been found on the Palau islands in the Pacific (Myles-Worsley *et al.*, 1999) and in Daghestan, Northern Caucasus (Bulayeva *et al.*, 2005). The lifetime prevalence of strictly diagnosed schizophrenia in Palau has been estimated at 2.8% in males and 1.2% in females. LMR for schizophrenia as high as 5% has been reported for some of the Daghestan isolates, The common factor accounting for such exceptionally high rates is the founder effect and gene drift over multiple generations of extended pedigrees, resulting in an aggregation of specific haplotypes with limited numbers of pathogenic alleles (Bulayeva *et al.*, 2005). At the other extreme, a virtual absence of schizophrenia has been observed amongst the Hutterites in South Dakota, a Protestant sect whose members live in closely knit endogamous communities, largely sheltered from the outside world (Eaton & Weil, 1955; Torrey, 1995; Nimgaonkar *et al.*, 2000). Negative selection for schizoid individuals who fail to adjust to the communal lifestyle and eventually migrate without leaving progeny has been suggested, but not definitively proven, as an explanation.

"Outlier" populations with unusually high or low incidence rates of schizophrenia are of considerable interest as potentially informative settings in the search for susceptibility genes, as well as for studies of culture–gene interactions over multiple successive generations.

The evidence for very high rates of schizophrenia in certain migrant groups is discussed later in this chapter.

Global variation in incidence

The widely commented WHO Ten-Country Study (Jablensky *et al.*, 1992) compared the incidence of both broadly and narrowly defined ICD-9 schizophrenia across 12 settings in 10 countries (both high and low income countries, and both rural and urban centers) using a standardized methodology. Whether schizophrenia was defined broadly or narrowly, there was an approximately two- to three-fold difference between the centers with the lowest and highest incidence rates. However, this only achieved statistical significance for broadly defined schizophrenia, leading, on occasions, to the erroneous interpretation of the WHO findings as evidence that the incidence of schizophrenia was invariant, regardless of place or population. More recently, a systematic review of the literature on the incidence of schizophrenia (McGrath *et al.*, 2004a) identified 147 studies in 33 countries and found a median incidence of 0.15 per 1000 and a range of variation from 0.70 to 0.43 per 1000 (not too dissimilar to the WHO-reported range of 0.16–0.42 per 1000). Compared to other complex or multifactorial diseases, this range of variation is noticeable, but is nowhere near the variation in the incidence of other complex or mutifactorial diseases, such as diabetes Type 1, where the difference between the highest rates in Sardinia and Finland and the lowest rate in China was more than 350 fold in 1990 (Karvonen *et al.*, 2000). Whether the apparently similar rates of manifestation of schizophrenia in different populations are primarily due to a uniformly distributed genetic liability, to some ubiquitous constellation of environmental factors interacting with it, or to a similar phenotypic expression of genetically different disorders, is an unresolved issue, to be addressed in future research.

Some recent studies, partly using published data from the WHO Ten-Country Study, have suggested that the incidence and prevalence of schizophrenia varies with degrees of latitude north of the equator (Saha *et al.*, 2006), or that the mean age at onset of disorder increases with higher latitudes (Shaner *et al.*, 2007). A more complex meta-analysis of prevalence studies (Kinney *et al.*, 2009) added low fish consumption, migrant groups with darker skin, and higher infant mortality to the latitude factor, and inferred a possible role of prenatal vitamin D deficiency in the etiology of schizophrenia. Although a latitude gradient of variation may be extracted statistically from published data, its reliability and validity as a risk indicator is far from being demonstrated (contrary to the latitude hypothesis, the highest incidence of schizophrenia in the WHO study was in a region in rural India, and the lowest in Denmark).

Rural–urban differences

There is a large literature on rural–urban differences in the incidence of schizophrenia, with the majority of studies reporting significantly higher rates in more urban areas. For instance, one early study of all first hospitalizations for schizophrenia over a 7-year period in Maryland, US (Eaton., 1974) found an almost three-fold higher incidence in urban Baltimore than in rural areas. However, this and other early studies relied exclusively on hospitalized or treated cases, and it is possible that the lower rates observed in rural areas could be associated with less access and utilization of healthcare services in these populations. More recent research has largely overcome this methodological flaw by using comprehensive case ascertainment procedures, including "leakage" studies which aim to identify cases missed by initial screening. The Aetiology and Ethnicity in Schizophrenia and Other Psychoses (ÆSOP) study, a large three-center population-based epidemiological study of first episode psychoses in the UK (Kirkbride *et al.*, 2006), identified all cases of schizophrenia, aged 16–64, presenting to services over a 2-year period in south-east London, Nottinghamshire, and Bristol—settings which provided a mix of urban, suburban, and rural environments. The study demonstrated that the incidence of schizophrenia was two to three times higher in the most urban area (south-east London) than in the less urban areas. The study was also able to adjust for other potential confounders that might explain these differences, such as age, sex, and ethnicity. This finding confirmed other reports of raised rates of schizophrenia in urban areas of the UK (Allardyce *et al.*, 2001).

Another issue which confounded early research was the difficulty in excluding social drift as a potential explanation of the higher rates of psychoses in urban areas. People in the prepsychotic prodromal stage of schizophrenia may find it increasingly difficult to remain in employment or in affordable housing, and move into inner city areas, traditionally the home of unskilled jobs or cheaper housing. This pattern of downward drift may be further compounded by a parallel upward drift by healthy individuals, better positioned to take advantage of labor and housing markets. Thus, it is possible that the concentration of people with schizophrenia in urban areas may reflect social and geographical drift, rather than etiologically relevant causal processes.

Recent studies have attempted to exclude the possible effects of social and geographical drift as an explanation for increased rates of schizophrenia in urban areas. These studies have mostly originated from Denmark and Sweden where it has been possible to link psychiatric case registers with large national registration databases covering the entire population. Such studies provide prospectively collected longitudinal data that enable the testing of hypotheses regarding the incidence of schizophrenia in relation to an array of social factors, including urban environments and ethnicity. One such study, based on a cohort of nearly 50 000 Swedish male army conscripts over a 13-year period (1970–1983), considered whether the incidence of schizophrenia was associated with urban residence at birth and during upbringing (Lewis *et al.*, 1992). Evidence that being born or raised in a more urban environment incurs an increased risk of schizophrenia in adult life would provide a strong argument against the social drift hypothesis. The conscripts' family and social background was evaluated with self-administered questionnaires at the start of the study; subjects with a pre-existing psychiatric illness were excluded. The participants were then linked to the Swedish National Register of Psychiatric Care which records all admissions to psychiatric services in Sweden. The authors tested whether urban birthplace or urban residence during upbringing was associated with an increased risk of schizophrenia. They found that the incidence of schizophrenia was 65% higher among men who were brought up in cities, relative to those who had had a rural upbringing. The excess incidence of schizophrenia attributable to city residence later in life was smaller (38%), but still statistically significant after adjustment for confounders, such as cannabis use, parental divorce, or family history of psychiatric disorder (Lewis *et al.*, 1992). In a similar analysis, of the place of birth of all first admissions for schizophrenia and other psychoses in The Netherlands between 1942 and 1978, Marcelis *et al.* (1999) found a nearly linear relationship between urban birth and moderate increases in the incidence of schizophrenia, affective psychoses, and other psychoses, with the effect size increasing in successive birth cohorts. A study on the incidence of schizophrenia in a cohort of 1.75 million people in Denmark, born between 1935 and 1978 (Mortensen *et al.*, 1999), also found a dose–response relationship between urban birthplace (scored on a five-point scale from rural area through to capital city) and later risk of schizophrenia. Controlling for confounders, the risk of schizophrenia was found to be over twice as high for those born in the capital city, compared with those born in rural areas. The finding of a linear dose–response relationship has been replicated in several settings (Harrison *et al.*, 2003; Spauwen *et al.*, 2004; Sundquist *et al.*, 2004) and provides strong support for the role of factors related to early exposure to "urbanicity" in conferring an increased risk of schizophrenia in later life. Such factors may operate from, or even before, birth (Mortensen *et al.*, 1999; Pedersen & Mortensen, 2006a),

during upbringing (Lewis *et al.*, 1992), and possibly close to the time of onset of schizophrenia (Kirkbride *et al.*, 2006).

Further discussion of the hypothetical nature of the "urban risk factor" is provided later in this chapter; see also Chapter 11.

Local (small-area) variation in incidence

The literature on rural–urban differences in the incidence of schizophrenia tends to overlook the variation *within* both urban and rural areas, which suggests that the environmental antecedents of schizophrenia may extend well beyond the ecologically inclusive factors of "urbanicity" or population density. This line of enquiry originates from one of the oldest and well-established findings in psychiatric epidemiology. Faris and Dunham (1939) demonstrated higher rates of first admission for schizophrenia in inner city census tracts of Chicago which followed a centripetal gradient towards the city center. This striking finding was in direct contrast to the affective psychoses (i.e., bipolar disorder) which followed no such pattern. The same pattern was observed in subsequent research (Pedersen & Mortensen, 2006b; Kirkbride *et al.*, 2007a). Similar findings have been reported from a variety of settings, including cities such as Mannheim in Germany (Löffler & Häfner, 1999) and Nottingham in the UK (Giggs, 1973, 1986; Giggs & Cooper, 1987; Cooper *et al.*, 1987), as well as rural communities in Ireland (Youssef *et al.*, 1999; Scully *et al.*, 2004). Recent studies have been able to quantify this variance more precisely. For instance, using hierarchical modelling on data from Maastricht (The Netherlands), one study estimated that around 12% of the variation in the incidence of schizophrenia across small administrative areas (median population, approx. 3000) can be best attributed to factors operating at the neighbourhood level (van Os *et al.*, 2000). A similar finding from the ÆSOP study in South-east London (UK) attributed 25% of variation in the incidence of schizophrenia across electoral wards (median population approx. 10 000) to neighborhood level factors (Kirkbride *et al.*, 2007b). The latter study was conducted in an exclusively urban setting, suggesting that not all urban areas have an equal distribution of the potential risk factors which presumably underpin schizophrenia onset. This has important implications for eliciting such factors in both between rural and urban settings, as well as within them.

Mortality

The first statistical investigation of mortality of the mentally ill was William Farr's "Report upon the Mortality of Lunatics", read before the Statistical Society of London in 1841. Farr's analysis revealed a six-fold excess of deaths among asylum inmates, relative to the general population of England and Wales. He concluded that, "the mortality of lunatics in asylums is much higher than the mortality of the general population, and the excess cannot be ascribed entirely, although it may partially, to the confinement, the unwholesomeness, or the usages of mad-houses"—in other words, it was mainly the result of lack of medical supervision and treatment. Nearly two centuries later, studies still provide compelling evidence for excess mortality associated with psychosis. In a systematic review of 37 studies emanating from 25 different countries, Saha *et al.* (2007) calculated a median standardized mortality ratio (SMR) of 2.58 for all-cause mortality in patients with schizophrenia. Using the UK's General Practice Research Database, Osborn *et al.* (2007) estimated a hazard ratio (HR) of 3.22 for increased risk of death from coronary heart disease and stroke in people with severe mental illness that could not be wholly explained by antipsychotic medication, smoking, or social deprivation. These recent findings point to a persisting "mortality gap" between people with schizophrenia and the general population (Chwastiak & Tek, 2009; see also Chapter 31). Excess mortality among patients with schizophrenia has indeed been documented over many decades by epidemiological studies of large cohorts. In Norway, national case register data indicated that while the total mortality of psychiatric patients decreased between 1926–41 and 1950–74, the relative mortality of patients with schizophrenia remained unchanged at a level more than twice that of the general population (Ødegaard, 1946a). Successive Danish national cohorts (Mortensen & Juel, 1993) have shown a trend of increasing mortality in first-admission patients with schizophrenia, with the 5-year cumulated SMR increasing from 5.30 (males) and 2.27 (females) in 1971–73 to 7.79 (males) and 4.52 (females) in 1980–82. More recent cohort and record linkage studies confirm the persistence and possible increase in excess mortality associated with schizophrenia (Lawrence *et al.*, 2000a; Ösby *et al.*, 2000). On average, SMRs for patients with schizophrenia are of the order of 2.60–3.00, which corresponds to a greater than 20% reduction in life-expectancy compared to the general population (Brown *et al.*, 2000). SMRs as high as 3.76 (men) and 3.14 (women) have been observed among homeless people with schizophrenia (Babidge *et al.*, 2001). Unnatural causes apart, there is a nearly five-fold increase (SMR 4.68) of "avoidable" natural deaths, due to hypertension, cerebrovascular disease, and smoking-related disease (Brown *et al.*, 2000; see Chapter 28). The phenomenon of "sudden unexplained death" among patients with schizophrenia (Appleby *et al.*, 2000) may be related to cardiotoxic effects of antipsychotic drugs, especially in patients receiving more than one antipsychotic concurrently (Waddington *et al.*, 1998; Lawrence *et al.*, 2003; Joukamaa *et al.*, 2006; Tilhonen *et al.*, 2009).

Unnatural causes, including suicide, accidents, and homicide (particularly high risk in men with schizophrenia), accounted for 25% of all deaths of people with psychoses over a 20-year period, according to a study based on the Danish Psychiatric Case Register (Hiroeh *et al.*, 2001). In recent decades, the suicide rate in patients with schizophrenia has become at least equal to, or possibly higher, than the suicide rate in major depression (SMR 9.60 in males, 6.80 in females; Mortensen & Juel, 1993). Data from Scotland (Geddes & Juszczak, 1995) and Australia (Lawrence *et al.*, 2001) point to an increasing suicide rate in patients with schizophrenia, mostly within the first year after discharge from hospital. Several risk factors have been suggested as relatively specific to schizophrenic suicide: being young and male, the experience of a disabling mental illness with multiple relapses and remissions, awareness of the deteriorating course of the condition, comorbid substance use, and loss of faith in treatment (Caldwell & Gottesman, 1990; Hawton *et al.*, 2005). Whether the trend of an increasing suicide mortality can be attributed to the transition from hospital to community management of schizophrenia, as some studies suggest (Heilä *et al.*, 2005), remains to be established.

Fertility

The low fertility of men and women diagnosed with schizophrenia has been extensively documented by Essen-Möller (1935), Larson and Nyman (1973), and Ødegaard (1980). The average number of children fathered by schizophrenic men was 0.9 in Sweden, and the average number of live births over the entire reproductive period of women treated for schizophrenia in Norway during 1936–75 was 1.8, compared with 2.2 for the general female population. Similar results have been reported from Germany (Hilger *et al.*, 1983) and Australia (McGrath *et al.*, 1999). Yet this phenomenon does not seem either to be universal or consistent over time. In the WHO Ten-Country Study (Jablensky *et al.*, 1992), the fertility of women with schizophrenia in India did not differ from that of women in the general population within the same age groups and geographical areas. An increase in the fertility of women with schizophrenia has been observed in recent decades (Nimgaonkar *et al.*, 1997) and is likely to be sustained as a result of the deinstitutionalization of the mentally ill. Although men with schizophrenia continue to be reproductively disadvantaged, at least one study (Lane *et al.*, 1995) has found a higher than average fertility among married schizophrenic men. Several studies on relatively small samples have examined the fertility of biological relatives of probands with schizophrenia and found higher than average fertility among their clinically asymptomatic parents and siblings (Faňanás & Bertranpetit, 1995; Waddington & Youssef, 1996; Srinivasan & Padmavati, 1997; Avila *et al.*, 2001). These studies suggest that increased reproductive fitness among the biological relatives of patients with schizophrenia may compensate for the reduced fertility of affected probands and thus explain the maintenance of a stable incidence of schizophrenia in the population. However, two large, population-based studies (Haukka et al., 2003; Svensson et al., 2007) failed to detect a compensation effect. Considering that schizophrenia is genetically complex, with locus heterogeneity and incomplete or variable expression of the phenotype, the loss of susceptibility alleles resulting from reduced reproductive fitness of affected individuals would have a negligible effect on the overall risk gene pool in the population (Jablensky & Kalaydjieva, 2003).

Age and sex

There is abundant evidence that schizophrenia may have its onset at almost any age—in childhood as well as past middle age—although the majority of onsets fall within the interval of 15–54 years of age (see Chapter 7). Neither childhood-onset schizophrenia (onset before age 12) nor late-onset schizophrenia (onset after age 50) presents with any clinical features or risk factors that are qualitatively distinct from those characterizing schizophrenia arising in young adults (Nicolson & Rapoport, 1999; Brodaty et al., 1999; Palmer et al., 2001), with the possible exception of psychotic disorganization symptoms being more likely to characterize early-onset cases and systematized paranoid delusions being predominant in late-onset cases (Häfner et al., 2001). The distribution of age at onset has been described as a continuum where variation is consistent with a model incorporating random genetic and developmental effects and environmental experiences unique to the individual (Kendler et al., 1996). This apparent continuum, however, may be masking underlying discontinuities, as suggested by admixture analysis of a series of prospectively recruited DSM-IV schizophrenia cases (Schürhoff et al., 2004). The best fitting model was a mixture of two normal distributions, one with a mean and standard deviation at 19.91 ± 3.56 years of age, and another with a mean and standard deviation at 33.48 ± 8.2 years. The early-onset subgroup was characterized by a predominance of male patients with a higher familial risk and non-paranoid symptom profiles; the smaller, late-onset subgroup included mainly females with a lower familial risk and paranoid symptomatology. This is consistent with much of the literature (reviewed in McGrath et al., 2004a) which broadly supports the view that onsets in men peak steeply in the age group 20–24; thereafter, the inception rate remains more or less constant at a lower level. In women, a less prominent peak in the age group 20–24 is followed by a moderate increase in incidence in age groups older than 35. However, this pattern of age and sex distribution of onsets is neither entirely consistent nor universal. Long-term observation studies point to an inversion of the male-to-female ratio with age, and cohorts followed up into old age exhibit a

higher cumulated lifetime risk in women compared to men (Helgason & Magnusson, 1989). A meta-analysis of studies published between 1980 and 2001 (Aleman et al., 2003) found a relatively modest increase in the incidence risk ratio for men to develop schizophrenia relative to women up to age 64 years (1.32; 95% confidence interval 1.13–1.55), but no sex differences in studies from developing countries. Lack of sex differences in age at onset has been reported for familial schizophrenia (Albus & Maier, 1995), and for all clinical subtypes (except for the paranoid form in which age at onset was lower in men) in a comprehensive study of hospital admissions in Finland (Salokangas et al., 2003). Attenuated or even inverted effect of sex, i.e., female preponderance of onsets in younger age groups, has been consistently reported from India (Murthy et al., 1998; Gangadhar et al., 2002) and China (Phillips et al., 2004). Data from the WHO Ten-Country Study (Jablensky & Cole, 1997) show that age at onset is influenced by multiple interacting factors, including sex, premorbid personality traits, family history of psychosis, and marital status. The unconfounding of such interactions resulted in a significant attenuation of the effect of sex on age at onset. Thus, the observed sex difference in age at onset is unlikely to be an invariant biological characteristic of the disease.

There is, also, no clear evidence of major or consistent sex differences in the symptoms of schizophrenia, including the frequency of positive and negative symptoms (Maric et al., 2003; Morgan et al., 2008a). Although sex differences have been described in relation to premorbid adjustment (better premorbid functioning in women); occurrence of brain abnormalities (more frequent in men); course (a higher percentage of remitting illness episodes and shorter hospital stay in women); and outcome (less disability and higher survival rate in the community in women), such differences are consistent with normal sexual dimorphism in brain development and a possible neuroprotective role of estrogen (Häfner, 2003; Hochman & Lewine, 2004; Kulkarni et al., 2008).

Marital status

Marital status is a strong predictor of psychiatric hospitalization (Jarman et al., 1992). In schizophrenia, it is significantly associated with measures of incidence, age at onset, course, and outcome. A study of a historical cohort of patients with schizophrenia first admitted to hospital in 1925 (Jönsson & Jonsson, 1992) found that marriage before index admission was the only predictor of a favorable outcome. Single men, and to a lesser degree single women, tend to be over-represented among first admissions or first contacts (68% and 39%, respectively in the WHO Ten-Country Study; Jablensky et al., 1992). Riecher-Rössler et al. (1992) found a 12-fold higher first admission rate for single men when compared to married men, and a 3.3 times higher rate for single women when compared to married women. Being single was associated with 50-fold higher odds of developing schizophrenia in males and 15-fold higher odds in women during the 1-year follow-up of the ECA study (Tien & Eaton, 1992). This is not sufficient to prove that being single is an independent, antecedent risk factor (or that being married is a protective risk modifier) since both overt schizophrenia and preschizophrenic traits and impairments reduce the chances of getting married (Agerbo et al., 2004). Patients with schizophrenia living in a stable marital or other partnership may be a positively selected group with a milder form of the disease (Ødegaard, 1946b). Evidence that being married (or living with a partner) can be a risk modifier delaying the onset of schizophrenia in males, but not in females, was obtained from the WHO Ten-Country Study after unconfounding the effects of gender, premorbid personality traits, family history of psychosis, and marital status on age at onset (Jablensky & Cole, 1997). An interaction between single marital status and a neighborhood environment characterized by a high degree of social isolation was significantly associated with incidence of schizophrenia in a Dutch study (van Os et al., 2000).

Comorbid association with other diseases and health problems

The concept of comorbidity (Lilienfeld et al., 1994) refers to the co-occurrence in an individual of two or more nosologically different disorders which may be either randomly associated or causally related. In schizophrenia, comorbidity comprises: (1) relatively common medical problems and diseases that tend to occur among patients with schizophrenia more frequently as a consequence of dysfunctional lifestyle, poor self-care or medical neglect; and (2) specific disorders that may have a pathogenetic relationship with schizophrenia itself or its treatment. For further discussion, see Chapter 31.

Comorbidity with medical problems and diseases

Physical disease is common among patients with schizophrenia but is rarely diagnosed. Between 46% and 80% of inpatients, and between 20% and 43% of outpatients with schizophrenia, have been found in different surveys to suffer from concurrent medical illnesses. In one study, physical illness was thought to aggravate the mental state in 46% of the patients, and in 7% it was life-threatening (Adler & Griffith, 1991). In a study of acute admissions of patients with schizophrenia, 10% were found to be dehydrated, 33% had hypokalemia, and 66% had elevated serum muscle enzymes (Hatta et al., 1999). Patients with schizophrenia have a dramatically increased risk of poisoning with psychotropic drugs (50-fold for men and 20-fold

for women; Mäkikirö et al., 1998). In addition to a generally increased susceptibility of patients with schizophrenia to infection, especially pulmonary tuberculosis (Baldwin, 1979; Ohta et al., 1988) and human immunodeficiency virus (HIV) (Sewell, 1996), they have significantly higher than expected rates of diabetes Type II, ischemic heart disease and myocardial infarction, chronic obstructive pulmonary disease, and acquired hypothyroidism (Dixon et al., 2000; Basu & Meltzer, 2006; Weber et al., 2009). Other conditions found to be more frequent in patients with schizophrenia than in the general population include middle ear disease (Mason & Winton, 1995); irritable bowel syndrome (Gupta et al., 1997); and some rare genetic or idiopathic disorders such as acute intermittent porphyria (Crimlisk, 1997). This heavy burden of medical morbidity remains largely under-recognized since patients with schizophrenia and comorbid conditions are usually excluded from research studies (Jeste et al., 1996).

A condition deserving special mention in this context is the cluster of interrelated health problems commonly referred to as the metabolic syndrome [central obesity, raised triglycerides, reduced high-density lipoprotein (HDL)-cholesterol, raised fasting plasma glucose, and hypertension; Alberti et al., 2005]. Patients with schizophrenia had a four-fold increased risk of metabolic syndrome in the Northern Finland 1996 birth cohort study (Saari et al., 2005), and a number of studies have reported prevalence rates as high as 36–51% in patients with schizophrenia samples (McEvoy et al., 2005; De Hert et al., 2006; John et al., 2009). There is growing evidence that the high prevalence of the metabolic syndrome among patients with schizophrenia might be explained by interactions between second-generation antipsychotic medications, lifestyle factors, and an inherent predisposition to diabetes and heart disease (Goff et al., 2005; McEvoy et al., 2005; see also Chapter 28).

Among central nervous system (CNS) conditions, a variety of rare organic brain disorders and anomalies have been described to occur in association with schizophrenia, including basal ganglia calcification (Francis & Freeman, 1984; Flint & Goldstein, 1992); aqueductus Sylvii stenosis (Roberts et al., 1983; Reveley & Reveley, 1983; O'Flaithbheartaigh et al., 1994); cerebral hemiatrophy (Puri et al., 1994; Honer et al., 1996); corpus callosum agenesis (Lewis et al., 1988); schizencephaly (Alexander et al., 1997); metachromatic leukodystrophy (Hyde et al., 1992); and septal cysts (Lewis & Mezey 1985); see Chapter 9. More common associations with schizophrenia involve epilepsy (odds ratio 11.1 in the 1966 North Finland general population birth cohort; Mäkikirö et al., 1998; review in Gaitatzis et al., 2004) and intellectual disability (in a population-based study, 3.7–5.2% of people with intellectual disability had also been diagnosed with schizophrenia; Morgan et al., 2008b).

In addition to such "positive" disease associations, "negative" comorbidity, i.e., a lower than expected rate of occurrence of diseases, has been often reported for rheumatoid arthritis in patients with schizophrenia (Österberg, 1978; Eaton et al., 1992; Gorwood et al., 2004). However, a large population study using the Danish Psychiatric Case Register (Mors et al., 1999) failed to confirm earlier findings and raised the possibility that the negative association might have resulted from a systematic underreporting of medical illness in smaller samples of patients with schizophrenia. A better replicated finding, originating in several population-based record linkage studies, is the lower incidence of some cancers in patients with schizophrenia relative to their occurrence in the general population, with particularly conspicuous reductions of respiratory cancer risk in males (Dupont et al., 1986; Mortensen, 1994; Lawrence et al., 2000b; Dalton et al., 2005; Barak et al., 2005; Hippisley-Cox et al., 2007). There is as yet no conclusive explanation for these observations. A protective effect of neuroleptic medication has been claimed for colorectal and prostate cancer, based on the findings of a population cohort study (Dalton et al., 2006), but the case remains unproven. Reduced cancer risk in unaffected biological parents and siblings of patients with schizophrenia, which might suggest a "protective gene", has been reported from two independent studies (Lichtermann et al., 2001; Levav et al., 2007), but this finding has not been replicated by other investigators (Dalton et al., 2004).

Comorbid substance use

Substance use disorders are the most commonly reported comorbid problem among patients with schizophrenia and involve alcohol, stimulants, anxiolytics, hallucinogens, antiparkinsonian drugs, as well as tobacco and caffeine. In the WHO Ten-Country Study (Jablensky et al., 1992), a history of alcohol use in the year preceding the first contact with mental health services was elicited in 57% of the male patients, and in three of the study areas, drug use (mainly cannabis and cocaine) was reported by 24–41% of the patients. Cannabis is by far the most widely used illicit substance among patients with schizophrenia. A review of 53 studies of clinical samples and five epidemiological surveys of people with non-affective psychoses (Green et al., 2005) produced prevalence estimates for current use at 23%, and for lifetime use at 42%. In an Australian epidemiological sample of 852 individuals with DSM-III-R diagnosed psychoses (Kavanagh et al., 2004), lifetime repeated use of cannabis (misuse or dependence) was reported by 40.9% of the participants, followed by amphetamines (17.8%), LSD (16.8%), heroin (14.3%), cocaine (12.3%), and PCP (10%). Trends in the joint incidence and prevalence of cannabis use and of schizophrenia between 1970 and 2002 in the UK were used by Hickman et al. (2007) to model the

population attributable fraction of cannabis-induced schizophrenia. They estimated that the marked increase of cannabis use in younger age groups may result, by 2010, in approximately 10% of schizophrenia cases being attributable to cannabis. Cannabis abuse was a significant predictor of poor 2-year outcome in the WHO study and has been shown to precipitate psychotic relapse or exacerbate the symptoms of schizophrenia (Linszen et al., 1994). Heavy cannabis use prior to the manifest onset of psychotic symptoms has been consistently reported. A Danish study on 535 patients, first treated for cannabis-induced psychotic symptoms, found that at 3-year follow-up 77.2% had experienced new schizophrenia-spectrum psychotic episodes (Arendt et al., 2005). Similar findings of a strong association between self-reported cannabis use and early onset of psychosis were reported from the West London First-Episode Schizophrenia Study (Barnes et al., 2006). In contrast to the exacerbation of psychotic symptoms attributable to cannabis use, several studies have found that significant cognitive impairment and personal disability were less common among cannabis users with schizophrenia-spectrum psychosis than in non-users with similar psychoses (Stirling et al., 2005; Baker et al., 2005; Potvin et al., 2008). These unexpected findings have not been fully explained, but the proposed interpretations focus on moderating factors, such as better social and cognitive skills, that may be required to sustain a drug habit (Potvin et al., 2008), or on a neuroprotective effect of cannabinoids (Ramírez et al., 2005). Overall, the question whether excessive cannabis use can precipitate or advance the onset of a schizophrenic illness in vulnerable individuals, or is a self-medication phenomenon analogous to nicotine abuse, has not been definitively answered. The analysis of the temporal sequence of cannabis use and psychosis onset is unlikely to resolve the causality issue without recourse to biological vulnerability markers, such as polymorphisms in the cannabinoid receptor type 1 (CNR1) gene that may characterize a "cannabis-sensitive" subset of patients with schizophrenia (Krebs et al., 2002). The evidence on cannabis as a causal risk factor for schizophrenia is reviewed later in this chapter.

Analytical epidemiology of schizophrenia: risk factors, exposures, and antecedents

Risk factors influence the probability of occurrence of a disease or its outcome without necessarily being direct causes. Since the strongest proof of causation is the experiment, the identification of risk factors that are modifiable by intervention and may result in a reduced incidence or a better outcome, is the ultimate aim of risk factor epidemiology. This is still a remote aim in schizophrenia but current research is beginning to address the issue. The epidemiological classification of initiating, pathogenetic, and interacting risk factors (Khoury *et al.*, 1993) is not readily applicable to schizophrenia, as the role of many putative risk factors is still insufficiently understood. A provisional grouping of such factors into biological, psychosocial, and broadly ecological variables may be more appropriate given the present state of knowledge.

Genetic risk

The contribution of genetic liability to the etiology of schizophrenia is one of the few firmly established facts about the disorder (see Chapter 12). As pointed out long ago by Shields (1977), "no environmental indicator predicts a raised risk of schizophrenia in small or moderate-sized samples of persons not already known to be genetically related to a schizophrenic". The genetic epidemiology of schizophrenia is underpinned by estimates of its *broad* heritability, generated from twin, adoptive, and family studies, and usually reported at 0.80 or higher (Gottesman *et al.*, 1987; Cardno *et al.*, 1999). Since the concordance rate in monozygotic twins does not exceed 50%, it is widely assumed that environmental factors also contribute to the pathogenesis of schizophrenia, but no single environmental variable has yet been demonstrated to be either necessary or sufficient for causation. Three models of the joint effects of genotype and environment have been proposed (Kendler & Eaves, 1986): (1) the effects of predisposing genes and environmental factors are additive and increase the risk of disease in a linear fashion; (2) genes control the sensitivity of the brain to environmental insults; and (3) genes influence the likelihood of an individual's exposure to environmental pathogens, e.g., by fostering certain personality traits.

Attempts at identifying major genetic loci by linkage analysis of multiply affected pedigrees or affected sib pairs have produced a plethora of results, but few of the positive findings have stood the test of replication (Ng *et al.*, 2009). Similarly, numerous genetic association studies have been beset with problems of Type I or Type II error due to population stratification, diagnostic misclassification, and uncertain biological plausibility of the candidate genes. Overall, a total of 24 genetic variants in 16 different genes have met statistical criteria for significance across 118 meta-analyses of association studies (Allen *et al.*, 2008). At present, the virtually undisputed view is that schizophrenia is a genetically complex disorder, characterized by multiple genes of small effect, incomplete penetrance, and likely locus and allelic heterogeneity. However, attempts to resolve this complexity by employing advances in genotyping technologies and pooling multiple case-control samples into "mega" databases have not resulted in a major breakthrough in understanding the genetics of the disorder. Recent genome-wide association studies (GWAS), typically using greater than 0.5 million single nucleotide polymor-

phisms (SNPs) in very large samples of cases and controls, have produced less than definitive evidence for the existence of common genetic variants that could explain a significant portion of schizophrenia risk (Mitchell & Porteus, 2009). For detailed discussion, see Chapter 13.

The relationship between genotype and phenotype in schizophrenia is likely to be mediated by complex causal pathways involving gene–gene and gene–environment interactions, "programmable" neural substrates, and stochastic events. Under such circumstances the gene effects might be too weak to be detectable through the clinical diagnostic phenotype in any but very large samples. In view of such constraints, alternative strategies have been proposed to circumvent the need for excessively large pooled samples (which may be confounded by latent population differences and by variations in ascertainment methods and diagnostic assessment). One such strategy proceeds from the assumption that the ICD-10 or DSM-IV clinical diagnoses of schizophrenia, based primarily on reported subjective symptoms and behavior changes, may not be sufficiently robust phenotypes for genetic research. Such clinical phenotypes may be the end-points of multiple and diverse developmental processes and pathogenetic pathways which make it hard for the currently available methods of genetic analysis to detect a common primary genetic basis or molecular mechanism. This has led to explorations of alternative, intermediate phenotypes (or "endophenotypes"; Gottesman & Gould, 2003; see Chapter 14), such as neurocognitive abnormalities, neurophysiological dysfunction, or brain imaging structural and functional features associated with schizophrenia and likely to be expressed in both affected individuals and their asymptomatic biological relatives. Such phenotypes have the advantage of being objectively and quantitatively measurable, and may allow a "deconstruction" of the heterogeneity of the disorder into components with higher penetrances and more clearly definable patterns of inheritance (Braff *et al.*, 2007).

Against this background, a new wave of studies focusing on genome rearrangements and rare mutations of potentially strong effect (copy number variation, CNV; microdeletions and microduplications) are generating evidence supporting the view that recurrent but rare deleterious variants in multiple, diverse genes may be cumulatively more important in schizophrenia risk than common polymorphisms (Xu *et al.*, 2008; Stefansson *et al.*, 2008; Need *et al.*, 2009). Importantly, such genome rearrangements and mutations seem to be shared across the conventional diagnostic boundaries between schizophrenia and bipolar disorder, and possibly extend also to autism, epilepsy, and some forms of intellectual disability. This signals the emergence of a novel conceptual perspective on CNS disorders, including schizophrenia. Considering the prospect of affordable new technologies for sequencing entire individual genomes in the not too distant future, the whole paradigm of schizophrenia genetics may undergo deep revision—with challenging implications for epidemiological research.

Paternal age

A number of studies, published in the last decade, and based on large databases of birth cohorts or record linkage, have reported significant associations between advanced paternal age and schizophrenia risk in the offspring (Malaspina *et al.*, 2001; Brown *et al.*, 2002; Byrne *et al.*, 2003; Zammit *et al.*, 2003; El-Saadi *et al.*, 2004; Sipos *et al.*, 2004; Torrey *et al.*, 2009). However, a minority of studies (Jung *et al.*, 2003; Pulver *et al.*, 2004) have not detected a paternal age effect. The positive findings typically refer to slight or moderate increases in relative risk, after adjusting for varying sets of possible confounding factors, such as socioeconomic status, birth order, or sibship size. The proposed interpretations focus almost exclusively on the hypothesis of transmission of *de novo* mutations in the paternal germ line, which tend to increase with age. While this mechanism is, in principle, biologically plausible but not disease-specific, as shown in a variety of disorders, e.g., acute lymphoblastic leukemia, low birthweight, osteogenesis imperfecta, and possibly Alzheimer disease, its significance in the pathogenesis of schizophrenia remains uncertain. Potential confounding factors, such as non-paternity, or colinearity between late marriage and paternal "schizotypal" traits, have rarely been considered or are difficult to control. Moreover, the statistical findings to date lack the essential support from molecular genetic studies of the frequency, penetrance, and effect sizes of actual paternal mutations. On present evidence, paternal age is a plausible but relatively weak risk factor contributing to schizophrenia, which is unlikely to provide important novel insights into its epidemiology.

Complications of pregnancy and childbirth

Maternal obstetric complications (OCs) have been a focus of research since the 1960s (Lane & Albee, 1964; Mednick, 1970; see Chapter 11). A large number of case-control studies, many reporting positive association between OC and schizophrenia, were published over two decades and became widely cited as evidence for OCs being an established risk factor in schizophrenia. Several explanatory models have been explored: (1) severe OCs, such as perinatal hypoxia and resulting hippocampal damage, can prepare the ground for adult schizophrenia even if genetic liability is weak; (2) genetic predisposition sensitizes the developing brain to lesions resulting from randomly occurring, less severe OCs; (3) genetic predisposition to schizophrenia leads to abnormal fetal development, which in turn causes OCs; and (4) maternal constitutional factors,

partially influenced by genes, such as small physique or proneness to risk behavior (drug use, smoking during pregnancy) increase the risk of OCs and fetal brain damage. However, most of the studies (reviewed by Geddes & Lawrie, 1995; Verdoux *et al.*, 1997a; McNeil *et al.*, 2000; Clarke *et al.*, 2006) were of small sample size and used parental interviews as the source of OC histories, which have been shown to have methodological limitations (Cantor-Graae *et al.*, 1998). Although significant associations have been found between complications in pregnancy and adult schizophrenia, the effects observed were inconsistent and indicated significant between-study heterogeneity. For these reasons, more rigorous standards for this type of research have more recently been adopted, requiring (1) birth cohorts or large populations samples; (2) prospectively recorded pregnancy and birth data; and (3) use of standardized scales enabling comparisons of data across studies. While a number of studies in the last decade have met the first two criteria, there is still no generally adopted framework for summarizing and reporting OC data; this limits the interpretation of findings.

Tentative risk factors emerging from population-based studies with prospectively collected OC data (reviewed by Cannon *et al.*, 2002a) include: (1) complications of pregnancy (bleeding, diabetes, pre-eclampsia, rhesus incompatibility); (2) abnormal fetal growth and development (low birthweight, congenital malformations, reduced head circumference); and (3) complications of delivery (asphyxia, uterine atonia, emergency cesarean section). Further possible risk factors are: gestation less than 37 weeks and/or small for gestational age; low maternal body mass index; non-attendance at antenatal appointments; and various combinations of the above (Sacker *et al.*, 1995; Jones *et al.*, 1998; Hultman *et al.*, 1999; Ichiki *et al.*, 2000; Kendell *et al.*, 2000; Cannon *et al.*, 2000; Wahlbeck *et al.*, 2001; Byrne *et al.*, 2007). Although many epidemiological studies report associations between one or more OC risk factors and subsequent schizophrenia, no obvious causal pathways have emerged, nor is it possible to conclude whether the effects of individual OCs are additive or interactive. A number of hypotheses focusing on aspects of neurodevelopment and gene–environment interactions have been proposed (reviewed by Abel, 2004), with some tentative support from neuroimaging (van Erp *et al.*, 2002) and gene association (Nicodemus *et al.*, 2008) studies. However, it remains difficult to answer conclusively questions about possible interactions between familial risk of schizophrenia and the contributions of OCs to the manifestation of the disease in adult life. One promising approach to analyzing such interactions is the study of developmental and disease outcomes in the offspring of women with schizophrenia or other severe mental disorder who have, or have not, experienced complications of pregnancy or childbirth. To date, several studies have found an increased risk of adverse pregnancy outcomes in women with schizophrenia, including preterm delivery, low birthweight, congenital malformations, and increased infant mortality (Bennedsen *et al.*, 1999, 2001: Nilsson *et al.*, 2002; Webb *et al.*, 2005, 2006). An Australian population-based study of 3174 births by women with schizophrenia or major affective disorders (Jablensky *et al.*, 2005) found overall increased risks of pregnancy, birth, and neonatal complications, and compared their occurrence in pregnancies before and after the first psychotic episode. While the majority of the adverse events were more frequent after the outbreak of psychosis, and possibly related to the behavioral concomitants of severe mental illness, two types of complication—low birthweight and congenital anomalies—occurred at the same frequency in pregnancies before and after the onset of psychosis, suggesting an intrinsic, possibly genetic vulnerability. While unqualified acceptance of OCs as a proven risk factor in schizophrenia is premature, further research aimed at clarifying their role remains an important priority for epidemiological research.

Maternal influenza and other pre- and post-natal infections

In utero exposure to influenza has been implicated as a risk factor since a report that an increased proportion of adult schizophrenia in Helsinki was associated with presumed second trimester *in utero* exposure to the 1957 A2 influenza epidemic (Mednick *et al.*, 1988). Over 50 studies have subsequently attempted to replicate the putative association between maternal influenza and schizophrenia, using designs ranging from interviews with mothers of probands with schizophrenia to statistical analyses of large databases linking the incidence of schizophrenia in birth cohorts to measures of mortality or morbidity associated with influenza epidemics. Ascertainment of influenza infection on the basis of recall has been shown to result in a high percentage of false-positive self-diagnoses when questionnaire responses were correlated with individual serological findings (Elder *et al.*, 1996). Therefore, it is not surprising that studies relating schizophrenia incidence rates to presumed prenatal exposure during documented epidemics have produced mixed results, some supporting the original Finnish findings (Barr *et al.*, 1990; Sham *et al.*, 1992; Adams *et al.*, 1993; Takei *et al.*, 1994; Kunugi *et al.*, 1995), and others failing to find such association (Morgan *et al.*, 1997; Grech *et al.*, 1997; Battle *et al.*, 1999; Selten *et al.*, 1999a; Mino *et al.*, 2000). While most of the population-based studies were ecological by design (information on individual exposures was not available), two studies (Crow & Done, 1992; Cannon *et al.*, 1996) with access to data on actually infected pregnant women found no increase in the risk of schizophrenia among the offspring. In a case-control study of a birth cohort 1959–1966 (Brown *et al.*, 2004), in which investigators assayed influenza antibodies in archived maternal

serum, the risk of schizophrenia was increased in the exposed subjects, but the association did not reach statistical significance, possibly due to a small sample size. The balance of evidence, therefore, does not provide unequivocal backing to the hypothesis of a significant contribution of *in utero* exposure to influenza to the etiology of schizophrenia. Indirectly, recent evidence from laboratory research, e.g., altered brain expression of schizophrenia-related genes in the offspring of mice infected with human influenza virus (Fatemi *et al.*, 2008), or a disruption of the fetal brain balance between pro- and anti-inflammatory cytokines (Meyer *et al.*, 2009), lends support to further investigations of neurodevelopmental risks associated with influenza pandemics.

The search for prenatal or postnatal exposures to infection as a risk factor has not been limited to influenza. In a follow-up study of the children of a cohort of women clinically and serologically documented with prenatal rubella, Brown *et al.* (2001) reported an increased risk of schizophrenia spectrum disorders. Postnatal CNS infections in children followed up to age 14 in the North Finland 1966 birth cohort was associated with a significant odds ratio of 4.8 for subsequent schizophrenia (Rantakallio *et al.*, 1997). An association between Borna disease virus and both schizophrenia and affective disorders has been suggested by several serological studies, but the clinical significance of this association remains to be elucidated (Taieb *et al.*, 2001; Nunes *et al.*, 2008). More recently, studies have focused on herpes simplex viruses 1 and 2, cytomegalovirus, and *Toxoplasma gondii* (Kim *et al.*, 2007; Mortensen *et al.*, 2007). Some tentative evidence for maternal toxoplasmosis has been presented in a meta-analysis of studies in 17 countries over five decades (Torrey *et al.*, 2007), but the variation in the seropositivity rates in the general population, and of the methods for their assessment, precludes any firm conclusions. The extent to which such research is capable of discovering true causal contributions to schizophrenia, in the absence of a more advanced pathogenetic understanding of the role of genetic factors, remains debatable.

Other prenatal exposures

A variety of other prenatal exposures has been explored in documented historical cohorts. Several studies have focused on prenatal nutritional deficiency as a risk factor for adult schizophrenia (Neugebauer, 2005). Fetal vulnerability to acute maternal starvation during the first trimester, with an increased subsequent risk of schizophrenia, has been suggested by a study of the offspring of Dutch women exposed to severe wartime famine in 1944–45. Severe food deprivation (<4200 kJ/day) was associated with an increased relative risk of 2.6 for narrowly defined schizophrenia in female offspring (Susser & Lin, 1992) and a relative risk of 2.0 for schizotypal personality disorder (Hoek *et al.*, 1996). A tentative replication of these findings using a much larger sample was reported by St Clair *et al.* (2005) in a study of psychiatric hospital admissions during 1971–2001 of individuals who had been prenatally exposed to the Chinese famine of 1959–1961. Among births during the famine year 1960, as compared to pre-famine births, the mortality-adjusted risk of schizophrenia in adulthood rose to 2.30 (95% confidence interval 1.99–2.23). A further replication, from a geographically distinct area of China, has recently been reported (Xu *et al.*, 2009). In a different type of study design, McGrath *et al.* (2004b) explored the association between the provision of vitamin D during the first year of life and the risk of adult schizophrenia in the Northern Finland 1966 Birth Cohort. A moderately reduced risk ratio was found for males on vitamin D supplementation compared to no supplementation.

The hypothesis that maternal psychological stress might affect the risk of schizophrenia in the offspring was explored by van Os & Selten (1998), using the 5-day German *blitzkrieg* against The Netherlands in May 1940 as a proxy measure of stress exposure during pregnancy. A small but statistically significant increase in relative risk (risk ratio 1.28) was found for first-trimester exposure. Another Dutch stress exposure study, using the 1953 flood catastrophe in the south-west of The Netherlands (Selten *et al.*, 1999b), failed to find a significant association between maternal stress and non-affective psychoses in the offspring. The lifetime prevalence of schizophrenia among 1867 people prenatally exposed to the 1945 atomic bomb explosion over Nagasaki was examined by Imamura *et al.* (1999) and found to be 0.96%, i.e., no different from the expected rate in non-exposed populations.

Season of birth

Seasonality of schizophrenic births was first described by Tramer (1929). The current interest in the phenomenon dates back to the 1960s (Barry & Barry, 1961). A 5–8% excess of schizophrenic births in winter–spring has been reported by a large number of studies The effect seems to be present in the Northern (reviewed by Davies *et al.*, 2003), but not in the Southern hemisphere, where studies (reviewed by McGrath & Welham, 1999) have failed to demonstrate a consistent seasonal variation. Seasonal fluctuations of births are not specific to schizophrenia and have been described in bipolar affective disorder, autism, attention deficit disorder, alcoholism, stillbirths, diabetes, Alzheimer disease, and Down syndrome. Many of the studies are methodologically vulnerable with regard to sample size, sampling bias, or statistical analysis. The evidence for a seasonal factor has been weakened, though not invalidated, by the argument that it could be an artifact of an age-incidence and age-prevalence bias (Lewis & Griffin, 1981); since the risk of onset of schizophrenia rises rapidly from age 15 on, "older" individuals born in the early months of each calendar year will have a higher rate of

onset of schizophrenia than "younger" individuals born late in the same year. Notwithstanding that, a marginally significant season of birth effect (schizophrenia relative risk 1.11; confidence interval 1.06–1.18 for births February–March) has been found after adjustment for possible confounders in a large Danish population cohort (Mortensen *et al.*, 1999). A similar relative excess of winter births has been reported by Kendell and Adams (1991) for all patients admitted to hospitals in Scotland since 1963, and by Suvisaari *et al.* (2001) for a national sample of patients with schizophrenia in Finland. A meta-analysis of southern hemisphere data (McGrath & Welham, 1999) suggests a weaker and less regular winter effect. No winter excess of schizophrenia births has been observed in Japan or Korea (Toguchi *et al.*, 2005).

Although a seasonality effect on schizophrenia births cannot be explained away as a statistical artifact, the understanding of its underlying causes has hardly progressed since the phenomenon was first described. Various explanations have been proposed, in terms of seasonal patterns of fertility or procreational habits; viral infections; extremes of temperature; and variation in nutrition or vitamin D levels, none of these hypotheses has been definitively confirmed or rejected. It is unlikely that the issue will be resolved by further studies of the effect itself. Seasonality of births may be a distant echo of the impact of other risk factors, including pregnancy and birth complications, immaturity, and low birthweight (Kendell *et al.*, 2002). Therefore, instead of focusing on seasonality of births, research could be more productive if risk factors known to disrupt normal fetal brain development were systematically examined for seasonal effects in their operation.

Children at high genetic risk

Studies of children born to parents diagnosed with schizophrenia (mothers in the majority of studies) have revealed a range of early developmental abnormalities that could be markers of increased risk of adult schizophrenia. Studies in the US (Fish, 1977; Goldstein, 1987; Erlenmeyer-Kimling *et al.*, 1997), Denmark (Schulsinger *et al.*, 1984), Sweden (McNeil & Kaij, 1987), and Israel (Mirsky *et al.*, 1995) have examined in prospective case-control designs a total of 230 high-risk children of a parent(s) with schizophrenia, 248 children of parents with other psychiatric disorders, and 392 control children born to parents with no psychiatric disorder. In reviewing these data, Fish *et al.* (1992) proposed a syndrome of "pandysmaturation" (PDM) as a marker of a neurointegrative defect, manifest as a transient retardation of motor and visual development, an irregular pattern of functional test scores on successive cross-sectional examinations, and a retardation of skeletal growth. PDM may develop *in utero* and in such cases it is associated with low birthweight, but obstetric complications do not lead to PDM in the absence of genetic risk. The PDM syndrome is relatively specific to the biological offspring of parent(s) with schizophrenia and remains a promising indicator of high risk for the disorder (Fish & Kendler, 2005). The effect of parental schizophrenia has been identified as the only "robust and direct predictor of adult psychiatric outcomes" in another high-risk study in which 18% of the offspring of a parent(s) with schizophrenia had developed schizophrenic illnesses after 19 years of follow-up, compared to 7% psychosis in the offspring of parent(s) with affective disorders and 2% in the control group (Erlenmeyer-Kimling *et al.*, 1991). Individuals at high genetic risk who developed schizophrenia as adults were more likely to manifest neurocognitive deficits and difficulties in social interaction during childhood and adolescence, compared to individuals at high risk who did not develop schizophrenia. Cognitive deficits in verbal learning and memory, social anxiety and "schizotypal cognition" in high-risk subjects who subsequently developed schizophrenia were reported from the Edinburgh High-Risk Study (Johnstone *et al.*, 2005), which included 163 young adults with two relatives with schizophrenia. In the framework of the Copenhagen High-Risk Study, brief videotape recordings of motor and social behavior were made in 1972 in a sample of 265 children aged 11–13 years, which included 81 children with a parent diagnosed with schizophrenia. In 1992, items of the children's non-verbal behavior were scored on a standard coding system by trained researchers who were blind to the children's psychiatric outcomes at ages 31–33 years. The analysis of this material revealed a markedly higher rate of general neuromotor signs, involuntary hand movements, and deficits in sociability among the 16 children who developed schizophrenia as adults (Schiffman *et al.*, 2004). In the more recent Helsinki High-Risk Study (Niemi *et al.* 2004, 2005), the offspring (n = 159) of women treated for schizophrenia-spectrum disorders were followed up to age 37. In this high-risk group, the cumulative incidences were 13.5% for any psychotic disorder and 6.7% for schizophrenia. The prospectively recorded childhood "health cards" revealed a high preschool- and school-age incidence of attentional deficits, soft neurological signs, and social inhibition in the children with later development of schizophrenia spectrum disorders. In a review of 16 major high-risk studies, Niemi *et al.* (2003) concluded that the early development characteristics which predict schizophrenia in the offspring of affected parents include neurological and motor abnormalities, verbal memory and attention deficits, poor social competence, and marked instability of the early rearing environment. Support for an effect of the early rearing environment on the risk of developing schizophrenia comes from a study involving a Finnish sample of 179 adopted-away children of parents with schizophrenia (a high-risk group) and a matched control sample of adoptees at no increased

genetic risk (Tienari, 1991; Wahlberg *et al.*, 1997). Psychosis or severe personality disorder was diagnosed in 34 of 121 high-risk subjects followed up for 5–7 years after the initial assessment, compared to 24 of 150 controls. While the rates of adult psychosis or severe personality disorder were significantly higher in the high-risk group compared to the control group, the difference was entirely attributable to the subset of high-risk children who grew up in dysfunctional adoptive families—a result consistent with the model of genetic control of sensitivity to the environment.

Early developmental precursors and markers of schizophrenia risk

While clearly demonstrating a parent-to-offspring transmission of schizophrenia risk, and presence of early neurobehavioral and cognitive deficits preceding by many years the onset of clinical symptoms, the results of high-risk studies may not generalize to larger populations where the majority of people who eventually develop schizophrenia do not have a parent or other first-degree relative with manifest schizophrenic illness. Furthermore, high-risk studies are not entirely conclusive as to whether the causation of the early developmental aberrations observed in such children is primarily genetic, environmental (e.g., due to parenting disrupted by psychosis), or involving an interaction between the two. A number of population cohort studies have partially addressed these issues. Evidence of early developmental peculiarities in children who develop schizophrenia as adults has been provided by prospectively collected data on a national birth cohort in the UK (Jones *et al.*, 1994). Pre-schizophrenic children had an excess (odds ratio 2.1–5.8) of speech and educational problems, social anxiety, and preference for solitary play. In a prospective cohort study of 9236 individuals born in Philadelphia from 1959 to 1966 and evaluated with tests of cognitive functioning at 4 and 7 years of age, Cannon *et al.* (2000) found that both those who developed schizophrenia or schizoaffective disorder and their unaffected siblings exhibited more deficits on verbal and non-verbal cognitive tests at these ages than non-psychiatric controls, thus supporting premorbid cognitive dysfunction as a relatively independent vulnerability indicator (the deficits were not associated with maternal obstetric complications or other confounding factors). However, the authors cautioned against using such deficits as screening criteria for predisposition to schizophrenia in general population samples, due to their limited positive prediction value (PPV). In the Swedish cohort study of 109 643 men conscripted into the army at age 18–20 and followed up over 15 years (Malmberg *et al.*, 1998; Gunnell *et al.*, 2002), poor performance at age 18 years on tests of verbal and non-verbal cognitive ability was associated with early-onset psychotic disorder. Poor social adjustment during childhood and adolescence was significantly more common among the individuals who subsequently developed schizophrenia than among the rest of the cohort. Similar results (deficits in social functioning and organizational ability, as well as low test scores on all measures) were reported from the Israeli conscript study (Davidson *et al.*, 1999). Impairments in cognitive and neuromotor development among children later diagnosed with schizophreniform disorder were also reported from the New Zealand Dunedin birth cohort of 1037 children born in 1972–1973 (Cannon *et al.*, 2002b); from a Danish cohort of 6923 men born in Copenhagen in 1953 (Osler *et al.*, 2007); and the Northern Finland 1966 Birth Cohort Study (Isohanni *et al.*, 2006).

On the balance of evidence to date, a cluster of early, subtle neurobehavioral and cognitive abnormalities may be a sensitive indicator of future risk of schizophrenia or schizophrenia spectrum disorders which is not restricted to the offspring of parents with manifest psychosis. However, the occurrence of such developmental signs in the general population of children is likely to be considerably higher than acceptable for the level of specificity that would warrant their potential use as predictors of individual risk of psychosis.

Premorbid intelligence (IQ)

The association between mental retardation and schizophrenia was first highlighted by Kraepelin (1919) who estimated that up to 7% of the cases of dementia praecox evolved on the basis of intellectual impairment, and introduced the term *Pfropfschizophrenie* (engrafted schizophrenia) for a subtype characterized by early onset, negativism, and stereotypies, likely resulting from a disruption in neurodevelopment (Mack *et al.*, 2002). A deficit in intellectual performance antedating the onset of schizophrenia by many years was first described by Lane and Albee (1964). The Kraepelinian concept has been revived and partially validated (Doody *et al.*, 1998; Sanderson *et al.*, 2001) in a study which identified a comorbid pattern of mild learning disability, neurological symptoms, and schizophrenia-like psychosis segregating in multiply affected families with high rates of chromosomal abnormalities. Independently of the notion of a discrete subtype of schizophrenia characterized by intellectual impairment, a consistent and strong relationship between low IQ and later development of schizophrenia has been demonstrated prospectively in the Swedish conscript study (David *et al.*, 1997; Gunnell *et al.*, 2002; Zammit *et al.*, 2004) and the Israeli conscript study (Davidson *et al.*, 1999; Reichenberg *et al.*, 2002; Caspi *et al.*, 2003). After controlling for confounding effects in the Swedish cohort, the risk of schizophrenia increased linearly with the decrement of IQ (compared to an IQ > 126 as the baseline, the odds ratio for schizophrenia increased from 3.5 for IQ 90–95 to 8.6 for IQ < 74). In a recent study (MacCabe *et al.*, 2008) of a Swedish national sample of 907

011 individuals born 1973–1983, prospectively recorded poor school performance at age 15–16 was found to be associated with a nearly four-fold increase of the risk of schizophrenia, independently of parental education level, socioeconomic status, and risk factors such as migrant status, low birthweight, and hypoxia at birth. Related evidence points to a significant association between borderline or mild intellectual disability and high risk of schizophrenia or other non-affective psychosis (Hassiotis *et al.*, 1999; Greenwood *et al.*, 2004; Morgan *et al.*, 2008b). Thus, the relationship between low IQ and risk of schizophrenia is among the most robust findings in the risk factor epidemiology of the disorder and merits further study. The balance of evidence favors a hypothesis of shared neurodevelopmental etiology for intellectual impairment and schizophrenia in a significant proportion of cases.

Pervasive developmental disorders and schizophrenia

Two recent studies draw attention to the co-occurrence of childhood-onset pervasive developmental disorders, including core autism, autism spectrum and Asperger disorder, and schizophrenia or schizophrenia spectrum disorder. In the National Institute of Mental Health (NIMH) childhood-onset schizophrenia sample, 19 (25%) of the 75 schizophrenia probands met DSM-IV lifetime diagnostic criteria for pervasive developmental disorder with early language, social and motor abnormalities; two of their siblings had been diagnosed with core autism (Sporn *et al.*, 2004). Independently, a Swedish study of 241 adults consecutively referred for evaluation of possible childhood-onset neuropsychiatric disorders, found that 7.8% of adults with autism spectrum disorders concurrently met criteria for schizophrenia or other non-affective psychosis. In adults with attention deficit hyperactive disorder (ADHD), the prevalence of schizophrenia (5%) or bipolar disorder (5%) was also higher than expected (Stahlberg *et al.*, 2004; Hofvander *et al.*, 2009). These findings, together with recent genetic evidence of a shared load of copy number variations (CNV) and rare mutations between probands with schizophrenia and autism (Szatmari *et al.*, 2007), suggest a possible continuum of risk and raise questions about the validity of the sharp distinction between pervasive developmental disorder and early-onset schizophrenia in current diagnostic classifications.

Substance abuse as risk exposure

There is good evidence that substance abuse is associated with an increased risk of schizophrenia. The majority of the literature has focused on the links between cannabis, one of the world's most popular illicit substances, and schizophrenia. The question as to whether this association is causal or due to confounding, reverse causality, common causality, or some combination of all these, remains unanswered. Most of the recent research has concluded that cannabis may contribute to causation but is neither a sufficient nor a necessary cause for schizophrenia (Arseneault *et al.*, 2004). The area remains contentious, not only because of the unresolved epidemiological issues, but also because of the political, social, and public health implications (Advisory Council on the Misuse of Drugs, 2008).

The possible confounding effect of recall or information bias has been largely excluded; studies based on longitudinal designs involving birth cohorts or military service conscripts have supported the association using prospectively collected data on cannabis exposure and independently ascertained outcomes. Henquet *et al.* (2005) reviewed the evidence from such studies and concluded that any prior cannabis use was associated with an approximate doubling of the risk of schizophrenia. The studies included in this meta-analysis controlled for potential confounders, such as age, sex, socioeconomic status, ethnicity, family history of psychiatric illness, urban residence, and use of other drugs, but the association remained significant, favoring causation as the likely explanation. Another systematic review (Moore *et al.*, 2007) came to a similar conclusion regarding the pooled effect size and reported a dose–response relationship between cannabis consumption and risk of psychotic disorder. This study noted that confounding was a problem in all studies, and where effects were relatively modest, residual confounding by unmeasured effects may remain. Moreover, the issue of reverse causation may also play a role. One study (Arseneault *et al.*, 2002) suggested that the risk of schizophrenia may be higher with earlier age at first cannabis use and that cannabis consumption may lead to abnormal neurodevelopment. However, such effect of age at first cannabis use has not been observed in all studies and adjustment for prior psychotic experiences in the Arseneault *et al.* (2002) study explained a quarter of the age effect.

Any increased risk of schizophrenia due to cannabis use may also be conditional on genetic vulnerability (gene–environment interaction). One study (Caspi *et al.*, 2005) observed that the risk of schizophrenia due to cannabis use was modified by the presence or absence of the valine allele at the Val158Met polymorphism of the catechol-O-methyltransferase (*COMT*) gene, which plays a role in the regulation of dopaminergic activity in the dorso-lateral prefrontal cortex and may influence the development of positive psychotic symptoms. However, this gene–environment interaction was only observed in a subset of the data and has yet to be replicated. It is likely that the links between cannabis use and the onset of psychosis are complex, and may involve a mix of causation, reverse causation, and confounding operating interactively and either simultaneously or consecutively. Further observational studies are unlikely to resolve this conundrum but, from a public health per-

spective, it is salient to remember that schizophrenia is a rare outcome and the increased risk associated with cannabis consumption may be statistically significant, but population-wise small. While there is ample evidence of harm from cannabis dependence in domains other than mental illness, which supports restricting its use (Advisory Council on the Misuse of Drugs, 2008), current evidence suggests that population-based interventions to reduce cannabis consumption may have only limited impact on preventing the occurrence of psychoses in the community. However, the complications that arise from cannabis use within clinical populations of people with schizophrenia are considerable and certainly worthy of interventions aiming to reduce harm (see Chapter 31).

Socioenvironmental factors

Socioeconomic status

Since the early report of higher rates of schizophrenia in the poorer areas of Chicago (Faris & Dunham, 1939), many studies have examined the relationships between socioeconomic status (SES) or social class and psychosis. Several studies (Hollingshead & Redlich, 1958; Dohrenwend & Dohrenwend, 1969), but not all (Goldberg & Morrison, 1963), have observed an inverse association between SES and schizophrenia, with the economically disadvantaged contributing disproportionately to the first episode admission rate for the disorder. Two explanatory hypotheses, of social causation ("breeder") and of social selection ("drift"), have been proposed (Mischler & Scotch, 1983) to account for these observations. According to the social causation theory, the socioeconomic adversity characteristic of lower class living conditions could precipitate psychosis in genetically vulnerable individuals who have a constricted capacity to cope with complex or stressful situations. In the 1960s this theory was considered refuted by a single study which found that the social class distribution of the fathers of patients with schizophrenia did not deviate from that of the general population, and that the excess of low SES among patients with schizophrenia was mainly attributable to individuals who had drifted down the occupational and social scale prior to the onset of psychosis (Goldberg & Morrison, 1963)—a tendency that has been confirmed in subsequent research (e.g., Jones *et al.*, 1993; Häfner *et al.*, 1999). There are indeed recent studies that have found evidence supporting the association between parental SES and risk of schizophrenia in offspring (e.g., Werner *et al.*, 2007), but this effect appears to be restricted to the very poorest socioeconomic groups and is typically small (Byrne *et al.*, 2004). Notably, these associations have not been observed in studies using prospectively collected longitudinal birth cohorts, which suggest that SES at birth is similar in those who do and do not go on to develop psychoses in adulthood (Jones *et al.*, 1994). It is possible that social class may only be a marker for other correlated socio-demographic factors, such as minority status or ethnicity (Bresnahan & Susser, 2003). Alternatively, SES may be important in the causation of schizophrenia in ways not anticipated by earlier theories. An example of this is the finding from the North Finland 1966 birth cohort (Mäkikirö et al., 1997) that the cumulative incidence of early-onset schizophrenia was higher among individuals whose fathers had attained status and achievement placing them into the highest social class. Upward occupational mobility in fathers was found to be associated with acculturation stress and high levels of psychopathology, which might exacerbate latent predisposition to psychosis in offspring. This, however, remains speculative and more refined research tools may be needed to tackle the issue. Part of the problem appears to be a difficulty in disentangling the effects of socioeconomic deprivation at the individual level and at the societal (ecological) level. A recent study (Werner et al., 2007) suggested that both individual SES and societal level socioeconomic deprivation at birth may independently increase the risk of schizophrenia. Some studies have been able to separate out the variance in incidence attributable to the individual and societal level. For example, van Os et al. (2000) and Kirkbride et al. (2007b) have demonstrated variance in the incidence of schizophrenia at the societal level which could not be explained by individual level factors such as age, sex, ethnicity, and marital status. Both studies found that measures which indexed individual level social isolation, such as being single or living in highly fragmented neighborhoods, were associated with an increased incidence of schizophrenia. Other studies, using ecological measures applied to neighborhoods, have shown that social fragmentation and adversity appear to increase the incidence of schizophrenia (Allardyce et al., 2005; Silver et al., 2002). Considering that societal level effects are notoriously difficult to measure, and that findings of ecological associations cannot be extrapolated to individuals, it will be important in future studies to incorporate individual level experiences of social isolation and adversity into societal level research designs.

Urban environment and schizophrenia

The 19th century hypothesis that urban environments increase the risk of psychosis (Freeman, 1994) has been revived in recent decades with numerous reports on statistical associations between the incidence of schizophrenia and urban environment, as introduced earlier. The "urban drift" phenomenon, resulting in a higher density of cases of psychosis residing in inner city areas, has been extensively documented since the 1930s (Faris & Dunham, 1939) and was mainly interpreted in socioeconomic and behavioral terms (availability of cheap accommodation, attraction of an anonymous lifestyle). In contrast, a critical distinction between urban residence and urban birth of

people with schizophrenia was introduced in the epidemiological literature by Astrup and Ødegaard (1961). More recently, Marcelis et al. (1999) analyzed by place of birth all first admissions for schizophrenia and other psychoses in The Netherlands between 1942 and 1978. Using a graded measure of urban exposure, they found a linear relationship between urban birth and moderate increases in the incidence of schizophrenia, affective psychoses, and other psychoses, with the effect size increasing in successive birth cohorts. In two studies using the Danish psychiatric case register, Mortensen et al. (1999) and Eaton et al. (2000) calculated a relative risk (RR) of 2.4–4.2 for schizophrenia prevalence in those born in the capital Copenhagen as compared with rural births. In terms of population attributable risk, urban birth accounted for 34.6% of all cases of schizophrenia in Denmark—in contrast to history of schizophrenia in a first-degree relative which, with a much higher RR of 9.3, accounted for only 5.5% of the cases in the population. A number of schizophrenia studies in the last decade, mainly in northern Europe, have reported similar associations with urban environments, so that taken at face value, "urbanicity" appears to be a fairly consistent covariate of the incidence of the disorder. However, the nature of the suspected "urban risk factor" remains cryptic and likely to be a proxy for multiple interacting factors yet to be identified. Attempts to disaggregate "urbanicity" into infectious or toxic insults on the developing brain (e.g., maternal viral infection during pregnancy), winter births, or household overcrowding facilitating the transmission of viral infections during upbringing have produced inconsistent or negative results (Murray & Lewis, 1987; Takei et al., 1995; Verdoux et al., 1997b; Mortensen et al., 1999; Agerbo et al., 2001). The possibility that the urban association may be an artifact of intergenerational rural–urban and urban–rural migration waves selectively involving individuals varying in their "load" of genes predisposing to schizophrenia has rarely been considered. A study of urban–rural variations in general health status in The Netherlands (Verheij et al., 1998) indicated that migration processes may cause in cross-sectional research spurious associations between urbanicity and health. Therefore, the existence of an independent urban risk factor for schizophrenia is yet to be demonstrated.

Migrant status and ethnicity

The exceptionally high incidence rate of schizophrenia and other psychoses in immigrant or ethnic minority groups in Western Europe is a consistently replicated, yet still controversial and challenging, finding in psychiatric epidemiology (Bhugra, 2004; Cantor-Graae & Selten, 2005; Singh & Burns, 2006). One of the earliest investigations of psychoses in immigrant populations was Ødegaard's (1932) study of Norwegian migrants to the US living in Minnesota. He demonstrated that these immigrants were twice as likely to develop schizophrenia as either native-born Americans or Norwegians in Norway, and proposed that selective migration of individuals with hereditary proneness to psychosis could account for the phenomenon.

European interest in the increase in psychoses in immigrant populations followed the influx of economic migrants to the UK and other Northern European countries since the 1950s. An early study reported increased rates of psychoses in black Caribbean migrants in the UK, compared with the native-born white British population (Hemsi, 1967). A four- to five-fold increased risk for schizophrenia in the black Caribbean group has since been replicated in a number of population-based studies (Littlewood & Lipsedge, 1981; McGovern & Cope, 1987; Harrison *et al.*, 1988; Castle *et al.*, 1991; Wessely *et al.*, 1991; Harrison *et al.*, 1996; Bhugra *et al.*, 1997; Eaton & Harrison, 2000; Fearon *et al.*, 2006). Notably, this excess morbidity is not restricted to recent immigrants and is, in fact, higher in the British-born second generation of migrants. Raised rates of psychoses have also been observed in people of black African origin in the UK (van Os *et al.*, 1996; Fearon *et al.*, 2006), but until recently the evidence regarding incidence rates in migrants from Asian populations has been inconsistent or contradictory (Bhugra *et al.*, 1997; King *et al.*, 1994). Since the Asian group is highly heterogeneous in terms of country of origin, cultures, religions, and patterns of migration, any variation in the risk of schizophrenia could have been masked by the treatment of these migrants as a single group in the literature (Bhopal *et al.*, 1991). In the largest study of schizophrenia in Asian immigrants to date, the East London First Episode Psychoses (ELFEP) project, incidence rates of schizophrenia were estimated separately for Indian, Pakistani, and Bangladeshi migrant groups. After adjustment for age and sex, the latter two ethnic groups, but not the Indian group, were found to have significantly raised rates of schizophrenia compared with the white British. Stratification by sex revealed that the effect was sex-specific, with Pakistani and Bangladeshi women having between four- and five-fold increased rates of schizophrenia compared with white British women, while incidence rates in their male counterparts did not differ from those in white British men (Kirkbride *et al.*, 2008b). Increased rates of psychoses in immigrants have also been reported from The Netherlands (Selten *et al.*, 1997, 2001; Veling *et al.*, 2006a), Denmark (Cantor-Graae *et al.*, 2003), and Sweden (Zolkowska *et al.*, 2001).

Since elevated rates of schizophrenia appear to be even more pronounced in second-generation immigrants (Harrison *et al.*, 1988, 1996; Sugarman & Craufurd, 1994; Coid *et al.*, 2008), post-migratory factors as possibly etiologically relevant have attracted attention (Cochrane & Bal, 1987). Early hypotheses proposed to explain this phenomenon have focused on sociodemographic differences; higher rates in the immigrants' country of origin; selective migration; misdiagnosis of psychotic disorders in the adoptive country; and a variety of risk exposures such as obstetric complications, substance use, and stressful life events. The possibility that immigrants may differ from the native born in terms of age and sex, being more likely younger and male, and thus at a higher risk for psychosis, has been largely discarded by studies controlling for these variables (Kirkbride *et al.*, 2006). Few studies have, thus far, adequately controlled for the confounding effects of SES, but two Swedish studies have found that a raised incidence of psychoses persisted in immigrants after adjustment for individual level SES, despite some attenuation (Hjern *et al.*, 2004; Leao *et al.*, 2006). This finding has recently been replicated in the ELFEP study in the UK (Kirkbride *et al.*, 2008b). The hypothesis that high rates of schizophrenia in the immigrants' country of origin may explain the higher rates in these groups when they moved to the UK has found no support from incidence studies conducted in Jamaica (Hickling & Rodgers-Johnson, 1995), Barbados (Mahy *et al.*, 1999), and Trinidad (Bhugra *et al.*, 1996). Each study found that the incidence of schizophrenia in the Caribbean was comparable to the incidence of schizophrenia in the white population in the UK. Other research, revisiting the selective migration hypothesis (Ødegaard, 1932), investigated whether individuals likely to eventually develop schizophrenia were more likely to migrate. An innovative research design was used to test this hypothesis on a quasi-hypothetical dataset of Surinamese immigrants to The Netherlands (Selten *et al.*, 2001, 2002). During the 1970s, more than one-third of the Surinamese population migrated to The Netherlands following political instability, and a study based on the Dutch psychiatric registry later found that these immigrants had roughly four to five times the rate of schizophrenia when compared with the native Dutch. The authors considered whether the excess of psychoses in Surinamese immigrants would remain evident under the hypothetical assumption that the entire population of Surinam, including those without a predilection to schizophrenia, had actually moved to the Netherlands. They found that the incidence of schizophrenia remained significantly higher in the Surinamese group, despite the enlarged population denominator, thus providing persuasive evidence against the selective migration hypothesis.

Little evidence has been presented for the hypothesis that a diagnostic bias may explain the excess rates of psychosis among immigrants. Misdiagnosis of cultural beliefs as psychotic experiences, or the possibility that these disorders might be better explained as acute transient psychoses or substance-induced episodes, have not found support. It seems that neither the psychopathology nor the course and outcome of these disorders presents any atypical features that would sufficiently set them apart from ICD-10 or DSM-IIIR schizophrenia (Hutchinson *et al.*, 1999; Harrison *et al.*, 1999), though one study found poor diagnostic agreement between a Jamaican and a British psychiatrist assessing the same cases (Hickling *et al.*, 1999). In this study, despite low inter-rater agreement, both psychiatrists diagnosed a similar proportion of the black Caribbean group with schizophrenia (52% *vs.* 55%), thus ruling out a "racial" bias. In more recent epidemiological studies, such as ÆSOP or ELFEP, the ethnicity of the subject is withheld from the clinical assessment panel prior to consensus diagnosis. This makes misdiagnosis an unlikely explanation (Bhugra, 2000). Furthermore, recent studies have also demonstrated that the elevated risk of psychoses for immigrants is not limited to schizophrenia but extends to the affective psychoses (Fearon *et al.*, 2006; Kirkbride *et al.*, 2008b), suggesting that immigrant groups are not more likely to receive a diagnosis of schizophrenia in preference to other diagnoses. Explanations in terms of biological risk factor exposures, such as an increased incidence of obstetric complications or maternal influenza (Hutchinson *et al.*, 1997; Selten *et al.*, 1998), have thus far found no support. Similarly, there is little evidence for substance use as a causal factor (McGuire *et al.*, 1995; Sandwijk *et al.*, 1995; Coulthard *et al.*, 2002; Veen *et al.*, 2002).

The failure of these hypotheses to explain the greater risk of psychoses for immigrants has led researchers to consider the hypothesis that psychosocial factors related to migration or the post-migratory experience are etiologically relevant. Migration itself is a major life event and may place considerable stress upon the individual. This is likely to be compounded by post-migratory experiences, including securing housing and employment, developing social relationships and networks, and understanding the norms, rules, and customs of the host culture. In a general population sample, it has been found that although the prevalence of psychotic symptoms is greater in black or ethnic minority (BME) groups, the risk of outbreak of psychosis may be explained by discrimination and stressful life events (Johns *et al.*, 2002). While the prevalence of stressful life events may be similar across ethnic groups, there is evidence that such events have a greater negative effect in ethnic minorities (Gilvarry *et al.*, 1999; Cooper *et al.*, 2008). Neighborhood-level factors such as deprivation, social fragmentation, and social capital may also have pronounced effects for migrants independent of, or interacting with, individual-level experiences, particularly given that migrants predominantly live in urban areas. Three studies, in different settings, have shown that the risk for migrants increases as they live in areas with a smaller proportion of minority residents, especially if the latter have darker skin color (Boydell *et al.*, 2001; Cantor-Graae & Selten, 2005; Veling *et al.*, 2006b; 2007; Kirkbride *et al.*, 2007b). Although psychosocial stress is a likely factor affecting migrants, there is at present no plausible mechanism linking such stress selectively to schizophrenia. Unexplored gene–environment interactions, involving various infectious, nutritional or toxic environmental factors, remain a possibility.

Childhood life events may be important in the genesis of psychoses in immigrant groups. In a study of childhood parental separation and loss in the ÆSOP study, Morgan *et al.* (2007) found that the risk for schizophrenia due to parental death or separation was similar for the white British, black Caribbean, and black African groups. However, parental separation events were almost twice as prevalent in the black Caribbean group, suggesting that this risk factor may have a greater impact in this population. Family disruption events are important as they may lead to, or be a marker for, a range of other adverse outcomes such as childhood behavior disorders, low educational achievement, and longer-term socioeconomic problems.

Other socioenvironmental factors

Several studies have considered the role of societal-level socioenvironmental factors. In an ecological study, Croudace *et al.* (2000) found a positive relationship between greater socioeconomic deprivation at the neighborhood level and predicted incidence of schizophrenia. However, this study was unable to adjust for individual-level variables which may have confounded some of this association. A recent study showed that both individual-level SES and societal-level socioeconomic deprivation at birth appear to independently increase the risk of schizophrenia (Werner *et al.*, 2007). Using similar statistical techniques, other studies have been able to separate out the variance in incidence attributable to the individual and societal level. For example, van Os *et al.* (2000) and Kirkbride *et al.* (2007b) have demonstrated variance in the incidence of schizophrenia at the societal level which cannot be explained by individual level factors such as age, sex, ethnicity, and marital status, or by societal level factors such as socioeconomic deprivation. Both studies found that measures which indexed social isolation, being single or living in highly fragmented neighborhoods, were associated with an increased incidence of schizophrenia. Other studies too have shown that social fragmentation and adversity appear to increase the incidence of schizophrenia (Allardyce *et al.*, 2005; Silver *et al.*, 2002). However, it should be noted that these societal level effects are notoriously difficult to measure. Furthermore, the current research base has largely used ecological measures applied to neighborhoods. Such findings cannot be extrapolated to individuals. It will be important for future designs to incorporate individual level experiences of social isolation and adversity into their studies.

Schizophrenia risk factors across multiple levels of causation

It is clear that the effects of socioenvironmental risk factors on the incidence of schizophrenia are complex, and it is likely that societal level effects interact with individual liability. For instance, the risk of psychosis for single persons has been shown to be increased when they live in areas with a higher proportion of married residents (van Os *et al.*, 2000). Similar effects regarding the risk of schizophrenia for BME individuals have been shown when they reside in primarily white neighborhoods (Boydell *et al.*, 2001; Kirkbride *et al.*, 2007b; Veling *et al.*, 2008). These studies all support Faris and Dunham's (1939) original assertion that social isolation is an important factor in the onset of disorder. The social isolation hypothesis may be extended into a broader hypothesis including both the social structure of the neighborhood and the notion of "social capital", which has been suggested as having a buffering effect on the risk of schizophrenia (Kirkbride *et al.*, 2007b, 2008a), though not all studies agree (Drukker *et al.*, 2006).

Prospects for epidemiology in the search for the causes of schizophrenia

After nearly a century of epidemiological research, essential questions about the nature and causes of schizophrenia still remain unanswered. Nevertheless, important insights into this complex disorder have been gained from population-based studies. Two major conclusions stand out. First, the clinical syndrome of schizophrenia is robust and can be identified reliably in diverse populations. Recent evidence, however, tends to undermine the belief that a common, single pathophysiology and common genetic predisposition are likely to explain the whole spectrum of manifestations of schizophrenia. There is now evidence to suggest that differences in incidence and disease risk can be found across populations at the global, national, and local level. Detailed study of these variations in the incidence of schizophrenia could provide novel clues to the etiology and pathogenesis of the disorder, complementary to the prospects of genetic research (McGrath & Richards, 2009). Notwithstanding the difficulties currently accompanying the genetic dissection of complex disorders, novel methods of genetic analysis will eventually reveal the complexity of the genetic architecture of schizophrenia and related disorders. Part of the solution is likely to be found in the domain of epidemiology since establishing the population frequency of both common and rare genetic variants and their associations with a variety of phenotypic expressions, including personality traits, is a prerequisite for understanding their causal role.

The second conclusion is that no single environmental risk factor of major effect on the incidence of schizophrenia has yet been discovered. Further studies using large samples are required to evaluate potential risk factors, antecedents, and predictors for which the present evidence is inconclusive. Assuming that the methodological pitfalls of risk factor epidemiology (such as the "ecological fallacy") can be avoided, and that a number of environmental variables of small to moderate effect will eventually be identified as risk factors, epidemiology will usefully complement genetic research. Current epidemiological research is making use of large existing databases, such as cumulative case registers or birth cohorts, to test hypotheses about risk factors in case-control designs. Methods and models of genetic epidemiology are increasingly being integrated within population-based studies. These trends predict an important role for epidemiology in the coming era of molecular biology of mental disorders. The complementarity between genetics and epidemiology will provide tools for unravelling the gene–environment interactions that are likely to be the key to the etiology of schizophrenia.

References

Abel, K.M. (2004) Foetal origins of schizophrenia: testable hypotheses of genetic and environmental influences. *British Journal of Psychiatry* **184**, 383–385.

Adams, W., Kendell, R.E., Hare, E.H. & Munk-Jørgensen, P. (1993) Epidemiological evidence that maternal influenza contributes to the aetiology of schizophrenia. *British Journal of Psychiatry* **163**, 522–534.

Adler, L.E. & Griffith, J.M. (1991) Concurrent medical illness in the schizophrenic patient. Epidemiology, diagnosis and management. *Schizophrenia Research* **4**, 91–107.

Advisory Council on the Misuse of Drugs (2008) *Cannabis: Classification and Public Health.* London: UK Government Home Office Report.

Agerbo, E., Torrey, E.F. & Mortensen, P.B. (2001) Household crowding in early adulthood and schizophrenia are unrelated in Denmark: A nested case-control study. *Schizophrenia Research*, **47**, 243–246.

Agerbo, E., Byrne, M., Eaton, W.W. & Mortensen, P.B. (2004) Marital and labor market status in the long run in schizophrenia. *Archives of General Psychiatry* **61**, 28–33.

Alberti K.G.M., Zummet P. & Shaw J., for the IDF Epidemiology Task Force Consensus Group (2005) The metabolic syndrome-a new worldwide definition. *Lancet* **366**, 1059–1062.

Albus, M. & Maier, W. (1995) Lack of gender differences in age at onset in familial schizophrenia. *Schizophrenia Research* **18**, 51–57.

Aleman, A., Kahn, R.S. & Selten, J.P. (2003) Sex differences in the risk of schizophrenia. Evidence from meta-analysis. *Archives of General Psychiatry* **60**, 565–571.

Alexander, R.C., Patkar, A.A., Lapointe, J.S. *et al.* (1997) Schizencephaly associated with psychosis. *Journal of Neurology, Neurosurgery and Psychiatry* **63**, 373–375.

Allardyce, J., Boydell, J., Van Os, J. *et al.* (2001) Comparison of the incidence of schizophrenia in rural Dumfries and Galloway and urban Camberwell. *British Journal of Psychiatry* **179**, 335–339.

Allardyce, J., Gilmour, H., Atkinson, J. *et al.* (2005) Social fragmentation, deprivation and urbanicity: Relation to first-admission rates for psychoses. *British Journal of Psychiatry* **187**, 401–406.

Allen, N.C., Bagade, S., McQueen, M.B. *et al.* (2008) Systematic meta-analyses and field synopsis of genetic association studies in schizophrenia: the SzGene database. *Nature Genetics* **40**, 827–834.

Andrews, G., Henderson, S. & Hall, W. (2001) Prevalence, comorbidity, disability and service utilisation. Overview of the Australian National Mental Health Survey. *British Journal of Psychiatry* **178**, 145–153.

Appleby, L., Thomas, S., Ferrier, N. *et al.* (2000) Sudden unexplained death in psychiatric in-patients. *British Journal of Psychiatry* **176**, 405–406.

Arajärvi, R., Suvisaari, J., Suokas, J. *et al.* (2005) Prevalence and diagnosis of schizophrenia based on register, case record and interview data in an isolated Finnish birth cohort born 1940–1969. *Social Psychiatry and Psychiatric Epidemiology* **40**, 808–816.

Arendt, M., Rosenberg, R., Foldager, L. *et al.* (2005) Cannabis-induced psychosis and subsequent schizophrenia-spectrum disorders: follow-up study of 535 incident cases. *British Journal of Psychiatry* **187**, 510–515.

Arseneault, L., Cannon, M., Poulton, R. *et al.* (2002) Cannabis use in adolescence and risk for adult psychosis: longitudinal prospective study. *British Medical Journal* **325**, 1212–1213.

Arseneault, L., Cannon, M., Whitten, J. & Murray R.M. (2004) Causal association between cannabis and psychosis: Examination of the evidence. *British Journal of Psychiatry* **184**, 110–117.

Astrup, C. & Ødegaard, Ø. (1961) Internal migration and mental illness in Norway. *Psychiatric Quarterly* **34**, 116–130.

Avila, M., Thaker, G. & Adami, H. (2001) Genetic epidemiology and schizophrenia: a study of reproductive fitness. *Schizophrenia Research* **47**, 233–241.

Ayuso-Mateos, J.L., Gutierrez-Recacha, P., Haro, J.M. & Chisholm, D. (2006) Estimating the prevalence of schizophrenia in Spain using a disease model. *Schizophrenia Research* **86**, 194–201.

Babidge, N.C., Buhrich, N. & Butler, T. (2001) Mortality among homeless people with schizophrenia in Sydney, Australia: a 10-year follow-up. *Acta Psychiatrica Scandinavica* **103**, 105–110.

Baker, A., Bucci, S., Lewin, T.J. *et al.* (2005) Comparisons between psychosis samples with different patterns of substance use recruited for clinical and epidemiological studies. *Psychiatry Research* **134**, 241–250.

Baldwin, J.A. (1979) Schizophrenia and physical disease. *Psychological Medicine* **9**, 611–618.

Bamrah, J.S., Freeman, H.L. & Goldberg, D.P. (1991) Epidemiology of schizophrenia in Salford, 1974–84. *British Journal of Psychiatry* **159**, 802–810.

Barak, Y., Achiron, A., Mandel, M. *et al.* (2005) Reduced cancer incidence among patients with schizophrenia. *Cancer* **104**, 2817–2821.

Barnes, T.R.E., Mutsatsa, S.H., Hutton, S.B. *et al.* (2006) Comorbid substance use and age at onset of schizophrenia. *British Journal of Psychiatry* **188**, 237–242.

Barr, C.E., Mednick, S.A. & Munk-Jorgensen, P. (1990) Exposure to influenza epidemics during gestation and adult schizophrenia. *Archives of General Psychiatry* **47**, 869–874.

Barry, H. & Barry, Jr., H. (1961) Season of birth. An epidemiological study in psychiatry. *Archives of General Psychiatry* **5**, 100–108.

Bash, K.W. & Bash-Liechti, J. (1969) Psychiatrische Epidemiologie in Iran. In: Ehrhard, H.E., ed. *Perspektiven der heutigen Psychiatrie*. Frankfurt: Gerhards, pp. 313–320.

Basu, A. & Meltzer, H.Y. (2006) Differential trends in prevalence of diabetes and unrelated general medical illness for schizophrenia patients before and after the atypical antipsychotic era. *Schizophrenia Research* **86**, 99–109.

Battle, Y.L., Martin, B.C., Dorfman, J.H. & Miller, L.S. (1999) Seasonality and infectious disease in schizophrenia: the birth hypothesis revisited. *Journal of Psychiatric Research* **33**, 501–509.

Bebbington, P. & Nayani, T. (1995) The psychosis screening questionnaire. *International Journal of Methods in Psychiatric Research* **5**, 11–19.

Bennedsen, B.E., Mortensen, P.B., Olesen, A.V. & Henriksen, T.B. (1999) Preterm birth and intra-uterine growth retardation among children of women with schizophrenia. *British Journal of Psychiatry* **175**, 239–245.

Bennedsen, B.E., Mortensen, P.B., Olesen, A.V. & Henriksen, T.B. (2001) Congenital malformations, stillbirths, and infant deaths among children of women with schizophrenia. *Archives of General Psychiatry* **58**, 674–679.

Bhopal, R.S., Phillimore, P. & Kohli, H.S. (1991) Inappropriate use of the term 'asian': An obstacle to ethnicity and health research. *Journal of Public Health Medicine* **13**, 244–246.

Bhugra, D. (2000) Migration and schizophrenia. *Acta Psychiatrica Scandinavica* **102**, 68–73.

Bhugra, D. (2004) Migration and mental health. *Acta Psychiatrica Scandinavica* **109**, 243–258.

Bhugra, D., Hilwig, M., Hossein, B. *et al.* (1996) First-contact incidence rates of schizophrenia in Trinidad and one-year follow-up. *British Journal of Psychiatry* **169**, 587–592.

Bhugra, D., Leff, J., Mallett, R. *et al.* (1997) Incidence and outcome of schizophrenia in Whites, African-Caribbeans and Asians in London. *Psychological Medicine* **27**, 791–798.

Bøjholm, S. & Strömgren, E. (1989) Prevalence of schizophrenia on the island of Bornholm in 1935 and in 1983. *Acta Psychiatrica Scandinavica* **79**, 157–166.

Böök, J.A., Wetterberg, L. & Modrzewska K. (1978) Schizophrenia in a North Swedish geographical isolate, 1900–1977: Epidemiology, genetics and biochemistry. *Clinical Genetics* **14**, 373–394.

Boydell, J., van Os, J., McKenzie, K. *et al.* (2001) Incidence of schizophrenia in ethnic minorities in London: Ecological study into interactions with environment. *British Medical Journal* **323**, 1336–1338.

Boydell, J., van Os, J., Lambri, M. *et al.* (2003) Incidence of schizophrenia in south-east London between 1965 and 1997. *British Journal of Psychiatry* **182**, 45–49.

Braff, D.L., Freedman, R., Schork, N.J. & Gottesman, I.I. (2007) Deconstructing schizophrenia: an overview of the use of endophenotypes in order to understand a complex disorder. *Schizophrenia Bulletin* **33**, 21–32.

Bremer, J. (1951) A social-psychiatric investigation of a small community in Northern Norway. *Acta Psychiatrica et Neurologica Scandinavica* **62** (Suppl.), 1–66.

Bresnahan, M. & Susser, E. (2003) Investigating socioenvironmental influences in schizophrenia: Conceptual and design issues. In: Murray, R.M., Jones, P.B., Susser E., van Os, J. & Cannon, M., eds. *The Epidemiology of Schizophrenia*. Cambridge: Cambridge University Press.

Brewin, J, Cantwell, R., Dalkin, T. *et al.* (1997) Incidence of schizophrenia in Nottingham. *British Journal of Psychiatry* **171**, 140–144.

Brodaty, H., Sachdev, P., Rose, N. *et al.* (1999) Schizophrenia with onset after age 50 years. I: Phenomenology and risk factors. *British Journal of Psychiatry* **175**, 410–415.

Brown, S., Inskip, H., & Barraclough, B. (2000) Causes of the excess mortality of schizophrenia. *British Journal of Psychiatry* **177**, 212–217.

Brown, A.S., Cohen, P., Harkavy-Friedman, J. *et al.* (2001) Prenatal rubella, premorbid abnormalities, and adult schizophrenia. *Biological Psychiatry* **49**, 473–486.

Brown, A.S., Schaefer, C.A., Wyatt, R.J. *et al.* (2002) Paternal age and risk of schizophrenia in adult offspring. *American Journal of Psychiatry* **159**, 1528–1533.

Brown A.S., Begg, M.D., Gravenstein S. *et al.* (2004) Serologic evidence of prenatal influenza in the etiology of schizophrenia. *Archives of General Psychiatry* **61**, 774–780.

Brugger, C. (1931) Versuch einer Geisteskrankenzählung in Thüringen. *Zeitschrift fur die gesamte Neurologie und Psychiatrie* **133**, 252–390.

Brugha, T.S., Nienhuis, F., Bagchi, D. *et al.* (1999) The survey form of SCAN: The feasibility of using experienced lay survey interviewers to administer a semi-structured systematic clinical assessment of psychotic and non-psychotic disorders. *Psychological Medicine* **29**, 703–711.

Bulayeva, K.B., Leal, S.M., Pavlova, T.A. *et al.* (2005) Mapping genes of complex psychiatric diseases in Daghestan genetic isolates. *American Journal of Medical Genetics Part B (Neuropsychiatric Genetics)* **132B**, 76–84.

Byrne, M., Agerbo, E., Ewald, H. *et al.* (2003) Parental age and risk of schizophrenia. *Archives of General Psychiatry* **60**, 673–678.

Byrne, M., Agerbo, E., Eaton, W.W. & Mortensen, P.B. (2004) Parental socio-economic status and risk of first admission with schizophrenia: A Danish national register based study. *Social Psychiatry and Psychiatric Epidemiology* **39**, 87–96.

Byrne, M., Agerbo, E., Bennedsen, B. *et al.* (2007) Obstetric conditions and risk of first admission with schizophrenia: a Danish national register based study. *Schizophrenia Research* **97**, 51–59.

Caldwell, C.B. & Gottesman, I.I. (1990) Schizophrenics kill themselves too: A review of risk factors for suicide. *Schizophrenia Bulletin* **16**, 571–589.

Cannon, M., Cotter, D., Coffey, V.P. *et al.* (1996) Prenatal exposure to the 1957 influenza epidemic and adult schizophrenia: A follow-up study. *British Journal of Psychiatry* **168**, 368–371.

Cannon, T.D., Rosso, I.M., Hollister, J.M. *et al.* (2000) A prospective cohort study of genetic and perinatal influences in the etiology of schizophrenia. *Schizophrenia Bulletin* **26**, 351–366.

Cannon, M., Jones, P.B. & Murray, R.M. (2002a) Obstetric complications and schizophrenia: historical and meta-analytic review. *American Journal of Psychiatry* **159**, 1080–1092.

Cannon, M., Caspi, A., Moffitt, T.E. *et al.* (2002b) Evidence for early-childhood, pan-developmental impairment specific to schizophreniform disorder. Results from a longitudinal birth cohort. *Archives of General Psychiatry* **59**, 449–456.

Cantor-Graae, E. & Selten, J.-P. (2005) Schizophrenia and migration: A meta-analysis and review. *American Journal of Psychiatry* **162**, 12–24.

Cantor-Graae, E., Cardenal, S., Ismail, B. & McNeil, T.F. (1998) Recall of obstetric events by mothers of schizophrenic patients. *Psychological Medicine* **28**, 1239–1243.

Cantor-Graae, E., Pedersen, C.B., McNeil, T.F. & Mortensen, P.B. (2003) Migration as a risk factor for schizophrenia: A Danish population-based cohort study. *British Journal of Psychiatry* **182**, 117–122.

Cardno, A.G., Marshall, E.J., Coid, B. *et al.* (1999) Heritability estimates for psychotic disorders: The Maudsley twin psychosis series. *Archives of General Psychiatry* **56**, 162–168.

Caspi, A., Reichenberg, A., Weiser, M. *et al.* (2003) Cognitive performance in schizophrenia patients assessed before and following the first psychotic episode. *Schizophrenia Research* **65**, 87–94.

Caspi, A., Moffitt, T. E., Cannon, M. *et al.* (2005) Moderation of the effect of adolescent-onset cannabis use on adult psychosis by a functional polymorphism in the catechol-O-methyltransferase gene: Longitudinal evidence of a gene x environment interaction. *Biological Psychiatry* **57**, 1117–1127.

Castle, D., Wessely, S., Der, G. & Murray, R.M. (1991) The incidence of operationally defined schizophrenia in Camberwell, 1965-84. *British Journal of Psychiatry* **159**, 790–794.

Chwastiak, L.A. & Tek, C. (2009) The unchanging mortality gap for people with schizophrenia. *Lancet* **374**, 590–592.

Clarke, M.C., Harley, M. & Cannon, M. (2006) The role of obstetric events in schizophrenia. *Schizophrenia Bulletin* **32**, 3–8.

Cochrane, R. & Bal, S.S. (1987) Migration and schizophrenia: An examination of five hypotheses. *Social Psychiatry and Psychiatric Epidemiology* **22**, 181–191.

Coid, J.W., Kirkbride, J.B., Barker, D. *et al.* (2008) Raised incidence of all psychoses among migrant groups: Findings from the East London First Episode Psychosis Study. *Archives of General Psychiatry* **65**, 1250–1258.

Cooper, J.E., Kendell, R.E., Gurland, B.J. *et al.* (1972) *Psychiatric Diagnosis in New York and London*. London: Oxford University Press.

Cooper, J.E., Goodhead, D., Craig, T. *et al.* (1987) The incidence of schizophrenia in Nottingham. *British Journal of Psychiatry* **151**, 619–626.

Cooper, C., Morgan, C., Byrne, M. *et al.* (2008) Perceptions of disadvantage, ethnicity and psychosis. *British Journal of Psychiatry* **192**, 185–190.

Coulthard, M., Farrell, M., Singleton, N. & Meltzer, H. (2002) *Tobacco, Alcohol and Drug Use and Mental Health*. London: HMSO.

Crimlisk, H.L. (1997) The little imitator-porphyria: A neuropsychiatric disorder. *Journal of Neurology, Neurosurgery and Psychiatry* **62**, 319–328.

Crocetti, G.J., Lemkau, P.V., Kulcar, Z. & Kesic, B. (1971) Selected aspect of the epidemiology of psychoses in Croatia, Yugoslavia. II. The cluster sample and the results of the pilot survey. *American Journal of Epidemiology* **94**, 126–134.

Croudace, T.J., Kayne, R., Jones, P.B. & Harrison, G.L. (2000) Non-linear relationship between an index of social deprivation, psychiatric admission prevalence and the incidence of psychosis. *Psychological Medicine* **30**, 177–185.

Crow, T.J. & Done, D.J. (1992) Prenatal exposure to influenza does not cause schizophrenia. *British Journal of Psychiatry* **161**, 390–393.

Dalton, S.O., Laursen, T.M., Mellemkjær, L. *et al.* (2004) Risk for cancer in parents of patients with schizophrenia. *American Journal of Psychiatry* **161**, 903–908.

Dalton, S.O., Mellemkjær, L., Thomassen, L., Mortensen, P.B. & Johansen, C. (2005) Risk for cancer in a cohort of patients hospitalized for schizophrenia in Denmark, 1969–1993. *Schizophrenia Research* **75**, 315–324.

Dalton S.O., Johansen C., Poulsen A.H. *et al.* (2006) Cancer risk among users of neuroleptic medication: a population-based cohort study. *British Journal of Cancer* **95**, 934–949.

David, A.S., Malmberg, A., Brandt, L., Allebeck, P. & Lewis, G. (1997) IQ and risk for schizophrenia: A population-based cohort study. *Psychological Medicine* **27**, 1311–1323.

Davidson, M., Reichenberg, A., Rabinowitz, J. *et al.* (1999) Behavioral and intellectual markers for schizophrenia in apparently healthy male adolescents. *American Journal of Psychiatry* **156**, 1328–1335.

Davies, G., Welham, J., Chant, D., Torrey, E.F. & McGrath, J. (2003) A systematic review and meta-analysis of northern hemisphere season of birth studies in schizophrenia. *Schizophrenia Bulletin* **29**, 587–593.

De Hert, M.A., van Winkel, R., Van Eyck, D. *et al.* (2006) Prevalence of the metabolic syndrome in patients with schizophrenia treated with antipsychotic medication. *Schizophrenia Research* **83**, 87–93.

Der, G., Gupta, S. & Murray, R.M. (1990) Is schizophrenia disappearing? *Lancet* **335**, 513–516.

Dixon, L., Weiden, P., Delahanty, J. *et al.* (2000) Prevalence and correlates of diabetes in national schizophrenia samples. *Schizophrenia Bulletin* **26**, 903–912.

Dohrenwend, B.P. & Dohrenwend, B.S. (1969) *Social Status and Psychological Disorder: A Causal Inquiry.* New York: John Wiley & Sons.

Done, D.J., Crow, T.J., Johnstone, E.C. & Sacker, A. (1994) Childhood antecedents of schizophrenia and affective illness: Social adjustment at ages 7 and 11. *British Medical Journal* **309**, 699–703.

Doody, G.A., Johnstone, E.C., Sanderson, T.L. *et al.* (1998) 'Pfropfschizophrenie' revisited. Schizophrenia in people with mild learning disability. *British Journal of Psychiatry* **173**, 145–153.

Drukker, M., Krabbendam, L., Driessen, G. & van Os, J. (2006) Social disadvantage and schizophrenia: A combined neighbourhood and individual-level analysis. *Social Psychiatry and Psychiatric Epidemiology* **41**, 595–604.

Dube, K.C. & Kumar, N. (1972) An epidemiological study of schizophrenia. *Journal of Biosocial Science* **4**, 187–195.

Dupont, A., Jensen, O.M., Strömgren, E. & Jablensky, A. (1986) Incidence of cancer in patients diagnosed as schizophrenic in Denmark. In: Horn, S.H., Giel, R. & Gulbinat, W., eds. *Psychiatric Case Registers in Public Health.* Amsterdam: Elsevier.

Eagles, J.M., Hunter, D. & McCance, C. (1988) Decline in the diagnosis of schizophrenia among first contacts with psychiatric services in North-East Scotland, 1969–1984. *British Journal of Psychiatry* **152**, 793–798.

Eaton, W.W. (1974) Residence, social class, and schizophrenia. *Journal of Health and Social Behavior* **15**, 289–299.

Eaton, J.W. & Weil, R.Y. (1955) *Culture and Mental Disorders.* Glencoe, IL: Free Press.

Eaton, W. & Harrison, G. (2000) Ethnic disadvantage and schizophrenia. *Acta Psychiatrica Scandinavica* **102**, 38–43.

Eaton, W.W., Romanoski, A., Anthony, J.C. & Nestadt, G. (1991) Screening for psychosis in the general population with a self-report interview. *Journal of Nervous and Mental Disease* **179**, 689–693.

Eaton, W.W., Hayward, C. & Ram, R. (1992) Schizophrenia and rheumatoid arthritis: A review. *Schizophrenia Research* **6**, 181–192.

Eaton, W.W., Mortensen, P.B. & Frydenberg, M. (2000) Obstetric factors, urbanization and psychosis. *Schizophrenia Research* **43**, 117–123.

Elder, A.G., O'Donnell, B., McCruden, E.A.B. *et al.* (1996) Incidence and recall of influenza in a cohort of Glasgow healthcare workers during the 1993-4 epidemic: Results of serum testing and questionnaire. *British Medical Journal* **313**, 1241–1242.

El-Saadi O., Pedersen C.B., McNeil T. *et al.* (2004) Paternal and maternal age as risk factors for psychosis: findings from Denmark, Sweden and Australia. *Schizophrenia Research* **67**, 227–236.

Erlenmeyer-Kimling, L., Rock, D., Squires-Wheeler, E. *et al.* (1991) Early life precursors of psychiatric outcomes in adulthood of subjects at risk for schizophrenia or affective disorders. *Psychiatry Research* **39**, 239–256.

Erlenmeyer-Kimling, L., Adamo, U.H., Rock, D. *et al.* (1997) The New York high-risk project. Prevalence and comorbidity of axis I disorders in offspring of schizophrenic patients at 25-year follow-up. *Archives of General Psychiatry* **54**, 1096–1102.

Essen-Möller, E. (1935) Untersuchungen über die Fruchtbarkeit gewisser gruppen von Geisteskranken. *Acta Psychiatrica et Neurologica Scandinavica* **8** (Suppl.).

Essen-Möller, E., Larsson, H., Uddenberg, C.E. & White, G. (1956) Individual traits and morbidity in a Swedish rural population. *Acta Psychiatrica et Neurologica Scandinavica* **100** (Suppl.).

Faňanás, L. & Bertranpetit, J. (1995) Reproductive rates in families of schizophrenic patients in a case-control study. *Acta Psychiatrica Scandinavica* **91**, 202–204.

Faris, R.E.L. & Dunham, H.W. (1939) *Mental Disorders in Urban Areas.* Chicago: University of Chicago Press.

Fatemi, S.H., Reutiman, T.J., Folsom, T.D. *et al.* (2008) Maternal infection leads to abnormal gene regulation and brain atrophy in mouse offspring: Implications for genesis of neurodevelopmental disorders. *Schizophrenia Research* **99**, 56–70.

Fearon, P., Kirkbride, J.B., Morgan, V. *et al.* (2006) Incidence of schizophrenia and other psychoses in ethnic minority groups: Results from the MRC AESOP Study. *Psychological Medicine* **36**, 1541–1550.

Fish, B. (1977) Neurobiologic antecedents of schizophrenia in children: Evidence for an inherited, congenital neurointegrative defect. *Archives of General Psychiatry* **34**, 1297–1313.

Fish, B. & Kendler, K.S. (2005) Abnormal infant neurodevelopment predicts schizophrenia spectrum disorders. *Journal of Child and Adolescent Psychopharmacology* **15**, 348–361.

Fish, B., Marcus, J., Hans, S.L., Auerbach, J.G. & Perdue, S. (1992) Infants at risk for schizophrenia: Sequelae of a genetic neurointegrative defect. *Archives of General Psychiatry* **49**, 221–235.

Flint, J. & Goldstein, L.H. (1992) Familial calcification of the basal ganglia: A case report and review of the literature. *Psychological Medicine* **22**, 581–595.

Francis, A. & Freeman, H. (1984) Psychiatric abnormality and brain calcification over four generations. *Journal of Nervous and Mental Disease* **172**, 166–170.

Freeman, H. (1994) Schizophrenia and city residence. *British Journal of Psychiatry* **164** (Suppl. 23), 39–50.

Fremming, K.H. (1947) *Sygdomsrisikoen for sindslidelser og andre sjaelige abnormtilstande i den Danske gennemshitbefolkning. Paa grundlag af en katamnestisk underøgelsse af 5500 personer født i 1883–87.* Copenhagen: Munksgaard.

Gaitatzis, A., Trimble, M.R. & Sander, J.W. (2004) The psychiatric comorbidity of epilepsy. *Acta Neurologica Scandinavica* **110**, 207–220.

Gangadhar, B.N., Selvan, C.P., Subbakrishna, D.K. *et al.* (2002) Age-at-onset and schizophrenia: reversed gender effect. *Acta Psychiatrica Scandinavica* **105**, 317–319.

Geddes, J.R. & Kendell, R.E. (1995) Schizophrenic subjects with no history of admission to hospital. *Psychological Medicine* **25**, 859–868.

Geddes, J.R. & Juszczak, E. (1995) Period trends in rate of suicide in first 28 days after discharge from psychiatric hospital in Scotland, 1968–92. *British Medical Journal* **311**, 357–360.

Geddes, J.R. & Lawrie, S.M. (1995) Obstetric complications and schizophrenia: A meta-analysis. *British Journal of Psychiatry* **167**, 786–793.

Giggs, J.A. (1973) Distribution of schizophrenics in Nottingham. *Transactions of the Institute of British Geographers* **59**, 5–76.

Giggs, J.A. (1986) Mental disorders and ecological structure in Nottingham. *Social Science and Medicine* **23**, 945–961.

Giggs, J.A. & Cooper, J.E. (1987) Ecological structure and the distribution of schizophrenia and affective psychoses in Nottingham. *British Journal of Psychiatry* **151**, 627–633.

Gilvarry, C.M., Walsh, E., Samele, C. *et al.* (1999) Life events, ethnicity and perceptions of discrimination in patients with severe mental illness. *Social Psychiatry and Psychiatric Epidemiology* **34**, 600–608.

Goff, D.C., Sullivan, L.M., McEvoy, J.P. *et al.* (2005) A comparison of ten-year cardiac risk estimates in schizophrenia patients from the CATIE study and matched controls. *Schizophrenia Research* **80**, 45–53.

Goldberg, E.M. & Morrison, S.L. (1963) Schizophrenia and social class. *British Journal of Psychiatry* **109**, 785–802.

Goldner, E.M., Hsu, L., Waraich, P. & Somers, J.M. (2002) Prevalence and incidence studies of schizophrenic disorders: a systematic review of the literature. *Canadian Journal of Psychiatry* **47**, 833–843.

Goldstein, M. (1987) The UCLA high-risk project. *Schizophrenia Bulletin* **13**, 505–514.

Gorwood, P., Pouchot, J., Vinceneux, P. *et al.* (2004) Rheumatoid arthritis and schizophrenia: a negative association at a dimensional level. *Schizophrenia Research* **66**, 21–29.

Gottesman, I.I. & Gould, T.D. (2003) The endophenotype concept in psychiatry: etymology and strategic intentions. *American Journal of Psychiatry* **160**, 636–645.

Gottesman, I.I., McGuffin, P. & Farmer, A.E. (1987) Clinical genetics as clues to the "real" genetics of schizophrenia (a decade of modest gains while playing for time). *Schizophrenia Bulletin* **13**, 23–47.

Grech, A., Takei, N. & Murray, R.M. (1997) Maternal exposure to influenza and paranoid schizophrenia. *Schizophrenia Research* **26**, 121–125.

Green, B., Young, R. & Kavanagh, D. (2005) Cannabis use and misuse prevalence among people with psychosis. *British Journal of Psychiatry* **187**, 306–313.

Greenwood, C.M.T., Husted, J., Bomba, M.D. *et al.* (2004) Elevated rates of schizophrenia in a familial sample with mental illness and intellectual disability. *Journal of Intellectual Disability Research* **48**, 531–539.

Gunnell, D., Harrison, G. Rasmussen, F. *et al.* (2002) Associations between premorbid intellectual performance, early-life exposures and early-onset schizophrenia. *British Journal of Psychiatry* **181**, 298–305.

Gupta, S., Masand, P.S., Kaplan, D., Bhandary, A. & Hendricks, S. (1997) The relationship between schizophrenia and irritable bowel syndrome (IBS). *Schizophrenia Research* **23**, 265–268.

Hagnell, O. (1966) *A Prospective Study of the Incidence of Mental Disorder.* Lund: Svenska Bokforlaget.

Häfner, H. (2003) Gender differences in schizophrenia. *Psychoneuroendocrinology* **28**, 17–54.

Häfner, H. & Reimann, H. (1970) Spatial distribution of mental disorders in Mannheim, 1965. In: Hare, E.H. & Wing, J.K., eds. *Psychiatric Epidemiology.* London: Oxford University Press, pp. 341–354.

Häfner, H., Maurer, K., Löffler, W. & Riecher-Rössler, A. (1993) The influence of age and sex on the onset and early course of schizophrenia. *British Journal of Psychiatry* **162**, 80–86.

Häfner, H., Löffler, W., Maurer *et al.* (1999) Depression, negative symptoms, social stagnation and social decline in the early course of schizophrenia. *Acta Psychiatrica Scandinavica* **100**, 105–118.

Häfner, H., Löffler, W., Riecher-Rössler, A. & Häfner-Ranabauer, W. (2001) Schizophrenie und Wahn im höheren und hohen Lebensalter. *Nervenarzt* **72**, 347–357.

Hagnell, O. (1966b) *A Prospective Study of the Incidence of Mental Disorder.* Lund: Svenska Bokforlaget.

Hare, E. (1983) Was insanity on the increase? *British Journal of Psychiatry* **142**, 439–445.

Harrison, G., Owens, D., Holton, A. *et al.* (1988) A prospective study of severe mental disorder in Afro-Caribbean patients. *Psychological Medicine* **18**, 643–657.

Harrison, G., Cooper, J.E. & Gancarczyk, R. (1991) Changes in the administrative incidence of schizophrenia. *British Journal of Psychiatry* **159**, 811–816.

Harrison, G., Brewin, J., Cantwell, R. *et al.* (1996) The increased risk of psychosis in African-Caribbean migrants to the UK: A replication. *Schizophrenia Research* **18**, 102.

Harrison, G., Amin, S., Singh, S. *et al.* (1999) Outcome of psychosis in people of African-Caribbean family origin. *British Journal of Psychiatry* **175**, 43–49.

Harrison, G., Fouskakis, D., Rasmussen, F. *et al.* (2003) Association between psychotic disorder and urban place of birth is not mediated by obstetric complications or childhood socio-economic position: A cohort study. *Psychological Medicine* **33**, 723–731.

Haslam, J. (1809) *Observations on madness and melancholy*, 2nd edn. London: Callow.

Hassiotis, A., Ukoumunne, O., Tyrer, P. *et al.* (1999) Prevalence and characteristics of patients with severe mental illness and borderline intellectual functioning. *British Journal of Psychiatry* **175**, 135–140.

Hatta, K., Takahashi, T., Nakamura, H. *et al.* (1999) Laboratory findings in acute schizophrenia. *General Hospital Psychiatry* **21**, 220–227.

Haukka, J., Suvisaari, J, Varilo, T. & Lönnqvist, J. (2001) Regional variation in the incidence of schizophrenia in Finland: a study of birth cohorts born from 1950 to 1969. *Psychological Medicine* **31**, 1045–1053.

Haukka, J., Suvisaari, J. & Lönnqvist, J. (2003) Fertility of patients with schizophrenia, their siblings, and the general population: A cohort study from 1950 to 1959 in Finland. *American Journal of Psychiatry* **160**, 460–463.

Hawton, K., Sutton, L. Haw, C. *et al.* (2005) Schizophrenia and suicide: systematic review of risk factors. *British Journal of Psychiatry* **187**, 9–10.

Heilä, H., Haukka, J., Suvisaari, J. & Lönnqvist, J. (2005) Mortality among patients with schizophrenia and reduced psychiatric hospital care. *Psychological Medicine* **35**, 725–732.

Helgason, T. (1964) Epidemiology of mental disorders in Iceland. *Acta Psychiatrica Scandinavica* **173** (Suppl.).

Helgason, T. & Magnusson, H. (1989) The first 80 years of life. A psychiatric epidemiological study. *Acta Psychiatrica Scandinavica* **79** (Suppl. 348), 85–94.

Hemsi, L.K. (1967) Psychiatric morbidity of West Indian immigrants. *Social Psychiatry* **2**, 95–100.

Henquet, C., Murray, R., Linszen, D. & van Os, J. (2005) The environment and schizophrenia: the role of cannabis use. *Schizophrenia Bulletin* **31**, 608–612.

Hickling, F.W. & Rodgers-Johnson, P. (1995) The incidence of first contact schizophrenia in Jamaica. *British Journal of Psychiatry* **167**, 193–196.

Hickling, F.W., McKenzie, K., Mullen, R. & Murray, R. (1999) A Jamaican psychiatrist evaluates diagnoses at a London psychiatric hospital. *British Journal of Psychiatry* **175**, 283–285.

Hickman M., Vuckerman P., Macleod J. *et al.* (2007) Cannabis and schizophrenia: model projections of the impact of the rise in cannabis use on historical and future trends in schizophrenia in England and Wales. *Addiction* **102**, 597–606.

Hilger, T., Propping, P. & Haverkamp, F. (1983) Is there an increase of reproductive rates in schizophrenics? *Archiv für Psychiatrie und Nervenkrankheiten* **233**, 177–186.

Hippisley-Cox, J., Vinogradova, Y., Coupland, C. & Parker, C. (2007) Risk of malignancy in patients with schizophrenia or bipolar disorder. Nested case-control study. *Archives of General Psychiatry* **64**, 1368–1376.

Hiroeh, U., Appleby, L., Mortensen, P.B. & Dunn, G. (2001) Death by homicide, suicide, and other unnatural causes in people with mental illness: a population-based study. *Lancet* **358**, 2110–2112.

Hjern, A., Wicks, S. & Dalman, C. (2004) Social adversity contributes to high morbidity in psychoses in immigrants -a national cohort study of two generations of Swedish residents. *Psychological Medicine* **34**, 1025–1033.

Hochman, K.M. & Lewine, R.R. (2004) Age of menarche and schizophrenia onset in women. *Schizophrenia Research* **69**, 183–188.

Hoek, H.W., Susser, E., Buck, K.A. *et al.* (1996) Schizoid personality disorder after prenatal exposure to famine. *American Journal of Psychiatry* **153**, 1637–1639.

Hofvander, B., Delorme, R., Chaste, P. *et al.* (2009) Psychiatric and psychosocial problems in adults with normal-intelligence autism spectrum disorders. *BMC Psychiatry* **9**, 35.

Hollingshead, A.B. & Redlich, F.C. (1958) *Social Class and Mental Illness*. New York: Wiley.

Honer, W.G., Kopala, L.C., Locke, J.J. & Lapointe, J.S. (1996) Left cerebral hemiatrophy and schizophrenia-like psychosis in an adolescent. *Schizophrenia Research* **20**, 231–234.

Hovatta, I., Varilo, T., Suvisaari, J. *et al.* (1999) A genomewide screen for schizophrenia genes in an isolated Finnish sub-population, suggesting multiple susceptibility loci. *American Journal of Human Genetics* **65**, 1114–1124.

Hultman, C.M., Sparén, P., Takei, N. *et al.* (1999) Prenatal and perinatal risk factors for schizophrenia, affective psychosis, and reactive psychosis of early onset: Case-control study. *British Medical Journal* **318**, 421–426.

Hutchinson, G., Takei, N., Bhugra, D. *et al.* (1997) Increased rate of psychosis among African-Caribbeans in Britain is not due to an excess of pregnancy and birth complications. *British Journal of Psychiatry* **171**, 145–147.

Hutchinson, G., Takei, N., Sham, P. *et al.* (1999) Factor analysis of symptoms in schizophrenia: Differences between White and Caribbean patients in Camberwell. *Psychological Medicine* **29**, 607–612.

Hyde, T.M., Ziegler, J.C. & Weinberger, D.R. (1992) Psychiatric disturbances in metachromatic leukodystrophy. *Archives of Neurology* **49**, 401–406.

Ichiki, M., Kunugi, H., Takei, N. *et al.* (2000) Intra-uterine physical growth in schizophrenia: Evidence confirming excess of premature birth. *Psychological Medicine* **30**, 597–604.

Imamura, Y., Nakane, Y., Ohta, Y. & Kondo, H. (1999) Lifetime prevalence of schizophrenia among individuals prenatally exposed to atomic bomb radiation in Nagasaki City. *Acta Psychiatrica Scandinavica* **100**, 344–349.

Indian Council of Mental Research (1988) *Multi-Centered Collaborative Study of Factors Associated with Course and Outcome of Schizophrenia*. New Delhi: ICMR.

Isohanni, M., Jones, P. B., Moilanen, K. *et al.* (2001) Early developmental milestones in adult schizophrenia and other psychoses. A 31-year follow-up of the Northern Finland 1966 Birth Cohort. *Schizophrenia Research* **52**, 1–19.

Isohanni, M., Miettunen, J., Mäki, P. *et al.* (2006) Risk factors for schizophrenia. Follow-up data from the Northern Finland Birth Cohort Study. *World Psychiatry* **5**, 168–171.

Jablensky, A. (1986) Epidemiology of schizophrenia: A European perspective. *Schizophrenia Bulletin* **12**, 52–73.

Jablensky, A. & Cole, S.W. (1997) Is the earlier age at onset of schizophrenia in males a confounded finding? Results from a cross-cultural investigation. *British Journal of Psychiatry* **170**, 234–240.

Jablensky, A. & Kalaydjieva, L. (2003) Genetic epidemiology of schizophrenia: phenotypes, risk factors and reproductive behavior. Editorial. *American Journal of Psychiatry* **160**, 425–429.

Jablensky, A., Sartorius, N., Ernberg, G. *et al.* (1992) Schizophrenia: Manifestations, incidence and course in different cultures. A World Health Organization Ten-Country Study. *Psychological Medicine* Monograph **20** (Suppl), 1–97.

Jablensky, A., Hugler, H., von Cranach, M. & Kalinov, K. (1993) Kraepelin revisited: A reassessment and statistical analysis of dementia praecox and manic-depressive insanity in 1908. *Psychological Medicine* **23**, 843–858.

Jablensky, A., McGrath, J., Herrman, H. *et al.* (2000) Psychotic disorders in urban areas: An overview of the Study of Low Prevalence Disorders. *Australian and New Zealand Journal of Psychiatry* **34**, 221–236.

Jablensky, A., Morgan, V., Zubrick, S.R. *et al.* (2005) Pregnancy, delivery, and neonatal complications in a population cohort of women with schizophrenia and major affective disorders. *American Journal of Psychiatry* **162**, 79–91.

Jarman, B., Hirsch, S., White, P. & Driscoll, R. (1992) Predicting psychiatric admission rates. *British Medical Journal* **304**, 1146–1151.

Jeffreys, S.E., Harvey, C.A., McNaught, A.S. *et al.* (1997) The Hampstead Schizophrenia Survey 1991. I. Prevalence and service use comparisons in an inner London health authority, 1986–91. *British Journal of Psychiatry* **170**, 301–306.

Jeste, D.V., Gladsjo, J.A., Lindamer, L.A. & Lacro, J.P. (1996) Medical comorbidity in schizophrenia. *Schizophrenia Bulletin* **22**, 413–430.

John, A.P., Koloth, R., Dragovic, M. & Lim, S.C.B. (2009) Prevalence of metabolic syndrome among Australians with severe mental illness. *The Medical Journal of Australia* **190**, 176–179.

Johns, L.C., Nazroo, J.Y., Bebbington, P. & Kuipers, E. (2002) Occurrence of hallucinatory experiences in a community sample and ethnic variations. *British Journal of Psychiatry* **180**, 174–178.

Johnstone E.C., Ebmeier K.P., Miller P. *et al.* (2005) Predicting schizophrenia: findings from the Edinburgh High-Risk Study. *British Journal of Psychiatry* **186**, 18–25.

Jones, P.B., Bebbington, P., Foerster, A. *et al.* (1993) Premorbid social underachievement in schizophrenia. Results from the Camberwell Collaborative Psychosis Study. *British Journal of Psychiatry* **162**, 65–71.

Jones, P., Rodgers, B., Murray, R. & Marmot, M. (1994) Child developmental risk factors for adult schizophrenia in the British 1946 birth cohort. *Lancet* **344**, 1398–1402.

Jones, P.B., Rantakallio, P., Hartikainen, A.L. *et al.* (1998) Schizophrenia as a long-term outcome of pregnancy, delivery, and perinatal complications: A 28-year follow-up of the 1966 North Finland general population birth cohort. *American Journal of Psychiatry* **155**, 355–364.

Jönsson, S.A.T. & Jonsson, H. (1992) Outcome in untreated schizophrenia: a search for symptoms and traits with prognostic meaning in patients admitted to a mental hospital in the preneuroleptic era. *Acta Psychaitrica Scandinavica* **85**, 313–320.

Joukamaa, M., Heliövaara, M., Knekt, P. *et al.* (2006) Schizophrenia, neuroleptic medication and mortality. *British Journal of Psychiatry* **188**, 122–127.

Joyce, P.R. (1987) Changing trends in first admissions and readmissions for mania and schizophrenia in New Zealand, 1974 to 1984. *Australian and New Zealand Journal of Psychiatry* **21**, 82–86.

Jung, A., Schuppe H.C. & Schill, W.B. (2003) Are children of older fathers at risk for genetic disorders? *Andrologia* **35**, 191–199.

Karvonen, M., Viik-Kajander, M., Moltchanova, E. *et al.* (2000) Incidence of childhood type 1 diabetes worldwide. *Diabetes Care* **23**, 1516–1526.

Kavanagh, D.J., Waghorn, G., Jenner, L. *et al.* (2004) Demographic and clinical correlates of comorbid substance use disorders in psychosis: multivariate analyses from an epidemiological sample. *Schizophrenia Research* **66**, 115–124.

Kebede, D. & Alem, A. (1999) Major mental disorders in Adis Ababa, Ethiopia. I. Schizophrenia, schizoaffective and cognitive disorders. *Acta Psychiatrica Scandinavica* **100**, 11–17.

Kendell, R.E. & Adams, W. (1991) Unexplained fluctuations in the risk for schizophrenia by month and year of birth. *British Journal of Psychiatry* **158**, 758–763.

Kendell, R.E., McInneny, K., Juszczak, E. & Bain, M. (2000) Obstetric complications and schizophrenia. Two case-control studies based on structured obstetric records. *British Journal of Psychiatry* **176**, 516–522.

Kendell, R.E., Boyd, J.H., Grossmith, V.L. & Bain M. (2002) Seasonal fluctuation in birthweight in schizophrenia. *Schizophrenia Research* **57**, 157–164.

Kendler, K.S. & Eaves, L.J. (1986) Models for the joint effect of genotype and environment on liability to psychiatric illness. *American Journal of Psychiatry* **143**, 279–289.

Kendler, K.S. & Walsh, D. (1995) Gender and schizophrenia: results of an epidemiologically based family study. *British Journal of Psychiatry* **167**, 184–192.

Kendler, K.S., Karkowski-Shuman, L. & Walsh, D. (1996) Age at onset in schizophrenia and risk of illness in relatives. *British Journal of Psychiatry* **169**, 213–218.

Kessler, R.C., McGonagle, K.A., Zhao, S. *et al.* (1994) Lifetime and 12-month prevalence of DSM-IIIR psychiatric disorders in the United States. *Archives of General Psychiatry* **51**, 8–19.

Khoury, M.J., Beaty, T.H. & Cohen, B.H. (1993) *Fundamentals of Genetic Epidemiology*. New York: Oxford University Press.

Kim, J.J., Shirts, B.H., Dayal, M. *et al.* (2007) Are exposure to cytomegalovirus and genetic variation on chromosome 6p joint risk factors for schizophrenia? *Annals of Medicine* **39**, 145–153.

King, M., Coker, E., Leavey, G., Hoare, A. & Johnson-Sabine, E. (1994) Incidence of psychotic illness in London: Comparison of ethnic groups. *British Medical Journal* **309**, 1115–1119.

Kinney, D.K., Teixeira, P., Hsu, D. *et al.* (2009) Relation of schizophrenia prevalence to latitude, fish consumption, infant mortality, and skin color: A role for prenatal vitamin D deficiency and infections? *Schizophrenia Bulletin* **35**, 582–595.

Kirkbride, J.B., Fearon, P., Morgan, C. *et al.* (2006) Heterogeneity in incidence rates of schizophrenia and other psychotic syndromes: Findings From the 3-center ÆSOP study. *Archives of General Psychiatry* **63**, 250–258.

Kirkbride, J.B., Fearon, P., Morgan, C. *et al.* (2007a) Neighbourhood variation in the incidence of psychotic disorders in Southeast London. *Social Psychiatry and Psychiatric Epidemiology* **42**, 438–445.

Kirkbride, J.B., Morgan, C., Fearon, P. *et al.* (2007b) Neighbourhood-level effects on psychoses: Re-examining the role of context. *Psychological Medicine* **37**, 1413–1425.

Kirkbride, J., Boydell, J., Ploubidis, G., *et al.* (2008a) Testing the association between the incidence of schizophrenia and social capital in an urban area. *Psychological Medicine* **38**, 1083–1094.

Kirkbride, J.B., Barker, D., Cowden F. *et al.* (2008b) Psychoses, ethnicity and socioeconomic status. *British Journal of Psychiatry* **193**, 18–24.

Klemperer, J. (1933) Zur Belastungsstatistik der Durchschnittsbevölkerung. Psychosehäufigkeit unter 1000 stichprobemässig ausgelesenen Probanden. *Zeitschrift für die gesamte Neurologie und Psychiatrie* **146**, 277–316.

Kraepelin, E. (1919) *Dementia Praecox and Paraphrenia*. Edinburgh: Livingstone.

Krebs, M.O., Leroy, S., Duaux, E. *et al.* (2002) Vulnerability to cannabis, schizophrenia and the (ATT)N polymorphism of the cannabinoid receptor type 1 gene (Abstract). *Schizophrenia Research* **53** (Suppl.), 72.

Kulkarni J., de Castella A., Fitzgerald P.B. *et al.* (2008) Estrogen in severe mental illness. A potential new treatment approach. *Archives of General Psychiatry* **65**, 955–960.

Kunugi, H., Nanko, S., Takei, N. *et al.* (1995) Schizophrenia following in utero exposure to the 1957 influenza epidemics in Japan. *American Journal of Psychiatry* **152**, 450–452.

Lane, E. & Albee, G.W. (1964) Early childhood intellectual differences between schizophrenic adults and their siblings. *Journal of Abnormal and Social Psychology* **68**, 193–195.

Lane, A., Byrne, M., Mulvany, F. *et al.* (1995) Reproductive behaviour in schizophrenia relative to other mental disorders: evidence for increased fertility in men despite decreased marital rate. *Acta Psychiatrica Scandinavica* **91**, 222–228.

Larson, C.A. & Nyman, G.E. (1973) Differential fertility in schizophrenia. *Acta Psychiatrica Scandinavica* **9**, 272–280.

Lawrence, D., Jablensky, A.V., Holman, C.D.J. & Pinder, T.J. (2000a) Mortality in Western Australian psychiatric patients. *Social Psychiatry and Psychiatric Epidemiology* **35**, 341–347.

Lawrence, D., Holman, C.D.J., Jablensky, A. *et al.* (2000b) Excess cancer mortality in Western Australian psychiatric patients due to higher case fatality rates. *Acta Psychiatrica Scandinavica* **101**, 382–388.

Lawrence D. Holman C.D.J., Jablensky A.V. *et al.* (2001) Increasing rates of suicide in Western Australian psychiatric patients: a record linkage study. *Acta Psychiatrica Scandinavica* **104**, 443–451.

Lawrence D.M., Holman C.D.J., Jablensky A.V. & Hobbs M.S.T. (2003) Death rate from ischaemic heart disease in Western Australian psychiatric patients 1980–1998. *British Journal of Psychiatry* **182**, 31–36.

Leao, T.S., Sundquist, J., Frank, G. *et al.* (2006) Incidence of schizophrenia or other psychoses in first- and second-generation immigrants: A national cohort study. *Journal of Nervous and Mental Disease* **194**, 27–33.

Lemkau, P., Tietze, C. & Cooper, M. (1943) A survey of statistical studies on the prevalence and incidence of mental disorder in sample populations. *Public Health Reports* **58**, 1909–1927.

Levav I., Lipshitz I., Novikov I. *et al.* (2007) Cancer risk among parents and siblings of patients with schizophrenia. *British Journal of Psychiatry* **190**, 156–161.

Lewis, M.S. & Griffin, T. (1981) An explanation for the season of birth effect in schizophrenia and certain other diseases. *Psychological Bulletin* **89**, 589–596.

Lewis, S.W. & Mezey, G.C. (1985) Clinical correlates of septum pellucidum cavities: An unusual association with psychosis. *Psychological Medicine* **15**, 43–54.

Lewis, S.W., Reveley, A.M., David, A.S. & Ron, M.A. (1988) Agenesis of the corpus callosum and schizophrenia. *Psychological Medicine* **18**, 341–347.

Lewis, G., David, A., Andreasson, S. & Allebeck, P. (1992) Schizophrenia and city life. *Lancet* **340**, 137–140.

Lichtenstein, P., Björk, C., Hultman, C. *et al.* (2006) Recurrence risks for schizophrenia in a Swedish national cohort. *Psychological Medicine* **36**, 1417–1425.

Lichtermann, D., Ekelund, J., Pukkala, E. *et al.* (2001) Incidence of cancer among persons with schizophrenia and their relatives. *Archives of General Psychiatry* **58**, 573–578.

Lieberman, Y.I. (1974) The problem of incidence of schizophrenia: material from a clinical and epidemiological study [in Russian]. *Zhurnal Nevropatologii i Psikhiatrii* **74**, 1224–1232.

Lilienfeld, S.O., Waldman, I.D. & Israel, A.C. (1994) A critical examination of the use and concept of comorbidity in psychopathology research. *Clinical Psychology Science and Practice* **1**, 71–83.

Lin, T.Y., Chu, H.M., Rin, H. *et al.* (1989) Effects of social change on mental disorders in Taiwan: observations based on a a15-year follow-up survey of general populations in three communities. *Acta Psychiatrica Scandinavica* **79** (Suppl. 348), 11–34.

Link, B. & Dohrenwend, B.P. (1980) Formulation of hypotheses about the ratio of untreated to treated cases in the true prevalence studies of functional psychiatric disorders in adults in the United States. In: Dohrenwend, B.P., Dohrenwend, B.S., Gould M.S., Link, B., Neugebauer, R. & Wunsch-Hitzig, R., eds. *Mental Illness in the United States: Epidemiologic Estimates*. New York: Praeger.

Linszen, D.H., Dingemans, P.M. & Lenior, M.E. (1994) Cannabis abuse and the course of recent-onset schizophrenic disorders. *Archives of General Psychiatry* **51**, 273–279.

Littlewood, R. & Lipsedge, M. (1981) Some social and phenomenological characteristics of psychotic immigrants. *Psychological Medicine* **11**, 289–302.

Löffler, W. & Häfner, H. (1999) Ecological patterns of first admitted schizophrenics to two German cities over 25 years. *Social Science and Medicine* **49**, 93–108.

MacCabe, J.H., Lambe, M.P., Cnattingius, S. *et al.* (2008) Scholastic achievement at age 16 and risk of schizophrenia and other psychoses: a national cohort study. *Psychological Medicine* **38**, 1133–1140.

Mack, A.H., Feldman, J.J, & Tsuang, M.T. (2002) A case of "pfropfschizophrenia": Kraepelin's bridge between neurodegenerative and neurodevelopmental conceptions of schizophrenia. *American Journal of Psychiatry* **159**, 1104–1110.

Mahy, E., Mallett, R., Leff, J. & Bhugra, D. (1999) First contact rate incidence of schizophrenia on Barbados. *British Journal of Psychiatry* **175**, 28–33.

Mäkikirö, T., Isohanni, M., Moring, J. *et al.* (1997) Is a child's risk of early onset schizophrenia increased in the highest social class? *Schizophrenia Research* **23**, 245–252.

Mäkikirö, T., Karvonen, J.T., Hakko, H. *et al.* (1998) Comorbidity of hospital-treated psychiatric and physical disorders with special reference to schizophrenia: A 28 year follow-up of the 1966 Northern Finland general population birth cohort. *Public Health* **112**, 221–228.

Malaspina, D., Harlap, S., Fennig, S. *et al.* (2001) Advancing paternal age and the risk of schizophrenia. *Archives of General Psychiatry* **58**, 361–367.

Malmberg, A., Lewsi, G., David, A. & Allebeck, P. (1998) Premorbid adjustment and personality in people with schizophrenia. *British Journal of Psychiatry* **172**, 308–313.

Marcelis, M., Takei, N. & van Os, J. (1999) Urbanization and risk for schizophrenia: Does the effect operate before or around the illness onset? *Psychological Medicine* **29**, 1197–1203.

Maric N., Krabbendam L., Vollebergh W. *et al.* (2003) Sex differences in symptoms of psychosis in a non-selected, general population sample. *Schizophrenia Research* **63**, 89–95.

Mason, P. R. & Winton, F. E. (1995) Ear disease and schizophrenia-a case-control study. *Acta Psychiatrica Scandinavica* **91**, 217–221.

McEvoy J.P., Meyer J.M., Goff D.C. *et al.* (2005) Prevalence of the metabolic syndrome in patients with schizophrenia: Baseline results from the Clinical Antipsychotic Trials of Intervention Effectiveness (CATIE) schizophrenia trial and comparison with national estimates from NHANES III. *Schizophrenia Research* **80**, 19–32

McGovern, D. & Cope, R.V. (1987) First psychiatric admission rates of first and second generation Afro Caribbeans. *Social Psychiatry and Psychiatric Epidemiology* **22**, 139–149.

McGrath, J.J. & Richards, L.J. (2009) Why schizophrenia epidemiology needs neurobiology- and vice versa. *Schizophrenia Bulletin* **35**, 577–581.

McGrath, J.J. & Welham, J.L. (1999) Season of birth and schizophrenia: A systematic review and meta-analysis of data from the Southern Hemisphere. *Schizophrenia Research* **35**, 237–242.

McGrath, J.J., Hearle, J., Jenner, L. *et al.* (1999) The fertility and fecundity of patients with psychoses. *Acta Psychiatrica Scandinavica* **99**, 441–446.

McGrath, J., Saha, S., Welham, J. *et al.* (2004a) A systematic review of the incidence of schizophrenia: the distribution of rates and the influence of sex, urbanicity, migrant status and methodology. *BMC Medicine* **2**, 13.

McGrath, J., Saari, K., Hakko, K. *et al.* (2004b) Vitamin D supplementation during the first year of life and risk of schizophrenia: a Finnish birth cohort study. *Schizophrenia Research* **67**, 237–245.

McGuire, P.K., Jones, P., Harvey, I. *et al.* (1995) Morbid risk of schizophrenia for relatives of patients with cannabis-associated psychosis. *Schizophrenia Research* **15**, 277–281.

McNaught, A., Jeffreys, S.E., Harvey, C.A. *et al.* (1997) The Hamstead Schizophrenia Survey 1991. II. Incidence and migration in inner London. *British Journal of Psychiatry* **170**, 307–311.

McNeil, T.F. & Kaij, L. (1987) Swedish high-risk study: Sample characteristics at age 6. *Schizophrenia Bulletin* **13**, 373–381.

McNeil, T.F., Cantor-Graae, E., & Ismail, B. (2000) Obstetric complications and congenital malformation in schizophrenia. *Brain Research Review* **31**, 166–178.

Mednick, S.A. (1970) Breakdown in individuals at high risk for schizophrenia. Possible predispositional perinatal factors. *Mental Hygiene* **54**, 50–63.

Mednick, S.A., Machon, R.A., Huttunen, M.O. & Bonett, D. (1988) Adult schizophrenia following prenatal exposure to an influenza epidemic. *Archives of General Psychiatry* **45**, 189v192.

Menezes, P.R., Scazufca, M., Busatto, G. *et al.* (2007) Incidence of first-contact psychosis in São Paulo, Brazil. *British Journal of Psychiatry* **51** (Suppl.), s102–s106.

Meyer U., Feldon J. & Yee B.K. (2009) A review of the fetal brain cytokine imbalance hypothesis of schizophrenia. *Schizophrenia Bulletin* **35**, 959–972.

Mino, Y., Oshima, I., Tsuda, T. & Okagami, K. (2000) No relationship between schizophrenic birth and influenza epidemics in Japan. *Journal of Psychiatric Research* **34**, 133–138.

Mirsky, A.F., Ingraham, L.J. & Kugelmass, S. (1995) Neuropsychological assessment of attention and its pathology in the Israeli cohort. *Schizophrenia Bulletin* **21**, 193–204.

Mischler, E.G. & Scotch, N.A. (1983) Sociocultural factors in the epidemiology of schizophrenia: A review. *Psychiatry* **26**, 315–351.

Mitchell, K.J. & Porteus, D.J. (2009) GWAS for psychiatric disease: is the framework built on a solid foundation? *Molecular Psychiatry* **14**, 740–741.

Moore, T.H.M., Zammit, S., Lingford-Hughes, A. *et al.* (2007) Cannabis use and risk of psychotic or affective mental health outcomes: A systematic review. *Lancet* **370**, 319–328.

Morgan, V., Castle, D., Page, A. *et al.* (1997) Influenza epidemics and incidence of schizophrenia, affective disorders and mental retardation in Western Australia: No evidence of a major effect. *Schizophrenia Research* **26**, 25–39.

Morgan, C., Kirkbride, J.B., Leff, J. *et al.* (2007) Parental separation, loss and psychosis in different ethnic groups: A case-control study. *Psychological Medicine* **37**, 495–503.

Morgan V.A., Castle D.J. & Jablensky A.V. (2008a) Do women express and experience psychosis differently from men? Epidemiological evidence from the Australian National Study of Low Prevalence (Psychotic) Disorders. *Australian and New Zealand Journal of Psychiatry* **42**, 74–82.

Morgan V.A., Leonard H., Bourke J. & Jablensky A. (2008b) Intellectual disability co-occurring with schizophrenia and other psychiatric illness: population-based study. *British Journal of Psychiatry* **193**, 365–372.

Mors, O., Mortensen, P.B. & Ewald, H. (1999) A population-based register study of the association between schizophrenia and rheumatoid arthritis. *Schizophrenia Research* **40**, 67–74.

Mortensen, P.B. (1994) The occurrence of cancer in first admitted schizophrenic patients. *Schizophrenia Research* **12**, 185–194.

Mortensen, P.B. & Juel, K. (1993) Mortality and causes of death in first admitted schizophrenic patients. *British Journal of Psychiatry* **163**, 183–189.

Mortensen, P.B., Pedersen, C.B., Westergaard, T. *et al.* (1999) Effects of family history and place and season of birth on the risk of achizophrenia. *New England Journal of Medicine* **340**, 603–608.

Mortensen P.B., Nørgaard-Pedersen B., Waltoft B.L. *et al.* (2007) *Toxoplasma gondii* as a risk factor for early-onset schizophrenia: Analysis of filter paper blood samples obtained at birth. *Biological Psychiatry* **61**, 688–693.

Munk-Jørgensen, P. (1986) Decreasing first-admission rates of schizophrenia among males in Denmark from 1970 to 1984. *Acta Psychiatrica Scandinavica* **73**, 645–650.

Munk-Jørgensen, P. & Mortensen, P.B. (1992) Incidence and other aspects of the epidemiology of schizophrenia in Denmark, 1971–87. *British Journal of Psychiatry* **161**, 489–495.

Murray, R.M. & Lewis, S.W. (1987) Is schizophrenia a neurodevelopmental disorder? *British Medical Journal (Clinical Research Edition)* **295**, 681–682.

Murthy, G.V.S., Janakiramaiah, N., Gangadhar, B.N. & Subbarrishna, D.K. (1998) Sex difference in age at onset of schizophrenia: Discrepant findings from India. *Acta Psychiatrica Scandinavica* **97**, 321–325.

Myles-Worsley, M., Coon, H., Tiobech, J. *et al.* (1999) Genetic epidemiological study of schizophrenia in Palau, Micronesia: prevalence and familiality. *American Journal of Medical Genetics Part B (Neuropsychiatric Genetics)* **88**, 4–10.

Need, A.C., Ge, D., Weale, M.E. *et al.* (2009) A genome-wide investigation of SNPs and CNVs in schizophrenia. *PLOS Genetics* **5**, e1000373.

Neugebauer, R. (2005) Accumulating evidence for prenatal nutritional origins of mental disorders. *JAMA* **294**, 621–623.

Ng, M.Y.M., Levinson, D.F., Faraone, S.V. *et al.* (2009) Meta-analysis of 32 genome-wide linkage studies of schizophrenia. *Molecular Psychiatry* **14**, 774–785.

Nicodemus, K.K., Marenco, S., Batten, A.J. *et al.* (2008) Serious obstetric complications interact with hypoxia-regulated/vascular-expression genes to influence schizophrenia risk. *Molecular Psychiatry* **13**, 873–877.

Nicole, L., Lesage, A. & Lalonde, P. (1992) Lower incidence and increased male:female ratio in schizophrenia. *British Journal of Psychiatry* **161**, 556–557.

Nicolson, R. & Rapoport, J.L. (1999) Childhood-onset schizophrenia: Rare but worth studying. *Biological Psychiatry* **46**, 1418–1428.

Niemi, L.T., Suvisaari, J.M., Tuulio-Henriksson, A. & Lönnqvist, J.K. (2003) Childhood developmental abnormalities in schizophrenia: evidence from high-risk studies. *Schizophrenia Research* **60**, 239–258.

Niemi, L.T., Suvisaari, J.M., Haukka, J.K. *et al.* (2004) Cumulative incidence of mental disorders among offspring of mothers with psychotic disorder. Results from the Helsinki High-Risk Study. *British Journal of Psychiatry* **185**, 11–17.

Niemi, L.T., Suvisaari, J.M., Haukka, J.K. & Lönnqvist, J.K. (2005) Childhood predictors of future psychiatric morbidity in offspring of mothers with psychotic disorder. Results from the Helsinki High-Risk Study. *British Journal of Psychiatry* **186**, 208–114.

Nilsson, E., Lichtenstein, P., Cnattingius, S. *et al.* (2002) Women with schizophrenia: pregnancy outcome and infant death among their offspring. *Schizophrenia Research* **58**, 221–229.

Nimgaonkar, V.L., Ward, S.E., Agarde, H. *et al.* (1997) Fertility in schizophrenia: Results from a contemporary US cohort. *Acta Psychiatrica Scandinavica* **95**, 364–369.

Nimgaonkar, V.L., Fujiwara, T.M., Dutta *et al.* (2000) Low prevalence of psychoses among the Hutterites, an isolated religious community. *American Journal of Psychiatry* **157**, 1065–1070.

Nunes, S.O.V., Itano, E.N., Amarante, M.K. *et al.* (2008) RNA from Borna disease virus in patients with schizophrenia, schizoaffective patients, and in their biological relatives. *Journal of Clinical Laboratory Analysis* **22**, 314–320.

Ødegaard, Ø. (1932) Emigration and insanity. *Acta Psychiatrica et Neurologica* **4** (Suppl.), 1–206.

Ødegaard, Ø. (1946a) A statistical investigation of the incidence of mental disorder in Norway. *Psychiatric Quarterly* **20**, 381–401.

Ødegaard, Ø. (1946b) Marriage and mental disease: A study in social psychopathology. *Journal of Mental Science* **92**, 35–59.

Ødegaard, Ø. (1980) Fertility of psychiatric first admissions in Norway, 1936-75. *Acta Pychiatrica Scandinavica* **62**, 212–220.

O'Flaithbheartaigh, S., Williams, P.A. & Jones, G.H. (1994) Schizophrenic psychosis and associated aqueduct stenosis. *British Journal of Psychiatry* **164**, 684–686.

Ohta, Y., Nakane, Y., Mine, M. *et al.* (1988) The epidemiological study of physical morbidity in schizophrenics- 2. Association between schizophrenia and incidence of tuberculosis. *The Japanese Journal of Psychiatry and Neurology* **42**, 41–47.

Osborn, D.P.J., Levy, G., Nazareth, I. *et al.* (2007) Relative risk of cardiovascular and cancer mortality in people with severe mental illness from the United Kingdom's General Practice Research Database. *Archives of General Psychiatry* **64**, 242–249.

Ösby, U., Correia, N., Brandt, L., Ekbom, A. & Sparén, P. (2000) Mortality and causes of death in schizophrenia in Stockholm County, Sweden. *Schizophrenia Research* **45**, 21–28.

Osler, M., Lawlor, D.A. & Nordentoft, M. (2007) Cognitive function in childhood and early adulthood and hospital admission for schizophrenia and bipolar disorders in Danish men born in 1953. *Schizophrenia Research* **92**, 132–141.

Österberg, E. (1978) Schizophrenia and rheumatic disease. *Acta Psychiatrica Scandinavica* **58**, 339–359.

Padmavathi, R., Rajkumar, S., Kumar, N., Manoharan, A. & Kamath, S. (1987) Prevalence of schizophrenia in an urban community in Madras. *Indian Journal of Psychiatry* **31**, 233–239.

Palmer, B.W., McClure, F.S. & Jeste, D.V. (2001) Schizophrenia in late life: Findings challenge traditional concepts. *Harvard Review of Psychiatry* **9**, 51–58.

Pedersen, C.B. & Mortensen, P.B. (2006a) Are the cause(s) responsible for urban-rural differences in schizophrenia risk rooted in families or in individuals? *American Journal of Epidemiology* **163**, 971–978.

Pedersen, C.B. & Mortensen, P.B. (2006b) Urbanicity during upbringing and bipolar affective disorders in Denmark. *Bipolar Disorders* **8**, 242–247.

Perälä J., Suvisaari, J. & Saarni, S.I. (2007) Lifetime prevalence of psychotic and bipolar I disorders in a general population. *Archives of General Psychiatry* **64**, 19–28.

Phillips, M., Yang, G., Li, S. & Li, Y. (2004) Suicide and unique prevalence pattern of schizophrenia in mainland China: a retrospective observational study. *Lancet* **364**, 1062–1068.

Pinel, P. (1803) *Nosographie Philosophique, ou la Methode de l'Analyse Apliquée a la Médecine*, Vol. **III**, 2nd edn. Paris: Brosson.

Potvin, S., Joyal, C.C., Pelletier, J. & Stip, E. (2008) Contradictory cognitive capacities among substance-abusing patients with schizophrenia: a meta-analysis. *Schizophrenia Research* **100**, 242–251.

Pulver, A.E., McGrath, J.A., Liang, K.Y. *et al.* (2004) An indirect test of the new mutation hypothesis associating advanced paternal age with the etiology of schizophrenia. *American Journal of Medical Genetics Part B (Neuropsychiatric Genetics)* **124B**, 6–9.

Puri, B.K., Hall, A.D. & Lewis, S.W. (1994) Cerebral hemiatrophy and schizophrenia. *British Journal of Psychiatry* **165**, 403–405.

Rajkumar, S., Padmavathi, R., Thara, R. & Sarada Menon, M. (1993) Incidence of schizophrenia in an urban community in Madras. *Indian Journal of Psychiatry* **35**, 18–21.

Raman, A.C. & Murphy, H.M.M. (1972) Failure of traditional prognostic indicators in Afro-Asian psychotics: results from a long-term follow-up study. *Journal of Nervous and Mental Disease* **154**, 238–247.

Ramírez B.G., Blázquez C., Gómez del Pulgar T. *et al.* (2005) Prevention of Alzheimer's disease pathology by cannabinopids: Neuroprotection mediated by blockade of microglial activation. *The Journal of Neuroscience* **25**, 1904–1913.

Rantakallio, P., Jones, P., Moring, J. & von Wendt, L. (1997) Association between central nervous system infections during childhood and adult onset schizophrenia and other psychoses: A 28-year follow-up. *International Journal of Epidemiology* **26**, 837–843.

Regier, D.A., Kaelber, C.T., Rae, D.S. *et al.* (1998) Limitations of diagnostic criteria and assessment instruments for mental disorders. Implications for research and policy. *Archives of General Psychiatry* **55**, 109–115.

Reid, D.D. (1960) *Epidemiological Methods in the Study of Mental Disorders*. Public Health Papers No.2. Geneva: World Health Organization.

Reichenberg, A., Weiser, M., Rabinowitz, J. *et al.* (2002) A population-based cohort study of premorbid intellectual, language, and behavioral functioning in patients with schizophrenia, schizoaffective disorder, and nonpsychotic bipolar disorder. *American Journal of Psychiatry* **159**, 2027–2035.

Reveley, A.M. & Reveley, M.A. (1983) Aqueduct stenosis and schizophrenia. *Journal of Neurology, Neurosurgery and Psychiatry* **46**, 18–22.

Riecher-Rössler, A., Fatkenheuer, B., Löffler, W. *et al.* (1992) Is age of onset in schizophrenia influenced by marital status? *Social Psychiatry and Psychiatric Epidemiology* **27**, 122–128.

Rin, H. & Lin, T.Y. (1962) Mental illness among Formosan aborittines as compared with the Chinese in Taiwan. *Journal of Mental Science* **198**, 134–146.

Roberts, J.K.A., Trimble, M.R. & Robertson, M. (1983) Schizophrenic psychosis associated with aqueduct stenosis in adults. *Journal of Neurology, Neurosurgery and Psychiatry* **46**, 892–898.

Robins, L.N. (1989) Diagnostic grammar and assessment: Translating criteria into questions. *Psychological Medicine* **19**, 57–68.

Robins, L.N. & Regier, D.A., eds. (1991) *Psychiatric Disorders in America. The Epidemiologic Catchment Area Study*. New York: The Free Press.

Robins, L.N., Helzer, J.E., Croughan, J. & Rarcliff, K.S. (1981) National Institute of Mental Health Diagnostic Interview Schedule: its history, characteristics, and validity. *Archives of General Psychiatry* **38**, 381–389.

Robins, L.N., Wing, J.K., Wittchen, H.U. *et al.* (1988) The Composite International Diagnostic Interview: An epidemiologic instrument suitable for use in conjunction with different diagnostic systems and in different cultures. *Archives of General Psychiatry* **45**, 1069–1077.

Rotstein, V.G. (1977) Material from a psychiatric survey of sample groups from the adult population in several areas of the USSR [in Russian]. *Zhurnal Nevropatologii i Psikhiatrii* **77**, 569–574.

Saari K.M., Lindeman S.M., Viilo K.M. *et al.* (2005) A 4-fold risk of metabolic syndrome in patients with schizophrenia: the Northern Finland 1966 birth cohort study. *Journal of Clinical Psychiatry* **66**, 559–563.

Sacker, A., Done, J., Crow, T.J. & Golding, J. (1995) Antecedents of schizophrenia and affective illness. Obstetric complications. *British Journal of Psychiatry* **166**, 734–741.

Saha, S., Chant, D., Welham, J. & McGrath, J. (2005) A systematic review of the prevalence of schizophrenia. *PLOS Medicine* **2**: issue 5/e141.

Saha, S., Chant, D.C., Welham, J.L. & McGrath, J.J. (2006) The incidence and prevalence of schizophrenia varies with latitude. *Acta Psychiatrica Scandinavica* **114**, 36–39.

Saha, S., Chant, D. & McGrath, J. (2007) A systematic review of mortality in schizophrenia. *Archives of General Psychiatry* **64**, 1123–1131.

Salan, R. (1992) Epidemiology of schizophrenia in Indonesia (the Tambora I study). *ASEAN Journal of Psychiatry* **2**, 52–57.

Salokangas, R.K.R., Honkonen, T. & Saarinen, S. (2003) Women have later onset than men in schizophrenia—but only in its paranoid form. Results of the DSP project. *European Psychiatry* **18**, 274–281.

Sanderson, T.L., Doody, G.A., Best, J. *et al.* (2001) Correlations between clinical and historical variables, and cerebral structural variables in people with mild intellectual disability and schizophrenia. *Journal of Intellectual Disability Research* **45**, 89–98.

Sandwijk, J.P., Cohen, P.D., Musterd, S. & Langemeijer, M.P. (1995) *Licit and Illicit Drug Use in Amsterdam. Report of a Household Survey in 1994 on the Prevalence of Drug Use Among the Population of 12 Years and Over*. Amsterdam: University of Amsterdam.

Sartorius, N., Jablensky, A., Korten, A. *et al.* (1986) Early manifestations and first-contact incidence of schizophrenia in different cultures. A preliminary report on the initial evaluation phase of the WHO Collaborative Study on Determinants of

Outcome of Severe Mental Disorders. *Psychological Medicine* **16**, 909–928.

Schiffman, J., Walker, E., Ekstrom, M. *et al.* (2004) Childhood videotaped social and neuromotor precursors of schizophrenia: A prospective investigation. *American Journal of Psychiatry* **161**, 2121–2027.

Schulsinger, F., Parnas, J., Petersen, E.T. *et al.* (1984) Cerebral ventricular size in the offspring of schizophrenic mothers. *Archives of General Psychiatry* **41**, 602–606.

Schürhoff, F., Golmard, J.L., Szöke, A. *et al.* (2004) Admixture analysis of age at onset in schizophrenia. *Schizophrenia Research* **71**, 35–41.

Scully, P.J., Quinn, J.F., Morgan, M.G. *et al.* (2002) First-episode schizophrenia, bipolar disorder and other psychoses in a rural Irish catchment area: incidence and gender in the Cavan-Monaghan study at 5 years. *British Journal of Psychiatry* **43** (Suppl.), s3–s9.

Scully, P.J., Owens, J.M., Kinsella, A. & Waddington, J.L. (2004) Schizophrenia, schizoaffective and bipolar disorder within an epidemiologically complete, homogeneous population in rural Ireland: small area variation in rates. *Schizophrenia Research* **67**, 143–155.

Selten, J.P., Slaets, J. & Kahn, R.S. (1997) Schizophrenia in Surinamese and Dutch Antillean immigrants to The Netherlands: Evidence of an increased incidence. *Psychological Medicine* **27**, 807–811.

Selten, J.P., Slaets, J. & Kahn, R. (1998) Prenatal exposure to influenza and schizophrenia in Surinamese and Dutch Antillean immigrants to The Netherlands. *Schizophrenia Research* **30**, 101–103.

Selten, J.P., Brown, A.S., Moons, K.G.M. *et al.* (1999a) Prenatal exposure to the 1957 influenza pandemic and non-affective psychosis in The Netherlands. *Schizophrenia Research* **38**, 85–91.

Selten, J.P., van der Graaf, Y., van Duursen, R., Gispen-de Wied, C. & Kahn, R.S. (1999b) Psychotic illness after prenatal exposure to the 1953 Dutch flood disaster. *Schizophrenia Research* **35**, 243–245.

Selten, J.P., Veen, N., Feller, W. *et al.* (2001) Incidence of psychotic disorders in immigrant groups to The Netherlands. *British Journal of Psychiatry* **178**, 367–372.

Selten, J.P., Cantor-Graae, E., Slaets, J. & Kahn, R.S. (2002) Ødegaard's selection hypothesis revisited: Schizophrenia in Surinamese immigrants to the Netherlands. *American Journal of Psychiatry* **159**, 669–671.

Sewell, D.D. (1996) Schizophrenia and HIV. *Schizophrenia Bulletin* **22**, 465–473.

Sham, P.C., O'Callaghan, E., Takei, N. *et al.* (1992) Schizophrenia following pre-natal exposure to influenza epidemics between 1939 and 1960. *British Journal of Psychiatry* **160**, 461–466.

Shaner, A., Miller, G. & Mintz, J. (2007) Evidence of a latitudinal gradient in the age at onset of schizophrenia. *Schizophrenia Research* **94**, 58–63.

Shields, J. (1977) High risk for schizophrenia: Genetic considerations. *Psychological Medicine* **7**, 7–10.

Silver, E., Mulvey, E.P. & Swanson, J.W. (2002) Neighborhood structural characteristics and mental disorder: Faris and Dunham revisited. *Social Science and Medicine* **55**, 1457–1470.

Singh, S.P. & Burns, T. (2006) Race and mental health: There is more to race than racism. *British Medical Journal* **333**, 648–651.

Sipos, A., Rasmussen, F., Harrison, G. *et al.* (2004) Paternal age and schizophrenia: a population based cohort study. *British Medical Journal* **329**, 1070.

Sjögren, T. (1948) Genetic-statistical and psychiatric investigations of a West Swedish population. *Acta Psychiatrica et Neurologica Scandinavica* **52** (Suppl.).

Spauwen, J., Krabbendam, L., Lieb, R. *et al.* (2004) Does urbanicity shift the population expression of psychosis? *Journal of Psychiatric Research* **38**, 613–618.

Sporn, A.L., Addington, A.M., Gogtay, N. *et al.* (2004) Pervasive developmental disorder and childhood-onset schizophrenia: Comorbid disorder or a phenotypic variant of a very early onset illness? *Biological Psychiatry* **55**, 989–994.

Srinivasan, T.N. & Padmavati, R. (1997) Fertility and schizophrenia: Evidence for increased fertility in the relatives of schizophrenic patients. *Acta Psychiatrica Scandinavica* **96**, 260–264.

Stahlberg, O., Soderstrom, H., Rastam, M. & Gillberg, C. (2004) Bipolar disorder, schizophrenia, and other psychotic disorders in adults with childhood onset AD/HD and/or autism spectrum disorders. *Journal of Neural Transmission* **111**, 891–902.

St Clair, D., Xu, M., Wang, P. *et al.* (2005) Rates of adult schizophrenia following prenatal exposure to the Chinese famine of 1959-1961. *JAMA* **294**, 557–562.

Stefansson, H., Rujescu, D., Cichon, S. *et al.* (2008) Large recurrent microdeletions associated with schizophrenia. *Nature* **455**, 232–236.

Stephens, J.H., Astrup, C., Carpenter, W.T. *et al.* (1982) A comparison of nine systems to diagnose schizophrenia. *Psychiatry Research* **6**, 127–143.

Stirling, J., Lewis, S., Hopkins, R. & White, C. (2005) Cannabis use prior to first onset psychosis predicts spared neurocognition at 10-year follow-up. *Schizophrenia Research* **75**, 135–137.

Strömgren, E. (1938) Beiträge zur psychiatrischen Erblehre, auf Grund von Untersuchungen an einer Inselbevölkerung. *Acta Psychiatrica et Neurologica Scandinavica* **19** (Suppl.).

Sugarman, P.A. & Craufurd, D. (1994) Schizophrenia in the Afro-Caribbean Community. *British Journal of Psychiatry* **164**, 474–480.

Sundquist, K., Frank, G. & Sundquist, J. (2004) Urbanisation and incidence of psychosis and depression: Follow-up study of 4.4 million women and men in Sweden. *British Journal of Psychiatry* **184**, 293–298.

Susser, E.S. & Lin, S.P. (1992) Schizophrenia after prenatal exposure to the Dutch hunger winter of 1944–1945. *Archives of General Psychiatry* **49**, 983–988.

Susser, E.S., Schaefer, C.A., Brown, A.S. *et al.* (2000) The design of the prenatal determinants of schizophrenia study. *Schizophrenia Bulletin* **26**, 257–273.

Susser, E. & Schwartz, S. (2006) Cohort designs in psychiatric epidemiology. In: Susser, E., Schwartz, S., Morabia, A. & Bromet, E.J., eds. *Psychiatric Epidemiology. Searching for the Causes of Mental Disorders*. New York: Oxford University Press, pp. 91–177.

Suvisaari, J.M., Haukka, J.K. & Lönnqvist, J.K. (2001) Season of birth among patients with schizophrenia and their siblings:

Evidence for the procreational habits hypothesis. *American Journal of Psychiatry* **158**, 754–757.

Svedberg, B., Mesterton, A. & Cullberg, J. (2001) First-episode non-affective psychosis in a total urban population: a 5-year follow-up. *Social Psychiatry and Psychiatric Epidemiology* **36**, 332–337.

Svensson A.C., Lichtenstein P., Sandin S. & Hultman C.M. (2007) Fertility of first-degree relatives of patients with schizophrenia: A three generation perspective. *Schizophrenia Research* **91**, 238–245.

Szatmari, P., Paterson, A.D., Zwaigenbaum, L. *et al.* (2007) Mapping autism risk loci using genetic linkage and chromosomal rearrangements. *Nature Genetics* **39**, 319–328.

Taieb, O., Baleyte, J.M., Mazet, P. & Fillet, A.M. (2001) Borna disease virus and psychiatry. *European Psychiatry* **13**, 3–10.

Takei, N., Sham, P., O'Callaghan, E. *et al.* (1994) Prenatal exposure to influenza and the development of schizophrenia: Is the effect confined to females? *American Journal of Psychiatry* **151**, 117–119.

Takei, N., Sham, P.C., O'Callaghan, E., Glover, G. & Murray, R.M. (1995) Early risk-factors in schizophrenia: Place and season of birth. *European Psychiatry* **10**, 165–170.

Tien, A.Y. & Eaton, W.W. (1992) Psychopathologic precursors and sociodemographic risk factors for the schizophrenia syndrome. *Archives of General Psychiatry* **49**, 37–46.

Tienari, P. (1991) Interaction between genetic vulnerability and family environment: The Finnish adoptive family study of schizophrenia. *Acta Psychiatrica Scandinavica* **84**, 460–465.

Tilhonen J., Lönnqvist J. Wahlbeck K. *et al.* (2009) 11-year follow-up of mortality in patients with schizophrenia: a population-based cohort study (FIN11 study). *Lancet* **374**, 620–627.

Toguchi, M., Onai, T., Narita, K. *et al.* (2005) Seasonality of schizophrenia births in the Japanese population: increased winter births possibly confined to the north area. *Schizophrenia Research* **75**, 433–438.

Torrey, E.F. (1995) Prevalence of psychosis among the Hutterites: A reanalysis of the 1950–53 study. *Schizophrenia Research* **16**, 167–170.

Torrey, E.F., Bartko, J.J. Lun, Z.R. & Yolken, R.H. (2007) Antibodies to *Toxoplasma gondii* in patients with schizophrenia: A meta-analysis. *Schizophrenia Bulletin* **33**, 729–736.

Torrey, E.F., Buka, S., Cannon, T.D. *et al.* (2009) Paternal age as a risk factor for schizophrenia: How important is it? *Schizophrenia Research* **114**, 1–5.

Tramer, M. (1929) Über die biologische Bedeutung des Geburtsmonats, insbesondere für die Psychosenerkrankung. *Schweizer Archiv für Neurologie, Neurochirurgie und Psychiatrie* **24**, 17–24.

van Erp, T.G.M., Saleh, P.A., Rosso, I.M. *et al.* (2002) Contributions of genetic risk and fetal hypoxia to hippocampal volume in patients with schizophrenia or schizoaffective disorder, their unaffected siblings, and healthy unrelated volunteers. *American Journal of Psychiatry* **159**, 1514–1520.

van Os, J. & Selten, J.P. (1998) Prenatal exposure to maternal stress and subsequent schizophrenia. *British Journal of Psychiatry* **172**, 324–326.

van Os, J., Castle, D.J., Takei, N. *et al.* (1996) Psychotic illness in ethnic minorities: Clarification from the 1991 census. *Psychological Medicine* **26**, 203–208.

van Os, J., Driessen, G., Gunther, N. & Delespaul, P. (2000) Neighbourhood variation in incidence of schizophrenia. Evidence for person-environment interaction. *British Journal of Psychiatry* **176**, 243–248.

Veen, N., Selten, J.P., Hoek, H.W. *et al.* (2002) Use of illicit substances in a psychosis incidence cohort: A comparison among different ethnic groups in the Netherlands. *Acta Psychiatrica Scandinavica* **105**, 440–443.

Veling, W., Selten, J-P., Veen, N. *et al.* (2006a) Incidence of schizophrenia among ethnic minorities in the Netherlands: A four-year first-contact study. *Schizophrenia Research* **86**, 189–193.

Veling, W.A., Selten, J-P., Van Hoeken, D. *et al.* (2006b) Ethnic density and incidence of schizophrenia in ethnic minorities in the Netherlands. *Schizophrenia Research* **81**, 174–174.

Veling, W., Susser, E., van Os, J. *et al.* (2008) Ethnic density of neighbourhoods and incidence of psychotic disorders among immigrants. *American Journal of Psychiatry* **165**, 66–73.

Verdoux, H., Geddes, J.R., Takei, N. *et al.* (1997a) Obstetric complications and age at onset in schizophrenia: An international collaborative meta-analysis of individual patient data. *American Journal of Psychiatry* **154**, 1220–1227.

Verdoux, H., Takei, N., de Saint-Mathurin, R.C. *et al.* (1997b) Seasonality of birth in schizophrenia: The effect of regional population density. *Schizophrenia Research* **23**, 175–180.

Verheij, R.A., van de Mheen, H.D., de Bakker, D.H. *et al.* (1998) Urban–rural variations in health in the Netherlands: Does selective migration play a part? *Journal of Epidemiology and Community Health* **52**, 487–493.

Waddington, J.L. & Youssef, H.A. (1996) Familial-genetic and reproductive epidemiology of schizophrenia in rural Ireland: Age at onset, familial morbid risk and parental fertility. *Acta Psychiatrica Scandinavica* **93**, 62–68.

Waddington, J.L., Youssef, H.A. & Kinsella, A. (1998) Mortality in schizophrenia. *British Journal of Psychiatry* **173**, 325–329.

Wahlbeck, K., Forsén, T., Osmond, C. *et al.* (2001) Association of schizophrenia with low maternal body mass index, small size at birth, and thinness during childhood. *Archives of General Psychiatry* **58**, 48–52.

Wahlberg, K.E., Lynne, L.C., Oja, H. *et al.* (1997) Gene-environment interaction in vulnerability to schizophrenia: Findings from the Finnish adoptive family study of schizophrenia. *Am.J.Psychiatry* **154**, 355–362.

Waldo, M.C. (1999) Schizophrenia in Kosrae, Micronesia: prevalence, gender ratios, and clinical symptomatology. *Schizophrenia Research* **35**, 175–181.

Webb, R., Abel, K., Pickles, A. & Appleby, L. (2005) Mortality of offspring of parents with psychotic disorders: A critical review and meta-analysis. *American Journal of Psychiatry* **162**, 1045–1056.

Webb, R.T., Abel, K.M., Pickles, A.R. *et al.* (2006) Mortality risk among offspring of psychiatric inpatients: A population-based follow-up study to early adulthood. *American Journal of Psychiatry* **163**, 2170–2177.

Weber, N.S., Cowan, D.N., Millikan, A.M. & Niebuhr, D.W (2009) Psychiatric and general medical conditions comorbid with schizophrenia in the National Hospital Discharge Survey. *Psychiatric Services* **60**, 1059–1067.

Weeke, A. & Strömgren E. (1978) Fifteen years later: A comparison of patients in Danish psychiatric institutions in 1957, 1962, 1967, and 1972. *Acta Psychiatrica Scandinavica* **57**, 129–144.

Weinberg, W. (1925) Methoden und Technik der Statistik mit besonderer Berücksichtigung der Sozialbiologie. *Handbuch der Sozialen Hygiene und Gesundheitsfursorge*, Band I. Berlin: Springer.

Welham, J., Isohanni, M., Jones, P. & McGrath, J. (2009) The antecedents of schizophrenia: A review of birth cohort studies. *Schizophrenia Bulletin* **35**, 603–623.

Werner, S., Malaspina, D. & Rabinowitz, J. (2007) Socioeconomic status at birth is associated with risk of schizophrenia: Population-based multilevel study. *Schizophrenia Bulletin* **33**, 1373–1378.

Wessely, S., Castle, D., Der, G. & Murray, R.M. (1991) Schizophrenia and Afro-Caribbeans. A case-control study. *British Journal of Psychiatry* **159**, 795–801.

Wing J.K., Cooper J.E. & Sartorius N. (1974) *The Measurement and Classification of Psychiatric Symptoms*. Cambridge: Cambridge University Press.

Wing J.K., Babor T., Brugha T. *et al.* (1990) SCAN. Schedules for Clinical Assessment in Neuropsychiatry. *Archives of General Psychiatry* **47**, 589–593.

Wing, J.K., Sartorius, N. & Üstün, T.B. (1998) *Diagnosis and Clinical Measutrement in Psychiatry. A reference manual for SCAN*. Cambridge: Cambridge University Press.

World Health Organization (1973) *Report of the International Pilot Study of Schizophrenia*, vol. **I**. Geneva: World Health Organization.

World Health Organization (1979) *Schizophrenia. An International Follow-up Study*. Chichester: Wiley.

Wu, E.Q., Shi, L., Birnbaum, H. *et al.* (2006) Annual prevalence of diagnosed schizophrenia in the USA: a claims data analysis approach. *Psychological Medicine* **36**, 1535–1540.

Xu, B., Roos, J.L., Levy, S. *et al.* (2008) Strong association of *de novo* copy number mutations with sporadic schizophrenia. *Nature Genetics* **40**, 880–885.

Xu, M.Q., Sun, W.S., Liu, B.X. *et al.* (2009) Prenatal malnutrition and adult schizophrenia: further evidence from the 1959–1961 Chinese Famine. *Schizophrenia Bulletin* **35**, 568–576.

Youssef, H.A., Scully, P.J., Kinsella, A. & Waddington, J.L. (1999) Geographical variation in rate of schizophrenia in rural Ireland by place at birth vs place at onset. *Schizophrenia Research* **37**, 233–243.

Zammit, S., Allebeck, P. Dalman, C. *et al.* (2003) Paternal age and risk of schizophrenia. *British Journal of Psychiatry* **183**, 405–408.

Zammit, S., Allebeck, P., David, A.S *et al.* (2004) A longitudinal study of premorbid IQ score and risk of developing schizophrenia, bipolar disorder, severe depression, and other nonaffective psychoses. *Archives of General Psychiatry* **61**, 354–360.

Zolkowska, K., Cantor-Graae, E. & McNeil, T.F. (2001) Increased rates of psychosis among immigrants to Sweden: is migration a risk factor for psychosis? *Psychological Medicine* **31**, 669–678.

Environmental risk factors for schizophrenia

John J. McGrath[1] and Robin M. Murray[2]

[1]Queensland Brain Institute, University of Queensland, Queensland, Australia
[2]Institute of Psychiatry, London, UK

Introduction

Biomedical science has long partitioned the causes of disease into headings such as "genetic" and "environmental". This convenient short-hand builds on long-standing cultural beliefs concerning nature *versus* nurture. However, the utility of this semantic division is increasingly doubtful as we learn more about the transactional nature of how inherited information meshes with non-inherited information (Meaney, 2001). The instructions that guide each step of the developmental trajectory emerge in a contingent fashion based on the previous set of conditions (Oyama *et al.*, 2001). Thus, while both "genetic" and "environmental" domains are continually integrated into the stream of developmental instructions, the emergent set of instructions become higher-order derivatives of many cycles of contingency. Attempting to separate out the relative contribution of isolated genetic and environmental factors from this dynamic matrix is a challenge. However, progress is being made and indeed the study of gene–environment

interactions is now one of the most productive fields in psychiatric epidemiology (Moffitt *et al.*, 2005). Before examining such interactions, one must first identify relevant factors in the environment, and the notion of environmental risk factors provides a useful heading under which to review the literature concerning the effect of the environment on liability to schizophrenia.

From conception to death, individuals are exposed to a range of non-inherited factors that are necessary for survival (e.g., requirements related to ambient temperature, provision of oxygen, etc.). Because these essential factors are usually highly predictable (they are, in a sense, the "wallpaper" of biology), their covert role in guiding development only attracts attention when they are disrupted (e.g., the absence of adequate oxygen around the time of birth can lead to hypoxia/ischemia injury). Events can disrupt the expected background of development, and the ability of an organism to recover is thus tested (Gluckman & Hanson, 2004). Evolution selects organisms that have the ability to buffer occasional perturbations (within limits). Furthermore, evolutionary developmental biology ("evo–devo") suggests that long-standing and essential biological functions are the most highly buffered, while more recent phylogenetic innovations may be more susceptible to per-

Schizophrenia, 3rd edition. Edited by Daniel R. Weinberger and Paul J Harrison © 2011 Blackwell Publishing Ltd.

turbation (put crudely "Last in, first to break"; Finlay, 2007; Waddington, 1953). This principle is helpful in understanding the vulnerability of functions related to the recently evolved, larger neocortex in humans and related primates (Finlay *et al.*, 2001). Evo–devo also points to the critical windows of development in early life. The potential impact of environmental factors during this period can have a disproportionately large impact compared to the same exposures in later periods of development.

Much of the research on the role of environmental factors in schizophrenia has been inspired by the neurodevelopmental hypothesis. In its original form, this hypothesis suggests that genetic or environmental factors, or more likely their interaction, during critical early periods of brain development, adversely impact on adult mental health (Murray & Lewis, 1987; Weinberger, 1987). Initially, this early disruption was thought to be clinically dormant ("silent") until after puberty, when maturational events lead to the emergence of the symptoms of schizophrenia. However, as we shall see, features of the original hypothesis have been refined in response to new data, to include the pathogenic effects of abuse of psychostimulants and cannabis, and also of chronic social adversity (Howes *et al.*, 2004; McDonald & Murray, 2000; McGrath *et al.*, 2003b). The evidence supporting the biological aspects of this hypothesis is covered in detail in Chapter 19.

In the 15 years since the first edition of this book was published, there have been some appreciable shifts in thinking about the epidemiology of schizophrenia. The wider research community has become more aware that the incidence of schizophrenia varies across time, between sites, and between groups. For example, new studies of the incidence of schizophrenia (Kirkbride *et al.*, 2006) and systematic reviews of existing data (McGrath *et al.*, 2004) have reminded us that schizophrenia, like all other complex and chronic disorders, shows prominent variations between sites. These data challenge the "equal incidence" notion promulgated after the publication of the World Health Organization (WHO) Ten-Country Study (Sartorius *et al.*, 1986). Such an occurrence would have made schizophrenia unique among diseases. Now this curious belief has been disproved by a raft of studies. In particular, a systematic review by McGrath *et al.* (2004) concluded that the incidence of schizophrenia shows prominent worldwide variation (up to five-fold), and that it is about 40% greater in men than women. The epidemiology of schizophrenia is no longer a flat and featureless horizon (McGrath, 2006).

Social biology has also become stronger in recent years. To a certain extent, the social biology of psychosis was over-shadowed by the advances in molecular biology and neuroimaging (Jarvis, 2007). However, convincing data concerning migration and urban living have drawn attention back to factors that originate in the social domain (Cantor-Graae, 2007). Factors that are best quantified at the

social level (e.g., the chronic stressors faced by some migrant groups), can translate to altered development via both cognitive and neurochemical pathways (Cougnard *et al.*, 2007; Selten & Cantor-Graae, 2005).

For convenience, we will discuss the non-genetic risk factors associated with schizophrenia under several overlapping headings. Where possible, we will separate out those exposures that are thought to impact in very early life from those that impact during childhood, adolescence, and adulthood. We will cite systematic reviews that include meta-analyses wherever possible. We aim to provide the reader with a concise summary of the field. Finally, we will reflect on how best to relate the data emerging from risk factor epidemiology to what we have learned from genetics and the broad field of neuroscience.

Risk factor epidemiology as a clue generator

Risk factor epidemiology generates clues that can help guide research. However, it is important to understand the taxonomy of risk factors. First, variables that correlate with an outcome, but do not precede the outcome, are sequelae and should not be labeled risk factors. Second, variables that precede an outcome, but are not causally related to that outcome, are defined as risk indicators or proxy markers; the nicotine-stained fingers of the individual with lung cancer is an example of a risk indicator which is not directly on the causal pathway to the illness. Many of the candidates described below are risk indicators of schizophrenia (e.g., season of birth). Third, the term "risk modifying factor" should be reserved for factors that appear to operate within the causal chain (contribute to the outcome). Risk factors can operate directly or indirectly. Migrant status, for example, is a proxy marker for a broad range of psychosocial, economic, and health-related variables. For example, social margination can be an "upstream" cause of stress, which then becomes a more proximal or direct cause for a wide range of altered neurobiological outcomes which may be component causes for a broad range of adverse mental health outcomes. Risk modifying factors can be fixed (e.g., gender) or variable (e.g., drug abuse), endogenous (e.g., genes) or exogenous (e.g., obstetric complications), protective or adverse.

In the absence of a thorough understanding of causal pathways, clues from observational epidemiology should be treated cautiously. Furthermore, without corroborating evidence from randomized controlled trials (which are not ethical and practical in many clinical scenarios), the level of proof provided by observational epidemiology is poor (Smith, 2001). Because of the potentially misleading nature of clues from observational epidemiology, when we consider schizophrenia, we must wherever possible incorporate evidence from a broader range of disciplines (e.g., clinical neuroscience, genetics, animal models) (McGrath, 2007). We will return to this issue at the end of the chapter.

Preschizophrenic characteristics as risk indicators

Children who go on to develop schizophrenia in adulthood appear to be subtly different from their peers in terms of motor, cognitive, and social functioning (Bearden *et al.*, 2000; Cannon *et al.*, 2001, 2006; Cornblatt *et al.*, 1999; Done *et al.*, 1994; Isohanni *et al.*, 1998; Jones *et al.*, 1994; Poulton *et al.*, 2000; Seidman *et al.*, 2006)

The Dunedin Birth Cohort Study, which followed the development of 1037 children through the ages of 3–15 years, and assessed them again at the ages of 18, 21, and 26 years (Cannon *et al.*, 2002a), has helped to identify early neurocognitive impairments in children who subsequently developed schizophrenia-like illnesses. This study found that poorer motor development, poorer receptive language, and a lower IQ all increased the risk of subsequently developing schizophreniform disorder. Other groups have reported that attention deficits (Cornblatt *et al.*, 1999; Oner & Munir, 2005) and deficits in executive function (Cannon *et al.*, 2006) are also more prevalent amongst children and adolescents who develop schizophrenia later in life.

The Dunedin cohort additionally provided clear evidence that many children who develop schizophrenia are already experiencing "quasi-psychotic" phenomena by the end of their first decade of life (Poulton *et al.*, 2000). These phenomena include beliefs that people are reading their minds or following or spying on them, or they are already hearing voices. Children with strong evidence of quasi-psychotic symptomatology were up to 16 times more likely to develop schizophreniform disorders by the age of 26 years; making these phenomena some of the most powerful early predictors of later psychosis.

Thus, it is now well established that children who go on to develop schizophrenia-like disorders are more likely to show neurocognitive difficulties and minor psychotic symptoms. However, there is no evidence that these characteristics are causal risk factors; rather they appear to be risk indicators.

Exposures to early biological hazards

Season of birth

One of the most consistently replicated epidemiological features of schizophrenia is the slight excess of births in the late winter and spring in the northern hemisphere (Torrey *et al.*, 1997). This winter–spring excess of births has been confirmed in a systematic review and meta-analysis, and the size of the effect increases at high latitudes (Davies *et al.*, 2003). A comprehensive Danish record-linkage study

(Mortensen *et al.*, 1999), found that the small seasonal excess of schizophrenia births (relative risk = 1.11) was associated with a sizeable (10.5%) population attributable fraction for the disorder. Candidate exposures that have been proposed as underlying the season of birth effect include perinatal viral exposures (Torrey *et al.*, 1997) and vitamin deficiencies (McGrath, 1999), both of which are postulated to be commoner during the winter months.

Prenatal nutrition

There has been considerable interest in recent years in the impact of prenatal nutrition and various adult-onset disorders such as diabetes, cardiovascular disease, and hypertension—the so-called "Barker hypothesis" (Barker *et al.*, 2002). Even in the absence of overt nutritional deficits, supplementing nutrition before and after birth warrants consideration. For example, supplementing folate to women periconceptually is associated with a reduction in the incidence of neural tube defects in their offspring (Pitkin, 2007). Even in those infants with pre-existing brain trauma, nutritional status can influence the eventual phenotype. For example, a randomized controlled trial of nutritional supplements for preterm infants found not only that cognitive outcomes (measured at age 7 years) were superior in the group allocated the enriched infant formulae, but this group also had less cerebral palsy (Lucas *et al.*, 1998).

Prenatal nutritional deprivation is a biologically plausible risk factor for schizophrenia (Brown *et al.*, 1996). While studies of the incidence of schizophrenia in developing nations (where more fetuses are exposed to poor nutrition) do not appear to show higher rates (Saha *et al.*, 2006), there remains the possibility that deficits in specific micronutrients may have a role. Two ecological studies have examined the association between prenatal exposure to famine and subsequent risk of schizophrenia. The Dutch Hunger Winter involved a well-documented restriction in food during World War II. Individuals who were *in utero* during this famine showed an increased risk of congenital anomalies of the central nervous system, but also of schizophrenia, depression, and schizophrenia spectrum personality disorders (Brown & Susser, 1997; Brown *et al.*, 2000b; Hoek *et al.*, 1998; Susser & Lin, 1992). The risk-increasing effect of maternal starvation on risk of schizophrenia in the offspring has recently been replicated twice in two regions exposed prenatally to catastrophic famine in China during the Cultural Revolution (St Clair *et al.*, 2005; Xu *et al.*, 2009).

Apart from these ecological studies, the association between risk of schizophrenia and two specific maternal micronutrients has been examined using banked maternal sera. Homocysteine, a marker of folate metabolism associated with a range of health outcomes, was found to be significantly elevated in the third trimester sera from mothers of individuals with schizophrenia (Brown *et al.*, 2007; Brown & Susser, 2005). Finally, low prenatal vitamin D has been proposed as a candidate risk factor underlying the season of birth effect (McGrath, 1999). There was a trend level association between very low vitamin D levels during the third trimester and an increased risk of schizophrenia (McGrath *et al.*, 2003a).

With respect to the general postnatal growth trajectory and risk of schizophrenia, the evidence is mixed. Low weight at birth and during infancy has been associated with schizophrenia (Wahlbeck *et al.*, 2001a). Some cohort studies have found altered growth trajectories in those who develop schizophrenia (compared to well cohort members; Gunnell *et al.*, 2003; Sorensen *et al.*, 2006), but altered growth has not been associated with schizophrenia in a consistent fashion (Haukka *et al.*, 2008).

Prenatal infection

One possible cause of the late winter–spring excess of births with schizophrenia is maternal exposure to winter-borne viruses. Many groups have followed up the early clues linking prenatal exposure to influenza to schizophrenia (Mednick *et al.*, 1988; O'Callaghan *et al.*, 1991). Most early studies were positive (McGrath & Castle, 1995), but in recent years, the evidence from ecological studies has generally weakened the case that prenatal exposure to influenza is associated with an increased risk of schizophrenia (Selten *et al.*, 1999; Westergaard *et al.*, 1999). Ecological studies have also found some evidence that exposure to various other viral epidemics (e.g., diphtheria, measles, varicella, polio) may be associated with an increased risk of schizophrenia (Suvisaari *et al.*, 1999; Torrey *et al.*, 1988; Watson *et al.*, 1984); but once again the evidence is inconsistent.

Access to biobanks has allowed stronger tests of the hypotheses linking prenatal infection and risk of schizophrenia. Maternal sera can be used to examine the seroprevalence against candidate exposures, and cord blood or neonatal dried blood spots more directly test the antibody status of the offspring. The results of these studies are summarized in Table 11.1.

Only one study has examined prenatal influenza (Brown *et al.*, 2004a). This study reported an association between the presence of antibodies to the influenza virus in first-trimester blood, but not during the other trimesters. A significant association was found between serologically-documented rubella exposure and an increased risk of non-affective psychosis [relative risk (RR) = 5.2; Brown *et al.*, 2000a].

Curiously, there is also preliminary evidence to suggest that prenatal exposure to herpes simplex virus type 2 (HSV2) may be associated with an increased risk of schizo-

phrenia (Buka *et al.*, 2001). This virus was identified in a screen for antibodies to several infectious agents based on banked maternal sera (27 cases of schizophrenia and other psychotic illnesses, and 54 matched unaffected controls). Mothers of cases had generally elevated IgG and IgM class immunoglobulins. IgG antibodies for toxoplasmosis were significantly elevated in the maternal sera of cases, while no group was significantly different on any IgA antibodies, nor on IgG antibodies to HSV1, cytomegalovirus, *Toxoplasma gondii*, rubella virus, human parvovirus B19, *Chlamydia trachomatis*, or human papillomavirus type 16. Another study with a similar design failed to confirm the specific finding on IgG against HSV2 (Brown *et al.*, 2006).

With respect to adult exposure to infectious agents as risk-modifying factors for schizophrenia, the body of evidence is mostly negative or unconvincing. Clearly, schizophrenia lacks a classical epidemiological profile suggestive of infective agents with short latencies (Yolken *et al.*, 2000; Yolken & Torrey, 1995). However, the discoveries linking *Helicobacter pylori* and peptic ulcer disease (Chan & Leung, 2002) reminds us of the importance of keeping an open mind with respect to these agents. Furthermore, because infectious agents offer avenues for potential intervention (e.g., public health measures, vaccinations, etc.), these candidates warrant continued scrutiny. One candidate exposure that has relatively consistent findings is *Toxoplasmosis gondii*. This relatively prevalent parasite is known to be associated with congenital abnormalities of the central nervous system. Studies based on banked maternal sera (Brown *et al.*, 2005) and neonatal dried blood spots (Mortensen *et al.*, 2007b) have supported an association. A systematic review and meta-analysis has also shown that those with schizophrenia have a significantly increased prevalence of antibodies to *Toxoplasmosis gondii* compared to well controls (Torrey *et al.*, 2007). These results cannot determine if exposure to this agent preceded the onset of psychosis (a necessary condition for a cause), or contributed to poorer outcomes in those with established schizophrenia (e.g., samples based on prevalent cases will be enriched with those who do not respond to treatment). The alternate explanation is that those with schizophrenia are more likely to be exposed to infections as a result of a wide range of consequences of the illness (e.g., poverty, impaired health status, etc.).

Despite the clues from epidemiology, evidence for an association between infective agents and schizophrenia based on postmortem brain tissue remains scant (Conejero-Goldberg *et al.*, 2003).

Pregnancy and birth complications

There is considerable evidence that pregnancy and birth complications (PBCs) are detrimental to the health of the developing fetus and, in particular, its

Table 11.1 Prenatal exposure to infection and risk of psychosis – studies based on biological samples.

Study (location)	Design and sample size	Findings
Brown et al. (2000a) (New York State, USA)	Two birth cohort studies: one with serologically confirmed prenatal exposure to rubella n = 70; one comparable "unexposed" group, n = 164	Rubella exposure associated with increased risk of non-affective psychosis (RR = 5.2; 95% CI = 1.9–14.3). Risk of psychosis in the exposed group also significantly higher than an age-matched subsample from a general population sample
Buka et al. (2001) (Providence, RI, USA)	Case–control study, nested within a birth cohort. Third trimester samples 27 cases (schizophrenia and other psychotic illnesses) 54 matched control subjects	Elevated IgG and IgM levels in mothers of cases. Increased antibodies to herpes simplex virus (HSV) Type 2 in mothers of cases. No group difference in IgA antibodies nor in specific IgG antibodies to HSV Type 1, cytomegalovirus, *Toxoplasma gondii*, rubella virus, human parvovirus B19, *Chlamydia trachomatis*, or human papillomavirus type 16
Brown et al. (2004) (Oakland, CA, USA)	Case–control study, nested within a birth cohort. Second-trimester samples 59 cases (schizophrenia and spectrum disorders) 105 matched controls	Elevated levels of second-trimester IL-8 levels in mothers of cases. No group differences with respect to maternal levels of IL-1β, IL-6, or TNF-α
Brown et al. (2004a)	Case–control study, nested within a birth cohort. First, second, and third trimester samples 64 cases of schizophrenia spectrum disorders 125 matched controls	Trend level significantly increased risk with influenza exposure during the first trimester (OR = 7.0; 95% CI 0.7–75.3; p = 0.08) No increased risk of schizophrenia with influenza during the second or third trimester
Brown et al. (2005)	Case–control study, nested within a birth cohort. Third trimester sample 63 cases (schizophrenia and spectrum disorders) 123 matched controls	Highest decile of *Toxoplasma gondii* IgG levels associated with a trend level increased risk of schizophrenia (OR = 2.42; 95% CI 0.94–6.25; p < 0.07). No association between moderate Toxoplasma Ig antibody titers and the risk of schizophrenia/spectrum disorders
Brown et al. (2006)	Case–control study, nested within a birth cohort. Third trimester sample 60 cases (schizophrenia and spectrum disorders) 110 matched controls	No associations between maternal IgG seropositivity or antibody levels to HSV Type 2 and risk of schizophrenia. No association between maternal IgG seropositivity to HSV Type 1, nor cytomegalovirus and risk of schizophrenia
Mortensen et al. (2007a) (Denmark)	Case–control study, nested within a population-based birth cohort. Neonatal blood samples 71 cases of schizophrenia, 186 cases of schizophrenia or related conditions. (Affective disorder groups not shown) 684 control subjects	Highest quartile of *Toxoplasma gondii* IgG levels significantly associated with increased schizophrenia risk (OR = 1.79; 95% CI 1.01–3.15) after adjustment for urbanicity of place of birth, year of birth, gender, and psychiatric diagnoses among first-degree relatives. No significant association between any marker of infection and other schizophrenia-like disorders or affective disorders

neurodevelopment (Low *et al.*, 1985; Paneth & Pinto-Martin, 1991). A substantial body of research is now available that examines the association between PBCs and schizophrenia. The studies have employed a range of designs (e.g., case–control studies, cohort studies), measures of the exposure (based on maternal recall, records, midwife notes, different scoring systems), and measures of the outcome (diagnosis confirmed on interview, register-based diagnosis). Several meta-analyses of these data are available (Cannon *et al.*, 2002b; Geddes *et al.*, 1999; Verdoux *et al.*, 1997). Overall, there is robust evidence that PBCs have a significant but modest effect in increasing the risk

of later schizophrenia [OR ~ 2]. Based on prospective population-based studies, Cannon *et al.* (2002b) reported that the following specific exposures were associated with increased risk: antepartum hemorrhage, diabetes, Rhesus incompatibility, pre-eclampsia, low birthweight, congenital malformations, reduced head circumference, uterine atony, asphyxia, and emergency cesarean section.

The interaction of PBCs and genetic risk on structural brain outcomes has also been examined. One study reported that the individuals with schizophrenia who had an obvious genetic predisposition were more prone to develop increased ventricular and decreased hippocampal volume in response to obstetric complications (Cannon *et al.*, 1989). McNeil *et al.* (2000) have shown that in monozygotic twins discordant for schizophrenia, the differences in brain structure are largely explained by exposure to delivery complications in the affected twins. More recently, magnetic resonance imaging (MRI) studies based on individuals with schizophrenia, their unaffected siblings, and healthy controls have shown that hippocampal volume differences occurred in a stepwise fashion with each increase in genetic load for schizophrenia (Van Erp *et al.*, 2002). The individuals with schizophrenia had smaller hippocampal volumes than did their full siblings, who in turn had smaller hippocampal volumes than did the healthy controls. Within the schizophrenia group, smaller hippocampal volumes were seen in those who experienced fetal hypoxia than in those who did not, a difference not noted within the other two groups. Thus, these findings suggest that hippocampal volume is influenced in part by schizophrenia susceptibility genes and an interaction of these genes with fetal hypoxia (a gene–environment interaction). The nature of these genes remains to be clarified (Schmidt-Kastner *et al.*, 2006). Evidence that several of the susceptibility genes interact with PBCs to increase schizophrenia risk has recently been presented (Nicodemus *et al.*, 2008).

Advanced paternal age

An interesting finding first noted 30 years ago is that schizophrenia is more common in those whose fathers were old at the time they were born (Hare & Moran, 1979). However, this had been largely forgotten until Malaspina *et al.* (2001) suggested that this might be related to the evidence that mutation rates increase as father's age at conception advances because of accumulating replication errors in sperm. They investigated whether the risk of schizophrenia was associated with advancing paternal age in a population-based birth cohort of 87 907 individuals born in Jerusalem by linking their records to the Israel Psychiatric Registry. Of the offspring, 658 were diagnosed as having schizophrenia and related psychoses. After controlling for maternal age and other confounding factors, they found that paternal age was a significant predictor of schizophrenia. Compared with offspring of fathers younger than 25 years, the relative risk of schizophrenia increased monotonically in each 5-year age group, reaching 2.02 and 2.96 in offspring of men aged 45–49 and 50 years or more, respectively. Categories of mother's age showed no significant effects, after adjusting for paternal age. These findings have been replicated by a number of other investigators (Table 11.2).

Table 11.2 Paternal age and risk of schizophrenia.

Study (location)	Design and sample size	Findings
Granville-Grossman (1966) (UK)	Case–control study 942 cases from hospital records 1949–62 (ICD-8) Controls from patient siblings	No association between paternal age and risk of schizophrenia when compared to paternal age of patient siblings
Hare & Moran (1979) (UK)	Case–control study 265 cases from hospital records 1967–72. 2000 controls from published normative data	Mean observed paternal age of cases 34.5 years compared to the general population mean paternal age of 32.0 years (p < 0.001)
Kinnell (1983) (UK)	Case–control study 320 cases from several hospitals 1788 controls from published normative data	Mean paternal age of cases 33.80 years compared to that of controls 32.01 years (p < 0.001)
Malama *et al.* (1988) (Greece)	Case–control study 221 cases (Feighner criterion) 221 control patients with non-psychiatric illness	No significant difference in paternal age between two groups
Raschka (1990) (Canada)	Unclear methodology 574 cases with schizophrenia.	Schizophrenia associated with increased paternal age. No data or statistics provided
Bertranpetit & Fananas (1993) (Spain)	Case–control study 120 cases from inpatient admission (DSM-III) 176 controls	No significant difference in paternal age
Malaspina *et al.* (2001) (Israel)	Case–control study, nested within a birth cohort 658 broad schizophrenia cases (including schizophrenia, schizotypal disorder, delusional disorder, non-affective psychoses and schizoaffective disorders)(ICD-8/9/10) Birth cohort n = 87 907	Compared to the offspring of fathers aged younger than 25 years, the risk of psychosis in the offspring of fathers aged 50 or more years was 2.96 (95% CI 1.60–5.47)

Continued

Table 11.2 *Continued*

Study (location)	Design and sample size	Findings
Brown *et al.* (2002) (USA)	Case–control study, nested within a birth cohort 68 cases with schizophrenia spectrum disorders (including schizophrenia, schizotypal disorder, delusional disorder, non-affective psychoses and schizoaffective disorders) (DSM-IV) Birth cohort n = 87 907	Trend level monotonic relationship between older fathers and increased risk of schizophrenia spectrum disorders (for every 10 years increase in paternal age, the risk increased 1.35; 95% CI 0.99–1.83; p = 0.053). Numerically but not statistically significant increase rate ratio when age bands 25–24, 35–44 and 45–68 were compared to 15–24 years
Dalman *et al.* (2002) (Sweden)	Case–control study 524 cases with schizophrenia 1043 controls	After adjustment for several confounders, the odds of schizophrenia in offspring of fathers 45 years old or older were 2.8 (95% CI 1.3–6.3) times as great as in offspring of fathers aged 20–24 years
Byrne *et al.* (2003) (Denmark)	Case–control study, nested within a population-based birth cohort 7704 cases with schizophrenia (ICD) Population cohort n = 192 590	After adjustment for socioeconomic status, maternal age and family history, the risk of schizophrenia with paternal age above 50 years increased to 2.10 (95% CI 1.35–3.28), between 50–54 was 2.22 (95% CI 1.44–3.44), and above 55 was 3.53 (95% CI 1.82–6.83). Effect slightly more prominent in female offspring
Zammit *et al.* (2003) (UK)	Military conscript cohort 362 cases with schizophrenia Cohort n = 50 053	After adjustment for several confounders, there was a significant linear relationship between paternal age and risk of schizophrenia (adjusted OR for linear trend = 1.3; 95% CI 1.0–1.5), but not for other psychotic disorders
El-Saadi *et al.* (2004) (Australia)	Case–control study 119 cases with schizophrenia and affective psychosis 141 controls	When adjusted for maternal age, no association between paternal age and risk of schizophrenia
El-Saadi *et al.* (2004) (Sweden)	Case–control study 134 cases with schizophrenia 8687 controls	Compared to the offspring of fathers aged 20–24, those with paternal age of at least 35 years were at significantly increased risk of schizophrenia (adjusted OR = 2.8, 95% CI 1.18–4.89)
El-Saadi *et al.* (2004) (Denmark)	Case–control study, nested within a population-based birth cohort 11 672 cases	Compared to the offspring of fathers aged between 20 and 24, the offspring of fathers 55 or older had a significant increased risk of schizophrenia (RR = 1.84; 95% CI 1.33–2.53)
Sipos *et al.* (2004) (Sweden)	Population-based birth cohort 639 cases with schizophrenia 1311 cases with non-affective psychosis Cohort n = 712 014	After adjustment for birth-related exposures, socioeconomic factors, family history of psychosis, and early parental death, the overall hazard ratio for each 10-year increase in paternal age was 1.47 (95% CI interval 1.23–1.76) for schizophrenia and 1.12 (95% CI 0.98–1.29) for non-schizophrenic non-affective psychosis. This association between paternal age and schizophrenia was restricted to cases with no family history of the disorder
Tsuchiya *et al.* (2005) (Japan)	Case–control study 99 cases with schizophrenia 381 controls	Compared to those with fathers aged 28 or younger, those with fathers aged at least 32 had an increased risk of schizophrenia (adjusted OR = 3.00; 95% CI 1.49–6.04)

One of the largest replications comes from Sipos *et al.* (2004) who studied the risk of schizophrenia in 754 330 people born in Sweden. The overall hazard ratio for developing schizophrenia for each 10-year increase in paternal age was 1.47. This association between paternal age and schizophrenia has been repeatedly shown to be present in those with no family history of the disorder, but not in those with a positive family history (Malaspina *et al.*, 2002; Sipos *et al.*, 2004). This stronger association between paternal age and schizophrenia in people without a family history raises the possibility that accumulation of *de novo* mutations in paternal sperm with aging contributes to the risk of schizophrenia.

The links between advanced paternal age and schizophrenia have been incorporated in a range of etiological theories of schizophrenia. For example, the persistence of schizophrenia in the population in spite of reduced fertility implicates a role for new genetic mutations. It has been suggested that advanced paternal age may be contributing to the transgenerational accumulation of copy error mutations, which in turn contributes to susceptibility to schizophrenia (Keller & Miller, 2006). Paternal exposure to micronutritional deficiencies such as folate may further amplify copy error mutations in the male germ cell lines (McClellan *et al.*, 2006). Finally, it is also feasible that epigenetic processes (e.g., chromatin folding, methylation of CpG bases, etc.) may be compromised in the sperm of older fathers, and that these mechanisms may contribute to the increased risk of schizophrenia in the offspring of older fathers (Perrin *et al.*, 2007).

Exposure to later biological candidate risk factors

Drug abuse

It has long been known that abuse of amphetamine can induce schizophrenia-like psychosis (Connell, 1958). Methamphetamine, a similar but more addictive compound, can also cause schizophrenia-like psychosis, which has become a major problem in Pacific countries and certain parts of the US. Chen *et al.* (2003) reported that methamphetamine psychosis mimics the positive symptoms of schizophrenia very closely. Genetic factors appeared to play a role in increasing susceptibility: individuals who had no family history of schizophrenia could abuse the drug without developing psychosis, whereas those with a greater familial predisposition to schizophrenia were more likely to experience psychotic symptoms. Those who developed psychosis were more likely to recover if they had no family history (Chen *et al.* 2004, 2005). With respect to more specific gene–environment interactions, studies based on variations in candidate genes involved in the dopaminergic pathways in those with methamphetine-related psychosis

have provided some interesting leads (Cheng *et al.*, 2005; Nakamura *et al.*, 2006)

It has long been accepted that cannabis intoxication (and exposure to its active ingredient tetrahydrocannabinol, THC) can cause brief psychotic episodes. Among patients with established psychosis, those who persisted in smoking cannabis had a worse outcome than those who did not (Grech *et al.*, 2005). In addition, numerous studies have shown that psychotic patients take more cannabis than the populations from which they are drawn (Kavanagh *et al.*, 2002).

But does cannabis actually *cause* psychosis? In an attempt to answer this question, researchers have performed longitudinal studies in general population samples and related cannabis consumption to subsequent onset of psychosis. Thus, Andreasson *et al.* (1987), who examined and followed-up almost 50 000 young Swedish male conscripts, found that men who had smoked cannabis by the age of conscription had double the risk of schizophrenia in the ensuing 15 years; those who had smoked cannabis on at least 50 occasions were six times more likely to later receive a diagnosis of schizophrenia. This association persisted after excluding polysubstance users and adjustments were made for possible confounders (cognitive deficits, nicotine use, urban childhood; Zammit *et al.*, 2002).

An Israeli cohort study also found that those hospitalized for schizophrenia were more likely to be cannabis-users during late adolescence (Weiser *et al.*, 2003). A study based on the Netherlands Mental Health Survey and Incidence Study (NEMESIS) found cannabis users with no psychotic disorder at baseline were at increased risk of clinically significant psychotic symptoms at follow-up after 3 years: this was independent of any baseline comorbid non-psychotic psychiatric disorder or other illegal drugs substances (van Os *et al.*, 2002). A large prospective population-based German study followed young people for 4 years (Henquet *et al.*, 2005a). Cannabis use at baseline was associated with an increased risk of psychotic symptoms at follow-up in a dose–response manner.

In the birth cohort study from Dunedin, New Zealand, noted earlier, individuals were asked about their drug consumption at the ages of 15 and 18, and then at 26 years; 96% were interviewed using a standardized psychiatric assessment (Arseneault *et al.*, 2002). Cannabis use at age 15 and 18 increased the risk of psychotic symptoms or schizophreniform disorder at age 26 (OR = 4.5 for those using cannabis before age 15).

The various studies that have related cannabis consumption to later psychosis are summarized in the Table 11.3 and have been extensively reviewed (Henquet *et al.*, 2005b; Moore *et al.*, 2007; Murray *et al.*, 2007; Semple *et al.*, 2005). The results of these reviews are broadly consistent with the findings from the primary data—the greater the exposure to cannabis, the greater the risk.

Table 11.3 General population studies of the effect of cannabis use on the risk of psychosis.

Study (location)	Design and sample size	Findings OR for psychosis outcome (95% CI)
Andreassen *et al.* (1987) Zammit *et al.* (2002) (Sweden)	Cohort of military conscripts n = 50 053	2.1 (1.2–3.7)
Tien & Anthony (1990) (USA)	Population-based sample n = 4494	2.4 (1.2–7.1)
Arseneault *et al.* (2002) (Dunedin, New Zealand)	Birth cohort n = 1253	3.1 (0.7–13.3)
van Os *et al.* (2002) (The Netherlands)	Population-based sample n = 4045	2.8 (1.2–6.5)
Weiser *et al.* (2003) (Israel)	Population-based sample n = 9724	2.0 (1.3–3.1)
Fergusson *et al.* (2005) (Christchurch, New Zealand)	Birth cohort n = 1265	2.8 (1.8–4.4)
Ferdinand *et al.* (2005) (The Netherlands)	Population-based sample n = 1580	2.8 (1.79–4.43)
Henquet *et al.* (2005a) (Germany)	Population-based sample n = 2436	1.7 (1.1–1.5)
Wiles *et al.* (2006) (UK)	Population-based sample n = 8580	1.5 (0.6–3.9)

Some have claimed that the studies discussed above may have been confounded by the effect of *other psychoactive drugs*, such as amphetamines and lysergic acid diethylamide (LSD), which are known to be psychotogenic. However, the association between cannabis use and later schizophrenia in the Dunedin, Dutch, and Swedish studies held even when the researchers adjusted for the use of other psychotogenic drugs.

A second criticism has been that the cannabis may have been taken in an *attempt to self-medicate* against psychotic symptoms (Ferdinand *et al.*, 2005). The best information concerning this comes from the Christchurch study in which data on both cannabis use and psychotic symptoms were collected on a cohort studied at the ages of 18, 21, and 25 (Fergusson *et al.*, 2005). The investigators were therefore able to study both the effects of cannabis use on later psychotic symptoms and also the effect of psychotic symptoms on later cannabis use. As expected, cannabis use at the age of 18 was associated with more psychotic symptoms 3 and 7 years later. However, the presence of psychotic symptoms at the age of 18 appeared to inhibit rather than encourage subsequent cannabis use. This suggests a causal link between cannabis use and the development of psychotic symptoms and does not support the idea that patients were taking the cannabis in an attempt at "self-medication".

Why do only a small minority of people who take cannabis, even in large quantities, develop psychosis? Individuals differ in their sensitivity to acute administration of THC, with a minority developing frank paranoia in response to doses that barely have an effect in others. Verdoux *et al.* (2003) studied the acute effects of cannabis in the everyday situation, and assessed their subjects using a questionnaire that measured subclinical psychotic experiences. Individuals without evidence of psychosis-proneness generally responded to cannabis by feeling more at ease with the world, and experienced only minor perceptual changes. However, those who were identified as psychosis-prone reported more marked perceptual changes and feelings of increased suspicion and hostility after taking cannabis.

Caspi *et al.* (2005) reasoned that this vulnerability might have a genetic basis. They therefore studied how the interaction between cannabis use and variation in the gene for catechol-O-methyltransferase (*COMT*) influences the risk of psychosis in volunteers from the Dunedin study that was discussed earlier. Due to a functional polymorphism that involves a Val-to-Met substitution at codon 158, this gene has two common allelic variants which influence the efficiency with which dopamine is broken down in the prefrontal cortex. Caspi *et al.* (2005) found that use of cannabis in adolescence had no effect on the subsequent risk of psychosis in individuals who were homozygous for the *COMT* Met allele. However, adolescent smokers with the Val/Val genotype were at least five times more likely to develop schizophreniform psychosis than people with the same genotype who did not take cannabis.

Head injury

For those who survive a head injury, there is an increased risk for a wide range of adverse neuropsychiatric outcomes (Deb *et al.*, 1999; Emanuelson *et al.*, 2003; Koponen *et al.*, 2002). With respect to schizophrenia, a study based on the Swedish register found no significant association with previous head injury, though a small association with other non-affective disorders was found (Harrison *et al.*, 2006). Other studies have found mixed evidence for the association (Nielsen *et al.*, 2002). A systematic review of the literature noted the methodological shortcomings of many studies, and concluded that there was some evidence suggesting that people with schizophrenia may be more prone to head injury, but it was unlikely that head injury contributed to schizophrenia (David & Prince, 2005).

Social biology

While some environmental risks can be modeled at the individual level (e.g., exposure to an infectious agent), other factors are best examined at the level of the family, neighborhood or society (March & Susser, 2006; Susser, 2004). Multilevel studies can capture both ecological-level variables (e.g., a neighborhood marker of social capital or poverty) and individual level variables (e.g., experience-sampling methodology to assess changes in individual stress levels). Social biology attempts to model risk factors from different categories of observation. Several of the risk factors associated with schizophrenia can be conceptualized within a social biology framework.

Place of birth and upbringing

There is now robust evidence linking place of birth and risk of schizophrenia. Those born and/or raised in urban regions have an increased risk of developing schizophrenia compared to rural regions (Lewis *et al.*, 1992; O'Callaghan *et al.*, 1992; Takei *et al.*, 1992). Two population-based studies, one from the Netherlands (Marcelis *et al.*, 1998) and one from Denmark (Mortensen *et al.*, 1999), found a relative risk of developing schizophrenia when born in the city *versus* being born in the country of about 2.4. However, as urban birth is relatively frequent, the two studies reported the population attributable risk for this variable to be substantial (about 30%). Place of birth could be a proxy marker for a risk-modifying variable operating at or before birth.

However, because most people who are born in a city are also brought up there, it is difficult to disentangle pre- and peri-natal effects from those operating later in childhood. There is evidence that the more years spent in an urban area during childhood, the greater the risk of developing schizophrenia (Pedersen & Mortensen, 2001), and that urban residence may operate prior to conception (Pedersen & Mortensen, 2006a,c).

The nature of the risk-modifying factor associated with urbanicity remains to be clarified (McGrath & Scott, 2006; Pedersen & Mortensen, 2006c). To date, studies have been unable to account for the finding by measuring overcrowding (as a proxy marker of increased risk of transmission of infectious agents) (Agerbo *et al.*, 2001; Wahlbeck *et al.*, 2001b) or by examining proximity to roads (as a proxy marker of petrol-related toxins) (Pedersen & Mortensen, 2006b). Lead exposure is more prevalent in urban settings. One study has used banked second-trimester maternal sera to examine (delta-aminolevulinic acid, a biomarker related to lead exposure) and later schizophrenia(Opler *et al.*, 2004). A trend level association between high prenatal delta-aminolevulinic acid and later schizophrenia was identified. It is also feasible that city residence acts as a proxy for a stress-related exposure, best captured by social biology and eco-epidemiology (Susser, 2004). Urban place of residence is associated with increased endorsement of minor psychotic symptoms in otherwise well individuals (Spauwen *et al.*, 2004). It is feasible that urban-related stressors may further contribute to the persistence of these psychotic symptoms in genetically susceptible individuals (Spauwen & van Os, 2006).

Migration

One of the most striking findings from schizophrenia epidemiology in recent decades has been the markedly increased risk found in some migrant groups. Despite initial concerns about methodological issues, recent systematic reviews have shown a consistent and coherent pattern (Cantor-Graae & Selten, 2005; McGrath *et al.*, 2004). In summary, the studies show that both first- and second-generation migrants have an increased risk of developing schizophrenia. The effect is most pronounced in dark-skinned migrants (Cantor-Graae & Selten, 2005). One of the most striking findings came from the ÆSOP study (Fearon *et al.*, 2006), a large incidence study based in three English cities. This study found a nine-fold increased risk of schizophrenia in African–Caribbean and a nearly six-fold increased risk in black Africans; increased risks of similar magnitude were found for risk of manic psychosis.

A report from a US birth cohort has also found an increased risk of schizophrenia in African–Americans (Bresnahan *et al.*, 2007), suggesting that factors related to race/ethnicity are operating independently of the stressors associated with recent migration. These results have triggered a search for possible candidate exposures that could explain these findings. Generally, the search for biological explanations for the high rates in migrants/ethnic minorities have proved negative, leading to a renaissance of research into other explanations, e.g., various forms of early childhood and adult adversity, neighborhood characteristics (e.g., social capital, ethnic density), and hypotheses related to social biology (Hoffman, 2007; Selten & Cantor-Graae, 2005).

Trauma and stress-related exposures

Extreme prenatal maternal stress is associated with adverse health outcomes in the offspring. For example, studies based on Danish registers have reported association between maternal life events (e.g., severe emotional stress such as bereavement, severe illness in a relative) and an increased risk of cranial–neural crest malformations (Hansen et al., 2000). Exposure to similar trauma in the year prior to the pregnancy carried an increased risk of being small for gestational age, suggesting that the mechanisms linking maternal stress and adverse health outcomes may have a longer latency than first thought (Precht et al., 2007).

With respect to schizophrenia, the evidence related to maternal (prenatal) stress is mixed. Huttunen and Niskanen (1978) reported an increased risk of schizophrenia in the offspring of women whose husbands had been killed in the Finnish–Russian war. Several studies have examined the risk of schizophrenia in those who were in utero during a war or natural disaster. A study based on Dutch data reported a significant association between exposure to stress during the first trimester and an increased risk of schizophrenia (van Os & Selten, 1998). However, studies based on wars in Israel (Selten et al., 2003) and a flood in the Netherlands (Selten et al., 1999) did not find any such association.

Two studies have examined unwantedness of pregnancy and risk of schizophrenia in the offspring. Based on the Northern Finish Birth Cohort, unwanted children had approximately a two-fold increased risk of schizophrenia (Myhrman et al., 1996), though this may have been confounded by parental psychiatric illness. A US study found a comparable effect size based on a birth cohort, but this finding was not statistically significant (Herman et al., 2006). Unwantedness may, of course, be a proxy measure for a range of adverse prenatal health behaviors (e.g. health-seeking behavior).

It has long been accepted that childhood trauma is associated with a broad range of adverse mental health outcomes. However, whether childhood trauma is associated with schizophrenia has been controversial (for review, see Read et al., 2005; Morgan & Fisher, 2007, also Chapter 29). Based on 20 studies that explored the prevalence of child-

hood abuse in those with a psychotic disorder, about half of both males and females report either childhood sexual or physical abuse (Morgan & Fisher, 2007). Population-based studies also suggest that those with prior exposure to trauma are more likely to have a psychotic disorder or report isolated symptoms of psychosis (e.g., delusions, hallucinations). A population-based UK study relying on retrospective recall found that individuals with psychosis had experienced a significant excess of victimizing experiences during childhood compared to the general population (Bebbington et al., 2004). Even in the general population, exposure to trauma (including childhood sexual abuse) was associated with delusional-like experiences, and those with more trauma exposures and/or associated post-traumatic stress disorder (PTSD) had an increased risk of delusional-like experience (Scott et al., 2007). Janssen et al. (2004) found an association between child abuse and psychotic symptoms whilst Sareen et al. (2005) reported an association between positive psychotic symptoms and PTSD. These studies are in keeping with the long-standing "diathesis–stress" hypothesis (Howes et al., 2004; Seedat et al., 2003; Walker & Diforio, 1997), where exposure to trauma may contribute to risk status in vulnerable individuals.

With respect to life event research in general, there is relatively good evidence linking life events and relapse in established schizophrenia (Hultman et al., 1997). There is also some evidence showing that individuals who develop schizophrenia may have had more life events prior to the onset of psychosis (Bebbington et al., 1993; Norman & Malla, 1993a,b).

Trauma clearly contributes to many adverse mental health outcomes. Understanding how stress impacts on different individuals, at different phases of life, to result in a broad spectrum of adverse mental health outcomes remains an important area of research (see Chapter 29 for further discussion).

Risk factors and dopamine dysregulation

In order to progress our understanding of candidate risk factors, we need to consider them in the light of what we know of the biology of psychosis. In other words, neuroscience is needed to evaluate the biological plausibility of candidate exposures (McGrath, 2007). The best established biological hypothesis concerning schizophrenia is the dopamine hypothesis (Toda & Abi-Dargham, 2007). Psychotic patients release excessive striatal dopamine in response to an amphetamine challenge, and the degree of dopamine release correlates positively with the severity of psychotic symptoms. The likely mechanism is that the increased dopamine results in increased attention and excessive significance ("salience") being attributed to everyday stimuli (Kapur, 2003). A number of the risk factors we have discussed above appear to impact upon the dopamine system.

Gender

Why should males be more prone to schizophrenia? Past speculations have included the possibly protective effects of estrogen and the greater fragility of the male brain during development (Castle & Murray, 1991). Munro *et al.* (2006) have now raised another possibility by showing that normal males respond to an amphetamine challenge by releasing more striatal dopamine than do normal females. It could well be that this greater sensitivity of the dopamine system renders males more prone to develop the striatal hyperdopaminergia which underlies psychosis.

Obstetric events

Exposure to a range of obstetric complications also increases risk, e.g., prematurity, low birthweight, and particularly hypoxia (Cannon *et al.*, 2002b; Gilmore *et al.*, 2006). Such hazards are known to be associated with hippocampal damage, and animal studies have shown that cesarean section and perinatal hippocampal damage can facilitate the development of dopamine sensitization once the animal matures (Boksa & El-Khodor, 2003; Lipska, 2004). Animal models of maternal immune activation (a consequence of prenatal infection) also implicate altered dopaminergic function in the adult offspring (Ozawa *et al.*, 2006; Zuckerman *et al.*, 2003).

Social adversity

There is evidence from a range of animal studies showing that methods of rearing, such as isolation (Hall *et al.*, 1999) and a submissive position in the social hierarchy (Morgan *et al.*, 2002), can increase the reactiveness of the mesolimbic dopamine system. Thus, a recent study showed that housing a mouse with a large "bully" mouse can induce brain-derived neurotrophic factor (BDNF) in the former, which of course controls the dopamine system (Berton *et al.*, 2006). As yet there are no human studies directly testing whether chronic social adversity can have a similar effect in humans. However, such a mechanism would provide a plausible way in which the social factors that are known to increase risk of schizophrenia might operate.

Drug abuse

It is well known that psychostimulants such as amphetamine and methamphetamine increase synaptic dopamine. Animal studies show that cannabis has a similar effect, though human studies are as yet lacking (Murray *et al.*, 2007). However, the evidence of a gene–environment interaction between the *COMT* gene and exposure to cannabis, discussed earlier, is compatible with such an effect since COMT has an important role in dopamine metabolism in the prefrontal cortex and other brain regions (Caspi *et al.*, 2005; Henquet *et al.*, 2006; Tunbridge *et al.*, 2006).

Conclusions and future directions

The epidemiology of schizophrenia is becoming more interesting and indeed surprising (McGrath, 2007). The list of candidate environmental risk factors for schizophrenia has lengthened considerably in recent years. While some of these candidates will turn out to be false leads, we should mentally prepare ourselves for the list of potential "environmental" risk factors for schizophrenia to lengthen even further in the years to come. In light of the marked variability in both the phenotype and genotype of schizophrenia, we must expect similar heterogeneity in environmental risk factors (McGrath, 2007). Like genetic risk factors (Sullivan, 2005), environmental risk factors will probably be of small effect, and will probably vary considerably between populations.

Epidemiological research can serve to "sharpen the focus", allowing candidate risk factors to be identified, but history has shown that risk factor epidemiology can sometimes enter cycles of uninformative replications (called "circular epidemiology") (Kuller, 1999). For example, "season of birth" has been studied as a risk factor for schizophrenia for 80 years, with little real progress in identifying the underlying risk-modifying exposure. Furthermore, epidemiology is a notoriously blunt and imprecise instrument. The danger of relying on observational studies alone has been reinforced in recent years (Davey Smith & Ebrahim, 2001). Associations that emerge from observational studies may operate via confounding factors that were not considered in the original research design. Thus, regardless of the strength and consistency of associations that emerge from observational studies, researchers must remain vigilant for residual and unidentified confounding.

It is worth contrasting what we know concerning the etiology of schizophrenia with that of another complex disorder, coronary artery disease. In both cases, we know a number of the environmental risk factors (in the case of coronary artery disease, smoking, lack of exercise). However, the major difference is that in coronary artery disease we understand the pathological mechanisms which such risk factors set in train, and we can trace the pathogenesis from the risk factor through to the clinical picture. We have no such knowledge of the pathogenetic mechanisms in schizophrenia other than the fact that dopamine dysregulation appears to be the final common pathway.

There is a case to broaden our categories of observation beyond narrow diagnostic criteria to explore symptoms associated with psychosis that can be found in otherwise-well individuals (Weiser *et al.*, 2005). Several large community-based samples have identified surprisingly high proportions of the general community who report hallucinations and delusional-like experiences (Scott *et al.*, 2006; van Os *et al.*, 2000). Furthermore, it has been shown that factors which are known to be associated with schizophrenia (e.g., poor education, urban living, belonging to an ethnic minority, cannabis dependence) are also associated with minor psychotic symptoms in the general populations (Johns *et al.*, 2004). This implies that it may be useful to think of the liability to schizophrenia being on a continuum which reaches into the general population, with risk factors acting (singly or more usually collectively) to push the individual towards, and eventually over a threshold, beyond which frank psychosis is expressed.

Wherever possible, we need to add value to future epidemiological studies. While incidence and prevalence studies can help service development and identify unmet needs, the return for the research dollar can be enriched by including blood for genotyping, and by adding neuroimaging and neurocognitive measures. In particular, where genetic factors are thought to influence or mediate candidate environmental exposures, then studies should seek to measure both (see recent reviews on Mendelian randomization; Smith & Ebrahim, 2004), as illustrated by the COMT–cannabis interaction mentioned above (Caspi *et al.*, 2005; Henquet *et al.*, 2006; van Winkel *et al.*, 2008).

While clinical research is clearly important, animal models remain the only practical tool for unraveling the mechanisms of action linking early life disruptions and later adult neuropsychiatric disorders. Animal models will never recapitulate the full phenotype of schizophrenia, but they are useful to focus on neurobiological correlates such as abnormal behavior or brain structure or function (Arguello & Gogos, 2006). For example, the impact of candidate exposures on neuronal development can be examined *in vitro* and in whole animal studies (with analyses ranging from gene expression to social behavior). Animal models in schizophrenia research have explored the impact of early life exposure to candidate risk factors and behavior. These include prenatal exposure to specific viruses such as influenza (Fatemi *et al.*, 2000), low prenatal vitamin D (Kesby *et al.*, 2006), and prenatal hypoxic/ischemic insults (Mallard *et al.*, 1999). The evidence linking prenatal infection has lead to rodent models of maternal immune activation. These models, which use non-infective viral (Poly I:C) or bacterial-like components (lipopolysaccharide, LPS) to trigger the innate immune systems, have produced behavioral phenotypes which are informative for schizophrenia (e.g., altered information processing, altered dopaminergic tone, etc.) and for developmental neurobiol-

ogy in general (Meyer *et al.*, 2006a,b; Ozawa *et al.*, 2006). Similarly, rodent models can explore the impact of exposures related to social defeat, and help explore the complex pathways linking social stress and neurobiology (Berton *et al.*, 2006; Carboni *et al.*, 2006). Access to transgenic mice also allows the potential to extend this type of research with the use of genetic "knock-out" mice (looking for gene–environment interactions). For further discussion of animal models, see Chapter 22.

Finally, the schizophrenia research community needs to generate a sense of urgency about unraveling the environmental risk factors contributing to the gradients. As discussed above, urban birth is associated with a substantial (30%) population attributable risk (Mortensen *et al.*, 1999). Considering that population demographics indicate increasing urbanization in both the developed and developing world (McMichael, 2001), it is feasible that the population attributable fraction of schizophrenia associated with urban birth will rise in the decades to come. In many developed societies, age of fatherhood is being delayed. Thus, it seems probable that this risk factor for schizophrenia will be amplified over successive generations. Similarly, if the prevalence of cannabis use continues to rise, we can predict an increase in the incidence and prevalence of active psychosis (Hickman *et al.*, 2007; McGrath & Saha, 2007). There is much work to be done in unraveling the hidden layers of complexity underpinning schizophrenia. In this quest we cannot afford to waste the valuable clues being generated by epidemiology.

Acknowledgements

Joy Welham and Sukanta Saha assisted in the identification of studies for this chapter.

References

Agerbo, E., Torrey, E.F. & Mortensen, P.B. (2001) Household crowding in early adulthood and schizophrenia are unrelated in Denmark: a nested case-control study. *Schizophrenia Research* **47**, 243–246.

Andreasson, S., Allebeck, P., Engstrom, A. & Rydberg, U. (1987) Cannabis and schizophrenia. A longitudinal study of Swedish conscripts. *Lancet* **2**, 1483–1486.

Arguello, P.A. & Gogos, J.A. (2006) Modeling madness in mice: one piece at a time. *Neuron* **5**, 179–196.

Arseneault, L., Cannon, M., Poulton, R. *et al.* (2002) Cannabis use in adolescence and risk for adult psychosis: longitudinal prospective study. *BMJ* **325**, 1212–1213.

Barker, D.J., Eriksson, J.G., Forsén, T. & Osmond, C. (2002) Fetal origins of adult disease: strength of effects and biological basis. *International Journal of Epidemiology* **31**, 1235–1239.

Bearden, C.E., Rosso, I.M., Hollister, J.M., *et al.* (2000) A prospective cohort study of childhood behavioral deviance and language abnormalities as predictors of adult schizophrenia. *Schizophrenia Bulletin* **26**, 395–410.

Bebbington, P., Wilkins, S., Jones, P. *et al.* (1993) Life events and psychosis: Initial results from the Camberwell Collaborative Psychosis Study. *British Journal of Psychiatry* **162**, 72–79.

Bebbington, P.E., Bhugra, D., Brugha, T. *et al.* (2004) Psychosis, victimisation and childhood disadvantage: evidence from the second British National Survey of Psychiatric Morbidity. *British Journal of Psychiatry* **185**, 220–226.

Berton, O., McClung, C.A., Dileone, R.J. *et al.* (2006) Essential role of BDNF in the mesolimbic dopamine pathway in social defeat stress. *Science* **311**, 864–868.

Bertranpetit, J. & Fananas, L. (1993) Parental age in schizophrenia in a case-controlled study. *British Journal of Psychiatry* **162**, 574.

Boksa, P. & El-Khodor, B.F. (2003) Birth insult interacts with stress at adulthood to alter dopaminergic function in animal models: possible implications for schizophrenia and other disorders. *Neuroscience Biobehavioural Reveiws* **27**, 91–101.

Bresnahan, M., Begg, M.D., Brown, A. *et al.* (2007) Race and risk of schizophrenia in a US birth cohort: another example of health disparity? *International Journal of Epidemiology* **36**, 751–758.

Brown, A.S. & Susser, E.S. (1997) Sex differences in prevalence of congenital neural defects after periconceptional famine exposure. *Epidemiology* **8**, 55–58.

Brown, A.S. & Susser, E.S. (2005) Homocysteine and schizophrenia: from prenatal to adult life. *Progress in Neuropsychopharmacology and Biological Psychiatry* **29**, 1175–1180.

Brown, A.S., Susser, E.S., Butler, P.D. *et al.* (1996) Neurobiological plausibility of prenatal nutritional deprivation as a risk factor for schizophrenia. *Journal of Nervous and Mental Disease* **184**, 71–85.

Brown, A.S., Cohen, P., Greenwald, S. & Susser, E. (2000a) Nonaffective psychosis after prenatal exposure to rubella. *American Journal of Psychiatry* **157**, 438–443.

Brown, A.S., van Os, J., Driessens, C. *et al.* (2000b) Further evidence of relation between prenatal famine and major affective disorder. *American Journal of Psychiatry* **157**, 190–195.

Brown, A.S., Schaefer, C.A., Wyatt, R.J. *et al.* (2002) Paternal age and risk of schizophrenia in adult offspring. *American Journal of Psychiatry* **159**, 1528–1533.

Brown, A.S., Begg, M.D., Gravenstein, S. *et al.* (2004a) Serologic evidence of prenatal influenza in the etiology of schizophrenia. *Archives of General Psychiatry* **61**, 774–780.

Brown, A.S., Hootonm J., Schaefer, C.A. *et al.* (2004b) Elevated maternal interleukin-8 levels and risk of schizophrenia in adult offspring. *American Journal of Psychiatry* **161**, 889–895.

Brown, A.S., Schaefer, C.A., Quesenberry, P. Jr. *et al.* (2005) Maternal exposure to toxoplasmosis and risk of schizophrenia in adult offspring. *American Journal of Psychiatry* **162**, 767–773.

Brown, A.S., Schaefer, C.A., Quesenberry, C.P. Jr. *et al.* (2006) No evidence of relation between maternal exposure to herpes simplex virus type 2 and risk of schizophrenia? *American Journal of Psychiatry* **163**, 2178–2180.

Brown, A.S., Bottiglieri, T., Schaefer, C.A. *et al.* (2007) Elevated prenatal homocysteine levels as a risk factor for schizophrenia. *Archives of General Psychiatry* **64**, 31–39.

Buka, S.L., Tsuang, M.T., Torrey, E.F. *et al.* (2001) Maternal infections and subsequent psychosis among offspring. *Archives of General Psychiatry* **58**, 1032–1037.

Byrne, M., Agerbo, E., Ewald, H. *et al.* (2003) Parental age and risk of schizophrenia: a case-control study. *Archives of General Psychiatry* **60**, 673–678.

Cannon, T.D., Mednick, S.A. & Parnas, J. (1989) Genetic and perinatal determinants of structural brain deficits in schizophrenia. *Archives of General Psychiatry* **46**, 883–889.

Cannon, M., Walsh, E., Hollis, C. *et al.* (2001) Predictors of later schizophrenia and affective psychosis among attendees at a child psychiatry department. *British Journal of Psychiatry* **178**, 420–426.

Cannon, M., Caspi, A., Moffitt, T.E. *et al.* (2002a) Evidence for early-childhood, pan-developmental impairment specific to schizophreniform disorder: results from a longitudinal birth cohort. *Archives of General Psychiatry* **59**, 449–456.

Cannon, M., Jones, P.B. & Murray, R.M. (2002b) Obstetric complications and schizophrenia: historical and meta-analytic review. *American Journal of Psychiatry* **159**, 1080–1092.

Cannon, M., Moffitt, T.E., Caspi, A. *et al.* (2006) Neuropsychological performance at the age of 13 years and adult schizophreniform disorder: prospective birth cohort study. *British Journal of Psychiatry* **189**, 463–464.

Cantor-Graae, E. (2007) The contribution of social factors to the development of schizophrenia: a review of recent findings. *Canadian Journal of Psychiatry* **52**, 277–286.

Cantor-Graae, E. & Selten, J.P. (2005) Schizophrenia and migration: a meta-analysis and review. *American Journal of Psychiatry* **162**, 12–24.

Carboni, L., Piubelli, C., Pozzato, C. *et al.* (2006) Proteomic analysis of rat hippocampus after repeated psychosocial stress. *Neuroscience* **137**, 1237–1246.

Caspi, A., Moffitt, T.E., Cannon, M. *et al.* (2005) Moderation of the effect of adolescent-onset cannabis use on adult psychosis by a functional polymorphism in the catechol-O-methyltransferase gene: longitudinal evidence of a gene X environment interaction. *Biological Psychiatry* **57**, 1117–11127.

Castle, D.J. & Murray, R.M. (1991) The neurodevelopmental basis of sex differences in schizophrenia. *Psychological Medicine* **21**, 565–575.

Chan, F.K. & Leung, W.K. (2002) Peptic-ulcer disease. *Lancet* **360**, 933–941.

Chen, C.K., Lin, S.K., Sham, P.C. *et al.* (2003) Pre-morbid characteristics and co-morbidity of methamphetamine users with and without psychosis. *Psychological Medicine* **33**, 1407–1414.

Chen, C.K., Hu, X., Lin, S.K. *et al.* (2004) Association analysis of dopamine D2-like receptor genes and methamphetamine abuse. *Psychiatric Genetics* **14**, 223–226.

Chen, C.K., Lin, S.K., Sham, P.C. *et al.* (2005) Morbid risk for psychiatric disorder among the relatives of methamphetamine users with and without psychosis. *American Journal of Medical Genetics Part B Neuropsychiatric Genetics* **136**, 87–91.

Cheng, C.Y., Hong, C.J., Yu, Y.W. *et al.* (2005) Brain-derived neurotrophic factor (Val66Met) genetic polymorphism is associated with substance abuse in males. *Brain Research Molecular Brain Research* **140**, 86–90.

Conejero-Goldberg, C., Torrey, E.F. & Yolken, R.H. (2003) Herpesviruses and *Toxoplasma gondii* in orbital frontal cortex of psychiatric patients. *Schizophrenia Research* **60**, 65–69.

Connell, P.H. (1958) *Amphetamine Psychosis*. London: Chapman and Hill.

Cornblatt, B., Obuchowski, M., Roberts, S. *et al.* (1999) Cognitive and behavioral precursors of schizophrenia. *Developmental Psychopathology* **11**, 487–508.

Cougnard, A., Marcelis, M., Myin-Germeys, I. *et al.* (2007) Does normal developmental expression of psychosis combine with environmental risk to cause persistence of psychosis? A psychosis proneness-persistence model. *Psychological Medicine* **37**, 513–527.

Dalman, C. & Allebeck, P. (2002) Paternal age and schizophrenia: further support for an association. *American Journal of Psychiatry* **159**, 1591–1592.

David, A.S. & Prince, M. (2005) Psychosis following head injury: a critical review. *Journal of Neurology, Neurosurgery and Psychiatry* **76** (Suppl 1), i53–60.

Davies, G., Welham, J., Chant, D., Torrey, E.F. & McGrath, J. (2003) A systematic review and meta-analysis of Northern Hemisphere season of birth studies in schizophrenia. *Schizophrenia Bulletin* **29**, 587–593.

Davey Smith, G. & Ebrahim, S. (2001) Epidemiology—is it time to call it a day? *International Journal of Epidemiology* **30**, 1–11.

Deb, S., Lyons, I., Koutzoukis, C. *et al.* (1999) Rate of psychiatric illness 1 year after traumatic brain injury. *American Journal of Psychiatry* **156**, 374–378.

Done, D.J., Crow, T.J., Johnstone, E.C. & Sacker, A. (1994) Childhood antecedents of schizophrenia and affective illness: social adjustment at ages 7 and 11. *BMJ* **309**, 699–703.

El-Saadi, O., Pedersen, C.B., McNeil, T.F. *et al.* (2004) Paternal and maternal age as risk factors for psychosis: findings from Denmark, Sweden and Australia. *Schizophrenia Research* **67**, 227–236.

Emanuelson, I., Andersson Holmkvist, E., Bjorklund, R. & Stalhammar, D. (2003) Quality of life and post-concussion symptoms in adults after mild traumatic brain injury: a population-based study in western Sweden. *Acta Neurologica Scandinavica* **108**, 332–338.

Fatemi, S.H., Cuadra, A.E., El Fakahany, E.E. *et al.* (2000) Prenatal viral infection causes alterations in nNOS expression in developing mouse brains. *Neuroreport* **11**, 1493–1496.

Fearon, P., Kirkbride, J.B., Morgan, C. *et al.* (2006) Incidence of schizophrenia and other psychoses in ethnic minority groups: results from the MRC AESOP Study. *Psychological Medicine* **36**, 1541–1550.

Ferdinand, R.F., Sondeijker, F., van der Ende, J. *et al.* (2005) Cannabis use predicts future psychotic symptoms, and vice versa. *Addiction* **100**, 612–618.

Fergusson, D.M., Horwood, L.J. & Ridder, E.M. (2005) Tests of causal linkages between cannabis use and psychotic symptoms. *Addiction* **100**, 354–366.

Finlay, B.L. (2007) Endless minds most beautiful. *Developmental Science* **10**, 30–34.

Finlay, B.L., Darlington, R.B. & Nicastro, N. (2001) Developmental structure in brain evolution. *Behavioural Brain Science* **24**, 263–278; discussion 278–308.

Geddes, J.R., Verdoux, H., Takei, N. *et al.* (1999) Schizophrenia and complications of pregnancy and labor: an individual patient data meta-analysis. *Schizophrenia Bulletin* **25**, 413–423.

Gilmore, J.H., Lin, W. & Gerig, G. (2006) Fetal and neonatal brain development. *American Journal of Psychiatry* **163**, 2046.

Gluckman, P. & Hanson, M. (2004) *The Fetal Matrix: Evolution, Development and Disease*. Cambridge: Cambridge University Press.

Granville-Grossman, K.L. (1966) Parental age and schizophrenia. *British Journal of Psychiatry* **112**, 899–905.

Grech, A., Van Os, J., Jones, P.B. *et al.* (2005) Cannabis use and outcome of recent onset psychosis. *European Psychiatry* **20**, 349–353.

Gunnell, D., Rasmussen, F., Fouskakis, D. *et al.* (2003) Patterns of fetal and childhood growth and the development of psychosis in young males: a cohort study. *American Journal of Epidemiology* **158**, 291–300.

Hall, F.S., Wilkinson, L.S., Humby, T. & Robbins, T.W. (1999) Maternal deprivation of neonatal rats produces enduring changes in dopamine function. *Synapse* **32**, 37–43.

Hansen, D., Lou, H.C. & Olsen, J. (2000) Serious life events and congenital malformations: a national study with complete follow-up. *Lancet* **356**, 875–880.

Hare, E.H. & Moran, P.A. (1979) Raised parental age in psychiatric patients: evidence for the constitutional hypothesis. *British Journal of Psychiatry* **134**, 169–177.

Harrison, G., Whitley, E., Rasmussen, F. *et al.* (2006) Risk of schizophrenia and other non-affective psychosis among individuals exposed to head injury: case control study. *Schizophrenia Research* **88**, 119–126.

Haukka, J., Suvisaari, J., Hakkinen, L. & Lonnqvist, J. (2008) Growth pattern and risk of schizophrenia. *Psychological Medicine* **38**, 63–70.

Henquet, C., Krabbendam, L., Spauwen, J. *et al.* (2005a) Prospective cohort study of cannabis use, predisposition for psychosis, and psychotic symptoms in young people. *BMJ* 330, 11.

Henquet, C., Murray, R., Linszen, D. & van Os, J. (2005b) The environment and schizophrenia: the role of cannabis use. *Schizophrenia Bulletin* **31**, 608–612.

Henquet, C., Rosa, A., Krabbendam, L. *et al.* (2006) An experimental study of catechol-o-methyltransferase Val158Met moderation of delta-9-tetrahydrocannabinol-induced effects on psychosis and cognition. *Neuropsychopharmacology* **31**, 2748–2757.

Herman, D.B., Brown, A.S., Opler, M.G. *et al.* (2006) Does unwantedness of pregnancy predict schizophrenia in the offspring? Findings from a prospective birth cohort study. *Social Psychiatry and Psychiatric Epidemiology* **41**, 605–610.

Hickman, M., Vickerman, P., Macleod, J. *et al.* (2007) Cannabis and schizophrenia: model projections of the impact of the rise in cannabis use on historical and future trends in schizophrenia in England and Wales. *Addiction* **102**, 597–606.

Hoek, H.W., Brown, A.S. & Susser, E. (1998) The Dutch famine and schizophrenia spectrum disorders. *Social Psychiatry and Psychiatric Epidemiology* **33**, 373–379.

Hoffman, R.E. (2007) A social deafferentation hypothesis for induction of active schizophrenia. *Schizophrenia Bulletin* **33**, 1066–1070.

Howes, O.D., McDonald, C., Cannon, M. *et al.* (2004) Pathways to schizophrenia: the impact of environmental factors. *International Journal of Neuropsychopharmacology* **7** (Suppl 1), S7–S13.

Hultman, C.M., Wieselgren, I.M. & Ohman, A. (1997) Relationships between social support, social coping and life events in the relapse of schizophrenic patients. *Scandinavian Journal of Psychology* **38**, 3–13.

Huttunen, M.O. & Niskanen, P. (1978) Prenatal loss of father and psychiatric disorders. *Archives of General Psychiatry* **35**, 429–431.

Isohanni, I., Jarvelin, M.R., Nieminen, P. *et al.* (1998) School performance as a predictor of psychiatric hospitalization in adult life. A 28-year follow-up in the Northern Finland 1966 Birth Cohort. *Psychological Medicine* **28**, 967–974.

Janssen, I., Krabbendam, L., Bak, M. *et al.* (2004) Childhood abuse as a risk factor for psychotic experiences. *Acta Psychiatrica Scandinavica* **109**, 38–45.

Jarvis, G.E. (2007) The social causes of psychosis in North American psychiatry: a review of a disappearing literature. *Canadian Journal of Psychiatry* **52**, 287–294.

Johns, L.C., Cannon, M., Singleton, N. *et al.* (2004) Prevalence and correlates of self-reported psychotic symptoms in the British population. *British Journal of Psychiatry* **185**, 298–305.

Jones, P., Rodgers, B., Murray, R. & Marmot, M. (1994) Child development risk factors for adult schizophrenia in the British 1946 birth cohort. *Lancet* **344**, 1398–1402.

Kapur, S. (2003) Psychosis as a state of aberrant salience: a framework linking biology, phenomenology, and pharmacology in schizophrenia. *American Journal of Psychiatry* **160**, 13–23.

Kavanagh, D.J., McGrath, J., Saunders, J.B. *et al.* (2002) Substance misuse in patients with schizophrenia: epidemiology and management. *Drugs* **62**, 743–755.

Keller, M.C. & Miller, G. (2006) Resolving the paradox of common, harmful, heritable mental disorders: which evolutionary genetic models work best? *Behavioral and Brain Sciences* **29**, 385–404; discussion 405–452.

Kesby, J.P., Burne, T.H., McGrath, J.J. & Eyles, D.W. (2006) Developmental vitamin D deficiency alters MK 801-induced hyperlocomotion in the adult rat: An animal model of schizophrenia. *Biological Psychiatry* **60**, 591–596.

Kinnell, H. (1983) Parental age in schizophrenia. *British Journal of Psychiatry* **142**, 204a.

Kirkbride, J.B., Fearon, P, Morgan, C. *et al.* (2006) Heterogeneity in incidence rates of schizophrenia and. other psychotic syndromes: findings from the 3-center AeSOP study. *Archives of General Psychiatry* **63**, 250–258.

Koponen, S., Taiminen, T., Portin, R. *et al.* (2002) Axis I and II psychiatric disorders after traumatic brain injury: a 30-year follow-up study. *American Journal of Psychiatry* **159**, 1315–1321.

Kuller, L.H. (1999) Circular epidemiology. *American Journal of Epidemiology* **150**, 897–903.

Lewis, G., David, A., Andreasson, S. & Allebeck, P. (1992) Schizophrenia and city life. *Lancet* **340**, 137–140.

Lipska, B.K. (2004) Using animal models to test a neurodevelopmental hypothesis of schizophrenia. *Journal of Psychiatry and Neuroscience* **29**, 282–286.

Low, J.A., Galbraith, R.S., Muir, D.W. *et al.* (1985) The contribution of fetal-newborn complications to motor and cognitive deficits. *Developmental Medicine and Child Neurology* **27**, 578–587.

Lucas, A., Morley, R. & Cole, T.J. (1998) Randomised trail of early diet in preterm babies and later intelligence quotient. *British Medical Journal* **317**, 1481–1487.

Malama, I.M., Papaioannou, D.J., Kaklamani, E.P. *et al.* (1988) Birth order sibship size and socio-economic factors in risk of schizophrenia in Greece. *British Journal of Psychiatry* **152**, 482–486.

Malaspina, D., Harlap, S., Fennig, S. *et al.* (2001) Advancing paternal age and the risk of schizophrenia. *Archives of General Psychiatry* **58**, 361–367.

Malaspina, D., Corcoran, C., Fahim, C. *et al.* (2002) Paternal age and sporadic schizophrenia: evidence for de novo mutations. *American Journal of Medical Genetics* **114**, 299–303.

Mallard, E.C., Rehn, A., Rees, S., *et al.* (1999) Ventriculomegaly and reduced hippocampal volume following intrauterine growth-restriction: implications for the aetiology of schizophrenia. *Schizophrenia Research* **40**, 11–21.

Marcelis, M., Navarro-Mateu, F., Murray, R. *et al.* (1998) Urbanization and psychosis: a study of 1942–1978 birth cohorts in The Netherlands. *Psychological Medicine* **28**, 871–879.

March, D. & Susser, E. (2006) The eco- in eco-epidemiology. *International Journal of Epidemiology* **35**, 1379–1383.

McClellan, J.M., Susser, E. & King, M.C. (2006) Maternal famine, de novo mutations, and schizophrenia. *JAMA* **296**, 582–584.

McDonald, C. & Murray, R.M. (2000) Early and late environmental risk factors for schizophrenia. *Brain Research Brain Research Reviews* **31**, 130–137.

McGrath, J. (1999) Hypothesis: is low prenatal vitamin D a risk-modifying factor for schizophrenia? *Schizophrenia Research* **40**, 173–177.

McGrath, J.J. (2006) Variations in the incidence of schizophrenia: data versus dogma. *Schizophrenia Bulletin* **32**, 195–197.

McGrath, J.J. (2007) The surprisingly rich contours of schizophrenia epidemiology. *Archives of General Psychiatry* **64**, 14–16.

McGrath, J. & Castle, D. (1995) Does influenza cause schizophrenia? A five year review. *Australian and New Zealand Journal of Psychiatry* **29**, 23–31.

McGrath, J.J. & Saha, S. (2007) Thought experiments on the incidence and prevalence of schizophrenia "under the influence" of cannabis. *Addiction* **102**, 514–515; discussion 516–518.

McGrath, J. & Scott, J. (2006) Urban birth and risk of schizophrenia: a worrying example of epidemiology where the data are stronger than the hypotheses. *Epidemiologia e Psichiatria Sociale* **15**, 243–246.

McGrath, J., Eyles, D., Mowry, B., *et al.* (2003a) Low maternal vitamin D as a risk factor for schizophrenia: a pilot study using banked sera. *Schizophrenia Research* **63**, 73–78.

McGrath, J., Feron, F., Burne, T.H.J., *et al.* (2003b) The neurodevelopmental hypothesis of schizophrenia; a review of recent developments. *Annals of Medicine* **35**, 86–93.

McGrath, J., Saha, S., Welham, J. *et al.* (2004) A systematic review of the incidence of schizophrenia: the distribution of rates and the influence of sex, urbanicity, migrant status and methodology. *BMC Medicine* **2**, 13.

McMichael, A.J. (2001) *Human Frontiers, Environments and Disease.* Cambridge: Cambridge University Press.

McNeil, T.F., Cantor-Graae, E. & Weinberger, D.R. (2000) Relationship of obstetric complications and differences in size of brain structures in monozygotic twin pairs discordant for schizophrenia. *American Journal of Psychiatry* **157**, 203–212.

Meaney, M.J. (2001) Nature, nurture, and the disunity of knowledge. *Annals of the New York Academy of Sciences* **935**, 50–61.

Mednick, S.A., Machón, R.A., Huttunen, M.O. & Bonett, D. (1988) Adult schizophrenia following prenatal exposure to an influenza epidemic. *Archives of General Psychiatry* **45**, 189–192.

Meyer, U., Feldon, J., Schedlowski, M. & Yee, B.K. (2006a) Immunological stress at the maternal-foetal interface: a link between neurodevelopment and adult psychopathology. *Brain, Behavior and Immunity* **20**, 378–388.

Meyer, U., Schwendener, S., Feldon, J. & Yee, B.K. (2006b) Prenatal and postnatal maternal contributions in the infection model of schizophrenia. *Experimental Brain Research* **173**, 243–257.

Moffitt, T.E., Caspi, A. & Rutter, M. (2005) Strategy for investigating interactions between measured genes and measured environments. *Archives of General Psychiatry* **62**, 473–481.

Moore, T.H., Zammit, S., Lingford-Hughes, A. *et al.* (2007) Cannabis use and risk of psychotic or affective mental health outcomes: a systematic review. *Lancet* **370**, 319–328.

Morgan, C. & Fisher, H. (2007) Environment and schizophrenia: environmental factors in schizophrenia: childhood trauma—a critical review. *Schizophrenia Bulletin* **33**, 3–10.

Morgan, D., Grant, K.A., Gage, H.D. *et al.* (2002) Social dominance in monkeys: dopamine D2 receptors and cocaine self-administration. *Nature Neuroscience* **5**, 169–174.

Mortensen, P.B., Pedersen, C.B., Westergaard, T. *et al.* (1999) Effects of family history and place and season of birth on the risk of schizophrenia. *New England Journal of Medicine* **340**, 603–608.

Mortensen, P.B., Nørgaard-Pedersen, B., Waltoft, B.L. *et al.* (2007a) *Toxoplasma gondii* as a risk factor for early-onset schizophrenia: analysis of filter paper blood samples obtained at birth. *Biological Psychiatry* **61**, 688–693.

Mortensen, P.B., Norgaard-Pedersen, B., Waltoft, B.L. *et al.* (2007b) Early infections of *Toxoplasma gondii* and the later development of schizophrenia. *Schizophrenia Bulletin* **33**, 741–744.

Munro, C.A., McCaul, M.E., Wong, D.F. *et al.* (2006) Sex differences in striatal dopamine release in healthy adults. *Biological Psychiatry* **59**, 966–974.

Murray, R.M. & Lewis, S.W. (1987) Is schizophrenia a neurodevelopmental disorder? *British Medical Journal (Clinical Research Edition)* **295**, 681–682.

Murray, R.M., Morrison, P.D., Henquet, C. & Di Forti, M. (2007) Cannabis, the mind and society: the hash realities. *Nature Reviews Neuroscience* **8**, 885–895.

Myhrman, A., Rantakallio, P., Isohanni, M. *et al.* (1996) Unwantedness of a pregnancy and schizophrenia in the child. *British Journal of Psychiatry* **169**, 637–640.

Nakamura, K., Chen, C.K., Sekine, Y. *et al.* (2006) Association analysis of SOD2 variants with methamphetamine psychosis in Japanese and Taiwanese populations. *Human Genetics* **120**, 243–252.

Nicodemus, K.K., Marenco, S., Batten, A.J. *et al.* (2008) Serious obstetric complications interact with hypoxia-regulated// vascular-expression genes to influence schizophrenia risk. *Molecular Psychiatry* **13**, 873–877.

Nielsen, A.S., Mortensen, P.B., O'Callaghan E. *et al.* (2002) Is head injury a risk factor for schizophrenia? *Schizophrenia Research* **55**, 93–98.

Norman, R.M. & Malla, A.K. (1993a) Stressful life events and schizophrenia. I: A review of the research. *British Journal of Psychiatry* **162**, 161–166.

Norman, R.M. & Malla, A.K. (1993b) Stressful life events and schizophrenia. II: Conceptual and methodological issues. *British Journal of Psychiatry* **162**, 166–174.

O'Callaghan, E., Sham, P., Takei, N. *et al.* (1991) Schizophrenia after prenatal exposure to 1957 A2 influenza epidemic. *Lancet* **337**, 1248–1250.

O'Callaghan, E., Colgan, K., Cotter, D. *et al.* (1992) Evidence for confinement of winter birth excess in schizophrenia to those born in cities. *Schizophrenia Research* **6**, 102.

Oner, O. & Munir, K. (2005) Attentional and neurocognitive characteristics of high-risk offspring of parents with schizophrenia compared with DSM-IV attention deficit hyperactivity disorder children. *Schizophrenia Research* **76**, 293–299.

Opler, M.G., Brown, A.S., Graziano, J. *et al.* (2004) Prenatal lead exposure, delta-aminolevulinic acid, and schizophrenia. *Environmental Health Perspectives* **112**, 548–552.

Oyama, S., Griffiths, P.E. & Gray, R.D., eds. (2001) *Cycles of Contingency: Developmental Systems and Evolution.* Cambridge, MA: MIT Press.

Ozawa, K., Hashimoto, K., Kishimoto, T. *et al.* (2006) Immune activation during pregnancy in mice leads to dopaminergic hyperfunction and cognitive impairment in the offspring: a neurodevelopmental animal model of schizophrenia. *Biological Psychiatry* **59**, 546–554.

Paneth, N. & Pinto-Martin, J. (1991) The epidemiology of germinal matrix/intraventricular hemorrhage. In: Kiely, M, ed. *Reproductive and Perinatal Epidemiology.* Boca Raton, FL, CRC Press, pp. 371–399.

Pedersen, C.B. & Mortensen, P.B. (2001) Evidence of a dose-response relationship between urbanicity during upbringing and schizophrenia risk. *Archives of General Psychiatry* **58**, 1039–1046.

Pedersen, C.B. & Mortensen, P.B. (2006a) Are the cause(s) responsible for urban-rural differences in schizophrenia risk rooted in families or in individuals? *American Journal of Epidemiology* **163**, 971–978.

Pedersen, C.B. & Mortensen, P.B. (2006b) Urbanization and traffic related exposures as risk factors for schizophrenia. *BMC Psychiatry* **6**, 2.

Pedersen, C.B. & Mortensen, P.B. (2006c) Why factors rooted in the family may solely explain the urban-rural differences in schizophrenia risk estimates. *Epidemiologia e Psichiatria Sociale* **15**, 247–251.

Perrin, M.C., Brown, A.S. & Malaspina, D. (2007) Aberrant epigenetic regulation could explain the relationship of paternal age to schizophrenia. *Schizophrenia Bulletin* **33**, 1270–1273.

Pitkin, R.M. (2007) Folate and neural tube defects. *American Journal of Clinical Nutrition* **85**, 285S–288S.

Poulton, R., Caspi, A., Moffitt, T.E., *et al.* (2000) Children's self-reported psychotic symptoms and adult schizophreniform disorder: a 15-year longitudinal study. *Archives of General Psychiatry* **57**, 1053–1058.

Precht, D.H., Andersen, P.K. & Olsen, J. (2007) Severe life events and impaired fetal growth: a nation-wide study with complete follow-up. *Acta Obstetricia et Gynecologica Scandinavica* **86**, 266–275.

Raschka, L.B. (1990) Genetic origins of pyschosis. *British Journal of Psychiatry* **157**, 781–782.

Read, J., van Os, J., Morrison, A.P. & Ross, C.A. (2005) Childhood trauma, psychosis and schizophrenia: a literature review with theoretical and clinical implications. *Acta Psychiatrica Scandinavica* **112**, 330–350.

Saha, S., Welham, J., Chant, D. & McGrath, J. (2006) Incidence of schizophrenia does not vary with economic status of the country: evidence from a systematic review. *Social Psychiatry and Psychiatric Epidemiology* **41**, 338–340.

Sareen, J., Cox, B.J., Goodwin, R.D. & Asmundson, G.J.G.A. (2005) Co-occurrence of posttraumatic stress disorder with positive psychotic symptoms in a nationally representative sample. *Journal of Traumatic Stress* **18**, 313–322.

Sartorius, N., Jablensky, A., Korten, A. *et al.* (1986) Early manifestations and first-contact incidence of schizophrenia in different cultures. A preliminary report on the initial evaluation phase of the WHO Collaborative Study on determinants of outcome of severe mental disorders. *Psychological Medicine* **16**, 909–928.

Schmidt-Kastner, R., van Os, J., Steinbusch, H.W.M. & Schmitz, C. (2006) Gene regulation by hypoxia and the neurodevelopmental origin of schizophrenia. *Schizophrenia Research* **84**, 253–271.

Scott, J., Chant, D., Andrews, G. & McGrath, J. (2006) Psychotic-like experiences in the general community: the correlates of CIDI psychosis screen items in an Australian sample. *Psychological Medicine* **36**, 231–238.

Scott, J., Chant, D., Andrews, G. *et al.* (2007) Association between trauma exposure and delusional experiences in a large community-based sample. *British Journal of Psychiatry* **190**, 339–343.

Seedat, S., Stein, M.B., Oosthuizen, P.P. *et al.* (2003) Linking posttraumatic stress disorder and psychosis: a look at epidemiology, phenomenology, and treatment. *Journal of Nervous and Mental Disease* **191**, 675–681.

Seidman, L.J., Buka, S.L., Goldstein, J.M. & Tsuang, M.T. (2006) Intellectual decline in schizophrenia: evidence from a prospective birth cohort 28 year follow-up study. *Journal of Clinical and Experimental Neuropsychology* **28**, 225–242.

Selten, J.P. & Cantor-Graae, E. (2005) Social defeat: risk factor for schizophrenia? *British Journal of Psychiatry* **187**, 101–102.

Selten, J.P., Brown, A.S., Moons, K.G. *et al.* (1999) Prenatal exposure to the 1957 influenza pandemic and non-affective psychosis in The Netherlands. *Schizophrenia Research* **38**, 85–91.

Selten, J.P., Cantor-Graae, E., Nahon, D. *et al.* (2003) No relationship between risk of schizophrenia and prenatal exposure to stress during the Six-Day War or Yom Kippur War in Israel. *Schizophrenia Research* **63**, 131–135.

Semple, D.M., McIntosh, A.M. & Lawrie, S.M. (2005) Cannabis as a risk factor for psychosis: systematic review. *Journal of Psychopharmacology* **19**, 187–194.

Sipos, A., Rasmussen, F., Harrison, G. *et al.* (2004) Paternal age and schizophrenia: a population based cohort study. *BMJ* **329**, 1070.

Smith, G.D. (2001) Reflections on the limitations to epidemiology. *Journal of Clinical Epidemiology* **54**, 325–331.

Smith, G.D. & Ebrahim, S. (2004) Mendelian randomization: prospects, potentials, and limitations. *International Journal of Epidemiology* **33**, 30–42.

Sorensen, H.J., Mortensen, E.L., Reinisch, J.M. & Mednick, S.A. (2006) Height, weight and body mass index in early adulthood and risk of schizophrenia. *Acta Psychiatrica Scandanavica* **114**, 49–54.

Spauwen, J. & van Os, J. (2006) The psychosis proneness: psychosis persistence model as an explanation for the association between urbanicity and psychosis. *Epidemoilogia e Psichiatria Sociale* **15**, 252–257.

Spauwen, J., Krabbendam, L., Lieb, R. *et al.* (2004) Does urbanicity shift the population expression of psychosis? *Journal of Psychiatric Research* **38**, 613–618.

St Clair, D., Xu, M., Wang, P. *et al.* (2005) Rates of adult schizophrenia following prenatal exposure to the Chinese famine of 1959–1961. *JAMA* **294**, 557–562.

Sullivan, P.F. (2005) The genetics of schizophrenia. *PLoS Medicine* **2**, e212.

Susser, E. (2004) Eco-epidemiology: thinking outside the black box. *Epidemiology* **15**, 519–20; author reply 527–528.

Susser, E.S. & Lin, S.P. (1992) Schizophrenia after prenatal exposure to the Dutch hunger winter of 1944-1945. *Archives of General Psychiatry* **49**, 938–988.

Suvisaari, J., Haukka, J., Tanskanen, A. *et al.* (1999) Association between prenatal exposure to poliovirus infection and adult schizophrenia. *American Journal of Psychiatry* **156**, 1100–1102.

Takei, N., Sham, P., O'Callaghan, E. & Murray, R.M. (1992) Cities, winter birth and schizophrenia. *Lancet* **340**, 558–559.

Tien, A.Y. & Anthony, J.C. (1990) Epidemiological analysis of alcohol and drug use as risk factors for psychotic experiences. *Journal of Nervous and Mental Disease* **178**, 473–480.

Toda, M. & Abi-Dargham, A. (2007) Dopamine hypothesis of schizophrenia: making sense of it all. *Current Psychiatry Reports* **9**, 329–336.

Torrey, E.F., Miller, J., Rawlings, R. & Yolken, R.H. (1997) Seasonality of births in schizophrenia and bipolar disorder: a review of the literature. *Schizophrenia Research* **28**, 1–38.

Torrey, E.F., Rawlings, R. & Waldman, I.N. (1988) Schizophrenic births and viral diseases in two states. *Schizophrenia Research* **1**, 73–77.

Torrey, E.F., Bartko, J.J., Lun, Z.R. & Yolken, R.H. (2007) Antibodies to Toxoplasma gondii in patients with schizophrenia: A meta-analysis. *Schizophrenia Bulletin* **33**, 729–736.

Tsuchiya, K.J., Takagai, S., Kawai, M. *et al.* (2005) Advanced paternal age associated with an elevated risk for schizophrenia in offspring in a Japanese population. *Schizophrenia Research* **76**, 337–342.

Tunbridge, E.M., Harrison, P.J. & Weinberger, D.R. (2006) Catechol-O-methyltransferase, cognition and psychosis: Val[158]Met and beyond. *Biological Psychiatry* **60**, 141–151.

Van Erp, T.G., Saleh, P.A., Rosso, I.M. *et al.* (2002) Contributions of genetic risk and fetal hypoxia to hippocampal volume in patients with schizophrenia or schizoaffective disorder, their unaffected siblings, and healthy unrelated volunteers. *American Journal of Psychiatry* **159**, 1514–1520.

van Os, J. & Selten, J.P. (1998) Prenatal exposure to maternal stress and subsequent schizophrenia. The May 1940 invasion of The Netherlands. *British Journal of Psychiatry* **172**, 324–326.

van Os, J., Hanssen, M., Bijl, R.V. & Ravelli, A. (2000) Strauss (1969) revisited: a psychosis continuum in the general population? *Schizophrenia Research* **45**, 11–20.

van Os, J., Bak, M., Hanssen, M., *et al.* (2002) Cannabis use and psychosis: a longitudinal population-based study. *American Journal of Epidemiology* **156**, 319–327.

van Winkel, R., Henquet, C., Rosa, A. *et al.* (2008) Evidence that the COMT(Val158Met) polymorphism moderates sensitivity to stress in psychosis: An experience-sampling study. *American Journal of Medical Genetics Part B Neuropsychiatric Genetics* **147B**, 10–17.

Verdoux, H., Geddes, J.R., Takei, N. *et al.* (1997) Obstetric complications and age at onset in schizophrenia: an international collaborative meta-analysis of individual patient data [see comments]. *American Journal of Psychiatry* **154**, 1220–1227.

Verdoux, H., Gindre, C., Sorbara, F. *et al.* (2003) Effects of cannabis and psychosis vulnerability in daily life: an experience sampling test study. *Psychological Medicine* **33**, 23–32.

Waddington, C.H. (1953) Genetic assimilation of an acquired character. *Evolution* **7**, 118–126.

Wahlbeck, K., Forsen, T., Osmond, C. *et al.* (2001a) Association of schizophrenia with low maternal body mass index, small size at birth, and thinness during childhood. *Archives of General Psychiatry* **58**, 48–52.

Wahlbeck, K., Osmond, C., Forsen, T. *et al.* (2001b) Associations between childhood living circumstances and schizophrenia: a population-based cohort study. *Acta Psychiatrica Scandinavica* **104**, 356–360.

Walker, E.F. & Diforio, D. (1997) Schizophrenia: a neural diathesis-stress model. *Psychological Review* **104**, 667–685.

Watson, C.G., Kucala, T., Tilleskjor, C. & Jacobs, L. (1984) Schizophrenic birth seasonality in relation to the incidence of infectious diseases and temperature extremes. *Archives of General Psychiatry* **41**, 85–90.

Weinberger, D.R. (1987) Implications of normal brain development for the pathogenesis of schizophrenia. *Archives of General Psychiatry* **44**, 660–669.

Weiser, M., Reichenberg, A., Rabinowitz, J. *et al.* (2003) Self-reported drug abuse in male adolescents with behavioral disturbances, and follow-up for future schizophrenia. *Biological Psychiatry* **54**, 655–660.

Weiser, M., van Os, J. & Davidson, M. (2005) Time for a shift in focus in schizophrenia: from narrow phenotypes to broad endophenotypes. *British Journal of Psychiatry* **187**, 203–205.

Westergaard, T., Mortensen, P.B., Pedersen, C.B. *et al.* (1999) Exposure to prenatal and childhood infections and the risk of schizophrenia: suggestions from a study of sibship characteristics and influenza prevalence. *Archives of General Psychiatry* **56**, 993–998.

Wiles, N.J., Zammit, S., Bebbington, P. *et al.* (2006) Self-reported psychotic symptoms in the general population: results from the longitudinal study of the British National Psychiatric Morbidity Survey. *British Journal of Psychiatry* **188**, 519–526.

Xu, M.Q., Sun, W.S., Liui, B.X. *et al.* (2009) Prenatal malnutrition and adult schizophrenia: further evidence from the 1959–1961 Chinese famine. *Schizophrenia Bulletin* **35**, 568–576.

Yolken, R.H. & Torrey, E.F. (1995) Viruses, schizophrenia, and bipolar disorder. *Clinical Microbiology Reviews* **8**, 131–145.

Yolken, R.H., Karlsson, H., Yee, F. *et al.* (2000) Endogenous retroviruses and schizophrenia. *Brain Research Brain Research Reviews* **31**, 193–199.

Zammit, S., Allebeck, P., Andreasson, S. *et al.* (2002) Self reported cannabis use as a risk factor for schizophrenia in Swedish conscripts of 1969: historical cohort study. *BMJ* **325**, 1199.

Zammit, S., Allebeck, P., Dalman, C. *et al.* (2003) Paternal age and risk for schizophrenia. *British Journal of Psychiatry* **183**, 405–408.

Zuckerman, L., Rehavi, M., Nachman, R. & Weiner, I. (2003) Immune activation during pregnancy in rats leads to a post-pubertal emergence of disrupted latent inhibition, dopaminergic hyperfunction, and altered limbic morphology in the offspring: a novel neurodevelopmental model of schizophrenia. *Neuropsychopharmacology* **28**, 1778–1789.

CHAPTER **12**

Classical genetic studies of schizophrenia

Brien Riley and Kenneth S. Kendler
Virginia Commonwealth University, Richmond, VA, USA

Introduction

Genetic study of schizophrenia is based on three key areas of research (specialist genetic terminology is shown in **bold** and defined throughout). First, **genetic epidemiology** asks whether there is risk in excess of the population baseline in the relatives of cases, and, if so, whether the excess risk is attributable to the genetic material or the environments they share. The answers to these questions explain why we are looking for schizophrenia liability genes and what we think we might find, both critical for appropriate study design. Study of the genetic epidemiology of schizophrenia has consistently demonstrated that (1) in aggregate, genetic effects are important risk factors for this disorder; (2) schizophrenia is not completely attributable to genetics: it is a **multifactorial trait**, with non-genetic (or **environmental**) factors also contributing to risk; and (3) patterns of transmission and linkage data in families are inconsistent with the action of individual genetic risk factors of large effect size (like Mendelian mutations) in one or a few single genes. Schizophrenia is a **complex trait**, one influenced by a large number of risk factors, most of which seem more likely to be within the range of normal human variation and to produce much more modest individual increases in risk.

There is substantial difference in DNA sequence between individuals at variable sites known as genetic **polymorphisms** or **markers**, which have multiple detectable specific forms, or **alleles** (the specific DNA sequence at

Schizophrenia, 3rd edition. Edited by Daniel R. Weinberger and Paul J Harrison © 2011 Blackwell Publishing Ltd.

such a variable position). The second area, **molecular genetics**, asks whether certain alleles are more common in affected than in unaffected individuals. The most common approaches in human molecular genetics are studies of **linkage** [which ask whether a trait and specific large chromosome segments **cosegregate** (or are inherited together) in families] and **association** (which ask whether DNA variation in specific smaller chromosome segments, often individual genes, is more common in affected than unaffected individuals in populations). We will discuss the underlying causes of these two genetic phenomena, the methods for detecting them and the limitations of each. These are essential for a critical assessment of the large body of evidence, as they describe how we attempt to identify liability genes, and how well we succeed.

Molecular genetic studies have, until very recently, been less successful in identifying the relationship between the aggregate genetic risks and specific DNA variants, protein molecules or biological processes for complex traits generally. A number of features of complex traits like schizophrenia contribute to an overall reduction in **power**, the probability that a true effect will be detected, particularly for linkage studies. First, schizophrenia is thought to be influenced by multiple common alleles of small effect. Both linkage and association study designs rely heavily on analytic approaches that assess single genes, which are less powerful for detecting multiple risk factors of small effect. Second, environmental factors and interactions appear necessary to account for patterns of risk. These remain unknown and generally untested. Third, the disorder is common, and genetic liability variants seem likely to be common, although increased rates of rare deletions and duplications (**structural or copy number variants**) in cases have been observed multiple times and suggest that rare variation may also contribute to disease in a proportion of cases. The common risk variants are expected to occur with relatively high frequency in the general population, reducing contrast between affected and unaffected individuals and reducing power. The impact of individual rare structural variants in the subset of cases where they are observed is harder to assess currently, but the observation of an aggregate increase appears robust, further increasing the apparent etiological complexity. Fourth, the expected frequency of risk alleles and the clinical variability in presentation, course, and outcome suggest that the etiology of individual cases may be **heterogeneous**, derived from different specific genes or alleles between individuals. Fifth, diagnostic boundaries are difficult to draw and there is some evidence for genes influencing risk of both schizophrenia and bipolar disorder, disease entities considered separate. Incorrect specification of affected status can substantially reduce power.

Linkage methods, which deliver relatively complete coverage of the genome, have great power to identify single genes causing Mendelian disorders, but are poorly suited to the genetic architecture of complex traits. Association methods are undeniably more powerful in such situations, but our limited understanding of the underlying disease neurobiology in the brain means that candidate gene selection has been weak, and such studies of schizophrenia have not generally produced robust and replicable results. Affordable technologies to deliver the higher density data required for unbiased genome-wide association testing have only recently become available and been applied to multiple large case–control samples.

In spite of these limitations, numerous regions of the human genome give consistent, though by no means unanimous, support for linkage. The precise nature of the linkage signals is not yet understood, and power to position the effects is poor, but meta-analyses show the co-occurrence is unlikely to be due to chance. Combined approaches utilizing linkage for genome-wide coverage and association for fine-scale follow-up have identified several promising positional candidate genes. A number of these reported associations have been widely, though again not unanimously, replicated. A clear definition of replication in a complex trait remains difficult to achieve, but the association data do not satisfy the most rigorous definition of replication, because the same alleles are not observed to have the same effect on risk across samples. The field is set to be further advanced by genome-wide association studies (GWAS), which are reviewed in detail in Chapter 13.

The third key area, **molecular biology**, undertakes functional studies of the effects of genes and gene variants to elucidate how a gene functions and is regulated normally, how specific DNA variants alter normal processes, and how these alterations contribute to specific disease states. This chapter provides a broad overview of the first two areas, an integration of the collected results of many studies, and a discussion of the most promising current areas. The details of specific genetic associations and the status of current molecular investigations of these genes and molecular biology of their protein products are addressed in Chapters 13.

Genetic epidemiology: Why are we looking for genes contributing to schizophrenia?

A large body of data collected from families, twins, and adoptees over many years has consistently supported the involvement of a major, complex genetic component in liability to schizophrenia and schizophrenia spectrum disorders. These results indicate only that genes contribute to risk in aggregate, and provide no information about the specific genes involved or their number.

Family studies: Does risk aggregate in relatives?

The first systematic family study, published by Rudin in 1916, found that dementia praecox was more common among the siblings of probands than in the general population. A large study of over a thousand porbands with schizophrenia, published by Kallman in 1938, showed that both siblings and offspring had increased rates of the disorder. There was early recognition of the need for **systematic ascertainment** (unselected sampling of cases, e.g., from consecutive admissions referred to a clinic) of **probands** (the index cases) for family studies so that the affected individuals sampled were maximally representative of schizophrenia as a whole, but some early studies lack this critical feature. In order to make accurate estimates of the lifetime morbid risk to various classes of relatives, family studies also need to correct for the age of the subjects. Only those who are beyond the age of risk can be unequivocally classified as unaffected, and some relatives unaffected at the time of study may develop the disorder in the future. Lifetime morbid risks are therefore calculated by dividing the number of affecteds by an age-corrected total of lifetimes at risk.

The combined results of many European studies published between 1921 and 1987 (Gottesman, 1991) are shown in Figure 12.1. The lifetime morbid risk in the general population is about 1%, but approximately 10 times that in the siblings or offspring of patients with schizophrenia. Smaller but consistent increases in risk are seen in second- and third-degree relatives. Two anomalies in the family data merit some discussion. Lower risk in parents (6%) com-

pared to siblings (9%), both of whom share 50% of their genetic material with probands, may be due to the substantial reduction in fertility observed in schizophrenia. If affected individuals are less likely to be parents, then they are less likely to be the parents of probands, thus reducing the estimated parental morbid risk. Lower risk in siblings (9%) compared to fraternal or dizygotic (DZ) twins (17%), again both of whom share 50% of their genetic material with probands, has not been explained, but suggests that some environmental factors that are more highly shared between twins than between singleton siblings, such as the intrauterine environment, may be involved. Neurodevelopment, a potential target of prenatal effects and a time of critical regulation of gene expression, has long been thought to be involved in the pathogenesis of schizophrenia.

Criticisms of the methodology of early family studies included the lack of systematic ascertainment discussed above, the lack of proper controls (since rates of schizophrenia were not assessed in the families of unaffected individuals), lack of standardized diagnostic criteria, and failure to diagnose family members blind to the status of the proband (which can produce bias in the diagnoses). A combined analysis of the data from seven studies designed to avoid these weaknesses yielded totals of 15 cases of schizophrenia in 3035 lifetimes at risk in the control families, and 116 cases of schizophrenia in 2418 lifetimes at risk in the patient families. These translate into average morbid risk for narrowly defined schizophrenia of 0.5% for relatives of controls and 4.8% for relatives of a proband with schizophrenia (Kendler & Diehl, 1993). The more recent,

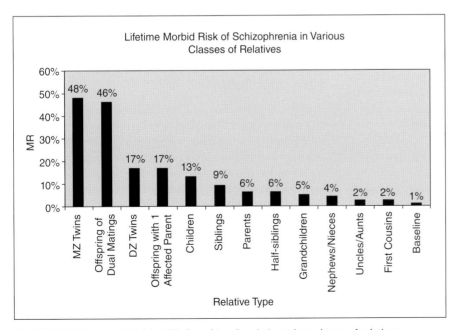

Fig. 12.1 Lifetime morbid risk (MR) for schizophrenia in various classes of relatives.

methodologically stronger studies replicate the early findings that a close relative of a patient with schizophrenia has an average 10 times the baseline population risk of the disorder.

Twin studies: How large is the genetic component of risk?

Studies of twins provide a way to estimate the relative importance of shared genetic material and shared environment in the development of a trait. The main strategy in twin studies is to compare the concordance for the disease between members of monozygotic (MZ) twin pairs and members of DZ twin pairs. Since MZ twins are genetically identical, whereas DZ twins share on average 50% of their genes, greater MZ than DZ concordance will reflect genetic influence, providing both MZ and DZ twins share their environment to approximately the same extent. Systematic ascertainment is also essential in twin studies, as bias here can result from the preferential selection of the most prominent twin pairs, which are likely to be MZ and concordant for the disorder. Since individual twins in a pair may be ascertained independently as two separate probands, the proband-wise concordance rate (where concordant pairs are counted twice if both co-twins are independently ascertained) is statistically preferable to the pair-wise concordance rate (where the pair is only counted once regardless of dual ascertainment), and provides an unbiased assessment of morbid risk for each co-twin that can be compared with the morbid risk to other relatives and the general population.

Twin studies of schizophrenia show consistent evidence of a genetic effect with higher concordance in MZ (35–58%) than DZ (9–27%) twins. Individual twin studies (Farmer et al., 1987; Cardno et al., 1999) and meta-analyses of twin studies (Sullivan et al., 2003) estimate the heritability of liability to schizophrenia to be approximately 80%. Twin studies of schizophrenia have been reviewed in detail by Cardno and Gottesman (2000), whose meta-analysis of rigorously conducted twin study data suggested somewhat lower overall concordance rates, but similarly high heritability.

Twin studies have been criticized for making the assumption that the environments are equal between members of MZ and DZ twin pairs because MZ twins are more likely to act and be treated more similarly, and so may have a greater degree of shared environment than DZ twins. However, a search for pairs of MZ twins reared apart in a review of all systematic twin studies of schizophrenia found that 7 of 12 (58%) such pairs of MZ twins (who do not share their environment) were concordant for schizophrenia, a rate similar to MZ twins reared together (Gottesman & Shields, 1982). This argues against MZ-specific increases in shared environment as the source of the increased concordance compared to DZ twins. The results from studies of twins argue that liability to schizophrenia is largely genetically *mediated*, because of the substantially higher risk in MZ compared to DZ co-twins, but not genetically *determined*, because the risk to an MZ co-twin of a proband is less than 100%.

Adoption studies: Is familial aggregation due to shared environment?

Family members share environments, in addition to sharing genetic material, so the effects of shared genes and shared environments are not truly separable. Adoption studies ask whether the increased risk observed in family members is still present when the relatives do not share their environments. Across all adoption studies performed, the increased risk of schizophrenia was present in the biological relatives of patients with schizophrenia (Prescott & Gottesman, 1993). The first adoption study found that 5 of 47 (16.6%) adopted-away offspring of mothers with schizophrenia had schizophrenia compared to 0 of 50 adopted-away offspring of control mothers (Heston, 1966). In Finland, a much larger study of adopted-away offspring of mothers with schizophrenia and control mothers found that 13 of 144 (9.1%) children of mothers with schizophrenia have a schizophrenia spectrum disorder and 7 of 144 (4.9%) have schizophrenia, while 2 of 178 control offspring (1.1%) have schizophrenia (Tienari, 1991). In studies of adoptees in Denmark, schizophrenia was found to be significantly more common in the biological relatives of adoptees with schizophrenia than in the biological relatives of control adoptees in both urban and non-urban samples (Kety, et al. 1968, 1994). The rates of schizophrenia were low and not different in the adoptive families of both affected and control groups.

Transmission models: How is the genetic risk transmitted?

Transmission models are mathematical expressions of a hypothetical genetic architecture for a trait and make specific predictions about risk in various classes of relatives. Such models are tested by assessing how well their predictions match observed patterns of risk. The risk patterns for single-gene Mendelian disorders are expressed using the generalized **single major locus** (SML) model, which assumes that a single gene is responsible for all liability. These two terms, **gene** and **locus** (pl. loci) are often used interchangeably, though they have specific meanings. A locus is simply a position on a chromosome (e.g., a polymorphic marker) which may or may not be within a gene, the specific DNA template for a polypeptide or functional RNA molecule. An analysis of the data from a carefully selected number of European studies demonstrated that the SML model is inadequate to explain observed patterns of risk (McGue *et al.* 1985). Both segregation analysis and the pattern of risk in families (~ 10% in first-degree relatives and ~50% in MZ co-twins of probands) are inconsistent with the action of highly penetrant mutations in single genes. The offspring of unaffected MZ co-twins have an elevated risk of illness, and there are no pedigrees in which schizophrenia is transmitted as a classical Mendelian disorder, unlike Alzheimer disease or breast cancer, where a well-recognized series of pedigrees exist in which the disorder segregates in a Mendelian manner.

In common with other complex traits, the conclusion has generally been that multiple **liability**, **susceptibility** or **predisposing** alleles seem most likely to account for the aggregate genetic effects observed in genetic epidemiology studies. One consequence of such a model is that, if the number of genes contributing to a trait rises, the frequencies of the risk alleles must also rise in the population in order to maintain the observed prevalence. Risk alleles for most complex traits are expected to be common, and to be found at appreciable frequencies in controls or in the population (and elevated frequencies in cases). Data from studies of numerous complex traits are consistent in showing little evidence for risk alleles of major effect size. Effect sizes of single-gene mutations are described by **penetrance** (the proportion of individuals with a mutation who develop a disease, often 1) while the odds ratio (OR) is widely used currently (Gottesman, 1991). Rather, individual complex trait risk alleles appear unlikely to have ORs greater than 1.1–1.5 (a 10–50% increase in risk relative to baseline). This has been well validated by the initial round of GWAS of complex traits (Altshuler & Daly, 2007; Petretto *et al.*, 2007). Thus, we expect the genetic risk for schizophrenia to be mediated by common alleles of small effect in multiple genes.

The mutations that cause most Mendelian disorders are sufficiently rare that for all practical purposes, the same disease gene will be responsible for all cases of illness in a family. Between families, the pattern with Mendelian disorders is variable. In most disorders, mutations at a single gene are responsible for all known cases of illness (e.g., Huntington disease, cystic fibrosis). However, for some Mendelian syndromes (e.g., limb-girdle muscular dystrophy and retinitis pigmentosa), a number of distinct genes, usually on different chromosomes, have been found in different subsets of families. Critically, within an individual family the same gene and mutation are responsible for all cases of disease. Epidemiological data from schizophrenia suggest that the population frequencies of liability variants are likely to be orders of magnitude greater than the frequency of even the most common single-gene mutations (like cystic fibrosis which has a high population allele frequency of 2.5%). Schizophrenia is much more common and clinically highly variable. It is widely believed that variants

in many genes can increase liability to schizophrenia (a **polygenic** model of total population risk). These are not thought to all be necessary for disease, but rather that a few of these genes predispose an individual to schizophrenia (an **oligogenic** model of individual risk). A consequence of this model is that the specific genetic risk factors are likely to differ between individuals. The implication is that between cases, even those within families, variants in both shared and distinct genes may predispose to illness. The expected frequency of risk alleles and the clinical variability in presentation, course, and outcome suggest that **heterogeneity** in etiology is likely at the level of the gene (different risk genes in different individuals) and possible at the level of the allele (different risk alleles in the same gene in different individuals).

The **multifactorial threshold** (MT) model is less genetically deterministic, and assumes a continuum of liability due to multiple genetic and environmental factors, based on the collected data above. Individuals with liability in the upper reaches of this continuum have substantial risk of developing schizophrenia. The segregation analysis above also demonstrated that the MT model is inadequate to explain observed patterns of risk (McGue *et al.*, 1985). The MT model, which has great intuitive appeal but poor predictive power, assumes that the effects of multiple genes on risk combine **additively** (the total liability from *n* genes is *equal to* the sum of the *n* individual liabilities) and that there is no interaction between them.

A key predictive failure of the MT model is that the observed concordance rate in MZ twins (~50%) is too high relative to the risk in siblings and DZ twins (9–27%). Such a pattern is more consistent with some degree of gene–gene (**GxG**) or **epistatic** interaction between genes, where the total liability from *n* genes is *greater than* the sum of the *n* individual liabilities. The fall-off in concordance rates for schizophrenia in first-, second- and third-degree relatives in the families of patients with schizophrenia is also most consistent with multiple epistatically interacting genes (Risch, 1990), although this study did not model the impact of reduced fertility, which is large in individuals with schizophrenia and could substantially bias the results. Conversely, if the inheritance model was fully epistatic, then the **tetrachoric correlation** (the correlation in the normally distributed liability to illness) in MZ twins should be substantially more than twice that seen in DZ twins, which is not observed. Additionally, recent studies have suggested that gene–environment interactions (**GxE**) are important components of the overall risk for conduct disorder (Caspi *et al.*, 2002; Foley *et al.*, 2004) and depression (Caspi *et al.*, 2003; Kendler *et al.*, 2005), and possibly for schizophrenia as well (Tienari *et al.*, 2004).

Although segregation analyses have not provided a definitive inheritance model for the genetic risk for schizophrenia, they suggest collectively that numerous kinds of influences (including additive and epistatic genetic risks, environmental risks, and GxE interactions) are involved, and substantially reduce the power of genetic study designs. Common risk alleles with small effect sizes reduce the contrast between affected and unaffected individuals, whether they are siblings in a linkage study or cases and controls in an association study. Large samples are needed to detect such effects, and many past studies have clearly been underpowered. Environmental risk factors also appear critical; several, including obstetric complications and intrauterine influenza infections, have been suggested to increase risk of illness, and some convincing epidemiological support for such risk factors is emerging. The evidence for one such factor is particularly compelling: subjects who were *in utero* during the very severe famine in the Netherlands in the winter of 1944–1945 had a twofold increase in their risk for schizophrenia (Susser & Lin, 1992). While intriguing, it was hard to see how such results could be easily verified. However, in 2005, using data from the severe famine in regions of China in 1959–1961, the results of the earlier Dutch study were robustly replicated (St Clair *et al.*, 2005).

We would expect the products of interacting genes (or their functions) to be biologically related, functionally (e.g., the subunits of heteromultimeric neurotransmitter receptors), temporally (e.g., in neurodevelopmental cascades) or spatially (e.g., co-localized cell surface receptors). Epistatic interaction is only possible if the risk allele or **genotype** (the pair of alleles at a variable site present on an individual's pair of chromosomes) at one gene moderates the effect of the genotype at another on the **phenotype** (the observable effect of the genotypes; here risk for schizophrenia). Where unbiased, genome-wide data are available for analysis, pathway and systems analysis approaches may help to isolate potentially interacting subsets of genes. It is less clear how environmental risk factors may interact with genetic vulnerabilities, and what kind of relationship we would expect between them.

Spectrum disorders: How broad is the range of psychiatric illness transmitted and who is considered affected?

Kendler and Diehl (1993) also reviewed results from studies of other illnesses in relatives of patients with schizophrenia. Again, only studies that used rigorous methodology, including personal interviews, structured diagnostic criteria, and blind diagnoses, were considered. The results are extremely variable across studies and different conditions examined. In five of seven studies, the risk of schizotypal or paranoid personality disorders in relatives of patients with schizophrenia are consistent at 4–4.5 times that in the control families. In studies (overlapping those above) which meet the same criteria and examine the risk of

schizoaffective, schizophreniform, and delusional disorders, and atypical psychosis in the relatives of patients, five of seven showed significantly higher risks of these conditions as well. The risk of psychotic spectrum disorders is clearly elevated in the relatives of schizophrenia probands. Two other studies, examining the converse of the question, found that the risk of schizophrenia is significantly higher in the relatives of individuals with schizoaffective and schizophreniform disorders than in controls (Kendler *et al.*, 1993, 1986).

Studies of wider spectra of psychopathology, including unipolar and bipolar affective illness, anxiety disorder, and alcoholism, show more ambiguous results. In studies examining the risk of affective disorders, six of nine find no significant difference between relatives of patients with schizophrenia or schizoaffective disorders and relatives of controls, consistent with the generally accepted dichotomy between psychotic and affective illness, but it is important to note that a third of studies do detect excess risk of affective disorders. There is evidence emerging from the molecular studies described below that individual genes associated with schizophrenia may also contribute to risk for other mental illness, particularly bipolar disorder. In studies of other conditions, five of six studies of anxiety disorder and four of five studies of alcoholism find no significant increase in risk in the relatives of schizophrenic probands. A twin study which explored the DSM-III definition of schizophrenia found evidence of an increased degree of genetic determination when concordance was broadened to include categories such as schizophreniform and atypical psychosis. However, when co-twins with a broader range of conditions, including major depression, were included as "affected", the evidence of a genetic effect, as reflected in the MZ-to-DZ concordance ratio, fell markedly (Farmer *et al.*, 1987).

Answers to this question are particularly important for molecular genetic investigation of schizophrenia, since they specify who is considered affected. Misclassification of affected individuals causes great loss in power to detect genetic effects. As is clear from the summary above, the boundaries of psychiatric illnesses are unclear, and consequently, we do not know exactly where to set definitions of illness for classifying individuals. There is obviously a great difference between calling a pair of siblings affected if both are diagnosed with schizophrenia and calling the same pair affected if one is diagnosed with schizophrenia and the other with a personality disorder, or one with schizophrenia and one with alcohol dependence. Though the field as a whole concurs that we do not know where to set the boundary, the approximation we choose in the meantime is the source of considerable controversy. It has become reasonably common to perform several analyses of data using a number of different definitions of illness. This has the benefits of allowing different genes to influence different ranges of pathology, and of making no assumptions about the range of pathology to which any gene predisposes a person.

Methods: Where and how will such genes be found?

Approaches: What are linkage and association?

Linkage and association are two fundamentally different genetic effects with quite different strategies for their detection. Both are widely used in the search for schizophrenia susceptibility genes, but because of the differences in the effects and their detection, they were applied to very different research questions, and so have generally been considered separately. Association studies tended in the past to focus on candidate genes, and the grounds on which candidates were selected were often relatively weak. Linkage studies have always collected data genome-wide and implicitly make no assumption about specific genes involved in etiology, but linkage is relatively weak when applied to complex traits. In the past 10 years, a first important shift in the field was that association studies have tended more and more to focus on chromosomal regions supported by multiple linkage studies. The sequential application of these two approaches has produced the most exciting current results, including a small but growing number of specific genes, which we will focus on, for which multiple groups have found support. (Note that additional genes may have been reported to be associated in the genomic regions we discuss below, but only those with substantial positive replication evidence are included here.) In a few cases, genes with known molecular interactions with the candidates have also generated replicated association evidence. A number of these best-supported candidate genes also provide some degree of evidence for association with other psychiatric phenotypes, particularly bipolar disorder, suggesting that there is some etiological overlap between conditions. It is only in the last 2 years that association studies of schizophrenia have begun to assess genome-wide data completely independent of linkage.

Linkage

Classical single-gene, or Mendelian, genetic illnesses are caused by mutations in a single gene, located at a single place on a chromosome. Because these illnesses are rare, the rare risk allele must segregate from parents with a family history into affected offspring, or arise as an even rarer *de novo* mutation. By following the segregation of marker alleles from the affected lineage into offspring, chromosome regions in which affected offspring inherit one marker allele and unaffected offspring the other can be identified. This phenomenon of chromosomal regions segregating with a trait in multiple families is called **linkage**. It is detectable because there is **cross-over**, a physical exchange of material, between the chromosome pairs during **meiosis**, the cell division resulting in the production of eggs or sperm. **Recombination**, the occurrence of chromosomes with new combinations of alleles, is observed genetically and is the result of this cross-over (Fig. 12.2). It also provides a common measure of genetic distance, the **centimorgan** (cM), which is equivalent to 1% recombination between two loci. If two genetic loci are on different chromosomes, the probability that they are inherited together will be 0.5. This means that the theoretical maximum genetic distance is 50 cM. This phenomenon of **independent assortment**, as Mendel described it, is also true for two loci far apart on the same chromosome when there is a 50% chance that they will be separated by cross-overs at meiosis. On the other hand, linkage is observed between two loci when they are in such close proximity on the same chromosome that their alleles are separated by cross-over less than half the time. This departure from independent assortment can be statistically tested for.

Linkage analysis methods

Two different forms of linkage analyses are in common use. **Parametric** analyses require the specification of a genetic model. Where these models can be specified accurately, parametric linkage is a powerful approach. However, the difficulties discussed above in defining a transmission model and specifying who should be considered affected suggest that it is much less powerful for analysis of schizophrenia. The parametric linkage statistic is the **LOD score** (the Logarithm of the Odds). A LOD score is the logarithm, to the base 10, of the ratio of the likelihood of the observed data given linkage divided by the likelihood of that same data given no linkage. A LOD score of +3 (which corresponds to a genome-wide significance level of p = 0.05; Morton, 1955; Lander & Kruglyak, 1995) thus means that the likelihood that the observed families are linked is 1000 times the likelihood that they are unlinked (and the likelihood ratio is 10^3 or 1000:1); a LOD score of −2 (which is generally accepted as significant evidence against linkage) means that the likelihood that the observed families are unlinked is 100 times the likelihood that they are linked (and the likelihood ratio is thus 10^{-2} or 0.01:1).

Because linkage analysis is likelihood-based and likelihood-based tests can be maximized over one or more parameters, a common technique is to vary parameters and use likelihood maximization to choose the best parameter value (e.g., the recombination fraction, Θ, which allows the assessment of the likelihood of linkage at several different genetic distances from a marker). Thus, the focus of linkage analysis is often comparison of the relative likelihood of the data under one parameter value compared to another.

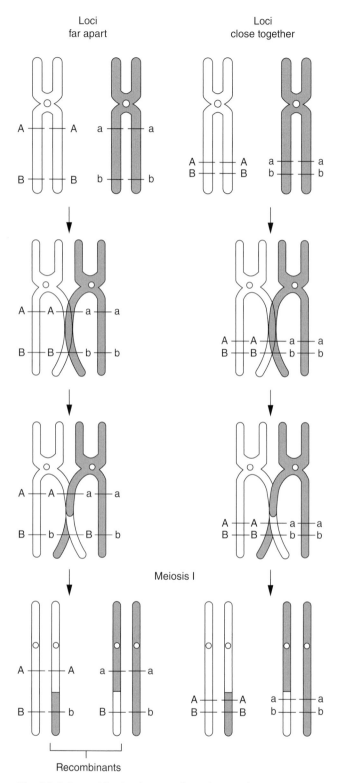

Loci far apart

Loci close together

Meiosis I

Recombinants

Fig. 12.2 Recombination between homologous chromosomes in meiosis. The left diagram illustrates two loci which are far apart on the same chromosome. These loci have an even chance that they will be separated by cross-overs at meiosis. On the right, the two loci are close together, so they are less likely to recombine.

Variations of the LOD score which allow for heterogeneity, or which assess only the affected individuals in a sample, have been applied to address some of the problems outlined above, but we will not distinguish between these in the discussion that follows.

An alternative approach, widely used in complex traits, is **non-parametric** linkage analysis (Kruglyak *et al.*, 1996). All classes of relatives have predefined probabilities of sharing zero, one, or two alleles at a random marker locus. These non-parametric statistics are based on testing for deviations from expected allele sharing distributions, and avoid the problem of specifying a transmission model, which as we saw above, is very difficult for schizophrenia.

Association

Association studies examine whether individuals affected by a disease more frequently have particular genetic variation in a gene than individuals not affected by the disease. This association can occur for two reasons: either the allele being studied directly influences risk for the disorder or, more commonly, the allele is in **linkage disequilibrium** (LD) with the disease-predisposing mutation. Linkage disequilibrium means that specific alleles at two nearby loci tend to occur together in an entire population. Linkage (the co-segregation of a chromosome region and a disease observed in families) occurs at scales of tens of millions of base pairs, while association (and LD) are seen at scales of tens of thousands of base pairs. LD is a reflection of an evolutionary history in which, because of these very small distances, recombination occurs very rarely between the two loci. LD occurs because a new variant (i.e., polymorphic marker or mutation) always arises on a specific background chromosome, and will, until separated by recombination, only exist in conjunction with the other alleles present on that background. Over time, the original LD (and thus the genetic association) between more distant loci decay as a result of recombination events, while the rarity of recombination between nearby loci preserves some or most of the original LD and association.

Association analysis methods

The simplest genetic association tests ask if specific alleles, genotypes or **haplotypes**, the combination of alleles on one of the pair of chromosomes, are more common in cases than in controls. Association approaches have two important advantages when compared to linkage. First, individual patients can be studied rather than families. Second, under many circumstances, a sample of equal size has considerably more power to detect association than to detect linkage for a gene of modest effect (Risch & Merikangas, 1996). However, they have two potential disadvantages. First, association studies have in the past only been able to examine much smaller regions of the genome than linkage studies. Because of the very different scales on which the two effects occur, association studies require more than 1000 times the density of data used in linkage studies. Practically, this means that association studies were used for the assessment of candidate genes or regions only, although this has changed dramatically with the arrival of affordable methods for collecting association data genome-wide. Second, association can occur for spurious reasons unrelated to disease etiology, such as **population stratification**, where the cases and controls come from different population groups or subgroups, and observed genotypic differences are due to this population difference, rather than to true association between marker and phenotype. This particular issue, although real, appears less significant than once thought provided controls are sampled from the same population as cases.

A number of analytical developments have improved association studies. **Transmission disequilibrium testing** (TDT) (Spielman & Ewens, 1996) assesses whether certain alleles or haplotypes are transmitted to affected individuals within families more often than expected by chance. **Pedigree disequilibrium testing** (PDT) (Martin *et al.*, 2000) and **family-based association testing** (FBAT) (Laird *et al.*, 2000) utilize both the "vertical" transmission information and the "horizontal" information in concordant and discordant siblings. Both of these have furthered the pursuit of association studies in family samples originally collected for linkage studies. The problems of **stochastic sampling variation,** the random variation of the predisposing genes represented in different family or case–control samples, and heterogeneity (among others) all suggest that the best place to follow-up a linkage finding is in the family sample which produced it.

Association studies in schizophrenia (and other psychiatric disorders) have tended in the past to focus on a limited set of "usual suspect" genes, generally those coding for receptors, transporters, and synthetic or degradatory enzymes in neurotransmitter pathways. Selection of candidate genes is often biased and results from these studies have generally not been particularly robust. While association studies remain a major interest in attempting to clarify the nature of the genetic liability to schizophrenia, only a few widely replicated findings have emerged from the older candidate gene association literature. It remains to be seen whether this will change with the analysis of several large GWAS datasets in schizophrenia, which avoid bias by assessing the entire genome.

Limitations of linkage and association

Linkage is a powerful method for Mendelian disorders where a small number of families can usually unambiguously produce strong evidence for linkage to a small chromosomal region. As we saw above, schizophrenia (in common with many complex traits) differs from Mendelian disorders in many critical ways, all of which reduce the power of linkage approaches: (1) risk cannot generally be explained by the action of rare highly penetrant alleles in single genes; (2) environmental factors are critical to account for observed patterns of risk, and GxG and/or GxE interactions seem likely; (3) risk variants generally seem likely to be common; (4) both locus and allelic heterogeneity seem likely; and (5) diagnostic boundaries are unclear and risk from a predisposing allele may not be limited to schizophrenia or schizophrenia spectrum disorders. Association is more powerful generally for detecting genes of small effect (Risch & Merikangas, 1996), but these features all also reduce the power of association studies. Current approaches analyze genes individually, but the risk associated with an individual gene is likely to be small and may depend on interactions with other genes. Replication studies are hampered by two additional issues. Inadequate sample sizes have been used in many studies: in replication, the follow-up sample must be larger than the original discovery sample to maintain power. Under a polygenic model of risk in the population, substantial stochastic sampling variation is expected: each sample tested will vary in the extent to which any specific risk factor is present (and association detectable). All of these issues should be borne in mind when assessing the evidence for specific chromosomal locations which follows.

DNA polymorphisms

Review of genetic marker types and their designations facilitates an understanding of the material that follows. Most linkage studies use a particular kind of DNA polymorphism, the **tandem repeat**. Tandem repeats are variable numbers of a repeating unit of nucleotides, from mononucleotides (rarely used due to the difficulty of accurate genotyping) through dinucleotides (the most common and most commonly used), tri-, tetra-, and penta-nucleotides. The frequency of polymorphisms of various unit sizes in the genome is generally inversely correlated with the length of the tandem repeat unit. They are referred to variously as microsatellites, short tandem repeats (STRs), simple sequence repeats (SSRs) or AC repeats (after the most common dinucleotide repeat sequence). The alleles of these markers are of different segment lengths due to different numbers of the tandemly repeated unit. This marker type is very common and tends to be extremely polymorphic (i.e., to have many alleles) and therefore to have high **heterozygosity** (the proportion of individuals who have two different alleles at the marker locus). As a result of the high heterozygosity, they also tend to be extremely **informative**, where information content is defined as the probability that the allele transmitted to a given offspring from a given parent can be unambiguously determined. Nomenclature for markers of this type are "D numbers" which identify the chromosome on which the marker locus maps and the historical order in which the marker was identified. Thus, the 278th microsatellite identified on chromosome 22 (discussed below) has the identifier D22S278.

In contrast, **single** or **simple nucleotide polymorphisms** (SNPs) are genetic variations involving common **transition** (purine to purine or pyrimidine to pyrimidine) or rarer **transversion** (purine to pyrimidine or pyrimidine to purine) changes at a single base or **insertion/deletion** variation up to a few nucleotides in size. SNPs generally have only two alleles, lower heterozygosity, and lower information content. Large numbers of alleles (and therefore high information content) are useful for linkage as they maximize the number of informative meioses. Association and LD studies tend, in general, to use SNPs as the marker of choice, because alleles of these markers evolve more slowly than microsatellites and preserve more of the evolutionary relationships on which LD and association are based. Standard nomenclature for these markers is the "rs number" catalog entry in dbSNP. The "common allele–position–rare allele" convention is common in older literature [e.g., the T102C polymorphism in the serotonin 2a-receptor (*5HT2A*) gene]. Where SNPs occur in coding sequence and alter amino acid sequence, the amino acid change and position (now in the polypeptide) are often used [e.g., Ser311Cys polymorphism in the dopamine receptor 2 (*DRD2*) gene]. We follow standard nomenclature for distinguishing between human genes and their protein products. Proteins are given as either the full name (e.g., catechol-O-methyltransferase) or the abbreviation (COMT) in upper case Roman font. Where a gene or protein has more than one name in current use in the literature [e.g., the approved nomenclature D-amino acid oxidase activator (*DAOA*) and the widely-used *G72*], both will be given. Gene symbols, usually the same as the protein abbreviations, are given in upper case italics (*COMT*).

Results: Where is the evidence strongest for schizophrenia susceptibility genes?

Through 2004, 25 complete or nearly complete genome linkage scans for schizophrenia (in which about 400 individual genetic markers are genotyped at regular intervals over the entire human genome) were published, and none revealed evidence for a gene of major effect for schizophrenia, consistent with the evidence reviewed above. A smaller number of genome scans examining specific clinical features of the illness (such as neuropsychological deficits, age at onset, and positive, negative, and disorganized symptoms) have been published. Finally, two meta-analyses of genome scan linkage data using different

statistical approaches and six meta-analyses of specific chromosomal regions have been published.

Some tentative evidence for replicated linkage for schizophrenia susceptibility genes has emerged from these studies. A number of promising genes have emerged from sequential linkage and association studies and multiple replication reports: in historical order, these are 22q12–q13, 8p22–p21, 6p24–p22, 13q14–q32, and 1q32–42. Two additional regions with little support in the primary literature, 2p11.1–q21.1 and 3p25.3–p22.1, were among the most significant in a meta-analysis of schizophrenia genome scans. A number of other regions (including 5q22–q31, 10p15–p11, 6q21–q22, and 15q13–q14) have less strong summary evidence but have been reported multiple times. We must note that the interpretation of these results is controversial, particularly as the definition of replication for linkage to a complex trait remains uncertain (Baron, 1996; Kendler *et al.*, 1996). In the interest of brevity, studies that do not find evidence for linkage in these selected regions have been omitted, but it is important to bear this selective bias in mind when considering the data that follow. More detailed information about putative linkage regions can be found elsewhere (Riley & McGuffin, 2000; Sullivan, 2005). The discussion of associated genes in these regions includes only those with substantial support from replication.

Chromosome 22q linkage studies

Initial evidence for linkage to chromosome 22q came from three markers spanning approx. 23 cM in the 22q13.1 region in the Maryland family sample (Pulver *et al.*, 1994a). A collaborative replication study in a total of 217 multiplex pedigrees did not confirm the linkage in the new samples (Pulver *et al.*, 1994b), but two other replication samples were positive (Coon *et al.*, 1994; Polymeropoulos *et al.*, 1994). Eleven groups contributed data from the most significant marker in the original sample and one replication, the dinucleotide repeat polymorphism, D22S278, to a large collaborative schizophrenia linkage study. There was excess sharing of alleles in these 620 affected sib pairs (p = 0.006), particularly in 296 pairs with data available from both parents (p = 0.001). It is important to note, however, that the authors calculated that this locus is likely to account for no more than 2% of total variance in liability (Gill *et al.*, 1996). The role of this region in liability to schizophrenia remains unclear, although the multiple positive findings seem unlikely to have occurred by chance.

Additional interest in this region of 22q came from a known chromosomal rearrangement. The cosegregation of chromosomal anomalies or rearrangements with phenotypes resembling a particular disease has provided useful clues to the locations of the gene(s) involved, most notably in the positional cloning of the dystrophin (or *DMD*) gene. Velo-cardio-facial syndrome (VCFS) is caused by deletions at 22q11, near to these linkage results for schizophrenia. Historically, about 10% of VCFS patients were thought to present with a psychotic phenotype, but more recent studies suggest much higher rates of 25–29% (Murphy et al., 1999; Pulver et al., 1994c). Conversely, preliminary results suggest that between 0.5% and 2% of adult-onset and up to 6% of childhood-onset patients with schizophrenia have microdeletions in this region, in excess of the estimated general population frequency of such deletions of 0.025% (Karayiorgou et al., 1995). Although statistically significant, this excess of deletions is probably not enough to explain significant **population attributable risk**, but variation in genes in this region in individuals without a deletion may contribute to liability (see also Structural variation below).

Chromosome 22q candidate genes

COMT

The VCFS critical region contains the gene for catechol-O-methyl transferase (COMT) located at 22q11, involved in the degradation of catecholamines, and is genetically and functionally polymorphic with a variable amino acid, Val158Met. Val and Met alleles are of almost identical frequency. Studies of the COMT gene show mixed results, recently reviewed by Williams et al. (2007). One study suggests that the high activity (Val) allele, through increased catabolism of dopamine in the prefrontal cortex, may slightly increase the risk of schizophrenia and may explain some of the observed differences in cognitive performance and prefrontal cortical functioning between cases and controls (Egan et al., 2001). Another study of COMT in a homogeneous population of Ashkenazi Jews used the largest case–control sample for schizophrenia then reported (Shifman et al., 2002). Three SNPs in the COMT gene showed significant association with schizophrenia in approx. 720 cases and 2000–4000 controls. In agreement with the study above, an association was found with the homozygous high activity genotype (Val/Val) and with the two other SNPs tested. A detailed discussion of COMT and studies of its association with schizophrenia is found in Chapter 13.

Chromosome 8p22–p21 linkage studies

The Maryland family sample also gave the first evidence of linkage to chromosome 8p22–p21 (Pulver et al., 1995). A multicenter collaborative linkage study supported this putative locus with excess allele sharing at D8S261 (Levinson et al., 1996). Data from pedigrees from numerous different ethnic backgrounds all support a locus on 8p, as did a statistically robust meta-analysis (Lewis et al., 2003). These replication results are spread across about 15 Mb of sequence. One of the key points to note is that although numerous samples support a locus on this chromosome,

comparison between individual studies is consistent with the possibility of multiple genes in the region, a feature of a number of linkage regions.

Chromosome 8p22–p21 candidate genes

NRG1

Following linkage evidence to chromosome 8p in Icelandic families, fine mapping with 50 markers across a 30 cM interval identified two risk haplotypes spanning a region of approx. 1 Mb within the gene for neuregulin 1 (NRG1) (Stefansson et al., 2002). Case–control samples from Scotland (Stefansson et al., 2003) and Ireland (Corvin et al., 2004) have provided additional support for this locus and for haplotypes identical or closely related to those identified in the Icelandic cases. In replication attempts, 13 independent studies in multiple populations have provided support for association (Williams et al., 2004a; Yang et al., 2003; Bakker et al., 2004; Li et al., 2004; Tang et al., 2004; Zhao et al., 2004; Petryshen et al., 2005; Fukui et al., 2006; Hall et al., 2006; Norton et al., 2006; Thomson et al., 2007; Turunen et al., 2007; Georgieva et al., 2008), though not always with the specific haplotypes originally reported, while nine studies have not supported involvement of NRG1 in schizophrenia (Hall et al., 2004; Iwata et al., 2004; Thiselton et al., 2004; Duan et al., 2005; Ingason et al., 2006; Walss-Bass et al., 2006; Rosa et al., 2007; Vilella et al., 2008; Ikeda et al., 2008). Studies of NRG1 have been recently reviewed (Tosato et al., 2005). A meta-analysis of studies of NRG1 supported involvement of the gene in schizophrenia liability, but did not provide evidence supporting association of the most prominent marker in the original studies (Munafo et al., 2006). In a pattern observed for a number of the best supported schizophrenia genes, several studies have also shown association between NRG1 and bipolar disorder (Green et al., 2005; Thomson et al., 2005; Georgieva et al., 2008). Functional evidence and discussion of the complex expression and functions of the NRG1 isoforms are included in Chapter 13.

NRG1 and ERBB4

ErbB4, encoded by the ERBB4 gene, is a receptor for NRG1 and has important roles in neurodevelopment and the modulation of NMDA receptor functioning. Both activation of ErbB4 and suppression of NMDA receptor activation by NRG1 are increased in the prefrontal cortex in individuals with schizophrenia compared to controls (Hahn et al., 2006). This functional relationship prompted assessment of ERBB4 for association with schizophrenia. Both primary association in ERBB4 and evidence of interaction with NRG1 have been reported (Norton et al., 2006, Nicodemus et al., 2006; Silberberg et al., 2006; Benzel et al., 2007). Associated alleles in ERBB4 alter splice-variant expression (Law et al., 2007) and both NRG1 and ErbB4 protein are increased in the brain in schizophrenia. These results confirming potential interaction between genes in schizophrenia may be of particular importance.

Chromosome 6p24–p22 linkage studies

The first evidence for linkage of schizophrenia to the 6p region came from studies of Irish families with a high density of disease (Straub et al., 1995). In data from 16 markers, evidence for linkage was modest under a narrow diagnostic model, but increased substantially as the diagnostic definition broadened to include spectrum disorders. Evidence for linkage fell when the definition was broadened further to include non-spectrum disorders, in keeping with the risk in relatives for these traits discussed above. Multiple independent reports of analyses of this region of 6p have been published. Studies of German and mixed German and Israeli pedigrees supported linkage to 6p24–p22 (Moises et al., 1995; Schwab et al., 1995). A family sample from Quebec found supportive evidence for a schizophrenia susceptibility locus in some, but not all, families (Maziade et al., 1997). A large, multigeneration family from Sweden supported this linkage in a single branch of the family; a haplotype of markers within the putative linked segment was found to segregate with schizophrenia (Lindholm et al., 1999). A large, multicenter collaboration detected significant excess allele sharing in this region (Levinson et al., 1996) as did the best meta-analysis (Lewis et al., 2003).

Chromosome 6p24–p22 candidate genes

DTNBP1

Follow-up work in the Irish family set demonstrated a positive association in the dystrobrevin binding protein 1 or dysbindin (DTNBP1) gene (Straub et al., 2002). Subsequent re-analysis of the association data revealed a risk haplotype of SNP markers in this gene (van den Oord et al., 2003). DTNBP1 has been widely associated with schizophrenia in samples from diverse ethnic backgrounds: 13 published studies of 15 independent samples reported significant positive associations with SNPs and/or haplotypes in the gene (Straub et al., 2002; van den Oord et al., 2003; Schwab et al., 2003; Van Den Bogaert et al., 2003; Tang et al., 2003; Funke et al., 2004; Kirov et al., 2004; Numakawa et al., 2004; Williams et al., 2004a; Li et al., 2005; Tochigi et al., 2006; Tosato et al., 2007; Vilella et al., 2008), while 14 studies of 18 independent samples showed no evidence for association of this gene with schizophrenia (Van Den Bogaert et al., 2003; Morris et al., 2003; Hall et al., 2004; DeLuca et al., 2005; Holliday et al., 2006; Joo et al., 2006; Turunen et al., 2007; Liu et al., 2007; Pedrosa et al., 2007; Wood et al., 2007; Bakker et al., 2007; Datta et al., 2007; Turunen et al., 2007; Peters et al., 2008; Sanders et al., 2008). One sample which showed no evidence in a first report (Morris et al., 2003) was positive

when additional SNPs were typed (Williams et al., 2004a). However, the specific details of reported associations have varied considerably with evidence for association on at least four different haplotype backgrounds. A further four studies have also provided positive evidence for association of DTNBP1 with bipolar disorder (Fallin et al., 2005; Breen et al., 2006; Joo et al., 2007; Pae et al., 2007).

The function of DTNBP1 protein in brain is unknown. It was first identified as a binding partner of both α- and β-dystrobrevins (Benson et al., 2001), which are binding partners of dystrophin, a large, membrane-associated protein expressed at highest levels in muscle and brain and mutated in Duchenne and Becker muscular dystrophy (Ray et al., 1985). In muscle, dystrophin is associated with the dystrophin-associated protein complex (DPC), which spans the membrane and links the cytoskeleton and the extracellular matrix. However, several lines of evidence suggest that the mechanisms of action for these molecules are different in neuronal and muscle tissue, and may be different in different regions of the brain. Some evidence suggests that the expression of DTNBP1 is reduced in certain brain regions of patients with schizophrenia at both the RNA (Weickert et al., 2004) and protein (Talbot et al., 2004) levels. Further details can be found in Chapter 13.

Chromosome 13q14–q32 linkage studies

Data from a mixed sample of UK and Japanese families initially suggested linkage to chromosome 13q14.1–q32 (Lin et al., 1995), of interest as the region contains the 5HT-2A receptor gene. Preliminary data from the Maryland and UK/Icelandic samples gave some initial support (Antonarakis et al., 1996; Kalsi et al., 1996). An attempt by the original group to replicate this in an independent sample of Taiwanese and UK families supported the finding only in the European families (Lin et al., 1997). Further analyses of the European sample using slightly different methods yielded positive data at two markers located at 13q32, but they were separated by a region where the values of the statistics dropped almost to zero.

Genome scan data from a mixed UK/US sample gave positive evidence, but extremely distant from other findings in the region (Shaw et al., 1998). The Maryland family sample gave modest evidence for linkage under a recessive model; non-parametric analysis of the same data was highly significant. Marker data in narrowly defined Canadian pedigrees gave fairly strong evidence for linkage (Brzustowicz et al., 1999). The results from chromosome 13 are particularly difficult to interpret because of the very large distances between positive markers. Unlike chromosome 6, where two distinct regions have been detected in different samples, there has been little agreement about the site of greatest evidence on 13q. Overall, the combined linkage reports are spread over a region of approx. 60 Mb, containing approx. 120 known or putative genes. On the other hand, although locations are much less certain on chromosome 13q than in other linkage regions, this chromosome has produced some of the most significant linkage evidence seen in the studies of schizophrenia.

Chromosome 13q14–q32 candidate genes

G72/DAOA

A study of approx. 200 SNPs tested across the distal 5 Mb of this broad linkage region and identified two regions of association (Chumakov *et al.*, 2002). In one of these regions, two genes [initially called *G72*, now D-amino acid oxidase activator (*DAOA*) and *G30*] were investigated. Of note, the exons of these genes could not be predicted by any computational method tested, suggesting that they are highly novel in their sequence and organization. Both genes show alternative transcripts in brain and other tissues. In 12 published association studies, SNPs within *G72/DAOA* have also provided substantial positive replication evidence (Addington *et al.*, 2004; Schumacher *et al.*, 2004; Korostishevsky *et al.*, 2004, 2006; Zou *et al.*, 2005; Hong *et al.*, 2006; Ma *et al.*, 2006; Yue *et al.*, 2006; Shin et al., 2007; Shinkai et al., 2007). A further seven studies have not provided supportive evidence of association (Hall *et al.*, 2004; Vilella *et al.*, 2008; Wood *et al.*, 2007; Sanders *et al.*, 2008; Mulle *et al.*, 2005; Liu *et al.*, 2006a; Goldberg *et al.*, 2006a). Three meta-analyses of the collected data showed weak positive (Li & He, 2007) and strong positive (Detera-Wadleigh & McMahon, 2006; Shi *et al.*, 2008) evidence of association between *G72/DAOA* and schizophrenia. *G72/DAOA* has also been associated with bipolar disorder in four studies (Hattori *et al.*, 2003; Chen *et al.*, 2004a; Goldberg *et al.*, 2006b; Prata *et al.*, 2007), and in one (Detera-Wadleigh & McMahon, 2006) but not a second (Shi *et al.*, 2008) meta-analysis.

G72/DAOA and DAO

D-amino acid oxidase (DAO) was identified as a binding partner of, and is activated by, the protein product of *G72/DAOA*. The *DAO* gene, on chromosome 12q24, was screened for association evidence in the original study (Chumakov *et al.*, 2002), and the four SNPs tested were significantly associated. Results of this kind (showing association in two interacting genes in the same sample) are rare, so this study provided a unique opportunity to test for an epistatic genetic interaction. Evidence for epistasis was observed for one pair of *DAO* and *G72/DAOA* genotypes, supporting a potential interaction between them in risk for schizophrenia. Fewer replication studies have assessed the role of *DAO*, and these are less clear in their support for the reported association, with four studies supporting (Wood *et al.*, 2007; Schumacher *et al.* 2004; Corvin *et al.*, 2007; Liu *et al.*, 2004) and four showing no support

for association with schizophrenia (Goldberg *et al.*, 2006b; Shinkai *et al.*, 2007; Liu *et al.*, 2007; Vilella *et al.*, 2008). One study of *DAO* suggested association with bipolar disorder (Fallin *et al.*, 2005).

Chromosome 1q32–q42 linkage studies

1q41–q42 and DISC1

Some of the strongest findings suggesting the involvement of genes on chromosome 1 in schizophrenia began with reports of a balanced 1:11 translocation segregating with serious mental illness in a large pedigree from Scotland (St Clair *et al.*, 1990). The chromosome 1 breakpoint lies at 1q42.1, and two groups reported suggestive linkage findings in this region, in national and population isolate samples from Finland (Hovatta *et al.*, 1999; Ekelund *et al.*, 2000) and in the Maryland sample. Ongoing work in the Scottish pedigree has now shown that the breakpoint directly disrupts a novel gene, Disrupted in Schizophrenia 1 (*DISC1*) (Millar *et al.*, 2000). There are now nine positive reports of association of *DISC1* with schizophrenia (Thomson *et al.*, 2005, Hennah *et al.*, 2003; Hodgkinson *et al.*, 2004; Callicott *et al.*, 2005; Cannon *et al.*, 2005; Liu *et al.*, 2006b; Palo et al., 2007; Qu *et al.*, 2007) and two of association with positive symptoms (De Rosse *et al.*, 2007; Szeszko *et al.*, 2008) suggesting that this gene is relevant to schizophrenia in the general population. However, as with the other genes noted above, SNP alleles and haplotypes have not been consistent across these studies. Other rare variants in this gene besides the breakpoint have also been reported to be associated with schizophrenia (Sachs *et al.*, 2005; Song *et al.*, 2008) and association has been reported for additional psychiatric diagnoses (reviewed by Hennah *et al.*, 2009) and for bipolar disorder (Perlis *et al.*, 2008). A smaller number of negative reports have also been published (Kockelkorn *et al.*, 2004; Zhang *et al.*, 2005a; Chen *et al.*, 2007a; Kim *et al.*, 2008; Sanders *et al.*, 2008).

1q23–q32 linkage and RGS4

Genome scan data in families from Canada (Brzustowicz *et al.*, 2000) and follow-up fine-mapping data in the population isolate samples from Finland (Ekelund *et al.*, 2001) have also provided evidence for linkage in a more centromeric position on chromosome 1, although the chromosomal position varies between these studies, making interpretation difficult. The latter provided very strong LOD scores but was not replicated by a large collaborative study (Levinson *et al.*, 2002).

Microarray studies of postmortem schizophrenic brain suggested that *RGS4*, the regulator of G-protein signalling 4 gene, showed altered expression in schizophrenia (Mirnics *et al.*, 2001). *RGS4* maps to the chromosome 1 linkage region, and in a subsequent study in mixed US pedigrees and samples from India, the same markers in the same 10 kb region were associated in both samples, although different specific marker haplotypes gave this evidence in the US compared to the Indian families (Chowdari *et al.*, 2002). In replication studies, six have provided supportive evidence for association of the RGS4 locus with schizophrenia liability (Chen *et al.*, 2004b; Morris *et al.*, 2004; Williams *et al.*, 2004b; Fallin *et al.*, 2005; Bakker *et al.*, 2007; So *et al.*, 2008) while nine have not (Cordeiro *et al.*, 2005; Sobell *et al.*, 2005; Guo *et al.*, 2006; Liu *et al.*, 2006c; Rizig *et al.*, 2006; Ishiguro *et al.*, 2007; Wood *et al.*, 2007; Sanders *et al.*, 2008; Vilella *et al.*, 2008). One study observed association in a Scottish sample but not in a Chinese sample (Zhang *et al.*, 2005b). Results of meta-analyses have both supported (Talkowski *et al.*, 2006) and failed to support (Li & He, 2006) the involvement of *RGS4* in schizophrenia.

Other chromosomal regions and genes

A number of additional chromosome regions have provided multiple signals, although the evidence for linkage to schizophrenia is less well replicated and less certain. These include: 5q22–q31, where association was recently reported in the interleukin-3 (*IL3*) gene (Chen *et al.*, 2007b), which awaits replication; 10p15–q21, where evidence of association in the phophatidyl inositol-phosphate 5 kinase 2a (*PIP5K2A*) gene (Schwab *et al.*, 2006) was followed by mixed positive (Bakker *et al.*, 2007; He *et al.*, 2007; Saggers-Gray *et al.*, 2008) and negative (Jamra *et al.*, 2006) replication results; 6q21–q22, where association with the trace amine associated receptor 6 (*TAAR6*, previously known as *TRAR4*) gene located at 6q23.2 (Duan *et al.*, 2004) has mixed positive (Vladimirov *et al.*, 2007; Pae *et al.*, 2008) and negative (Ikeda *et al.*, 2005; Duan *et al.*, 2006; Sanders *et al.*, 2008) replications; and 15q13–q14, where evidence for linkage to an evoked potential abnormality common in patients and relatively rare in controls (Freedman *et al.*, 1997) was supported by five additional studies reporting positive linkage evidence for schizophrenia in the same narrow region (Riley *et al.*, 2000; Liu *et al.*, 2001; Tsuang *et al.*, 2001; Xu *et al.*, 2001; Gejman *et al.*, 2001).

A number of other high profile candidate genes, such as *PRODH1* (Liu *et al.*, 2002) and *PPP3CC* (Gerber *et al.*, 2003), identified through other means, have not replicated well. One exception to this pattern is the evidence for involvement of the *AKT1* gene in schizophrenia (Emamiam *et al.*, 2004), which has similar numbers of positive (Ikeda *et al.*, 2004; Schwab *et al.*, 2005; Bajestan *et al.*, 2006; Xu *et al.*, 2007; Thiselton *et al.*, 2008) and negative (Turunen *et al.*, 2007; Sanders *et al.*, 2008; Ohtsuki *et al.*, 2004; Ide *et al.*, 2006; Liu *et al.*, 2006d; Norton *et al.*, 2007) replications.

Meta-analyses of linkage and association data

Meta-analysis of whole genome screen data offers a different kind of insight into the mechanisms of complex trait genetics: because many samples, and therefore more data, are included, they represent a first approximation of a very large, multi-sample genome screen. Two different statistical approaches for such meta-analyses have been published. One combines the significance levels reported in the original genome screens after correcting each value for the size of the suggested region. Results from the first approach were significant for chromosomes 8p, 13q, and 22q (Badner & Gershon, 2002). The major limitations of this analysis are that it relies on published results, which prevents critical standardization across studies, and, unlike the second approach below, no new information about potential regions of interest can be extracted with it.

The second method ranks 30 cM bins of the genome from most positive to least positive for each study, and then sums the ranks for each bin. Significance levels are calculated by simulation. Since this method uses not significance levels but the actual marker LOD scores, it is possible to identify regions of the genome which are of potential interest on the basis of modest positive results occurring in the same region across many studies but which may have been overlooked due to stronger signals in the individual sample analyses. Results of the second approach, which is methodologically the stronger of the two, supported linkage to chromosomes 6p, 8p, and 10p of the previously identified regions discussed above (Lewis *et al.*, 2003). However, the strongest evidence for a potential locus was on chromosome 2p11.1–q21.1, a region suggested by only a few studies and not widely followed up, and on 3p, the site of an early linkage finding in the Maryland sample which could never be replicated by subsequent studies. Finally, significant evidence of linkage was also detected for two regions never previously implicated by an individual study, on chromosomes 11q and 14p.

Meta-analyses of association data have tended to assess one gene at a time. A recent effort has been made to systematize the collection and archiving of association data from studies of schizophrenia, and to provide a framework for continuous updating of both the data and the meta-analytic results (Allen *et al.*, 2008). The resulting SzGene database (http://www.szgene.org/) is regularly updated and publicly available. Meta-analyses of the data contained in this resource provided support of varying degrees for 24 SNPs in 16 previously reported genes, including older candidate genes (e.g., *DRD2*), those resulting from association-based follow-up of linkage data (e.g., *DTNBP1*), and those suggested by more recent genome-wide studies (e.g., *PLXNA2*).

Summary of current gene findings

Currently, all of the regions and candidate genes discussed above remain promising, but further assessment of each is still needed, to identify additional associated genes, clarify patterns of association, and elucidate their contribution to the neurobiology of schizophrenia. The reported associations for several of the current candidates, *DTNBP1*, *NRG1*, *DAOA/G72*, *DAO*, *DISC1*, and *RGS4* have been replicated in multiple samples, and positive replications outnumber negative ones for most. Other candidates, such as *IL3*, await the collection of sufficient data to interpret the validity of the original findings. Still others, like *TAAR6*, already have substantial data collected, but without strong or widespread replication.

One particularly exciting shared feature of many of the candidates discussed above is that they can be related to potential pathophysiology through dysfunction in glutamatergic neurotransmission, which may be an important systemic element in the etiology of schizophrenia. Although a detailed discussion of this theory is outside the scope of this chapter, recent reviews of the genetic (Harrison and Owen, 2003) and neuroscience (Moghaddam, 2003) data and evidence from other studies highlight the positions of the gene products of *NRG1*, *COMT*, *DAO*, *DAOA/G72*, *RGS4*, and possibly *DTNBP1*, among others, in the biochemical and functional pathways influencing the glutamatergic system (see also Chapter 21).

Genome-wide association studies

The field has been advanced further by the current round of GWAS, which have a number of distinct advantages over previous methods and have already revolutionized the understanding of other complex traits such as Type 2 diabetes (Sladek *et al.*, 2007; Saxena *et al.*, 2007; Zeggini *et al.*, 2007; Scott *et al.*, 2007; Steinthorsdottir *et al.*, 2007; Frayling *et al.*, 2007). By assaying 500 000–1 000 000 DNA variants in a single experiment, these provide unbiased genome-wide coverage and so avoid the weakness of selecting candidate genes when little is known about underlying disease processes. They use an association framework for analysis and so avoid the weaknesses of linkage in complex traits. They impose stringent criteria due to the number of tests performed ($p < 10^{-7}$ for genome-wide significance, although in practice $p < 10^{-5}$ is often considered strong enough to replicate or report). Finally, they hold enormous potential to move beyond the identification of single genes (which may show small effects and be difficult to detect individually) toward the simultaneous identification of multiple genes and their functional involvement in pathways, systems or processes. These studies are discussed in detail in Chapter 13.

Rare structural variation in schizophrenia

This chapter is written from the perspective of investigators who favor the common disease/common variant hypothesis of the genetic risks for complex traits, based on the epidemiological and genetic data outlined throughout the chapter. The current results of GWAS in other complex traits provided a major validation of this model. The alternative common disease/rare variant hypothesis of genetic risks for complex traits has been proposed recently in autism (Zhao *et al.*, 2007) and schizophrenia (McClellan *et al.*, 2007), largely based on the reduction in fertility observed in cases. A key focus of research in this area has been the deletions and duplications (or copy-number variation, CNV) and inversions of a few thousand (kb) to a few million (Mb) base pairs, collectively known as structural variation, an area of intense research interest generally since 2004 (Sebat *et al.*, 2004; Iafrate *et al.*, 2004; Tuzun *et al.*, 2005). The most common mechanism by which these variants arise is recombination occurring between two distinct but highly similar repeat sequences physically close to each other on a chromosome, called non-allelic homologous recombination (Plate 12.1).

As a class, this type of variation is common, but the individual deletion, duplication, and inversion events giving rise to the structural variation are rare. Genomic survey studies estimate that as much as 360 Mb or 12% of the genome is included in structural variation; 50% of variants were observed in more than one individual, consistent with stable inheritance in the population (Redon *et al.*, 2006). No study has yet been published assessing these common structural variants in disease. A few such variants occur at high frequency due to apparent selection in certain populations or contexts, e.g. increases in copy number of the *CCL3L1* gene [protective against human immunodeficiency virus (HIV) infection] in African primates, including humans (Gonzalez *et al.*, 2005), and the amylase (*AMY1*) gene in cereal farming groups, but not their pastoralist neighbors (Perry *et al.*, 2007).

However, studies of large samples are consistent in showing that the majority of structural variants are rare, often occurring in only one individual. This is broadly consistent with the widespread occurrence of repeat sequences in the human genome, which provide a basis for large numbers of randomly distributed, individually rare events. The aggregate rate of such rare structural variants is significantly increased in individuals with schizophrenia in all four studies reported (Xu *et al.*, 2008; Walsh *et al.*, 2008; Stefansson *et al.*, 2008; International Schizophrenia Consortium, 2008). Critically, there is substantial overlap between studies in the regions where structural variation is observed in excess in cases, most notably on chromosomes 22q11, 15q13.3, and 1q21.1, with some evidence that regions containing genes expressed in neurodevelopment are overrepresented, as in Rujescu *et al.* (2009). The most extreme test of this hypothesis based on fertility argues that *de novo* events in affected individuals are the most likely to represent highly penetrant genetic lesions because they are not present in the parents of affected individuals, who have successfully reproduced. *De novo* events are also observed at significantly higher frequency both in cases of autism (Sebat *et al.*, 2007) and schizophrenia (Xu *et al.*, 2008; Stefansson *et al.*, 2008). A few relatively rare structural variants have been observed to be recurrent: one example is the VCFS deletion on chromosome 22q discussed above, which is present at elevated frequency in individuals with schizophrenia. However, even considered in aggregate, rare structural variants are observed in at most 15%, and *de novo* structural variants in at most only 10%, of schizophrenia cases at the resolution and genomic coverage of experiments in 2010. The variants detected so far thus cannot account for a substantial fraction of the total population risk, and *de novo* events cannot account for any of the observed familial risk. A more difficult problem is that, because most are rare, the true impact of individual structural variants on schizophrenia is difficult to validate and interpret. The true importance of these findings in schizophrenia in the population is unclear at this time, although the replication of excess structural variation in cases on chromosomes 22q11, 15q13.3, and 1q21.1 is extremely encouraging.

Discussion

As is clear from the final two sections above, the field of genetic studies of schizophrenia continues to change rapidly and may have altered considerably by the time this chapter is read. Certainly the most important development in the last several years has been the emergence of a number of replicated positional candidate genes in target regions. Given the vast number of statistical tests that are now performed in most studies (multiple markers, diagnostic or genetic models, and analytical approaches), the true type I (or false-positive) error rate emerging from any individual study is nearly impossible to quantify. It remains a major concern that highly statistically significant results could occur by chance alone because so many tests are performed.

Therefore, replication is critical. However, there are many reasons why a "true" finding might not be replicated, including variation between populations or samples and differences in statistical power, diagnostic methods, and statistical approaches. Given the evidence of replication for linkage to a number of regions and association with genes in those regions, it seems increasingly unlikely that all of these results represent false positives. It is difficult to conceive of an inherent bias that would produce spuriously positive results across multiple groups (especially given the wide differences between the studies described above) in the same gene or chromosomal region.

In results from whole genome linkage scans for other complex disorders, including Type 1 (Hashimoto *et al.*, 1994) and Type 2 (Vionnet et al., 2000; Wiltshire *et al.*, 2001; Busfield *et al.*, 2002) diabetes mellitus, multiple sclerosis

(Sawcer *et al.*, 1996; Coraddu *et al.*, 2001), inflammatory bowel disease (Ogura *et al.*, 2001; Hugot *et al.*, 2001), and asthma (Laitinen *et al.*, 2001), non-replication across groups is as frequent as replication. These results suggest that the difficulties in detecting replicable linkages for schizophrenia may not be unique to the psychiatric disorders, but rather may reflect a general pattern of problems associated with linkage studies in complex traits. However, there appears to be cause for some optimism, as the candidates currently under most intense scrutiny have provided positive evidence across multiple samples. The results from GWAS of other complex traits have produced much better replicated initial results, but replication design may be critical to this success.

Conclusions

The evidence is strong that schizophrenia is a familial disorder and that the familial aggregation of schizophrenia is due largely, although probably not entirely, to genetic factors. Whatever the familial predisposition that operates for schizophrenia, it not only influences the classical, deteriorating psychotic disorder, but also increases liability to schizophrenia spectrum personality disorders and probably some other non-schizophrenic non-affective psychoses. Two decades of research using statistical methods have failed to clearly delineate the mode of transmission of schizophrenia, a result which is understandable given its likely complexity.

In generalizing to other psychiatric and complex phenotypes, the broad conclusions from the study of schizophrenia seem likely to hold: (1) such phenotypes are genetically influenced but not genetically determined; (2) a number of genes (which may even vary between individual family members) are likely to be involved; (3) the liability variants in these genes are generally expected to be common, within the range of normal human variation and to have low risk associated with them individually; (4) some of the variants may interact with others or with environmental risk factors; and (5) some of the variants may predispose individuals to wider spectra of psychopathology.

Advances in molecular and statistical genetics have opened up realistic opportunities to localize on the human genome the specific genes that influence the liability to schizophrenia. Association studies have yet to provide convincing evidence for the role of a range of candidate genes in the etiology of schizophrenia. Genome scan strategies have produced several regions, where multiple groups have found evidence for linkage, and more importantly, association in specific genes. While false-positive findings cannot be ruled out, it seems likely than one or more of these are true susceptibility genes for schizophrenia. Further, given the power of genome-wide association designs, it seems increasingly likely that within several years, the field may have widely replicated susceptibility genes for schizophrenia. This would represent a true watershed event in the history of schizophrenia research.

While unambiguous gene identification will itself represent a major advance, it is the identification of specific variants in these genes and their impact on disease which will initiate the most critical phase, that of translational research, including (1) rational drug design based on knowledge of basic pathophysiology and personalized medicine; (2) characterization of genotype–phenotype relationships based on knowledge of specific pathogenic mutations; (3) identification of environmental risk factors that interact with specific genes; and (4) realistic prevention research given our ability to identify high-risk individuals.

References

Addington, A.M., Gornick, M., Sporn, A.L. *et al.* (2004) Polymorphisms in the 13q33.2 gene G72/G30 are associated with childhood-onset schizophrenia and psychosis not otherwise specified. *Biological Psychiatry* **55**, 976–980.

Allen, N.C., Bagade, S., McQueen, M.B. *et al.* (2008) Systematic meta-analyses and field synopsis of genetic association studies in schizophrenia: the SzGene database. *Nature Genetics* **40**, 827–834.

Altshuler, D. & Daly, M. (2007) Guilt beyond a reasonable doubt. *Nature Genetics* **39**, 813–815.

Antonarakis, S.E., Blouin, J.L., Curran, M. *et al.* (1996) Linkage and sib-pair analysis reveal a potential schizophrenia susceptibility gene on chromosome 13q32. *American Journal of Human Genetics* **59**, A210.

Badner, J.A. & Gershon, E.S. (2002) Meta-analysis of whole-genome linkage scans of bipolar disorder and schizophrenia. *Molecular Psychiatry* **7**, 405–411.

Bajestan, S.N., Sabouri, A.H., Nakamura, M. *et al.* (2006) Association of AKT1 haplotype with the risk of schizophrenia in Iranian population. *American Journal of Medical Genetics Neuropsychiatric Genetics* **141**, 383–386.

Bakker, S.C., Hoogendoorn, M.L., Selten, J.P. *et al.* (2004) Neuregulin 1: genetic support for schizophrenia subtypes. *Molecular Psychiatry* **9**, 1061–1063.

Bakker, S.C., Hoogendoorn, M.L., Hendriks, J. *et al.* (2007) The PIP5K2A and RGS4 genes are differentially associated with deficit and non-deficit schizophrenia. *Genes, Brain and Behavior* **6**, 113–119.

Baron, M. (1996) Linkage results in schizophrenia. *American Journal of Medical Genetics* **67**, 121–123.

Benson, M.A., Newey, S.E., Martin-Rendon, E., Hawkes, R. & Blake, D.J. (2001) Dysbindin, a novel coiled-coil-containing protein that interacts with the dystrobrevins in muscle and brain. *Journal of Biological Chemistry* **276**, 24232–24241.

Benzel, I., Bansal, A., Browning, B.L. *et al.* (2007) Interactions among genes in the ErbB-Neuregulin signalling network are associated with increased susceptibility to schizophrenia. *Behavioural and Brain Functions* **3**, 31.

Breen, G., Prata, D., Osborne, S. *et al.* (2006) Association of the dysbindin gene with bipolar affective disorder. *American Journal of Psychiatry* **163**, 1636–1638.

Brzustowicz, L.M., Honer, W.G., Chow, E.W.C., Little, D., Hodgkinson, K. & Bassett, A. (1999) Linkage of familial schizophrenia to chromosome 13q32. *American Journal of Human Genetics* **65**, 1096–1103.

Brzustowicz, L.M., Hodgkinson, K.A., Chow, E.W.C., Honer, W.G. & Bassett, A.S. (2000) Location of a major susceptibility locus for familial schizophrenia on chromosome 1q21–q22. *Science* **288**, 678–682.

Busfield, F., Duffy, D.L., Kesting, J.B. *et al.* (2002) A genomewide search for type 2 diabetes-susceptibility genes in indigenous Australians. *American Journal of Human Genetics* **70**, 349–357.

Callicott, J.H., Straub, R.E., Pezawas, L. *et al.* (2005) Variation in DISC1 affects hippocampal structure and function and increases risk for schizophrenia. *Proceedings of the National Academy of Science USA* **102**, 8627–8632.

Cannon, T.D., Hennah, W., van Erp, T.G. *et al.* (2005) Association of DISC1/TRAX haplotypes with schizophrenia, reduced prefrontal gray matter, and impaired short- and long-term memory. *Archives of General Psychiatry* **62**, 1205–1213.

Cardno, A.G. & Gottesman, I.I. (2000) Twin studies of schizophrenia: From bow-and-arrow concordances to Star Wars Mx and functional genomics. *American Journal of Medical Genetics* **97**, 12–17.

Cardno, A.G., Marshall, E.J., Coid, B. *et al.* (1999) Heritability estimates for psychotic disorders: the Maudsley twin psychosis series. *Archives of General Psychiatry* **56**, 162–168.

Caspi, A., McClay, J. & Moffitt, T.E. *et al.* (2002) Role of genotype in the cycle of violence in maltreated children. *Science* **297**, 851–854.

Caspi, A., Sugden, K., Moffitt, T.E. *et al.* (2003) Influence of life stress on depression: moderation by a polymorphism in the 5-HTT gene. *Science* **301**, 386–389.

Chen, Y.S., Akula, N. & tera-Wadleigh, S.D. *et al.* (2004a) Findings in an independent sample support an association between bipolar affective disorder and the G72/G30 locus on chromosome 13q33. *Molecular Psychiatry* **9**, 87–92.

Chen, X., Dunham, C., Kendler, S. *et al.* (2004b) Regulator of G-protein signaling 4 (RGS4) gene is associated with schizophrenia in Irish high density families. *American Journal of Medical Genetics* **129B**, 23–26.

Chen, Q.Y., Chen, Q., Feng, G.Y. *et al.* (2007a) Case-control association study of Disrupted-in-Schizophrenia-1 (DISC1) gene and schizophrenia in the Chinese population. *Journal of Psychiatric Research* **41**, 428–434.

Chen, X., Wang, X., Hossain, S. *et al.* (2007b) Interleukin 3 and schizophrenia: the impact of sex and family history. *Molecular Psychiatry* **12**, 273–282.

Chowdari, K.V., Mirnics, K., Semwal, P. *et al.* (2002) Association and linkage analyses of RGS4 polymorphisms in schizophrenia. *Human Molecular Genetics* **11**, 1373–1380.

Chumakov, I., Blumenfeld, M., Guerassimenko, O. *et al.* (2002) Genetic and physiological data implicating the new human gene G72 and the gene for D-amino acid oxidase in schizophrenia. *Proceedings of the National Academy of Science USA* **99**, 13675–13680.

Coon, H., Holik, J., Hoff, M. *et al.* (1994) Analysis of chromosome 22 markers in nine schizophrenia pedigrees. *American Journal of Medical Genetics* **54**, 72–79.

Coraddu, F., Sawcer, S., D'Alfonso, S. *et al.* (2001) A genome screen for multiple sclerosis in Sardinian multiplex families. *European Journal of Human Genetics* **9**, 621–626.

Cordeiro, Q., Talkowski, M.E., Chowdari, K.V., Wood, J., Nimgaonkar, V. & Vallada, H. (2005) Association and linkage analysis of RGS4 polymorphisms with schizophrenia and bipolar disorder in Brazil. *Genes, Brain and Behaviour* **4**, 45–50.

Corvin, A.P., Morris, D.W., McGhee, K. *et al.* (2004) Confirmation and refinement of an "at-risk" haplotype for schizophrenia suggests the EST cluster, Hs.97362, as a potential susceptibility gene at the Neuregulin-1 locus. *Molecular Psychiatry* **9**, 208–213.

Corvin, A., McGhee, K.A., Murphy, K. *et al.* (2007) Evidence for association and epistasis at the DAOA/G30 and D-amino acid oxidase loci in an Irish schizophrenia sample. *American Journal of Medical Genetics B Neuropsychiatric Genetics* **144B**, 949–953.

Datta, S.R., McQuillin, A., Puri, V., *et al.* (2007) Failure to confirm allelic and haplotypic association between markers at the chromosome 6p22.3 dystrobrevin-binding protein 1 (DTNBP1) locus and schizophrenia. *Behavioural and Brain Functions* **3**, 50.

DeLuca, V., Voineskos, D., Shinkai, T., Wong, G. & Kennedy, J.L. (2005) Untranslated region haplotype in dysbindin gene: analysis in schizophrenia. *Journal of Neural Transmitters* **112**, 12163–12167.

DeRosse, P., Hodgkinson, C.A., Lencz, T. *et al.* (2007) Disrupted in schizophrenia 1 genotype and positive symptoms in schizophrenia. *Biological Psychiatry* **61**, 1208–1210.

Detera-Wadleigh, S.D. & McMahon, F.J. (2006) G72/G30 in schizophrenia and bipolar disorder: review and meta-analysis. *Biological Psychiatry* **60**, 106–114.

Duan, J., Martinez, M., Sanders, A.R. *et al.* (2004) Polymorphisms in the trace amine receptor 4 (TRAR4) gene on chromosome 6q23.2 are associated with susceptibility to schizophrenia. *American Journal of Human Genetics* **75**, 624–638.

Duan, J., Martinez, M., Sanders, A.R. *et al.* (2005) Neuregulin 1 (NRG1) and schizophrenia: analysis of a US family sample and the evidence in the balance. *Psychological Medicine* **35**, 1599–1610.

Duan, S., Du, J., Xu, Y. *et al.* (2006) Failure to find association between TRAR4 and schizophrenia in the Chinese Han population. *Journal of Neural Transmitters* **113**, 381–385.

Egan, M.F., Goldberg, T.E., Kolachana, B.S. *et al.* (2001) Effect of COMT Val108/158 Met genotype on frontal lobe function and risk for schizophrenia. *Proceedings of the National Academy of Sciences USA* **98**, 6917–6922.

Ekelund, J., Lichtermann, D., Hovatta, I. *et al.* (2000) Genome-wide scan for schizophrenia in the Finnish population: Evidence for a locus on chromosome 7q22. *Human Molecular Genetics* **9**, 1049–1057.

Ekelund, J., Hovatta, I., Parker, A. *et al.* (2001) Chromosome 1 loci in Finnish schizophrenia families. *Human Molecular Genetics* **10**, 1611–1617.

Emamian, E.S., Hall, D., Birnbaum, M.J., Karayiorgou, M. & Gogos, J.A. (2004) Convergent evidence for impaired AKT1-GSK3beta signaling in schizophrenia. *Nature Genetics* **36**, 131–137.

Fallin, M.D., Lasseter, V.K., Avramopoulos, D. *et al.* (2005) Bipolar I disorder and schizophrenia: a 440-single-nucleotide polymorphism screen of 64 candidate genes among Ashkenazi Jewish case-parent trios. *American Journal of Human Genetics* **77**, 918–936.

Farmer, A.E., McGuffin, P. & Gottesman, I.I. (1987) Twin concordance for DSM-III schizophrenia. Scrutinizing the validity of the definition. *Archives of General Psychiatry* **44**, 634–640.

Foley, D.L., Eaves, L.J., Wormley, B. *et al.* (2004) Childhood adversity, monoamine oxidase a genotype, and risk for conduct disorder. *Archives of General Psychiatry* **61**, 738–744.

Frayling, T.M., Timpson, N.J., Weedon, M.N. *et al.* (2007) A common variant in the FTO gene is associated with body mass index and predisposes to childhood and adult obesity. *Science* **316**, 889–894.

Freedman, R., Coon, H., Myles-Worsley, M. *et al.* (1997) Linkage of a neurophysiological deficit in schizophrenia to a chromosome 15 locus. *Proceedings of the National Academy of Sciences USA* **94**, 587–592.

Funke, B., Finn, C.T., Plocik, A.M., *et al.* (2004) Association of the DTNBP1 Locus with Schizophrenia in a U.S. Population. *American Journal of Human Genetics* **75**, 891–898.

Fukui, N., Muratake, T., Kaneko, N., Amagane, H. & Someya, T. (2006) Supportive evidence for neuregulin 1 as a susceptibility gene for schizophrenia in a Japanese population. *Neuroscience Letters* **396**, 117–120.

Gejman, P.V., Sanders, A.R., Badner, J.A., Cao, Q. & Zhang, J. (2001) Linkage analysis of schizophrenia to chromosome 15. *American Journal of Medical Genetics* **105**, 789–793.

Georgieva, L., Dimitrova, A., Ivanov, D. *et al.* (2008) Support for neuregulin 1 as a susceptibility gene for bipolar disorder and schizophrenia. *Biological Psychiatry* **64**, 419–427.

Gerber, D.J., Hall, D., Miyakawa, T. *et al.* (2003) Evidence for association of schizophrenia with genetic variation in the 8p21.3 gene, PPP3CC, encoding the calcineurin gamma subunit. *Proceedings of the National Academy of Science USA* **100**, 8993–8998.

Gill, M., Vallada, H., Collier, D. *et al.* (1996) A combined analysis of D22S278 marker alleles in affected sib-pairs: Support for a susceptibility locus for schizophrenia at chromosome 22q12. *American Journal of Medical Genetics Neuropsychiatric Genetics* **67**, 40–45.

Goldberg, T.E., Straub, R.E., Callicott, J.H. *et al.* (2006a) The G72/G30 gene complex and cognitive abnormalities in schizophrenia. *Neuropsychopharmacology* **31**, 2022–2032.

Goldberg, T.E., Straub, R.E., Callicott, J.H. *et al.* (2006b) The G72/G30 gene complex and cognitive abnormalities in schizophrenia. *Neuropsychopharmacology* **31**, 2022–2032.

Gonzalez, E., Kulkarni, H., Bolivar, H. *et al.* (2005) The influence of CCL3L1 gene-containing segmental duplications on HIV-1/AIDS susceptibility. *Science* **307**, 1434–1440.

Gottesman, I.I. (1991) *Schizophrenia Genesis*. New York: WH Freeman.

Gottesman, I.I. & Shields, J. (1982) *Schizophrenia: The Epigenetic Puzzle*. Cambridge: Cambridge University Press.

Green, E.K., Raybould, R., Macgregor, S. *et al.* (2005) Operation of the schizophrenia susceptibility gene, neuregulin 1, across traditional diagnostic boundaries to increase risk for bipolar disorder. *Archives of General Psychiatry* **62**, 642–648.

Guo, S., Tang, W., Shi, Y. *et al.* (2006) RGS4 polymorphisms and risk of schizophrenia: an association study in Han Chinese plus meta-analysis. *Neuroscience Letters* **406**, 122–127.

Hahn, C.G., Wang, H.Y., Cho, D.S. *et al.* (2006) Altered neuregulin 1-erbB4 signaling contributes to NMDA receptor hypofunction in schizophrenia. *Nature Medicine* **12**, 824–828.

Hall, D., Gogos, J.A. & Karayiorgou, M. (2004) The contribution of three strong candidate schizophrenia susceptibility genes in demographically distinct populations. *Genes Brain Behavior* **3**, 240–248.

Hall, J., Whalley, H.C., Job, D.E. *et al.* (2006) A neuregulin 1 variant associated with abnormal cortical function and psychotic symptoms. *Nature Neuroscience* **9**, 1477–1478.

Harrison, P.J. & Owen, M.J. (2003) Genes for schizophrenia? Recent findings and their pathophysiological implications. *Lancet* **361**, 417–419.

Hashimoto, L., Habita, C., Beressi, J.P. *et al.* (1994) Genetic mapping of a susceptibility locus for insulin-dependent diabetes mellitus on chromosome 11q. *Nature* **371**, 161–164.

Hattori, E., Liu, C., Badner, J.A. *et al.* (2003) Polymorphisms at the G72/G30 gene locus, on 13q33, are associated with bipolar disorder in two independent pedigree series. *American Journal of Human Genetics* **72**, 1131–1140.

He, Z., Li, Z., Shi, Y. *et al.* (2007) The PIP5K2A gene and schizophrenia in the Chinese population—a case-control study. *Schizophrenia Research* **94**, 359–365.

Hennah, W., Varilo, T., Kestila, M. *et al.* (2003) Haplotype transmission analysis provides evidence of association for DISC1 to schizophrenia and suggests sex-dependent effects. *Human Molecular Genetics* **12**, 3151–3159.

Hennah, W., Thomson, P., McQuillin, A. *et al.* (2009) DISC1 association, heterogeneity and interplay in schizophrenia and bipolar disorder. *Molecular Psychiatry* **14**, 863–873.

Heston, L.L. (1966) Psychiatric disorders in foster home reared children of schizophrenic mothers. *British Journal of Psychiatry* **112**, 819–825.

Hodgkinson, C.A., Goldman, D., Jaeger, J. *et al.* (2004) Disrupted in schizophrenia 1 (DISC1): association with schizophrenia, schizoaffective disorder, and bipolar disorder. *American Journal of Human Genetics* **75**, 862–872.

Holliday, E.G., Handoko, H.Y., James, M.R. *et al.* (2006) Association study of the dystrobrevin-binding gene with schizophrenia in Australian and Indian samples. *Twin Research and Human Genetics* **9**, 531–539.

Hong, C.J., Hou, S.J., Yen, F.C., Liou, Y.J. & Tsai, S.J. (2006) Family-based association study between G72/G30 genetic polymorphism and schizophrenia. *Neuroreport* **17**, 1067–1069.

Hovatta, I., Varilo, T., Suvisaari, J. *et al.* (1999) A genome-wide screen for schizophrenia genes in an isolated Finnish subpopulation suggesting multiple susceptibility loci. *American Journal of Human Genetics* **65**, 1114–1124.

Hugot, J.P., Chamaillard, M., Zouali, H. *et al.* (2001) Association of NOD2 leucine-rich repeat variants with susceptibility to Crohn's disease. *Nature* **411**, 599–603.

Iafrate, A.J., Feuk, L., Rivera, M.N. *et al.* (2004) Detection of large-scale variation in the human genome. *Nature Genetics* **36**, 949–951.

Ide, M., Ohnishi, T., Murayama, M. *et al.* (2006) Failure to support a genetic contribution of AKT1 polymorphisms and altered AKT signaling in schizophrenia. *Journal of Neurochemistry* **99**, 277–287.

Ikeda, M., Iwata, N., Suzuki, T. *et al.* (2004) Association of AKT1 with schizophrenia confirmed in a Japanese population. *Biological Psychiatry* **56**, 698–700.

Ikeda, M., Iwata, N., Suzuki, T. *et al.* (2005) No association of haplotype-tagging SNPs in TRAR4 with schizophrenia in Japanese patients. *Schizophrenia Research* **78**, 127–130.

Ikeda, M., Takahashi, N., Saito, S. *et al.* (2008) Failure to replicate the association between NRG1 and schizophrenia using Japanese large sample. *Schizophrenia Research* **101**, 1–8.

Ingason, A., Soeby, K., Timm, S. *et al.* (2006) No significant association of the 5′ end of neuregulin 1 and schizophrenia in a large Danish sample. *Schizophrenia Research* **83**, 1–5.

International Schizophrenia Consortium (2008) Rare chromosomal deletions and duplications increase risk of schizophrenia. *Nature* **455**, 237–241.

Ishiguro, H., Horiuchi, Y., Koga, M. *et al.* (2007) RGS4 is not a susceptibility gene for schizophrenia in Japanese: association study in a large case-control population. *Schizophrenia Research* **89**, 161–164.

Iwata, N., Suzuki, T., Ikeda, M. *et al.* (2004) No association with the neuregulin 1 haplotype to Japanese schizophrenia. *Molecular Psychiatry* **9**, 126–127.

Jamra, R.A., Klein, K., Villela, A.W. *et al.* (2006) Association study between genetic variants at the PIP5K2A gene locus and schizophrenia and bipolar affective disorder. *American Journal of Medical Genetics B Neuropsychiatric Genetics* **141B**, 663–665.

Joo, E.J., Lee, K.Y., Jeong, S.H., Ahn, Y.M., Koo, Y.J. & Kim, Y.S. (2006) The dysbindin gene (DTNBP1) and schizophrenia: no support for an association in the Korean population. *Neuroscience Letters* **407**, 101–106.

Joo, E.J., Lee, K.Y., Jeong, S.H. *et al.* (2007) Dysbindin gene variants are associated with bipolar I disorder in a Korean population. *Neuroscience Letters* **418**, 272–275.

Kalsi, G., Chen, C.H., Smyth, C. *et al.* (1996) Genetic linkage analysis in an Icelandic/British sample fails to exclude the putative chromosome 13q14.1–q32 schizophrenia susceptibility locus. *American Journal of Human Genetics* **59**, A388.

Karayiorgou, M., Morris, M.A., Morrow, B. *et al.* (1995) Schizophrenia susceptibility associated with interstitial deletions of chromosome 22q11. *Proceedings of the National Academy of Sciences USA* **92**, 7612–7616.

Kendler, K.S. & Diehl, S.R. (1993) The genetics of schizophrenia: A current, genetic-epidemiologic perspective. *Schizophrenia Bulletin* **19**, 261–285.

Kendler, K.S., Gruenberg, A.M. & Tsuang, M.T. (1986) A DSM-III family study of the nonschizophrenic psychotic disorders. *American Journal of Psychiatry* **143**, 1098–1105.

Kendler, K.S., McGuire, M., Gruenberg, A.M., Spellman, M., O'Hare, A. & Walsh, D. (1993) The Roscommon family study: II. The risk of nonschizophrenic nonaffective psychoses in relatives. *Archives of General Psychiatry* **50**, 645–652.

Kendler, K.S., Straub, R.E., MacLean, C.J. & Walsh, D. (1996) Reflections on the evidence for a vulnerability locus for schizophrenia on chromosome 6p24–22. *American Journal of Medical Genetics* **67**, 124–126.

Kendler, K.S., Kuhn, J.W., Prescott, C.A., Vittum, J. & Riley, B. (2005) The interaction of stressful life events and a serotonin transporter polymorphism in the prediction of episodes of major depression: a replication. *Archives of General Psychiatry* **62**, 529–535.

Kety, S.S., Rosenthal, D., Wender, P.H., Schulsinger, F. & Jacobsen, B. (1968) The types and prevalence of mental illness in the biological and adoptive families of adopted schizophrenics. *Journal of Psychiatric Research* **6**, 345–362.

Kety, S.S., Wender, P.H., Jacobsen, B. *et al.* (1994) Mental illness in the biological and adoptive relatives of schizophrenic adoptees: Replication of the Copenhagen study in the rest of Denmark. *Archives of General Psychiatry* **51**, 442–455.

Kim, H.J., Park, H.J., Jung, K.H. *et al.* (2008) Association study of polymorphisms between DISC1 and schizophrenia in a Korean population. *Neuroscience Letters* **430**, 60–63.

Kirov, G., Ivanov, D., Williams, N.M. *et al.* (2004) Strong evidence for association between the dystrobrevin binding protein 1 gene (DTNBP1) and schizophrenia in 488 parent-offspring trios from Bulgaria. *Biological Psychiatry* **55**, 971–975.

Kockelkorn, T.T., Arai, M., Matsumoto, H. *et al.* (2004) Association study of polymorphisms in the 5' upstream region of human DISC1 gene with schizophrenia. *Neuroscience Letters* **368**, 41–45.

Korostishevsky, M., Kaganovich, M., Cholostoy, A. *et al.* (2004) Is the G72/G30 locus associated with schizophrenia? single nucleotide polymorphisms, haplotypes, and gene expression analysis. *Biological Psychiatry* **56**, 169–176.

Korostishevsky, M., Kremer, I., Kaganovich, M. *et al.* (2006) Transmission disequilibrium and haplotype analyses of the G72/G30 locus: Suggestive linkage to schizophrenia in Palestinian Arabs living in the North of Israel. *American Journal of Medical Genetics B Neuropsychiatric Genetics* **141B**, 91–95.

Kruglyak, L., Daly, M.J., Reeve-Daly, M.P. & Lander, E.S. (1996) Parametric and nonparametric linkage analysis: a unified multipoint approach. *American Journal of Human Genetics* **58**, 1347–1363.

Laird, N.M., Horvath, S. & Xu, X. (2000) Implementing a unified approach to family-based tests of association. *Genetic Epidemiology* **19** (Suppl. 10), S36–S42.

Laitinen, T., Daly, M.J., Rioux, J.D. *et al.* (2001) A susceptibility locus for asthma-related traits on chromosome 7 revealed by genome-wide scan in a founder population. *Nature Genetics* **28**, 87–91.

Lander, E. & Kruglyak, L. (1995) Genetic dissection of complex traits: Guidelines for interpreting and reporting linkage results. *Nature Genetics* **11**, 241–247.

Law, A.J., Kleinman, J.E., Weinberger, D.R. & Weickert, C.S. (2007)Disease-associated intronic variants in the ErbB4 gene are related to altered ErbB4 splice-variant expression in the brain in schizophrenia. *Human Molecular Genetics* **16**, 129–141.

Levinson, D.F., Wildenauer, D.B., Schwab, S.G. *et al.* (1996) Additional support for schizophrenia linkage on chromo-

somes 6 and 8: A multicenter study. *American Journal of Medical Genetics Neuropsychiatric Genetics* **67**, 580–594.

Levinson, D.F., Holmans, P.A., Laurent, C., *et al.* (2002) No major schizophrenia locus detected on chromosome 1q in a large multicenter sample. *Science* **296**, 739–741.

Lewis, C.M., Levinson, D.F., Wise, L.H. *et al.* (2003) Genome scan meta-analysis of schizophrenia and bipolar disorder, part II: Schizophrenia. *American Journal of Human Genetics* **73**, 34–48.

Li, D. & He, L. (2006) Association study of the G-protein signaling 4 (RGS4) and proline dehydrogenase (PRODH) genes with schizophrenia: a meta-analysis. *European Journal of Human Genetics* **14**, 1130–1135.

Li, D. & He, L. (2007) G72/G30 genes and schizophrenia: a systematic meta-analysis of association studies. *Genetics* **175**, 917–122.

Li, T., Stefansson, H., Gudfinnsson, E. *et al.* (2004) Identification of a novel neuregulin 1 at-risk haplotype in Han schizophrenia Chinese patients, but no association with the Icelandic/Scottish risk haplotype. *Molecular Psychiatry* **9**, 698–704.

Li, T., Zhang, F., Liu, X. *et al.* (2005) Identifying potential risk haplotypes for schizophrenia at the DTNBP1 locus in Han Chinese and Scottish populations. *Molecular Psychiatry* **10**, 1037–1044.

Lin, M.W., Curtis, D., Williams, N. *et al.* (1995) Suggestive evidence for linkage of schizophrenia to markers on chromosome 13q14.1–q32. *Psychiatric Genetics* **5**, 117–126.

Lin, M.W., Sham, P., Hwu, H.G., Collier, D., Murray, R. & Powell, J.F. (1997) Suggestive evidence for linkage of schizophrenia to markers on chromosome 13 in Caucasian but not Oriental populations. *Human Genetics* **99**, 417–420.

Lindholm, E., Ekholm, B., Balciuniene, J. *et al.* (1999) Linkage analysis of a large Swedish kindred provides further support for a susceptibility locus for schizophrenia on chromosome 6p23. *American Journal of Medical Genetics* **88**, 369–377.

Liu CM, Hwu HG, Lin M.W. *et al.* (2001) Suggestive evidence for linkage of schizophrenia to markers at chromosome 15q13-14 in Taiwanese families. *American Journal of Medical Genetics* **105**, 658–661.

Liu, H., Heath, S.C., Sobin, C. *et al.* (2002) Genetic variation at the 22q11 PRODH2/DGCR6 locus presents an unusual pattern and increases susceptibility to schizophrenia. *Proceedings of the National Academy of Science USA* **99**, 3717–3722.

Liu, X., He, G., Wang, X. *et al.* (2004) Association of DAAO with schizophrenia in the Chinese population. *Neuroscience Letters* **369**, 228–233.

Liu, Y.L., Fann, C.S., Liu, C.M. *et al.* (2006a) No association of G72 and D-amino acid oxidase genes with schizophrenia. *Schizophrenia Research* **87**, 15–20.

Liu, Y.L., Fann, C.S., Liu, C.M. *et al.* (2006b) A single nucleotide polymorphism fine mapping study of chromosome 1q42.1 reveals the vulnerability genes for schizophrenia, GNPAT and DISC1: Association with impairment of sustained attention. *Biological Psychiatry* **60**, 554–562.

Liu, Y.L., Shen-Jang, F.C., Liu, C.M. *et al.* (2006c) Evaluation of RGS4 as a candidate gene for schizophrenia. *American Journal of Medical Genetics B Neuropsychiatric Genetics* **141**, 418–420.

Liu, Y.L., Fann, C.S., Liu, C.M. *et al.* (2006d) Absence of significant associations between four AKT1 SNP markers and schizophrenia in the Taiwanese population. *Psychiatric Genetics* **16**, 39–41.

Liu, C.M., Liu, Y.L., Fann, C.S. *et al.* (2007) No association evidence between schizophrenia and dystrobrevin-binding protein 1 (DTNBP1) in Taiwanese families. *Schizophrenia Research* **93**, 391–398.

Ma, J., Qin, W., Wang, X.Y. *et al.* (2006) Further evidence for the association between G72/G30 genes and schizophrenia in two ethnically distinct populations. *Molecular Psychiatry* **11**, 479–487.

Martin, E.R., Monks, S.A., Warren, L.L. & Kaplan, N.L. (2000) A test for linkage and association in general pedigrees: The Pedigree Disequilibrium Test. *American Journal of Human Genetics* **67**, 146–154.

Maziade, M., Bissonnette, L., Rouillard, E. *et al.* (1997) 6p24-22 region and major psychoses in the Eastern Quebec population. Le Groupe IREP. *American Journal of Medical Genetics* **74**, 311–318.

McClellan, J.M., Susser, E. & King, M.C. (2007) Schizophrenia: a common disease caused by multiple rare alleles. *British Journal of Psychiatry* **190**, 194–199.

McGue, M., Gottesman, I. & Rao, D.C. (1985) Resolving genetic models for the transmission of schizophrenia. *Genetic Epidemiology* **2**, 99–110.

Millar, J.K., Wilson-Annan, J.C., Anderson, S. *et al.* (2000) Disruption of two novel genes by a translocation co-segregating with schizophrenia. *Human Molecular Genetics* **9**, 1415–1423.

Mirnics, K., Middleton, F.A., Lewis, D.A. & Levitt, P. (2001) Analysis of complex brain disorders with gene expression microarrays: schizophrenia as a disease of the synapse. *Trends in Neuroscience* **24**, 479–486.

Moghaddam, B. (2003) Bringing order to the glutamate chaos in schizophrenia. *Neuron* **40**, 881–884.

Moises, H.W., Yang, L., Kristbjarnarson, H. *et al.* (1995) An international two-stage genome-wide search for schizophrenia susceptibility genes. *Nature Genetics* **11**, 321–324.

Morris, D.W., McGhee, K.A., Schwaiger, S. *et al.* (2003) No evidence for association of the dysbindin gene [DTNBP1] with schizophrenia in an Irish population-based study. *Schizophrenia Research* **60**, 167–172.

Morris, D.W., Rodgers, A., McGhee, K.A. *et al.* (2004) Confirming RGS4 as a susceptibility gene for schizophrenia. *American Journal of Medical Genetics* **125B**, 50–53.

Morton, N.E. (1955) Sequential tests for the detection of linkage. *American Journal of Human Genetics* **7**, 277–318.

Mulle, J.G., Chowdari, K.V., Nimgaonkar, V. & Chakravarti, A. (2005) No evidence for association to the G72/G30 locus in an independent sample of schizophrenia families. *Molecular Psychiatry* **10**, 431–433.

Munafo, M.R., Thiselton, D.L., Clark, T.G. & Flint, J. (2006) Association of the NRG1 gene and schizophrenia: a meta-analysis. *Molecular Psychiatry* **11**, 539–546.

Murphy, K.C., Jones, L.A. & Owen, M.J. (1999) High rates of schizophrenia in adults with velo-cardio-facial syndrome. *Archives of General Psychiatry* **56**, 940–945.

Nicodemus, K.K., Luna, A., Vakkalanka, R. *et al.* (2006) Further evidence for association between ErbB4 and schizophrenia and influence on cognitive intermediate phenotypes in healthy controls. *Molecular Psychiatry* **11**, 1062–1065.

Norton, N., Moskvina, V., Morris, D.W. *et al.* (2006) Evidence that interaction between neuregulin 1 and its receptor erbB4 increases susceptibility to schizophrenia. *American Journal of Medical Genetics B Neuropsychiatric Genetics* **141**, 96–101.

Norton, N., Williams, H.J., Dwyer, S. *et al.* (2007) Association analysis of AKT1 and schizophrenia in a UK case control sample. *Schizophrenia Research* **97**, 271–276.

Numakawa, T., Yagasaki, Y., Ishimoto, T. *et al.* (2004) Evidence of novel neuronal functions of dysbindin, a susceptibility gene for schizophrenia. *Human Molecular Genetics* **13**, 2699–2708.

Ogura, Y., Bonen, D.K., Inohara, N. *et al.* (2001) A frameshift mutation in NOD2 associated with susceptibility to Crohn's disease. *Nature* **411**, 603–606.

Ohtsuki, T., Inada, T. & Arinami, T. (2004) Failure to confirm association between AKT1 haplotype and schizophrenia in a Japanese case-control population. *Molecular Psychiatry* **9**, 981–983.

Pae, C.U., Serretti, A., Mandelli, L. *et al.* (2007) Effect of 5-haplotype of dysbindin gene (DTNBP1) polymorphisms for the susceptibility to bipolar I disorder. *American Journal of Medical Genetics B Neuropsychiatric Genetics* **144B**, 701–703.

Pae, C.U., Yu, H.S., Amann, D. *et al.* (2008) Association of the trace amine associated receptor 6 (TAAR6) gene with schizophrenia and bipolar disorder in a Korean case control sample. *Journal of Psychiatric Research* **42**, 35–40.

Palo, O.M., Antila, M., Silander, K. *et al.* (2007) Association of distinct allelic haplotypes of DISC1 with psychotic and bipolar spectrum disorders and with underlying cognitive impairments. *Human Molecular Genetics* **15**, 2517–2528.

Pedrosa, E., Ye, K., Nolan, K.A. *et al.* (2007) Positive association of schizophrenia to JARID2 gene. *American Journal of Medical Genetics B Neuropsychiatric Genetics* **144B**, 45–51.

Perlis, R.H., Purcell, S., Fagerness, J. *et al.* (2008) Family-based association study of lithium-related and other candidate genes in bipolar disorder. *Archives of General Psychiatry* **65**, 53–61.

Perry, G.H., Dominy, N.J., Claw, K.G. *et al.* (2007) Diet and the evolution of human amylase gene copy number variation. *Nature Genetics* **39**, 1256–1260.

Peters, K., Wiltshire, S., Henders, A.K. *et al.* (2008) Comprehensive analysis of tagging sequence variants in DTNBP1 shows no association with schizophrenia or with its composite neuro-cognitive endophenotypes. *American Journal of Medical Genetics B Neuropsychiatric Genetics* **147B**, 1159–1166.

Petretto, E., Liu, E.T. & Aitman, T.J. (2007) A gene harvest revealing the archeology and complexity of human disease. *Nature Genetics* **39**, 1299–1301.

Petryshen, T.L., Middleton, F.A., Kirby, A. *et al.* (2005) Support for involvement of neuregulin 1 in schizophrenia pathophysiology. *Molecular Psychiatry* **10**, 366–374.

Polymeropoulos, M.H., Coon, H., Byerley, W. *et al.* (1994) Search for a schizophrenia susceptibility locus on human chromosome 22. *American Journal of Medical Genetics* **54**, 93–99.

Prata, D., Breen, G., Osborne, S., Munro, J., St Clair, D. & Collier, D. (2007) Association of DAO and G72(DAOA)/G30 genes with bipolar affective disorder. *American Journal of Medical Genetics B Neuropsychiatric Genetics* **147B**, 914–917.

Prescott, C.A. & Gottesman, I.I. (1993) Genetically mediated vulnerability to schizophrenia. *Psychiatric Clinics of North America* **16**, 245–267.

Pulver, A.E., Karayiorgou, M., Wolyniec, P.S. *et al.* (1994a) Sequential strategy to identify a susceptibility gene for schizophrenia: Report of potential linkage on chromosome 22q12-q13.1: Part 1. *American Journal of Medical Genetics* **54**, 36–43.

Pulver, A.E., Karayiorgou, M., Lasseter, V.K., *et al.* (1994b) Follow-up of a report of a potential linkage for schizophrenia on chromosome 22q12–q13.1: Part 2. *American Journal of Medical Genetics* **54**, 44–50.

Pulver, A.E., Nestadt, G., Goldberg, R. *et al.* (1994c) Psychotic illness in patients diagnosed with velo-cardio-facial syndrome and their relatives. *Journal of Nervous & Mental Disease* **182**, 476–478.

Pulver, A.E., Lasseter, V.K., Kasch, L. *et al.* (1995) Schizophrenia: A genome scan targets chromosomes 3p and 8p as potential sites of susceptibility genes. *American Journal of Medical Genetics Neuropsychiatric Genetics* **60**, 252–260.

Qu, M., Tang, F., Yue, W. *et al.* (2007) Positive association of the Disrupted-in-Schizophrenia-1 gene (DISC1) with schizophrenia in the Chinese Han population. *American Journal of Medical Genetics B Neuropsychiatric Genetics* **144**, 266–270.

Ray, P.N., Belfall, B., Duff, C. *et al.* (1985) Cloning of the breakpoint of an X;21 translocation associated with Duchenne muscular dystrophy. *Nature* **318**, 672–675.

Redon, R., Ishikawa, S., Fitch, K.R. *et al.* (2006) Global variation in copy number in the human genome. *Nature* **444**, 444–454.

Riley, B.P. & McGuffin, P. (2000) Linkage and associated studies of schizophrenia. *American Journal of Medical Genetics Seminars in Medical Genetics* **97**, 23–44.

Riley, B.P., Makoff, A., Mogudi-Carter, M. *et al.* (2000) Haplotype transmission disequilibrium and evidence for linkage of the CHRNA7 gene region to schizophrenia in southern African Bantu families. *American Journal of Medical Genetics Neuropsychiatric Genetics* **96**, 196–201.

Risch, N. (1990) Linkage strategies for genetically complex traits. I. Multilocus models. *American Journal of Human Genetics* **46**, 222–228.

Risch, N. & Merikangas, K. (1996) The future of genetic studies of complex human diseases. *Science* **273**, 1516–1517.

Rizig, M.A., McQuillin, A., Puri, V. *et al.* (2006) Failure to confirm genetic association between schizophrenia and markers on chromosome 1q23.3 in the region of the gene encoding the regulator of G-protein signaling 4 protein (RGS4). *American Journal of Medical Genetics B Neuropsychiatric Genetics* **141**, 296–300.

Rosa, A., Gardner, M., Cuesta, M.J. *et al.* (2007) Family-based association study of neuregulin-1 gene and psychosis in a Spanish sample. *American Journal of Medical Genetics B Neuropsychiatric Genetics* **144**, 954–957.

Rujescu, D., Ingason, A., Cichon, S. *et al.* (2009) Disruption of the neurexin 1 gene is associated with schizophrenia. *Human Molecular Genetics* **18**, 988–996.

Sachs, N.A., Sawa, A., Holmes, S.E., Ross, C.A., DeLisis L.E. & Margolis, R.L. (2005) A frameshift mutation in Disrupted in Schizophrenia 1 in an American family with schizophrenia and schizoaffective disorder. *Molecular Psychiatry* **10**, 758–764.

Saggers-Gray, L., Heriani, H., Handoko, H.Y. *et al.* (2008) Association of PIP5K2A with schizophrenia: A study in an indonesian family sample. *American Journal of Medical Genetics B Neuropsychiatric Genetics* **147B**, 1310–1313.

Sanders, A.R., Duan, J., Levinson, D.F. *et al.* (2008) No significant association of 14 candidate genes with schizophrenia in a large European ancestry sample: implications for psychiatric genetics. *American Journal of Psychiatry* **165**, 497–506.

Sawcer, S., Jones, H.B., Feakes, R. *et al.* (1996) A genome screen in multiple sclerosis reveals susceptibility loci on chromosome 6p21 and 17q22. *Nature Genetics* **13**, 464–468.

Saxena, R., Voight, B.F., Lyssenko, V. *et al.* (2007) Genome-wide association analysis identifies loci for type 2 diabetes and triglyceride levels. *Science* **316**, 1331–1336.

Schumacher, J., Jamra, R.A., Freudenberg, J. *et al.* (2004) Examination of G72 and D-amino-acid oxidase as genetic risk factors for schizophrenia and bipolar affective disorder. *Molecular Psychiatry* **9**, 203–207.

Schwab, S.G., Albus, M. & Hallmayer, J. *et al.* (1995) Evaluation of a susceptibility gene for schizophrenia on chromosome 6p by multipoint affected sib-pair linkage analysis. *Nature Genetics* **11**, 325–327.

Schwab, S.G., Knapp, M., Mondabon, S. *et al.* (2003) Support for association of schizophrenia with genetic variation in the 6p22.3 gene, dysbindin, in sib-pair families with linkage and in an additional sample of triad families. *American Journal of Human Genetics* **72**, 185–190.

Schwab, S.G., Hoefgen, B., Hanses, C. *et al.* (2005) Further Evidence for Association of Variants in the AKT1 gene with schizophrenia in a sample of European sib-pair families. *Biological Psychiatry* **58**, 446–450.

Schwab, S.G., Knapp, M., Sklar, P. *et al.* (2006) Evidence for association of DNA sequence variants in the phosphatidylinositol-4-phosphate 5-kinase IIalpha gene (PIP5K2A) with schizophrenia. *Molecular Psychiatry* **11**, 837–846.

Scott, L.J., Mohlke, K.L., Bonnycastle, L.L. *et al.* (2007) A genome-wide association study of type 2 Ddabetes in Finns detects multiple susceptibility variants. *Science* **316**, 1341–1345.

Sebat, J., Lakshmi, B., Troge, J. *et al.* (2004) Large-scale copy number polymorphism in the human genome. *Science* **305**, 525–528.

Sebat, J., Lakshmi, B., Malhotra, D. *et al.* (2007) Strong association of *de novo* copy number mutations with autism. *Science* **316**, 445–449.

Shaw, S.H., Kelly, M., Smith, A.B. *et al.* (1998) A genome-wide search for schizophrenia susceptibility genes. *American Journal of Medical Genetics Neuropsychiatric Genetics* **81**, 364–376.

Shi, J., Badner, J.A., Gershon, E.S. & Liu, C. (2008) Allelic association of G72/G30 with schizophrenia and bipolar disorder: a comprehensive meta-analysis. *Schizophrenia Research* **98**, 89–97.

Shifman, S., Bronstein, M., Sternfeld, M. *et al.* (2002) A highly significant association between a COMT haplotype and schizophrenia. *American Journal of Human Genetics* **71**, 1296–1302.

Shin, H.D., Park, B.L., Kim, E.M. *et al.* (2007) Association analysis of G72/G30 polymorphisms with schizophrenia in the Korean population. *Schizophrenia Research* **96**, 119–124.

Shinkai, T., De, L.V., Hwang, R. *et al.* (2007) Association analyses of the DAOA/G30 and D-amino-acid oxidase genes in schizophrenia: further evidence for a role in schizophrenia. *Neuromolecular Medicine* **9**, 169–177.

Silberberg, G., Darvasi, A., Pinkas-Kramarski, R., Navon, R. (2006) The involvement of ErbB4 with schizophrenia: association and expression studies. *American Journal of Medical Genetics B Neuropsychiatric Genetics* **141B**, 142–148.

Sladek, R., Rocheleau, G., Rung, J. *et al.* (2007) A genome-wide association study identifies novel risk loci for type 2 diabetes. *Nature* **445**, 881–885.

So, H.C., Chen, R.Y., Chen, E.Y., Cheung, E.F. & Li, T. (2008) Sham PC. An association study of RGS4 polymorphisms with clinical phenotypes of schizophrenia in a Chinese population. *American Journal of Medical Genetics B Neuropsychiatric Genetics* **147B**, 77–85.

Sobell, J.L., Richard, C., Wirshing, D.A. & Heston, L.L. (2005) Failure to confirm association between RGS4 haplotypes and schizophrenia in Caucasians. *American Journal of Medical Genetics B Neuropsychiatric Genetics* **139**, 23–27.

Song, W., Li, W., Feng, J., Heston, L.L., Scaringe, W.A. & Sommer, S.S. (2008) Identification of high risk DISC1 structural variants with a 2% attributable risk for schizophrenia. *Biochemical and Biophysics Research Communications* **367**, 700–706.

Spielman, R.S. & Ewens, W.J. (1996) The TDT and other family-based tests for linkage disequilibrium and association. *American Journal of Human Genetics* **59**, 983–989.

St Clair, D., Blackwood, D., Muir, W. *et al.* (1990) Association within a family of a balanced autosomal translocation with major mental illness. *Lancet* **336**, 13–16.

St Clair, D. Xu, M., Wang, P. *et al.* (2005) Rates of adult schizophrenia following prenatal exposure to the Chinese famine of 1959–1961. *JAMA* **294**, 557–562.

Stefansson, H., Sigurdsson, E., Steinthorsdottir, V. *et al.* (2002) Neuregulin 1 and susceptibility to schizophrenia. *American Journal of Human Genetics* **71**, 877–892.

Stefansson, H., Sarginson, J., Kong, A. *et al.* (2003) Association of neuregulin 1 with schizophrenia confirmed in a Scottish population. *American Journal of Human Genetics* **72**, 83–87.

Stefansson, H., Rujescu, D., Cichon, S. *et al.* (2008) Large recurrent microdeletions associated with schizophrenia. *Nature* **455**, 232–236.

Steinthorsdottir, V., Thorleifsson, G., Reynisdottir, I. *et al.* (2007) A variant in CDKAL1 influences insulin response and risk of type 2 diabetes. *Nature Genetics* **39**, 770–775.

Straub, R.E., MacLean, C.J., O'Neill, F.A. *et al.* (1995) A potential vulnerability locus for schizophrenia on chromosome 6p24–22: Evidence for genetic heterogeneity. *Nature Genetics* **11**, 287–93.

Straub, R.E., Jiang, Y., MacLean, C.J. *et al.* (2002) Genetic variation in the 6p22.3 gene DTNBP1, the human ortholog of mouse dysbindin, is associated with schizophrenia. *American Journal of Human Genetics* **71**, 337–348.

Sullivan, P.F. (2005) The genetics of schizophrenia. *PLoS Medicine* **2**, e212.

Sullivan, P.F., Kendler, K.S. & Neale, M.C. (2003) Schizophrenia as a complex trait: evidence from a meta-analysis of twin studies. *Archives of General Psychiatry* **60**, 1187–1192.

Susser, E.S. & Lin, S.P. (1992) Schizophrenia after prenatal exposure to the Dutch Hunger Winter of 1944–1945. *Archives of General Psychiatry* **49**, 983–988.

Szeszko, P.R., Hodgkinson, C.A., Robinson, D.G. *et al.* (2008) DISC1 is associated with prefrontal cortical gray matter and positive symptoms in schizophrenia. *Biological Psychology* **79**, 103–110.

Talbot, K., Eidem, W.L., Tinsley, C.L. *et al.* (2004) Dysbindin-1 is reduced in intrinsic, glutamatergic terminals of the hippocampal formation in schizophrenia. *Journal of Clinical Investigation* **113**, 1353–1363.

Talkowski, M.E., Seltman, H., Bassett, A.S. *et al.* (2006) Evaluation of a susceptibility gene for schizophrenia: genotype based meta-analysis of RGS4 polymorphisms from thirteen independent samples. *Biological Psychiatry* **60**, 152–162.

Tang, J.X., Zhou, J., Fan, J.B. *et al.* (2003) Family-based association study of DTNBP1 in 6p22.3 and schizophrenia. *Molecular Psychiatry* **8**, 717–718.

Tang, J.X., Chen, W.Y., He, G. *et al.* (2004) Polymorphisms within 5' end of the Neuregulin 1 gene are genetically associated with schizophrenia in the Chinese population. *Molecular Psychiatry* **9**, 11–12.

Thiselton, D.L., Webb, B.T., Neale, B.M. *et al.* (2004) No evidence for linkage or association of neuregulin-1 (NRG1) with disease in the Irish study of high-density schizophrenia families (ISHDSF). *Molecular Psychiatry* **9**, 777–783.

Thiselton, D.L., Vladimirov, V.I., Kuo, P.H. *et al.* (2008) AKT1 is associated with schizophrenia across multiple symptom dimensions in the Irish study of high density schizophrenia families. *Biological Psychiatry* **63**, 449–457.

Thomson, P.A., Wray, N.R. & Millar, J.K. *et al.* (2005) Association between the TRAX/DISC locus and both bipolar disorder and schizophrenia in the Scottish population. *Molecular Psychiatry* **10**, 657–668.

Thomson, P.A., Christoforou, A., Morris, S.W. *et al.* (2007) Association of Neuregulin 1 with schizophrenia and bipolar disorder in a second cohort from the Scottish population. *Molecular Psychiatry* **12**, 94–104.

Tienari, P. (1991) Interaction between genetic vulnerability and family environment: The Finnish adoptive family study of schizophrenia. *Acta Psychiatrica Scandinavica* **84**, 460–465.

Tienari, P., Wynne, L.C., Sorri, A. *et al.* (2004) Genotype-environment interaction in schizophrenia-spectrum disorder. Long-term follow-up study of Finnish adoptees. *British Journal of Psychiatry* **184**, 216–222.

Tochigi, M., Zhang, X., Ohashi, J. *et al.* (2006) Association study of the dysbindin (DTNBP1) gene in schizophrenia from the Japanese population. *Neuroscience Research* **56**, 154–158.

Tosato, S., Dazzan, P. & Collier, D. (2005) Association between the neuregulin 1 gene and schizophrenia: A systematic review. *Schizophrenia Bulletin* **31**, 613–617.

Tosato, S., Ruggeri, M., Bonetto, C. *et al.* (2007) Association study of dysbindin gene with clinical and outcome measures in a representative cohort of Italian schizophrenic patients. *American Journal of Medical Genetics B Neuropsychiatric Genetics* **144B**, 647–659.

Tsuang, D.W., Skol, A.D., Faraone, S.V. *et al.* (2001) Examination of genetic linkage of chromosome 15 to schizophrenia in a large Veterans Affairs Cooperative Study sample. *American Journal of Medical Genetics* **105**, 662–668.

Turunen, J.A., Peltonen, J.O., Pietilainen, O.P. *et al.* (2007) The role of DTNBP1, NRG1, and AKT1 in the genetics of schizophrenia in Finland. *Schizophrenia Research* **91**, 27–36.

Tuzun, E., Sharp, A.J., Bailey, J.A. *et al.* (2005) Fine-scale structural variation of the human genome. *Nature Genetics* **37**, 727–732.

Van Den Bogaert, A., Schumacher, J., Schulze, T.G. *et al.* (2003) The DTNBP1 (dysbindin) gene contributes to schizophrenia, depending on family history of the disease. *American Journal of Human Genetics* **73**, 1438–1443.

van den Oord, E., Sullivan, P.F., Chen, X., Kendler, K.S. & Riley, B. (2003) Identification of a high risk haplotype for the dystrobrevin binding protein 1 (DTNBP1) gene in the Irish study of high density schizophrenia families. *Molecular Psychiatry* **8**, 499–510.

Vilella, E., Costas, J., Sanjuan, J. *et al.* (2008) Association of schizophrenia with DTNBP1 but not with DAO, DAOA, NRG1 and RGS4 nor their genetic interaction. *Journal of Psychiatric Research* **42**, 278–288.

Vionnet, N., Hani, E., Dupont, S. *et al.* (2000) Genomewide search for type 2 diabetes-susceptibility genes in French whites: evidence for a novel susceptibility locus for early-onset diabetes on chromosome 3q27-qter and independent replication of a type 2-diabetes locus on chromosome 1q21–q24. *American Journal of Human Genetics* **67**, 1470–1480.

Vladimirov, V., Thiselton, D.L., Kuo, P.H. *et al.* (2007) A region of 35 kb containing the trace amine associate receptor 6 (TAAR6) gene is associated with schizophrenia in the Irish study of high-density schizophrenia families. *Molecular Psychiatry* **12**, 842–853.

Walsh, T., McClellan, J.M., McCarthy, S.E. *et al.* (2008) Rare structural variants disrupt multiple genes in neurodevelopmental pathways in schizophrenia. *Science* **320**, 539–543.

Walss-Bass, C., Raventos, H., Montero, A.P. *et al.* (2006) Association analyses of the neuregulin 1 gene with schizophrenia and manic psychosis in a Hispanic population. *Acta Psychiatrica Scandinavica* **113**, 314–321.

Weickert, C.S., Straub, R.E., McClintock, B.W. *et al.* (2004) Human dysbindin (DTNBP1) gene expression in normal brain and in schizophrenic prefrontal cortex and midbrain. *Archives of General Psychiatry* **61**, 544–555.

Williams, N.M., Preece, A., Morris, D.W. *et al.* (2004a) Identification in 2 independent samples of a novel schizophrenia risk haplotype of the dystrobrevin binding protein gene (DTNBP1). *Archives of General Psychiatry* **61**, 336–344.

Williams, N.M., Preece, A., Spurlock, G. *et al.* (2004b) Support for RGS4 as a susceptibility gene for schizophrenia. *Biological Psychiatry* **55**, 192–195.

Williams, H.J., Owen, M.J. & O'Donovan, M.C. (2007) Is *COMT* a susceptibility gene for schizophrenia? *Schizophrenia Bulletin* **33**, 635–641.

Wiltshire, S., Hattersley, A.T., Hitman, G.A. *et al.* (2001) A genomewide scan for loci predisposing to type 2 diabetes in a U.K. population (the Diabetes UK Warren 2 Repository): analysis of 573 pedigrees provides independent replication of a susceptibility locus on chromosome 1q. *American Journal of Human Genetics* **69**, 553–569.

Wood, L.S., Pickering, E.H. & Dechairo, B.M. (2007) Significant support for DAO as a schizophrenia susceptibility locus: examination of five genes putatively associated with schizophrenia. *Biological Psychiatry* **61**, 1195–1199.

Xu, J., Pato, M.T., Torre C.D. *et al.* (2001) Evidence for linkage disequilibrium between the alpha 7-nicotinic receptor gene (CHRNA7) locus and schizophrenia in Azorean families. *American Journal of Medical Genetics* **105**, 669–674.

Xu, M.Q., Xing, Q.H., Zheng, Y.L. *et al.* (2007) Association of AKT1 gene polymorphisms with risk of schizophrenia and with response to antipsychotics in the Chinese population. *Journal of Clinical Psychiatry* **68**, 1358–1367.

Xu, B., Roos, J.L., Levy, S., van Rensburg, E.J., Gogos, J.A. & Karayiorgou, M. (2008) Strong association of *de novo* copy number mutations with sporadic schizophrenia. *Nature Genetics* **40**, 880–885.

Yang, J.Z., Si, T.M., Ruan, Y. *et al.* (2003) Association study of neuregulin 1 gene with schizophrenia. *Molecular Psychiatry* **8**, 706–709.

Yue, W., Liu, Z., Kang, G. *et al.* (2006) Association of G72/G30 polymorphisms with early-onset and male schizophrenia. *Neuroreport* **17**, 1899–1902.

Zeggini, E., Weedon, M.N., Lindgren, C.M. *et al.* (2007) Replication of genome-wide association signals in U.K. samples reveals risk loci for type 2 diabetes. *Science* **316**, 1336–1341.

Zhao, X., Shi, Y., Tang, J. *et al.* (2004) A case control and family based association study of the neuregulin1 gene and schizophrenia. *Journal of Medical Genetics* **41**, 31–34.

Zhang, X., Tochigi, M., Ohashi, J. *et al.* (2005a) Association study of the DISC1/TRAX locus with schizophrenia in a Japanese population. *Schizophrenia Research* **79**, 175–180.

Zhang F, St CD, Liu X, *et al.* (2005b) Association analysis of the RGS4 gene in Han Chinese and Scottish populations with schizophrenia. *Genes, Brain and Behavior* **4**, 444–448.

Zhao, X., Leotta, A., Kustanovich, V. *et al.* (2007) A unified genetic theory for sporadic and inherited autism. *Proceedings of the National Academy of Science USA* **104**, 12831–12836.

Zou, F., Li, C., Duan, S. *et al.* (2005) A family-based study of the association between the G72/G30 genes and schizophrenia in the Chinese population. *Schizophrenia Research* **73**, 257–261.

CHAPTER 13

Genetic associations in schizophrenia

Michael C. O'Donovan and Michael J. Owen

Basis of genetic association

Genetic association studies involve comparisons between affected individuals and some sort of control group. In the simplest and most common design, allele or genotype counts are compared between unrelated cases and controls using standard contingency table analysis. For a given marker, if the test statistic surpasses a given threshold, this suggests that marker is associated with the disorder. In most studies, multiple markers are tested, and therefore usually, an uncorrected test statistic of $p \leq 0.05$ is inadequate to conclude in favor of a true association. For categorical disorders such as diagnostic status, the strength of the association is usually expressed as an odds ratio (OR) or relative risk (RR).

Statistical issues aside, it is necessary to understand how *true* genetic associations arise in order to interpret the results of such studies (Plate 13.1). At some point in history when the population is relatively small, consider an indi-

vidual who has two **haplotypes** at a chromosomal region that can be distinguished by a number of **single nucleotide polymorphisms** (**SNPs**) (haplotypes are stretches of DNA defined by more than one polymorphism). One ancestral haplotype (ancestral red haplotype in Plate 13.1) is defined by allele 1 at all SNPs, the other (ancestral blue haplotype) by allele 2. In this individual, imagine a new mutation (M) that influences susceptibility to disease has arisen on the red haplotype. Although that person is the only case with the susceptibility variant, technically, all alleles on the red haplotype are associated with the risk variant and therefore with disease.

For most diseases, many genes *could* impact on risk, and so the above scenario will probably occur at multiple regions of the genome innumerable times in history. Sometimes, the new risk allele will rapidly vanish from the population either because of selection or because by chance that allele is not transmitted to subsequent generations. However, provided negative selection is not strong, sometimes a risk allele may also rise in frequency to become fairly common, provided the original population is small enough for chance fluctuation to have a perceptible effect on the allele frequency. As the population expands through

Schizophrenia, 3rd edition. Edited by Daniel R. Weinberger and Paul J Harrison © 2011 Blackwell Publishing Ltd.

successive generations, random fluctuations progressively impact less on allele frequencies and so, in the absence of selection, allele frequencies become fixed in the population. Those with frequencies greater than 1% are termed common alleles or polymorphisms. In some cases, alleles will increase in frequency if, despite their contribution to susceptibility, they confer benefits regarding reproductive fitness in unaffected carriers or even in affected individuals.

If in the example above, the risk allele is retained in the population, association between it and many of the alleles defining the red ancestral haplotype will be degraded by recombination in successive generations (Plate 13.1). In this way, the uninterrupted associated haplotype becomes progressively shorter. Since the probability of recombination is (roughly) proportionate to physical distance, a marker that is close to a disease allele is more likely to remain associated with it than one that is further away. Genetic variants that are associated with each other by virtue of insufficient recombination between them are said to be in **linkage disequilibrium (LD)**. The age of the mutation event is also important; newer mutations have fewer historical opportunities to be separated from alleles on the ancestral haplotype by recombination (compare generation 2 with generation 100). Note that unless they are positively selected for, fairly recent mutations (in population history terms) are also unlikely to achieve appreciable frequencies given that random fluctuations make little overall impact.

Given enough generations and a random distribution of recombination events, it would be expected that eventually, all ancestral haplotypes would become degraded, and that LD would cease to exist, even between adjacent markers. However, recombination events are not random. Instead, there are areas of the genome where recombination is very frequent, so-called "recombination hotspots", in which there is effectively no LD between markers. These are interspersed with regions where recombination events are so uncommon that few if any recombination events have occurred in the modern human lineage. As a result, much of the genome can be parsed into segments with an average size of about 10–20 kb where no recombination has occurred between alleles on ancestral chromosomes. In such segments, which are sometimes called **haplotype blocks**, all alleles are in LD with each other. A haplotype block surrounded by two recombination hotspots is depicted in Plate 13.1. In this example, the allele at one locus (red or blue) predicts the status of all other alleles within that block.

Now consider a study in which a SNP is reported to be associated with a disease. One interpretation is that the associated allele itself is involved in susceptibility to the disease. This is called **direct association**. Alternatively, it may simply be one of several ancestral markers in LD with the disease locus, and hence the disease. This is called **indirect association**. It is virtually impossible to distinguish between the two using association data alone, but with current study designs, it is usually reasonable to assume that the association is indirect. It is also important to keep in mind that associations point to all regions of the genome in LD with the associated SNP, not the gene which happens either to span, or be nearest to, the associated SNP. While LD is in some respects an obstacle to the functional interpretation of association studies, it is an asset in locating risk alleles because within regions of LD, a few SNPs can capture through indirect association most of the information concerning all the SNPs in the region. This considerably reduces the effort required to detect disease associations, and is responsible for allowing the recent generation of genome-wide association scans.

The extent to which one SNP captures information from another is usually estimated by r^2 or the square of the correlation between them. Rather arbitrarily, r^2 values of 0.8 or above are considered to be useful levels of LD. Where two SNPs are in LD, one is often denoted as redundant, since much of the information at that locus can be inferred by genotyping the other. The genotyped marker is said to **tag** the ungenotyped marker.

False positives

Statistical

In addition to true association, direct or indirect, it is important to consider causes of false association. First, false-positive associations may occur as a consequence of multiple testing. The conventional approach to multiple testing is to correct the best p-value for the number of statistical comparisons undertaken, preferably using some permutation test that allows for non-independence of markers due to LD. But what should one correct for? Consider two groups, each studying 100 genes. One publishes 100 papers, one on each gene, the other a single paper. The multiple testing burdens are identical but the correction reported will almost certainly not be. Moreover, if we simply correct for tests performed, this fails to recognize that as more genes are tested, the probability that at least one of the genes is a true susceptibility gene also increases.

Suppose there are approximately 1 million common independent SNPs and that 100 of these are genuinely associated with schizophrenia, each with a frequency of 0.25 and an OR of 1.15. *Regardless of how many SNPs* are to be tested, the probability that any *random* SNP will generate a false association is the product of the proportion of SNPs *in the genome* that are not associated with disease (F) and the significance level (A) for claiming association. The probability that any observation will be true is the product of the power (P) of the study to make an observation at the

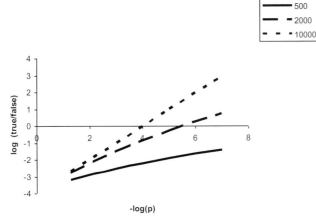

Fig. 13.1 Ratio of true-to-false associations. The expected ratio of true-to-false associations are provided for association samples containing 500, 2000, and 10 000 each of cases and controls. It is assumed there are 1 million independent SNPs, 100 true loci, minor allele frequency 0.25, and OR 1.15. Axes are plotted as log(10) of the ratio and –log(10) of the p value. The first data point corresponds to p = 0.05.

designated level A and the proportion of true (T) associated SNPs *in the genome*. None of the factors dictating the probabilities of observing true and false associations depends on the number of markers tested and so neither does the confidence (ratio of true to false) that any one finding is true. Based upon this Bayesian approach, the key to increasing confidence in a finding is not to type fewer markers but to increase the prior probability of a true observation, which depends largely on power, *and* to increase the threshold for statistical significance. This is illustrated in Figure 13.1 where, for several sample sizes and based upon the assumptions above, we plot the log(10) of the ratio of probabilities for any association being true and false for a range of observed p-values [expressed as the negative log(10)P]. For all sample sizes, p values in the order of 0.05 are approx. 1000 times more likely to be false than true. Even at an association p-value of 10^{-7} [–log(10) = 7], the findings from the smaller sample of 500 cases and controls are about 20 times more likely to be false than to be true. In contrast, for much larger sizes (2000 cases and controls), associations at $p \sim 1 \times 10^{-6}$ are slightly more likely to be true than false, a situation reached at $p \sim 1 \times 10^{-4}$ for the largest sample illustrated.

There are other approaches to increasing the prior probability of a true association other than increasing sample size. Instead of selecting SNPs at random, they can be selected because they map within genes for which there is a prior case for their involvement based on position or function. Another is to consider SNPs as higher priority based upon prior reports of association with disease, a principle that essentially provides the basis for accepting much less stringent statistical evidence in replication studies. However, while replication is a key step in the acceptance of an association as true, how one interprets replication is not always straightforward. This is because the extent to which a previous association has actually altered the prior probability is not equal for all studies, but is instead dependent on the expected ratio of true to false associations for the earlier study. Moreover, what actually constitutes replication is, as we shall see, at least debatable. For example, does a prior report of association to a SNP alter the prior probability for other SNPs that are localized in the same candidate gene, even if they are not LD with the "associated" SNP. Assuming that many genes contain multiple functional variants, association to *any* SNP within a gene must to some extent increase the prior probability for all SNPs within that gene, and even to SNPs in genes whose functions are related to that gene. It is clear that how one assesses the statistical evidence for an association to a SNP or a gene, and subsequent replications, depends to a considerable extent on the assumptions one is willing to make. Consequently, as we shall discuss at greater length below, there is considerable potential for valid disagreements in how individual reports of association should be interpreted.

Stratification

Since many SNP allele frequencies differ between ethnic groups, poor matching of cases to controls can result in allele frequency differences between cases and controls that are not relevant to affected status. Such associations are said to be due to **population stratification** or **substructure**. Genome-wide association studies (see below) have shown that in studies constrained within national boundaries, the impact of stratification is limited, and can easily be adjusted for statistically. Nevertheless, in the past, the potential impact of stratification has been used as an argument for abandoning case–control designs in favor of **family-based** designs in which genetic information from the parents (or other relatives) is used to generate a perfectly matched "internal" control group. There are many variations on this theme, but the most commonly used is the transmission disequilibrium test (TDT). Under the null hypothesis of no association, the basic Mendelian transmission probability is that an allele from a heterozygous individual will be transmitted to 50% of their offspring. However, if an allele is (directly or indirectly) associated with a disorder, it will be more frequently transmitted to affected offspring than expected. It is a simple matter of comparing the number of observed transmissions from heterozygous parents with that expected under the null hypothesis. The TDT has been refined to allow its application to families with missing parents, with only siblings available, and with multiple affected members, as well as for examining quantitative traits.

Application of association

Association has long been considered *potentially* the most promising approach to complex disorders because it is more powerful than other approaches, principally linkage, for detecting the alleles of small effect that are widely thought to contribute to most of the genetic variance for most complex disorders. However, a major obstacle is that in outbred populations (i.e., those without significant inbreeding), common genetic variation is so old that in the region of 500 000 markers are required to tag most of the common variation in the genome. The enormity of this has meant that association studies have focused on genes suspected as being involved in a disorder by virtue of a functional hypothesis, a **candidate gene approach,** or on regions suspected to harbor a disease gene because of linkage or because of a relationship between a chromosome abnormality and disorder, a **positional approach.** Often a hybrid of these has been adopted where the focus is specific genes within the linkage regions, a **positional candidate gene approach**. Recently (since around 2005), so-called **genome-wide association studies (GWAS)** have become feasible, and it is here we start our discussion. The reason for starting here is that because GWAS are systematic, the findings that have emerged provide a useful standpoint from which to revisit some of the earlier work.

Genome-wide association studies

The key developments that have enabled GWAS are the assembly of the human genome sequence, the creation of genome-wide maps of millions of SNPs, the development of methods allowing up to about 1 million (at the time of writing) SNPs to be genotyped simultaneously, and the assembly of large enough samples to exploit those technologies. Based on these developments, a number of standardized commercial products have been released that allow association analysis to be conducted either based upon SNPs scattered across the genome randomly (more or less) or with a bias towards genes. The capacity of these products now permits association analyses that can tag most common variation in the genome. The use of "off-the-shelf" GWAS tools has dramatically driven down the cost of genotyping relative to that attainable with custom-made products and consequently, most genetic investigators have favored the former type of product. This has led to much greater cross-study comparability with regard to methodology, quality control, analytic methodology, transparency about multiple testing, and the information finally extracted than would otherwise have been achieved, all of which facilitate subsequent efforts to combine datasets in meta-analysis. These benefits come in addition to the greatest perceived advantage of GWAS; the ability to harness the power advantage of association to detect small effects (relative to linkage) in the context of the whole genome and therefore with no prior requirement for specific knowledge of pathogenesis.

GWAS are transforming our knowledge of genetic susceptibility for many phenotypes. An early success was the identification of the gene encoding complement factor H (*CFH*) as a risk locus for age-related macular degeneration (AMD). This finding was highly atypical for complex diseases; the risk variant had a large effect (OR > 4) and so was detectable in a small sample of only 96 cases and 50 controls (Klein *et al.*, 2005). Subsequently, GWAS have confidently associated SNPs with many common diseases, including coronary artery disease, atrial fibrillation, asthma, Crohn disease, rheumatoid arthritis, Types 1 and 2 diabetes, obesity, prostate cancer, breast cancer, and celiac disease, but the effect sizes are typically much smaller than for *CFH* and AMD. For example, in a landmark GWAS study of seven common diseases by the Wellcome Trust Case Control Consortium (WTCCC, 2007), the median OR was 1.34, and even this is likely inflated, a phenomenon known as the so-called "winner's curse". The winner's curse arises because for a small effect to be discovered in underpowered samples, the measured effect size must be amplified by a favorable constellation of factors that maximize the distinction between case and control groups. These include spurious fluctuations in measured allele frequencies that arise by sampling variance, minor uncorrected degrees of stratification, or genotyping errors, as well as genuine fluctuations that may arise as a result of inter-sample heterogeneity.

The issues of effect size and sample requirements are underscored by meta-analyses of Type 2 diabetes (T2D). Whereas the WTCCC using 2000 cases and 3000 controls identified only three susceptibility loci for T2D at the most stringent threshold, a follow-up meta-analysis (Zeggini *et al.*, 2007) of around 32 000 subjects identified nine associated SNPs (p = $1.2 \times 10^{-7} - 1 \times 10^{-48}$). Small genetic effects were the rule; all but one had an OR ≤ 1.20. Since the majority of risk loci were not detected even in samples of this size, we can assume most effect sizes are smaller, a hypothesis supported by an even larger study based upon an effective sample size of around 64 000 subjects where the median OR of novel strongly implicated loci was 1.1 (Zeggini *et al.*, 2008). If the findings are typical, a series of failures to replicate findings in modestly-sized replication samples cannot be considered the equivalent of refutation. Indeed in the latter study, the median sample size required to replicate the findings at p = 0.05 was 16 350 subjects.

Another lesson is that a major source of false association is systematic differences in genotyping between cases and controls (or parents). Genotyping is not a perfect science, e.g., subjects who are in fact heterozygous for a SNP might tend to be misclassified as homozygous for a particular allele or even to have no genotype called at all. Classification errors that occur at equal rates in cases and controls will tend to obscure true differences in allele frequencies and generate false negatives. However, if there is a systematic difference in error rates (misclassification or drop out) between cases and controls, spurious differences in allele frequencies (i.e., association) can be generated. There are many fairly commonly applicable reasons why genotyping quality might systematically differ between populations. For example, DNA from cases and controls may have been processed several years apart, or in multiple laboratories, or have come from different sources (blood, postmortem tissues, etc.) with the relative proportions varying between patients and controls. Another situation which is increasingly common is to combine case genotype data from one laboratory with population reference data genotyped in a different laboratory. These issues are not trivial; indeed it appears so far that in reasonably well-controlled GWAS studies, the *unadjusted* contribution from technical error is much greater than that from stratification. Ironically, the family-based studies brought in to solve the problem of stratification are actually more susceptible to the effects of technical error than case–control studies, and might therefore be more prone to generate false positives. The lessons from GWAS studies have important implications for interpreting smaller-scale candidate gene studies which have, in the past, paid insufficient attention to reporting quality control metrics.

Studies of schizophrenia

Two early GWAS studies (Kirov *et al.*, 2009a; Shifman *et al.*, 2008) were based on pooling, in which cases are mixed together in a single quantitative assay, as are controls, and the differences in allele frequencies estimated. Neither identified associations at genome-wide significant levels, but of particular note, the latter suggested a female-specific association between *reelin* (*RELN*) and schizophrenia, a finding that could be replicated in samples from Europe and the US. *Reelin* is a gene with strong biological plausibility in schizophrenia since it plays an important role in the formation of the cerebral cortex, and its expression has been shown to be reduced in schizophrenia (see Shifman, *et al.*, 2008). In the light of testing multiple genetic models, more support is required before this strong finding can be considered definitive.

The first two GWAS studies (Lencz *et al.*, 2007; Sullivan *et al.*, 2008) to be based on individual genotyping were also fairly small, and like the pooling studies, did not convincingly implicate specific loci. The third GWAS with individual genotypes was our own (O'Donovan *et al.*, 2008). We undertook an initial GWAS of 479 UK cases and 2937 UK controls, and followed up 12 loci surpassing a threshold of $p < 10^{-5}$ in up to 6829 cases and 9897 controls from multiple groups from Europe, the US, Australia, Israel,

Japan, and China. Strong replicated support ($p < 5 \times 10^{-4}$) was observed to the same allele as we observed in the GWAS for three of the loci. Moreover, when we considered the distribution of test statistics in the follow-up data, the probability that the SNPs selected for follow-up represented a random set of SNPs was negligible ($p = 9 \times 10^{-8}$). The best supported locus was on chromosome 2 in the vicinity of *zinc finger protein 804A* (*ZNF804A*). Moreover, the same marker in *ZNF804A* also shows evidence for association to bipolar disorder (combined schizophrenia and bipolar disorder, $p = 9 \times 10^{-9}$), suggesting it influences a broader psychosis phenotype. A number of follow-up studies, including a large meta-analysis (Williams *et al.*, 2010) comprising around 60 000 subjects have confirmed that the association at the *ZNF804A* locus is genuine ($p_{meta} = 2.5 \times 10^{-11}$ for schizophrenia; $p_{meta} = 4.1 \times 10^{-13}$ for combined schizophrenia and bipolar datasets).

A landmark development in schizophrenia genetics was the simultaneous publication in 2009 of three GWAS in *Nature*. The studies, each containing more than 2000 cases and up to 13 500 controls, were from three consortia; the Molecular Genetics of Schizophrenia (Shi *et al.*, 2009b), the International Schizophrenia Consortium (2009) and SGENE (Stefansson *et al.*, 2009). The consortia also exchanged data for the top 1000 or so SNPs from their studies to enable meta-analysis. In the combined datasets, along with additional subjects giving a total of 12 945 cases and 34 591 controls, four loci emerged as genome-wide significant (Stefansson *et al.*, 2009). Two ($p = 2.3 \times 10^{-10}$ and $p = 1.4 \times 10^{-14}$) map to a broad region of chromosome 6 that includes the major histocompatibility complex (MHC) region, one is adjacent to *neurogranin* (*NRGN*) and the other is in an intron of *transcription factor 4* (*TCF 4*).

In addition to the single locus findings, using a novel multilocus method for analyzing GWAS data, the International Schizophrenia Consortium (2009) was able to demonstrate a substantial polygenic component to the disorder. In essence, it observed that a summary score derived from top sets of hundreds to thousands of alleles that were more common in the cases (but mostly not significantly more common) in a discovery schizophrenia GWAS could weakly, but highly significantly, discriminate case status in independent schizophrenia GWAS datasets. Remarkably, the International Schizophrenia Consortium also found that the same sets of alleles also discriminated (again weakly but highly significantly) people with bipolar disorder from controls. After considering and rejecting several potential sources of bias, the authors came to the following conclusions. First, a large number, probably in the thousands, of loci of small effect (OR < 1.1) contribute to the etiology of schizophrenia. Second, these together account for at least a third of the total variance (genetic and non-genetic) in liability to the disorder, and quite possibly much more than this. Third, as we reported for the schizophrenia susceptibility allele at *ZNF804A*, this poly-genic risk is substantially shared with bipolar disorder.

Regarding the robust findings that exist now, additional work will be required to show that the associations point to the specific genes mentioned above, rather than to as yet uncharacterized functional elements that colocalize with those genes. Nevertheless the findings offer potentially important new clues into the pathogenesis of schizophre-nia. For example, the protein neurogranin, encoded by *NRGN*, is particularly highly expressed in the dendritic spines of hippocampal neurons where it binds to, and reg-ulates the availability of, free calmodulin. Upon *N*-methyl-D-aspartate (NMDA) receptor activation by glutamate, a local increase in the concentration of calcium induces dis-sociation of neurogranin from calmodulin, allowing the latter to activate a number of downstream effectors. These in turn regulate the development of synaptic plasticity and long-term potentiation (Zhong *et al.*, 2009). Association at this locus is therefore consistent with hypotheses of aber-rant synaptic function in schizophrenia (see Chapter 21). As for the other loci, TCF4 is a transcription factor involved in neuronal precursor development (Blake *et al.*, 2010), whereas the function of ZNF804A is unknown, although based upon sequence similarity to other proteins, it may also be a transcription factor. The implications of the asso-ciations at these two loci for the pathophysiology of schizo-phrenia must await better characterization of the functions of these proteins, and in particular a better understanding of the genes that are regulated by them. Nevertheless, in the absence of knowledge of cellular function, robust genetic associations can be used to identify alterations in brain function of relevance to schizophrenia. One example is the recent report (Esslinger *et al.*, 2009) that the risk variant at *ZNF804A* is associated with enhanced patterns of correlation between measures of task-induced activation in the hippocampus and prefrontal cortex, a finding that supports the hypothesis that altered connectivity between brain structures is of pathogenic relevance in schizophrenia.

While novel findings are emerging from GWAS, and we would anticipate that many more will come in the near future from larger studies, we end this section with comment on the limitations of the GWAS approach, limita-tions which also apply to the more focused studies we discuss below. First, power is relatively low if there are multiple risk variants within a single region of high LD, or if the same mutation event occurs multiple times. This is because risk variants arise on more than one ancestral hap-lotype, weakening the relationship between risk of disease and tagging alleles. Second, where a tagging allele is in relatively low LD with a risk allele, or where there are multiple risk variants at a locus, the identity of a tagging allele can reverse, or an entirely different tag marker can emerge as associated in different samples (Moskvina &

O'Donovan, 2007). Where this occurs, associations may be obscured by combining multiple samples. The same phe-nomenon can also occur as a result of ethnic variation in LD and allele frequencies. Third, while current platforms tag a high proportion of common sequence variation, they do not capture it all. Low frequency variants (minor allele frequency < 1%) are particularly poorly tagged and, even when tagged, require samples many times larger to detect equivalent effect sizes. Fourth, the GWAS imperative for large samples might by confounded by the use of more relaxed inclusion criteria and thereby the introduction of greater clinical and genetic heterogeneity. Examples of how this might affect true associations are given in the candidate gene sections below. These considerations mean that GWAS cannot "exclude" a gene from involvement in susceptibility to illness.

As noted above, the prior probabilities of true associa-tions are not equal for all loci and it follows that a single statistical threshold for all SNPs in a GWAS is arguably not appropriate. Less stringent thresholds may be applicable to markers in linked genomic positions or in particular genes where there is good knowledge of some aspects of pathophysiology. GWAS should be seen as another phase in molecular genetics, albeit an important one, but one that does not supersede all that has gone before it. There remains the need for detailed analyses of positional and functional candidates and it is to these studies that we now turn.

Functional candidate genes

Prior to the year 2000 or so, genotyping technology in most laboratories could generate only a few hundred genotypes per day, curtailing sample sizes and the number of variants examined. Moreover, without the large scale catalogs of SNPs and of the LD relationships between them in (e.g., the HapMap; www.hapmap.org), systematic examination of any gene was a major challenge. As a result, the func-tional candidate gene literature, comprising thousands of studies, largely consists of either direct association studies based upon a single functional variant, or indirect associa-tion studies based upon a small subset of variants selected without regard to the amount of the genetic variation extracted. Even studies based upon systematic mutation scanning to uncover all common variation have focused on subsets of the functional elements of genes, typically exons and promoter regions. These considerations, allied with likely small genetic effects and our limited understanding of pathophysiology have no doubt contributed to the current situation with the functional candidate gene litera-ture. Negative findings abound as do positive findings that have either not been replicated, or have seemed insuffi-ciently convincing that there have been few attempts to replicate them. To what extent any extant data in the functional candidate literature represent true positives is sufficiently debatable for there to be a wide spectrum of opinion concerning their interpretation. So first, what can be said with reasonable confidence?

First, nothing has emerged with support on a par with, for example, the evidence for *HLA* in Type I diabetes or *APOE* in Alzheimer disease. Indeed most schizophrenia researchers would agree that no *fully convincing robustly replicated* findings have emerged from candidate gene studies. [The issue of replication is discussed further below but in the present context, we are using a very stringent definition. Thus, by fully convincing robustly replicated, we mean that the same allele or haplotype broadly shows the same pattern of association across studies—the significance of individual studies will of course vary with sample size—and that meta-analysis provides statistical support that is at least one order of magnitude better than genome-wide significance (i.e., $\sim 5 \times 10^{-9}$)]. Second, while most of the reported positives are unlikely to stand the test of time, no functional candidate has been excluded from containing common risk alleles, much less rare alleles, that contribute with the sort of effect sizes that might be typical. Third, for power reasons, failure to replicate does not refute a previous finding. It simply does not support it. Fourth, the search for rare high penetrance SNPs has barely begun and at the time of writing, no gene has been sequenced in sufficient detail to exclude rare highly penetrant alleles.

It is then self-evident that definitive answers cannot be provided regarding any given gene. Nevertheless, it is worth discussing a few that have provoked considerable interest as themes have emerged with respect to interpreting those studies and these will, without doubt, continue to emerge for genetic findings in the near future. Readers with a particular interest in specific genes might also care to look at a web-based resource called SZgene (http://www.schizophreniaforum.org/res/sczgene/default.asp), a useful resource established to collate the results of candidate gene studies and, where appropriate, perform meta-analyses (Allen *et al.*, 2008).

Dopamine genes

The dopamine hypothesis of schizophrenia is discussed in detail in Chapter 20. For our discussion, we need simply note that there is a large and convincing body of evidence that altered dopaminergic function is involved in the pathophysiology of schizophrenia and few would disagree that genes closely related to dopamine function are among those with the highest prior probability of being involved in disease. Genes less proximal to dopamine function are also candidates, but the promiscuous nature of protein–protein interactions is such that as one moves less proximal to the hypothesis, the number of potential candidates

rapidly rises, and so the prior probability of any one candidate must diminish.

Catechol-O-methyl transferase (COMT), encoded by the *COMT* gene, is a catabolic enzyme involved in the degradation of a number of bioactive molecules including dopamine and other catecholamines (see Chapter 20). Moreover, *COMT* (along with 47 other genes) is located in a region of chromosome 22q11 which, when deleted, results in a complex 22q11 deletion syndrome (22q11DS), the psychiatric manifestations of which include schizophrenia (see below). Allied with its involvement in dopamine catabolism, this positional information places *COMT* near the top of almost any list of candidate genes for schizophrenia.

Within the coding sequence of *COMT* is a common polymorphism that produces a valine-to-methionine (Val/Met) substitution. The polymorphism is usually referred to as the Val/Met locus, but also by the reference sequence code rs4680 (previously also rs165688). The amino acid change is functional, Val conferring higher enzyme activity and stability. The polymorphism has generally been thought of as the main source of genetic variation in COMT activity (see Chapter 20). The constellation of affairs comprising an excellent functional and positional candidate which contains a variant with a known functional effects is rare, and represents the optimum scenario for a targeted candidate gene approach. Moreover, the recent demonstration of additional functional variants, including rs4818 which has profound effects on enzyme activity by inhibiting the rate of translation (Nackley *et al.*, 2006), and in Korean and Japanese populations, a functional alanine-to-serine polymorphism (rs6267) (Lee *et al.*, 2005) adds additional complexity to this gene. We will therefore discuss *COMT* in detail because there are important lessons to be learned.

Since the earliest study (Daniels *et al.*, 1996), *COMT* has become an irresistible target in almost every imaginable psychiatric and behavioral disorder. In schizophrenia, by June 2010, *COMT* had been tested in over 100 association samples, though some are updates of earlier studies. The studies include positive and negative findings at Val/Met (Williams *et al.*, 2007) *potentially* consistent with a true association of small effect but where replication is hampered by lack of power. However, against this interpretation, recent meta-analyses find no significant effect at the Val/Met locus, with an overall OR of 0.99 (95% CI, 0.95–1.04) for the low activity Met allele (SZgene, June 2010). The combined data do not then support a general effect of the Val/Met polymorphism on schizophrenia risk. So, what does this tells us about the dopamine hypothesis of schizophrenia? The answer depends upon whether (1) the Val/Met polymorphism is a significant determinant of dopamine availability in at least one brain region with a function relevant to schizophrenia; *and* (2) there is a predictable relationship between dopamine availability and that brain function. If both criteria are met, the data would *seem* to undermine the dopamine hypothesis of schizophrenia.

COMT does have a role in dopamine clearance in some regions of plausible relevance to schizophrenia, including prefrontal and other cortical regions (Gogos, *et al.* 1998; Turnbridge, *et al.* 2004). What is less clear is whether the Val/Met polymorphism results in a functionally significant difference in dopamine availability, although there is indirect evidence that makes such a relationship likely. For example, a recent positron emission tomography (PET) study (Slifstein *et al.*, 2008) reported that compared with Met carriers, Val/Val homozygotes had higher dopamine D_1 receptor binding in the cortex as indexed by labeled ligand binding. This is compatible with the Val/Val genotype resulting in low dopamine availability and a homeostatic increase in D_1 receptors. The notion that the Val/Met locus is associated with physiologically relevant variation in dopamine activity is also supported by studies of cognition. The first of these reported the high activity allele was associated with poor executive function (Egan *et al.*, 2001). Others have subsequently related the Val/Met locus to variable performance in a range of cognitive tasks. Although the effects are small (Barnett *et al.*, 2008), these observations imply the Val/Met locus influences dopamine at physiologically relevant levels. Thus, it would appear that the criteria above are likely to be correct, and that in the absence of association, the dopamine hypothesis of schizophrenia is not correct at a primary causal level.

Unfortunately, the complexities of the schizophrenia phenotype, of human biology, and of population genetics defy simple interpretations. As similar issues are likely to be applicable to many true susceptibility genes, we deal with each in turn below.

The first issue is phenotypic complexity. Positive symptoms are generally regarded as related to excess dopamine in subcortical structures. Since COMT does not play much of a role in dopamine bioavailability in these structures, we cannot use the negative association data to conclude against the dopamine hypothesis of positive symptoms. What about cognitive symptoms? If the cognitive impairments that have been associated with the Val/Met locus are causal for some forms of schizophrenia, we would expect to find some degree of association between Val/Met and schizophrenia, although the effect size would vary between samples depending upon the degree to which ascertainment was biased for cognitively impaired subjects. A limiting factor is, as always, effect size. The meta-analysis of cognitive function referred to above suggested only a weak relationship between the Val/Met locus and IQ. If in turn low IQ (or any other cognitive measure) was itself only modestly associated with certain forms of schizophrenia, the sample size of cases required to demonstrate an association could be prohibitive. Moreover, the issue of association to disorder is also one of nomenclature. If the cognitive impairments that have been associated with COMT are reclassified as core features of schizophrenia, the Val/Met polymorphism would become *de-facto* associated with risk of schizophrenia.

Given repeated reports of association between COMT and almost every imaginable psychiatric phenotype, another phenotypic issue concerns overlaps and comorbidities between schizophrenia and other disorders. These include reports of association between COMT and treatment response or to unconventionally labeled psychosis-mood spectrum disorders, which may influence ascertainment and therefore patterns of observed association (Craddock *et al.*, 2006). Interestingly, work on genetically manipulated mice points to a divergence between the impact of COMT activity on cognition and on stress reactivity, lower COMT activity being associated with better cognitive function but also greater stress reactivity and increased anxiety-like traits (Papaleo *et al.*, 2008). If schizophrenia comprises a set of disorders in which, for example, cognitive, mood, anxiety, and other groups of symptoms are variable features upon which COMT may have divergent effects, the overall directionality of any association could be sensitive to the phenotypic composition of any given sample.

The second potential complexity relates to biology. Rather than a linear relationship between dopamine and brain function (as indexed by tests of cognition), there is evidence for an inverted "U"-shaped relationship. Under this model, too little or too much dopamine has relatively deleterious effects (Mattay *et al.*, 2003; Papaleo *et al.*, 2008). It follows that, at the individual level, whether the low activity allele enhances or impairs function depends upon whether that individual has, respectively, too little or too much dopamine. While true at the individual level, we would still expect the direction of association to be dictated (within broadly similar populations) by the population mean position on the curve, and therefore a consensus for a particular allele. Moreover, there is sufficient homogeneity in population mean positions to demonstrate directional associations as testified by association between Val/Met and certain measures of cognition. In our view, it does not seem that biological complexity alone (as manifest by a U-shaped curve) can readily explain the overall negative findings in schizophrenia, unless it is allied with COMT-related phenotypic complexity as discussed in the previous paragraph.

The third complexity is genetic. Although the focus has largely been on the Val/Met locus, several studies have shown that variants that do not change the amino acid sequence of COMT can influence COMT mRNA expression (Bray *et al.*, 2003), enzyme activity (Chen *et al.*, 2004), and the rate of COMT mRNA translation (Nackley *et al.*, 2006). As explained above in the GWAS section, the existence of multiple risk variants within a single locus can result in largely unpredictable patterns of association, and the potential for this to influence the direction of a reported association has specifically been demonstrated using *COMT* (Lin *et al.*, 2007).

Aiming to overcome the impact of non-linear relationships between dopamine availability and brain function, and also some of the genetic complexities underpinning association, researchers have adopted approaches that *might* allow for these. These can be divided into haplotype-based approaches, tests of gene–gene interaction, and tests of gene–environment interaction.

Haplotype tests

In the context of a direct association study of a *known* functional variant, haplotype association approaches are based on the premise that the impact of functional alleles may be modified by another variant on the same DNA strand. Such studies would be most powerful if the additional functional variants are also directly tested, but since a full catalog of functional variation is not available, this is not possible. Haplotype-based studies at *COMT* are then hybrids of direct and indirect association. Interpretation is therefore likely to be confounded by the unpredictable nature of LD, so unsurprisingly, the data are not easy to interpret. Very strong statistical evidence for a haplotype of *COMT* was reported in a large sample of Ashkenazi Jews (Shifman *et al.*, 2002) in which only modest evidence for association was found with the Val allele alone. Gender effects were also reported, although these are difficult to interpret because much of the effect was driven by differences in the controls, not the cases. Since then, several studies have reported evidence for association at COMT that appears stronger with haplotypes than with the Val/Met locus alone (Craddock *et al*, 2006), although the specific associated haplotypes vary considerably between studies.

The issues of directionality in indirect studies make it tenable to suspend the requirement that replication studies must implicate the same alleles and haplotypes to provide support for association, but it is also important not to regard any study with a nominally significant marker/halotype as supportive of an earlier finding. So how can we avoid being cavalier in claiming support for association? This is unresolved in genetics but we have suggested (Georgieva *et al.*, 2008) that a follow-up study is supportive where the finding (1) survives correction for multiple testing; (2) is based upon a coherent study design in which it is clear that the results could not have arisen by ceasing genotyping at the point a marker was found that met the first criterion; and (3) cannot be attributed to poor matching of cases and controls (i.e., stratification). It also goes without saying there should be good quality control, particularly in haplotype-based studies where trivial amounts of genotyping error can considerably inflate the false-positive rate (Moskvina *et al.*, 2006). If these criteria are genuinely met across more studies than chance or publication bias allows, then the failure to replicate association to single alleles or haplotypes means that we do not understand what is driving the association, not, as some would have it, that the results are spurious.

Unfortunately with respect to *COMT* few have addressed these issues so we can only gain an impression of "significance". Our own judgment is that the haplotype findings keep *COMT* in the list of risk genes with some support, but there are insufficient studies that would be clearly significant when corrected for multiple testing to draw stronger conclusions.

Gene–gene interaction

It seems reasonable to postulate that more consistent association findings with regard to the Val/Met locus might emerge when factors are allowed for that are extrinsic to the *COMT* gene but which make contributions to an individual's position in a non-linear dopamine dose–response curve, or alternatively, are known to influence risk of disorder. One such approach is to undertake analysis of gene–gene interactions. Several gene–gene interactions have been reported for *COMT*, including *RGS4*, *G72*, *GRM3*, and *DISC1* (Nicodemus *et al.*, 2007), selected primarily as possible candidate genes for schizophrenia, and also the dopamine transporter *DAT1* (Talkowski *et al.*, 2008). However, unless there are compelling functional polymorphisms in candidate interacting genes, the prior-probability advantage that is conferred by the candidacy of the Val/Met locus may be lost amid a multiplicity of reasonable, but nevertheless weak, hypotheses. This is exacerbated when polymorphisms other than Val/Met are tested, and imposes a requirement for strong statistical support, including subsequent independent replication. So far, none of the individual interaction data yet achieves this.

Gene–environment interaction

A second class of extrinsic variables that might influence the influence the Val/Met locus is environmental. Similar comments about multiple testing and prior probabilities that were made above with respect to gene–gene interactions also apply; indeed, the problem may be worse since there are few, if any, environmental variables robustly implicated in the etiology of schizophrenia. Moreover, most environmental exposures can be measured in multiple ways. Nevertheless, evidence for gene–environment interaction involving the Val/Met polymorphism and schizophrenia symptoms has been obtained from a birth cohort study. Adult carriers of the Val allele were at increased risk of psychotic symptoms and of schizophreniform disorder if they used cannabis, whereas cannabis users with two copies of the Met allele had no increase in risk (Caspi *et al.*, 2005). This observation is consistent with *COMT* modulating the psychotogenic effects of cannabis exposure, but at least one fairly large study involving schizophrenia rather than the above softer phenotypes is negative (Zammit *et al.*, 2007). Additional studies of this potentially important observation are eagerly awaited.

The potential complexities we have discussed and their impact on interpreting negative association studies in particular apply to most of the remainder of the chapter, which is why we have devoted so much space to this one gene. We will not repeat them below, but ask readers to bear them in mind in all that follows.

DRD2

Genes encoding dopamine receptors are also among the highest plausibility candidate genes, and among these, given the strong correlation between the therapeutic efficacy of antipsychotic drugs (see Chapter 25) and their affinity for dopamine 2 receptors (encoded by *DRD2*), *DRD2* is the best candidate.

Like *COMT*, most studies of *DRD2* (n > 50) have focused on a small number of SNPs for which there is some evidence for functionality (usually n = 1). Arinami *et al.* (1996) provided evidence for association between a serine to cysteine polymorphism in *DRD2* in Japanese people with schizophrenia without negative symptoms. The associated cysteine allele has also been reported to impair the function of the encoded receptor (Cravchik *et al.*, 1996). Although subsequent individual studies have not provided much support, meta-analysis of about 3700 cases and nearly 5500 controls (Glatt & Jönsson, 2006) provides a somewhat more encouraging picture (0.001 < p < 0.01) for association, as does the meta-analysis in the SZgene database (June 2010). The same Japanese group (Arinami *et al.*, 1997) also reported that a −141G insertion/deletion variant (141 bases upstream of the gene) both reduced *DRD2* expression and was associated with schizophrenia. However, despite some positive studies, including one large study (900 subjects) in which the opposite allele was associated (Breen *et al.*, 1999), meta-analyses (Glatt *et al.*, 2004; SZgene database, June 2010) do not support association.

A third functional variant that has received attention in multiple studies is rs6277, a synonymous SNP which alters mRNA stability and translational efficiency (Duan *et al.*, 2003). Following the first positive report of Lawford *et al.* (2005), several independent studies have now supported association to the allele that confers higher mRNA stability and translational efficiency. A recent meta-analysis of 885 cases and 1485 controls also provides fairly impressive (p < 0.00005) statistical support (Monakhov *et al.*, 2008), as does an unpublished meta-analysis (SZgene, June 2010) of 4000 cases and 4500 controls with the estimated effect size

being larger than typical disease susceptibility alleles (OR = 1.27). This certainly suggests that this variant warrants further study.

As discussed above, instead of a direct association approach based upon functional alleles, it is also possible to conduct an indirect association study with the aim of tagging most or all known common genetic variation at a locus. Based upon the HapMap (February 2009), a detailed indirect study of *DRD2* requires 16 SNPs to achieve coverage of *DRD2* based upon tagging all known SNPs with a minor allele frequency (MAF) of 0.05 at $r^2 > 0.9$ (we will use these values as our standard definition of intensive coverage for *common* variants). Few studies have examined *DRD2* at anything like the depth required. Sanders *et al.* (2008) examined 31 SNPs in about 1900 cases and 2000 controls of European ancestry; although a few showed weak evidence (p < 0.05), at a gene-wide level the study provided no support. The other systematic study (Glatt *et al.*, 2009) examined 24 SNPs in just over 600 Taiwanese families. Multiple significant SNPs were observed, two at a threshold that just survived at a gene-wide level (p = 0.05). A complex pattern of association with haplotypes was also observed, probably no better than that observed from SNPs alone.

To summarize, the findings from two functional polymorphisms provides some support for the hypothesis that variation at *DRD2* influences susceptibility to schizophrenia. Given that the existence of multiple functional SNPs is precisely the scenario predicted to give rise to complex patterns of association, clearer data might emerge from tests of specific combinations of the functional variants for evidence of co-action or interaction rather simple tests based upon LD structure alone.

DRD3

Apart from its general candidacy as a dopamine receptor gene, *DRD3* was thought to be particularly interesting because of its pattern of limbic expression. Moreover, the expression of *DRD3* was known to be altered by a range of antipsychotic drugs, typical and atypical (Buckland *et al.*, 1992). The first association study (Crocq *et al.*, 1992) was typical of studies of that generation; analysis was restricted to a single non-synonymous variant (Ser–Gly), though there is little evidence that it is functionally important. Although large for its time, there were only a total of 141 cases and 139 controls. Despite this, the authors reported modest evidence for association with homozygosity for the Ser genotype (p < 0.008) and, more significantly, homozygosity for either genotype (combined p = 0.0001). As for *DRD2*, there have been more than 50 follow-up studies with the vast majority focusing on just this one polymorphism. Findings have been mixed, but a series of meta-analyses culminating in 8000 subjects provided significant support for the original finding (Jönsson *et al.*, 2003). However, as the worldwide dataset has doubled, the meta-analysis has become non-significant (Ma *et al.*, 2008). Provisionally, the original findings must be considered false positives and, based upon the Bayesian considerations discussed above and with the benefit of hindsight with regard to likely effect sizes, this is no surprise.

A small number of groups have examined the gene more systematically. Anney *et al.* (2002) systematically studied putative regulatory elements upstream to (or **5′ flanking**) *DRD3*, but failed to find evidence for association. Domínguez *et al.* (2007) also observed no evidence for any of 17 SNPs in about 500 subjects. Although they reported association to rare haplotypes, there is a special concern here as rare haplotypes are highly prone to the influence of genotyping error (Moskvina *et al.*, 2006). Finally, Talkowski *et al.* (2008) examined *DRD3* methodically by typing 18 SNPs spanning the gene in US, Indian, and Bulgarian samples. Nominally significant evidence was found for several SNPs in the US samples, but the combined analysis was not strongly supportive. Thus, currently, *DRD3* cannot be considered to have much support.

Other dopamine genes

DRD1, *DRD4*, and *DRD5* have also been the subject of investigation, though not to the same extent as *DRD2* and *DRD3*. To the authors' knowledge, no study has provided evidence for association to *DRD1*. There are a mixture of positive and negative studies of *DRD4* and *DRD5*, but none alone or in combination provides a strong case for association. Meta-analysis of about 2000 cases and controls (Allen *et al.*, 2008) does provide some support (p = 0.003) for a variant in the vicinity of *DRD4*, but this must be considered weak since it is no longer significant after exclusion of the initial sample. The situation with *DRD4* contrasts with that in attention deficit hyperactivity disorder (ADHD) where a 48bp repeat polymorphism has been convincingly associated (Thapar *et al.*, 2005). Given this must reflect association between the repeat and altered function, one might expect that, if *DRD4* is involved in schizophrenia, some association would be observed. However, meta-analysis does not support this hypothesis (Glatt *et al.*, 2003).

Among the other key dopaminergic genes, probably the best prior candidates are the *tyrosine hydroxylase* gene (*TH*), encoding the rate-limiting enzyme for dopamine synthesis, and genes encoding both the dopamine transporter and monoamine oxidase enzymes, which are responsible in most brain regions for synaptic clearance and catabolism of dopamine (Chapter 20). Although there are reports of *post-hoc* associations based upon, for example, one of many possible genetic models or gender-specific associations, the evidence for any of *TH*, *MAO-A*, or *MAO-B* is scant at best.

Being obvious candidates, dopamine-related genes were among the earliest genes studied and therefore, as we have seen, they tend not to have been subjected to adequately powered detailed studies. Recognizing this, Talkowski *et al.* (2008) screened 95 SNPs in 18 dopamine-related genes in up to approximately 500 US cases and controls. For genes showing evidence for association, they increased the SNP coverage in the US sample and also an additional 637 Bulgarian trios. It should be noted that the first stage was not exhaustive, and only for those genes with at least one SNP with p < 0.05 was a more complete evaluation undertaken. In the context of multiple testing, no gene was strongly endorsed by combined analyses, but of those genes for which there was evidence, the strongest ($p_{min} = 0.0004$) was the *dopamine transporter* (*DAT1* or *SLCA63*), which hitherto has not been much supported in schizophrenia. Additional weaker associations were reported for *COMT*, *DRD3*, and *SLC18A2* (0.01 < p < 0.05), encoding vesicular monoamine transporter 2.

Given a single pathway with plausible functional interactions, Talkowski *et al.* (2008) tested SNPs showing trends in the US sample for interactions. Of 29 positive interactions in the US sample, seven showed evidence for interaction effects in the Bulgarian sample, with *DAT1* showing interaction with each of *COMT*, *DRD3*, and *SLC18A2*. Although it is not clear that the qualitative nature of the interaction terms was exactly replicated, the number of significant interactions was unlikely to occur by chance (p ~ 0.001). This study and the promising findings in *DRD2* underscore the need for further detailed investigation of dopamine genes using large samples and, preferably, approaches powered to detect rare effects as well.

Serotonergic genes

Many atypical antipsychotic drugs modulate the serotonergic (5-HT) system (see Chapter 23). Based largely upon this, genes encoding key proteins involved in this system have a claim as candidates for schizophrenia. Among those studied, *SLC6A4* (encoding the 5-HT transporter) and *HTR2A* (encoding the 5-HT$_{2A}$ receptor) have attracted most attention.

According to the current HapMap, *HTR2A* requires 36 SNPs for coverage; no one has yet studied this gene in this depth but neither of the most detailed studies so far (Domínguez, *et al.* 2007; Sanders *et al.*, 2008) provides gene-wide evidence for association. Most of the remaining 50 or so samples in which this gene has been examined have focused on a SNP known as T102C or rs6313. There is no clear evidence for functionality for this polymorphism, although there are contradictory reports that it is associated with altered *HTR2A* expression (Polesskaya & Sokolov, 2002; Bray *et al.*, 2004). Early studies (Inayama *et al.*, 1996; Williams *et al.*, 1996) have provided evidence for association, but despite a number of favorable meta-analyses, this variant is not supported by the most recent update of over 19 000 subjects (SZgene, June 2010).

The *serotonin transporter* has been systematically studied by Ikeda *et al.* (2006; 600 subjects) who found no evidence for association. Most of the remaining 30 or so samples that have been studied have focused on one or two common polymorphic sites; a variable number tandem repeat (VNTR) polymorphism in intron 2 and a 44 base insertion/deletion in the promoter region. The long (insertion) variant of the latter confers higher expression of the mRNA and protein (Lesch *et al.*, 1996). The findings have been mixed but meta-analysis of approximately 6500 subjects (Fan & Sklar, 2005) found no effect of the insertion/deletion but fairly significant evidence (p = 0.0001) for the VNTR 12 repeat allele (called STin2.12) in about 4500 case–control subjects and also in 784 families (p = 0.02). The family finding is not robust, being substantially driven by a single study. Moreover, where the finding becomes difficult to interpret is that the VNTR has no known function. Since most associations are indirect, this is not a major problem *per se*. What is difficult is to reconcile that finding in the context of the insertion/deletion variant which is functional yet not associated. This does not mean the VNTR association is false, but it is enough to suggest caution.

One other gene in the 5-HT system deserves mention as this is starting to receive more than the usual degree of attention. *TPH1* is one of two enzymes encoding tryptophan hydroxylase, the rate-limiting enzyme in the synthesis of 5-HT. Zaboli *et al.* from Sweden (2006) and Watanabe *et al.* from Japan (2007) both conducted systematic assessments of *TPH1*, albeit in moderate sized samples. The Swedish group (~400 subjects) reported association to a polymorphism in the promoter region of *TPH1* polymorphism in their sample and also in a meta-analysis of over 1500 cases and controls. Although there was no support in the Japanese sample for any variant at the gene (~850 subjects), meta-analysis of about 1200 cases and 1700 controls revealed evidence for association to an intronic SNP (rs1800532; p < 0.001). At present the evidence supporting this variant, which has no known function, is interesting, and the most recent meta-analysis in SZGene is also supportive (OR 1.16, June 2010). However, the numbers studied are still rather small (approx. 2500 cases and 3500 controls). As with *DRD3* and *HTR2A*, there is at least the possibility that findings might yet reverse as samples sizes are increased.

Positional candidate genes

Positional candidate genes are genes that have been implicated on the basis of initial clues about location in the genome based on linkage (Chapter 12) and/or chromosomal abnormalities. Here, we discuss some of the more prominent examples, excepting those discussed elsewhere [*neuregulin* (*NRG1*; see Chapter 21) and *dysbindin* (*DTNBP1*; see Chapter 12)].

D-amino acid oxidase activator and D-amino oxidase

D-amino acid oxidase activator (*DAOA*) was first implicated in schizophrenia by Chumakov *et al.* (2002) after association analysis across a putative schizophrenia and bipolar linkage region on 13q22–34. Evidence for association was obtained in two populations, French–Canadian and Russian, the signal spanning two novel genes they called *G72* and *G30*. Neither was of known function but using techniques that can identify novel protein interactions, they reported evidence for physical and functional interactions between the G72 protein and D-amino acid oxidase (DAO). DAO oxidizes D-serine which in turn is an activator of NMDA glutamate receptors. Since G72 enhances DAO function, it has subsequently been named DAOA. In the same study, *DAO* was also shown to be associated with schizophrenia in one of the samples, while analysis of *DAOA* and *DAO* variants revealed modest evidence for a statistical interaction. Given the evidence for physical, biochemical, and statistical interaction, the authors concluded *DAOA* and *DAO* influence risk of schizophrenia through an NMDA-receptor related function.

Early support for *DAOA* was obtained in samples from Germany (Schumacher *et al.*, 2004) and China (Wang *et al.*, 2004), and while the results now from around 30 samples are mixed, most conclude in favor of association. Given the wealth of data, a number of meta-analyses have been performed. Those that have been published are positive but unfortunately, given the potential functional insights, the status of *DAOA* as a schizophrenia susceptibility gene is not quite compelling. In the most recent and largest published meta-analysis based on 19 schizophrenia samples comprising 4304 cases, 5423 controls, and 1384 families (Shi *et al.*, 2008), there was evidence for association (corrected p < 10^{-4}) but only in Asian, not European, samples. While statistically strong, the original observation was made not in Asian but in European samples (Chumakov *et al.*, 2002). Moreover, the evidence for association came from only three Asian samples, and while still significant, has diminished with the addition of more samples (Shi *et al.*, 2009a). Nevertheless, there is a clear excess of studies with associations at statistical levels that would be significant after correction for multiple testing.

Possible explanations for the mixed findings at *DAOA* relate to the precise nature of the associated phenotype. For example, *DAOA* has also been implicated in bipolar disorder (Hattori *et al.*, 2003; Schumacher *et al.*, 2004), mood symptomatology in both schizophrenia and bipolar disorder (Williams *et al.*, 2006), and in major depression and neuroticism (Rietschel *et al.*, 2008). While none of these findings is robustly confirmed, as discussed in more detail above for *COMT*, if association varies with aspects of the phenotype, patterns of association might vary with the predominant clinical pictures of subjects in any given study.

DAO itself has received much less attention, but several studies have reported evidence that would survive correction (e.g., Schumacher *et al.*, 2004; Corvin *et al.*, 2007) for multiple testing and, as for *DAOA*, it appears there are more gene-wide significant studies than expected. However, with the small number of studies published, there is a greater possibility of publication bias. Notwithstanding a small meta-analysis of about 1500 cases and controls that found nominally significant results for one marker (Allen *et al.*, 2008), the current level of evidence is weak.

DISC1

DISC1 is an example of gene identified through the co-occurrence of a chromosomal abnormality and disorder. St Clair *et al.* (1990) reported a Scottish family in which a balanced t(1;11)(q42.1;q14.3) translocation involving chromosomes 1 and 11 cosegregated with major mental illnesses. In a clear example of the lack of validity of psychiatric diagnoses, the maximum evidence for linkage is obtained when the affected status includes both schizophrenia and major mood disorders (bipolar and recurrent major depression) (Blackwood *et al.*, 2001). Further studies (Millar *et al.*, 2000) localized the translocation breakpoint on chromosome 1 to two genes, subsequently called *Disrupted In Schizophrenia 1* (*DISC1*) and *Disrupted In Schizophrenia 2* (*DISC2*). The translocation interrupts the coding sequence of *DISC1*, potentially resulting in a truncated protein, and also in reduced *DISC1* expression in family members. *DISC2* appears to specify a non-coding RNA which may regulate *DISC1* expression.

While the translocation event is unique to this family, linkage studies suggest that *DISC1* or a gene in the same region operates more generally as a susceptibility gene for psychiatric illness, including schizophrenia, schizoaffective disorder, and bipolar disorder (see Hennah *et al.*, 2009). However, attributing the linkages to *DISC1* has proven difficult. Promising support was obtained with the report of a nonsense mutation in a second family affected by schizophrenia, which initially had the appearance of a rare highly penetrant mutation, but subsequent observations of the same variant in controls (Green *et al.*, 2006) makes this unlikely.

An impediment to interpreting the growing *DISC1* association literature is the size of the gene. At 414 000 bases, over 150 SNPs are required to interrogate the known common variation, posing both a strong multiple testing

burden and difficulties tackling it systematically. Currently, the typical number of SNPs in a study is less than 20. Moreover, different SNPs generally appear in different studies and the reported association signals span the whole gene (see Hennah *et al.*, 2009). Aiming to obtain consistency in the data, a consortium from Finland and the UK examined 75 SNPs that met appropriate levels of quality control in combined samples of 1263 schizophrenia cases, 1008 bipolar cases, and 1275 controls (Hennah *et al*, 2009). Many of the samples had been included in previous positive studies by the collaborating groups. Across all samples there were a number of nominally significant findings, but none that survived correction for multiple testing; nor was there uncorrected support for a non-synonymous SNP (Ser–Cys) that had previously been associated with schizophrenia, brain structure, and brain function (Callicott *et al.*, 2005). Analyses by subgroupings based on site, disorder, and gender, and tests of SNP–SNP interaction also revealed several nominally significant findings, but again, these would not remain significant after correction. While this study does not provide significant support for common susceptibility variation in *DISC1*, the nominally significant findings with respect to particular associations and SNP–SNP interactions provides a number of hypotheses that merit attention in other datasets. As yet no clear replications have been reported in clinical samples, but several of the SNPs have been reported to show complex patterns of association to self-reported social anhedonia in a population cohort (Tomppo *et al.*, 2009). While intriguing and in line with the hypothesis of multiple variants with independent effects on *DISC1* function, the relevance of these findings with respect to the earlier findings in schizophrenia and psychosis (Hennah *et al.*, 2009) is not yet clear.

Most of the other relatively systematic studies (here we restrict to samples independent of those used by Hennah and colleagues) have also been negative in the context of multiple testing, including those of Sanders *et al.* (2008), Sullivan *et al.* (2008), and Schumacher *et al.* (2009). However, the relatively detailed studies are not all negative; indeed a recent large meta-analysis provided weak support for association (p = 0.046) after correction for multiple testing (Schumacher *et al.*, 2009), although it is not quite clear that the correction was appropriately stringent. Moreover, an association between schizoaffective disorder and *DISC1* survived correction for 39 SNPs (Hodgkinson *et al.*, 2004) and for multiple phenotypes, and is of particular interest given the mixture of phenotypes observed in the translocation family and the report of a genome-wide significant linkage to schizoaffective disorder at the *DISC1* region (Hamshere *et al.*, 2005).

Overall, the evidence from population-based studies does not strongly support association between *DISC1* and schizophrenia, but this does not mean *DISC1* is not involved in schizophrenia. The most compelling evidence remains that from cosegregation between the translocation and major mental disorders, an observation most likely explained by risk being conferred through *DISC1* itself. Even if common variation at *DISC1* does not operate in the general population, rare phenomena (the translocation) can still contribute to knowledge of pathogenesis for the generality of cases. In this respect, *DISC1* has no shortage of biological plausibility. A discussion of the biology of *DISC1* is beyond the scope of this chapter (see Ross *et al.*, 2006, also Chapter 22), but there is strong evidence that DISC1 plays a role in numerous processes relevant to brain development, including neural migration, neurite extension, neural progenitor proliferation, and neurogenesis, as well as synaptic transmission and plasticity. Moreover, there is evidence that variation in the gene may be associated with performance in neurocognitive tests, including working memory and also with various structural and functional brain neuroimaging (Callicott *et al.*, 2005; DiGiorgio *et al.*, 2008) and neuropathological (Eastwood *et al.*, 2010) variables.

Indirect genetic support for *DISC1* has also been provided by a number of published analyses of genes of encoding proteins known to interact with DISC1. The most interesting example concerns the gene *phosphodiesterase 4B* (*PDE4B*), identified as a candidate as a result of another translocation carried by a person with schizophrenia and his cousin who had a prolonged but unclassified psychiatric disorder (Millar *et al.*, 2005). The translocation disrupted two genes, *cadherin-8* and *PDE4B* on chromosome 1, the latter being of particular interest since it physically interacts with DISC1. Subsequently, a small number of associations between *PDE4B* and schizophrenia have been reported, as has decreased *PDE4B* expression in schizophrenia (Fatemi *et al.*, 2008), but there are too few findings yet to be confident of a genuine association. Further analyses of genes with which DISC1 interacts offers the possibility of discriminating between those myriad functions of DISC1 that are relevant to disease and those that are not.

RGS4

A *positional* candidate mapping to a putative linkage region on 1q21–q22 (see Chapter 12), *RGS4*, was also proposed as a functional candidate gene for schizophrenia. *RGS* genes encode guanine triphosphate (GTP)ase-activating proteins, which dampen the effects of neurotransmitter–receptor interaction at G protein-coupled receptors, including, for example, dopamine receptors. More specifically, *RGS4* is down-regulated in the brains of patients with schizophrenia (Chowdari *et al.*, 2002). For these reasons, Chowdari *et al.* (2002) targeted *RGS4* in samples from the US and India. Across all samples, they observed significant evidence for association, although as we have seen for other candidate genes, the associated haplotypes differed even between two samples from the US.

A series of studies followed, some supportive of *RGS4* (Williams *et al.*, 2004; Morris *et al.*, 2004), but with levels of support far short of unequivocal. Aiming to resolve some of the discrepancies, the original group coordinated a meta-analysis comprising 10 family-based association datasets and eight case-control datasets; a total of almost 14 000 subjects (Talkowski *et al.*, 2006). Across all samples, the authors found no support for association to a single specific haplotype, but they did observe significant overtransmission of two haplotypes at levels that survive correction for multiple testing. In each of the case–control and the family-based association samples, they also observed a significant excess of association signals. As discussed above, this is compatible with true association at the locus but other possible explanations cannot be fully discounted. Therefore, whilst this analysis lends credence to *RGS4* as a susceptibility gene, it does not convincingly implicate it. Additional studies have failed to resolve the complexity, with So *et al.* (2008) reporting association to one of the two main haplotypes implicated by Talkowski *et al.* (2006), and the large study of Sanders *et al.* (2008) finding nominally significant association to one of the original SNPs. In contrast, other large or fairly large studies are completely negative (Ishiguro *et al.*, 2007; Vilella *et al.*, 2008). Nevertheless, the most recent meta-analysis (June 2010) reported in the SZgene database provides nominally significant association to *RGS4*, which must therefore be considered another gene for which there is some overall evidence, albeit not definitive.

Some (Nicodemus *et al.*, 2007) have observed evidence for interaction between *RGS4* and *COMT*, and have offered the hypothesis that the differences in results across samples relate to allele frequencies at multiple interacting loci. This is a plausible explanation, but it is not as yet replicated.

On the theme of positional candidates, we should note that *RGS4* was not identified after a screen of the whole linked region, and other genes in this general linkage peak have been reported to be associated. These include *U2AF homology motive kinase 1* (*UHMK1*) (Puri *et al.*, 2007, 2008) and the *neuronal nitric oxide synthase 1 adaptor protein* (also known as *CAPON*) (Brzustowicz *et al.*, 2004). These have yet to be widely tested in other samples.

Structural genomic variation

Structural genomic variation exists in a variety of forms, including deletion, duplication, sequence inversion, and chromosomal translocation. There are several ways by which these can alter gene function, but one that is currently the subject of much interest is by altering the number of copies of genes. Structural genomic variants that are (by current convention) at least 1000 bases (1 kb) in size and which change the number of copies of a given stretch of DNA sequence are called copy number variants (CNVs).

The idea that a proportion of schizophrenia might be caused by structural variation (or indeed aneuploidy) has been around for some time. Indeed until recently, structural variants were the only class of DNA variation where a pathogenic role could have been considered virtually undisputed. This refers to 22q11DS, otherwise known as velo-cardio-facial syndrome (VCFS), DiGeorge syndrome, or Shprintzen syndrome. This syndrome involves small (most commonly ~ 3 Mb) deletions of chromosome 22q11, giving rise to a variable phenotype that involves a dramatic increase in the risk of psychosis, especially schizophrenia (Lindsay *et al.*, 1995; Murphy *et al.*, 1999), in addition to characteristic core features of dysmorphology and congenital heart disease.

With an estimated prevalence of 1 in 4000 live births, VCFS cannot be responsible for more than a small fraction (~0.05%) of cases of schizophrenia. Nevertheless, this raises the question of whether a gene within the deleted region is involved in susceptibility to schizophrenia more generally, a hypothesis supported somewhat by linkage to schizophrenia and 22q (see Chapter 12). To date, several specific schizophrenia risk genes within the deleted region have been suggested including *COMT* (see above), *proline dehydrogenase (PRODH), zinc finger, DHHC domain containing 8 (ZDHHC8)* (see Ross *et al.*, 2006), and, more recently, multiple samples support *guanine nucleotide binding protein (G protein)* and *beta polypeptide 1-like (GNB1L)* (Williams *et al.*, 2008). However, none is supported by multiple independent replications.

New technologies permit systematic genome-wide CNV scanning at increasing resolution, and it now appears CNVs are ubiquitous in the population and account for more sequence variation than SNPs. The first generation of genome-wide CNV scans have demonstrated that new CNV mutation events (so-called *denovos*) of about 100 kb or more contribute to about 10% of cases of idiopathic mental retardation (MR) and also of sporadic autism (e.g., Autism Genome Project Consortium, 2007; Sebat *et al.*, 2007). Several studies have also recently shown that CNVs play a role in schizophrenia, although the scale of their involvement and the magnitude of the associated genetic effects are both as yet unclear.

One clear line of evidence for the involvement of CNVs in schizophrenia is that genome wide, cases have a greater load of low-frequency CNVs than controls (Walsh *et al.*, 2008; International Schizophrenia Consortium, 2008; Xu *et al.*, 2008, Kirov *et al.*, 2009b). Most studies are in agreement concerning this, but there is marked variation in the magnitude of the observed effect. Currently, CNV measurement is an imprecise art, the assay platforms being very sensitive to measurement error. Thus, some of variance in the estimated effect may reflect differences in the specificity and sensitivity of CNV assays. Another potential source is the phenotypic composition of the samples, cases with early-onset or lower IQ being particularly enriched for CNVs in one study (Walsh *et al.*, 2008). Whatever the explanation, assuming for now that the largest study probably provides the best estimate across the disorder as a whole, the increase in CNV burden in schizophrenia is probably quite modest. Thus, in the International Schizophrenia Consortium study (2008) of over 6000 subjects, cases had a 1.15-fold excess of low-frequency CNVs, rising to 1.6-fold for deletions greater than 500 kb, the latter being the CNV category most enriched in cases.

Very large samples are required to unambiguously demonstrate association to specific rare events, but two genome-wide CNV studies were large enough to do exactly that (International Schizophrenia Consortium, 2008; Stefansson *et al.*, 2008). More importantly, they were in agreement regarding specific loci, namely, deletions mapping to 1q21.1 and 15q13.3. Each deletion is rare, with control frequencies less than 0.1%, and that in cases of less than 1%. However, their effect sizes are large, with an estimated OR of about 10 (Kirov *et al.*, 2009b). A third deletion at 15q11.2 was highlighted by only one of the studies (Stefansson *et al.*, 2008), but a recent re-analysis of the International Schizophrenia Consortium data confirms this locus is indeed associated with schizophrenia (Kirov *et al.*, 2009), but with a much smaller effect size (OR ~ 3) than for the other two loci. Since these landmark genome-wide CNV studies were published, targeted studies of selected loci have additionally provided very strong evidence for association between schizophrenia and microduplication at 16p11.2 (McCarthy *et al.*, 2009), and somewhat weaker, but still strong, evidence for association with microduplication at 16p13.1 (Ingason *et al.*, 2009).

The data suggest the excess CNV burden in schizophrenia reflects variants with a range of effect sizes, and there is no reason to suppose this does not include much weaker effects than have been detected so far. Some effect sizes are clearly large, but so far, none is sufficient to cause disease. Moreover, the associations between individual CNVs are not specific to schizophrenia; for example, the locus at 1q21.1 that confers high risk of schizophrenia increases risk of MR, autism, and ADHD (Mefford *et al.*, 2008), while that at 15q13.3 has been additionally implicated in idiopathic generalized epilepsy (Helbig *et al.*, 2009). Other genes or environmental factors are therefore evidently involved in the phenotypic manifestations of these CNVs. A question that has been raised before in the context of whole chromosomal abnormalities, e.g., Klienfelter and Turner syndromes, and regarding 22q11DS, which is also associated with MR and autism, is whether the CNV-related psychoses represent true forms of schizophrenia. Schizophrenia is a diagnosis based solely on clinical criteria, and since those criteria are met by individuals with the CNVs, the diagnosis is as "true" as it is in any other person with the disorder. It is also the case that in people with the CNVs, schizophrenia can occur in the absence of MR or epilepsy, and therefore it is not simply a non-specific manifestation of those disorders that can easily be placed in a separate diagnostic category. However, whether these disorders represent "true schizophrenia" in the sense that there is pathophysiological overlap between forms of disorder with and without CNVs cannot be answered until we have greater understanding about how they increase risk, how risk is raised in the wider schizophrenia population, and whether there is overlap in the pathophysiologies operating in each group. Currently, at the genetic level, there is no evidence for association between common variation within genes mapping to the CNV regions and schizophrenia (Stefansson *et al.*, 2008) indicative of overlapping pathophysiology, but this does not preclude the existence of such alleles.

Another line of enquiry based on CNVs is based upon the hypothesis that as in autism, a proportion of cases can be attributed to *denovo* CNV mutation events. Kirov *et al*, (2008) detected only a single *denovo* event after scanning 93 subjects; a duplication of 1.4 Mb of chromosome 15. They also observed a rare deletion that affects part of *neurexin 1* (*NRXN1*). Although not *de novo*, it was also carried by an affected sibling and was of interest since deletions of *NRXN1* had been observed in both autism and MR (e.g., Autism Genome Project Consortium, 2007). Moreover, NRXN1 interacts with amyloid beta A4 precursor protein-binding (APBA2), which is encoded by one of three genes in the *denovo* 1.4 Mb duplicated region of chromosome 15. Together, NRXN1 and APBA2 play a role in the development of normal synaptic function, processes that are likely fundamental to schizophrenia etiology. While firm conclusions are difficult to draw from what are effectively case reports, the case for *NRXN1* in schizophrenia is now much more convincing, with a meta-analysis of around 9000 cases and 42 000 controls (Kirov *et al.*, 2009c) reporting strong evidence for association.

As in the study of Kirov *et al.* (2008), *de novo* events were also uncommon in a study of childhood-onset schizophrenia, occurring in only two of 83 individuals (Walsh *et al.*, 2008), but a third study reached a different conclusion (Xu *et al.*, 2008), the rate of *de novo* events being about 10% in schizophrenic cases, compared with 2% in controls. More studies of parent–offspring trios (cases and controls) are therefore required to establish the extent to which *de novo* events contribute to schizophrenia. The design of one of the studies was likely to result in underestimation of the *de novo* rate (Kirov *et al.*, 2008), and as before, one can speculate that the differences between studies might reflect technical and phenotypic variation between studies. One potentially relevant phenotype highlighted by Xu *et al.* (2008) was that the increased rate of *denovos* was restricted to "sporadic" cases (no family history of schizophrenia in first- or second-degree relatives). The robustness of this

observation is limited by the small sample size of familial cases (n = 48), but intuitively, it does not seem surprising that the *de novo* introduction of a CNV with a substantial impact on risk might manifest as an apparently sporadic cases. It should be stressed that the use of sporadic here does imply the *de novo* event is causal (in the sense that it is sufficient) in such cases since, as we have seen, there are no known CNVs that occur only in cases. Even in the case of the longest established schizophrenia-related CNV (22q11DS), most carriers do not have schizophrenia.

Currently, CNVs for which there is very strong evidence for involvement in schizophrenia occur in only about 2% of cases, although there are other loci with strong but less compelling evidence (Kirov *et al.*, 2009b) and the figure will probably rise as better resolution platforms and more samples are deployed. Despite some of the uncertainties outlined above, the early work shows CNV analysis to have the potential to pinpoint novel pathogenic mechanisms, and provides a strong rationale for further work in this area as a complementary approach to more traditional SNP-based analyses.

Conclusions

Association studies in schizophrenia have gone through several phases. The first comprised studies of functional candidate genes. These have been bedeviled by methodological and interpretation difficulties, and despite the large numbers of studies reported there is no compelling evidence implicating any functional candidate gene. However, none has been studied with sufficient rigor to exclude the possibility that common variation confers susceptibility, let alone rare variation. The second wave focused upon positional candidates and here, the evidence is stronger. Currently the best supported genes are *NRG1*, *DTNBP1*, and *DISC1*, though in no case has specific risk alleles or haplotypes been robustly identified as causal, and in no case does the strength and consistency (same alleles or haplotypes across studies) of the genetic evidence equal that for genes now known to be involved in other complex disorders, or implicated in schizophrenia by GWAS.

Some of the more robust findings for other disorders doubtless reflect the fact that for some loci the effect sizes are at the larger end of the spectrum seen in common disease. However, most of the success is recent, and has come from GWAS applied to large patient and control samples and, of vital importance, follow-up analyses in even larger samples. Such approaches are currently being applied to schizophrenia and results are promising. The application of new genome-wide approaches has also revealed that submicroscopic chromosomal abnormalities play a role in at least some cases, and it seems likely that this figure will rise with the use of technologies with higher resolution. CNVs with large effect sizes will likely contribute to a minority of cases, but their identification has the potential to inform pathophysiology, and as has been the case in *VCFS* and *DISC1*, offer enticing genetic targets for animal models. As more becomes known about the involvement of specific CNV loci, it may become clinically important to detect such cases, and offer genetic counseling.

The foregoing suggests that efforts in the genetics of schizophrenia are bearing fruit, and there are strong grounds for being optimistic that research in these disorders is poised to benefit further from the same advances in genomics and post-genomics that are being successfully applied to other common non-psychiatric disorders. At present, these consist of whole genome studies aimed at detecting genetic association with SNPs and the involvement of CNVs in pathogenesis. In the near future, we can look forward to the ability to detect rare variants by pangenomic resequencing. The success of this work will depend, amongst other things, upon the assembly of large, well-phenotyped patient samples, effective collaboration, and sharing of patient resources, and the ability to handle and analyze increasingly large and complex datasets. Moreover, as more risk loci are identified, there will be an increasing imperative to focus upon translating genetic findings into clinical benefit via a greater understanding of pathogenic mechanisms, improved classification, and the development of new interventions.

References

Allen, N.C., Bagade, S., McQueen, M.B. *et al.* (2008) Systematic meta-analyses and field synopsis of genetic association studies in schizophrenia: the SzGene database. *Nature Genetics* **40**, 827–834.

Anney, R.J., Rees, M.I., Bryan, E. *et al.* (2002) Characterisation, mutation detection, and association analysis of alternative promoters and 5′ UTRs of the human dopamine D3 receptor gene in schizophrenia. *Molecular Psychiatry* **7**, 493–502.

Arinami, T., Itokawa, M., Aoki, J. *et al.* (1996) Further association study on dopamine D2 receptor variant S311C in schizophrenia and affective disorders. *American Journal of Medical Genetics* **67**, 133–138.

Arinami, T., Gao, M, Hamaguchi, H. & Toru, M. (1997) A functional polymorphism in the promoter region of the dopamine D2 receptor gene is associated with schizophrenia. *Human Molecular Genetics* **6**, 577–582.

Autism Genome Project Consortium (2007) Mapping autism risk loci using genetic linkage and chromosomal rearrangements. *Nature Genetics* **39**, 319–328.

Barnett, J.H., Scoriels, L. & Munafò, M.R. (2008) Meta-analysis of the cognitive effects of the catechol-O-methyltransferase gene Val158/108Met polymorphism. *Biological Psychiatry* **64**, 137–144.

Blackwood, D.H., Fordyce, A., Walker, M.T., St Clair, D.M., Porteous, D.J. & Muir, W.J. (2001) Schizophrenia and affective disorders-cosegregation with a translocation at chromosome 1q42 that directly disrupts brain-expressed genes: clinical and

P300 findings in a family. *American Journal of Human Genetics* **69**, 428–433.

Blake, D.J., Forrest, M., Chapman, R.M., Tinsley, C.L., O'Donovan, M.C. & Owen, M.J. (2010) TCF4, schizophrenia, and Pitt-Hopkins Syndrome. *Schizophrenia Bulletin* **36**, 443–447.

Bray, N.J., Buckland, P.R., Williams, N.M. *et al.* (2003) A haplotype implicated in schizophrenia susceptibility is associated with reduced COMT expression in human brain. *American Journal of Human Genetics* **73**, 152–161.

Bray, N.J., Buckland, P.R., Hall, H., Owen, M.J. & O'Donovan, M.C. (2004) The serotonin-2A receptor gene locus does not contain common polymorphism affecting mRNA levels in adult brain. *Molecular Psychiatry* **9**, 109–114.

Breen, G., Brown, J., Maude, S. *et al.* (1999) −141 C del/ins polymorphism of the dopamine receptor 2 gene is associated with schizophrenia in a British population. *American Journal of Medical Genetics* **88**, 407–410.

Brzustowicz, L.M., Simone, J., Mohseni, P. *et al.* (2004) Linkage disequilibrium mapping of schizophrenia susceptibility to the CAPON region of chromosome 1q22. *American Journal of Human Genetics* **74**, 1057–1063.

Buckland, P.R., O'Donovan, M.C. & McGuffin, P. (1992) Changes in dopamine D1, D2 and D3 receptor mRNA levels in rat brain following antipsychotic treatment. *Psychopharmacology (Berlin)* **106**, 479–483.

Callicott, J.H., Straub, R.E., Pezawas, L. *et al.* (2005) Variation in DISC1 affects hippocampal structure and function and increases risk for schizophrenia. *Proceedings of the National Academy of Science of the USA* **102**, 8627–8632.

Caspi, A., Moffitt, T.E., Cannon, M. *et al.* (2005) Moderation of the effect of adolescent-onset cannabis use on adult psychosis by a functional polymorphism in the catechol-O-methyltransferase gene: longitudinal evidence of a gene × environment interaction. *Biological Psychiatry* **57**, 1117–1127.

Chen, J., Lipska, B.K., Halim, N. *et al.* (2004) Functional analysis of genetic variation in catechol-O-methyltransferase (COMT): effects on mRNA, protein, and enzyme activity in postmortem human brain. *American Journal of Human Genetics* **75**, 807–821.

Chowdari, K.V., Mirnics, K., Semwal, P. *et al.* (2002) Association and linkage analyses of RGS4 polymorphisms in schizophrenia. *Human Molecular Genetics* **11**, 1373–1380.

Chumakov, I., Blumenfeld, M., Guerassimenko, O. *et al.* (2002) Genetic and physiological data implicating the new human gene G72 and the gene for D-amino acid oxidase in schizophrenia. *Proceedings of the National Academy of Science of the USA* **99**, 13675–13680.

Corvin, A., McGhee, K.A., Murphy, K. *et al.* (2007) Evidence for association and epistasis at the DAOA/G30 and D-amino acid oxidase loci in an Irish schizophrenia sample. *American Journal of Medical Genetics Part B Neuropsychiatric Genetics* **144B**, 949–953.

Craddock, N., Owen, M.J. & O'Donovan, M.C. (2006) The catechol-O-methyl transferase (COMT) gene as a candidate for psychiatric phenotypes: evidence and lessons. *Molecular Psychiatry* **11**, 446–458.

Cravchik, A., Sibley, D.R. & Gejman, P.V. (1996) Functional analysis of the human D2 dopamine receptor missense variants. *Journal of Biological Chemistry* **271**, 26013–26017.

Crocq, M.A., Mant, R., Asherson, P. *et al.* (1992) Association between schizophrenia and homozygosity at the dopamine D3 receptor gene. *Journal of Medical Genetics* **29**, 858–860.

Daniels, J.K., Williams, N.M., Williams, J. *et al.* (1996) No evidence for allelic association between schizophrenia and a polymorphism determining high or low catechol O-methyltransferase activity. *American Journal of Psychiatry* **153**, 268–270.

Di Giorgio, A., Blasi, G., Sambataro, F. *et al.* (2008) Association of the SerCys DISC1 polymorphism with human hippocampal formation gray matter and function during memory encoding. *European Journal of Neuroscience* **28**, 2129–136.

Domínguez, E., Loza, M.I., Padín, F. *et al.* (2007) Extensive linkage disequilibrium mapping at HTR2A and DRD3 for schizophrenia susceptibility genes in the Galician population. *Schizophrenia Research* **90**, 123–129.

Duan, J., Wainwright, M.S., Comeron, J.M. *et al.* (2003) Synonymous mutations in the human dopamine receptor D2 (DRD2) affect mRNA stability and synthesis of the receptor. *Human Molecular Genetics* **12**, 205–216.

Eastwood, S.L., Walker, M., Hyde, T.M., Kleinman, J.E. & Harrison, P.J. (2010) The DISC1 Ser704Cys substitution affects centrosomal localisation of its binding partner PCM1 in glia in human brain. *Human Molecular Genetics* **19**, 2487–2496.

Egan, M.F., Goldberg, T.E., Kolachana, B.S. *et al.* (2001) Effect of COMT Val108/158 Met genotype on frontal lobe function and risk for schizophrenia. *Proceedings of the National Academy of Sciences of the USA* **98**, 6917–6922.

Esslinger, C., Walter, H., Kirsch, P. *et al.* (2009) Neural mechanisms of a genome-wide supported psychosis variant. *Science* **324**, 605.

Fan, J.B. & Sklar, P. (2005) Meta-analysis reveals association between serotonin transporter gene STin2 VNTR polymorphism and schizophrenia. *Molecular Psychiatry* **10**, 928–938.

Fatemi, S.H., King, D.P., Reutiman, T.J. *et al.* (2008) PDE4B polymorphisms and decreased PDE4B expression are associated with schizophrenia. *Schizophrenia Research* **101**, 36–49.

Georgieva, L., Dimitrova, A., Ivanov, D. *et al.* (2008) Support for neuregulin 1 as a susceptibility gene for bipolar disorder and schizophrenia. *Biological Psychiatry* **64**, 419–427.

Glatt, S.J. & Jönsson, E.G. (2006) The Cys allele of the DRD2 Ser311Cys polymorphism has a dominant effect on risk for schizophrenia: evidence from fixed- and random-effects meta-analyses. *American Journal of Medical Genetics B Neuropsychiatric Genetics* **141B**, 149–154.

Glatt, S.J., Faraone, S.V. & Tsuang, M.T. (2003) Schizophrenia is not associated with DRD4 48-base-pair- repeat length or individual alleles: results of a meta-analysis. *Biological Psychiatry* **54**, 629–635.

Glatt, S.J., Faraone, S.V. & Tsuang, M.T. (2004) DRD2 -141C insertion/deletion polymorphism is not associated with schizophrenia: results of a meta-analysis. *American Journal of Medical Genetics B Neuropsychiatric Genetics* **128B**, 21–23.

Glatt, S.J., Faraone, S.V., Lasky-Su, J.A. *et al.* (2009) Family-based association testing strongly implicates DRD2 as a risk gene for schizophrenia in Han Chinese from Taiwan. *Molecular Psychiatry* **14**, 885–893.

Gogos, J.A., Morgan, M., Luine, V. *et al.* (1998) Catechol-O-methyltransferase-deficient mice exhibit sexually dimorphic changes in catecholamine levels and behavior. *Proceedings of the National Academy of Science of the USA* **95**, 9991–9996.

Green, E.K., Norton, N., Peirce, T. *et al.* (2006) Evidence that a DISC1 frame-shift deletion associated with psychosis in a single family may not be a pathogenic mutation. *Molecular Psychiatry* **11**, 798–799.

Hamshere, M.L., Bennett, P., Williams, N. *et al.* (2005) Genomewide linkage scan in schizoaffective disorder: significant evidence for linkage at 1q42 close to DISC1, and suggestive evidence at 22q11 and 19p13. *Archives of General Psychiatry* **62**, 1081–1088.

Hattori, E., Liu, C., Badner, J.A. *et al.* (2003) Polymorphisms at the G72/G30 gene locus, on 13q33, are associated with bipolar disorder in two independent pedigree series. *American Journal of Human Genetics* **72**, 1131–1140.

Helbig, I., Mefford, H.C., Sharp, A.J. *et al.* (2009) 15q13.3 microdeletions increase risk of idiopathic generalized epilepsy. *Nature Genetics* **41**, 160–162.

Hennah, W., Thomson, P., McQuillin, A. *et al.* (2009) DISC1 association, heterogeneity and interplay in schizophrenia and bipolar disorder. *Molecular Psychiatry* **14**, 863–873.

Hodgkinson, C.A., Goldman, D., Jaeger, J. *et al.* (2004) Disrupted in schizophrenia 1 (DISC1): association with schizophrenia, schizoaffective disorder, and bipolar disorder. *American Journal of Human Genetics* **75**, 862–872.

Ikeda, M., Iwata, N., Suzuki, T. *et al.* (2006) No association of serotonin transporter gene (SLC6A4) with schizophrenia and bipolar disorder in Japanese patients: association analysis based on linkage disequilibrium. *Journal of Neural Transmission* **113**, 899–905.

Inayama, Y., Yoneda, H., Sakai, T. *et al.* (1996) Positive association between a DNA sequence variant in the serotonin 2A receptor gene and schizophrenia. *American Journal of Medical Genetics* **67**, 103–105.

Ingason, A., Rujescu, D., Cichon, S. *et al.* (2009) Copy number variations of chromosome 16p13.1 region associated with schizophrenia. *Molecular Psychiatry* 2009 Sept 29 [Epub ahead of print].

International Schizophrenia Consortium (2008) Rare chromosomal deletions and duplications increase risk of schizophrenia. *Nature* **455**, 237–241.

International Schizophrenia Consortium (2009) Common polygenic variation contributes to risk of schizophrenia and bipolar disorder. *Nature* **460**, 748–752.

Ishiguro, H., Horiuchi, Y., Koga, M. *et al.* (2007) RGS4 is not a susceptibility gene for schizophrenia in Japanese: association study in a large case-control population. *Schizophrenia Research* **89**, 161–164.

Jönsson, E.G., Flyckt, L., Burgert, E. *et al.* (2003) Dopamine D3 receptor gene Ser9Gly variant and schizophrenia: association study and meta-analysis. *Psychiatric Genetics* **13**, 1–12.

Kirov, G., Gumus, D., Chen, W. *et al.* (2008) Comparative genome hybridization suggests a role for NRXN1 and APBA2 in schizophrenia. *Human Molecular Genetics* **17**, 458–465.

Kirov, G., Zaharieva, I., Georgieva, L. *et al.* (2009a) A genomewide association study in 574 schizophrenia trios using DNA pooling. *Molecular Psychiatry* **14**, 796–803.

Kirov, G., Grozeva, D., Norton, N. *et al.* (2009b) Support for the involvement of large copy number variants in the pathogenesis of schizophrenia. *Human Molecular Genetics* **18**, 1497–1503.

Kirov, G., Rujescu, D., Ingason, A., Collier, D.A., O'Donovan, M.C. & Owen MJ. (2009c) Neurexin 1 (NRXN1) deletions in schizophrenia. *Schizophrenia Bulletin* **35**, 851–854.

Klein, R.J., Zeiss, C., Chew, E.Y. *et al.* (2005) Complement factor H polymorphism in age-related macular degeneration. *Science* **308**, 385–389.

Lawford, B.R., Young, R.M., Swagell, C.D. *et al.* (2005) The C/C genotype of the C957T polymorphism of the dopamine D2 receptor is associated with schizophrenia. *Schizophrenia Research* **73**, 31–37.

Lee, S.G., Joo, Y., Kim, B. *et al.* (2005) Association of Ala72Ser polymorphism with COMT enzyme activity and the risk of schizophrenia in Koreans. *Human Genetics* **116**, 319–328.

Lencz, T., Morgan, T.V., Athanasiou, M. *et al.* (2007) Converging evidence for a pseudoautosomal cytokine receptor gene locus in schizophrenia. *Molecular Psychiatry* **12**, 572–580.

Lesch, K.P., Bengel, D., Heils, A. *et al.* (1996) Association of anxiety-related traits with a polymorphism in the serotonin transporter gene regulatory region. *Science* **274**, 1527–1531.

Lin, P.I., Vance, J.M. Pericak-Vance, M.A. & Martin, E.R. (2007) No gene is an island: the flip-flop phenomenon. *American Journal of Human Genetics* **80**, 531–538.

Lindsay, E.A., Morris, M.A., Gos, A. *et al.* (1995) Schizophrenia and chromosomal deletions within 22q11.2. *American Journal of Human Genetics* **56**, 1502–1503.

Ma, G., *et al.* (2008) The Ser9Gly polymorphism of the dopamine D3 receptor gene and risk of schizophrenia: an association study and a large meta-analysis. *Schizophrenia Research* **101**, 26–35.

Mattay, V.S., Goldberg, T.E., Fera, F. *et al.* (2003) Catechol O-methyltransferase val158-met genotype and individual variation in the brain response to amphetamine. *Proceedings of the National Academy of Science of the USA* **100**, 6186–6191.

McCarthy, S.E., Makarov, V., Kirov, G. *et al.* (2009) Microduplications of 16p11.2 are associated with schizophrenia. *Nature Genetics* **41**, 1223–1227.

Mefford, H.C., Sharp, R.J., Baker, C. *et al.* (2008) Recurrent rearrangements of chromosome 1q21.1 and variable pediatric phenotypes. *New England Journal of Medicine* **359**, 1685–1699.

Millar, J.K., Wilson-Annan, J.C., Anderson, S. *et al.* (2000) Disruption of two novel genes by a translocation co-segregating with schizophrenia. *Human Molecular Genetics* **9**, 1415–1423.

Millar, J.K., Pickard, B.S., Mackie, S. *et al.* (2005) DISC1 and PDE4B are interacting genetic factors in schizophrenia that regulate cAMP signaling. *Science* **310**, 1187–1191.

Monakhov, M., Golimbet, V., Abramson, L., Kaleda, V. & Karpov, V. (2008) Association study of three polymorphisms in the dopamine D2 receptor gene and schizophrenia in the Russian population. *Schizophrenia Research* **100**, 302–307.

Morris, D.W., Rodgers, A., McGhee, K.A. *et al.* (2004) Confirming RGS4 as a susceptibility gene for schizophrenia. *American Journal of Medical Genetics* **125B**, 50–53.

Moskvina, V. & O'Donovan, M.C. (2007) Detailed analysis of the relative power of direct and indirect association studies and the implications for their interpretation. *Human Heredity* **64**, 63–73.

Moskvina, V., Craddock, N., Holmans, P., Owen, M.J. & O'Donovan, M.C. (2006) Effects of differential genotyping error rate on the type I error probability of case-control studies. *Human Heredity* **61**, 55–64.

Murphy, K.C., Jones, L.A. & Owen, M.J. (1999) High rates of schizophrenia in adults with velo-cardio-facial syndrome. *Archives of General Psychiatry* **56**, 940–945.

Nackley, A.G., Shabalina, S.A., Tchivileva, I.E. *et al.* (2006) Human catechol-O-methyltransferase haplotypes modulate protein expression by altering mRNA secondary structure. *Science* **314**, 1930–1933.

Nicodemus, K.K., Callicott, J.H., Higier, R.G. *et al.* (2007) Evidence for statistical epistasis between catechol-O-methyl-transferase (COMT) and polymorphisms in RGS4, G72 (DAOA), GRM3, and DISC1: influence on risk of schizophrenia. *Human Genetics* **120**, 889–906.

O'Donovan, M.C., Craddock, N., Norton, N. *et al.* (2008) Identification of novel schizophrenia loci by genome-wide association and follow-up. *Nature Genetics* **40**, 1053–1055.

Papaleo, F., Crawley, J.N., Song, J. *et al.* (2008) Genetic dissection of the role of catechol-O-Methyltransferase in cognition and stress reactivity in mice. *The Journal of Neuroscience* **28**, 8709–8723.

Polesskaya, O.O. & Sokolov, B.P. (2002) Differential expression of the C and T alleles of the 5-HT2A receptor gene in the temporal cortex of normal individuals and schizophrenics. *Journal of Neuroscience Research* **67**, 812–822.

Puri, V., McQuillin, A, Choudhury, K. *et al.* (2007) Fine mapping by genetic association implicates the chromosome 1q23.3 gene UHMK1, encoding a serine/threonine protein kinase, as a novel schizophrenia susceptibility gene. *Biological Psychiatry* **61**, 873–879.

Puri, V., McQuillan, A., Datta, S. *et al.* (2008) Confirmation of the genetic association between the U2AF homology motif (UHM) kinase 1 (UHMK1) gene and schizophrenia on chromosome 1q23.3. *European Journal of Human Genetics* **16**, 1275–1282.

Rietschel, M., Beckmann, L., Strohmaier, J. *et al.* (2008) G72 and its association with major depression and neuroticism in large population-based groups from Germany. *American Journal of Psychiatry* **165**, 753–762.

Ross, C.A., Margolis, R.L., Reading, S.A., Pletnikov, M. & Coyle, J.T. (2006) Neurobiology of schizophrenia. *Neuron* **52**, 139–153.

Sanders, A.R., Duan, J., Levinson, D.F. *et al.* (2008) No significant association of 14 candidate genes with schizophrenia in a large European ancestry sample: implications for psychiatric genetics. *American Journal of Psychiatry* **165**, 497–506.

Schumacher, J., Jamra, R.A., Freudenberg, J. *et al.* (2004) Examination of G72 and D-amino-acid oxidase as genetic risk factors for schizophrenia and bipolar affective disorder. *Molecular Psychiatry* **9**, 203–207.

Schumacher, J., Laje, G., Abou Jamra, R. *et al.* (2009) The DISC locus and schizophrenia: evidence from an association study in a central European sample and from a meta-analysis across different European populations. *Human Molecular Genetics* **18**, 2719–2727.

Sebat, J., Lakshmi, B., Malhotra, D. *et al.* (2007) Strong association of de *novo* copy number mutations with autism. *Science* **316**, 445–449.

Shi, J., Badner, J.A., Gershon, E.S. & Liu, C. (2008) Allelic association of G72/G30 with schizophrenia and bipolar disorder: a comprehensive meta-analysis. *Schizophrenia Research* **98**, 89–97.

Shi, J., Badner, J.A., Gershon, E.S. *et al.* (2009a) Further evidence for an association of G72/G30 with schizophrenia in Chinese. *Schizophrenia Research* **107**, 324–326.

Shi, J., Levinson, D.F., Duan, J. *et al.* (2009b) Common variants on chromosome 6p22.1 are associated with schizophrenia. *Nature* **460**, 753–757.

Shifman, S., Bronstein, M., Sternfeld, M. *et al.* (2002) A highly significant association between a COMT haplotype and schizophrenia. *American Journal of Human Genetics* **71**, 1296–1302.

Shifman, S., Johannesson, M., Bronstein, M. *et al.* (2008) Genome-wide association identifies a common variant in the reelin gene that increases the risk of schizophrenia only in women. *Public Library of Science Genetics* **4**, e28.

Slifstein, M., Kolachana, B., Simpson, E.H. *et al.* (2008) COMT genotype predicts cortical-limbic D1 receptor availability measured with [11C]NNC112 and PET. *Molecular Psychiatry* **13**, 821–827.

So, H.C., Chen, R.Y., Chen, E.Y., Cheung, E.F. & Li, T. (2008) Sham PC. An association study of RGS4 polymorphisms with clinical phenotypes of schizophrenia in a Chinese population. *American Journal of Medical Genetics B Neuropsychiatric Genetics* **147B**, 77–85.

St Clair, D., Blackwood, D., Muir, W. *et al.* (1990) Association within a family of a balanced autosomal translocation with major mental illness. *Lancet* **336**, 13–16.

Stefansson, H., Rujescu, D., Cichon, S. *et al.* (2008) Large recurrent microdeletions associated with schizophrenia. *Nature* **455**, 232–236.

Stefansson, H., Ophoff, R.A., Steinberg, S. *et al.* (2009) Common variants conferring risk of schizophrenia. *Nature* **460**, 744–747.

Sullivan, P.F., de Guess, E.J., Willemsen, G. *et al.* (2008) Genomewide association for schizophrenia in the CATIE study: results of stage 1. *Molecular Psychiatry* **13**, 570–584.

Talkowski, M.E., Seltman, H., Bassett, A.S. *et al.* (2006) Evaluation of a susceptibility gene for schizophrenia: genotype based meta-analysis of RGS4 polymorphisms from thirteen independent samples. *Biological Psychiatry* **60**, 152–162.

Talkowski, M.E., Kirov, G., Bamne, M. *et al.* (2008) A network of dopaminergic gene variations implicated as risk factors for schizophrenia. *Human Molecular Genetics* **17**, 747–758.

Thapar, A., O'Donovan, M. & Owen, M.J. (2005) The genetics of attention deficit hyperactivity disorder. *Human Molecular Genetics* **14** (Spec No. 2), R275–282.

Tomppo, L., Hennah, W., Miettunen, J. *et al.* (2009) Association of variants in DISC1 with psychosis-related traits in a large population cohort. *Archives of General Psychiatry* **66**, 134–141.

Tunbridge, E.M., Bannerman, D.M., Sharp, T. & Harrison, P.J. (2004) Catechol-o-methyltransferase inhibition improves set-shifting performance and elevates stimulated dopamine release in the rat prefrontal cortex. *Journal of Neuroscience* **24**, 5331–5335.

Vilella, E., Costas, J., Sanjuan, J. *et al.* (2008) Association of schizophrenia with DTNBP1 but not with DAO, DAOA, NRG1 and RGS4 nor their genetic interaction. *Journal of Psychiatric Research* **42**, 278–288.

Walsh, T., McClellan, J.M., McCarthy, S.E. *et al.* (2008) Rare structural variants disrupt multiple genes in neurodevelopmental pathways in schizophrenia. *Science* **320**, 539–543.

Wang, X., He, G., Gu, N. *et al.* (2004) Association of G72/G30 with schizophrenia in the Chinese population. *Biochemistry and Biophysics Research Communications* **319**, 1281–1286.

Watanabe, Y., Nunokawa, A., Kaneko, N. & Someya, T. (2007) The tryptophan hydroxylase 1 (TPH1) gene and risk of schizophrenia: a moderate-scale case-control study and meta-analysis. *Neuroscience Research* **59**, 322–326.

Wellcome Trust Case Control Consortium (2007) Genome-wide association study of 14000 cases of seven common diseases and 3,000 shared controls. *Nature* **447**, 661–678.

Williams, J., *et al.* (1996) Association between schizophrenia and T102C polymorphism of the 5-hydroxytryptamine type 2a-receptor gene. European Multicentre Association Study of Schizophrenia (EMASS) Group. *Lancet* **347**, 1294–1296.

Williams, N.M., Preece, A., Spurlock, G. *et al.* (2004) Support for RGS4 as a susceptibility gene for schizophrenia. *Biological Psychiatry* **55**, 192–195.

Williams, N.M., Green, E.K., Macgregor, S. *et al.* (2006) Variation at the DAOA/G30 locus influences susceptibility to major mood episodes but not psychosis in schizophrenia and bipolar disorder. *Archives of General Psychiatry* **63**, 366–373.

Williams, H.J., Owen, M.J. & O'Donovan, M.C. (2007) Is *COMT* a susceptibility gene for schizophrenia? *Schizophrenia Bulletin* **33**, 635–641.

Williams, N.M., Glaser, B., Norton, N. *et al.* (2008) Strong evidence that GNB1L is associated with schizophrenia. *Human Molecular Genetics* **17**, 555–566.

Williams, H.J., Norton, N., Dwyer, S. *et al.* (2010) Fine mapping of ZNF804A and genome-wide significant evidence for its involvement in schizophrenia and bipolar disorder. *Molecular Psychiatry* Apr 6 [Epub ahead of print].

Xu, B., Roos, J.L., Levy, S., van Rensburg, E.J., Gogos, J.A. & Karayiorgou, M. (2008) Strong association of de novo copy number mutations with sporadic schizophrenia. *Nature Genetics* **40**, 880–885.

Zaboli, G., Jönsson, E.G., Gizatullin, R. *et al.* (2006) Tryptophan hydroxylase-1 gene variants associated with schizophrenia. *Biological Psychiatry* **60**, 563–569.

Zammit, S., Spurlock, G., Williams, H. *et al.* (2007) Genotype effects of CHRNA7, CNR1 and COMT in schizophrenia: interactions with tobacco and cannabis use. *British Journal of Psychiatry* **191**, 402–407.

Zeggini, E., Weedon, M.N., Lindgren, C.M. *et al.* (2007) Replication of genome-wide association signals in U.K. samples reveals risk loci for type 2 diabetes. *Science* **316**, 1336–1341.

Zeggini, E., Scott, L.J., Saxena, R. *et al.* (2008) Meta-analysis of genome-wide association data and large-scale replication identifies additional susceptibility loci for type 2 diabetes. *Nature Genetics* **40**, 638–645.

Zhong, L., Cherry, T., Bies, C.E., Florence, M.A. & Gerges, N.Z. (2009) Neurogranin enhances synaptic strength through its interaction with calmodulin. *EMBO Journal* **28**, 3027–3039.

14

Intermediate phenotypes in genetic studies of schizophrenia

Michael F. Egan[1] and Tyrone D. Cannon[2]

[1]Merck Research Laboratories, Merck & Co, Inc; North Wales, PA, USA
[2]Departments of Psychology and Psychiatry and Biobehavioral Sciences, Staglin Center for Cognitive Neuroscience, and Semel Institute for Neuroscience and Human Behavior University of California, Los Angeles, Los Angeles, CA, USA

Introduction

Intermediate phenotypes, or "endophenotypes", generally refer to clinical or biological measures related to genetic risk for schizophrenia. The concept was initially introduced by Shields and Gottesman (1972) and referred specifically to unobserved "internal" traits. Since then, many views on the definition and properties of intermediate phenotypes have been put forward. These views generally share the notion that endophenotypes are heritable, biological abnormalities that have a simpler genetic architecture compared to schizophrenia itself. Furthermore, they lie in an intermediate position between genes and clinical symptoms (Plate 14.1). As such, they should provide substantially more power for finding disease genes. Some geneticists, however, have suggested that the intermediate phenotype approach is misguided and unlikely to inform the discovery of schizophrenia genes. One concern is that they may be just as complex from a genetic standpoint as schizophrenia itself (e.g., Flint & Munafo, 2007).

From an historical perspective, interest in intermediate phenotypes was fueled by the seemingly intractable obstacles that confounded early linkage studies. Despite evidence that schizophrenia is largely genetic, initial linkage studies were unsuccessful. Problems included unknown mode of inheritance, genetic heterogeneity, phenocopies, and incomplete penetrance (e.g., Lander & Schork, 1994). Furthermore, the exact phenotype was uncertain, as family studies have suggested that heritability increased when the affected status included some personality disorders. The intermediate phenotype strategy offered hope of identifying elemental, genetically tractable traits related to risk which could be used as a primary phenotype, in lieu of diagnosis, in linkage studies.

As biological abnormalities were first identified in schizophrenia, follow-up family studies found that first-degree relatives sometimes had similar abnormalities, suggesting they could be heritable traits. These early studies included measures of eye tracking dysfunction, sensory gating, and cognition. To further qualify these measures as valid intermediate phenotypes, investigators evaluated other properties, such as stability over time, response to neuroleptic treatment, and, critically, genetic architecture. Regarding the latter, some traits appeared at first to have an autosomal dominant mode of transmission, ideal for linkage studies. Unfortunately, later studies suggested that, by and large, these traits were most likely polygenic, for which linkage approaches are not well suited. More

Schizophrenia, 3rd edition. Edited by Daniel R. Weinberger and Paul J Harrison © 2011 Blackwell Publishing Ltd.

recently, advances in genetics have led largely to the abandonment of linkage in favor of association designs, which are substantially more powerful and flexible. As a result, intermediate phenotypes have been included in many association studies, where they have played an increasingly prominent role in providing convergent evidence for the role of specific genes in the biology of schizophrenia.

The list of putative intermediate phenotypes has become quite extensive and includes a variety of eye tracking, cognitive, neurophysiological, and neuroimaging measures. Many of these meet generally agreed criteria for good intermediate phenotypes, such as being stable, quantitative traits related to genetic risk for schizophrenia. Increasingly, however, the qualifying studies that demonstrate such properties are being bypassed. Because of the ease of genotyping and the development of large clinical datasets, it is now possible to look directly at the effects of genetic polymorphisms on biological measures related to schizophrenia. Significant genotype–phenotype associations are becoming *ipso facto* evidence that a measure has genetic determinants. For example, a promising single nucleotide polymorphism (SNP) rs1344706, in the schizophrenia candidate gene, *ZNF804A*, is significantly associated with the functional coupling of the dorso-lateral prefrontal cortex [DLPFC; assessed with functional magnetic resonance imaging (fMRI)] across hemispheres and with the hippocampus (Esslinger *et al.*, 2009). This functional coupling phenotype, recently shown to be abnormal in schizophrenia, had not been previously examined in family studies to assess heritability but could now be viewed as an intermediate phenotype. This example, and others like it, may be a harbinger of things to come, where prequalified intermediate phenotypes will not simply be used as phenotypes *in lieu* of diagnosis to find genes in association studies. Rather, a wide variety of biological measures will be used to explore and understand the biology of specific candidate genes, which themselves may only be weakly associated with schizophrenia.

In this chapter, we review the existing literature on intermediate phenotypes associated with schizophrenia. The primary focus is on studies that have taken a traditional approach to qualifying putative traits. We also include examples of measures whose primary qualification is a positive association study. In the first section, we describe methodological issues pertinent to the use of intermediate phenotypes in genetic studies. In subsequent sections we review studies that attempt to qualify specific measures and group them based on methodology (e.g., eye tracking, imaging, electrophysiology). Where relevant, we include results of genetic studies using these phenotypes. Overall, the data show that a number of stable, neurobiological abnormalities are present in unaffected family members and are related to genetic risk for schizophrenia. Some

measures, particularly those linked closely to disease pathophysiology, have been associated with specific gene variants and have provided compelling, convergent data implicating specific genetic mechanisms. Critical challenges for the future will be sorting out which putative phenotypes merit intensive genetic investigation and which genotype–phenotype associations are truly relevant to the pathophysiology of schizophrenia.

Methodological issues

Characteristics of valid intermediate phenotypes

As mentioned above, various criteria have been proposed for validating measures as intermediate phenotypes (e.g., Cannon & Keller, 2006). These have included, first and most obviously, that intermediate phenotypes should be heritable. Approaches to demonstrate heritability are reviewed in the next section. Second, intermediate phenotypes should be associated with causes rather than effects of a disorder or its treatment. Putative traits should be abnormal in patients and present from before illness onset. Ideally, an intermediate phenotype should not be impacted by treatment with neuroleptics and other drugs, as this adds environmental variance and reduces genetic variance. Third, as traits, intermediate phenotypes should vary continuously in the general population and can therefore be studied in non-affected populations, greatly simplifying the sampling process. Population-based studies on such intermediate phenotypes circumvent some of the problems associated with ascertainment biases and illness-related factors that confound assessments in patients. Finally, intermediate phenotypes likely to be of greatest use in psychiatric genetics are those that reflect different levels of analysis of an abnormally functioning neural system (Cannon & Rosso, 2002). In this model, a specific set of genetic variants gives rise to emergent abnormalities at progressively higher levels of analysis, such as cellular function, local neural system activity, and the interaction of multiple neural systems (Plate 14.1). A critical by-product of traversing these multilevel intermediate phenotypes in humans is the facilitation of their translation into animal models of these diseases.

Determining genetic variance for intermediate phenotypes

Many biological findings in patients with schizophrenia may be related to environmental factors, such as chronic illness, head injury, substance abuse, or neuroleptic treatment, rather than to schizophrenia genes. An essential feature for intermediate phenotypes is that they have a significant genetic component related to risk for schizophrenia. Such a relationship can be established in genetic epidemiological studies of relatives who vary in genetic resemblance (i.e., twins, first and second degree), as well as spouses and adoptees, to infer the genetic and environmental components of total phenotypic variance (Plomin *et al.*, 1990). Such studies are lacking for most candidate intermediate phenotypes; the majority of studies have included only one class of relatives—siblings or parents. Correlations between first-degree relatives set an upper limit on heritability. Studies of first-degree relatives are unable, however, to exclude shared environment as a cause for family correlations. Nevertheless, at least for some phenotypes, shared environment is likely to play only a small role, and much of the variance in familial correlations is likely brought about by genetic factors that increase risk for schizophrenia. Data from twin and family studies, for example, suggest that familial aggregation of schizophrenia in general is largely accounted for by genetic and not shared environmental factors (McGue & Gottesman, 1989).

Most investigations of intermediate phenotypes begin by looking for a difference between first-degree relatives, typically unaffected by psychiatric illness, and controls. One advantage to studying unaffected relatives is that they do not share illness-related environmental factors, such as neuroleptic treatment, poor medical care, etc. The strength of genetic effect can be estimated using the intraclass correlation coefficient (ICC) or relative risk measures. The former is the classical method used with quantitative traits. Relative risk (percentage sibs "affected"/percentage controls " affected"), on the other hand, looks specifically for heritability of *impairment* (e.g., 1 SD below the control mean) (Egan *et al.*, 2000, 2001a). A few notable studies have used monozygotic (MZ) and dizygotic (DZ) twin pairs and matched control pairs (e.g., (Cannon *et al.*, 2000; Glahn *et al.*, 2003; Johnson *et al.*, 2003; McNeil *et al.*, 2000). In this design, the intermediate phenotype can be evaluated for dose dependency with genetic risk by comparing the unaffected MZ co-twins, who share 100% of their genes with an affected individual, the unaffected DZ co-twins, who share 50% of their genes, and normal controls. In addition, the non-genetic component can be isolated by subtracting the value of the unaffected from the affected co-twin among MZ pairs (Cannon & Rosso, 2002).

Despite substantial efforts to measure the heritability of candidate traits, replication has sometimes been challenging. Several factors may be involved. First, initial reports of putative traits typically include small numbers of subjects who are not systematically ascertained. Second, control groups are poorly matched, and often "supernormal" with no psychopathology or higher IQs than relatives. In contrast, family cohorts are frequently mixtures of parents and siblings with a variety of psychiatric disorders.

Both age and psychiatric comorbidity could spuriously increase abnormalities in family members.

Design of genetic studies using intermediate phenotypes

The two traditional approaches to finding genes for complex disorders are linkage and association (see Chapter 12). Linkage, which uses two or more members from the same family, may be underpowered relative to association studies for complex traits (Risch & Merikangas, 1996), although for phenotypes with a simple mode of inheritance this may not be the case. For example, one study suggested that abnormal sensory gating, assessed using the P50 wave, could have a simple Mendelian inheritance pattern (Siegel *et al.*, 1984). For most of the intermediate phenotypes described below, however, the genetic architecture is uncertain and likely polygenic. Therefore, linkage may not be optimal. A second issue with linkage is that using either elderly or very young subjects in multigenerational families can introduce additional variance from aging. Using age as a covariate may not adequately adjust biological or cognitive measures because they may have a non-linear relationship to age. An alternative linkage design, which uses affected sib pairs, could also be problematic given the high rates of drug and alcohol abuse that confound most phenotypic measures described below. Excluding such subjects makes recruiting adequate numbers extremely difficult and also raises questions concerning representativeness of samples.

Some of the limitations of linkage are avoided using association methods, which include case–control and family-based designs. Family-based designs use genotypes of family members as controls, including parents (for qualitative phenotypes; Spielman *et al.*, 1993) or siblings (for qualitative or quantitative measures; Allison *et al.*, 1999). Given the issues related to age mentioned above, using sibs may provide an advantage over multigenerational designs. A recent popular method is the whole genome association study, where case–control samples are compared across the entire genome using chip-based SNPs. Concerns about population stratification can be addressed with genomic controls. Given their many advantages, association designs will likely remain the method of choice for the foreseeable future. Association studies have been used, for example, with single groups alone, such as control groups, where one can assess association between candidate genes and specific traits, such as fMRI-derived regional brain activation (Hariri *et al.*, 2002), dopamine release (Slifstein *et al.*, 2008), or gene expression levels in human brain tissue (e.g., Egan *et al.*, 2004). Association designs combined with advances in genetics have thus greatly expanded the scope of traits amenable to genetic dissection.

Eye tracking dysfunction

Abnormalities in eye tracking are one of the first and most extensively studied candidate intermediate phenotypes in schizophrenia and thus serve as a good starting point for a review of the subject. Decades of research on eye tracking illustrate the problems that face efforts to use intermediate phenotypes. Overall, the data suggest that eye tracking dysfunction (ETD) is present and familial in schizophrenia but its suitability as an intermediate phenotype remains uncertain. As illustrated in subsequent sections, interest in other phenotypes, such as cognitive impairment and brain imaging measures, have supplanted ETD.

Observed early in the 20th century, ETD was rediscovered by Holzman *et al.* (1973) who also noted impairment in unaffected relatives (Holzman *et al.*, 1974). The initial excitement that ETD may identify a simple Mendelian trait related to risk for schizophrenia (Holzman *et al.*, 1988) gradually gave way as additional studies produced conflicting findings. A review of this extensive literature highlights many of the issues that confront and confound studies of intermediate phenotypes. For example, precisely which measures should be used in genetic studies? To what degree is ETD genetic, and how is it related to risk for schizophrenia? Is ETD affected by neuroleptics? Unfortunately, despite many years of intensive effort, it remains uncertain how useful ETD may be for finding and understanding the effects of susceptibility genes for schizophrenia.

Over 100 studies have been published on ETD in patients with schizophrenia, addressing issues ranging from frequency, specificity, medication effects, familial pattern, and underlying neurobiology. These studies have used a variety of methods to record eye movements as well as different tasks and outcome measures. Electro-oculography and, more recently, high-resolution infrared oculography, have been the most commonly used methods to assess and quantify ETD. Qualitative ratings of how closely the eye tracks the target have been recommended by some, but such measures do little to clarify the mechanisms underlying global impairment. Consequently, most recent studies include quantitative parameters. The two frequently studied aspects of eye tracking are the smooth pursuit and saccade systems (for review, see Levy *et al.*, 1993). Gain, or speed of the eye, is a measure of the smooth pursuit system and is slowed in patients. Saccades are very rapid movements used to move the eye quickly toward a target, such as when one hears a voice and rapidly turns the eye to the estimated position of the speaker. Patients with schizophrenia, during smooth pursuit, follow the target slowly and often show compensatory saccades to catch-up to the target (Levy *et al.*, 1994). Subjects may also move ahead of the target ("anticipatory saccades"). Thus, the most commonly reported pattern in patients is reduced gain, with a compensatory increase in "catch-up" saccades to correct the increasing error in eye position (Levy *et al.*, 1994). Some studies have reported normal gain and a primary deficit in intrusive saccades (Levin *et al.*, 1982). Another frequently used outcome measure is root mean square (RMS) error, which captures how closely the eye remains foveated on the target. Estimates of the frequency of ETD (typically using qualitative ratings, gain, and/or RMS error) in patients with schizophrenia range from 20% to 80%. Reasons for this large range are unclear but may be related to differences in methodology, the measures used, and/or ascertainment issues (see below).

A variety of other abnormalities in eye movements have also been found. For example, fixation, or the ability to stay focused on a fixed target, may be impaired (Amador *et al.*, 1995). Patients also simply spend less time engaged in pursuit tasks. A second variation is "predictive" gain, where eye movements predicting the movement of an unseen target are measured (Hong *et al.*, 2008). In a promising "antisaccade" task, subjects must produce a "volitional" saccade in the direction opposite to the target (McDowell & Clementz, 1996). Patients and relatives perform poorly relative to controls (Clementz, 1998), although a recent meta-analysis suggests that heritability may be small (Levy *et al.*, 2008). A further modification of ETD is the memory-guided saccade generated during an oculomotor delayed response task (Park *et al.*, 1995; McDowell & Clementz, 1996). Overall, many of these additional phenotypes appear to involve more than simple eye movements. For example, the delayed response tasks involve the spatial working memory system. Performance of these additional tasks may also be impaired in relatives.

A number of studies have examined whether various measures of ETD are secondary to factors related to psychiatric illness, such as medications (for review, see Reilly *et al.*, 2008), as well as the relationship of ETD to illness onset, severity, and stability over time. Dozens of studies using a variety of different designs suggest that neuroleptics produce a slight, deleterious effect on ETD. Other medications, such as lithium, may be more liable to worsen ETD. Overall, this extensive literature suggests that that several parameters related to eye movements are abnormal in schizophrenia, including gain, intrusive saccades, predictive gain, fixation, inhibitory control, and overall attentional capacity for task engagement. This may not be surprising given the deficits seen in schizophrenia using other modalities (e.g., neuroimaging) assessing parietal, temporal, and prefrontal function and their involvement in modulating eye tracking. Some environmental factors also have a significant impact on ETD. Despite the uncertainties about which measures and methods are most useful for family and genetic studies of ETD, many measures have been examined in family studies in an effort to estimate heritability.

Family ETD studies began in the early 1970s, when a series of studies by (Holzman *et al.*, 1973) suggested that ETD was common in family members, unique to schizophrenia and due to a single dominant gene. Subsequent studies steadily eroded the strength of these findings. Most investigators have used the smooth pursuit paradigm and measures derived from it, including RMS error and gain. Unfortunately, a common strategy was to use "supernormal" control groups, which likely overestimated the frequency of abnormalities in family members. A second methodological problem relates to age. ETD increases in normal subjects with increasing age, and initial family studies often compared parents of probands with younger controls, leading to further overestimations of ETD in families. Data from the first 15 years of family studies suggested that ETD was present in 27–43% of first-degree relatives, while the only reported rate in a single "supernormal" control group of 72 subjects was 8%. Studies using quantitative measures found that ETD was present in a much smaller percentage of patients and relatives. However, they too often employed younger "supernormal" control groups. Twin studies have also been employed to assess the heritability of ETD but because of the small sample sizes, the results are difficult to interpret. Family data have been used to develop genetic models relating ETD to risk for schizophrenia. Holzman *et al.* (1974) first suggested that a single dominant gene could account for their data, supported by some subsequent analyses (e.g., Iacono *et al.*, 1992), but this seems unlikely. A recent meta-analysis concluded that several ETD measures show a moderate effect size, supporting their use as possible endophenotypes (Calkins *et al.*, 2008). These included memory-guided saccade accuracy and error rate, global smooth pursuit dysfunction, intrusive saccades during fixation, antisaccade error rate, and smooth pursuit closed-loop gain. However, given the problems with many of the studies included in the meta-analysis, these conclusions are difficult to have confidence in. In summary, it remains uncertain to what degree relatives have increased rates of ETD, which measures and paradigms are best to capture this, what the genetic architecture is, and how useful it might be as an intermediate phenotype.

Despite these many issues, ETD measures have been included in several genetic studies. Arolt *et al.* (1996, 1999) used gain and saccade frequency as phenotypes and reported credible linkage to the 6p21–23 region, where prior studies had reported linkage with schizophrenia (near the gene for dysbindin). Matthysse *et al.* (2004) subsequently provided some evidence for replication using a nearby marker. Remarkably, there have not yet been follow-up association studies looking at ETD and genes in this region, such as dysbindin. Association studies have looked at other genes, including catechol-O-methyltransferase (*COMT*), e.g., Thaker *et al.*, 2004), the dopamine D$_3$

receptor, and phospholipase A(2) (PLA2) (Rybakowski *et al.*, 2001, 2003). In general, these studies use small sample sizes, different ETD parameters, and multiple testing. The results have been statistically weak and unreplicated. Perhaps a major drawback to the use of ETD is the uncertainty about the clinical relevance of ETD in patients with schizophrenia. Would a drug designed to improve ETD show any clinically detectable beneficial effects? In contrast, based on current knowledge, many of the other candidate phenotypes reviewed below seem to be more directly related to disease biology (e.g., frontal lobe function, hyperdopaminergia) or outcome (e.g., cognition).

Electrophysiological/sensorimotor gating phenotypes (see also Chapter 15)

Electrophysiological measures were first used to investigate information processing deficits in schizophrenia in the early 1970s. Since then, a variety of subtle abnormalities have been discovered in patients, many of which have also been found in family members. These include event-related potentials (ERPs), derived from electroencephalography (EEG), as well as gating of the startle response (e.g., to an unexpected, loud noise). Most ERP studies have used auditory stimuli to generate ERP waveforms. Abnormalities in visually-evoked ERPs have also been described but have not been studied as extensively. The primary outcome measures in studies of ERPs have included amplitude, latency, and/or topography of specific waveforms which are time locked to auditory stimuli. A number of different paradigms have been used. For example, studies of the P50, a "mid latency" waveform which occurs 50 ms after a stimulus, have used pairs of repeated auditory inputs. Healthy subjects show a reduced P50 amplitude to the second auditory stimulus, a response attributed to "sensory gating" of an irrelevant (or redundant) stimulus, while patients with schizophrenia have impaired gating. Other studies have evaluated later occurring ERPs, such as the N100 (and the related "mismatch negativity") and P300. These studies have focused on responses elicited by an infrequent auditory tone (e.g., 20% frequency) in a series of repetitive standard tones (80% frequency), referred to as the "oddball" task. The N100 waveform generated following the "rare" (or oddball) stimulus in an oddball task is the first ERP that discriminates between different sensory inputs. As such, it is thought to reflect the analysis of the physical parameters of sensory stimuli. The P300 waveform is related to the post-perceptual updating of short-term working memory traces of expected environmental stimuli (Donchin & Isreal, 1980). In addition to ERPs, inhibition of the startle response to loud noise has been investigated in schizophrenia. Startle reactions can be inhibited when preceded by a soft noise (prepulse inhibition); deficits in prepulse inhibition in schizophrenia may reflect deficits in sensorimotor gating, perhaps analogous at a general level to gating deficits seen with the P50 paradigm, though these two measures tend not to correlate. Overall, electrophysiological and sensorimotor gating phenotypes appear to be promising brain phenotypes representing discreet information processing steps with relatively straightforward translation into animal studies (for recent reviews, see Turetsky *et al.*, 2007; Thaker, 2007). Nevertheless, they too have been plagued by the methodological issues similar to those seen with ETD, including questions about medication and illness effects, the use of differing methodologies and outcome measures, and uncertain heritability estimates from small sample sizes.

Of all the electrophysiological measures, the P50 waveform has generated perhaps the most enthusiasm as an intermediate phenotype. This is due, in part, to promising translational studies suggesting that P50 deficits in schizophrenia are due to impaired nicotinic α7 receptor function in the hippocampus. The P50 paradigm examines gating of the amplitude of the P50 wave to consecutive, simple, auditory clicking noises separated by 500 ms (Freedman *et al.*, 1983). P50 sensory gating is reported as a ratio of the amplitude of the second wave to the first wave; larger ratios indicating less suppression are seen in schizophrenia. An interesting recent variation of this paradigm has focused on gating of theta–alpha frequency power around 50 ms. The neurobiology of sensory gating has been examined in rodent models and is critically dependent on cholinergic input to the hippocampus, mediated by the nicotinic α7 receptor. In clinical studies, the P50 sensory gating ratio has been shown to be relatively stable over time, but may be normalized by atypical antipsychotics and, at least transiently, with nicotine intake (e.g., from cigarettes). Abnormal P50 gating has also been reported in acutely manic patients, where it appears to be state-dependent (Baker *et al.*, 1987). Some researchers have not replicated the P50 deficit in schizophrenia or have reported that the amplitude from the second click is the same in patients and controls, while the amplitude and/or latency of the first click is altered in patients and accounts for the decreased ratio (e.g., Jin & Potkin, 1996; Jin *et al.*, 1997). Nevertheless, a meta-analysis of 20 P50 studies including 421 patients and 401 controls reported a large effect size for the P50 ratio of −1.56 (Bramon *et al.*, 2004).

Patients with schizophrenia and roughly 50% of their first-degree relatives were found to have impaired sensory gating in an initial family study using the P50 paradigm (Siegel *et al.*, 1984). This suggested an autosomal dominant genetic architecture, favorable for linkage studies. On the other hand, later studies have not found such a strong genetic component. For example, Greenwood *et al.* (2007) found that the traditionally used P50 ratio was not itself significantly heritable; however, a *post hoc* analysis using

the difference between the first and second P50 amplitude did show a significant heritability of 0.28. Despite the uncertainties about heritability, a linkage study was initiated and, remarkably, found the P50 phenotype linked to markers on 15q13. A follow-up association study found a significant relationship between P50 and SNPs in the promoter region of the α7 receptor gene (Freedman *et al.*, 1997; Leonard *et al.*, 2002). These reports were particularly credible given prior rodent data implicating α7 with P50 gating and postmortem findings of reduced α7 receptors in schizophrenia. Subsequently, clinical trials have been performed with an α7 agonist in normal subjects and patients with schizophrenia. The data here are mixed, however, and await the results of more definitive trials. One concern has been raised about what clinical benefit would be provided by normalizing P50 deficits (for discussion, see Potter *et al.*, 2006). On the other hand, preclinical data from rodent studies and data from normal humans suggest that α7 plays a significant role in modulating cognition. Overall, P50 deficits constitute one of the most successful uses of the intermediate phenotype strategy to date.

Mismatch negativity (MMN), a second promising ERP, is related to the N100, a cortical evoked potential. The MMN is the difference in the N100 amplitude generated by common and rare stimuli during an oddball task. N100 amplitude to a rare stimulus is larger and is thought to reflect the pre-attentive detection of a change in auditory input. N100 and MMN are generated by auditory and frontal cortices and trigger involuntary attention shifting towards deviant or novel stimuli (Naatanen & Kahkonen, 2009). In addition to MMN, several other aspects of the N100 have been examined, including amplitude after single tone and gating with paired stimuli, although these studies are much less common. Regarding MMN, several methods have been used by different investigators. For example, the rare stimulus in the oddball task can differ by duration, pitch, or intensity, relative to the frequent stimulus. Deficits have been observed in schizophrenia for all three (Naatanen & Kahkonen, 2009; Turetsky *et al.*, 2007). Overall, differences in stimulus duration may generate a larger difference in MMN between patients and controls, while frequency differences may track more closely to illness progression and severity (Naatanen & Kahkonen, 2009; Umbricht & Krljes, 2005). Visual stimuli elicit an occipital N100 and MMN, which may also be altered in schizophrenia (e.g. Yeap *et al.*, 2006). The basis of reduced auditory MMN could be secondary to impaired processing of the primary auditory inputs, perhaps related to impaired generation of gamma activity (Thaker, 2007). Pharmacological studies suggest N-methyl-D-aspartate (NMDA) plays a role in MMN, as antagonists diminish MMN (e.g. Javitt *et al.*, 1996).

MMN offers several advantages as a potential trait but there are disadvantages as well. Regarding the former, because MMN does not require significant attention, assessment is not confounded by impaired attention and motivation, in contrast to some measures (e.g. P300). Second, the effects of neuroleptics appear to be limited (Turetsky *et al.*, 2007). Third, N100 appears to be highly stable over time (Light & Braff, 2005). On the other hand, MMN deficits may not be present early in the illness but appear to emerge over time (Magno *et al.*, 2008; Salisbury *et al.*, 2002), although one study found MMN deficits in high-risk subjects (Shin *et al.*, 2009). Most concerning, the heritability of MNM is uncertain. A small twin study suggested significant heritability of MMN related to genetic risk for schizophrenia, but possibly less so than P50 or P300 (Hall *et al.*, 2007), while a similar study suggested N100 amplitude but not MMN was heritable (Ahveninen *et al.*, 2006). Overall, data on the heritability and genetics of MMN are very limited.

A third cortical ERP, the P300, is perhaps the most widely studied waveform in schizophrenia and has many characteristics of an ideal intermediate phenotype. Most investigations of the P300 have used auditory stimuli in an oddball task. It is thought to reflect several cognitive processes, including context updating, working memory, and related attentional control. The neurobiology of the P300 is, consequently, complex, and there are likely many cortical generators. Some studies have distinguished between the earlier P3a and later P3b, which have different generators. Despite some differences in methods and measures, many groups have reported reduced P300 amplitude and, less commonly, increased latency, in schizophrenia (Friedman & Squires-Wheeler, 1994; Turetsky *et al.*, 2007). Several meta-analyses have reported substantial effect sizes: 0.65–1.05 for amplitude and −0.38 to −0.75 for latency (Bramon *et al.*, 2004; Jeon & Polich, 2003). Furthermore, the standard auditory P300 amplitude appears to be a stable trait with little evidence of an effect of neuroleptic medication or clinical state. Reduced P300 amplitude has also been reported in several studies of subjects at high risk for schizophrenia and first-episode patients. Reduced P300 is not specific to schizophrenia and has been found in dementia, alcoholism, depression, and bipolar disorder.

Regarding the critical issue of heritability, the data from healthy families suggest P300 amplitude has a substantial genetic component (0.4–0.6). While studies of first-degree relatives of subjects with schizophrenia have been mixed, a meta-analysis found a moderate effect size for both amplitude and latency (Bramon *et al.*, 2005). Subsequent studies have largely supported this finding (e.g. Groom *et al.*, 2008). Similarly, twin studies have reported substantial correlations between P300 amplitude and genetic risk for schizophrenia (e.g., (Hall *et al.*, 2007). P300 has been used in association studies where positive findings have been reported with several candidate genes. These include the D₃ dopamine receptor (Mulert *et al.*, 2006) and *COMT*.

Reduced P300 amplitude was also found in the Scottish pedigree with the DISC1 translocation (Blackwood & Muir, 2004). While replication of these genetic associations is important, the implications for understanding the neurobiology of schizophrenia are not clear, compared, for example, to P50. The degree of biological and genetic complexity of P300 may be comparable to that of schizophrenia itself, and the clinical effects of normalizing P300 are unclear.

Prepulse inhibition (PPI) is another trait, like P50, related perhaps to inhibition and gating of sensory inputs. An intense sensory stimulus, such as a loud noise, elicits a whole body startle response. This response is reduced when a weak stimulus (prepulse) precedes the intense one by 30–300 ms. The startle response is typically measured with electromyographic measures of the eye blink response. One advantage of PPI is that extensive studies in rodents have delineated its pharmacology and neurobiology (Swerdlow *et al.* 2001). PPI deficits can be induced by D₂ agonists and NMDA antagonists, and are reversed by antipsychotic drugs. Consequently, it has become a common screening model in the development of novel antipsychotic drugs. Human studies have shown that the magnitude of PPI appears to be dependent on the time between the prepulse and the startle stimulus. Habituation to startle, differences between the right and left eye, and the effects of age and gender have all been reported and complicate comparisons between studies. Nevertheless, several studies have shown that patients with schizophrenia have impaired PPI. These deficits are seen at an inter-stimulus interval of 60 ms but not 30 ms or 120 ms (Swerdlow *et al.*, 2006). PPI is stable in normal subjects and perhaps in patients. As with rodents, antipsychotic drugs can normalize PPI deficits in patients, a potential problem for genetic studies. PPI deficits have been correlated with several clinical features, including cognitive impairment and thought disorder. Regarding heritability, first-degree relatives have been evaluated in only a few studies and appear to have deficits similar to those seen in patients (e.g., Cadenhead *et al.*, 2000; Kumari *et al.*, 2005). Heritability of PPI has ranged from 0.32 to 0.38 (Greenwood *et al.*, 2007; Aukes *et al.*, 2008). Genetic studies are limited but PPI measures have been used to identify a promising genetic association with schizophrenia and the *Fabp7* gene (Watanabe *et al.*, 2007).

Finally, an electrophysiological measure emerging as a potentially interesting phenotype is gamma band power. Oscillations in the gamma frequency (30–100 Hz) derived from quantitative EEG are high frequency, locally generated oscillations. Gamma band oscillations are an emergent cortical feature hypothesized to underlie a variety of cognitive processes, such as those underlying binding of sensory input to form a perception of an object. While its neurobiology is complex, gamma oscillations involve synchronized, recurrent gamma-aminobutyric acid (GABA) neuronal inhibition of pyramidal neurons. Evoked gamma band power may be reduced in schizophrenia (for review, see van der Stelt & Belger, 2007). Although heritability has not been studied, gamma band power has been used as a phenotype in association studies, and several positive findings have been reported (e.g., with *DRD4*, *DAT*, and *COMT*) (Demiralp *et al.*, 2007). Given data implicating deficits in cortical GABAergic function in schizophrenia, gamma band power will likely continue to play a role in genetic studies of schizophrenia.

Overall, the studies reviewed above suggest that the use of electrophysiological measures appears promising. These measures could potentially provide tools to parse specific information processing steps that underlie impaired cortical function and cognition. However, many questions remain about their use in genetic studies. Beyond the details related to methodology (e.g., which parameters and methods should be used, how should neuroleptic effects be managed), it is unclear which specific measures should be the focus of genetic studies. While it seems likely that many associations between different measures and different genes will be found, deciding which are most critical for the pathophysiology of schizophrenia will be challenging.

Neuroimaging phenotypes (see also Chapters 16 and 17)

Neuroimaging techniques hold significant promise in unraveling the genetic complexity of schizophrenia, as such measures appear, at least *prima facie*, to index phenomena closer to the biological effects of genes than many other intermediate phenotypes. In addition, structural and metabolic neuroimaging procedures are likely to be less subject to confounders related to understanding task instructions, motivation, and other vicissitudes of testing that might affect, for example, eye tracking and neuropsychological tests. One of the first demonstrations of the power of neuroimaging measures in genetics research on schizophrenia came from a study of the effects of *COMT* genotype on prefrontal function (Egan *et al.*, 2001b). In that study, the effects of the Val108/158Met polymorphism, which has a profound effect on enzyme activity and prefrontal dopamine catabolism, could be detected using fMRI measures of prefrontal efficiency during a working memory task with as few as 15 subjects. In contrast, several hundred subjects were needed to detect this effect using scores from the working memory task, and several thousand may be needed to show an effect related to schizophrenia diagnosis. This pattern indicates that *COMT* genotype has a larger effect on the fMRI-derived measures of frontal lobe function than on test scores or syndromal status.

Efforts to uncover other neuroimaging phenotypes have generated promising leads. By far the most intensive efforts have been directed towards structural measures derived from MRI scans. fMRI and magnetic resonance spectroscopy (MRS) have also been used in several studies, while methods involving radioactive ligands, such as positron emission tomography (PET), have been evaluated in only a few studies.

Structural measures derived from MRI seem prime candidates to serve as intermediate phenotypes, given their high heritabilities and hypothesized roles in the pathophysiology of schizophrenia (see Chapter 16). Twin studies using traditional volumetric approaches have reported moderate to high heritabilities for major neuroanatomic features. Additive genetic influences appear to account for 52–91% of the total variance in intracranial volume (Carmelli *et al.*, 1998; Pfefferbaum *et al.*, 2000; Posthuma *et al.* 2000), 62–94% for total brain volume (Bartley *et al.*, 1997; Carmelli *et al.*, 1998; Wright *et al.*, 2002), 82–87% for gray and white matter volumes (Baare *et al.*, 2001), 40–69% for hippocampal volume (Sullivan *et al.*, 2001), and 79–94% for corpus callosum areas (Pfefferbaum *et al.*, 2000; Scamvougeras *et al.* 2003). However, because many aspects of cortical surface geometry differ between individuals, and even between pairs of genetically identical co-twins, quantification techniques that do not account for individual differences in sulcal–gyral patterning and other landmarks may be misleading. These limitations can be overcome using computational methods for cortical surface modeling and cortical pattern matching (Fischl & Dale, 2000; Thompson *et al.*, 2004; Hurdal & Stephenson, 2004; Van Essen, 2004).

Thompson *et al.* (2001)) reported the first such cortical maps of genetic influences on human brain structure in twins. These maps revealed a non-uniform genetic continuum, in which brain structure was increasingly similar in subjects with increasing genetic affinity, more so in heteromodal association areas than in other regions. Genetic factors significantly influenced cortical structure in Broca's and Wernicke's language areas, as well as frontal brain regions (rMZ > 0.8). Heritability estimates indicated that localized middle frontal cortical regions, near Brodmann areas 9 and 46, displayed a 90–95% genetic determination of structure. Further, frontal gray matter differences were linked to Spearman's g, which measures successful test performance across multiple cognitive domains and is itself highly heritable. The findings were subsequently replicated in independent volumetric studies (Baare *et al.*, 2001; Wright *et al.*, 2002), which examined heritabilities of Brodmann area volumes using variance components analysis.

The demonstration that brain structure is highly heritable in general is necessary but not sufficient for demonstrating relevance of structural brain abnormalities to the genetics of schizophrenia, for which studies of relatives of patients are also required. Early work using computed tomography (CT), which is sensitive only to brain *versus* cerebrospinal fluid (CSF) contrast, strongly implicated enlargement of the third and lateral ventricles and cortical sulci in patients with schizophrenia, but was less consistent on the question of CSF-space expansion in relatives of patients, though the sample sizes in studies investigating relatives were small. MRI is sensitive to gray *versus* white matter contrast in addition to brain *versus* CSF contrast and has significantly improved spatial resolution compared with CT. Initial studies using this technique were encouraging but were difficult to interpret because of small sample sizes and the exclusive reliance on region of interest (rather than voxel-based) approaches. Several larger and better-designed MRI studies followed. Cannon *et al.* (1998) reported reduced cortical gray volume in 60 non-psychotic siblings largely past the age of risk compared with a well-matched control group. In contrast, in a study by Sharma *et al.* (1998) of 57 unaffected relatives (parents and siblings) from 16 families with at least two affected subjects, no difference in cortical gray or white matter volume was observed between patients, relatives, and a younger "supernormal" control group. Lawrie *et al.* (1999) found reduced thalamic as well as amygdala–hippocampal volume in 100 subjects at "high risk" (two relatives with schizophrenia) compared with a "supernormal" control group. A weak trend ($p = 0.09$) was found for reduced left prefrontal volume. Many of these young at-risk subjects are likely to later develop schizophrenia, suggesting that these findings could be antecedents to the illness itself. In a follow-up study with an expanded sample size, similar findings were reported (Lawrie *et al.*, 2001). Reduced amygdala–hippocampal volume was also reported in a small sample of healthy adult siblings (n = 20) compared with a well-matched control group (O'Driscoll *et al.*, 2001), and in a cohort (n = 28) of healthy parents, sibs and adult children (Seidman *et al.*, 1999). Finally, Staal *et al.* (1998, 2000) found only reduced thalamic volume in 16 healthy siblings compared with a carefully matched control group, but no differences for volumes of a number of other structures, including the hippocampi and prefrontal gray or white matter.

Cannon and Rosso (2002) reported the first three-dimensional cortical surface maps in MZ and DZ twins discordant for schizophrenia compared with demographically-matched control twins. A map encoding gray matter variation associated with genetic proximity to a patient (MZ co-twins > DZ co-twins > control twins) isolated deficits primarily in the polar and dorso-lateral prefrontal cortex, indicating substantial (and dose-dependent) genetic influence on these cortical regions. A map encoding differences between affected and unaffected MZ co-twins detected gray matter reductions of 5–8% in the DLPFC, Broca's area, premotor cortex and frontal eye fields, superior parietal lobule, Heschl's gyrus, and middle

temporal gyrus in the probands. The observed disease-related deficits in gray matter did not appear to reflect secondary phenomena, as they were associated with increased severity of negative and positive symptoms and with cognitive dysfunction, but not with duration of illness or antipsychotic drug treatment. In a variance components analysis of hippocampal volumes, additive genetic effect on hippocampal volume (corrected for cortical gray matter volume) was 71% in the healthy twins, but only 42% in the discordant twins, indicating that while hippocampal volume in healthy subjects is under substantial genetic control, hippocampal volume in patients with schizophrenia and their relatives appears to be influenced to a greater extent by unique and shared environmental factors (van Erp *et al.*, 2004). A similar pattern of results was observed in a Dutch twin sample (van Haren *et al.*, 2004).

Only a handful of studies have looked at neuroimaging parameters other than structural measures. Klemm *et al.* (2001) used ^{31}PMRS to study 14 first-degree relatives (sibs and offspring) compared with 14 age-matched controls. Relatives had increased phosphodiesters, interpreted by the authors as suggesting increased breakdown of phospholipids in thePFC. Keshavan *et al.* (1997) found a trend for reduced cingulate *N*-acetylaspartate (NAA) measures in a small group (n = 10) of young offspring of mothers with schizophrenia. Callicott *et al.* (1998), in by far the largest cohort of siblings studied with MRS to date, looked at 60 healthy siblings compared with 66 controls. Siblings had significantly reduced hippocampal NAA measures, with relative risk estimates ranging from 3.8 to 9, depending on the criteria to define abnormal NAA (e.g., 1 or 2 SD below the control mean). Block *et al.* (2000) found no differences in NAA levels in a cohort of 35 non-psychotic family members, but they only looked in the PFC. Of note, Callicott *et al.* (1998) also found no reductions in sib PFC. In a twin study, NAA, creatine + phosphocreatine (Cr), glycerophosphocholine + phosphocholine (Cho), and myo-inositol (mI) did not differ significantly between patients with schizophrenia, their unaffected co-twins, or healthy controls in a mesial prefrontal gray matter voxel (Lutkenhoff *et al.*, 2010). However, glutamate (Glu) was significantly lower in patients with schizophrenia (31% difference) and unaffected co-twins (21%) than in healthy controls. In a left hippocampus voxel, levels of NAA, Cr, and Cho were higher in patients with schizophrenia compared with controls and their unaffected co-twins, who did not differ.

Abnormalities in prefrontal physiology have also been reported in family members of patients with schizophrenia. Blackwood *et al.* (1999) noted reduced prefrontal blood flow in a cohort of 36 first-degree relatives using SPECT. Similarly, abnormalities in prefrontal blood flow ("inefficiency") were seen by Callicott *et al.* (2003) using fMRI and a working memory paradigm, the n-back. As noted above, this phenotype was useful in demonstrating the effect of

COMT Val158Met genotype on prefrontal function. Subsequent studies have confirmed that prefrontal activation during working memory tasks is under significant genetic control (Koten *et al*, 2009; Blokland *et al.*, 2008), and that relatives exhibit abnormal activation similar to patients, replicating the Callicott finding (e.g., MacDonald *et al.*, 2006; for review, see MacDonald *et al.*, 2009). Regarding default network activity, Whitfield-Gabrieli *et al.* (2009) found in an fMRI study that controls exhibited task-related suppression of activation in the default network, including the medial prefrontal cortex (MPFC) and posterior cingulate cortex/precuneus. Patients and relatives exhibited significantly reduced task-related suppression in the MPFC, and these reductions remained after controlling for performance. Increased task-related MPFC suppression correlated with better working memory performance in patients and relatives and with less psychopathology in all three groups (patients, relatives, and controls). Hyperactivity of the default network may therefore mark risk for schizophrenia, a possibility that requires evaluation in a study incorporating subjects with multiple degrees of genetic relationship.

Although in principle whole genome approaches could be used to detect genetic associations with neuroimaging phenotypes, given the large sample sizes required for whole genome analyses and the relatively high costs of neuroimaging assessments, their use has thus far been mostly limited to smaller-scale studies of candidate genes (Cannon *et al.*, 2006). SNP markers and haplotypes of a number of such genes have been found to associate with neuroimaging phenotypes for schizophrenia. While the particular SNPs and haplotypes often vary considerably across studies, the detected associations have proven useful as additional validation of particular signaling pathways thought to play a role in the pathophysiology of the disorder. Despite limitations in sample size, one whole genome study has been published using DLPRC activation elicited by a working memory task as the phenotype (Potkin *et al.*, 2009). Interestingly, the authors reported six genes, all of which may play a role in neurodevelopment and/or stress response, showing suggestive evidence of association. While further replication will be important, this study may presage future whole genome studies using larger cohorts and fMRI phenotypes.

Schizophrenia-related variations in brain structure have been associated with polymorphisms in *COMT* (e.g., Crespo-Facorro *et al.*, 2007), *DISC1* (Callicott *et al.*, 2005; Cannon *et al.* 2005), *BDNF* (Agartz *et al.*, 2006; Bueller *et al.*, 2006; Ho *et al.*, 2006, 2007; Nemoto *et al.*, 2006; Szeszko *et al.*, 2005), *NRG1* (McIntosh *et al.*, 2008; Gruber *et al.*, 2008), and RSG4 (Buckholtz *et al.*, 2007). The associations with *DISC1* and *NRG1* may implicate specific mechanistic effects of aberrant gene function in relation to gray and white matter development, respectively, as reviewed briefly below.

The DISC1 protein forms a functional complex with the developmentally regulated proteins Nudel and Lis1 (Brandon *et al.*, 2004; Morris *et al.*, 2003; Ozeki *et al.*, 2003) and is involved in cell migration, neurite outgrowth, and synaptogenesis (Kamiya *et al.*, 2005; Millar *et al.*, 2003; Ozeki *et al.*, 2003). In human samples, DISC1 variants associated with schizophrenia are also related to reduced gray matter thickness in the PFC and hippocampus, as well as decreased gray matter volume in the superior frontal gyrus and cingulate (Callicott *et al.*, 2005; Cannon *et al.*, 2005; Szeszko *et al.*, 2008). Postmortem studies indicate that cortical gray matter reduction in schizophrenia reflects reduced dendritic elaboration and synaptic contacts rather than loss of cell bodies (Selemon *et al.*, 1995; Glantz & Lewis, 1997). Using an inducible transgenic mouse model Li *et al.* (2007) showed that induction of a mutant C-terminal fragment of the DISC1 protein early in postnatal development, but not during adulthood, results in a number of phenotypic changes, including decreased dendritic complexity, impaired spatial working memory, sociability, and depressive-like traits, paralleling the pattern of phenotypic associations with DISC1 variants in humans (Cannon *et al.*, 2005; Hennah *et al.*, 2005).

Neuregulin (NRG1) influences neuronal migration, neurite formation and outgrowth, and oligodendrocyte development and proliferation (Gamett *et al.*, 1995; Vaskovsky *et al.*, 2000; Villegas *et al.*, 2000; Liu *et al.*, 2001; Vartanian*et al.*, 1999). Individuals with the schizophrenia-related *NRG1* genotype have white matter abnormalities in the fronto-thalamic connections as assessed by MRI and diffusion-tensor imaging (DTI) (McIntosh *et al.*, 2008), as well as decreased hippocampal volume (Gruber *et al.*, 2008). Among childhood-onset cases, risk allele carriers showed a steeper decline in white and gray matter volume from childhood to adolescence than non-risk allele carriers; unaffected controls with the risk allele showed a similar but attenuated effect, indicating a possible interaction of disease state and genotype (Addington *et al.*, 2007).

Following the findings with *COMT* (see above), fMRI has been used in a variety of subsequent genetic studies. Similar alterations in fMRI signals elicited during cognitive activation paradigms have been seen with SNPs in a number of schizophrenia candidate genes, including *GRM3, DISC1, DAOA, DTNBP1, ZNF804A, PRODH, RGS4,* and *KCNH2*. One potential advantage to fMRI phenotypes is that they serve as a link between cognition, physiology, and underlying molecular neurobiological abnormalities observed in brain tissue from patients with schizophrenia. For example, SNPs in the *GAD1* gene, whose expression is reduced in PFC tissue, predict fMRI-based measures of prefrontal efficiency during working memory tasks (Straub *et al.*, 2007). For *KCNH2*, whose expression is also altered in schizophrenia postmortem brain tissue, an SNP impacting hippocampal mRNA expression and risk for schizophrenia predicted fMRI-based abnormal hippocampal activation during a cognitive challenge (Huffaker *et al.*, 2009). These two examples highlight the utility of an integrated systems approach using intermediate phenotypes from several biological levels, including fMRI, in providing convergent data implicating specific pathophysiological mechanisms. While genetic studies of fMRI-based phenotypes are in their infancy, this class of phenotypes appears promising.

In summary, neuroimaging methods have been used to elucidate several intermediate phenotypes for schizophrenia. Among these, structural measures from MRI studies have been most clearly validated from the perspectives of having high heritabilities in general and showing deviation in relatives of patients with schizophrenia. Moreover, variants of a number of putative schizophrenia-related genes, including *DISC1* and *NRG1*, associate with alterations in gray and white matter that parallel those seen in patients with schizophrenia, effects that are consistent with the roles of these genes in brain development and plasticity. However, apart from a few interesting leads (Law *et al.*, 2006), it remains to be determined whether any of the inherited variants studied thus far in humans have functional impact on gene expression and related signaling pathways. Further, given the relative expense of neuroimaging, these approaches have thus far not been employed in genome-wide association studies, although in principle such studies would be extremely valuable. Several other neuroimaging phenotypes, including neurochemical measurements from MRS and physiological measures from fMRI, seem very promising but require replications of case–control and relative–control differences in large samples with well-matched control groups and additional work on basic heritability.

Cognitive phenotypes

Neuropsychological deficits are a prominent dimension of schizophrenia and may account for a substantial portion of the functional impairments in daily living (see Chapter 7). These deficits are enduring and stable features of the disorder, persisting even among patients who respond well to antipsychotic drugs. An impressive number of studies of first-degree relatives also indicate that cognitive impairments may be familial and that the pattern of such deficits is similar to, albeit less severe than, that seen in patients themselves (Cannon *et al.*, 1994; Kremen *et al.*, 1994). Furthermore, tests of different cognitive domains do not tap into completely overlapping variation, suggesting that there may be several cognitive phenotypes suitable for use as intermediate phenotypes (Egan *et al.*, 2001a). Studies of neuropsychological deficits share some of the same problems described above for studies of other intermediate phenotypes, such as the use of "supernormal" controls and

inconsistent results. However, overall matching with controls is generally better than that seen in other studies: subjects with Axis I disorders are excluded but siblings with Axis II disorders are included, whereas controls with these disorders are not. Such studies of "healthy" sibs and their matched "supernormal" controls therefore are less likely to overestimate differences between sibs and controls. Furthermore, while inconsistencies exist, the majority of studies are positive, suggesting that the differences are robust.

The earliest family studies focused on "at-risk" children of mothers with schizophrenia. These children exhibited a variety of behavioral abnormalities, including impaired attention (Fish, 1977). Studies using more rigorous neuropsychological testing, such as the Continuous Performance Tests (CPT), soon followed (Cornblatt & Keilp, 1994; Nuechterlein & Dawson, 1984). "At-risk" children do poorly on these tests, particularly on harder versions (e.g., Rutschmann *et al.*, 1977, 1986). The type of CPT used may be important, because more difficult CPT tasks are likely to involve cognitive demands beyond pure attention. Some versions [e.g., the identical pairs (IP) version] have significant working memory loads, which may therefore confound impaired attention with impaired working memory. Adult siblings largely past the age of risk for schizophrenia have also shown impairment on CPT performance, again primarily with more difficult versions (e.g., Cornblatt & Keilp, 1994). Results of studies using simpler versions of the CPT have been mixed. One large study using well-matched controls found no overall differences between sibs (n = 193) and controls (n = 47) (Egan *et al.*, 2001b), although sibs of probands with impaired attention were worse as a group compared with controls. Two studies have reported a trend for impaired attention in sibs (Keefe *et al.*, 1997; Laurent *et al.*, 2000), while five have reported marked impairments (Maier *et al.*, 1992; Cannon *et al.*, 1994; Finkelstein *et al.*, 1997; Chen *et al.*, 1998; Saoud *et al.*, 2000). The reasons for discrepancies between studies are unclear. Some studies used "supernormal" control groups (Finkelstein *et al.*, 1997; Keefe *et al.*, 1997) and have included sib groups with relatively high rates of schizophrenia spectrum disorders, such as personality disorders (Cannon *et al.*, 1994; Finkelstein *et al.*, 1997; Keefe *et al.*, 1997). Some studies included both parents and siblings, leading to possible bias as a result of age effects (Chen *et al.*, 1998).

Several studies have tried to quantify the magnitude of the familial effect on impaired attention. Grove *et al.* (1991) estimated heritability of CPT performance in 61 first-degree relatives using the ICC and found $h^2 = 0.79$, suggesting a substantial genetic component. A study of a Taiwanese cohort (parents and siblings, n = 148; Chen *et al.*, 1998) found very high rates of impairment in relatives compared with controls. Relative risk of "impaired attention" was 18–130, depending on the cut-off criteria, which is dramatically higher than the relative risk for schizophrenia itself. In contrast, a second large study of 193 siblings in a US cohort (Egan *et al.*, 2001b) found only slightly increased relative risk in a subgroup of siblings. The marked differences in these relative risk values could be a result of confounds such as ethnicity, recruitment biases, education, and type of relatives (parent or sib) studied. Overall, it remains possible that subtle deficits in attention are present in siblings, or at least in a subgroup, that these deficits are not simply antecedents of illness and that CPT measures could serve as a useful intermediate phenotype, but the effect seems weak.

Soon after impaired attention was noted, a variety of additional cognitive deficits were reported in family members. In general, these include cognitive tasks referable to prefrontal and medial temporal structures. Prefrontal deficits were seen using several tests, most notably the Wisconsin Card Sort Test (WCST), but also tests of verbal fluency and the "n-back" working memory task. Second, tests of declarative memory, such as the Wechsler Memory Scale, revised version (WMS-R) or the California Verbal List Test (CVLT), have also tended to be abnormal in first-degree family members. Third, scores on the Trail Making tests, including A and B versions, are reduced, implicating oculomotor scanning/psychomotor speed. Poor Trails B performance, while a crude measure sensitive to many neurological insults, is also seen with prefrontal deficits. Other abnormalities have also been reported, although less consistently (Kremen *et al.*, 1994).

Studies employing fairly comprehensive neuropsychological batteries, while somewhat inconsistent, suggest the effect size in the moderate range for several tests, with abnormalities seen even in healthy relatives. First, Pogue-Geile *et al.* (1991), in 40 sibs without schizophrenia, and then Franke *et al.* (1992), in 33 healthy sibs, both found impaired performance on the WCST, Trails B, and verbal fluency compared with well-matched control groups. On the other hand, Scarone *et al.* (1993) found no differences in WCST in 35 well siblings compared with matched but "supernormal" controls. In contrast, Cannon *et al.*, (1994) found impaired performance on a large battery of tests, including attention, working memory/executive function, and verbal memory in 16 siblings without schizophrenia, but six of 16 had definite or likely schizotypal personality disorder compared with "supernormal" controls. Larger studies have more consistently found differences. Keefe *et al.* (1994), in a cohort of 54 first-degree relatives without psychosis, found impaired performance on Trails B and verbal fluency (both letter and category), but not on the WCST, compared with "supernormal" controls. Faraone *et al.* (1995) found impairments in abstraction, verbal memory, and attention in a group of 35 non-psychotic first-degree relatives, similar to the results of Toomey *et al.*, (1998), who found impaired working memory (WCST) and

verbal memory in an overlapping sample of 54 first-degree healthy relatives. Both studies apparently used the same well-matched control group, screened using the Minnesota Multiphasic Personality Inventory (MMPI). Egan *et al.* (2001a), in a study of 193 siblings compared with a closely matched control group, found deficits on WCST, Trails B, and CVLT, whether or not subjects with schizophrenia spectrum disorders were included in these groups. Thus, as studies have included larger groups of siblings, more consistent differences have emerged and implicate the same brain regions and cognitive functions that are typically seen in patients with schizophrenia, including the PFC/working memory and ventral temporal lobe/declarative memory.

Two major studies have examined cognitive deficits in twins. In the first study of discordant twins (Goldberg *et al.*, 1993, 1994, 1995), using a wide neuropsychological battery, found that unaffected MZ twins have subtle cognitive deficits for the WMS-R, with trends for impairment on WCST perseverative errors (PE) and Trails A (p = 0.05) (Goldberg *et al.*, 1995). A second study of 18 MZ and 34 DZ discordant twin pairs examined the relationship between cognitive deficits and genetic risk for schizophrenia using canonical discriminant analysis (Cannon *et al.*, 2000). Four tests contributed unique genetic variance to increased risk for schizophrenia. These tests were spatial working memory (visual span test of the WMS-R), divided attention (using a Brown–Peterson dual-task paradigm), intrusions during recall of a word list (CVLT), and choice reaction time (using a Posner paradigm related to the CPT). It is unclear whether the same group differences were seen with these MZ twins compared with the Goldberg sample. In Cannon *et al.*'s analysis, verbal memory was more impaired in affected MZ subjects, relative to co-twins, suggesting an effect of unique environmental variance related to illness, paralleling the results with respect to hippocampal volume in the same twin pairs. While these data leave open the question of which tests are most informative for genetic studies, the conclusions are similar to those of other relatives in one important respect: several domains of cognition are impaired, including working memory/executive function and some aspects of verbal recall and attention, which are related to genetic risk for schizophrenia.

Finding deficits on several neuropsychological tests does not necessarily mean that these measure independent traits. An alternative possibility is that impairments are found on different tests because of one underlying abnormality. Attempts to address this question, using several statistical approaches, suggest that this is not the case. For example, correlations between measures are generally low in these groups (e.g. Keefe, *et al.*, 1994). On the other hand, (Toomey *et al.*, 1998) found fairly high correlations between attention and verbal memory, and between attention and abstraction in a cohort of 54 first-degree relatives, but no significant correlation between WCST and memory measures (on the WMS-R). Egan *et al.* (2001a), using multiple regression, found only modest shared variance (<15% in siblings) between measures of working memory, verbal memory, and psychomotor speed. Using factor analysis, Mirsky *et al.* (1991) and Kremen *et al.* (1992) found that WCST and Trails B load on different factors, similar to Egan *et al.* (2001a). Cannon *et al.* (2000), in a critical analysis of MZ and DZ twins, found evidence for four distinct independent cognitive deficits using canonical discriminant analysis. In non-patient populations, factor analysis has consistently shown that most of the variance on tests of different cognitive domains load significantly on the first factor, often referred to as "g". In contrast, analyses of patient and sib groups, which include subjects with a variety of impairments, tend to find somewhat less loading on the first factor and more evidence of additional orthogonal factors where both patients and siblings have lower scores than controls. Overall, these results suggest that several independent domains of cognitive dysfunction are related to genetic risk for schizophrenia, and that correlation and factor analytical studies could show different results because of different patterns of impairments. On the other hand, in a multivariate twin analysis, Toulopoulou *et al.* (2007) found that genetic influences contributed substantially to all cognitive domains, but intelligence and working memory were the most heritable. A significant correlation was found between intelligence and schizophrenia (r = –0.61; 95% CI –0.71 to –0.48), with shared genetic variance accounting for 92% of the covariance between the two. Genetic influences also explained most of the covariance between working memory and schizophrenia. Significant but lesser portions of covariance between the other cognitive domains and schizophrenia were also found to be genetically shared. Environmental effects, although separately linked to neurocognition and schizophrenia, did not generally contribute to their covariance. The authors concluded that genome-wide searches using factorial designs stratifying for levels of intelligence and working memory will assist in the search for quantitative trait loci for schizophrenia.

Is it plausible to use neuropsychological phenotypes to find schizophrenia genes? Support for this approach comes from a finding by Egan *et al.* (2001b) using working memory and the WCST as the phenotype. One attractive aspect of using working memory is that the neurobiology is increasingly well understood (Williams & Goldman-Rakic, 1995; Goldman-Rakic *et al.*, 1996). Specifically, D_1-mediated dopamine neurotransmission at glutamatergic neurons in the PFC is critical. Prefrontal COMT activity is critical for inactivating released dopamine (Karoum *et al.*, 1994) and knock-outs show increased prefrontal dopamine (Gogos *et al.*, 1998), a regional specificity that is likely to be caused by the paucity of the dopamine transporter in the PFC

(Sesack *et al.*, 1998). Also, remarkably, several studies in animals and humans suggest that reduced COMT activity improves working memory (Kneavel *et al.*, 2000). The human Val/Met polymorphism produces a dramatic effect on COMT enzyme activity (Weinshilboum & Dunnette, 1981). Thus, the Val allele would be expected to be related to relatively reduced working memory. In a cohort of 175 patients, 200 siblings, and 45 controls (Egan *et al.*, 2001b) found that the *COMT* genotype was associated with working memory; subjects with the Val allele had worse scores. Furthermore, the Val allele was associated with schizophrenia using the transmission disequilibrium test (TDT). Thus, this intermediate phenotype pointed to gene and mechanism of action, making the weak association much more plausible. Subsequently, many studies have found evidence for an effect of *COMT* genetic variants on cognition or risk for schizophrenia, although some have not. Attempts at meta-analyses have suggested that the effects of COMT may not be robust (Barnett *et al.*, 2008), although this has raised further controversy (Goldman *et al.*, 2009). At the very least, the difficulties and controversies in conclusively demonstrating COMT's effects on risk for schizophrenia by altering dopamine neurotransmission, frontal lobe biology, and cognition highlight the challenges and opportunities facing the use of intermediate phenotypes.

Since then, a number of studies have reported associations between genes and cognition in schizophrenia. Many of these have not been replicated and should thus be considered preliminary. Examples of genes and the cognition measures they may impact include: (1) *DISC1* and spatial working memory, (2) *GRM3* and verbal memory and verbal fluency, (3) *GAD1* and declarative memory, attention, and working memory, and (4) DARPP-32 (encoded by the gene, *PPP1R1B*) and processing speed and IQ. Evidence for replication has been provided for some gene and cognition associations. For example, following an initial report of an association between SNPs in dysbindin and IQ and cognitive decline (e.g., Burdick *et al.*, 2006), follow-up studies reported associations with spatial working memory in one study, episodic memory in a second, and IQ in a third in either patient or normal control cohorts. Alleles associated with schizophrenia in G72 (or DAOA) were originally reported to have a negative effect on working memory and attention in patients but not controls. Later studies showed that these alleles: (1) impaired attention in a normal cohort; (2) improved semantic fluency in a cohort of patients with schizophrenia; and (3) improved verbal memory in healthy subjects. Reasons for these discrepant results are unclear. Finally, risk alleles in AKT1 predicted impaired executive function and processing speed in one study, and verbal learning and memory in a second. In evaluating replication studies, several factors should be considered, including whether the same or different alleles affect the same or different cognitive tests or domains. Differences between populations (e.g., Scandinavian *vs.* Chinese) could also impact findings and produce apparent discrepancies.

Receptors, neurotransmitters, and cell-based phenotypes

Biological phenotypes proximal to the output of genes, such as levels of mRNA, protein, neurotransmitters, and receptors, are potentially the most basic of all intermediate phenotypes. While some may be difficult to access and measure, particularly in family samples, demonstrating heritability may be unnecessary in contrast to more distal measures. Levels of mRNA transcripts and splice variants related to SNPs in specific candidate genes are obviously important to assess for all candidate genes. Most are unlikely to be used beyond the relevant candidate gene and its related canonical pathway. Exceptions may be mRNA expression and/or protein levels of genes hypothesized to be related to a final common pathophysiological mechanism, such as GAD1, dysbindin, KCNH2, or D1. mRNA studies have provided substantial convergent evidence for SNPs in several candidate genes (see Kleinman *et al.*, 2011). For example, a non-coding SNP in the promoter region for *NRG1*, reported by several groups to increase risk for schizophrenia, appears to impact splicing of *NRG1* in the human brain (Law *et al.*, 2006). Cellular phenotypes are also emerging as potential candidates for genetic studies. For example, lymphoblasts exhibit several properties that are in part mediated by genes also expressed in the brain, including schizophrenia-risk genes like *NRG1* and *COMT* (Sei *et al.*, 2007).

Proteins and molecules related to neurotransmission represent another set of potential phenotypes. Given the evidence for dopamine abnormalities in schizophrenia, it is not surprising that the earliest of such studies looked at measures related to dopamine. As described in Chapter 17, *in vivo* neuroimaging methods have been used to explore dopamine indices in patients with schizophrenia. Regarding D_2 receptor density, no clear consensus has emerged, as some studies have reported slight increases but many have found no differences between patients and controls. One small PET study of MZ and DZ twins discordant for schizophrenia reported increased D_2 density in the caudate associated with genetic risk for schizophrenia (Hirvonen *et al.*, 2005). More consistent abnormalities have been reported for measures of presynaptic striatal dopamine. Increased presynaptic dopamine has been seen in medicated and unmedicated patients, first-break patients, and subjects in the prodromal phase. In a study using 6-^{18}F-fluorodopa (FDOPA) PET imaging to measure striatal dopamine synthesis, first-degree relatives were found to have increased levels, similar to patients (Huttunen *et al.*, 2008). Alterations

of D_1 binding have also been suggested (both increased and reduced). A twin study found high D_1 receptor density in the MPFC associated with increasing genetic risk for schizophrenia (Hirvonen *et al.*, 2006). Remarkably, an association study found that increased D_1 density was associated with the *COMT* Val/Met SNP, with Val/Val subjects showing higher D_1 levels (Slifstein *et al.*, 2008). This is consistent with cognition results (see above) and what might be expected based on higher COMT activity with the Val allele resulting in relatively less synaptic dopamine and downstream up-regulation of D_1. Overall, these studies suggest that dopamine abnormalities seen in schizophrenia are present in relatives and are viable phenotypes for genetic studies, as well as potential biomarkers for illness. Although other neurotransmitter systems have not yet been studied using genetic techniques, the widespread availability of genotyping may change this in the near future.

Other phenotypes

A variety of other abnormalities found in patients with schizophrenia have also been examined in relatives. These include measures such as handedness, neurological signs (Egan *et al.*, 2001c), minor physical anomalies (Ismail *et al.*, 1998), finger ridge counts, and others. In general, these studies are relatively small and inconclusive. Clinical measures of ratings of symptoms, such as positive and negative symptoms, have also been studied as candidate intermediate phenotypes. Odd personalities among the biological relatives of subjects with schizophrenia were observed both by Kraepelin and Bleuler. Using standardized scales, first-degree family members have been reported to have increased ratings on anhedonia scales and, less commonly, on measures of perceptual aberrations. Family studies of affected patients have also shown evidence that there may be a familial component for ratings of positive or negative symptoms, although studies are not conclusive. These symptom dimensions have also been used in linkage studies (e.g., Brzustowicz *et al.*, 1997) and association studies. One problem with these studies is that symptoms vary over time for a variety of reasons, including changes in medication, stress, etc., suggesting that symptom measures may not be stable traits. Therefore, they may not meet many of the criteria for the ideal intermediate phenotype (see above).

Conclusions

Do intermediate phenotypes exist and can they be used to find genes that increase risk for schizophrenia? The substantial body of research reviewed above suggests that some measures do meet many of the criteria for a valid intermediate phenotype. Studies of first-degree relatives, for example, have found abnormalities in a wide range of traits assessed using electrophysiological, cognitive, and neuroimaging methods. Candidate traits have been incorporated into genetic studies and several credible, replicated associations have emerged. In some cases, intermediate phenotypes have provided substantial, convergent evidence implicating specific mechanisms that increase risk for schizophrenia. Most compelling are studies that include traits from several biological levels related to specific neural systems (Plate 14.1), such as the relationship between SNPs in *COMT* and cognition, prefrontal function, and prefrontal dopamine metabolism. On the other hand, the use of intermediate phenotypes as a substitute for the diagnosis of schizophrenia in linkage and whole genome association studies has had limited success. This use of intermediate phenotypes to find genes remains controversial due to concerns that they may be as genetically complex as schizophrenia.

Assessing the viability of a trait for use as an intermediate phenotype has traditionally involved qualifying studies to assess such properties as stability, reliability, and relationship to genetic risk for schizophrenia. Methodological issues have often complicated attempts to qualify specific measures, as illustrated by the literature on eye tracking dysfunction (ETD). Differing methods and outcome measures have been used by different investigators, resulting in a limited database for concluding that any one specific ETD measure robustly meets all of the qualifications for a compelling intermediate phenotype. Furthermore, issues with ascertainment in family studies have often resulted in poor matching between relatives and controls on age, gender, psychopathology, and IQ. This can overestimate the frequency of abnormalities in relatives and heritability. For most methods and measures, evidence for heritability is uncomfortably limited and/or inconsistent. Overall, it remains unclear whether finding genes for some phenotypes, such as ETD, will enhance our understanding of the biology of schizophrenia. Similar methodological issues pertain, more or less, to phenotypes derived using other techniques, including imaging, cognitive testing, and electrophysiology. Estimates of heritability, for example, are often derived only from studies of first-degree family members, which are unable to distinguish environmental from genetic sources of variance. Even if the latter is small, heritability estimates are usually substantially lower than that seen for schizophrenia itself.

Despite these problems, some phenotypes appear relatively promising, such as neuroimaging phenotypes. Neuroanatomical volumetric measures have been shown to be highly heritable (~0.90 or higher) and abnormalities in several brain regions vary according to degree of genetic relationship to an affected individual. Credible associations have been found between volumetric phenotypes and SNPs within several putative schizophrenia genes, including *COMT*, *DISC1*, and *NRG1*. fMRI phenotypes have pro-

duced several stunning results. For example, prefrontal dysfunction has been widely linked to schizophrenia pathophysiology, and fMRI measures of prefrontal function are abnormal in patients and relatives. These measures have been included in studies of candidate genes, such as *COMT*, *DISC1*, *GRM3*, and *KCNH2*, where they have provided convergent data implicating working memory networks. Electrophysiological markers, such as those related to MMN, sensorimotor gating, and the P300, are conceptually attractive given their potential to parse different steps of information processing, but genetic findings have been limited. One bright spot has been the use of the P50 waveform and the sensory gating paradigm where both animal modeling and human genetic data implicate the α7 nicotinic receptor. Cognitive abnormalities, widely found in relatives, provide another level beyond imaging and electrophysiology and are attractive because of their close relationship with both specific neural systems and, clinically, with functional outcome. Cognition phenotypes have provided convergent evidence for genes weakly associated with schizophrenia (e.g. *DTNBP1*, *DISC1*, *GRM3*, *DAOA*, *COMT*, *AKT1*, *KCNH2*), often in conjunction with MRI and fMRI measures assaying the underlying neural systems. Nevertheless, while many of the measures reviewed above are promising, further work is needed to identify more elementary phenotypes. For example, deficits in episodic memory could be due to abnormal encoding, early or late phases of long-term potentiation (LTP), or other factors related to dendrite formation and stabilization (see, for example, Milner *et al.*, 1998). Deficits in prefrontal function may be related to processes such as reduced GABA-mediated inhibition of glutamate neurons, alterations in neuronal migration, or reduced presynaptic dopamine input. Unfortunately, at present, methods to study such phenotypes in human subjects have not been fully developed.

The genetics of schizophrenia remain a challenging problem. Recent results from genome-wide associations studies (GWAS) suggest that perhaps hundreds to thousands of genes may make miniscule contributions to risk. It is not clear whether identifying these genes will shed significant light on disease biology or pathophysiology. Using intermediate phenotypes, particularly those clearly related to risk and disease biology, may be a viable alternative but is controversial. Some phenotypes are undoubtedly polygenic and offer little apparent advantage in GWAS over the diagnosis of schizophrenia. Furthermore, many genes impacting such traits may be irrelevant for schizophrenia (e.g., prepulse inhibition impairments and genes for deafness). On the other hand, some intermediate phenotypes are linked and span several levels of biology, from cellular and physiological abnormalities to systems level and cognition. For example, a set of phenotypes, including reduced GAD expression, fMRI-derived prefrontal activation, and working memory, span several biological levels and are all themselves implicated in the biology of schizophrenia. Finding a specific gene (e.g., *GAD1*) that has an effect on these many levels of biology offers important evidence that mitigates the relatively weak statistical association with clinical diagnosis. Other examples of such convergent evidence are available for a number of genes, including the nicotinic α7 receptor, *COMT*, *KCNH2*, *DISC1*, and *NRG1*. A key issue with such an integrative approach is how to evaluate statistical significance. While a rigorous statistical approach to human genetics might require a correction for a large number of genes and phenotypes, prior biological research often implicates specific genes and pathways and allow for less stringent statistical testing. The level of this *a priori* support may be convincing to some, but not all. Overall, the future of research on the genetics of neurobiological intermediate phenotypes promises to be exceptionally rich and exciting, if not controversial.

References

Addington, A.M., Gornick, M.C., Shaw, P. *et al.* (2007) Neuregulin 1 (8p12) and childhood-onset schizophrenia: susceptibility haplotypes for diagnosis and brain developmental trajectories. *Molecular Psychiatry* **12**, 195–205.

Agartz, I., Sedvall, G.C., Terenius, L. *et al.* (2006) BDNF gene variants and brain morphology in schizophrenia. *American Journal of Genetics B Neuropsychiatric Genetics* **141B**, 513–523.

Ahveninen, J., Jaaskelainen, I.P., Osipova, D. *et al.* (2006) Inherited auditory-cortical dysfunction in twin pairs discordant for schizophrenia. *Biological Psychiatry* **60**, 612–620.

Allison, D.B., Heo, M., Kaplan, N. & Martin, E.R. (1999) Sibling-based tests of linkage and association for quantitative traits. *American Journal of Human Genetics* **64**, 1754–1763.

Amador, X.F., Malaspina, D., Sackeim, H.A. *et al.* (1995) Visual fixation and smooth pursuit eye movement abnormalities in patients with schizophrenia and their relatives. *Journal of Neuropsychiatry and Clinical Neuroscience* **7**, 197–206.

Arolt, V., Lencer, R., Nolte, A. *et al.* (1996) Eye tracking dysfunction is a putative phenotypic susceptibility marker of schizophrenia and maps to a locus on chromosome 6p in families with multiple occurrence of the disease. *American Journal of Medical Genetics* **67**, 564–579.

Arolt, V., Lencer, R., Purmann, S. *et al.* (1999) Testing for linkage of eye tracking dysfunction and schizophrenia to markers on chromosomes 6, 8, 9, 20, and 22 in families multiply affected with schizophrenia. *American Journal of Medical Genetics* **88**, 603–606.

Aukes, M.F., Alizadeh, B.Z., Sitskoorn, M.M. *et al.* (2008) Finding suitable phenotypes for genetic studies of schizophrenia: heritability and segregation analysis. *Biological Psychiatry* **64**, 128–136.

Baare, W.F., van Oel, C.J., Hulshoff Pol, H.E. *et al.* (2001) Volumes of brain structures in twins discordant for schizophrenia. *Archives of General Psychiatry* **58**, 33–40.

Baker, N., Adler, L.E., Franks, R.D. *et al.* (1987) Neurophysiological assessment of sensory gating in psychiatric inpatients: comparison between schizophrenia and other diagnoses. *Biological Psychiatry* **22**, 603–617.

Barnett, J.H., Scoriels, L. & Munafo, M.R. (2008) Meta-analysis of the cognitive effects of the catechol-O-methyltransferase gene Val158/108Met polymorphism. *Biological Psychiatry* **64**, 137–144.

Bartley, A.J., Jones, D.W. & Weinberger, D.R. (1997) Genetic variability of human brain size and cortical gyral patterns. *Brain* **120**, 257–269.

Blackwood, D.H. & Muir, W.J. (2004) Clinical phenotypes associated with DISC1, a candidate gene for schizophrenia. *Neurotoxicology Research* **6**, 35–41.

Blackwood, D.H., Glabus, M.F., Dunan, J. *et al.* (1999) Altered cerebral perfusion measured by SPECT in relatives of patients with schizophrenia. Correlations with memory and P300. *British Journal of Psychiatry* **175**, 357–366.

Block, W., Bayer, T.A., Tepest, R. *et al.* (2000) Decreased frontal lobe ratio of N-acetyl aspartate to choline in familial schizophrenia: a proton magnetic resonance spectroscopy study. *Neuroscience Letters* **289**, 147–151.

Blokland, G.A., McMahon, K.L., Hoffman, J. *et al.* (2008) Quantifying the heritability of task-related brain activation and performance during the N-back working memory task: a twin fMRI study. *Biological Psychology* **79**, 70–79.

Bramon, E., Rabe-Hesketh, S., Sham, P., Murray, R.M. & Frangou, S. (2004) Meta-analysis of the P300 and P50 waveforms in schizophrenia. *Schizophrenia Research* **70**, 315–329.

Bramon, E., McDonald, C., Croft, R.J. *et al.* (2005) Is the P300 wave an endophenotype for schizophrenia? A meta-analysis and a family study. *Neuroimage* **27**, 960–968.

Brandon, N.J., Handford, E.J., Schurov, I. *et al.* (2004) Disrupted in Schizophrenia 1 and Nudel form a neurodevelopmentally regulated protein complex: implications for schizophrenia and other major neurological disorders. *Molecular and Cellular Neuroscience* **25**, 42–55.

Brzustowicz, L.M., Honer, W.G., Chow, E.W., Hogan, J., Hodgkinson, K. & Bassett, A.S. (1997) Use of a quantitative trait to map a locus associated with severity of positive symptoms in familial schizophrenia to chromosome 6p. *American Journal of Human Genetics* **61**, 1388–1396.

Buckholtz, J.W., Meyer-Lindenberg, A., Honea, R.A. *et al.* (2007) Allelic variation in RGS4 impacts functional and structural connectivity in the human brain. *Journal of Neuroscience* **27**, 1584–1593.

Bueller, J.A., Aftab, M., Sen, S., Gomez-Hassan, D., Burmeister, M. & Zubieta, J.K. (2006) BDNF Val66Met allele is associated with reduced hippocampal volume in healthy subjects. *Biological Psychiatry* **59**, 812–815.

Burdick, K.E., Lencz, T., Funke, B. *et al.* (2006) Genetic variation in DTNBP1 influences general cognitive ability. *Human Molecular Genetics* **15**, 1563–1568.

Cadenhead, K.S., Swerdlow, N.R., Shafer, K.M., Diaz, M. & Braff, D.L. (2000) Modulation of the startle response and startle laterality in relatives of schizophrenic patients and in subjects with schizotypal personality disorder: evidence of inhibitory deficits. *American Journal of Psychiatry* **157**, 1660–1668.

Calkins, M.E., Iacono, W.G. & Ones, D.S. (2008) Eye movement dysfunction in first-degree relatives of patients with schizophrenia: a meta-analytic evaluation of candidate endophenotypes. *Brain and Cognition* **68**, 436–461.

Callicott, J.H., Egan, M.F., Bertolino, A. *et al.* (1998) Hippocampal N-acetyl aspartate in unaffected siblings of patients with schizophrenia: a possible intermediate neurobiological phenotype. *Biological Psychiatry* **44**, 941–950.

Callicott, J.H., Egan, M.F., Mattay, V.S. *et al.* (2003) Abnormal fMRI response of the dorsolateral prefrontal cortex in cognitively intact siblings of patients with schizophrenia. *American Journal of Psychiatry* **160**, 709–719.

Callicott, J.H., Straub, R.E., Pezawas, L. *et al.* (2005) Variation in DISC1 affects hippocampal structure and function and increases risk for schizophrenia. *Proceedings of the National Academy of Science USA* **102**, 8627–8632.

Cannon, T.D. & Keller, M.C. (2006) Endophenotypes in the genetic analyses of mental disorders. *Annual Review of Clinical Psychology* **2**, 267–290.

Cannon, T.D. & Rosso, I.M. (2002) Levels of analysis in etiological research on schizophrenia. *Developmental Psychopathology* **14**, 653–666.

Cannon, T.D., Zorrilla, L.E., Shtasel, D. *et al.* (1994) Neuropsychological functioning in siblings discordant for schizophrenia and healthy volunteers. *Archives of General Psychiatry* **51**, 651–661.

Cannon, T.D., van Erp, T.G., Huttunen, M. *et al.* (1998) Regional gray matter, white matter, and cerebrospinal fluid distributions in schizophrenic patients, their siblings, and controls. *Archives of General Psychiatry* **55**, 1084–1091.

Cannon, T.D., Huttunen, M.O., Lonnqvist, J. *et al.* (2000) The inheritance of neuropsychological dysfunction in twins discordant for schizophrenia. *American Journal of Human Genetics* **67**, 369–382.

Cannon, T.D., Hennah, W., van Erp, T.G. *et al.* (2005) Association of DISC1/TRAX haplotypes with schizophrenia, reduced prefrontal gray matter, and impaired short- and long-term memory. *Archives of General Psychiatry* **62**, 1205–1213.

Cannon, T.D., Thompson, P.M., van Erp, T.G. *et al.* (2006) Mapping heritability and molecular genetic associations with cortical features using probabilistic brain atlases: methods and applications to schizophrenia. *Neuroinformatics* **4**, 5–19.

Carmelli, D., DeCarli, C., Swan, G.E. *et al.* (1998) Evidence for genetic variance in white matter hyperintensity volume in normal elderly male twins. *Stroke* **29**, 1177–1181.

Chen, W.J., Liu, S.K., Chang, C.J. *et al.* (1998) Sustained attention deficit and schizotypal personality features in non-psychotic relatives of schizophrenic patients. *American Journal of Psychiatry* **155**, 1214–1220.

Clementz, B.A. (1998) Psychophysiological measures of (dis) inhibition as liability indicators for schizophrenia. *Psychophysiology* **35**, 648–668.

Cornblatt, B.A. & Keilp, J.G. (1994) Impaired attention, genetics, and the pathophysiology of schizophrenia. *Schizophrenia Bulletin* **20**, 31–46.

Crespo-Facorro, B., Roiz-Santianez, R., Pelayo-Teran, J.M. *et al.* (2007) Low-activity allele of Catechol-O-Methyltransferase (COMTL) is associated with increased lateral ventricles in patients with first episode non-affective psychosis. *Progress in Neuropsychopharmacology and Biological Psychiatry* **31**, 1514–1518.

Demiralp, T., Herrmann, C.S., Erdal, M.E. *et al.* (2007) DRD4 and DAT1 polymorphisms modulate human gamma band responses. *Cerebral Cortex* **17**, 1007–1019.

Donchin, E. & Isreal, J.B. (1980) Event-related potentials and psychological theory. *Progress in Brain Research* **54**, 697–715.

Egan, M.F., Goldberg, T.E., Gscheidle, T., Weirich, M., Bigelow, L.B. & Weinberger, D.R. (2000) Relative risk of attention deficits in siblings of patients with schizophrenia. *American Journal of Psychiatry* **157**, 1309–1316.

Egan, M.F., Goldberg, T.E., Gscheidle, T. *et al.* (2001a) Relative risk for cognitive impairments in siblings of patients with schizophrenia. *Biological Psychiatry* **50**, 98–107.

Egan, M.F., Goldberg, T.E., Kolachana, B.S. *et al.* (2001b) Effect of COMT Val108/158 Met genotype on frontal lobe function and risk for schizophrenia. *Proceedings of the National Academy of Science USA* **98**, 6917–6922.

Egan, M.F., Hyde, T.M., Bonomo, J.B *et al.* (2001c) Relative risk of neurological signs in siblings of patients with schizophrenia. *American Journal of Psychiatry* **158**, 1827–1834.

Egan, M.F., Straub, R.E., Goldberg, T.E. *et al.* (2004) Variation in GRM3 affects cognition, prefrontal glutamate, and risk for schizophrenia. *Proceedings of the National Academy of Science USA* **101**, 12604–12609.

Esslinger, C., Walter, H., Kirsch, P. *et al.* (2009) Neural mechanisms of a genome-wide supported psychosis variant. *Science* **324**, 605.

Faraone, S.V., Seidman, L.J., Kremen, W.S., Pepple, J.R., Lyons, M.J. & Tsuang, M.T. (1995) Neuropsychological functioning among the nonpsychotic relatives of schizophrenic patients: a diagnostic efficiency analysis. *Journal of Abnormal Psychology* **104**, 286–304.

Finkelstein, J.R., Cannon, T.D., Gur, R.E., Gur, R.C. & Moberg, P. (1997) Attentional dysfunctions in neuroleptic-naive and neuroleptic-withdrawn schizophrenic patients and their siblings. *Journal of Abnormal Psychology* **106**, 203–212.

Fischl, B. & Dale, A.M. (2000) Measuring the thickness of the human cerebral cortex from magnetic resonance images. *Proceedings of the National Academy of Science USA* **97**, 11050–11055.

Fish, B. (1977) Neurobiologic antecedents of schizophrenia in children. Evidence for an inherited, congenital neurointegrative defect. *Archives of General Psychiatry* **34**, 1297–1313.

Flint, J. & Munafo, M.R. (2007) The endophenotype concept in psychiatric genetics. *Psychological Medicine* **37**, 163–180.

Franke, P., Maier, W., Hain, C. & Klingler, T. (1992) Wisconsin Card Sorting Test: an indicator of vulnerability to schizophrenia? *Schizophrenia Research* **6**, 243–249.

Freedman, R., Adler, L.E., Waldo, M.C., Pachtman, E. & Franks, R.D. (1983) Neurophysiological evidence for a defect in inhibitory pathways in schizophrenia: comparison of medicated and drug-free patients. *Biological Psychiatry* **18**, 537–551.

Freedman, R., Coon, H., Myles-Worsley, M. *et al.* (1997) Linkage of a neurophysiological deficit in schizophrenia to a chromosome 15 locus. *Proceedings of the National Academy of Science USA* **94**, 587–592.

Friedman, D. & Squires-Wheeler, E. (1994) Event-related potentials (ERPs) as indicators of risk for schizophrenia. *Schizophrenia Bulletin* **20**, 63–74.

Gamett, D.C., Greene, T., Wagreich, A.R., Kim, H.H., Koland, J.G. & Cerione, R.A. (1995) Heregulin-stimulated signaling in rat pheochromocytoma cells. Evidence for ErbB3 interactions with Neu/ErbB2 and p85. *Journal of Biological Chemistry* **270**, 19022–19027.

Glahn, D.C., Therman, S., Manninen, M. *et al.* (2003) Spatial working memory as an endophenotype for schizophrenia. *Biological Psychiatry* **53**, 624–626.

Glantz, L.A. & Lewis, D.A. (1997) Reduction of synaptophysin immunoreactivity in the prefrontal cortex of subjects with schizophrenia. Regional and diagnostic specificity. *Archives of General Psychiatry* **54**, 943–952.

Gogos, J.A., Morgan, M., Luine, V. *et al.* (1998) Catechol-O-methyltransferase-deficient mice exhibit sexually dimorphic changes in catecholamine levels and behavior. *Proceedings of the National Academy of Science USA* **95**, 9991–9996.

Goldberg, T.E., Torrey, E.F., Gold, J.M., Ragland, J.D., Bigelow, L.B. & Weinberger, D.R. (1993) Learning and memory in monozygotic twins discordant for schizophrenia. *Psychological Medicine* **23**, 71–85.

Goldberg, T.E., Torrey, E.F., Berman, K.F. & Weinberger, D.R. (1994) Relations between neuropsychological performance and brain morphological and physiological measures in monozygotic twins discordant for schizophrenia. *Psychiatry Research* **55**, 51–61.

Goldberg, T.E., Torrey, E.F., Gold, J.M. *et al.* (1995) Genetic risk of neuropsychological impairment in schizophrenia: a study of monozygotic twins discordant and concordant for the disorder. *Schizophrenia Research* **17**, 77–84.

Goldman, D., Weinberger, D.R., Malhotra, A.K., & Goldberg, T.E. (2009) The role of COMT Val158Met in cognition. *Biological Psychiatry* **65**, e1–e2.

Goldman-Rakic, P.S., Bergson, C., Mrzljak, L. & Williams, G.V. (1996) Dopamine receptors and cognitive function in nonhuman primates. In: Neve, K.A. & Neve, R.L., eds. *The Dopamine Receptors.* Totowa, NJ: Human Press, pp. 499–522.

Greenwood, T.A., Braff, D. L., Light, G. A. *et al.* (2007) Initial heritability analyses of endophenotypic measures for schizophrenia: the consortium on the genetics of schizophrenia. *Archives of General Psychiatry* **64**, 1242–1250.

Groom, M.J., Bates, A.T., Jackson, G.M., Calton, T.G., Liddle, P.F. & Hollis, C. (2008) Event-related potentials in adolescents with schizophrenia and their siblings: a comparison with attention-deficit/hyperactivity disorder. *Biological Psychiatry* **63**, 784–792.

Grove, W.M., Lebow, B.S., Clementz, B.A., Cerri, A., Medus, C. & Iacono, W.G. (1991) Familial prevalence and coaggregation of schizotypy indicators: a multitrait family study. *Journal of Abnormal Psychology* **100**, 115–121.

Gruber, O., Falkai, P., Schneider-Axmann, T., Schwab, S.G., Wagner, M. & Maier, W. (2008) Neuregulin-1 haplotype HAP(ICE) is associated with lower hippocampal volumes in schizophrenic patients and in non-affected family members. *Journal of Psychiatric Research* **43**, 1–6.

Hall, M.H., Rijsdijk, F., Picchioni, M. *et al.* (2007) Substantial shared genetic influences on schizophrenia and event-related potentials. *American Journal of Psychiatry* **164**, 804–812.

Hariri, A.R., Mattay, V.S., Tessitore, A. *et al.* (2002) Serotonin transporter genetic variation and the response of the human amygdala. *Science* **297**, 400–403.

Hennah, W., Tuulio-Henriksson, A., Paunio, T. *et al.* (2005) A haplotype within the DISC1 gene is associated with visual memory functions in families with a high density of schizophrenia. *Molecular Psychiatry* **10**, 1097–1103.

Hirvonen, J., van Erp, T.G., Huttunen, J. *et al.* (2005) Increased caudate dopamine D2 receptor availability as a genetic marker for schizophrenia. *Archives of General Psychiatry* **62**, 371–378.

Hirvonen, J., van Erp, T.G., Huttunen, J. *et al.* (2006) Brain dopamine d1 receptors in twins discordant for schizophrenia. *American Journal of Psychiatry* **163**, 1747–1753.

Ho, B.C., Milev, P., O'Leary, D.S., Librant, A., Andreasen, N.C. & Wassink, T.H. (2006) Cognitive and magnetic resonance imaging brain morphometric correlates of brain-derived neurotrophic factor Val66Met gene polymorphism in patients with schizophrenia and healthy volunteers. *Archives of General Psychiatry* **63**, 731–740.

Ho, B.C., Andreasen, N.C., Dawson, J.D. & Wassink, T.H. (2007) Association between brain-derived neurotrophic factor Val66Met gene polymorphism and progressive brain volume changes in schizophrenia. *American Journal of Psychiatry* **164**, 1890–1899.

Holzman, P.S., Proctor, L.R. & Hughes, D.W. (1973) Eye-tracking patterns in schizophrenia. *Science* **181**, 179–181.

Holzman, P.S., Proctor, L.R., Levy, D.L., Yasillo, N.J., Meltzer, H.Y. & Hurt, S.W. (1974) Eye-tracking dysfunctions in schizophrenic patients and their relatives. *Archives of General Psychiatry* **31**, 143–151.

Holzman, P.S., Kringlen, E., Matthysse, S. *et al.* (1988) A single dominant gene can account for eye tracking dysfunctions and schizophrenia in offspring of discordant twins. *Archives of General Psychiatry* **45**, 641–647.

Hong, L.E., Turano, K.A., O'Neill, H. *et al.* (2008) Refining the predictive pursuit endophenotype in schizophrenia. *Biological Psychiatry* **63**, 458–464.

Huffaker, S.J., Chen, J., Nicodemus, K.K. *et al.* (2009) A primate-specific, brain isoform of KCNH2 affects cortical physiology, cognition, neuronal repolarization and risk of schizophrenia. *Nature Medicine* **15**, 509–518.

Hurdal, M.K. & Stephenson, K. (2004) Cortical cartography using the discrete conformal approach of circle packings. *Neuroimage* **23** (Suppl. 1), S119–S128.

Huttunen, J., Heinimaa, M., Svirskis, T. *et al.* (2008) Striatal dopamine synthesis in first-degree relatives of patients with schizophrenia. *Biological Psychiatry* **63**, 114–117.

Iacono, W.G., Moreau, M., Beiser, M., Fleming, J.A. & Lin, T.Y. (1992) Smooth-pursuit eye tracking in first-episode psychotic patients and their relatives. *Journal of Abnormal Psychology* **101**, 104–116.

Ismail, B., Cantor-Graae, E. & McNeil, T.F. (1998) Minor physical anomalies in schizophrenic patients and their siblings. *American Journal of Psychiatry* **155**, 1695–1702.

Javitt, D.C., Steinschneider, M., Schroeder, C.E. & Arezzo, J.C. (1996) Role of cortical N-methyl-D-aspartate receptors in auditory sensory memory and mismatch negativity generation: implications for schizophrenia. *Proceedings of the National Academy of Science USA* **93**, 11962–11967.

Jeon, Y.W. & Polich, J. (2003) Meta-analysis of P300 and schizophrenia: patients, paradigms, and practical implications. *Psychophysiology* **40**, 684–701.

Jin, Y. & Potkin, S.G. (1996) P50 changes with visual interference in normal subjects: a sensory distraction model for schizophrenia. *Clinical Electroencephalography* **27**, 151–154.

Jin, Y., Potkin, S.G., Patterson, J.V., Sandman, C.A., Hetrick, W.P. & Bunney, W.E., Jr. (1997) Effects of P50 temporal variability on sensory gating in schizophrenia. *Psychiatry Research* **70**, 71–81.

Johnson, J.K., Tuulio-Henriksson, A., Pirkola, T. *et al.* (2003) Do schizotypal symptoms mediate the relationship between genetic risk for schizophrenia and impaired neuropsychological performance in co-twins of schizophrenic patients? *Biological Psychiatry* **54**, 1200–1204.

Kamiya, A., Kubo, K., Tomoda, T. *et al.* (2005) A schizophrenia-associated mutation of DISC1 perturbs cerebral cortex development. *Nature Cell Biology* **7**, 1167–1178.

Karoum, F., Chrapusta, S.J. & Egan, M.F. (1994) 3-Methoxytyramine is the major metabolite of released dopamine in the rat frontal cortex: reassessment of the effects of antipsychotics on the dynamics of dopamine release and metabolism in the frontal cortex, nucleus accumbens, and striatum by a simple two pool model. *Journal of Neurochemistry* **63**, 972–979.

Keefe, R.S., Silverman, J.M., Roitman, S.E. *et al.* (1994) Performance of nonpsychotic relatives of schizophrenic patients on cognitive tests. *Psychiatry Research* **53**, 1–12.

Keefe, R.S., Silverman, J.M., Mohs, R.C. *et al.* (1997) Eye tracking, attention, and schizotypal symptoms in nonpsychotic relatives of patients with schizophrenia. *Archives of General Psychiatry* **54**, 169–176.

Keshavan, M.S., Montrose, D.M., Pierri, J.N. *et al.* (1997) Magnetic resonance imaging and spectroscopy in offspring at risk for schizophrenia: preliminary studies. *Prog. Neuropsychopharmacol. Biological Psychiatry* **21**, 1285–1295.

Kleinman, J.E., Law, A.J., Lipska, B.K. *et al.* (2011) Genetic neuropathology of schizophrenia: new approaches to an old question, and new uses for post mortem human brains. *Biological Psychiatry* (in press).

Klemm, S., Rzanny, R., Riehemann, S. *et al.* (2001) Cerebral phosphate metabolism in first-degree relatives of patients with schizophrenia. *American Journal of Psychiatry* **158**, 958–960.

Kneavel, M., Gogas, J., Karayiorgou K. & Luine, V. (2000) Interaction of COMT gene deletion and environment on cognition. Society for Neuroscience, 30th Annual Meeting, 2000.

Koten, J.W., Jr., Wood, G., Hagoort, P. *et al.* (2009) Genetic contribution to variation in cognitive function: an FMRI study in twins. *Science* **323**, 1737–1740.

Kremen, W.S., Tsuang, M.T., Faraone, S.V. & Lyons, M.J. (1992) Using vulnerability indicators to compare conceptual models of genetic heterogeneity in schizophrenia. *Journal of Nervous and Mental Disease* **180**, 141–152.

Kremen, W.S., Seidman, L.J., Pepple, J.R., Lyons, M.J., Tsuang, M.T. & Faraone, S.V. (1994) Neuropsychological risk indicators for schizophrenia: a review of family studies. *Schizophrenia Bulletin* **20**, 103–119.

Kumari, V., Das, M., Zachariah, E., Ettinger, U. & Sharma, T. (2005) Reduced prepulse inhibition in unaffected siblings of schizophrenia patients. *Psychophysiology* **42**, 588–594.

Lander, E.S. & Schork, N.J. (1994) Genetic dissection of complex traits. *Science* **265**, 2037–2048.

Laurent, A., Biloa-Tang, M., Bougerol, T. *et al.* (2000) Executive/attentional performance and measures of schizotypy in patients with schizophrenia and in their non-psychotic first-degree relatives. *Schizophrenia Research* **46**, 269–283.

Law, A.J., Lipska, B.K., Weickert, C.S. *et al.* (2006) Neuregulin 1 transcripts are differentially expressed in schizophrenia and regulated by 5′ SNPs associated with the disease. *Proceedings of the National Academy of Science USA* **103**, 6747–6752.

Lawrie, S.M., Whalley, H., Kestelman, J.N. *et al.* (1999) Magnetic resonance imaging of brain in people at high risk of developing schizophrenia. *Lancet* **353**, 30–33.

Lawrie, S.M., Whalley, H.C., Abukmeil, S.S. *et al.* (2001) Brain structure, genetic liability, and psychotic symptoms in subjects at high risk of developing schizophrenia. *Biological Psychiatry* **49**, 811–823.

Leonard, S., Gault, J., Hopkins, J. *et al.* (2002) Association of promoter variants in the alpha7 nicotinic acetylcholine receptor subunit gene with an inhibitory deficit found in schizophrenia. *Archives of General Psychiatry* **59**, 1085–1096.

Levin, S., Jones, A., Stark, L., Merrin, E.L., & Holzman, P.S. (1982) Identification of abnormal patterns in eye movements of schizophrenic patients. *Archives of General Psychiatry* **39**, 1125–1130.

Levy, D.L., Holzman, P.S., Matthysse, S. & Mendell, N.R. (1993) Eye tracking dysfunction and schizophrenia: a critical perspective. *Schizophrenia Bulletin* **19**, 461–536.

Levy, D.L., Holzman, P.S., Matthysse, S. & Mendell, N.R. (1994) Eye tracking and schizophrenia: a selective review. *Schizophrenia Bulletin* **20**, 47–62.

Levy, D.L., Bowman, E.A., Abel, L., Krastoshevsky, O., Krause, V. & Mendell, N.R. (2008) Does performance on the standard antisaccade task meet the co-familiality criterion for an endophenotype? *Brain and Cognition* **68**, 462–475.

Li, W., Zhou, Y., Jentsch, J.D. *et al.* (2007) Specific developmental disruption of disrupted-in-schizophrenia-1 function results in schizophrenia-related phenotypes in mice. *Proceedings of the National Academy of Science USA* **104**, 18280–18285.

Light, G.A. & Braff, D.L. (2005) Mismatch negativity deficits are associated with poor functioning in schizophrenia patients. *Archives of General Psychiatry* **62**, 127–136.

Liu, Y., Ford, B., Mann, M.A., & Fischbach, G.D. (2001) Neuregulins increase alpha7 nicotinic acetylcholine receptors and enhance excitatory synaptic transmission in GABAergic interneurons of the hippocampus. *Journal of Neuroscience* **21**, 5660–5669.

Lutkenhoff, E.S., van Erp, T.G., Thomas, M.A. *et al.* (2010) Proton MRS in twin pairs discordant for schizophrenia. *Molecular Psychiatry* **15**, 308–318.

MacDonald, A.W., III, Becker, T.M., & Carter, C.S. (2006) Functional magnetic resonance imaging study of cognitive control in the healthy relatives of schizophrenia patients. *Biological Psychiatry* **60**, 1241–1249.

MacDonald, A.W., III, Thermenos, H.W., Barch, D.M. & Seidman, L.J. (2009) Imaging genetic liability to schizophrenia: systematic review of FMRI studies of patients' nonpsychotic relatives. *Schizophrenia Bulletin* **35**, 1142–1162.

Magno, E., Yeap, S., Thakore, J.H., Garavan, H., De Sanctis, P. & Foxe, J.J. (2008) Are auditory-evoked frequency and duration mismatch negativity deficits endophenotypic for schizophrenia? High-density electrical mapping in clinically unaffected first-degree relatives and first-episode and chronic schizophrenia. *Biological Psychiatry* **64**, 385–391.

Maier, W., Franke, P., Hain, C., Kopp, B. & Rist, F. (1992) Neuropsychological indicators of the vulnerability to schizophrenia. *Progress in Neuropsychopharmacology and Biological Psychiatry* **16**, 703–715.

Matthysse, S., Holzman, P.S., Gusella, J.F. *et al.* (2004) Linkage of eye movement dysfunction to chromosome 6p in schizophrenia: additional evidence. *American Journal of Medical Genetics B Neuropsychiatric Genetics* **128B**, 30–36.

McDowell, J.E. & Clementz, B.A. (1996) Ocular-motor delayed-response task performance among schizophrenia patients. *Neuropsychobiology* **34**, 67–71.

McGue, M. & Gottesman, I.I. (1989) Genetic linkage in schizophrenia: perspectives from genetic epidemiology. *Schizophrenia Bulletin* **15**, 453–464.

McIntosh, A.M., Moorhead, T.W., Job, D. *et al.* (2008) The effects of a neuregulin 1 variant on white matter density and integrity. *Molecular Psychiatry* **13**, 1054–1059.

McNeil, T.F., Cantor-Graae, E. & Weinberger, D.R. (2000) Relationship of obstetric complications and differences in size of brain structures in monozygotic twin pairs discordant for schizophrenia. *American Journal of Psychiatry* **157**, 203–212.

Millar, J.K., Christie, S. & Porteous, D.J. (2003) Yeast two-hybrid screens implicat–e DISC1 in brain development and function. *Biochemisry and Biophysics Research Communications* **311**, 1019–1025.

Milner, B., Squire, L.R. & Kandel, E.R. (1998) Cognitive neuroscience and the study of memory. *Neuron* **20**, 445–468.

Mirsky, A.F., Anthony, B.J., Duncan, C.C., Ahearn, M.B. & Kellam, S.G. (1991) Analysis of the elements of attention: a neuropsychological approach. *Neuropsychology Reviews* **2**, 109–145.

Morris, J.A., Kandpal, G., Ma, L. & Austin, C.P. (2003) DISC1 (Disrupted-In-Schizophrenia 1) is a centrosome-associated protein that interacts with MAP1A, MIPT3, ATF4/5 and NUDEL: regulation and loss of interaction with mutation. *Human Molecular Genetics* **12**, 1591–1608.

Mulert, C., Juckel, G., Giegling, I. *et al.* (2006) A Ser9Gly polymorphism in the dopamine D3 receptor gene (DRD3) and event-related P300 potentials. *Neuropsychopharmacology* **31**, 1335–1344.

Naatanen, R. & Kahkonen, S. (2009) Central auditory dysfunction in schizophrenia as revealed by the mismatch negativity (MMN) and its magnetic equivalent MMNm: a review. *International Journal of Neuropsychopharmacology* **12**, 125–135.

Nemoto, K., Ohnishi, T., Mori, T. *et al.* (2006) The Val66Met polymorphism of the brain-derived neurotrophic factor gene affects age-related brain morphology. *Neuroscience Letters* **397**, 25–29.

Nuechterlein, K.H. & Dawson, M.E. (1984) Information processing and attentional functioning in the developmental course of schizophrenic disorders. *Schizophrenia Bulletin* **10**, 160–203.

O'Driscoll, G.A., Florencio, P.S., Gagnon, D. *et al.* (2001) Amygdala-hippocampal volume and verbal memory in first-degree relatives of schizophrenic patients. *Psychiatry Research* **107**, 75–85.

Ozeki, Y., Tomoda, T., Kleiderlein, J. *et al.* (2003) Disrupted-in-Schizophrenia-1 (DISC-1): mutant truncation prevents binding to NudE-like (NUDEL) and inhibits neurite outgrowth. *Proceedings of the National Academy of Science USA* **100**, 289–294.

Park, S., Holzman, P.S., & Goldman-Rakic, P.S. (1995) Spatial working memory deficits in the relatives of schizophrenic patients. *Archives of General Psychiatry* **52**, 821–828.

Pfefferbaum, A., Sullivan, E.V., Swan, G.E. & Carmelli, D. (2000) Brain structure in men remains highly heritable in the seventh and eighth decades of life. *Neurobiology of Aging* **21**, 63–74.

Plomin, R., DeFries, J.C. & McClearn, G.E. (1990) *Behavioral Genetics*, 2nd edn. New York: W.H. Freeman.

Pogue-Geile, M.F., Garrett, A.H., Brunke, J.J. & Hall, J.K. (1991) Neuropsychological impairments are increased in siblings of schizophrenic patients. *Schizophrenia Research* **4**, 390.

Posthuma, D., de Geus, E.J., Neale, M.C. *et al.* (2000) Multivariate genetic analysis of brain structure in an extended twin design. *Behavioral Genetics* **30**, 311–319.

Potkin, S.G., Turner, J.A. Guffanti, G. *et al.* (2009) A genome-wide association study of schizophrenia using brain activation as a quantitative phenotype. *Schizophrenia Bulletin* **35**, 96–108.

Potter, D., Summerfelt, A., Gold, J. & Buchanan, R.W. (2006) Review of clinical correlates of P50 sensory gating abnormalities in patients with schizophrenia. *Schizophrenia Bulletin* **32**, 692–700.

Reilly, J.L., Lencer, R., Bishop, J.R., Keedy, S. & Sweeney, J.A. (2008) Pharmacological treatment effects on eye movement control. *Brain and Cognition* **68**, 415–435.

Risch, N. & Merikangas, K. (1996) The future of genetic studies of complex human diseases. *Science* **273**, 1516–1517.

Rutschmann, J., Cornblatt, B. & Erlenmeyer-Kimling, L. (1977) Sustained attention in children at risk for schizophrenia. Report on a continuous performance test. *Archives of General Psychiatry* **34**, 571–575.

Rutschmann, J., Cornblatt, B. & Erlenmeyer-Kimling, L. (1986) Sustained attention in children at risk for schizophrenia: findings with two visual continuous performance tests in a new sample. *Journal of Abnormal Child Psychology* **14**, 365–385.

Rybakowski, J.K., Borkowska, A., Czerski, P.M. & Hauser, J. (2001) Dopamine D3 receptor (DRD3) gene polymorphism is associated with the intensity of eye movement disturbances in schizophrenic patients and healthy subjects. *Molecular Psychiatry* **6**, 718–724.

Rybakowski, J.K., Borkowska, A., Czerski, P.M., Dmitrzak-Weglarz, M. & Hauser, J. (2003) The study of cytosolic phospholipase A2 gene polymorphism in schizophrenia using eye movement disturbances as an endophenotypic marker. *Neuropsychobiology* **47**, 115–119.

Salisbury, D.F., Shenton, M.E., Griggs, C.B., Bonner-Jackson, A. & McCarley, R.W. (2002) Mismatch negativity in chronic schizophrenia and first-episode schizophrenia. *Archives of General Psychiatry* **59**, 686–694.

Saoud, M., d'Amato, T., Gutknecht, C. *et al.* (2000) Neuropsychological deficit in siblings discordant for schizophrenia. *Schizophrenia Bulletin* **26**, 893–902.

Scamvougeras, A., Kigar, D.L., Jones, D., Weinberger, D.R., & Witelson, S.F. (2003) Size of the human corpus callosum is genetically determined: an MRI study in mono and dizygotic twins. *Neuroscience Letters* **338**, 91–94.

Scarone, S., Abbruzzese, M. & Gambini, O. (1993) The Wisconsin Card Sorting Test discriminates schizophrenic patients and their siblings. *Schizophrenia Research* **10**, 103–107.

Sei, Y., Ren-Patterson, R., Li, Z. *et al.* (2007) Neuregulin1-induced cell migration is impaired in schizophrenia: association with neuregulin1 and catechol-o-methyltransferase gene polymorphisms. *Molecular Psychiatry* **12**, 946–957.

Seidman, L.J., Faraone, S.V., Goldstein, J.M. *et al.* (1999) Thalamic and amygdala-hippocampal volume reductions in first-degree relatives of patients with schizophrenia: an MRI-based morphometric analysis. *Biological Psychiatry* **46**, 941–954.

Selemon, L.D., Rajkowska, G. & Goldman-Rakic, P.S. (1995) Abnormally high neuronal density in the schizophrenic cortex. A morphometric analysis of prefrontal area 9 and occipital area 17. *Archives of General Psychiatry* **52**, 805–818.

Sesack, S.R., Hawrylak, V.A., Matus, C., Guido, M.A., & Levey, A.I. (1998) Dopamine axon varicosities in the prelimbic division of the rat prefrontal cortex exhibit sparse immunoreactivity for the dopamine transporter. *Journal of Neuroscience* **18**, 2697–2708.

Sharma, T., Lancaster, E., Lee, D. *et al.* (1998) Brain changes in schizophrenia. Volumetric MRI study of families multiply affected with schizophrenia – the Maudsley Family Study 5. *British Journal of Psychiatry* **173**, 132–138.

Shields, J. & Gottesman, I.I. (1972) Cross-national diagnosis of schizophrenia in twins. The heritability and specificity of schizophrenia. *Archives of General Psychiatry* **27**, 725–730.

Shin, K.S., Kim, J.S., Kang, D.H. *et al.* (2009) Pre-attentive auditory processing in ultra-high-risk for schizophrenia with magnetoencephalography. *Biological Psychiatry* **65**, 1071–1078.

Siegel, C., Waldo, M., Mizner, G., Adler, L.E. & Freedman, R. (1984) Deficits in sensory gating in schizophrenic patients and their relatives. Evidence obtained with auditory evoked responses. *Archives of General Psychiatry* **41**, 607–612.

Slifstein, M., Kolachana, B., Simpson, E.H. *et al.* (2008) COMT genotype predicts cortical-limbic D1 receptor availability measured with [11C]NNC112 and PET. *Molecular Psychiatry* **13**, 821–827.

Spielman, R.S., McGinnis, R.E. & Ewens, W.J. (1993) Transmission test for linkage disequilibrium: the insulin gene region and insulin-dependent diabetes mellitus (IDDM). *American Journal of Human Genetics* **52**, 506–516.

Staal, W.G., Hulshoff Pol, H.E., Schnack, H., van der Schot, A.C. & Kahn, R.S. (1998) Partial volume decrease of the thalamus in relatives of patients with schizophrenia. *American Journal of Psychiatry* **155**, 1784–1786.

Staal, W.G., Hulshoff Pol, H.E., Schnack, H.G., Hoogendoorn, M.L., Jellema, K. & Kahn, R.S. (2000) Structural brain abnormalities in patients with schizophrenia and their healthy siblings. *American Journal of Psychiatry* **157**, 416–421.

Straub, R.E., Lipska, B.K., Egan, M.F. *et al.* (2007) Allelic variation in GAD1 (GAD67) is associated with schizophrenia and influences cortical function and gene expression. *Molecular Psychiatry* **12**, 854–869.

Sullivan, E.V., Pfefferbaum, A., Swan, G.E., & Carmelli, D. (2001) Heritability of hippocampal size in elderly twin men: equivalent influence from genes and environment. *Hippocampus* **11**, 754–762.

Swerdlow, N.R., Geyer, M.A. & Braff, D.L. (2001) Neural circuit regulation of prepulse inhibition of startle in the rat: current knowledge and future challenges. *Psychopharmacology (Berlin)* **156**, 194–215.

Swerdlow, N.R., Light, G.A., Cadenhead, K.S., Sprock, J., Hsieh, M.H. & Braff, D.L. (2006) Startle gating deficits in a large cohort of patients with schizophrenia: relationship to medications, symptoms, neurocognition, and level of function. *Archives of General Psychiatry* **63**, 1325–1335.

Szeszko, P. R., Lipsky, R., Mentschel, C. *et al.* (2005) Brain-derived neurotrophic factor val66met polymorphism and volume of the hippocampal formation. *Molecular Psychiatry* **10**, 631–636.

Szeszko, P.R., Hodgkinson, C.A., Robinson, D.G., *et al.* (2008) DISC1 is associated with prefrontal cortical gray matter and positive symptoms in schizophrenia. *Biological Psychology* **79**, 103–110.

Thaker, G.K. (2007) Schizophrenia endophenotypes as treatment targets. *Expert Opinion in Therapeutic Targets* **11**, 1189–1206.

Thaker, G.K., Wonodi, I., Avila, M.T., Hong, L.E. & Stine, O.C. (2004) Catechol O-methyltransferase polymorphism and eye tracking in schizophrenia: a preliminary report. *American Journal of Psychiatry* **161**, 2320–2322.

Thompson, P.M., Cannon, T.D., Narr, K.L. *et al.* (2001) Genetic influences on brain structure. *Nature Neuroscience* **4**, 1253–1258.

Thompson, P.M., Hayashi, K.M., Sowell, E.R. *et al.* (2004) Mapping cortical change in Alzheimer's disease, brain development, and schizophrenia. *Neuroimage* **23** (Suppl. 1), S2–18.

Toomey, R., Faraone, S.V., Seidman, L.J., Kremen, W.S., Pepple, J.R. & Tsuang, M.T. (1998) Association of neuropsychological vulnerability markers in relatives of schizophrenic patients. *Schizophrenia Research* **31**, 89–98.

Toulopoulou, T., Picchioni, M., Rijsdijk, F. *et al.* (2007) Substantial genetic overlap between neurocognition and schizophrenia: genetic modeling in twin samples. *Archives of General Psychiatry* **64**, 1348–1355.

Turetsky, B.I., Calkins, M.E., Light, G.A., Olincy, A., Radant, A.D. & Swerdlow, N.R. (2007) Neurophysiological endophenotypes of schizophrenia: the viability of selected candidate measures. *Schizophrenia Bulletin* **33**, 69–94.

Umbricht, D. & Krljes, S. (2005) Mismatch negativity in schizophrenia: a meta-analysis. *Schizophrenia Research* **76**, 1–23.

van der Stelt, O. & Belger, A. (2007) Application of electroencephalography to the study of cognitive and brain functions in schizophrenia. *Schizophrenia Bulletin* **33**, 955–970.

van Erp, T.G., Saleh, P.A., Huttunen, M. *et al.* (2004) Hippocampal volumes in schizophrenic twins. *Archives of General Psychiatry* **61**, 346–353.

Van Essen, D.C. (2004) Surface-based approaches to spatial localization and registration in primate cerebral cortex. *Neuroimage* **23** (Suppl. 1), S97–107.

van Haren, N.E., Picchioni, M.M., McDonald, C. *et al.* (2004) A controlled study of brain structure in monozygotic twins concordant and discordant for schizophrenia. *Biological Psychiatry* **56**, 454–461.

Vartanian, T., Fischbach, G. & Miller, R. (1999) Failure of spinal cord oligodendrocyte development in mice lacking neuregulin. *Proceedings of the National Academy of Science USA* **96**, 731–735.

Vaskovsky, A., Lupowitz, Z., Erlich, S. & Pinkas-Kramarski, R. (2000) ErbB-4 activation promotes neurite outgrowth in PC12 cells. *Journal of Neurochemistry* **74**, 979–987.

Villegas, R., Villegas, G.M., Longart, M. *et al.* (2000) Neuregulin found in cultured-sciatic nerve conditioned medium causes neuronal differentiation of PC12 cells. *Brain Research* **852**, 305–318.

Watanabe, A., Toyota, T., Owada, Y. *et al.* (2007) Fabp7 maps to a quantitative trait locus for a schizophrenia endophenotype. *PLoS Biology* **5**, e297.

Weinshilboum, R. & Dunnette, J. (1981) Thermal stability and the biochemical genetics of erythrocyte catechol-O-methyltransferase and plasma dopamine-beta-hydroxylase. *Clinical Genetics* **19**, 426–437.

Whitfield-Gabrieli, S., Thermenos, H.W., Milanovic, S. *et al.* (2009) Hyperactivity and hyperconnectivity of the default network in schizophrenia and in first-degree relatives of persons with schizophrenia. *Proceedings of the National Academy of Science USA* **106**, 1279–1284.

Williams, G.V. & Goldman-Rakic, P.S. (1995) Modulation of memory fields by dopamine D1 receptors in prefrontal cortex. *Nature* **376**, 572–575.

Wright, I.C., Sham, P., Murray, R.M., Weinberger, D.R. & Bullmore, E.T. (2002) Genetic contributions to regional variability in human brain structure: methods and preliminary results. *Neuroimage* **17**, 256–271.

Yeap, S., Kelly, S.P., Sehatpour, P. *et al.* (2006) Early visual sensory deficits as endophenotypes for schizophrenia: high-density electrical mapping in clinically unaffected first-degree relatives. *Archives of General Psychiatry* **63**, 1180–1188.

CHAPTER 15

Electrophysiology of schizophrenia

Georg Winterer[1] and Robert W. McCarley[2]

[1]Cologne Center for Genomics, Cologne, Germany
[2]VA Boston Healthcare System, Brockton, MA, USA

Introduction

The electroencephalogram (EEG) was the first physiological technique used to examine brain activity in schizophrenia and has evolved into a powerful method for studying brain information processing activity. In today's world of multimodal imaging it is unsurpassed in providing real-time, millisecond resolution of normal and pathological brain processing, literally at the speed of thought. In this chapter, we will discuss the application of this technique to schizophrenia research. The first section is for the reader unfamiliar with electrophysiology who wishes an introduction to the basics. The reader desiring more information regarding EEG and event-related potential (ERP) theory and techniques is referred to Handy (2004).

The electroencephalogram

Cognitive events are subserved by neurons in the brain. This activity is reflected in the EEG or alternatively in the magnetoencephalogram (MEG), the electromagnetic activity recorded from the surface of the scalp. In general, the EEG derives from summated postsynaptic activity in many neurons. When the dendritic fields of neurons are aligned,

as is true of pyramidal cells in the cortex, the voltages generated by simultaneously occurring dendritic postsynaptic potentials (PSPs, either hyper- or de-polarizations) summate and produce the EEG field. It is important to emphasize that EEG does not typically reflect neuronal discharges, since they are usually too brief and also too asynchronous. [As an aside, we note blood-oxygen-level-dependent (BOLD) functional magnetic resonance imaging (fMRI) "activation" similarly mainly reflects PSP activity, which is metabolically most demanding and necessitates the increased blood flow, but not action potential activity, which is metabolically much less demanding.]

The EEG reflects all of the activity in the brain that reaches the scalp. Thus, the EEG reflects the activity of many groups of nerve cells, and this activity represents brain operations related to many different ongoing events, such as breathing, seeing, hearing, and thinking, as well as different processing modes of large groups of nerve cells. (The reader is cautioned that neurotransmitter signals not only have consequences of ion channel modulation, but also may set off internal signal cascades in second messenger systems, which may bring about more lasting changes, a topic beyond the scope of this chapter.)

Event-related potentials

One of the important advances in EEG-based research was the development of a technique to isolate brain activity

Schizophrenia, 3rd edition. Edited by Daniel R. Weinberger and
Paul J Harrison © 2011 Blackwell Publishing Ltd.

related to specific events from the background EEG. Using averaging techniques, small potentials related to one of the many different brain operations reflected in the EEG can be visualized. Typically these events are related to the specific processing of certain stimuli in the stimulus field, i.e., the events in the environment impinging upon the individual. Signal averaging seeks to isolate the brain activity to specific events by recording small portions of the EEG each time a specific stimulus is presented. The stimulus is presented many times, with a number of EEG epochs thus recorded. Each of these epochs is recorded relative to the presentation of the stimulus, which might be a tone, and might last one second after the presentation of the tone. For each epoch, there will be two types of activity: (1) the activity specifically related to the tone; and (2) the activity related to everything else going on in the brain. The former activity, which is related to the tone, is said to be time-locked, with all the activity in sensory system relay and processing areas occurring at roughly the same time after each tone is presented. Hence, at any specific point in time after the presentation of the stimulus, time-locked event-related activity will be temporally stable from one trial to the next (for limitations of this assumption, see Spencer, 2004). The latter activity, which is not specifically related to the stimulus, will be, by definition, random with respect to the tone. By averaging together all the epochs, the time-locked event-related activity will remain stable, since it occurs at roughly the same time from trial to trial, but the non-time-locked EEG activity will be averaged out—since it is sometimes negative and sometimes positive at the same point in time from one trial to the next. The time-locked brain activity that remains is referred to as the event-related potential (ERP) waveform, and each of the various positive or negative events that comprise it are referred to as event-related potentials (Jervis *et al.*, 1983; Hillyard & Picton, 1987). The ERP technique in cognitive neuroscience allows scientists to observe human brain activity that reflects specific cognitive processes in the time and spatial domains.

A complementary approach driven by biophysical and neurocomputational concepts is termed time-frequency analysis. This approach views brain activity as a sum of superimposed oscillations maintained within and between brain regions giving rise to spontaneous or event-related/ induced oscillations. This approach states that the sensory stimulus induces a "phase resetting" of ongoing EEG rhythms in each trial and that averaging these reset, phase-coherent rhythms is important in producing the ERP (see, for example, Winterer *et al.*, 1999; Makeig *et al.*, 2002). It seems obvious that both summated sensory-driven neural events and phase resetting may play a role in the observed ERPs, although the relative importance of each is still a matter of debate and needs empirical resolution.

Depending on the types of interaction that occur in a specific behavioral condition, cortical networks may dis-play different states of synchrony, causing their ERPs to oscillate in different frequency bands, designated delta (0–4 Hz), theta (5–8 Hz), alpha (9–12 Hz), beta (13–30 Hz), and gamma (31–100 Hz). The inverse of synchrony in all or any of these frequency bands can be called "noise" (see below). A related, but distinct, approach to assessment of neural synchrony has been evaluation of auditory steady-state response (ASSR) or steady-state visual evoked potential (ssVEP). In this approach, sensory systems are driven at the frequency of interest, and amplitude of the cortical response is assessed as a function of stimulation rate. Thus, activity is not generated endogenously, but is driven exogenously.

The place of electrophysiology in the neuroimaging spectrum

In recent years, many new means of measuring brain structure and function have been developed. Some image the structure of the brain. Structural imaging includes X-ray-based techniques, e.g., computerized axial tomography (CAT) scans, and nuclear magnetic field-based techniques, e.g., MRI. These structural techniques have high spatial resolution and provide detailed information about the static structure of the brain (see Chapter 16). However, they provide little information about brain activity, as they provide only a snapshot of brain tissue rather than a series of measures of brain physiology. A second class of brain imaging techniques measure brain functional activity, e.g., fMRI (see Chapter 17). These functional techniques assay brain activity based on such measures as blood oxygenation level, an indirect measure of brain activity (BOLD fMRI), or on positron emission tomography (PET), which uses radioactive-labeled substances to measure metabolism (^{18}fludeoxyglucose, [^{18}F]2DG), blood flow (^{15}O water), or receptor occupancy (labeled ligands), as well as single photon emission tomography (SPECT). It is an important point that fMRI hemodynamic signals and [^{15}O]H$_2$O PET, as well as [^{18}F]2DG PET metabolic measures, all primarily derive from PSP activity and not neuronal discharge, since PSP activity is metabolically most demanding on the neuron and also evokes most of the blood flow changes (cf. Logothetis *et al.*, 2001). Thus "activation" as is commonly used in neuroimaging mainly reflects PSPs (often from input to the region) and not neuronal discharge. These techniques provide relatively good spatial resolution (although not as good as structural MRI). However, in current psychiatric imaging the temporal resolutions of fMRI are in the second range, although new advances in modeling the BOLD response (Hermandez *et al.*, 2002) and in multiple channel acquisition (Lin *et al.* 2006) suggest the as yet unrealized possibility of resolutions in the hundred millisecond range in the future. This current temporal resolution is several thousand-fold less than electrophysiological measures, which provide resolution within a few milliseconds (ms). The interested reader is referred to Toga and Mazziotta (2002) for further information regarding different imaging modalities, as well as to other chapters in this volume.

In contrast to its superior temporal resolution, the EEG's spatial resolution is limited, since the source of the voltage fluctuations at the scalp cannot be precisely identified as coming from particular brain regions (the so-called "inverse-problem"). This temporal sensitivity and spatial insensitivity of the EEG is nicely complemented by the exquisitely detailed spatial information from structural MRI. Structural MRI provides detailed information on which brain regions show pathological reduction in gray matter in many diseases, including schizophrenia. To combine EEG and MRI information, McCarley and collaborators have determined the association of structural volumetric abnormalities in particular regions with particular evoked potentials. This resembles the classical "lesion" approach to behavior and disturbed physiology, where disease-caused lesions are associated with disturbed behavior or physiological processing. This methodology has advantages over some other source localization methods in that the associations are not subject to the caveat that dipole source localization techniques do not have unique solutions. This method has been fruitfully applied using the P300 evoked potential and the mismatch negativity ERPs in schizophrenia. Historically this method has been productively used by many investigators (citations in McCarley *et al.*, 2002).

Over the past decade, however, increasingly sophisticated source analysis approaches have been developed that evaluate the electromagnetic sources of scalp-derived activity within the brain. Still, validation of these methods must be through some other method, such as intracranial recording, association with structural MRI "lesions" or with functional MRI. Validation of an ERP source solution with fMRI is best achieved by varying a task such that a particular ERP component in a sequence of ERPs is selectively emphasized. The corresponding local change(s) of the BOLD response—ideally under identical task conditions—would be the validation of the source, although the BOLD response will occur seconds after the electrical event. In many cases, however, reliance on combined ERP/fMRI—or alternatively MEG/fMRI measurements—will not be sufficient for validation requiring expert knowledge taking into account intracranial recordings and/or lesion studies. Even so, good spatial agreement is typically obtained between fMRI and ERP or oscillation-based measures (Bledowski *et al.*, 2004; Bénar *et al.*, 2007; Winterer *et al.*, 2007a). In particular, an accurate agreement is achieved during early rather than late stages of information processing when the number of simultaneously active sources is still limited. MEG usually offers the advantage over EEG that localization of electromagnetic sources is not

distorted by volume conduction of the magnetic fields, which provides higher accuracy than EEG. A disadvantage of MEG over EEG is that it is only sensitive to tangential (and superficial) components of the electromagnetic field, while EEG is sensitive to both the tangential and radial component. Even intracranial recording, although key in localizing sources from the perspective of a restricted brain region, cannot definitively state whether or how much these sources contribute to the scalp-recorded ERP.

Electrophysiology in schizophrenia

Here we will discuss some key issues in patient selection in schizophrenia research, provide a brief account of the history of electrophysiological research in schizophrenia, and then focus on four electrophysiological features of particular relevance to current schizophrenia research [mismatch negativity, P300, gamma band and slow-frequency oscillations ("noise")]. We conclude this section with a brief overview of other ERPs that have been studied in patients with schizophrenia. While we focus on ERP and event-related oscillation measures in schizophrenia in this chapter, we note that other EEG measures have been studied extensively. For example, measures of resting level EEG and techniques for analyzing that data, such as measuring the relative amounts of activity in each constituent frequency band, called quantitative electroencephalography (Q-EEG) or EEG microstate syntax analysis, have been frequently used to study brain–behavior relationships in schizophrenia. The interested reader is referred to John *et al.* (1988, 2007) or Lehmann *et al.* (2005); see also Chapter 14.

Patient selection

The vast majority of electrophysiological studies of pathology in schizophrenia have measured abnormalities in chronically-ill patients. By chronically-ill we mean patients who have had persistent symptoms for many years. The study of chronically-ill patients is confounded by the fact that being chronically ill may itself lead to secondary effects on brain physiology due to poor diet, an understimulating environment, and comorbidity due to the use of illicit drugs, nicotine and alcohol, or poor health, as well as the possible effects of long-term medication on brain structure. Such factors could affect the brain independently of any disease process and it is difficult to identify which effects arise from chronicity factors as opposed to those directly related to a schizophrenic disease process.

A physiological abnormality in chronically-ill patients that is also present at the onset of the disease cannot be caused by the secondary effects associated with chronicity. Whatever abnormal brain process gives rise to schizophrenia at the time of first overt psychosis should give clues as to the primary brain pathology of schizophrenia. Extending this approach, subjects who are at risk for schizophrenia can be studied, including patients in the prodromal state or clinically unaffected family members of patients with schizophrenia. The investigation of the latter population is particularly useful when adopting an "endophenotyping" approach for genetic analyses based on the fact that EEG and ERPs are highly heritable.

History

Since the discovery of the EEG by Hans Berger in the 1920s, numerous qualitative studies have indicated abnormal conventional EEG findings in 20–60% of patients with schizophrenia. The vast majority of electrophysiological research in schizophrenia over the past decades, however, has been conducted on ERPs, although the investigation of resting-state EEG (and resting-state fMRI) has recently gained renewed interest due to recent evidence for the importance of abnormal brain oscillations in schizophrenia (Winterer et al., 2000).

The technique for signal averaging the EEG to reveal ERPs was developed in the late 1950s, and the brain potentials related to the stimulus parameters, the so-called sensory potentials, were being recorded in patients with schizophrenia as early as 1959 (Shagass, 1968). Much of the early ERP work in schizophrenia focused on the N100, a negative-going brain potential arising approximately 100 ms after the onset of a stimulus. This was initially thought to be abnormally large due to filtering deficiencies or abnormally small due to a defensive reduction to compensate for the abnormal filter. Later work with technically improved equipment indicated the N100 amplitude was, in general, reduced in schizophrenia, and the field's interest shifted from the early sensory-evoked potentials to the P300 amplitude, which was robustly reduced in patients and clearly linked to the operations of selective attention and processing of infrequent stimuli. (For more historical detail the reader is referred to earlier reviews of ERP research by Shagass, by Buchsbaum, and by Roth in *Schizophrenia Bulletin*, 1977.)

The P300 is an ERP that occurs 300 ms after a rare stimulus embedded in a train of more frequent stimuli that a subject actively detects and processes. Work on this ERP began in 1965, when Sutton et al. (1965) used a prediction paradigm wherein subjects tried to guess which of two stimuli was going to be presented. The P300 potential was exciting because it was clearly related to internal cognitive processing rather than the sensory characteristics of the stimulus, as was the N100. The P300 is sometimes termed the P3, because it is the third positive potential after the stimulus. Roth and Cannon (1972) were the first to examine P300 in schizophrenia, and reported that P300 was reduced relative to controls. This finding has subsequently been termed the most robust physiological finding of any abnor-

mality in schizophrenia, but reduction of P300 at central electrodes, however, is not pathognomonic to schizophrenia as it is also reduced in other psychiatric diseases, such as bipolar disorder and Alzheimer dementia. More specific alterations of the total scalp field, or regionally specific topographic differences, by contrast, may be specifically associated with different psychiatric diseases, as discussed below in the section P300, which also discusses the important topic of P300 in schizophrenia in detail.

Mismatch negativity

Mismatch negativity (MMN) is a relatively short-latency brain event occurring after the presentation of a deviant stimulus in a train of preceding repetitive "standard" stimuli: for example, a 1.2 kHz tone ("pitch") is presented 5% of the time among 1.0 kHz tones, or alternatively a 1.0 kHz tone of 100 ms duration is presented 10% of the time among 1.0 kHz tones of 50 ms duration. The MMN occurs in the interval approx. 100–220 ms following the deviant stimulus, and is calculated by subtracting the ERP to deviant stimuli from that to standard stimuli. It is important to emphasize that the P300 depends on attentive, conscious processing of the deviant stimuli (often by counting), whereas attentive processing is not needed or used for the MMN, where often a distractor task is used to minimize conscious attention; the MMN is thus often referred to as "pre-attentive". Näätänen et al. (2007) summarize evidence differentiating the MMN from the sensory N100 and indicating the pre-eminence of a pre-attentive, supratemporal component from a weaker frontal process associated with an attention shift caused by auditory stimulus change. The supratemporal component is primarily evoked automatically, pre-attentively and pre-consciously, and is thus thought to reflect the operations of sensory ("echoic") memory, a kind of memory of past stimuli used by the auditory cortex in analysis of temporal patterns. The scalp-recorded MMN has its largest amplitude over the fronto-central scalp areas.

The modeling of the generator sources of the MMN with equivalent current dipoles (ECDs) suggests that the fronto-centrally predominant scalp distribution of the MMN could be explained by the sum of the activity bilaterally generated in the supratemporal cortices, a conclusion consistent with MEG source localization (reviewed in Näätänen et al., 2007). However, it should be kept in mind that MEG—as compared to EEG—is well known to be insensitive to the radial and deep components of an electromagnetic source (Huang et al., 2007), thus possibly leading to an underestimation of the contribution of radial prefrontal sources detected by EEG source analyses. Currently, it can be said, however, that the frontal lobe generator and its functional role in MMN generation remains less well researched and understood, as is true for postulated

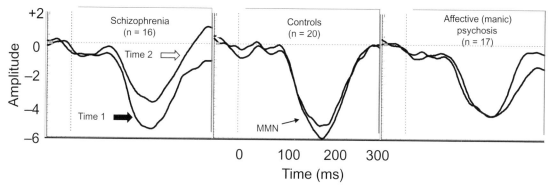

Fig 15.1 Pitch mismatch negativity (MMN) is normal at first hospitalization in patients with schizophrenia [Time 1, arrow indicates this event-related potential (ERP)], but becomes abnormal 1.5 years later (Time 2). In contrast subjects with affective (manic) psychosis and healthy controls do not show a reduction 1.5 years later. [Adapted from Salisbury *et al.* (2007).]

generators in the thalamus and hippocampus which have less supporting evidence (Näätänen *et al.*, 2007). Depth recordings of humans, monkeys, and cats have found sources in the primary auditory cortex (e.g., Javitt, *et al.* 2000a), although comparable studies have not been conducted in the prefrontal cortex (PFC). Laminar analysis in the auditory cortex indicates that MMN reflects the activity of glutamatergic N-methyl-D-aspartate (NMDA)-channel mediated influx of current flow in supragranular cortical layers. Javitt *et al.* (1996, 2000b, 2008) showed in monkeys that deviants elicited MMN-like activity in the supragranular (surface) layers of primary auditory cortex and further, that this activity was obliterated by application of NMDA-specific antagonists (Javitt *et al.*, Umbricht *et al.* (2000) showed reduced MMN in normal subjects following ketamine administration.

Mismatch negativity in schizophrenia

This evoked potential component has attracted great interest in schizophrenia because of its abnormality in this disorder and evidence that it may track progression of the disorder. With respect to schizophrenia, Todd *et al.* (2008) have systematically studied the similarities and differences to MMN elicited by duration, pitch, and intensity deviants to patients tested within 5 years of illness onset ("short" illness, mean duration 2.6 years) and after long duration illness (>5 years, mean 18.9 years). In short duration illness, a clear reduction was evident in MMN to duration and intensity but not frequency deviants, while longer duration illness was associated with a reduction in frequency and in duration to a lesser degree, but not intensity MMN. That frequency deviants were not reduced early in the illness but were reduced later is consistent with the findings of Javitt *et al.* (2000b) and Salisbury *et al.* (2002). However, these three studies were cross-sectional, i.e., different groups of patients were studied for the "early" and "late" groups, and are subject to the potential objection of a "cohort effect", that is, the changes observed might be

explained by the early and late groups having differences in severity, with the "late" groups having sicker patients. Thus, Salisbury *et al.* (2007) examined frequency deviants in the same group of patients studied longitudinally at first hospitalization for psychosis and a mean 1.5 years later. The longitudinal comparison for pitch MMN included 16 subjects with schizophrenia, 17 subjects with psychotic bipolar disorder in a manic phase, and 20 psychiatrically-well control subjects, with samples matched on age, parental socioeconomic status (SES), and handedness. Although all groups were similar in MMN at protocol entrance, patients with schizophrenia showed progressive reductions of MMN compared with the other groups (p = 0.011) (Fig. 15.1).

Combined structural MRI and ERP investigations were undertaken because of the strong evidence for the supratemporal origin of the MMN in the auditory cortex, notably the work of Wible *et al.* (2001) suggesting a localization of the pitch MMN as within Heschl's gyrus and nearby the posterior superior temporal gyrus, and reduced fMRI activation (BOLD) in schizophrenia. Consequently, Salisbury *et al.* (2007) also evaluated the association of MMN alterations with alterations in MRI volumetric measurements of left and right Heschl's gyrus, which contains the primary and some secondary auditory cortex. Although at initial testing patients with schizophrenia and control subjects did not differ in MMN amplitude, patients with schizophrenia showed reduced Heschl's gray matter volumes compared with bipolar and control subjects. Moreover, within the schizophrenia group there was a significant correlation between left hemisphere Heschl's gyrus gray matter volume and MMN amplitude at the midfrontal site (p = 0.02), suggesting the possibility that a pathological process reduces volume in the left Heschl's gyrus and that this process causes the within-group association, although the pathological process is not yet sufficiently far advanced to cause a reduction in mean MMN amplitude.

This hypothesis was consistent with evidence for both an initial and a progressive volume reduction in the left Heschl's gyrus in schizophrenia (Kasai *et al.*, 2003), but longitudinal data were needed for definitive testing. Of the subjects who tolerated both MMN and MRI initial testing at first hospitalization, retest comparison after approximately 1.5 years was performed. As with the larger group with longitudinal testing on MMN alone, the schizophrenia group showed significant MMN reduction over time (p < 0.004) but there was no MMN reduction in either the bipolar group (p > 0.9) or healthy control group (p > 0.4). The left Heschl's gyrus was significantly reduced in volume over time in all subjects in the schizophrenia group (p < 0.005, 6% reduction), but not in the bipolar or control groups, where reductions were essentially at chance level. Of primary importance, the reductions in amplitude of the MMN and the reductions in the left Heschl gyrus volume were tightly coupled in the schizophrenia group (r = 0.62;

p = 0.04), but there was no such associations between Heschl's gyrus volume and MMN in the other two groups.

The authors concluded that these interrelated functional and structural measures supported the presence of a post-onset progression in schizophrenia. Pitch MMN amplitude in schizophrenia, even when within the normal range at first hospitalization, was tightly coupled to the volume of the underlying left temporal auditory cortex, showing progressive reductions coupled with ongoing cortical gray matter reduction of the left temporal auditory cortex (Fig. 15.2), and thus might serve as a measure of successful interventions in halting such peri-onset progressive abnormalities. Several possible caveats to these conclusions should be discussed. First, the subject number in the combined MMN–MRI longitudinal group, although sufficient for robust significance, was relatively small and results need to be confirmed. There was no evidence for medication effects on either MRI or MMN and, furthermore, any

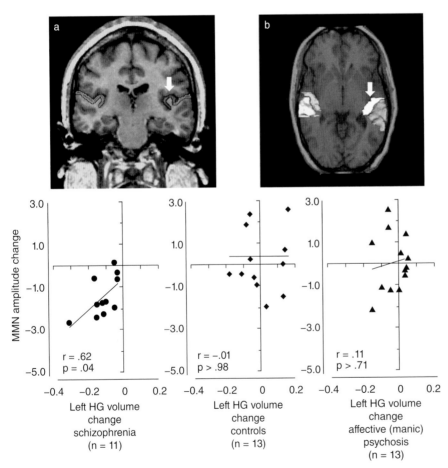

Fig. 15.2 Conjoint progression of gray matter loss in the left Heschl's gyrus (HG) and reduction of mismatch negativity (MMN) in the 1.5 years after first hospitalization in schizophrenia but not in affective (manic) psychosis. (a)Coronal MRI and (b) axial MRI, with the left HG indicated by arrow. In the lower panel, note the strong association between degree of HG gray matter volume reduction over time and the degree of abnormality of MMN in schizophrenia, but not in the healthy controls or affective (manic) psychosis. [Adapted from Salisbury *et al.* (2007).]

MRI medication effects would be expected to be observed across the whole brain, while the observed changes were present only in the left, but not in the right, Heschl's gyrus in schizophrenia. Differential disease effects of subjects lost to follow-up also were considered, but, at initial evaluation, returned and lost subjects showed no difference in age, Brief Psychiatric Rating Scale (BPRS) scores, medication dosages, SES or parental SES, while the small differences in IQ and Global Assessment Scale (GAS) were worse in the lost to follow-up group, suggesting that, if anything, this lost to follow-up group might have an even poorer MMN and MRI outcome than the follow-up group. Also, MRI volumetric changes in other brain regions were not evaluated with respect to MMN association, although, for example, Nakamura et al. (2007) showed progressive post-onset changes in both the temporal and prefrontal neocortex in schizophrenia. Thus, it would be interesting to evaluate the PFC for association with MMN change since recent MMN source analysis studies have provided evidence for altered electromagnetic activity in the PFC of patients with schizophrenia (Baldeweg et al., 2002; Oknina et al., 2005).

Duration mismatch negativity and schizophrenia prodrome

In contrast to the pitch MMN, the duration MMN shows evidence of being abnormal at onset of schizophrenia, as reviewed by Todd et al. (2008). This of course raises the question of whether this duration MMN might show a progression of abnormality in individuals prodromal for schizophrenia or might indicate those individuals destined for progression. Published data are sparse but Mathalon et al. (2006) have presented preliminary data indicating a reduction in combined pitch and duration deviants in prodromes destined for conversion. Thus, investigation of the time course of duration change is one of the high priorities in current MMN research in schizophenia.

Reliability and heritability

Turetsky et al. (2007) summarize reliability data for healthy controls as moderate for the "pitch'" deviant (~ 0.5) but high for the duration deviant (>0.8). In chronic schizophrenia, Light and Braff (2005) found duration MMN reliability to be 0.87, while Salisbury et al. (2007) found pitch MMN reliability to be 0.74 in first-episode schizophrenia, but lower in healthy controls (0.52) and still lower in patients with a first-episode bipolar disorder (0.22). Of note, the reduction of MMN in patients chronically-ill with schizophrenia appears to be trait-like and not ameliorated by either typical (haloperidol) or atypical (clozapine) medication (Umbricht et al., 1998). Heritability of the duration MMN is substantial (h^2 = 60–70) and comparable to the heritability of the P300 amplitude (Hall et al., 2006). Of the three family studies that have been conducted with MMN

to date, two found a reduction in MMN generation in unaffected family members of patients with schizophrenia (Jessen et al., 2001; Michie et al., 2002), while the third did not (Bramon et al., 2004).

Specificity to schizophrenia

Umbricht et al. (2003) reported specificity of duration MMN reduction in schizophrenia, compared with affective disorder and healthy controls. Salisbury et al. (2007) found specificity of progression of pitch abnormalities in schizophrenia compared with bipolar disorder and healthy controls. Of note, the progression in Heschl gyrus volume reduction has similarly been reported in schizophrenia, but not in controls or bipolar disorder (Kasai et al., 2003), suggesting that diseases with loss of Heschl gyrus volume will similarly show reduction of MMN.

Because MMN may reflect, in part, NMDA-mediated activity and this receptor plays an important role not only in cortical excitation but also in brain development, it is tempting to speculate about an NMDA-related abnormality being related to developmental abnormalities as well as to further changes in the course of the illness. Based on the data of Salisbury et al. (2007) indicating the MMN undergoes a process of active reduction during the first few years after symptom onset, there is the possibility that the MMN, especially the pitch MMN, might serve as an index of disease progression in the superior temporal gyrus. Further, the presence of an active phase of gray matter loss and electrophysiologial impairment around the time of first hospitalization would immediately underline the need for pharmacological treatment, especially if the neurodegeneration were dependent on hyperactivation, as a number of theories suggest (see review in McCarley et al., 1996, 1999).

P300

The P300 is an ERP that occurs to a stimulus that a subject actively detects and processes. Similar to MMN, P300 is elicited most commonly in the context of the auditory oddball paradigm. However, when P300 is to be elicited, subjects are instructed to selectively attend to the sequence of tones, and either count the deviants, or press a button in response to the deviants. Under such conditions, P300 occurs approximately 300 ms following deviant tone presentation, while the visual "P300" actually occurs nearer 400 ms after a target visual stimulus. Thus, as opposed to MMN with its pre-attentive component generated in the primary auditory cortex, P300 is clearly dependent on selective attention. Typically, P300 is divided into two subcomponents, an early P3-like potential ("P3a"), which is topographically located relatively frontally, and a later, more parietal component "P3b". While the P3b amplitude is larger when the stimulus is rarer, the amplitude of the P3a is increasing when a third novel stimulus is accompanied by an orienting response of the subject.

P300 reflects the activity of several, mostly simultaneously active bilateral generators. There is clear evidence from multisite intracortical recordings (Halgren *et al.*, 1995ab; Baudena *et al.*, 1995), neuroimaging experiments (Linden *et al.*, 1999; Winterer *et al.*, 2007b), and electromagnetic source localization studies (Winterer *et al.*, 2001; Pae *et al.*, 2003) for a network of distributed activity in at least half a dozen cortical locations—most notably in the inferior parietal lobule and posterior superior temporal gyrus—corresponding to the scalp-recorded P3b. These studies also suggest a contribution from the dorso-lateral PFC (DLPFC) and anterior cingulate cortex (ACC) to the scalp-recorded P3a. It is also likely that many of the deep sources that generate P300-like activity do not propagate to the scalp (e.g., the hippocampus). Vector-based spatial decomposition of the corresponding BOLD response further indicates that the associated behavioral response (reaction time speed) does not only depend on the overall level of cortical activation, but also on the degree of activity distribution within the participating network of generators (Musso *et al.*, 2006).

From the theoretical considerations on the generation of ERPs (see above), one would expect P300 to be modulated by glutamatergic mechanisms in an analogous way to MMN. However, there are remarkably few data available (Gallinat *et al.*, 2007). Nevertheless, over the past few years, our understanding of the molecular, genetic, and pharmacological basis of P300 has improved considerably. Preliminary evidence associates the late temporo-parietal P300 component with specific genetic variations in the dopamine D_3 and D_2 receptor genes (Hill *et al.*, 1998; Anokhin *et al.*, 1999; Mulert *et al.*, 2004; Berman *et al.*, 2006), whereas variations in the gene that codes for the dopamine catabolizing enzyme catechol-O-methyltransferase (*COMT*) have been associated with fronto-central and centro-parietal P300 amplitude variations (Gallinat *et al.*, 2003; Golimbet *et al.*, 2006; Ehlis *et al.*, 2007). However, negative genetic association findings also have been described for P300 amplitude (Lin *et al.*, 2001; Tsai *et al.*, 2003; Bramon *et al.*, 2006). To some extent, conflicting results have also been reported for the pharmacological effects on P300 amplitude. Oranje *et al.* (2006) did not find an effect of L-dopa or bromocriptine treatment on P300-amplitude. In contrast, acute challenge with D-amphetamine was reported to increase P300 amplitude (López *et al.*, 2004). In this context, a study conducted by Niznikiewicz *et al.* (2005) also deserves mention. They found a significant increase in the P300 amplitude in patients treated with clozapine relative to baseline, off-medication status. The P300 amplitude improvement was not found in chlorpromazine-treated patients.

Involvement of cholinergic mechanisms in auditory evoked P300 has also been observed. Acetylcholine and cholinergic drugs appear to strongly increase P300 amplitude. The opposite observation, i.e., a decrease of P300 amplitude is made for anticholinergic substances. Both effects are likely to be mediated by muscarinic and perhaps also nicotinergic receptors (Hollander *et al.*, 1987; Dierks *et al.*, 1994; Anokhin *et al.*, 2000; Thomas *et al.*, 2000; Knott *et al.*, 2002; Neuhaus *et al.*, 2006; Werber *et al.*, 2001). In line with these observations in humans, septal cholinergic lesions abolish P300 in cats (Harrison *et al.*, 1988). More recently, an association of the α4 subunit nicotinergic acetylcholine receptor gene and the parietal and prefrontal BOLD response during oddball task conditions has also been reported (Winterer *et al.*, 2007b). Therefore, and since abnormal cholinergic transmission appears to be involved in aspects of schizophrenia pathophysiology, in particular cognitive deficits including memory and attentional deficits (Tamminga, 2006), and because rodent models of the P300 ERP have been developed (Slawecki *et al.*, 2000; Ehlers & Somes, 2002), P300 may be considered a useful translational biomarker to track pharmacological interventions with cholinergic drugs, not only in schizophrenia but in any neuropsychiatric disorder involving the cholinergic system, including Alzheimer dementia, addiction, and attention deficit disorder (Javitt *et al.*, 2008).

P300 in schizophrenia

Roth and Cannon (1972) were the first to report a reduction in schizophrenia of P300 (P3b) amplitude in recording sites over the sagittal midline of the head. Since then, nearly all studies have reported a reduction of central P300 amplitude in subjects with chronic schizophrenia. Delays in the onset of P300 are less commonly reported. A meta-analysis by Bramon *et al.* (2004) of studies with Cz or Pz recordings found an effect size for schizophrenia of 0.85 for amplitude and 0.57 for latency (for both, p < 0.001) with no significant influence of antipsychotic medication or duration of illness. Latency differences were an important feature of the cross-sectional study of O'Donnell *et al.* (1995), which found a greater rate of decrease in latency with age in schizophrenia compared with controls, a finding compatible with progression; more definitive evidence about progression, however, would require longitudinal studies.

The amplitude reduction of P300 is not related to a lack of motivation to adhere to the task in the patients, as it remains reduced relative to controls even when the patients' performance in detecting the tones is as good as that of controls (Ford *et al.*, 1994; Salisbury *et al.*, 1994a). Furthermore, the latency of P300 in patients with schizophrenia does vary with task difficulty as in controls, but the amplitude remains reduced. Thus, P300 amplitude is robustly reduced in patients chronically-ill with schizophrenia.

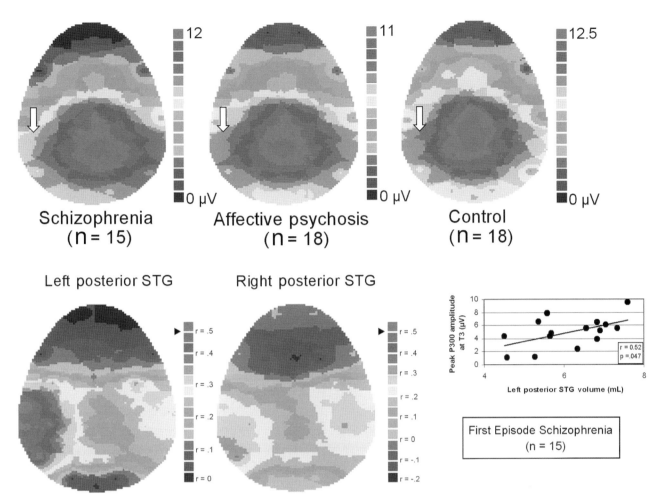

Fig. 15.3 P300 left lateralization in schizophrenia is associated with left posterior superior temporal gyrus (STG) gray matter reduction. Top, Topography of P300 to target tones. Note the lateralized amplitude reduction at over left temporal scalp areas (arrows) in schizophrenia compared with affective psychosis and controls. Bottom, Pearson correlation r-values between posterior STG and P300 in schizophrenia. The gray matter volume of the left posterior STG (left image) shows a left temporal regionally selective association with P300 amplitude, but the gray matter volume of the right posterior STG (right image) does not show any selective P300 amplitude association. Scattergram plot of the association between the left posterior STG volume and P300 amplitude at an electrode in the left temporal region (T3). (In all images the frontal dark areas in this black and white rendering of a color map represent low correlations.) [After McCarley et al. (2002).]

P300 topographic differences in schizophrenia

In addition to the broad reductions of P300 over both left and right hemispheres, ill subjects first-hospitalized with schizophrenia display an asymmetry in P300 with smaller voltage over the left *versus* the right temporal lobe (Fig. 15.3). This finding was first observed in chronic schizophrenia where this left temporal P300 amplitude abnormality was found to be correlated negatively with the extent of psychopathology as reflected in thought disorder, delusions, and auditory hallucinations (e.g., McCarley et al., 1993; Turetsky et al., 1998; Gallinat et al., 2001; Frodl et al., 2002). There is also evidence that this left temporal amplitude reduction is diagnostically relatively specific for schizophrenia, at least as contrasted with affective (manic) psychosis (Morstyn et al., 1983; Strik et al., 1993; Salisbury et al., 1999; O'Donnell et al., 2004), although more studies, and in different disease entities, are needed. It may, however, turn out that diagnostic specificity can be further improved when taking into account not only topographic information but also single evoked potential characteristics of the P300 wave. For instance, there is some evidence— although still controversial—that increased latency variably may contribute to the overall amplitude reduction of the averaged P300 ERP, rather than an amplitude reduction of single evoked potential amplitudes *per se* (Donchin et al., 1970; Callaway et al., 1970; Roth et al., 1981, 2007; Ford et al., 1994; Röschke et al., 1996). In order to obtain a clearer picture in this regard, it will probably be necessary to

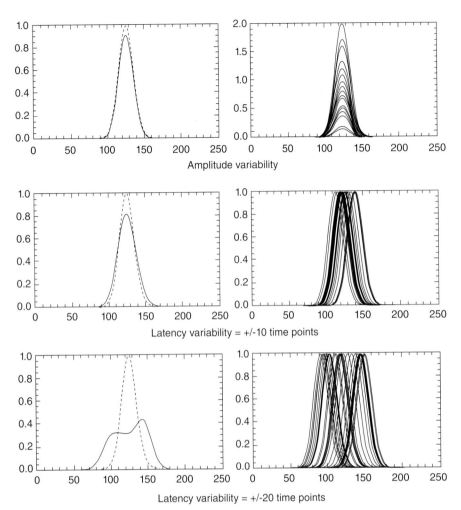

Fig. 15.4 Effect of amplitude variability and latency variability (jitter) on event-related potential (ERP) waveforms. Left panels, Dotted line is the simulated ERP and solid line is the average. Right panels, single trial values. Note the reduced amplitude of the average can come from either variability in amplitude or variability in latency. Longer duration latency variation (bottom panel) markedly distorts the ERP shape. [Adapted from Spencer (2004).]

further improve P300 single trial analysis procedures (Fig. 15.4; Spencer, 2004). In particular, it needs to be taken into account that any single trial analysis of ERPs depends on its signal-to-noise ratio which is diminished in schizophrenia (see below).

In both first-hospitalized and chronic schizophrenia, the left temporal P300 amplitude reduction correlates positively with the gray matter volume of the left posterior superior temporal gyrus (STG), one of the generator sites of P300, and an area also intimately related to language processing and thinking (McCarley *et al.*, 1993). The volume of cortical gray matter in the left STG volume, in turn, correlates negatively with measures of thought disorder (Shenton *et al.*, 1992) and the severity of auditory hallucinations (Barta *et al.*, 1990). Therefore, abnormal left temporal P300 may reflect—to a considerable extent—underlying STG abnormality, index the severity of psychopathology,

and serve as a physiological tie between underlying brain pathology and behavioral psychopathology.

However, chronic patients are subject to potential confounders from chronic medication and chronic illness. Accordingly, Salisbury, McCarley and colleagues have conducted a series of studies in patients with first-episode schizophrenia, with first-episode affective psychosis (mainly bipolar), and healthy controls, group-matched on age, gender, handedness, and parental SES. Comparison with patients with first-episode affective psychosis not only is useful to test diagnostic specificity, but also helps rule out medication confounders since they and patients with schizophrenia patients often are taking the same medication. In the combined ERP and MRI study, McCarley *et al.* (2002) evaluated P300 in first-episode subjects with schizophrenia (n = 15) or affective psychosis (n = 18; 17 bipolar in a manic phase, and statistical conclusions remained the same when only patients with bipolar disorder were included) or control subjects (n = 18), as they silently counted infrequent target tones amid standard tones. MRI provided quantitative measures of temporal lobe gray matter regions of interest, including the anterior STG, hippocampus, Heschl's gyrus, and planum temporal components in the posterior STG. Patients with first-episode schizophrenia displayed smaller P300 amplitudes than controls along the sagittal midline, but there were no statistically significant group differences (schizophrenia, affective psychosis, controls, p > 0.7), suggesting this dimension is not a good diagnostic differentiator. However, the patients with schizophrenia displayed a reversed P300 temporal area asymmetry (smaller on the left) compared with controls and patients with affective psychosis (p = 0.002). MRI showed smaller gray matter volumes of the left posterior STG in the patients with schizophrenia relative to control subjects and patients with affective psychosis (15.4% and 11.0%, respectively), smaller gray matter volumes of the left planum temporale (21.0% relative to both), and a smaller total Heschl's gyrus volume (14.6% and 21.1%, respectively). For this left temporal feature in schizophrenia, it was the left posterior STG and the left planum temporale, but not other regions of interest, that were specifically and positively correlated (r > 0.5) with T3 left temporal P300 voltage, but there was no correlation with patients with affective psychosis or control subjects. Neither dose nor duration of medication was significantly correlated with P300 amplitudes or MRI volumes in any group. We note the finding of smaller volume of the STG in schizophrenia is one of the most replicated MRI findings in the field, although not all studies have agreed on findings of smaller volumes of its components (the Heschl's gyrus and planum temporale).

Thus, interrelated, regionally restricted P300 voltage abnormality and reduction in the left posterior STG and planum temporale volume appear selective for schizophrenic *versus* manic psychosis and are seen at first hospitalization, even in the presence of relatively large and normal midline P300 amplitudes. The McCarley *et al.* (2002) study used the classical method of correlating an anatomical abnormality ("lesion", see above) in a disorder with functional information such as the left temporal P300 deficit. This method suggests that the left STG is a major source of the left temporal deficit in schizophrenia, although the possible contributions of other cortical regions, such as frontal and parietal, were not determined. It is therefore of interest that a recent structural/functional MRI study found that group differences between patients with schizophrenia and controls in bilateral parietal and frontal, as well as posterior, temporal regions in gray matter were associated with bilateral temporal regions activated by the auditory oddball target stimuli (Calhoun *et al.*, 2006).

The frontally generated P3a is also abnormally altered in schizophrenia. Of note, both increased amplitudes (Winterer *et al.*, 2003) and decreased amplitudes (Mathalon *et al.*, 2000) have been described. However, under standard auditory oddball conditions, the P3a peak amplitude is difficult to detect reliably and, as has been pointed out (Winterer *et al.*, 2004), an abnormally altered P3a amplitude—particularly when found to be increased—may reflect an increased amplitude of "noise power" (see below) rather than a true abnormality of this P300 subcomponent.

Reliability and heritability

Measurement stability and heritability of the P300b amplitude is about as high as for the duration deviant MMN (Turetsky *et al.*, 2007), i.e., test–retest reliability is in the range of 0.8–0.9 with heritability (h^2) around 0.6. As a trait-like characteristic, because of the relatively high heritability and since P300 amplitude reduction is also found in family members of patients with schizophrenia patients, P300 amplitude is generally accepted as a marker of the genetic risk for schizophrenia (Winterer *et al.*, 2003; Hall *et al.*, 2007; Turetsky *et al.*, 2007; see Chapter 14). A meta-analysis by Bramon *et al.* (2004) on P300 in relatives of individuals with schizophrenia showed a significant reduction in P300 amplitude (effect size = 0.61). On the other hand, Frodl *et al.* (2002) described a negative correlation of P300 amplitude and illness duration. Turetsky *et al.* (1998) found a trend toward normalization of the left temporal P300 subcomponent that correlated with change in BPRS score, which was observed in a similar way by Mathalon *et al.* (2000). While the latter group found a correlation with changes in positive and negative symptoms, Gallinat *et al.* (2001) related this P300 amplitude change to positive but not negative symptoms. Ford *et al.* (1994) demonstrated that, although P300 showed moderate amplitude increases with symptom resolution, it did not approach normal values during these periods of remission. Currently, it appears (Hall *et al.*, 2007) that while MMN and P300 amplitude reductions have both state- and trait-like components, the trait aspect, i.e., the genetic component, may be more pronounced for P300 than for MMN, whereas the opposite may be true for the state aspect related to the course of the illness.

Neural synchrony and oscillation measures

One of the exciting developments in human electrophysiological work has been its linking with basic neuroscience discoveries about the role of neural synchrony or oscillations in neuronal communication. We first discuss gamma frequency band oscillations (31–100Hz), a topic of current very high interest and research (138 PubMed-cited papers in 2007 alone). Subsequently, we will highlight low-frequency or "theta" synchrony and its inverse, called "noise", which captures synchrony of brain oscillations in the frequency range 0.5–10 Hz. The concept of "noise" has recently attracted considerable interest in schizophrenia research because it was demonstrated to be a strong endophenotype for schizophrenia (see below).

Gamma oscillations

Gamma-band synchronization appears to be one of the fundamental modes of neuronal activity: that activated neuronal groups engage in rhythmic synchronization in the gamma-frequency band has been documented in the cortex of many brain regions, including the visual, auditory, somatosensory, motor, parietal, and entorhinal regions, as well as in hippocampus (see relevant citations in the review by Fries *et al.*, 2007). It is present in many species, from insects to mammals, including humans, and during conditions ranging from simple sensory stimulation to attentional selection, working memory maintenance, and perceptual integration (citations in Fries *et al.*, 2007). At the cognitive level, work in humans suggests that gamma activity reflects the convergence of multiple processing streams in the cortex, this "feature binding" giving rise to a unified percept. A simple example is a "firetruck", where a particular combination of features of form perception, motion perception, and auditory perception are melded to form this percept. It is disturbed in many pathological conditions, including schizophrenia (see below).

What is the neuronal interplay generating gamma activity? Basically it involves an interaction between pyramidal projection neurons (glutamatergic, excitatory, and regular spiking) and, in the cortex, a particular kind of gamma-aminobutyric acid (GABA)ergic inhibitory neuron, one that is fast spiking (high-frequency spikes following current injection), containing the calcium-binding protein parvalbumin (PARV), and comprised of basket and chandelier cells, and found to be abnormal in postmortem work in schizophrenia. In response to excitatory input from the pyramidal neurons, the group of GABAergic neurons tends to discharge synchronously, as a result of interconnections mediated by both neurotransmitter (GABAergic) and electrical (gap junction) activity. This GABAergic synchronous activity, in turn, synchronizes the population of pyramidal cells to which they project. The timing of the discharges and the time course of resultant alterations in membrane polarization result in the gamma frequency activity.

There is now considerable evidence supporting this model of the substrate for gamma oscillations in the cortex with interaction of GABAergic interneurons with glutamatergic neurons in the upper cortical layers, layers II and II (see, for example, Cunningham *et al.*, 2006). This abnormality of glutamatergic–GABAergic interaction in the production of gamma band oscillations is congruent with accumulating postmortem evidence of reduced inhibition of pyramidal neurons in schizophrenia (Lewis *et al.*, 2005) and with basic *in vitro* studies indicating an increased sensitivity of the NMDA synapse on GABAergic neurons to inhibition by psychotomimetics and, consequently, to disinhibition of the pyramidal targets of the GABA neurons (Grunze *et al.*, 1996; Rujescu *et al.*, 2006).

An important theoretical question is whether rhythmic activity in the high beta range (20–30 Hz) is generated by the same cortical mechanisms as gamma band activity. Work by the Newcastle group indicates that high beta activity is generated in layer V and is independent of gamma oscillation since it survives a cut separating layer V and II and a blockade of GABA$_A$ receptors sufficient to suppress gamma (Roopun *et al.*, 2006; M.A. Whittington, M.A., presentation at 2007 American College of Neuropsychopharmacology, ACNP).

Gamma oscillations and schizophrenia

One way to view studies of the gamma band in schizophrenia is to determine if there is a basic circuit abnormality, such as a deficiency in recurrent and feed forward inhibition, postulated by a number of workers (see review in McCarley *et al.*, 1996, 1999). Kwon *et al.* (1999) began the study of the gamma band in schizophrenia using an exogenous input of 40 Hz auditory clicks, leading to a steady-state gamma response. The magnitude of the brain response was measured by power, the amount of EEG energy at a specific frequency, with the degree of capability of gamma driving being reflected in the power at and near 40 Hz.

Patients with schizophrenia had, compared with healthy controls, a markedly reduced power at 40 Hz input, although showing normal driving at slower frequencies between 20 Hz and 40 Hz, which indicated this was not a general reduction in power, but one specific to the gamma band. Moreover, the phase—response curve, a description of the relationship between the timing of each stimulus and the EEG response, suggested that it was an intrinsic oscillator that was being driven. This was because the time duration between the stimulus and the EEG response, as the 40 Hz stimulation continued, was reduced to a duration too short to be explained by simple conduction to the auditory cortex. This phase response curve is very common when an external signal drives a "tuned oscillator", much as auditory stimuli can set in motion a tuning fork, which oscillates (resonates) at a particular frequency. The abnormal amplitude and phase response in patients with schizophrenia raised the possibility that there was an intrinsic deficit in the brain circuitry supporting 40 Hz oscillations.

However, it remained to be determined if this deficiency in externally driven gamma implies a deficiency in gamma band synchronization that occurs endogenously in the course of perception as when, for example, a certain pattern of spots embedded in a field of spots is suddenly perceived to be a Dalmatian dog. Since gamma band synchrony has been classically linked to perceptual feature-binding, Spencer *et al.* (2003) investigated gamma oscillations in schizophrenia using a task designed to invoke visual feature-binding mechanisms. In this experiment, subjects discriminated between squares formed by illusory contours (illusory square condition) and a control condition (no square). As can be seen in Plate 15.1, the stimuli in each condition are physically identical, but the rotation of the "pac-men" determines whether or not observers perceive a coherent object. In healthy control subjects, illusory squares but not the no squares elicited a gamma oscillation phase-locked to the stimuli at occipital electrodes (Plate 15.15, left). [A key methodological point is that, while evoked power and phase-locking factor both reflect synchrony of activity, phase-locking factor is independent of the amplitude of the signal, while evoked power depends on it. Hence gamma band phase coherence is a more sensitive measure of oscillation than gamma band power. Consequently, healthy controls often show differences in phase locking with schizophrenia when amplitude is not significant (Ford *et al.*, 2007; Spencer *et al.*, 2003).] For patients with schizophrenia, however, neither stimulus elicited an oscillation even though the stimuli were correctly identified. A follow-up study examined response-locked gamma oscillations in the same paradigm (Spencer *et al.*, 2004). The authors reasoned that the neural mechanisms underlying conscious perception might be more correlated with reaction time (measured by button press) than stimulus onset, as has been found in animal single-unit recording studies. In healthy subjects illusory squares elicited a response-locked gamma oscillation at around 250 ms before the reaction time button press, also at occipital electrodes. No such oscillation was elicited by no-square stimuli. Thus, the response-locked oscillation may be a correlate of visual feature-binding processes involved in conscious perception.

For the schizophrenia group, a response-locked oscillation at occipital electrodes was also elicited by illusory squares. However, this response-locked oscillation occurred in a lower frequency range for patients with schizophrenia (22–24 Hz) than healthy subjects (34–40 Hz). This difference in synchronization frequency suggests that synchrony was necessary for the coherent object to be perceived, but the cell assemblies coding the object were unable to synchronize in the normal gamma range for patients with schizophrenia. One possible cause of this effect is reduced cortical connectivity. Selemon and Goldman-Rakic (1999) have suggested that reduced connectivity is an important neural substrate of schizophrenia, and a study modeling gamma oscillations found that increased conduction delays lowered the synchronization frequency of a cell assembly (Kopell *et al.*, 2000). Evidence for a close relationship between the response-locked oscillation and core cognitive and neural

abnormalities in schizophrenia was found in the strong correlations between positive symptoms (visual hallucinations, thought disorder, and disorganization) and the degree of phase coherence. These data are consistent with studies by Uhlhaas *et al.* (2004), who have found correlations between thought disorder and disorganization symptoms and psychophysical measures of visual perception. Notably, gamma band abnormalities may not reflect drug effects since they have also been observed in unmedicated patients (Gallinat *et al.*, 2004) and new-generation antipsychotics may even reverse pre-existing gamma abnormalities (Hong *et al.*, 2004).

In addition, gamma deficits may already be present at the onset of illness. Spencer *et al.* (2006) have recently shown in first-episode patients that gamma abnormalities in schizophrenia have a left-sided bias, compatible with structural MRI findings, whereas those in affective (bipolar) psychosis do not have a hemispheric bias. Thus, gamma band abnormalities *per se* may not be specific to schizophrenia but the source of the abnormalities may differ according to the pathophysiology of the disorder, which includes structural alterations in schizophrenia not present in bipolar disorder. Gamma abnormalities may occur in other conditions affecting the neural circuit involved in their generation, including attention-deficit hyperactivity disorder, autism, epilepsy, and Alzheimer disease (Van der Stelt *et al.*, 2004; Herrmann & Demiralp, 2005). Results have been mixed as to whether the gamma deficits observed in patients with schizophrenia are also present in persons with schizotypal personality traits or with increased genetic risk for schizophrenia (Brenner *et al.*, 2003; Winterer *et al.*, 2004; Hong *et al.*, 2004). It also remains to be determined if there is evidence for progression of gamma abnormalities in schizophrenia, as has been observed for the MMN and MRI abnormalities. Further investigations in this currently very active topic of study are needed to specify further how gamma oscillation abnormalities in schizophrenia are relevant to its clinical features and whether certain features may be diagnostically specific.

Low frequency oscillations and "noise"

Over the past decades, the neurophysiological and pharmacological basis of synchronous low-frequency oscillations has been extensively investigated in animal models and more recently in humans during various task conditions. By low-frequency oscillations we mean oscillations in the delta (1–4 Hz) and theta (4–8 Hz) band, according to our clinical definitions of frequency bands. Theta activity in animals, primarily rodents, has been extensively investigated and reviewed (e.g., Buzsaki, 2002; Hasselmo, 2005; Vertes, 2005). In studies of rodents, (hippocampal) oscillations across a broad range of frequencies between 5 and 12 Hz are termed theta. Theta is prominent during motor behavior, variously described as "voluntary," "preparatory," "orienting," or "exploratory", and during rapid eye movement sleep (REM) sleep. An acceleration of frequency within the theta band is seen, for instance, with stronger orienting responses or stronger exploratory behavior, i.e., slow and fast theta (for overview, see Miller, 1991). In larger animals, including cats, dogs and primates, the frequency range of theta is usually lower than in rodents, ranging from 3 to 8 Hz. In addition, theta activity can be quite different from that in the rodent in terms of state- and site-dependency. For instance, in intracranial recordings in the human hippocampus, there is no constant theta oscillation during REM sleep, but rather short bursts of 4–7 Hz waves appear in this state and during transitions to wakefulness.

Whether neocortical theta oscillations exist that are completely or partly independent of the hippocampal formation is a matter under investigation. So far, evidence for independent theta oscillations has been obtained in the rabbit cingulate cortex (Leung & Borst, 1987; Borst et al., 1987; Talk et al., 2004) and more recently in primates. Tsujimoto et al. (2006) identified with intracortical recordings a slow-wave oscillation source (5–6 Hz) in primate ACC during an executive attentional task whereby synchrony (coherence between electrodes) increased with task performance. In another investigation using subdural and depth recordings, conducted by Cantero et al. (2003), theta waves (4–7 Hz) were observed in the basal temporal lobe and frontal cortex during transitions from sleep to wake, but not in REM. Importantly, Cantero et al. found theta activity in the human hippocampus and neocortex was not correlated (coherent), supporting the notion of cortical theta generators being independent of hippocampal generators. In this context, an investigation of Guderian and Düzel (2005) in human subjects is of considerable interest. Using whole-head magnetoencephalography, they found that recollection of personal events is associated with an induced activity increase in a distributed synchronous theta (4.5–7 Hz) network, including prefrontal, mediotemporal, and visual areas. This would suggest that independent theta generators may cooperate under certain task conditions.

Scalp EEG recordings in humans have suggested for some years the existence of a frontal midline slow-wave oscillator during tasks that require selective attention (0.5–5 Hz) (Winterer et al., 1999), problem-solving or working memory (5–7 Hz) (Ishihara & Yoshii, 1972; Gevins et al., 1997), i.e., in cognitive conditions that are typically impaired in schizophrenia. Gevins and Smith (2000) reported that subjects with stronger frontal midline slow-wave oscillations (5–7 Hz) have higher cognitive ability. Winterer et al. (2004) found that lower prefrontal slow-wave synchrony, i.e., higher slow-wave variability ("noise") during an oddball task condition predicts attentional performance (for details, see below). It is, however, not yet resolved how synchronized slow-wave oscillations contribute to task performance. Jensen and colleagues (Jensen & Lisman, 2005; Jensen & Colgin, 2007) suggested on the basis of electrophysiological recordings in animals and humans that the power of fast gamma oscillations is modulated by the phase of slow-wave oscillations, whereby coupled slow-wave oscillations might mediate a dynamic link between hippocampal and neocortical, including prefrontal, areas, thereby allowing the recruitment and binding of distributed cortical representations. A similar suggestion was made by Jones and Wilson (2005) who proposed that the coordination of slow-wave oscillations between prefrontal and hippocampal sites may constitute a general mechanism through which the relative timing of disparate neural activities during cognitive operations can be controlled. In agreement with this notion is a recent report of Jacobs et al. (2007), who investigated the temporal relationship between brain oscillations and single-neuron activity in humans during a virtual navigation task with recordings from 1924 neurons in various brain regions. They found that neuronal activity in various brain regions increases at specific phases of brain oscillations. Neurons in widespread brain regions were phase-locked to oscillations in the theta- (4–8 Hz) and gamma- (30–90 Hz) frequency bands. In the hippocampus, phase locking was prevalent in the delta- (1–4 Hz) and gamma-frequency bands. Individual neurons were phase locked to various phases of theta and delta oscillations, but they only were active at the trough of gamma oscillations. The authors proposed that slow-wave oscillations facilitate phase coding and that gamma oscillations help to decode combinations of simultaneously active neurons. In this context, it is of interest that Hyman et al. (2005) recently showed that the majority of the medial prefrontal cells with a significant correlation of firing rate changes with behavior were entrained to slow-wave oscillations in the hippocampus, which leaves, however, open the question whether entrainment is also present with prefrontal slow-wave oscillations.

For many years, theta oscillations have been the topic of extensive investigations because of their association with memory processing and gating of neuronal discharge: they are believed to be critical for temporal coding/decoding of active neuronal ensembles and neuroplasticity, i.e., the modification of synaptic weights underlying memory (long-term potentiation and long-term depression; Buzsaki, 2002). In the rodent, a model of theta generation has been proposed (reviewed by Vertes, 2005; see his Fig. 1). In this model, neural activity underlying theta originates in tonic discharges in rostral pontine reticular formation and propagates to the supramammilary nucleus, where it is converted to a rhythmic discharge projecting to the medial septum, onto both hippocampal-projecting cholinergic and GABAergic neurons. Medial septal GABAergic neurons connect with and inhibit GABAergic cells of the hippocampus, thereby exerting a disinhibitory action on pyramidal neurons. Medial septal cholinergic pacemaking neurons simultaneously excite hippocampal pyramidal cells and GABAergic interneurons. In the hippocampus, it is thought that the hippocampal GABAergic neurons are the chief theta pacemaker, and theta rhythm in field potentials is highly correlated with pyramidal cell discharges.

Dopamine apparently also has an impact on slow-wave oscillations. In rodents, Fitch *et al.* (2006) found that the dopamine D_1 receptor stimulation provides a state-dependent bi-directional modulation of the theta burst (4–7 Hz) occurrence. The effect of dopamine on task-related slow-wave oscillations (0.5–4.6 Hz) was also investigated in humans by Winterer *et al.* (2006a). In order to test the hypothesis whether dopamine affects synchrony of prefrontal slow-wave oscillations during an auditory oddball task, the effect of the Val/Met *COMT* genotype was investigated. COMT is an enzyme critically involved in the catabolism of cortical dopamine. A number of neuroimaging investigations, underpinned by a host of basic research studies (both reviewed by Tan *et al.*, 2007), have suggested that Val allele carriers–as opposed to Met carriers–would have relatively greater inactivation of prefrontal synaptic dopamine and therefore less effective prefrontal dopamine signaling during working or short-term memory and attentional requiring tasks. Winterer *et al.* (2006a) found in a Caucasian sample comprising unrelated normal subjects, and probands with schizophrenia and their unaffected siblings that homozygous Val carriers, who are thought to have less synaptic dopamine available in the PFC, have greatest prefrontal electrophysiological "noise" values during an auditory oddball task. In a subsequently conducted fMRI study (Winterer *et al.*, 2006b), analogous results were obtained. In this study, event-related fMRI was conducted during a visual oddball task (checkerboard reversal). As compared to Val carriers, stronger and more extended BOLD responses were observed in homozygous Met carriers in the left supplementary motor area (SMA) extending to the ACC and DLPFC. *Vice versa*, increased levels of "noise" were seen in Val carriers surrounding the peak activation maximum. Thus, this work suggests that dopamine decreases "noise", i.e., increases slow-wave synchrony in the PFC. More generally, one could say that dopamine stabilizes cortical microcircuits by suppressing "noise" in cortical (prefrontal) networks (Winterer & Weinberger, 2004).

Slow-wave oscillations and schizophrenia

In 2000, Winterer *et al.* first reported, based on electrophysiological investigations, that information processing in schizophrenia might be characterized by a diminished cortical signal-to-noise ratio resulting from a poor low-frequency (0.5–5.5 Hz) phase-synchrony (i.e., increased "noise") of event-related fronto-central brain oscillations.

In this study, electrophysiological recordings from the scalp were obtained during a two-choice reaction time task with a randomized checkerboard presentation in the left and right hemifield requiring subjects to respond accordingly by button press. "Noise" was calculated as the power (μV^2) of the averaged event-related EEG subtracted from the mean power (μV^2) of the single evoked EEG responses. The noise power formula is:

$$\text{Noise power} = \frac{1}{N}\sum_{i=1}^{N}\left(u_i^2\right) - \left(\frac{1}{N}\sum_{i=1}^{N}u_i\right)^2$$

where N is the number of trials and u_i is the EEG signal of trial i.

Accordingly, this "noise" measure is related to the latency variability measure of ERPs (see above; Spencer, 2004). However, the two measures are not identical: "noise"—as an oscillatory-based measure—does not exclusively consider the peak latency variability, but also the amplitude variability of an evoked EEG response. In addition, it is not limited to a narrow time window around the peak of an ERP, but takes into account the entire evoked response. Several noteworthy findings were obtained in this study: test–retest reliability of the noise measure turned out to be highly stable (Cronbach's alpha > 0.9); patients with schizophrenia (n = 14) were unmedicated (>1 year); a comparable trend for increased "noise" was also seen in subjects at risk for schizophrenia (schizotypal subjects, n = 18); and in those patients (n = 16) who had received antipsychotic drug treatment (typical and atypical) within a few days (>3 days) before investigation, "noise" was diminished as compared to that in long-term drug-free patients. In addition, it was found that patients with a diagnosis of depression (n = 62) do not show increased "noise", suggesting diagnostic specificity of the "noise" measure. Referring to computational neural network models, the authors then proposed that this (synchrony) deficit may lead to specific changes of the attractor properties within cortical networks, most notably a decrease of attractor stability, which ultimately may account for the clinical symptoms observed in schizophrenia. Winterer *et al.* (2004) followed up on this finding in a series of electrophysiological and fMRI studies. As part of the National Institute of Mental Health (NIMH) schizophrenia sibling study, they explored whether this particular physiological abnormality predicts working memory and attentional performance (n-back task) and whether the "noise" is related to the genetic risk for schizophrenia. "Noise" was calculated for discrete frequency components across a broad frequency range (0.5–45.0 Hz) during processing of an auditory oddball paradigm in patients with schizophrenia (n = 66), their clinically unaffected siblings (n = 115), and healthy comparison subjects (n = 89). As predicted, frontal "noise" was highest in patients (mostly medicated), intermediate in their siblings, and lowest in the control subjects

(Plate 15.2), suggesting that increased prefrontal "noise" is associated with genetic risk for schizophrenia. Of note, increased "noise" in patients and their siblings was found across the entire frequency spectrum (0.5–45 Hz), suggesting that the synchronization deficit in schizophrenia may not be limited to low-frequency oscillations but is a more general and perhaps frequency-independent feature—a finding which has been recently confirmed by several groups using different task conditions, i.e., visual steady-state evoked responses (Krishnan *et al.*, 2005; Uhlhaas *et al.*, 2007). In the study of Winterer *et al.* (2004), intraclass correlations (ICC) within sibpairs (patients with schizophrenia *vs.* unaffected siblings) were in the range between 0.6 and 0.9, but lower in the higher beta/gamma frequencies (0.05–0.1), which may indicate that high-frequency oscillations are under less genetic control. In addition, it was observed that prefrontal "noise" (0.5–4.0 Hz) is negatively correlated with attention/working memory performance across all subjects (1-back r = −0.49, p < 0.0001; 2-back r = −0.34; p < 0.0002; 3-back r = −0.40, p < 0.0001). Interestingly, similar correlations were also seen for the alpha freqeuncy band (8.5–12.5 Hz). On the basis of these results, the authors concluded that frontal lobe-related cognitive function may depend on the ability of a subject to synchronize cortical pyramidal neurons, which is in part genetically controlled, and that increased prefrontal "noise" is an intermediate phenotype related to genetic susceptibility for schizophrenia.

Since both the EEG and BOLD responses depend on postsynaptically generated field potentials (see above), it was a logical step to investigate whether prefrontal BOLD-response variability is also increased in schizophrenia (Winterer *et al.*, 2006c). In this study, the authors used fMRI during a visual two-choice reaction task in order to measure, with higher topographic accuracy, signal stability in patients with schizophrenia (n =12) compared to controls (n = 16). They also assessed the relationship with more traditional measures of BOLD activation. In patients with schizophrenia, an increased cortical (prefrontal) BOLD-response variability ("BOLD noise") was found (Plate 15.2), which predicted the level of prefrontal activation in these subjects. An additional independent component analysis (ICA) revealed a "fractionized" and unfocused pattern of activation in patients. In the left hemisphere, residual noise variance strongly correlated with psychotic symptoms (r = 0.7, p < 0.05). The authors proposed that these findings may suggest unstable cortical signal processing underlying classical abnormal cortical activation patterns as well as psychosis in schizophrenia. Of interest in this context is that a recent simultaneous fMRI/EEG study found that "EEG noise" is strongly correlated with "BOLD noise" (Mobascher *et al.*, 2007).

While these "noise" findings appear to be promising, there is still considerable work ahead to be done. First, it will be necessary to further establish diagnostic specificity of "noise". In addition, it will be required to obtain a better understanding of the relationships between single neuron activity, local field potentials, and their impact on EEG and BOLD response variability ("noise") (Rolls *et al.*, 2008). Moreover, the precise nature of the mutual dependencies of low- and high-frequency oscillations across different brain regions—in particular between the frontal and temporal lobes—is far from understood. Ultimately, it will be necessary to explore the molecular, genetic, and pharmacological basis of synchrony in humans.

Other ERPs in schizophrenia

Other ERPs are the focus of intense research in patients with schizophrenia, but space limitations preclude extensive discussion of them here. Several of these potentials have been related to the search for an electrophysiological concomitant of an early sensory gating deficit in schizophrenia. These include, for example, the startle response, where the size of a blink to an acoustic probe is measured. Patients with schizophrenia appear to be unable to modify their large startle response when forewarned that a probe is coming, by contrast with controls (e.g., Braff *et al.*, 1978).

Another ERP thought to be sensitive to an early sensory gating abnormality in schizophrenia is the P50. In the sensory gating paradigm, an auditory click is presented to a subject, eliciting a positive deflection about 50 ms after stimulus onset, the P50 component. After a brief interval (about 500 ms), a second click elicits a much smaller amplitude P50 in normal adult subjects, who are said to show normal gating: the first stimulus inhibits, or closes the gate, to neurophysiological processing of the second stimulus. Patients with schizophrenia, on the other hand, show less reduction in P50 amplitude to the second click, which is referred to as a failure in gating (Adler *et al.*, 1982; Freedman *et al.*, 1983). This putative gating deficit occurs in about half the first-degree relatives of a patient with schizophrenia, suggesting that it may index a genetic factor in schizophrenia in the absence of overt psychotic symptoms (Waldo *et al.*, 1991). However, there have been concerns regarding the test–retest reliability of this measure which would limit it's utility as an endophenotype—at least in smaller samples (Rentzsch *et al.*, 2008; Turetsky *et al.*, 2007). While patients with affective disorder may show a gating deficit, the deficit does not persist after successful treatment, whereas in patients with schizophrenia the deficit occurs in both medicated and unmedicated patients, and persists after symptom remission (Adler & Waldo, 1991; Freedman *et al.*, 1983).

The putative gating effect is thought to take place in temporal lobe structures, possibly the medial temporal lobe (Adler *et al.*, 1985). However, more recently it has been suggested that while the temporal lobe is the main generator of the P50 component, the frontal lobe seems to be a substantial contributor to the process of sensory gating as observed from scalp recordings (Korzyukov *et al.*, 2007). P50 gating is enhanced by nicotinic cholinergic mechanisms, and it is possible that smoking in patients with schizophrenia is a form of self-medication (McCarley *et al.*, 1996). Freedman *et al.* (1994) have shown that blockade of the α7 nicotinic receptor causes loss of the inhibitory gating response to auditory stimuli in an animal model. The failure of inhibitory mechanisms to gate sensory input to higher-order processing may result in "sensory flooding", which Freedman suggests may underlie many of the symptoms of schizophrenia.

The N100 has recently received renewed interest in schizophrenia. These newer studies have been interested in behavior of the responses as stimulus parameters change. Adler *et al.* (1990) showed that N100 in patients with schizophrenia was less influenced by intensity and inter-stimulus interval (ISI) than N100 in controls. This effect was also demonstrated by Shelley *et al.* (1999), who suggested this effect was related to a deficit in current flow in underlying neurons. This hypothesis was tested in monkeys, where applications of PCP (phencyclidine), an NMDA receptor antagonist, blocked the normal increase in N100 amplitude with increasing ISI (Javitt *et al.*, 2000b). Interestingly, Katsanis *et al.* (1996) measured visual ERPs in first-episode patients, and reported no evidence of reductions in N100. However, source localization differences were found in drug-naïve and -free patients, mostly in the prefrontal midline, but also in the secondary auditory cortex (Mulert *et al.*, 2001; Gallinat *et al.*, 2002).

One other potential, the N200, is thought to relate to the initial categorization of stimuli in the selective attention stream, and is reduced in schizophrenia (e.g., Salisbury *et al.*, 1994b). Overall, however, there has been relatively little examination of N200, and the factors that affect it, in schizophrenia.

Magnetoencephalography: a complement to electroencephalography

Magnetoencephalography (MEG) is the measure of magnetic fields generated by the brain. A key difference in the physical source of the MEG as contrasted to the EEG is that the MEG is sensitive to cells which lie tangential to the brain surface and consequently have magnetic fields oriented tangentially. Cells with a radial orientation (perpendicular to the brain surface) do not generate signals detectable with MEG. The EEG and MEG are complementary in that the EEG is most sensitive to radially oriented neurons and fields. This distinction arises, of course, because magnetic fields are generated at right angles to electrical fields. One major advantage magnetic fields have over electrical potentials is that, once generated, they are

relatively invulnerable to intervening variations in the media they traverse (i.e., the skull, gray and white matter, and cerebrospinal fluid), unlike electrical fields, which are "smeared" by different electrical conductivities. This has made MEG a favorite for use in source localization, where attention has been especially focused on early potentials.

Perhaps because of the expense and non-mobility of the recording equipment needed for MEG, there has been relatively little work using MEG in schizophrenia to replicate and extend the findings of ERPs. A search of Medline revealed only 23 published studies using MEG measures of brain activity in schizophrenia. The most recent review currently available by Reite *et al.* (1999) should be consulted for details of the work on MEG in schizophrenia.

To summarize the studies to date, most have focused on M100 (N100m), the magnetic analog of N100. Results show a great degree of consistency across laboratories. The M100 shows abnormalities particularly in the left hemisphere, with an altered dipole location (shifted anteriorly), and reduced asymmetry for right-ear stimuli in schizophrenia patients.

Conclusions

ERPs provide the greatest temporal resolution of all the current functional imaging techniques. When coupled with information about likely generator sites from intracortical recordings, lesion studies, and fMRI, and with spatially accurate measures of brain structure from high-resolution MRI, ERPs greatly contribute to the elucidation of brain function, essentially detecting physiology at the speed of thought. Further, ERPs allow for the elucidation of information processing long before any overt behavior on the part of the subject. Both exogenous and endogenous ERPs are abnormal in patients chronically-ill with schizophrenia. As was demonstrated, these ERPs have helped to direct investigations of specific cortical regions, which has identified pathophysiology specific to schizophrenia compared with affective psychosis. The concurrent investigation of ERPs and MRI in chronically-ill and first-episode patients has allowed for the detection of those abnormalities that are present at disease onset and those that appear to develop with disease course. For the latter abnormalities, such a demonstration immediately suggests the importance of developing psychopharmacological and psychosocial interventions, which might counter at least some of the symptoms that develop with the disease course.

References

Adler, L.E. & Waldo, M.C. (1991) Counterpoint: sensory gating-hippocampal model of schizophrenia. *Schizophrenia Bulletin* **17**, 19–24.

Adler, L.E., Pachtman, E., Franks, R.D., Pecevich, M., Waldo, M.C. & Freedman, R. (1982) Neurophysiological evidence for a defect in neuronal mechanisms involved in sensory gating in schizophrenia. *Biological Psychiatry* **17**, 639–654.

Adler, L.E., Waldo, M.C. & Freedman, R. (1985) Neurophysiologic studies of sensory gating in schizophrenia: comparison of auditory and visual responses. *Biological Psychiatry* **20**, 1284–1296.

Adler, L.E., Waldo, M.C., Tatcher, A., Cawthra, E., Baker, N. & Freedman, R. (1990) Lack of relationship of auditory gating defects to negative symptoms in schizophrenia. *Schizophrenia Research* **3**, 131–138.

Anokhin, A.P., Todorov, A.A., Madden, P.A., Grant, J.D. & Heath, A.C. (1999) Brain event-related potentials, dopamine D2 receptor gene polymorphism, and smoking. *Genetic Epidemiology* **17** (Suppl. 1), S37–42.

Anokhin, A.P., Vedeniapin, A.B., Sirevaag, E.J. *et al.* (2000) The P300 brain potential is reduced in smokers. *Psychopharmacology (Berlin)* **149**, 409–413.

Baldeweg, T., Klugman, A., Gruzelier, J.H. & Hirsch, S.R. (2002) Impairment in frontal but not temporal components of mismatch negativity. *International Journal of Psychophysiology* **43**, 111–122.

Barta, P.E., Pearlson, G.D., Powers, R.E., Richards, S.S. & Tune, L.E. (1990) Auditory hallucinations and smaller superior temporal gyral volume in schizophrenia. *American Journal of Psychiatry* **147**, 1457–1462.

Baudena, P., Halgren, E., Heit, G. & Clarke, J.M. (1995) Intracerebral potentials to rare target and distractor auditory and visual stimuli. III. Frontal cortex. *Electroencephalography and Clinical Neurophysiology* **94**, 251–264.

Bénar,C.G., Schön, D., Grimault, S. *et al.* (2007) Single-trial analysis of oddball event-related potentials in simultaneous EEG-fMRI. *Human Brain Mapping* **28**, 602–613.

Berman, S.M., Noble, E.P., Antolin, T., Sheen, C., Conner, B.T. & Ritchie, T. (2006) P300 development during adolescence: effects of DRD2 genotype. *Clinical Neurophysiology* **117**, 649–659.

Bledowski, C., Hoechstetter, K., Scherg, M., Wibral, M., Goebel, R. & Linden, D.E. (2004) Localizing P300 generators in visual target and distractor processing: a combined event-related potential and functional magnetic resonance imaging study. *Journal of Neuroscience* **24**, 9353–9360.

Borst, J.G.G., Leung, L.-W.S. & MacFabe, D.F. (1987) Electrical activity of the cingulate cortex. II. Cholinergic modulation. *Brain Research* **407**, 81–93.

Braff, D., Stone, C., Callaway, E., Geyer, M., Glick, I. & Bali, L. (1978) Prestimulus effects on human startle reflex in normals and schizophrenics. *Psychophysiology* **15**, 339–343.

Bramon, E., Rabe-Hesketh, S., Shama, P., Murray, R.M. & Frangou, S. (2004) Meta-analysis of the P300 and P50 waveforms in schizophrenia. *Schizophrenia Research* **70**, 315–329.

Bramon, E., Dempster, E., Frangou, S. *et al.* (2006) Is there an association between the COMT gene and P300 endophenotypes? *European Psychiatry* **21**, 70–73.

Brenner, C.A., Sporns, O., Lysaker, P.H. & O'Donnell, B.F. (2003) EEG synchronization to modulated auditory tones in schizophrenia, schizoaffective disorder, and schizotypal personality disorder. *American Journal of Psychiatry* **160**, 2238–2240.

Buzsaki, G. (2002) Theta oscillations in the hippocampus. *Neuron* **33**, 325–340.

Calhoun, V.D., Adali, T., Giuliani, N.R., Pekar, J.J., Kiehl, K.A. & Pearlson, G.D. (2006) Method for multimodal analysis of independent source differences in schizophrenia: combining gray matter structural and auditory oddball functional data. *Human Brain Mapping* **27**, 47–62.

Callaway, E., Jones, R.T. & Donchin, E. (1970) Auditory evoked potential variability in schizophrenia. *Electroencephalography and Clinical Neurophysiology* **29**, 421–428.

Cantero, J.L., Atienza, M., Stickgold, R., Kahana, M.J., Madsen, J.R. & Kocsis, B. (2003) Sleep dependent theta oscillations in the human hippocampus and neocortex. *Journal of Neuroscience* **23**, 10897–10903.

Cunningham, M.O., Hunt, J., Middleton, S. *et al.* (2006) Region-specific reduction in entorhinal gamma oscillations and parvalbumin-immunoreactive neurons in animal models of psychiatric illness. *Journal of Neuroscience* **26**, 2767–2776.

Dierks, T., Frölich, L., Ihl, R. & Maurer, K. (1994) Event-related potentials and psychopharmacology. Cholinergic modulation of P300. *Pharmacopsychiatry* **27**, 72–74.

Donchin, E., Callaway, E. & Jones, R.T. (1970) Auditory evoked potential variability in schizophrenia. II. The application of discriminant analysis. *Electroencephalography and Clinical Neurophysiology* **29**, 429–440.

Ehlers, C.L. & Somes, C. (2002) Long latency event-related potentials in mice: effects of stimulus characteristics and strain. *Brain Research* **957**, 117–128.

Ehlis, A.C., Reif, A., Herrmann, M.J., Lesch, K.P. & Fallgatter, A.J. (2007) Impact of catechol-O-methyltransferase on prefrontal brain functioning in schizophrenia spectrum disorders. *Neuropsychopharmacology* **32**, 162–170.

Fitch, T.E., Sahr, R.N., Eastwood, B.J., Zhou, F.C. & Yang, C.R. (2006) Dopamine D1/D5 receptor modulation of firing rate and bidirectional theta burst firing in medial septal/vertical limb of diagonal band neurons *in vivo*. *Journal of Neurophysiology* **95**, 2808–2820.

Ford, J.M., White, P., Lim, K.O. & Pfefferbaum, A. (1994) Schizophrenics have fewer and smaller P300s: a single-trial analysis. *Biological Psychiatry* **35**, 96–103.

Ford, J.M., Roach, B.J., Faustman, W.O. & Mathalon, D.H. (2007) Out-of-Synch and Out-of-Sorts: Dysfunction of Motor-Sensory Communication in Schizophrenia. Available online 5 November 2007, *Biological Psychiatry*.

Freedman, R., Adler, L.E., Waldo, M.C., Pachtman, E. & Franks, R.D. (1983) Neurophysiological evidence for a defect in inhibitory pathways in schizophrenia: comparison of medicated and drug-free patients. *Biological Psychiatry* **18**, 537–551.

Freedman, R., Adler, L.E., Bickford, P. *et al.* (1994) Schizophrenia and nicotinic receptors. *Harvard Reviews of Psychiatry* **2**, 179–192.

Fries, P., Nikolic, D. & Singer, W. (2007) The gamma cycle. *Trends in Neuroscience* **30**, 309–316.

Frodl, T., Meisenzahl, E.M., Müller, D. *et al.* (2002) P300 subcomponents and clinical symptoms in schizophrenia. *International Journal of Psychophysiology* **43**, 237–246.

Gallinat, J., Riedel, M., Juckel, G. *et al.* (2001) P300 and symptom improvement in schizophrenia. *Psychopharmacology (Berlin)* **158**, 55–65.

Gallinat, J., Mulert, C., Bajbouj, M. *et al.* (2002) Frontal and temporal dysfunction of auditory stimulus processing in schizophrenia. *Neuroimage* **17**, 110–127.

Gallinat, J., Bajbouj, M., Sander, T. *et al.* (2003) Association of the G1947A COMT (Val(108/158)Met) gene polymorphism with prefrontal P300 during information processing. *Biological Psychiatry* **54**, 40–48.

Gallinat, J., Winterer, G., Herrmann, C.S. & Senkowski, D. (2004) Reduced oscillatory gamma-band responses in unmedicated schizophrenic patients indicate impaired frontal network processing. *Clinical Neurophysiology* **115**, 1863–1874.

Gallinat, J., Götz, T., Kalus, P., Bajbouj, M., Sander, T. & Winterer, G. (2007) Genetic variations of the NR3A subunit of the NMDA receptor modulate prefrontal cerebral activity in humans. *Journal of Cognitive Neuroscience* **19**, 59–68.

Gevins, A. & Smith, M.E. (2000) Neurophysiological measures of working memory and individual differences in cognitive ability and cognitive style. *Cerebral Cortex* **10**, 829–839.

Gevins, A., Smith, M.E., McEvoy, L. & Yu. D. (1997) High-resolution EEG mapping of cortical activation related to working memory: effects of task difficulty, type of processing, and practice. *Cerebral Cortex* **7**, 374–385.

Golimbet, V., Gritsenko, I., Alfimova, M. *et al.* (2006) Association study of COMT gene Val158Met polymorphism with auditory P300 and performance on neurocognitive tests in patients with schizophrenia and their relatives. *World Journal of Biological Psychiatry* **7**, 238–245.

Grunze, H.C., Rainnie, D.G., Hasselmo, M.E. *et al.* (1996) NMDA-dependent modulation of CA1 local circuit inhibition. *Journal of Neuroscience* **16**, 2034–2043.

Guderian, S. & Düzel, E. (2005) Induced theta oscillations mediate large-scale synchrony with mediotemporal areas during recollection in humans. *Hippocampus* **15**, 901–912.

Halgren, E., Baudena, P., Clarke, J.M. *et al.* (1995a) Intracerebral potentials to rare target and distractor auditory and visual stimuli. I. Superior temporal plane and parietal lobe. *Electroencephalography and Clinical Neurophysiology* **94**, 191–220.

Halgren, E., Baudena, P., Clarke, J.M. *et al.* (1995b) Intracerebral potentials to rare target and distractor auditory and visual stimuli. II. Medial, lateral and posterior temporal lobe. *Electroencephalography and Clinical Neurophysiology* **94**, 229–250.

Hall, M.H., Schulze, K., Rijsdijk, F. et al. (2006) Heritability and reliability of P300, P50 and duration mismatch negativity. *Behavioural Genetics* **36**, 845–857.

Hall, M.H., Rijsdijk, F., Picchioni, M. *et al.* (2007) Substantial shared genetic influences on schizophrenia and event-related potentials. *American Journal of Psychiatry* **164**, 804–812.

Handy, T.C. (2004) *Event-Related Potentials: A Methods Handbook.* Cambridge, MA: MIT Press.

Harrison, J.B., Buchwald, J.S., Kaga, K., Woolf, N.J. & Butcher, L.L. (1988) "Cat P300" disappears after septal lesions. *Electroencephalography and Clinical Neurophysiology* **69**, 55–64.

Hasselmo, M.E. (2005) What is the function of hippocampal theta rhythm? Linking behavioral data to phasic properties of field potential and unit recording data. *Hippocampus* **15**, 936–949.

Hermandez, L., Badre, D., Noll, D. & Jonides, J. (2002) Temporal sensitivity of event-related fMRI. *Neuroimage* **17**, 1018–1026.

Herrmann, C.S. & Demiralp, T. (2005) Human EEG gamma oscillations in neuropsychiatric disorders. *Clinical Neurophysiology* **116**, 2719–2733.

Hill, S.Y., Locke, J., Zezza, N. *et al.* (1998) Genetic association between reduced P300 amplitude and the DRD2 dopamine receptor A1 allele in children at high risk for alcoholism. *Biological Psychiatry* **43**, 40–51.

Hillyard, S.A. & Picton, T.W. (1987) Electrophysiology of cognition. In: Plum, F., ed. *Handbook of Physiology. Section 1. The Nervous System*, vol. **5**. Oxford: Oxford University Press, pp. 519–584.

Hollander, E., Davidson, M., Mohs, R.C. *et al.* (1987) RS 86 in the treatment of Alzheimer's disease: cognitive and biological effects. *Biological Psychiatry* **22**, 1067–1078.

Hong, L., Summerfelt, A., McMahon, R. *et al.* (2004) Evoked gamma band synchronization and the liability for schizophrenia. *Schizophrenia Research* **70**, 293–302.

Huang, M.X., Song, T., Hagler, D.J. *et al.* (2007) A novel integrated MEG and EEG analysis method for dipolar sources. *Neuroimage* **37**, 731–748.

Hyman, J.M., Zilli, E.A., Paley, A.M. & Hasselmo, M.E. (2005) Medial prefrontal cortex cells show dynamic modulation with the hippocampal theta rhythm dependent on behavior. *Hippocampus* **15**, 739–749.

Ishihara, T. & Yoshii, N. (1972) Multivariate analytic study of EEG and mental activity in juvenile delinquents. *Electroencephalography and Clinical Neurophysiology* **33**, 71–80.

Jacobs, J., Kahana, M.J., Ekstrom, A.D. & Fried, I. (2007) Brain oscillations control timing of single-neuron activity in humans. *Journal of Neuroscience* **27**, 3839–3844.

Javitt, D.C. (2000) Intracortical mechanisms of mismatch negativity dysfunction in schizophrenia. *Audiology and Neurootology* **5**, 207–215.

Javitt, D.C., Steinschneider, M., Schroeder, C.E. & Arezzo, J.C. (1996) Role of cortical N-methyl-D-aspartate receptors in auditory sensory memory and mismatch negativity generation: implications for schizophrenia. *Proceedings of the National Academy of Science USA* **93**, 11962–11967.

Javitt, D.C., Shelley, A.-M., Silipo, G. & Lieberman, J.A. (2000a) Deficits in auditory and visual context-dependent processing in schizophrenia: Defining the pattern. *Archives of General Psychiatry* **57**, 1131–1137.

Javitt, D.C., Jayachandra, M., Lindsley, R.W., Specht, C.M. & Schroeder, C.E. (2000b) Schizophrenia-like deficits in auditory P1 and N1 refractoriness induced by the psychomimetic agent phencyclidine (PCP). *Clinical Neurophysiology* **111**, 833–836.

Javitt, D.C., Spencer, K.M., Thaker, G.K., Winterer, G. & Hajós, M. (2008) Neurophysiological biomarkers for drug development in schizophrenia. *Nature Reviews Drug Discovery* **7**, 68–83.

Jensen, O. & Colgin, L.L. (2007) Cross-frequency coupling between neuronal oscillations. *Trends in Cognitive Science* **11**, 267–269.

Jensen, O. & Lisman, J.E. (2005). Hippocampal sequence-encoding driven by a cortical multi-item working memory buffer. *Trends in Neuroscience* **28**, 67–72.

Jervis, B.W., Nichols, M.J., Johnson, T.E., Allen, E. & Hudson, N.R. (1983) A fundamental investigation of the composition of auditory evoked potentials. *IEEE Transactions in Biomedical Engineering* **30**, 43–50.

Jessen, F., Fries, T., Kucharski, C. *et al.* (2001) Amplitude reduction of the mismatch negativity in first-degree relatives of patients with schizophrenia. *Neuroscience Letters* **309**, 185–188.

John, E.R., Prichep, L.S., Firdman, J. & Easton, P. (1988) Neurometrics: Computer-assisted differential diagnosis of brain dysfunctions. *Science* **239**, 162–169.

John, E.R., Prichep, L.S., Winterer, G. *et al.* (2007) Electrophysiological subtypes of psychotic states. *Acta Psychiatrica Scandinavica* **116**, 17–35.

Jones, M.W. & Wilson, M.A. (2005). Theta rhythms coordinate hippocampal-prefrontal interactions in a spatial memory task. *PLoS Biology* **3**, e402.

Kasai, K., Shenton, M.E., Salisbury, D.F. *et al.* (2003) Progressive decrease of left Heschl's gyrus and planum temporale gray matter volume in schizophrenia: a longitudinal MRI study of first-episode patients. *Archives of General Psychiatry* **60**, 766–775.

Katsanis, J., Iacono, W.G. & Beiser, M. (1996) Visual event-related potentials in first-episode psychotic patients and their relatives. *Psychophysiology* **33**, 207–217.

Knott, V., Mohr, E., Mahoney, C., Engeland, C. & Ilivitsky, V. (2002) Effects of acute nicotine administration on cognitive event-related potentials in tacrine-treated and non-treated patients with Alzheimer's disease. *Neuropsychobiology* **45**, 156–160.

Kopell, N., Ermentrout, G.B., Whittington, M.A. & Traub, R.D. (2000) Gamma rhythms and beta rhythms have different synchronization properties. *Proceedings of the National Academy of Science USA* **97**, 1867–1872.

Korzyukov, O., Pflieger, M.E., Wagner, M. *et al.* (2007) Generators of the intracranial P50 response in auditory sensory gating. *Neuroimage* **35**, 814–826.

Krishnan, G.P., Vohs, J.L., Hetrick, W.P. *et al.* (2005) Steady state visual evoked potential abnormalities in schizophrenia. *Clinical Neurophysiology* **116**, 614–624.

Kwon, J.S., O'Donnell, B.F., Wallenstein, G.V. *et al.* (1999) Gamma Frequency Range Abnormalities to Auditory Stimulation in Schizophrenia. *Archives of General Psychiatry* **56**, 1001–1005.

Lehmann, D., Faber, P.L., Galderisi, S. *et al.* (2005) EEG microstate duration and syntax in acute, medication-naïve, first-episode schizophrenia: a multi-center study. *Psychiatry Research* **28**, 141–156.

Leung, L.-W.S. & Borst, J.G.G. (1987) Electrical activity of the cingulate cortex. 1. generating mechanisms and relations to behavior. *Brain Research* **407**, 68–80.

Lewis, D.A., Hashimoto, T. & Volk, D.W. (2005) Cortical inhibitory neurons and schizophrenia. *Nature Reviews Neuroscience* **6**, 312–324.

Light, G.A. & Braff, D.L. (2005) Stability of mismatch negativity deficits and their relationship to functional impairments in chronic schizophrenia. *American Journal of Psychiatry* **162**, 9.

Lin, C.H., Yu, Y.W., Chen, T.J., Tsa, S.J. & Hong, C.J. (2001) Association analysis for dopamine D2 receptor Taq1 polymorphism with P300 event-related potential for normal young females. *Psychiatric Genetics* **11**, 165–168.

Lin, F.H., Wald, L.L., Ahlfors, S.P., Hämäläinen, M.S., Kwong, K.K. & Belliveau, J.W. (2006) Dynamic magnetic resonance inverse imaging of human brain function. *Magnetic Resonance Medicine* **56**, 787–802.

Linden, D.E., Prvulovic, D., Formisano, E. *et al.* (1999) The functional neuroanatomy of target detection: an fMRI study of visual and auditory oddball tasks. *Cerebral Cortex* **9**, 815–823.

Logothetis, N.K., Pauls, J., Augath, M., Trinath, T. & Oeltermann, A. (2001) Neurophysiological investigation of the basis of the fMRI signal. *Nature* **412**, 150–157.

López, J., López, V., Rojas, D. *et al.* (2004). Effect of psychostimulants on distinct attentional parameters in attentional deficit/hyperactivity disorder. *Biological Research* **37**, 461–468.

Makeig, S., Westerfield, M., Jung, T.P. *et al.* (2002) Dynamic brain sources of visual evoked responses. *Science* **295**, 690–694.

Mathalon, D.H., Ford, J.M. & Pfefferbaum, A. (2000) Trait and state aspects of P300 amplitude reduction in schizophrenia: a retrospective longitudinal study. *Biological Psychiatry* **47**, 434–449.

Mathalon, D.H., McGlashan, T.H., Miller, T.J. & Woods, S.W. (2006) Frequency and duration mismatch negativity in the prodromal and early illness stages of schizophrenia. *Biological Psychiatry* **59**, 264S.

McCarley, R.W., Shenton, M.E., O'Donnell, B.F. *et al.* (1993) Auditory P300 abnormalities and left posterior superior temporal gyrus volume reduction in schizophrenia. *Archives of General Psychiatry* **50**, 190–197.

McCarley, R.W., Hsiao, J., Freedman, R., Pfefferbaum, A. & Donchin, E. (1996) Neuroimaging and the cognitive neuroscience of schizophrenia. *Schizophrenia Bulletin* **22**, 703–726.

McCarley, R.W., Niznikiewicz, M.A., Salisbury, D.F. *et al.* (1999) Cognitive dysfunction in schizophrenia: unifying basic research and clinical aspects. *European Archives of Psychiatry and Clinical Neuroscience* **249** (Suppl. IV), 69–82.

McCarley, R.W., Salisbury, D.F., Hirayasu, Y. *et al.* (2002) Association between smaller left posterior superior temporal gyrus MRI volume and smaller left temporal P300 amplitude in first-episode schizophrenia. *Archives of General Psychiatry* **59**, 321–331.

Michie, P.T., Innes-Brown, H., Todd, J. & Jablensky, A.V. (2002) Duration mismatch negativity in biological relatives of patients with schizophrenia spectrum disorders. *Biological Psychiatry* **52**, 749–758.

Miller, R. (1991) Discovery and general behavioural correlates of the hippocampal theta rhythm in several species. In: Miller, R., ed. *Corticohippocampal Interplay and the Representation of Context in the Brain.* Berlin: Springer.

Mobascher, A., Brinkmeyer, J., Musso, F. *et al.* (2007) Event-related EEG synchronization predicts BOLD residual noise variance. Human Brain Mapping Meeting, Chicago (poster presentation).

Morstyn, R.M., Duffy, F.H. & McCarley, R.W. (1983) Altered P300 topography in schizophrenia. *Archives of General Psychiatry* **40**, 729–734.

Mulert, C., Gallinat, J., Pascual-Marqui, R. *et al.* (2001) Reduced event-related current density in the anterior cingulate cortex in schizophrenia. *Neuroimage* **13**, 589–600.

Mulert, C., Juckel, G., Giegling, I. *et al.* (2004) A Ser9Gly polymorphism in the dopamine D3 receptor gene (DRD3) and event-related P300 potentials. *Neuropsychopharmacology* **31**, 1335–1344.

Musso, F., Konrad, A., Vucurevic, G. *et al.* (2006) Distributed BOLD-response in association cortex vector state space predicts reaction time during selective attention. *Neuroimage* **29**, 1311–1318.

Näätänen, R., Paavilainen, P., Rinne, T. & Alho, K. (2007) The mismatch negativity (MMN) in basic research of central auditory processing: A review. *Clinical Neurophysiology* **118**, 2544–2290.

Nakamura, M., Salisbury, D.F., Hirayasu, Y. *et al.* (2007) Neocortical gray matter volume in first episode schizophrenia and first episode affective psychosis: a cross-sectional and longitudinal MRI study. *Biological Psychiatry* **62**, 773–783.

Neuhaus, A., Bajbouj, M., Kienast, T. *et al.* (2006) Persistent dysfunctional frontal lobe activation in former smokers. *Psychopharmacology (Berlin)* **186**, 191–200.

Niznikiewicz, M.A., Patel, J.K., McCarley, R. *et al.* (2005) Clozapine action on auditory P3 response in schizophrenia. *Schizophrenia Research* **76**, 19–21.

O'Donnell, B.F., Faux, S.F., McCarley, R.W. *et al.* (1995) Increased rate of P300 latency prolongation with age in schizophrenia. Electrophysiological evidence for a neurodegenerative process. *Archives of General Psychiatry* **52**, 544–549.

O'Donnell, B.F., Vohs, J.L., Hetrick, W.P., Carroll, C.A. & Shekhar, A. (2004) Auditory event-related potential abnormalities in bipolar disorder and schizophrenia. *International Journal of Psychophysiology* **53**, 45–55.

Oknina, L.B., Wild-Wall, N., Oades, R.D. *et al.* (2005) Frontal and temporal sources of mismatch negativity in healthy controls, patients at onset of schizophrenia in adolescence and others at 15 years after onset. *Schizophrenia Research* **76**, 25–41.

Oranje, B., Gispen-de Wied, C.C., Westenberg, H.G., Kemner, C., Verbaten, M.N. & Kahn, R.S. (2006) No effects of l-dopa and bromocriptine on psychophysiological parameters of human selective attention. *Journal of Psychopharmacology* **20**, 789–98.

Pae, J.S., Kwon, J.S., Youn, T. *et al.* (2003) LORETA imaging of P300 in schizophrenia with individual MRI and 128-channel EEG. *Neuroimage* **20**, 1552–1560.

Reite, M., Teale, P. & Rojas, D.C. (1999) Magnetoencephalography: applications in psychiatry. *Biological Psychiatry* **45**, 1553–1563.

Rentzsch, J., Jockers-Scherübl, M.C., Boutros, N.N. & Gallinat, J. (2008) Test-retest reliability of P50, N100 and P200 auditory sensory gating in healthy subjects. *International Journal of Psychophysiology* **67**, 81–90.

Rolls, E.T., Loh, M., Deco, G. & Winterer, G. (2008) Computational models of schizophrenia and dopamine modulation in the prefrontal cortex. *Nature Reviews Neuroscience* **9**, 696–709.

Roopun, A.K., Middleton, S.J., Cunningham, M.O. *et al.* (2006) A beta2-frequency (20-30 Hz) oscillation in nonsynaptic networks of somatosensory cortex. *Proceedings of the National Academy of Science USA* **103**, 15646–15650.

Röschke, J., Wagner, P., Mann, K., Fell, J., Grözinger, M. & Frank, C. (1996) Single trial analysis of event related potentials: a comparison between schizophrenics and depressives. *Biological Psychiatry* **40**, 844–852.

Roth, W.T. (1977) Late event-related potentials and psychopathology. *Schizophrenia Bulletin* **3**, 105–120.

Roth, W.T. & Cannon, E.H. (1972) Some features of the auditory evoked response in schizophrenics. *Archives of General Psychiatry* **27**, 466–471.

Roth, W.T., Pfefferbaum, A., Kelly, A.F., Berger, P.A. & Kopell, B.S. (1981) Auditory event-related potentials in schizophrenia and depression. *Psychiatry Research* **4**, 199–212.

Roth, A., Roesch-Ely, D., Bender, S., Weisbrod, M. & Kaiser, S. (2007) Increased event-related potential latency and amplitude variability in schizophrenia detected through wavelet-based single trial analysis. *International Journal of Psychophysiology* **66**, 244–254.

Rujescu, D., Bender, A., Keck, M. *et al.* (2006) A pharmacological model for psychosis based on N-methyl-D-aspartate receptor hypofunction: Molecular, cellular, functional and behavioral abnormalities. *Biological Psychiatry* **59**, 721–729.

Salisbury, D.F., O'Donnell, B.F., McCarley, R.W., Nestor, P.G., Faux, S.F. & Smith, R.S. (1994a) Parametric manipulations of auditory stimuli differentially affect P3 amplitude in schizophrenics and controls. *Psychophysiology* **31**, 29–36.

Salisbury, D.F., O'Donnell, B.F., McCarley, R.W., Shenton, M.E. & Benavage, A. (1994b) The N2 event-related potential reflects attention deficit in schizophrenia. *Biological Psychology* **39**, 1–13.

Salisbury, D.F., Shenton, M.E. & McCarley, R.W. (1999) P300 topography differs in schizophrenia and manic psychosis. *Biological Psychiatry* **45**, 98–106.

Salisbury, D.F., Shenton, M.E., Griggs, C.B., Bonner-Jackson, A. & McCarley, RW. (2002) Mismatch Negativity in chronic schizophrenia and first-episode schizophrenia. *Archives of General Psychiatry* **59**, 686–694.

Salisbury, D.F., Kuroki, N., Kasai, K., Shenton, M.E. & McCarley, R.W. (2007) Progressive and interrelated functional and structural evidence for post-onset brain reduction in schizophrenia. *Archives of General Psychiatry* **64**, 521–529.

Selemon, L.D. & Goldman-Rakic, P.S. (1999) The reduced neuropil hypothesis: a circuit based model of schizophrenia. *Biological Psychiatry* **45**, 17–25.

Shagass, C. (1968) Cerebral evoked responses in schizophrenia. *Conditional Reflex* **3**, 205–216.

Shagass, C. (1977) Early evoked potentials. *Schizophrenia Bulletin* **3**, 80–92.

Shelley, A.M., Silipo, G. & Javitt, D.C. (1999) Diminished responsiveness of ERPs in schizophrenic subjects to changes in auditory stimulation parameters: implications for theories of cortical dysfunction. *Schizophrenia Research* **37**, 65–79.

Shenton, M.E., Kikinis, R., Jolesz, F.A. *et al.* (1992) Abnormalities of the left temporal lobe and thought disorder in schizophrenia. A quantitative magnetic resonance imaging study. *New England Journal of Medicine* **327**, 604–612.

Slawecki, C.J., Thomas, J.D., Riley, E.P. & Ehlers, C.L. (2000) Neonatal nicotine exposure alters hippocampal EEG and event-related potentials (ERPs) in rats. *Pharmacology Biochemisty and Behavior* **65**, 711–718.

Spencer, K.M. (2004) Averaging, detection, and classification of single-trial ERPs. In: Handy, T., ed. *Event-Related Potentials: A Methods Handbook*. Cambridge, MA: The MIT Press, pp. 209–227.

Spencer, K.M., Nestor, P.G., Niznikiewicz, M.A., Salisbury, D.F., Shenton, M.E. & McCarley, R.W. (2003) Abnormal neural synchrony in schizophrenia. *Journal of Neuroscience* **23**, 7407–7411.

Spencer, K.M., Nestor, P.G., Perlmutter, R. *et al.* (2004) Neural synchrony indexes disordered perception and cognition in schizophrenia. *Proceedings of the National Academy of Science USA* **101**, 17288–17293.

Spencer, K.M., Salisbury, D.F., Shenton, M.E. & McCarley, R.W. (2006) Gamma-band steady-state responses are impaired in first episode psychosis. *Social Neuroscience Abstracts* **36**, 122.

Strik, W.K., Dierks, T., Franzek, E., Maurer, K. & Beckmann, H. (1993) Differences in P300 amplitudes and topography between cycloid psychosis and schizophrenia in Leonhard's classification. *Acta Psychiatrica Scandinavica* **87**, 179–183.

Sutton, S., Braren, M., Zubin, J. & John, E.R. (1965) Evoked-potential correlates of stimulus uncertainty. *Science* **150**, 1187–1188.

Talk, A., Kang, E. & Gabriel, M. (2004) Independent generation of theta rhythm in the hippocampus and posterior cingulate cortex. *Brain Research* **1015**, 15–24.

Tamminga, C.A. (2006) The neurobiology of cognition in schizophrenia. *Journal of Clinical Psychiatry* **67** (Suppl 9), 9–13.

Tan, H.Y., Callicott, J.H. & Weinberger, D.R. (2007) Dysfunctional and compensatory prefrontal cortical systems, genes and the pathogenesis of schizophrenia. *Cerebral Cortex* **1** (Suppl.), 171–181.

Thomas, A., Iacono, D., Bonanni, L., D'Andreamatteo, G. & Onofrj, M. (2000) Donepezil, rivastigmine, and vitamin E in Alzheimer disease: a combined P300 event-related potentials/neuropsychologic evaluation over 6 months. *Clinical Neuropharmacology* **24**, 31–42.

Todd, J., Michie, P.T., Schall, U., Karayanidis, F., Yabe, H. & Näätänen, R. (2008) Deviant matters: Duration, frequency, and intensity deviants reveal different patterns of mismatch negativity reduction in early and late schizophrenia. *Biological Psychiatry* **63**, 58–64.

Toga, A.W. & Mazziotta, J.C. (2002) *Brain Mapping: the Methods*. Orlando: Academic Press.

Tsai, S.J., Yu, Y.W., Chen, T.J., Chen, M.C. & Hong, C.J. (2003) Association analysis for dopamine D3 receptor, dopamine D4 receptor and dopamine transporter genetic polymorphisms and P300 event-related potentials for normal young females. *Psychiatric Genetics* **13**, 51–53.

Tsujimoto, T., Shimazu, H. & Isomura, Y. (2006) Direct recording of theta oscillations in primate prefrontal and anterior cingulate cortices. *Journal of Neurophysiology* **95**, 2987–3000.

Turetsky, B., Colbath, E.A. & Gur, R.E. (1998) P300 subcomponent abnormalities in schizophrenia: II. Longitudinal stability and relationship to symptom change. *Biological Psychiatry* **43**, 31–39.

Turetsky, B.I., Calkins, M.E., Light, G.A., Olincy, A., Radant, A.D. & Swerdlow, N.R. (2007) Neurophysiological endophenotypes of schizophrenia: the viability of selected candidate measures. *Schizophrenia Bulletin* **33**, 69–94.

Uhlhaas, P., Silverstein, S.M., Phillips, W.A. & Lovell, P.G. (2004) Evidence for impaired visual context processing in schizotypy with thought disorder. *Schizophrenia Research* **68**, 249–260.

Uhlhaas, P., Rodriguez, R., Roux, F., Haenschel, C., Maurer, K. & Singer, W. (2007) Neuronal synchrony as a pathophysiological mechanism in schizophrenia. 1st European Conference on Schizophrenia Research (oral presentation).

Umbricht, D., Javitt, D., Novak, G. *et al.* (1998) Effects of clozapine on auditory event-related potentials in schizophrenia. *Biological Psychiatry* **44**, 716–725.

Umbricht, D., Schmid, L., Koller, R., Vollenweider, F.X., Hell, D. & Javitt, D.C. (2000) Ketamine-induced deficits in auditory and visual context-dependent processing in healthy volunteers: implications for models of cognitive deficits in schizophrenia. *Archives of General Psychiatry* **57**, 1139–1147.

Umbricht, D., Koller, R., Schmid, L. *et al.* (2003) How specific are deficits in mismatch negativity generation to schizophrenia? *Biological Psychiatry* **53**, 1120–1131.

Van der Stelt, O., Belger, A. & Lieberman, J.A. (2004) Macroscopic fast neuronal oscillations and synchrony in schizophrenia. *Proceedings of the National Academy of Science USA* **101**, 17567–17568.

Vertes, R.P. (2005) Hippocampal theta rhythm: a tag for short-term memory. *Hippocampus* **15**, 923–935.

Waldo, M.C., Carey, G., Myles-Worsley, M. *et al.* (1991) Codistribution of a sensory gating deficit and schizophrenia in multi-affected families. *Psychiatry Research* **39**, 257–68.

Werber, A.E., Klein, C. & Rabey, J.M. (2001) Evaluation of cholinergic treatment in demented patients by P300 evoked related potentials. *Neurologie Neurochirugie Pol* **35** (Suppl 3), 37–43.

Wible, C.G., Kubicki, M., Yoo, S.S. *et al.* (2001) A functional magnetic resonance imaging study of auditory mismatch in schizophrenia. *American Journal of Psychiatry* **158**, 938–943.

Winterer, G. & Weinberger, D.R. (2004) Genes, dopamine and cortical signal-to-noise ratio in schizophrenia. *Trends in Neuroscience* **27**, 683–690.

Winterer, G., Ziller, M., Dorn, H. *et al.* (1999) Cortical activation, signal-to-noise ratio and stochastic resonance during information processing in man. *Clinical Neurophysiology* **110**, 1193–1203.

Winterer, G., Ziller, M., Dorn, H. *et al.* (2000) Schizophrenia: reduced signal-to-noise ratio and impaired phase-locking during information processing. *Clinical Neurophysiology* **111**, 837–849.

Winterer, G., Mulert, C., Mientus, S. *et al.* (2001) P300 and LORETA: comparison of normal subjects and schizophrenic patients. *Brain Topography* **13**, 299–313.

Winterer, G., Egan, M.F., Raedler, T. *et al.* (2003) P300 and genetic risk for schizophrenia. *Archives of General Psychiatry* **60**, 1158–1167.

Winterer, G., Coppola, R., Goldberg, T.E. *et al.* (2004) Prefrontal broadband noise, working memory, and genetic risk for schizophrenia. *American Journal of Psychiatry* **161**, 490–500.

Winterer, G., Egan, M.F., Kolachana, B.S., Goldberg, T.E., Coppola, R. & Weinberger, D.R. (2006a) Prefrontal electrophysiologic "noise" and catechol-O-methyltransferase genotype in schizophrenia. *Biological Psychiatry* **60**, 578–584.

Winterer, G., Musso, F., Vucurevic, G. *et al.* (2006b) COMT genotype predicts BOLD signal and noise characteristics in prefrontal circuits. *Neuroimage* **32**, 1722–1732.

Winterer, G., Musso, F., Beckmann, C. *et al.* (2006c) Instability of prefrontal signal processing in schizophrenia. *American Journal of Psychiatry* **163**, 1960–1968.

Winterer, G., Carver, F.W., Musso, F., Mattay, V., Weinberger, D.R. & Coppola, R. (2007a) Complex relationship between BOLD signal and synchronization/desynchronization of human brain MEG oscillations. *Human Brain Mapping* **28**, 805–816.

Winterer, G., Musso, F., Konrad, A. *et al.* (2007b) Association of attentional network function with exon 5 variations of the CHRNA4 gene. *Human Molecular Genetics* **16**, 2165–2174.

CHAPTER 16

Structural brain imaging in schizophrenia and related populations

Stephen M. Lawrie[1] and Christos Pantelis[2]

[1]University of Edinburgh, Edinburgh, UK
[2]The University of Melbourne & Melbourne Health, Melbourne, Australia

The idea that schizophrenia is a manifestation of disturbances in brain structure and function has received considerable support over the past 30 years from an increasing array of sophisticated and complementary neuroimaging techniques. There are now substantial structural and functional imaging literatures and several consistently replicated findings. Refinements of techniques and their application to particular populations, such as those at high risk for genetic or symptomatic reasons, are likely to help further delineate phenotypes, facilitate the application of molecular biological techniques, and provide insight into the pathophysiology of schizophrenia.

In this chapter we will consider the gains in our knowledge from the main structural neuroimaging techniques that have been and are being used to study schizophrenia. We will briefly describe the principles of the main methods used for brain imaging—computerized tomography (CT), structural magnetic resonance imaging (sMRI), magnetic resonance spectroscopy (MRS), and diffusion tensor-MRI (DT-MRI or DTI), as well as methods of image analysis, and consider the etiopathophysiological correlates of signal changes in patients and related populations.

Historical techniques

The first attempts at imaging brain structure *in vivo* were conducted using pneumoencephalography, which was introduced by the American neurosurgeon Dandy in 1919. After lumbar puncture, cerebrospinal fluid (CSF) was withdrawn and replaced with air to outline the cerebral ventricles and cortical surface on X-ray roentography. The technique was first applied to psychiatric patients by Jacobi and Winkler in 1927, who described an apparent loss of brain tissue in schizophrenia. Enlarged lateral and third ventricles, as well as widened cortical sulci, proved to be widely replicated findings despite substantial variations in methods (see Johnstone & Owens, 2004). Many early reports were, however, based on visual assessments and confounded by the fact that most assessments were not made blind to the subjects' diagnosis. In view of the considerable morbidity and small but definite mortality associated with pneumoencephalography, the American Roentgen Ray Society decreed in 1929 that it was not appropriate to use normal subjects for control purposes.

Schizophrenia, 3rd edition. Edited by Daniel R. Weinberger and Paul J Harrison © 2011 Blackwell Publishing Ltd.

This led to greater interest in comparing different psychiatric populations and changes over time—with several accounts of apparently progressive abnormalities in studies of patients with schizophrenia—but ultimately sounded the death-knell for the technique.

The method necessary to take structural brain imaging forward was provided by Hounsfield, working for Electrical and Musical Industries in London, who first demonstrated his technique of computerized axial tomography (CAT) in 1973. This was a relatively safe method of visualizing internal body structures, including soft tissues, without the need for injecting contrast media, and because it was sensitive and had minimal requirements for patient cooperation, it was ideal for intracranial imaging, especially in psychiatric patients. CAT soon came to mean computer-assisted tomography and then computerized tomography (CT). The procedure involved an X-ray source that rotated in a specified plane around the circumference of a cross-section of the head. Transmitted X-rays were detected using various methods, e.g., sodium iodide crystals and photomultiplier tubes. As the source rotated, voltages were computed for X-ray paths traversing the brain from various angles. The voltage readings were then mathematically reconstructed, from multiple projections around the object of interest, generally with a "back projection" technique, into an image that represented the distribution of densities within that tissue slice. As the procedure was non-invasive, normal controls could be compared with patients and the range of appearances in normal subjects could be related to variables such as age.

In the first CT scan study in schizophrenia, Johnstone *et al.* (1976) hand-traced the outline of the ventricles and the brain by planimetry (on to graph paper) and found the lateral ventricular area to be increased in a group of chronically institutionalized patients with schizophrenia in comparison to an age-matched group of normal controls. This finding met with a mixed and sometimes skeptical response, but was soon replicated (Weinberger *et al.*, 1979). Weinberger *et al.* also demonstrated cerebral "atrophy". The great majority of the studies conducted after these confirmed the findings of lateral ventricular enlargement and widened cortical sulci. Clinical correlates were less consistently demonstrated but greater levels of these abnormalities tended to be associated with neuropsychological impairment, negative rather than positive symptoms, poor premorbid adjustment, relatively poor outcome, and the presence of spontaneous involuntary movements (Lewis, 1991). The possibility that the findings could have been due to the effects of treatment was raised early on, but similar findings are evident in first-episode psychosis and even to some extent in the unaffected relatives of patients. The repeated lack of association between duration of illness and ventricular enlargement (Lewis, 1991) also provided additional indirect evidence against any medication-mediated progression of abnormalities. On the other hand, quantitative summaries of the literature have found correlations between the number and cumulative length of hospitalizations and the extent of ventricular enlargement (Raz & Raz, 1990) and a relationship between illness duration and lateral ventricular enlargement (van Horn & McManus, 1992). These are, however, relatively weak statistical associations that cannot clarify cause or effect. In the final analysis, the lack of longitudinal studies with adequate standardization procedures for repeat scans and the relatively poor spatial resolution of CT scanning mean that questions about possible progression of abnormalities and antipsychotic medication effects were never satisfactorily resolved with this technique. Moreover, ventricular enlargement presumably reflects tissue loss in one or more neighboring brain regions which CT could not really distinguish because of limited gray–white matter contrast. For these reasons, CT was superseded by MRI.

Structural magnetic resonance imaging

MRI was initially referred to as nuclear magnetic resonance by the research groups of Bloch and Purcell to describe the phenomenon whereby certain atoms can be made to absorb or emit radiation when placed in a magnetic field. The application of this technique to man and reconstructing the data to create an image was developed during the 1970s, with pioneering work being conducted by Mansfield in Nottingham and Lauterbur in New York. It became widely available during the 1980s.

MRI uses signals from protons—usually the hydrogen nucleus in water—which can be considered as a charge rotating about a randomly orientated axis. When an external magnetic field (B0) is applied, the axis of rotation aligns along the axis of the field (so-called precession or resonance). The resonance frequency is the product of the magnetic field strength (B0) and the "gyromagnetic ratio" of particular atoms. Different tissues, with different atomic compositions, have different resonance frequencies and these can be used to provide image contrast. The magnetic fields from the protons sum to produce a measurable signal, but because this signal is much less than B0, only the component at right angles to B0 (in the transverse plane) is measurable. Even this requires a temporary tilt (or flip) of the individual proton axes further away from B0, by a certain "flip angle", through the brief application of a radiofrequency (RF) pulse. Following the RF pulse, transverse magnetization returns to the longitudinal plane (axis of B0) over a period of time known as the T1 relaxation time (also known as the *spin-lattice* or longitudinal relaxation time). It is usually necessary to repeatedly apply RF pulses in a series, each tailored to a given position in the static field gradient, to obtain spatial information in three dimensions. The time between each pulse is called

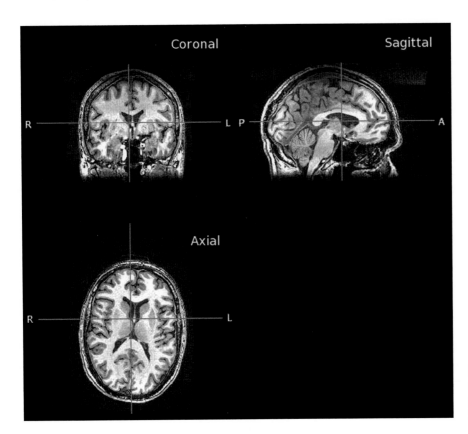

Fig. 16.1 A high-resolution T1-weighted structural MRI scan of the brain, in three planes, from a 3T scanner (courtesy of J.T.O. Cavanagh and J. McLean).

the repetition time (TR) and for any tissue with a particular T1, there is an optimal TR that produces best image contrast. Additionally, for any given TR there is an optimal flip angle, which maximizes signal strength. T1 images provide good gray–white matter contrast within the brain, and tend to be used to delineate small structures for research purposes (Fig. 16.1). Tilting or flipping the proton magnetic field results in a rotational component in the transverse plane, an "echo" which is measurable. Initially, all the proton axes are essentially rotating at the same time (in phase), but rapidly begin to rotate at different speeds (dephasing), resulting in a loss of transverse signal over a period termed the T2 relaxation time (also known as the transverse magnetization time or *spin–spin* relaxation time). Note that T2 is less than or equal to T1. The interval between the creation of transverse magnetization and its measurement is the echo time (TE). Not all tissues exhibit differences in T2 but for those that do, an optimal TE exists and provides the best image contrast. T2-weighted images are particularly useful for distinguishing brain from CSF and for imaging pathological processes in the brain, such as white matter hyperintensities and demyelination.

Structural MRI (sMRI) images are of very much higher resolution compared with CT, particularly at the high magnetic fields of 3 Tesla machines, and much more able to image the temporal lobes and other structures near bone.

Greater magnetic strength has the effect of increasing signal-to-noise ratio (SNR) and provides greater tissue contrast. These factors, together with reduced slice thickness and acquisition of the data as contiguous slices, all serve to reduce "partial volume" errors or artifacts (derived from sampling the signal in one part of brain tissue that is contaminated by signal from one or more adjacent regions). However, magnetic field strength also has the potential problem of inhomogeneous contrast across the image. Thus, field strength is usually maximal at the center or core of the magnet and decays slightly at distances further away from the center. This "field inhomogeneity" can lead to differences in tissue contrast and quality, which increase noise, but which are usually controlled for by scanning an object of homogeneous density and correcting the images for any inhomogeneity observed in that object.

Analyzing sMRI data

The image itself is created from the measurement of energy "released" from tissue by several radiofrequency detectors located in a coil placed around the head of the subject. Images are created using Fourier analysis of this information to make a "back projection" of the properties of the tissue which gave rise to the signal in the first place. The decay constants T1 and T2, as well as the overall proton density (PD), at each unit of brain volume (voxel) can be presented as a gray-scale image with the highest signals represented as white voxels and low signals as black.

Until about 10 years ago, studies almost exclusively used semi-automated methods to extract the brain from the surrounding tissues, followed by manual tracing around regions of interest (ROI) with the aid of a tissue contrast facility, and this remains the "gold standard" approach to analysis. Tracings are usually made by one or more experienced operators, blind to subject details, with the aid of an anatomical atlas and using detailed operationalized criteria for identifying anatomical landmarks and delineating brain structures. Volumes are then calculated by multiplying each regional area by the slice thickness, and summing all slice volumes over the brain region in question. This technique is, however, laborious, somewhat subjective, and it is essential to first establish adequate interrater and/or intrarater reliability. Large structures (e.g., whole brain, temporal and prefrontal lobes) tend to have high measurement reliability, whereas smaller structures (e.g., hippocampus, amygdala, caudate) are generally subject to greater measurement error. In an attempt to measure smaller volumes more reliably, parcelation techniques have been developed. These generally involve tracing in three dimensions simultaneously, but this technique is also very time-consuming and subjective judgments continue to be necessary.

Alternative automated approaches to sMRI analysis have been developed and can be collectively termed "computational morphometry". Probably the most commonly used technique is voxel based morphometry (VBM) as implemented in the Statistical Parametric Mapping (SPM) software developed by Friston and colleagues (Ashburner & Friston, 2000). All of these techniques involve the transformation of each brain into a common three-dimensional space ("spatial normalization"). The normalized images can then be partitioned or "segmented" into gray and white matter and CSF using automated (e.g., Bayesian) methods for separate analyses of each compartment. The next stage is usually spatial smoothing (blurring) of the image. This reduces the spatial resolution of the image but maximizes the probability of signal detection, and ensures the validity of subsequent statistical methods. Differences in, for example, gray matter density, are then computed by comparing the normalized, segmented, and smoothed brains from each group on a voxel by voxel basis. It is worth noting that VBM detects changes in the surfaces or boundaries between different parts of the brain (e.g., gray–white matter interfaces) and therefore, systematic shape differences between populations and/or differential "brain averaging" at the spatial normalization stage can produce artifacts and false-positive results. Another concern is that there are typically tens of thousands of voxels in such analyses, so correction for multiple testing is required, usually

Table 16.1 Comparison of region of interest (ROI) and voxel-based morphometry (VBM) approaches to the analysis of structural magnetic resonance imaging data.

	ROI	VBM
Region selection	A prerequisite, and the region must have definable boundaries	Not required, but can be included
Technique	Hand-drawn	Automatic
Variability in application	Can vary within and between raters	Can vary within software (according to preprocessing steps and thresholding) and between different software programs
Imaging plane	One or more	Any
Labor	Intensive	Relatively quick
Reliability	Reliable for large regions; less so for small regions	Highly reliable, but less suited to analyses at the whole brain level
Validity	Gold standard but basis of signal change unclear	Validity questioned but some concurrent validity with ROI established
Effective spatial resolution	Limited by human eye	Limited by technical factors
Major limitations	Subjective and time-consuming	Brain averaging is problematic and can cause artifacts

with reference to false discovery or family-wise error rates—as a straightforward Bonferoni correction is too conservative because adjacent voxels are not independent after image blurring. Overall, VBM is a relatively conservative technique, avoids subjective judgments about where a region of interest begins and ends, and can be used to investigate very small structures, but the results obtained reflect the statistical probability of differences in tissue density or volume and cannot be interpreted with the same ease as a mean difference in volume. Fortunately, studies and reviews of both ROI analysis and VBM suggest that the results obtained are generally similar (see McIntosh & Lawrie, 2004), and the two bodies of evidence provide a complementary picture of the abnormalities in patients.

The limitations of both ROI and VBM approaches (see Table 16.1) has meant that more sophisticated approaches to brain mapping have become of increasing interest to the neuroimaging community. High dimensional non-linear transformations of computerized brain templates can precisely locate morphological changes and accommodate individual variation at both specific and more general scales. To give some successful examples, hippocampal surface modeling (Csernansky et al., 1998), deformation-based morphometry (Gaser et al., 1999), and cortical thickness mapping (Kuperberg et al., 2003; Fornito et al., 2008) have all provided detailed assessments of consistently replicated schizophrenia-related changes, and sometimes show clinical correlations (see below). Other methods seek to make more use of the richness of sMRI data in other ways. Techniques that have been developed for pattern classification and data mining in other domains (e.g., handwriting recognition) have been productively applied to quantify the degree of separation between patients and controls, and may prove to be an aid to early diagnostic procedures (Koutsouleris et al., 2009). Automated parcelation strategies to isolate subregional volumes may ultimately remove the need for brain averaging and facilitate individual *versus* group analyses of value to the clinician. Similar approaches have been able to extract measures of sulcal depth and/or cortical folding and demonstrate increased folding in the right prefrontal cortex (PFC) in genetic high-risk samples but reduced cortical complexity in the left hemisphere in established cases (e.g., Harris et al., 2007). In contrast, studies of cortical folding in the region of the anterior cingulate cortex (ACC) have identified (para)cingulate sulcus discontinuity and a loss of normal laterality in established schizophrenia (Yücel et al., 2002), while in a clinical high-risk group such abnormality was present but did not discriminate those developing psychosis from non-converters (Yücel et al., 2003). Importantly, such differences in folding patterns need to be taken into account when comparing groups volumetrically, as differences in density, volume or thickness may relate to such sulcal/gyral variations or abnormalities (Fornito et al., 2006). There is also an intriguing account of qualitative abnormalities of the orbito-frontal cortex (Nakamura et al., 2007) that awaits external replication.

All of these computationally intensive techniques should, however, not blind us to the possibility that there are gross abnormalities of the brain in schizophrenia, or perhaps in subgroups according to particular risk or clinical strata, which the unaided human eye can both detect and "automatically" adjust for variability in human neuroanatomy.

Findings in patients with schizophrenia

The first controlled MRI study in schizophrenia was published in 1984, but it was several years before researchers took full advantage of the technique to measure regional and subregional brain volumes. There are now well over 100 controlled MRI studies of various regional volumes in schizophrenia and numerous narrative and quantitative reviews of them. As a general rule, reduced volume of the PFC and temporal lobe by approximately 5%, and by 5–10% in some of their constituent parts, are the best rep-

licated findings (Lawrie & Abukmeil, 1998; Wright et al., 2000). The lateral and third ventricles are approximately 20–30% larger in patients with schizophrenia compared to controls and this difference is greater still for the body of the lateral ventricles, which are approximately 50% larger. These are all disproportionate to reductions of approximately 3% in the whole brain, but it is worth noting that many individual studies do not find statistically significant differences, probably due to low power as a result of relatively small numbers of patients and measurement variability (Lawrie & Abukmeil, 1998; Shenton et al., 2001). Importantly, CT, sMRI, and postmortem studies generally agree about these large-scale abnormalities (Harrison, 1999; Harrison et al., 2003; see Chapter 18).

Both ROI and VBM studies suggest that whole brain gray matter volumes are preferentially reduced, by approximately 3–4%, compared to white matter on sMRI. There is also good agreement between these techniques that parts of the anterior cingulate, superior temporal gyri, and the medial temporal lobe complex, including amygdala, hippocampus, and parahippocampus are all substantially reduced (Gaser et al., 1999; Job et al., 2002; Fornito et al., 2009b). A smaller number of parcelation studies suggest particular deficits in the fusiform gyrus as well as orbital and dorso-lateral PFC (DLPFC) (e.g., Goldstein et al., 1999; Zhou et al., 2005). There is also impressive agreement between sMRI (especially ROI) and postmortem studies that the thalamus, and the medio-dorsal and pulvinar nuclei in particular, are smaller in schizophrenia than one would expect from global tissue reductions (Harrison, 1999; Konick & Friedman, 2001). There are also intriguing, albeit inconsistent, findings of more frequently absent adhesio interthalamica (or massa intermedia) in people with schizophrenia, with recent evidence of such abnormality in a clinical high-risk group (Takahashi et al., 2008). This midline structure is formed in the first trimester and similar qualitative abnormalities, such as the increased prevalence of a cavum septum pellucidum between the lateral ventricles and the disturbances in PFC and ACC morphology described above, also suggest early disruption of brain development (Shenton et al., 2001). The basal ganglia, on the other hand, are increased in volume (e.g., see recent VBM meta-analysis, Glahn et al., 2008) and this appears to be the only structural abnormality in schizophrenia that can be confidently attributed to antipsychotic medication, given that the volume correlates with (first-generation) antipsychotic dose and tends to regress on second-generation treatment (Chakos et al., 1995). The increases are maximal, approaching 20%, in the globus pallidus (Wright et al., 2000).

It remains unclear whether other regions such as the parietal lobes and cerebellum, which are likely to be involved in schizophrenia, are structurally abnormal (e.g., Tanskanen et al., 2008). Gender may have a moderating

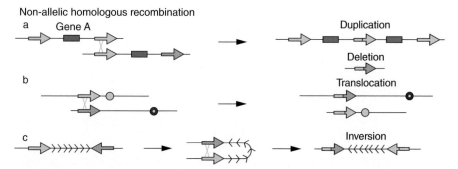

Plate 12.1 Repeat-mediated mechanisms of non-allelic homologous recombination (NAHR) and their results. (a) NAHR between adjacent repeat sequences produces duplications and deletions, depending on the specific pairing involved in the NAHR. (b) NAHR between repeats on non-homologous chromosomes can produce translocations. In both cases, the copies created are in the same orientation as the original repeats. (c) By contrast, inversions can occur as a consequence of recombination between inverted intrachromosomal repeat sequences.

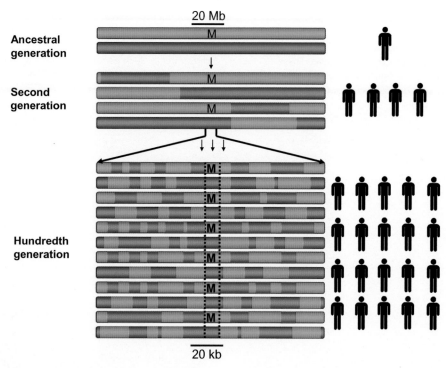

Plate 13.1 Effect of recombination on association. A population founder is depicted who carries two ancestral haplotypes which differ in sequence at a number of positions. A new mutation (M) has arisen on the red haplotype; all red alleles are now associated or in linkage disequilibrium (LD) with that mutation. The size of the haplotype in LD with the mutation is reduced in the next generation as a result of recombination between blue and red haplotypes. This process continues through successive generations until typically, only markers that are close to the mutation, usually 20 kb or less, remain strongly associated with the mutation. Recombination hotspots are indicated by dotted lines between which no recombination events have occurred during population expansion. In this example, the allele at one locus predicts the status of all other alleles within that block. Mb (million bases) and kb (thousand bases) scale lines are given.

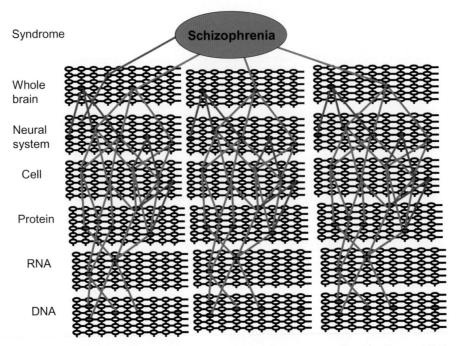

Syndrome

Whole
brain

Neural
system

Cell

Protein

RNA

DNA

Plate 14.1 Intermediate phenotypes are biological traits more closely related to the effects of genes that increase risk for illness in complex genetic disorders such as schizophrenia. These measures can increase the power for finding disease genes because of their simpler genetic architecture and because often their underlying molecular biology is more certain, providing a stronger basis for selecting candidate genes. The causative path from genetic variant through effects on RNA, protein, cell, neural system, to whole brain is shown in red for genes affecting risk for schizophrenia. Such genes may also cause other changes at various levels that are not related to the pathophysiology of schizophrenia (e.g., green paths). It is also possible that schizophrenia itself could produce changes (in blue) at various levels that are not related to disease pathophysiology.

Plate 15.2 Cortical response variability ("noise") is increased in patients with schizophrenia. Left, Frequency domain analyses showing increased prefrontal noise, that is, increased variability of slow-wave oscillations, in patients with schizophrenia and their clinically unaffected siblings (Winterer et al., 2004). Increased variability of slow-wave oscillations results from impaired phase-locking of these oscillations in schizophrenia (Winterer et al., 2000). Right, An analogous increase in variability of blood-oxygen-level-dependent (BOLD) response is observed in patients with schizophrenia (Winterer et al., 2006c). Prefrontal noise is modulated by synaptic dopamine modulation [catechol-O-methyltransferase (COMT) genotype] as measured by electrophysiology and functional magnetic resonance imaging (Winterer & Weinberger, 2004; Winterer et al., 2006a,b; reproduced with permission from Nature Reviews Drug Discovery.)

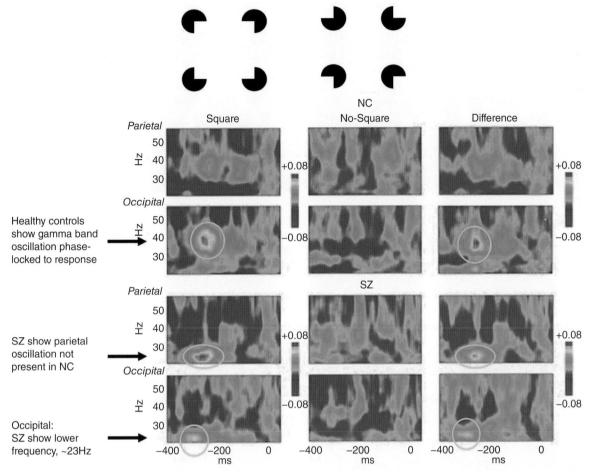

NC

| Parietal | Square | No-Square | Difference |

Healthy controls show gamma band oscillation phase-locked to response →

Occipital

SZ

SZ show parietal oscillation not present in NC →

Occipital: SZ show lower frequency, ~23Hz →

Plate 15.1 Response-locked gamma band oscillation. Subject responses indicate the presence of an illusory square (pac man-like figures oriented as shown) or its absence (different orientation of pac man-like figures). Prior to the onset of a response (Time 0) to the presence or absence of illusory squares, healthy controls (NC) show occipital gamma band activity (~40 Hz, circle) phase-locked to the response to perception of a square ("square" column label) but not to the response when an illusory square is not present. Right panel, Square minus no-square responses. In contrast,

patients with schizophrenia (SZ) show only a lower frequency band response (~23 Hz, circle) and an abnormal parietal oscillation. Both the lower frequency of the response-locked oscillation and the abnormal parietal oscillation suggest difficulties in efficiently integrating information in schizophrenia. The presence of a response-locked oscillation may represent a re-activation of the percept to guide a response. [Adapted from Spencer *et al.* (2004).]

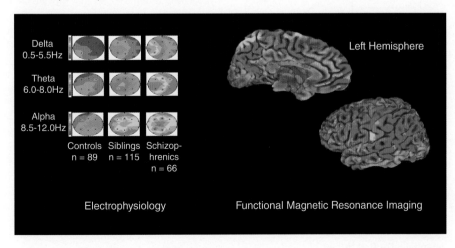

Plate 15.2

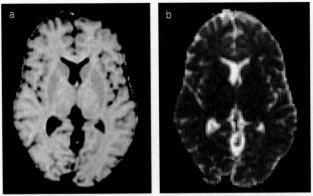

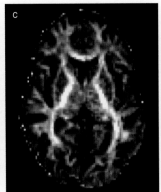

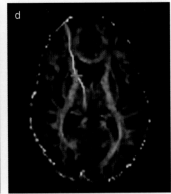

Plate 16.1 Axial parametric maps of: (a) magnetization transfer ratio, (b) mean diffusivity, (c) fractional anisotropy, and (d) tractography of the right anterior limb of the internal capsule (ALIC). The three-dimensional representations of the ALIC were generated using a modified version of the BEDPOSTX/ProbTrack algorithm, by automatically placing tractography seed points within a voxel neighborhood centered on a seed point. The seed point was transferred from the center of the ALIC in standard space to the corresponding location in native space, and the software chooses the tract which best represents a previously chosen ALIC reference tract, allowing the ALIC to be reliably segmented from subject to subject. Values of fractional anisotropy (FA) averaged over the segmented ALIC can then be calculated for each subject (courtesy of Drs Mark Bastin and Jon Clayden).

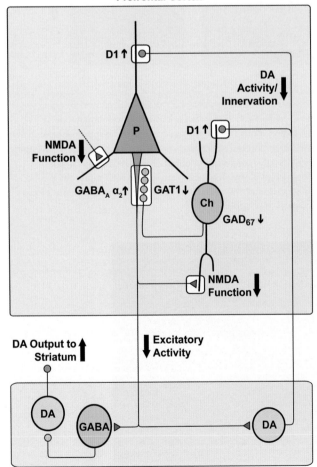

Prefrontal Cortex

Mesencephalic DA Cell Nuclei

Plate 18.1 Circuitry diagram illustrating some of the putative alterations in glutamate, GABA, and dopamine (DA) signaling in the dorso-lateral prefrontal cortex (DLPFC) in schizophrenia, and one schema by which they may be interrelated. A decrease in glutamatergic excitatory input onto mesencephalic DA cells could result from pyramidal cell (P) hypoactivity, perhaps secondary to NMDA receptor hypofunction or a reduction in the number of pyramidal neuron dendritic spines (see Plate 18.2, also Plate 21.3). This reduced excitatory input might produce sustained hypoactivity of the DA cells that provide DA input to the DLPFC, leading to morphological and biochemical changes in the DA cells. For instance, in schizophrenia, reductions have been reported in the size of DA neuron cell bodies and the amount of tyrosine hydroxylase (TH) in the DA mesencephalic nuclei; these changes are accompanied by evidence for a decreased DA innervation of the DLPFC in terms of TH and dopamine transporter (DAT) immunoreactive DA axons. The decrease in DA innervation and putatively lower DA levels in the DLPFC might lead to compensatory, but functionally insufficient, up-regulation of D_1 receptors in pyramidal cells or GABA neurons or both. Because D_1 receptor activation increases the activity of parvalbumin (PV)-positive, fast-spiking GABA neurons, reduced D_1-mediated signaling may reduce the activity of these neurons and lead to activity-dependent down-regulation of the expression of glutamic acid decarboxylase 67 (GAD_{67}) and PV. Ch, chandelier cells; GAT, GABA transporter (adapted from Lewis & Gonzalez-Burgos, 2008).

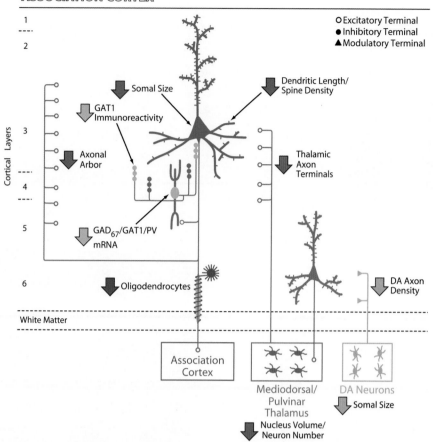

○ Excitatory Terminal
● Inhibitory Terminal
▲ Modulatory Terminal

Cortical Layers

1

2

3

4

5

6

Somal Size

GAT1 Immunoreactivity

Axonal Arbor

GAD$_{67}$/GAT1/PV mRNA

Oligodendrocytes

White Matter

Dendritic Length/ Spine Density

Thalamic Axon Terminals

DA Axon Density

Association Cortex

Mediodorsal/ Pulvinar Thalamus

DA Neurons

Somal Size

Nucleus Volume/ Neuron Number

Plate 18.2 Schematic diagram summarizing schizophrenia-associated disturbances in the canonical circuitry of the association neocortex. Many of these alterations have been reported in the dorso-lateral prefrontal cortex, but are unlikely to be restricted to this cortical region. Not all of these observations have been sufficiently replicated, or demonstrated to be specific to the disease process of schizophrenia, to be considered established "facts." Thus, this summary should be viewed as a working model of the cortical neuropathology of schizophrenia. See text for additional details and references, and see also Plate 21.2 for a more detailed view of inhibitory circuitry alterations. GAD, glutamic acid decarboxylase; GAT, GABA transporter (adapted from Lewis & Lieberman, 2000).

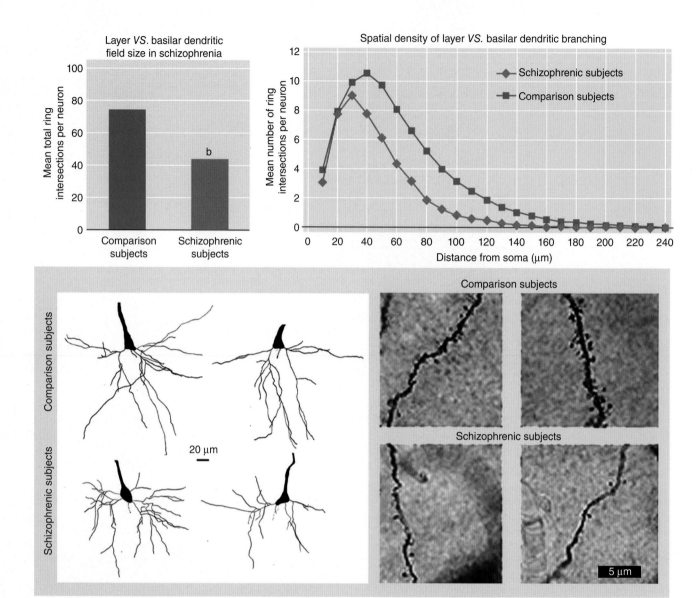

Plate 21.1 Characterization of the reduction in size of the basilar dendritic fields of pyramidal neurons in layer 5 of area 10 of the prefrontal cortex. Schizophrenia is associated with the size of the dendritic field, as suggested by the reduced numbers of ring interactions (upper left) and reduced dendritic branching, as suggested by the number of ring intersections per neuron (upper right). The reduction in dendritic branching is supported by a camera lucida drawing of neurons from Golgi-stained sections (lower left), and a high power field photograph showing reduced dendritic spines (lower right) (reproduced from Black *et al.*, 2004, with permission).

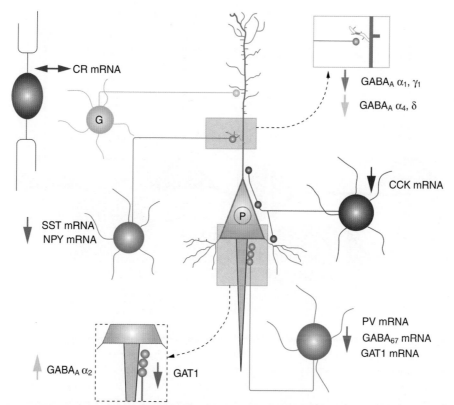

Plate 21.2 Schematic summary of alterations in GABA-mediated circuitry in the dorso-lateral prefrontal cortex (DLPFC) of subjects with schizophrenia. Altered GABA neurotransmission by parvalbumin (PV)-containing neurons (green) is indicated by gene expression deficits in these neurons and associated changes in their synapses, a decrease in GAT1 expression in their terminals, and an up-regulation of the GABA$_A$ receptor α2-subunit at the axon initial segments of pyramidal neurons (lower enlarged square). Decreased gene expression for both somatostatin (SST) and neuropeptide Y (NPY) indicates alterations in SST and/or NPY-containing neurons (blue) that target the distal dendrites of pyramidal neurons. Decreased cholecystokinin (CCK) mRNA levels indicate an alteration of CCK-containing large basket neurons (purple) that represent a separate source of perisomatic inhibition from PV-containing neurons. Gene expression in CR-containing GABA neurons (red) does not seem to be altered. Other neurons, such as PV-containing basket neurons, are not shown because the nature of their involvement in schizophrenia is unclear. G, generic GABA neuron; P, pyramidal neuron (reproducded from Lewis & Gonzalez-Burgos, 2008, with permission).

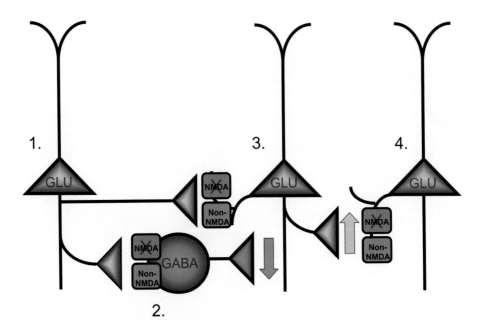

Plate 21.3 Depiction of the impact of NMDA receptor antagonist administration on the function of cortical networks. When neuron 1 is activated, glutamate (GLU) that is released by this neuron activates a GABA neurons (neuron 2) via both NMDA and non-NMDA glutamate receptors. Subanesthetic doses of NMDA receptor antagonists preferentially block receptors on GABA neurons, illustrated by the "X" in the NMDA receptor box on neuron 2. As a result, there is less GABA is released by neuron 2, resulting in disinhibition of glutamatergic neuron 3. Glutamate released by neuron 3 binds to postsynaptic receptors with an imbalance of NMDA (some blocked by the NMDA receptor antagonist) and non-NMDA glutamate receptors. The collective implications of the changes in network activity are: (1) NMDA receptor antagonists increase cortical network activation, (2) the impairment in NMDA receptors and the reduction in GABA release reflect disruption of two critical mechanisms for coordinating network activity, consistent with the emergence of chaotic network activity and disruption of network oscillations (modified from Krystal *et al.*, 2003c; Lewis & Moghaddam, 2006, with permission).

influence on the neuroanatomy of schizophrenia, although the reviews already cited make it clear that this is far from confirmed. As there is now a well-established series of neuroanatomical correlates of schizophrenia, recent sMRI studies in schizophrenia are focused on subregional examinations, whether abnormalities are progressive, and what genetic and environmental factors may underlie these effects. These are increasingly conducted with automated parcelation schedules and at high magnetic fields. Arguably the greatest insights could accrue from studies which are able to compare gray and white matter disturbances in key subregions by acquiring high quality images along their long axes, such as para-axially through the hippocampal subfields.

Time course and drug effects

As with CT, sMRI studies have found similar abnormalities in first-episode cases as in chronic patients (Steen *et al.*, 2006; Vita *et al.*, 2006; Ellison-Wright *et al.*, 2008). These are usually interpreted as evidence of developmental effects and do not favor the view of progressive changes. On the other hand, the fact that at least some of the deficits at psychosis presentation are of greater magnitude than those found in unaffected relatives at risk of the disorder (Boos *et al.*, 2007), suggests some possible longitudinal change as schizophrenia develops and after onset (Lawrie *et al.*, 2008). Further, there is evidence from the clinical high-risk groups suggesting progression (e.g., Velakoulis *et al.*, 2006; Takahashi *et al.*, 2009; for discussion: Pantelis *et al.*, 2005; Wood *et al.*, 2008a,b, 2009).

The whole brain volume literature in relatives with sMRI is equivocal, but most studies suggest that the lateral ventricles are larger in patients than relatives and that they in turn probably have larger lateral ventricles as compared to controls (Lawrie *et al.*, 2008). Third ventricle increases and/or thalamus reductions in relatives may be almost as marked as the abnormalities in patients. Early ROI studies tended to examine the amygdala and hippocampus together, and consistently found reductions in relatives compared to controls, but most relatives did not have volume reductions to pathological levels (Lawrie *et al.*, 2001). The most consistent evidence is for hippocampal reductions in relatives, with an effect size of about 0.3, and additional differences between relatives and patients (Boos *et al.*, 2007). There are also replicated computational morphometry studies demonstrating PFC density reductions in the relatives of patients with schizophrenia (Cannon *et al.*, 2002).

Hippocampal findings at baseline do not consistently predict psychosis in relatives at high genetic risk or in prodromal patients with an "at-risk mental state" (e.g., Velakoulis *et al.*, 2006). In contrast, PFC volumes, ACC thickness, as well as morphology and gyral folding, all look

to have stronger and more consistent predictive effects (Yücel *et al.*, 2002; Pantelis *et al.*, 2003; Harris *et al.*, 2007; Fornito *et al.*, 2008). The two main studies to have addressed these issues to date are the Edinburgh High Risk Study (EHRS) and the study conducted in the Personal Assessment and Crisis Evaluation (PACE) clinic in Melbourne, Australia. These pioneering studies have examined large populations of people at risk, for genetic or clinical reasons, over almost 10 years. Pantelis *et al.* (2003) demonstrated longitudinal reductions in gray matter density in the left parahippocampal and fusiform gyri, as well as in the left PFC and left cerebellar cortex, over approximately a year in 11 people as they developed a diagnosis of psychosis, usually schizophrenia. Job *et al.* (2005) revealed reductions in gray matter density in the left (para) hippocampal uncus, fusiform gyrus, and right cerebellar cortex in eight individuals at genetic high risk who developed schizophrenia on average 2.5 years after the first of two scans, obtained approximately 18 months apart. More recently, surface retraction involving thinning of gray matter over the PFC was reported in the clinical high-risk (PACE) cohort and over the first 2–4 years following psychosis onset (Sun *et al.* 2009a,b). These and other studies suggest there are reductions in PFC and/or temporal lobe structure around the time of transition to a diagnosis of psychosis, offering opportunities for early detection and intervention (Koutsouleris *et al.*, 2009). The next generation of high-risk studies needs to use more sophisticated methods, such as tensor-based morphometry to detect change, and be large enough to compare subgroups according to putative pathological processes underpinning these changes. The EHRS has already shown medication is not responsible, as none of the participants was medicated until after their second scan and the diagnosis had been established.

Changes in brain structure during the transition to psychosis could at least in theory continue and generate progressive abnormality after onset. This has been quite extensively studied over the past 10 years or so and the balance of the available evidence is clearly in favor of progressive loss of brain tissue and ventricular expansion beyond the first episode of schizophrenia, and that this can be related to symptom severity, neurocognitive impairment, and poor outcome (Lieberman *et al.*, 2001; Thompson *et al.*, 2001; Cahn *et al.*, 2002; Pantelis *et al.*, 2005; Salisbury *et al.*, 2007; Wood *et al.*, 2008b; Sun *et al.*, 2009a,b). The same process(es) appear to continue for 10–20 years in established cases, with the greatest changes apparently being in PFC and temporal lobe gray matter (Hulshoff Pol & Kahn, 2008). There are however inconsistencies in the literature about the principal location of the changes and which clinical features of the illness they relate to, as well as issues about the extent of the changes and their interpretation (Weinberger & McClure, 2002). Typical annual changes reported around onset are about 2–3% in patients and

0.5–1% in controls, and 0.5% per year in chronic cases compared to 0.2% in similarly aged healthy controls. Apart from the first figure, which clearly could not continue for long given overall reductions in gray matter of about 2–3% at postmortem, these are around the likely measurement error in the techniques used. The challenge for researchers is to quantify and reduce this measurement error so as to be able to detect and distinguish between potential explanations, such as the effects of risk genes (Ho *et al.*, 2007), alcohol excess (Mathalon *et al.*, 2003), cannabis use (Rais *et al.*, 2008; Yücel *et al.*, 2008), and various aspects of the impoverished lifestyle that is so frequent in schizophrenia.

Alcohol certainly has neuroanatomical effects, even when drinking does not reach the level of psychological or physical dependence, but the effects on the brain are usually generalized, or show a PFC rather than temporal lobe bias. Further, the abnormalities in schizophrenia noted above are present in patients with no history of alcohol abuse and the best available evidence is that comorbid alcohol problems exaggerate patient–control differences rather than account for them (Mathalon *et al.*, 2003). Nicotine use is even more common in schizophrenia and can certainly impact on gray matter density, but is unlikely to be a major confounder; whereas the better recognized and greater impact of illicit "hard drugs" such as cocaine and ecstasy are unlikely confounders as they are infrequently used by patients. An alternative possible explanation for apparently progressive neuroanatomical changes is that antipsychotic medication is responsible. It is certainly true that first-generation antipsychotic medication status and indeed dose is associated with enlargement of parts of the basal ganglia and increases in the volume of the globus pallidus in particular (Chakos *et al.*, 1994; Wright *et al.*, 2000). It is also true that "typical antipsychotics" have been associated with cortical gray matter decreases, apparently even after only a few weeks' treatment (Lieberman *et al.*, 2005), but repeated demonstrations of effects in particular regions are few and far between. Most of the studies have been observational comparisons that seemingly seek to establish that the second-generation ("atypical") antipsychotics have beneficial or at least less harmful effects. Indeed, Hulshoff Pol and Kahn (2008) recently concluded that, "higher daily cumulative dose of antipsychotic medication intake is either not associated with brain volume changes or with less prominent brain volume changes". Even though intriguing animal studies using chronic antipsychotic administration have shown reductions in brain volumes and glial cell numbers (see Chapter 18), these could represent species effects as seems to apply with alcohol and ecstasy neurotoxicity (Harrison, 1999). Further, the fact that similar patterns of neuroanatomical disturbance are found in many neuropsychiatric disorders with vastly different epidemiological associations and treatments argues against these effects being prominent in patients with schizophrenia.

Clinical correlations

Even though there is what could be called a neuroanatomy of schizophrenia, it is non-specific. Though more work is needed, the abnormalities in bipolar disorder show qualitative similarities but of lesser magnitude (though see Fornito *et al.*, 2009a). If there are differences, these may prove to be relatively greater in "emotional" parts of the PFC, such as the subgenual anterior cingulate and orbito-frontal cortex, with lesser effects in "cognitive" DLPFC, while the amygdalae may even be enlarged (e.g. Velakoulis *et al.*, 2006; Fornito *et al.*, 2009a). Volume reductions in the medial temporal lobe are also reported in depression and anxiety states, such as post-traumatic stress disorder (PTSD), and it is speculated, on the basis of animal studies, that these decreases may be related to hypercortisolemia. Alzheimer disease begins in the hippocampus, where volumes fall by about 5% each year, with a 10-fold increase in the age-related rate of ventricular dilation (at approximately 15% per year) as progressive atrophy affects the temporo-parietal cortex and then the PFC. There are also fairly consistent findings from neuroimaging studies in the different dementias, of reasonably strong correlations between generalized neuronal pathology and clinical characteristics such as cognitive impairment, and between temporal lobe pathology and psychotic features. These commonalities in regional anatomy disruptions could mean that they are manifestations of final common pathways across a variety of neuropsychiatric disorders rather than specific processes.

The search for associations between particular symptoms and regional brain volumes in patients with schizophrenia has only been partly successful. Studies focusing on hallucinations or delusions have shown a tendency to implicate the temporal lobes, particularly on the left side (Barta *et al.*, 1990; Shapleske *et al.*, 1999). Auditory hallucinations have been repeatedly linked to the superior temporal gyrus (STG), and especially the left anterior STG, while reductions in left posterior STG gray matter have been found in association with thought disorder (Shenton *et al.*, 1992). Negative symptoms, on the other hand, tend to show an association with smaller PFC volumes (Gur *et al.*, 2000). There are, however, many negative findings for each of these ROI associations, and VBM studies are similarly inconsistent. The sMRI associations of neuropsychological deficits in schizophrenia are less consistent than those found with CT. Various explanations are possible. The studies tend to be small and lack anatomical detail. Symptom severity is difficult to measure reliably and can fluctuate over hours and even minutes, whereas neuronal number and density is relatively static over those time frames. The clinical manifestations of psychosis may be more attributable to tendencies for disruptions in distributed networks over time periods rather than isolated lesions at particular time points, while cognitive deficits may reflect more generalized processes.

Etiological associations and pathophysiological basis

Structural abnormality could therefore be more closely related to etiological risk factors for schizophrenia and pathophysiological factors than the clinical features of the current episode, and there is a fair amount of supportive evidence that this is the case. Twin (Cannon *et al.*, 2002) and other relative studies (Lawrie *et al.*, 2001) demonstrate that there are genetic contributions to PFC volumes in schizophrenia (see Chapter 14). The Val allele at a particular locus of the catechol-O-methyl-transferase (*COMT*) gene has been repeatedly linked to PFC volumes, perhaps reflecting its impact on PFC function throughout development (McIntosh *et al.*, 2007). Variation in the brain-derived neurotrophic factor (*BDNF*) gene is another plausible candidate for other effects on sMRI, given that it is a neurotrophin and widely expressed in the temporal lobes, and a number of studies have been published relating *BDNF* Met allele status to reduced size of the temporal lobe and apparently progressive changes in established patients (Ho *et al.*, 2007).

Hippocampal and ventricular volumes appear to be attributable to an interaction between genetic risk and environmental factors, such as obstetric complications (OCs). CT studies show associations between OCs and ventriculomegaly in patients and sibs (Lawrie *et al.*, 2008), with a range of adverse neurodevelopmental outcomes. McNeil *et al.* (2000) examined an extended sample of discordant twin pairs from the original study by Suddath *et al.* (1990) and found that those with schizophrenia and large (right and total) ventricles were more likely to have had labor and neonatal problems, and that intra-pair differences in volumes of rostral hippocampi between discordant monozygotic (MZ) twins were related to prolonged labor. Using original hospital records, and focusing on hypoxic events and "blue babies", van Erp *et al.* (2002) found that 72 Finnish patients had smaller hippocampi than 58 siblings, who in turn had smaller volumes than healthy controls, but only patients with documented OCs had smaller hippocampi. The fact that OC frequency was equal across groups in most of these studies argues against gene–environment covariation, and the results as a whole suggest gene–environment interaction—a sensitivity to the effects of OCs in those with genetic risk factors for schizophrenia as they render the brain more sensitive to the effects of hypoxia. Polymorphisms in the *BDNF* gene are plausible candidates for this effect, but no such interaction study has yet been reported.

Stress and specifically hypercortisolemia-mediated dendritic shrinkage has been repeatedly demonstrated in several different animals and is in keeping with the known neuropathological changes in schizophrenia of preserved neuronal numbers but reduced neuropils (Harrison, 1999). There are, however, no direct demonstrations that stress can be related to the characteristic sMRI findings in schizophrenia. Interestingly, studies of pituitary size (a measure of hypothalamic-pituitary-adrenal axis function) have identified increased size of the pituitary immediately before and following psychosis onset independent of medication (Garner *et al.*, 2005; Pariante *et al.*, 2005). Although a number of studies in anxiety and depression suggest that predisposing and precipitating stressors are associated with reduced volumes of the hippocampus, it is difficult to imagine that sufficient numbers of dendrites could be reduced to the point where regional volumes are reduced to the extent observed in patients. They could however, perhaps account for a proportion of state- or disease-associated abnormalities over and above developmental or trait effects.

Summary of sMRI findings

It is beyond doubt that there are gross neuroanatomical changes in patients with schizophrenia, but these are probably non-specific, weakly related to the cardinal manifestations of the disorder, and of largely unknown cause. Even so, there are tantalizing glimpses of the clinical potential of sMRI in picking up progressive changes before and after onset. The principal challenge now is to identify this phenotype more precisely, and relate it to the pathophysiology of the disorder.

Magnetic resonance spectroscopy

Spectroscopy measures the relative concentrations of certain chemicals in an object of interest. *In vivo* magnetic resonance spectroscopy (MRS) of the brain exploits the magnetic field induced by spinning nuclei such as hydrogen (^{1}H) and phosphorus (^{31}P). In essence, it is possible to identify different chemical molecules as different peaks in a spectrum, in which each peak corresponds to one or more molecules and the area under the peak is proportional to the concentration of the molecule.

Basic principles and methodology

Applying RF waves, or "excitation pulses", at a specific frequency (the frequency of precession of the particular nucleus one wants to image, also called the Larmor frequency) modifies the alignment of spinning nuclei as they absorb energy from the radio waves and then release it. This energy can be measured and the signal can then be

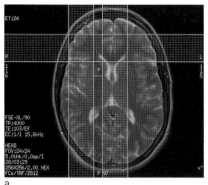
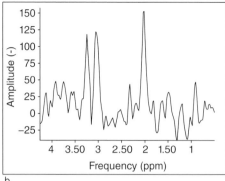

a

b

Fig. 16.2 Magnetic resonance spectroscopy scan from a test subject. (a) Position of volume of interest marked by a cross on a T2-weighted sMRI localizer, and (b) resulting spectrum, with prominent peaks of (from left to right) choline, creatine and N-acetyl-aspartate (NAA) (courtesy of Dr Katherine Lymer and Professor Ian Marshall).

mathematically transformed into different frequencies—the Fourier transform—which yield estimates of power for each frequency measured. At each image element, the power in a certain frequency band reflects the concentration of the compound that emits that particular frequency. Several chemical moieties can usually be distinguished by having peaks of different amplitudes. The amplitude of the spectra is modulated by relaxation and chemical exchange. The position of the peaks in the spectrum (measured in parts per million, or ppm, relative to a reference frequency, usually that of tetramethylsilane for proton spectra) is caused by the phenomenon of "chemical shift"—electron clouds produce their own small magnetic field that "shields" the nucleus, causing it to resonate at a slightly lower frequency. Figure 16.2 shows a typical sampling procedure and the resultant spectrum.

For molecules to be "visible" with MRS, they have to be naturally abundant and the molecule must be in solution, i.e., mobile. Phosphorus (^{31}P) spectroscopy quantifies the resonances of phosphomonoesters (PMEs), phosphodiesters (PDEs), inorganic orthophosphate (Pi), phosphocreatine (PCr), and the nucleoside adenosine triphosphate (ATP), producing a total of seven peaks in a typical spectrum, of which three correspond to ATP. It therefore provides a means of directly assessing membrane phospholipids and high-energy metabolism (Malhi *et al.*, 2002). The principal metabolites of interest for proton (^{1}H) MRS studies of schizophrenia are: water at 4.7 ppm, which is by far the strongest signal in tissue; N-acetyl-aspartate (NAA) at 2 ppm; creatine-containing compounds (Cre) at 3 ppm, and choline-containing compounds (Cho) at 3.2 and 3.9 ppm (Marenco *et al.*, 2004). Table 16.2 lists some of the chemicals imaged in MRS and their biological significance.

Biological role of measured compounds

The PME resonance reflects the concentrations of membrane phospholipid precursors (e.g. phosphorylcholine), while the PDE resonance reflects the concentrations of the

Table 16.2 Chemical elements commonly detected in phosphorus (^{31}P) and proton (^{1}H) magnetic resonance spectroscopy and their biological significance.

Type	Chemical	Significance
^{31}P	Phosphomonoester (PME)	Membrane phospholipid precursors
	Phosphodiester (PDE)	Membrane phospholipid breakdown products
	Inorganic phosphate (Pi)	Reflects intracellular pH
	Adenosine triphosphate (ATP)	High-energy reservoir for carbohydrate, protein and lipid metabolism
	Phosphocreatine (PCR)	Buffers ATP levels, shuttles cellular energy
^{1}H	N-acetyl-aspartate (NAA)	Detected mainly in pyramidal glutamatergic neurons
	Choline (Cho)	Increases indicate excessive membrane breakdown
	Creatine (Cre)	Precursor and reserve for high energy phosphates
	Glutamate (Glu)	Excitatory neurotransmitter
	Glutamine (Gln)	Substrate for Glu synthesis

products of membrane phospholipid breakdown (e.g., glycerylphosphorylcholine and glycerylphosphorylinositol). The relative concentrations of PME and PDE metabolites are closely related to the metabolic activity of membrane phospholipids. With increasing age during neurodevelopment, precursor levels fall and the concentration of breakdown products increases, resulting in a gradual reduction in PME/PDE levels, which level off as the brain matures.

The resonances of ATP, PCr, and Pi provide information about high-energy phosphate metabolism. In the Krebs' cell cycle, ATP acts as a high-energy reservoir and levels within the brain are buffered by high-energy PCr. When energy consumption increases or there is reduced production of PCr, the level of PCr falls and Pi increases. The Pi resonance peak reflects the equilibrium between phosphate ions with two or four negative charges and is therefore used to calculate intracellular pH. In ^{31}P-spectra, ATP has three peaks that correspond to its three high-energy phosphate bonds. Two of these bind a magnesium ion and their chemical shift is affected by the *in vivo* concentration of magnesium. Lithium also affects the chemical shifts of ATP as it competes with magnesium in binding to ATP (Malhi *et al.*, 2002).

NAA is produced primarily in mitochondria of neurons from aspartate and acetyl-CoA by the enzyme l-aspartate N-acetyltransferase (Jacobson, 1959) and can be detected mainly in pyramidal glutamatergic neurons in the PFC. The main enzyme responsible for NAA's degradation is, however, predominantly found in oligodendrocytes. Therefore, NAA concentrations may index mitochondrial metabolism in gray and white matter in addition to neuronal survival. The precise physiological role of NAA remains undetermined but probably includes roles in transporting water molecules produced during oxidative metabolism outside of the neuron, as an acetyl donor for the formation of membranes, supporting glutamate production (Moffett *et al.*, 2007).

The Cho peak includes several other metabolites, especially glycerophosphocholine and phosphocholine, and to a lesser extent phosphatidylcholine and acetylcholine. Cho peak increases are generally interpreted as indicating excessive membrane breakdown, but the degree to which the choline peak is sensitive to dietary intake is unclear.

The Cre peak includes creatine and creatine phosphate, which serve as a precursor and a reserve for high energy phosphates and buffer ATP/ADP reservoirs. Generally, Cre is thought to be unaffected in several pathological processes, and it is used as a reference to normalize other metabolites, but this assumption is rarely tested. It would obviously be preferable to have absolute measurements of metabolites rather than ratios, but these measurements *in vivo* have important limitations.

Glutamate (Glu) is an excitatory neurotransmitter that is found in abundance in the cortex. Following synaptic release it is converted to glutamine (Gln) by adjacent glia, which then forms the substrate of mitochondrial Glu synthesis. Glu–Gln cycling is closely coupled to glial glucose use and lactate production, and Gln is probably a more sensitive indicator of glutamatergic neurotransmission than Glu itself. The spectral peaks of Gln and Glu overlap considerably, and are often indistinguishable, such that they are sometimes regarded collectively as the "Glx" peak

(Malhi *et al.*, 2002). Techniques such as short echo times can identify peaks containing glutamate and gamma-amino-butyric-acid (GABA), but these are not easily differentiated from the background and corrections for unsuppressed water and other macromolecules become critical (Stanley *et al.*, 2000).

Findings in schizophrenia

^{31}P-MRS studies of membrane metabolism in patients with schizophrenia have repeatedly found a decrease in the ratio of PME/PDE in fronto-temporal brain regions (after Stanley *et al.*, 1995), suggestive of decreased synthesis and increased degradation of membrane phospholipids that is perhaps the result of increased phospholipase activity or diminished phosphodiesterase activity. Similar changes probably precede the clinical manifestation of the illness given that they have been observed in young first-degree relatives of patients with schizophrenia (Klemm *et al.*, 2001). This is in keeping with the neurodevelopmental theory of schizophrenia in that the observed changes may be an exaggeration of the normal synaptic pruning that occurs in late childhood and early adolescence (Keshavan *et al.*, 1994). PMEs and PDEs do not, however, consist solely of phospholipid precursors and products, and changes in their concentrations in schizophrenia could be attributable to, for example, alterations of neuronal membrane structure. Other studies have reported changes in the concentrations of high-energy phosphate metabolites, choline-containing compounds, and myoinositol, but the findings have been inconsistent, at least in part because of variability in clinical methods and MRS applications (Keshavan *et al.*, 2000; Stanley *et al.*, 2000). Higher field strength magnet systems will, however, deliver enhanced resolution and the opportunity to assay molecules of direct genetic and pharmacological relevance that cannot be obtained from other *in vivo* technologies.

Most of the ^{1}H-MRS literature on schizophrenia agrees that NAA/Cre is reduced in the hippocampus and other parts of the temporal lobe. Hippocampal reductions were first shown by Nasrallah *et al.* (1994) in chronic patients treated with antipsychotics. This has been replicated numerous times with single and multiple voxel techniques in chronic and first-episode patients treated with antipsychotics (Renshaw *et al.*, 1995). A more recent study corrected for CSF contributions to the imaging voxels and estimated reduced absolute concentrations of NAA (Weber-Fahr *et al.*, 2002). Reductions have also been found in medication-free patients (Bertolino *et al.*, 1998) and in the siblings of patients (Keshavan *et al.*, 1997), suggesting that this too is a genetically inherited trait that may predispose to the illness (Jessen *et al.*, 2006), although other studies report normal NAA at the earliest stages of schizophrenia (Wood *et al.*, 2003, 2008a). Intriguingly, Egan *et al.* (2003)

found a reduction in left hippocampal NAA/Cre associated with the presence of a variation of the gene encoding BDNF. This variation consists of the substitution of a single amino acid (a methionine for a valine) in the BDNF proprotein. The authors show that this mutation has important implications in the trafficking of the protein and probably disrupts its depolarization-induced secretion, which may be critical for the effects of this molecule on long-term potentiation (and other forms of synaptic plasticity) in the medial temporal lobe.

Bertolino et al. (1996, 1998a) have also reported reduced NAA/Cre in the DLPFC in patients on and off medications, and correlations have emerged between these reductions and increased negative symptoms (Bertolino et al., 2000a), reduced functional activation on executive tasks (Bertolino et al., 2000b), increased dopamine release in the basal ganglia as measured by the displacement of ^{11}C raclopride by amphetamine (Bertolino et al., 2000a), and increased D_2 receptor availability in the basal ganglia as measured by binding potential for iodobenzamide (Bertolino et al., 1999). Other studies largely agree—even negative NAA/Cre studies tend to find NAA/Cho reductions in the DLPFC. Reduced NAA in the DLPFC at psychosis onset has also been linked to impaired functional outcome (Wood et al., 2006). Results for other parts of the PFC are however more mixed, but this may reflect the wide variety of methodological approaches taken, and the balance of the evidence favors reduced NAA in the medial PFC and white matter (Stanley et al., 2000; Keshavan et al., 2000; Marenco et al., 2004). Intriguing reports have also emerged of increased glutamine in the medial PFC in unmedicated patients, which may indicate reduced glutamate transmission, but there are concerns about measurement variability (Bartha et al., 1997) and a lack of NAA deficits in these studies (Theberge et al., 2002).

NAA studies of the thalamus are evenly balanced between positive and negative findings, but most have not corrected for partial voluming of gray and white matter in voxels (4–6 ml), which are typically larger than key substructures, such as the mediodorsal nucleus, where any deficits could actually reflect reduced volumes or cell counts, as reported in some postmortem studies (see Chapter 18). However, Theberge et al. (2002) have found an increase in left thalamic glutamine similar to their finding in the anterior cingulate region.

MRS summary, conclusions, and future directions

MRS is an important tool in the study of the complex abnormalities of brain structure and function associated with schizophrenia. It is, however, more technically demanding and therefore less commonly used than sMRI, and fewer definitive conclusions can yet be drawn as a result. Current limitations of MRS include relatively poor spatial resolution with consequent partial volume effects, long data acquisition times, and the susceptibility artifact. Nonetheless, a systematic review and meta-analysis of 64 published studies involving 1209 patients with schizophrenia and 1256 controls found consistent evidence of NAA reductions in the PFC and the hippocampus (Steen et al., 2005). Studies of euthymic patients with bipolar disorder also suggest decreases in NAA in the PFC and hippocampus in that disorder, as reported in a review of 22 studies involving 328 adults with bipolar disorder and 349 control subjects (Yildiz-Yesiloglu & Ankerst, 2006a). Another systematic review and meta-analysis by the same authors indicated increased choline-containing metabolites in the basal ganglia but no alteration of NAA in depression (Yildiz-Yesiloglu & Ankerst, 2006b). Choline and PMEs also appear to be increased in the PFC of affective disorders, in contrast to reductions in schizophrenia.

MRS could make even more important contributions to understanding the pathophysiology of schizophrenia, not least as it has the ability to measure the concentrations of compounds of importance in fundamental cell processes such as oxidative metabolism. As our understanding of the function of NAA increases, so will our ability to interpret those findings in the literature. One key area for development that will likely improve understanding will derive from studying the associations of NAA and phosphorus imaging measures such as ADP/ATP with genetic variants that may influence the schizophrenia phenotype (c.f. Egan et al., 2003). Moreover, improvements in the image acquisition techniques and in absolute quantification of metabolites in vivo will advance our understanding further, especially when complemented by the study of new cellular metabolites. Spectroscopic techniques able to study the metabolic cycle of glutamate and glutamine (by administering ^{13}C-labeled glucose that is incorporated into glutamate and rapidly exchanged with glutamine proportionally to excitatory metabolism) and GABA metabolism are under development. All of this information will be complemented by an increased understanding of the structure and function of white matter tracts that connect the PFC and temporal lobes.

Diffusion tensor MRI

Diffusion tensor MRI (DT-MRI) allows the direct mapping of white matter connectivity in vivo by measuring the three-dimensional mobility of water molecules from sets of diffusion-weighted MR images. Since water molecules diffuse preferentially along axons rather than across them, the measurement of diffusion "anisotropy" from the diffusion tensor can provide detailed information on fiber-tract orientation and other architectural features.

Principles

Diffusion (D) in fluid systems is usually described by the probability of a particle moving a certain distance over a measurement time. The microscopic random motions of each molecule, caused by repeated collisions with other molecules, are driven by the ambient thermal energy of the fluid. These molecular motions are termed "random walks", as the magnitude and direction of each trajectory are unrelated to those of the previous path. In biological tissue, the presence of multiple cellular compartments with semipermeable barriers causes the diffusion of water protons to depart significantly from that seen in unrestricted isotropic diffusion in an infinite medium. Thus, they must travel tortuous paths to cover any given distance. D has a smaller value than that measured for free diffusion. For example, typical measured values for the diffusion coefficient of water in brain parenchyma range from 700 to $1000 \times 10^{-6} \, mm^2/s$, while D of pure water is $3080 \times 10^{-6} \, mm^2/s$ at $37.4°C$. To reflect the fact that water diffusion is governed both by temperature and interactions with the cellular microstructure, the diffusion coefficient of water measured by MRI is termed the apparent diffusion coefficient (ADC; Bastin & Lawrie, 2004).

The measurement of brain water diffusion *in vivo* is typically achieved using a fast pulsed gradient spin-echo sequence designed to generate two-dimensional diffusion-weighted (DW) MR images in the axial, coronal or sagittal plane. Diffusion sensitivity is achieved by inserting two strong magnetic field gradient pulses around the $180°$ refocusing pulse and measurements of water diffusion are then obtained along the direction in which the diffusion sensitizing gradient is applied. These gradient pulses magnetically label protons attached to diffusing molecules, which then act like endogenous tracers whose motion can be monitored, as diffusing protons do not experience the same net gradient field during the two pulses due to their random motions. This results in imperfect refocusing of the spin-echo leading to signal attenuation. The extended duration of these diffusion sensitizing pulses means that long echo times (TE) are needed to achieve adequate diffusion-related signal attenuation and DW images are therefore inherently also T2-weighted.

Imaging methods

In the typical DW imaging experiment, the measured signal intensity is assumed to be a monotonic function of the applied gradient, and estimates of T2-weighted signal intensity and the ADC are determined by fitting a straight line to values obtained at two different gradient factors (or b-values), b_{max} and b_{min}. Usually, these "two-point sampling schemes" involve acquiring a baseline T2-weighted image ($b_{min} \sim 0 \, s/mm^{-2}$) and one or more DW images at b_{max}. The

choice of b_{max} is, however, complicated by the fact that the signal is in reality a bi-exponential function, with a fast diffusion component in the range $b \sim 0$–$1500 \, s/mm^{-2}$, and a slow diffusion component in the range $b \sim 2500$–$4000 \, s/mm^2$. The exact origin of these is unclear, but it is likely that the fast diffusion component originates from extracellular water and the slow component from intracellular water. Regardless, to avoid underestimating the fast diffusion component by including data from the slow component, most studies use sampling schemes with b_{max} from 1000 to $1500 \, s/mm^{-2}$.

The addition of large diffusion-encoding gradients into a spin-echo sequence makes it highly sensitive to involuntary patient motion. By far the most common single-shot DW acquisition is that based on spin-echo echo-planar imaging (EPI), as it provides rapid, high spatial resolution, with good SNR characteristics; although it also suffers from artifacts caused by susceptibility changes at tissue boundaries, and from geometric image distortions created by the significant eddy currents arising from the diffusion sensitizing gradients. The removal of eddy current distortions can, however, be combined with image registration to remove bulk scan-to-scan patient motion, although care must be taken that the original orientational information in DW images is not lost when these various image warps are applied. These EPI artifacts can also be significantly reduced by other image acquisition approaches, such as line scan diffusion MRI (Buchsbaum *et al.*, 1998). This acquisition method makes the sequence largely insensitive to bulk patient motion, chemical shift, and susceptibility artifacts, but it takes longer and is not commonly available on clinical scanners. Pulsatile brain motion artifacts from the cardiac cycle can affect posterior brain regions in EPI-based acquisitions, but these can be removed by gating the acquisition to the cardiac cycle using a peripheral-gating device attached to the subject's finger.

The tendency of axonal membranes to bias the random motion of water molecules along the principal axes of white matter fiber bundles means that diffusion can only be fully characterized if both its magnitude and directionality can be determined. In the simplest possible DT-MRI experiment, a T2-weighted EP image ($b_{min} \sim 0 \, s/mm^{-2}$) and six DW-EP images ($b_{max} \sim 1000$–$1500 \, s/mm^{-2}$) are collected for each slice location. This provides quick estimations of D, but if the variance of D is required, as it is for group studies, then additional measurements of the DW signal intensity can be obtained either by acquiring DW images at two or more non-zero b-values or by collecting DW images in which diffusion gradients are applied in more than six non-colinear directions. Since white matter fibers are orientated in a three-dimensional space, diffusion *in vivo* can be represented mathematically by a second-order symmetric tensor. Diffusion anisotropy can be measured quantitatively from the diffusion tensor (see Tractography below), but it is important to remove these anisotropy effects when calculating the ADC. This is usually done by determining the ADC in three orthogonal directions and calculating a mean rotationally invariant ADC (<ADC>; Bastin & Lawrie, 2004).

D does not provide quantitative measures of diffusion that can be used to compare different patient populations. The simplest scalar parameter of quantitative diffusion indices is the mean diffusivity (<D>). This parameter is the tensor equivalent of <ADC> obtained from the three orthogonal gradient encodings. However, <D> provides no indication of the shape of the diffusion, which must be obtained from diffusion anisotropy indices. These show that CSF has high <D> and low fractional anisotropy (FA) values; gray and white matter have similar values of <D>, but the diffusion anisotropy of white matter is significantly greater than gray matter. Group comparisons of scalar DT-MRI data can be achieved using manual placement of ROIs on parametric maps obtained from individual subjects, or from voxel-by-voxel and ROI analysis of group-averaged datasets (Buchsbaum *et al.*, 1998; Burns *et al.*, 2003).

There are, however, substantial concerns about the effects of smoothing on the integrity of DT-MRI data, and how differing neuroanatomies may complicate the registration used for spatial normalization, even more so than for VBM studies of sMRI data. There are also specific concerns about using SPM voxel-based methods to analyze DT-MRI as SPM assumes that the data have a Gaussian distribution (Ashburner & Friston 2000), which is not the case for diffusion anisotropy data, and the operations of spatial normalization and Gaussian smoothing performed by SPM alter the orientational information contained within the original diffusion anisotropy maps. The ROI approach is probably a more reliable method of detecting changes in white matter fiber tracts, especially if these are large enough for the ROI to be reliably placed. A specific software package called Tract-Based Spatial Statistics (TBSS) aims to get round the problems with SPM; a carefully tuned non-linear registration is followed by projection onto an alignment-invariant tract representation (the "mean FA skeleton"), which represents the centers of all tracts common to the group. Each subject's aligned FA data are then projected onto this skeleton and the resulting data fed into voxelwise cross-subject statistics (Smith *et al.*, 2006). Tractography approaches have, however, attracted even more interest.

Between-group differences could in theory arise from disturbances in any longitudinally orientated neuronal structure that provides a barrier to water molecules in directions perpendicular to the principal axonal axis. Three such structures are the myelin sheath around the axons, the axonal membrane, and the three-dimensional axonal cytoskeleton consisting of microtubules, neurofilaments,

and interconnecting microfilaments. Diffusion parallel to the length of the axon could also be aided by fast axonal transport. However, extensive *in vivo* and *in vitro* experiments on various non-myelinated neuronal fibers, axons with large axoplasmic spaces, and neurons in which fast axonal transport has been inhibited indicate that the primary determinant of anisotropic water diffusion is the dense packing of axonal membranes hindering water mobility, with myelin playing an important, but secondary, role. Therefore, at the low values of diffusion-weighting used in most human studies ($b < 1500 \text{ s/mm}^{-2}$), differences in diffusion anisotropy probably arise directly from the altered anisotropic tortuosity of the extracellular space.

Findings in schizophrenia

There are now more than 30 controlled studies published which have used DT-MRI to investigate whether the brains of patients with schizophrenia exhibit abnormal white matter structure compared with healthy controls. These studies are predicated on the assumption that diffusion parameters derived from D are sensitive indices of axonal integrity. Thus, reduced FA suggests structural damage and disrupted organization of white matter fiber tracts, while increased <D> suggests edema, demyelination, and/or axonal loss.

In the first of these studies, Buchsbaum *et al.* (1998) acquired both line scan DT-MRI and fluoro-2-deoxy-D-glucose positron-emission tomography (PET) data from five patients and six controls. They found that the patients with schizophrenia had significantly reduced FA in PFC white matter and significantly lower glucose metabolic rates both in this region and in the striatum. Lim *et al.* (1999) found widespread, generalized reductions in white matter FA in 10 male patients who had no white matter volume deficits. Defining small ROIs in the genu and splenium, Foong *et al.* (2000) investigated whether there were any structural abnormalities in the corpus callosum of 20 patients with schizophrenia. They found that <D> was significantly increased while the FA was significantly reduced in the splenium but not the genu in the group with schizophrenia compared with the controls. In 15 male patients, Kubicki *et al.* (2002) found reduced FA and a lack of the normal left-greater-than-right asymmetry in the FA of the uncinate fasciculus. Burns *et al.* (2003) found significantly reduced FA in the left uncinate fasciculus (at a trend level) and left arcuate fasciculus in 30 (15 men, 15 women) patients without any corresponding reduction in white matter density. Kubicki *et al.* (2003) also found reduced FA in the cingulum bundle, caudal to the genu of the corpus callosum. In an intriguing combined DT/magnetization transfer (MT)-MRI study, Kubicki *et al.* (2005) found evidence for joint abnormalities in frontal regions, but DT-MRI differences only in the arcuate fasciculus and corpus callosum. The MT-MRI reductions are similar to those previously reported by another group and implicate overlapping neuropathology (Bagary *et al.*, 2003).

Subsequent ROI and VBM studies have replicated each of these findings of abnormal white matter tract integrity several times, but different studies tend to highlight one or other finding and negative studies for particular regions are quite common. These inconsistent findings are probably attributable to a combination of factors, including lower study power due to small numbers, highly variable methods for both image acquisition (e.g., imaging sequence, *b* values) and analysis (artifact correction, ROI placement), and even some genuine anatomical uncertainty, for example, about where the uncinate and inferior fronto-occipital fasciculi can be distinguished (Kanaan *et al.*, 2005). More recent studies have used the TBSS method and examined components of FA to assess, for example, radial *versus* axial diffusivity (e.g., Seal *et al.*, 2008), which may provide more detailed information and may improve consistency across studies. As is often the case, however, power may be the single greatest consideration. Certainly, recent large studies and a meta-analysis have clearly demonstrated widespread reductions in white matter tract FA in schizophrenia (Ellison-Wright & Bullmore, 2009). It is clear that these are evident in first-episode cases, but it is not yet established whether subjects at high risk show such abnormalities and whether or not there is any progression in chronic patients (Friedman *et al.*, 2008; Kanaan *et al.*, 2009).

Tractography

DT-MRI data not only provide scalar measures of diffusion anisotropy, but can also map white matter fiber tract trajectories *in vivo*. The three-dimensional tracking of white matter fibers, or "tractography", can be achieved using the information contained within the eigenvectors of D. Tractography is based on the assumption that the eigenvector associated with the largest diffusivity (eigenvalue) lies parallel to the local fiber direction in large white matter fiber bundles. However, tracking fibers in three dimensions is complex, requiring the component DW images to have good spatial resolution, be relatively free from artifacts, and have a high SNR so that algorithms can track the direction of principal eigenvectors through many contiguous slices. Furthermore, the image voxels should be near-isotropic (e.g., $2.5 \times 2.5 \times 2.5$ mm) to remove any bias in the diffusion anisotropy measurements that could arise from the orientation of the imaging plane (Bastin & Lawrie, 2004).

A number of different approaches have been suggested which allow white matter fibers to be followed *in vivo*. In the simplest terms, tractography algorithms work by propagating a continuous streamline from an initial seed point in the direction of the principal eigenvector of a set of voxels whose diffusion anisotropy is above a certain empirically determined threshold (Plate 16.1). If over a certain specified distance the track breaks or its curvature becomes too great, then it is terminated. More advanced algorithms determine the connectivity between brain regions using probabilistic methods (Behrens *et al.*, 2003). Such approaches use probability density functions defined at each point in the brain to delineate the underlying fiber structure, thereby identifying regions of crossing fibers, which are not well described by the single tensor model.

Jones *et al.* (2002) have described an elegant method for generating a generic map of brain connectivity or "connectogram" from a group of subjects, i.e., performing tractography on population-averaged diffusion tensor data, to facilitate group contrasts. Their method involves the generation of a diffusion tensor template in standard space, the coregistration of each individual dataset to the template whilst preserving the principal eigenvector direction, and then creating metrics of the central tendency of the distribution of tensors for each voxel within the standard space. The problem is that each laboratory has developed its own solution to these issues and we are again at the stage of individual studies implicating different regions in particular populations. More positively, the size of studies has increased and the rise of "translational medicine" appears to have increased interest in relating abnormalities to clinical features and pathophysiologies. We have, for example, described similar abnormalities in tractography of the uncinate fasciculus and anterior thalamic radiation in 25 patients with schizophrenia and 40 with bipolar disorder as compared to 49 healthy controls (McIntosh *et al.*, 2008). These reductions in FA were unrelated to age, duration of illness, current medication, or current psychiatric symptoms in all patients or the lifetime presence of psychotic symptoms in subjects with bipolar disorder, suggesting that they might be related to shared genetic/environmental risk factors and disease mechanisms common to both disorders.

Future of DT-MRI

It is clear that DT-MRI is a very valuable tool for investigating possible white matter structural abnormalities in schizophrenia. It has great potential to interrogate the pathophysiology of schizophrenia because it measures anatomical or structural connectivity. Much greater attention needs to be given to whether abnormalities are evident in unmedicated patients and relatives, in schizophrenia and other disorders, and if there is any relationship with the clinical features of schizophrenia. The full potential of this exciting new imaging modality will, however, only be unlocked once the field has matured to the point where most researchers can agree on the best available data acquisition and image processing methodologies.

Overall conclusions and challenges

The sMRI, MRS, DT-MRI, and neuropathological literature in schizophrenia all support a relative structural and functional deficiency of temporal and especially hippocampal circuits (Weinberger, 1999), as well as PFC and especially DLPFC networks (Weinberger *et al.*, 2001), associated with small neurons and reduced neuropil (Harrison, 1999). The demonstration of structural brain abnormalities in psychiatric disorders adds weight to arguments that they are diseases or at least disruptions of the central nervous system. To date, however, structural imaging has provided limited information about the fundamental nature of schizophrenia. Although replicated and occasionally detailed patterns of abnormality are beginning to emerge for what was once thought to be a "functional psychosis", until they can be related to specific diagnoses, symptoms or causes, these reports remain vulnerable to the argument that they are artifactual, confounded or incidental epiphenomena. It could be that the pathophysiological disruptions of schizophrenia are better characterized at the synaptic or systems level, and that these are better captured by functional indices such as cerebral perfusion and receptor binding, but thus far at least these techniques have not been conspicuously more successful at distinguishing disorders or underlying processes. Regardless, the structural deficits require explanation, and MRS and DT-MRI may provide just as much and complementary insight into fundamental cellular events and relevant disconnectivities. As resolution increases it may be, for example, that DTI is the best method of evaluating the integrity of both fronto-temporal tracts and the major organizing influences of basal ganglia-thalamo-cortical re-entrant loops. Increasingly focused sMRI examinations, including inter-regional associations in small brain networks and attempts to establish exactly what is reduced (with reference to complementary animal and human postmortem and sMRI examinations) are also important.

Causal processes, and sometimes diagnoses, are best established by prospective longitudinal studies. Clinical researchers have established structural imaging studies that prospectively examine patients with first-episode psychosis, established schizophrenia and bipolar disorder, and individuals at elevated risk for genetic or symptomatic reasons. It is a truism that larger studies are generally better, but study number is inevitably restricted by the size of local populations, the ability of researchers to re-engage participants, funding constraints, and advances in technology that leave previous methods outdated every 5 years or so. These constraints mean that some questions which will inevitably require hundreds of images, e.g. whether there are gene by group by time interactions, and whether subjects at high genetic risk of different disorders differ from each other and from those who become ill with each disor-der, will need to be conducted by several collaborating research groups in multicenter studies in order to obtain sufficiently large samples.

Brain imaging researchers therefore need to standardize their approach to data acquisition, processing, and analyses in what could be called a "human brain mapping" project. Combining large datasets will enable the derivation of "four-dimensional brains" (three-dimensional brains over time), construction of normal and abnormal brain development "atlases", and perhaps even a "human brain connectome" (Gur *et al.* 2007). This will require methods which can accurately combine scans from different people and yet ensure that normalized data remain valid at a single subject level. These developments are certainly a prerequisite for the "1-*versus*-n" studies required if brain imaging is to have direct clinical impact. Despite the substantial overlap between patients and controls on sMRI, MRS, and DT-MRI, and the fact that abnormalities that have been replicated are demonstrable only at the level of the group, and not at an individual level, there are now several demonstrations of the feasibility of using sMRI as a diagnostic aid of schizophrenia in specific contexts (Suddath *et al.*, 1990; Job *et al.*, 2006; Koutsouleris *et al.*, 2009). It is, however, perhaps more realistic, and certainly more realizable in the short term, to state that these initiatives would at the very least demand advances in neuroimaging databases, scanner calibration, and multicenter harmonization that will accurately establish the reliability and power of our principle techniques for imaging the structure of the human brain, and its involvement in disorders such as schizophrenia.

References

Ashburner, J. & Friston, K.J. (2000) Voxel-based morphometry—the methods. *Neuroimage* **11**, 805–821.

Bagary, M.S., Symms, M.R., Barker, G.J., Mutsatsa, S.H., Joyce, E.M. & Ron, M.A. (2003) Gray and white matter brain abnormalities in first-episode schizophrenia inferred from magnetization transfer imaging. *Archives of General Psychiatry* **60**, 779–788.

Barta, P.E., Pearlson, G.D., Powers, R.E., Richards, S.S. & Tune, L.E. (1990) Auditory hallucinations and smaller superior temporal gyral volume in schizophrenia. *American Journal of Psychiatry* **147**, 1457–1462.

Bartha, R., Williamson, P.C., Drost, D.J. *et al.* (1997) Measurement of glutamate and glutamine in the medial prefrontal cortex of never-treated schizophrenic patients and healthy controls by proton magnetic resonance spectroscopy. *Archives of General Psychiatry* **54**, 959–965.

Bastin, M.E. & Lawrie, S.M. (2004) Diffusion tensor magnetic resonance imaging. In: Lawrie, S.M., Johnstone, E.C. & Weinberger, D.R., eds. *Schizophrenia: From Neuroimaging to Neuroscience*. Oxford: Oxford University Press, pp. 93–118.

Behrens, T.E., Johansen-Berg. H., Woolrich, M.W. *et al.* (2003) Non-invasive mapping of connections between human thalamus and cortex using diffusion imaging. *Nature Neuroscience* **6**, 750–757.

Bertolino, A., Nawroz, S., Mattay, V.S. *et al.* (1996) Regionally specific pattern of neurochemical pathology in schizophrenia as assessed by multislice proton magnetic resonance spectroscopic imaging. *American Journal of Psychiatry* **153**, 1554–1563.

Bertolino, A., Callicott, J.H., Elman, I. *et al.* (1998) Regionally specific neuronal pathology in untreated patients with schizophrenia: a proton magnetic resonance spectroscopic imaging study. *Biological Psychiatry* **43**, 641–648.

Bertolino, A., Knable, M.B., Saunders, R.C. *et al.* (1999) The relationship between dorsolateral prefrontal N-acetylaspartate measures and striatal dopamine activity in schizophrenia. *Biological Psychiatry* **45**, 660–667.

Bertolino, A., Breier, A., Callicott, J.H. *et al.* (2000a) The relationship between dorsolateral prefrontal neuronal N-acetylaspartate and evoked release of striatal dopamine in schizophrenia. *Neuropsychopharmacology* **22**, 125–132.

Bertolino, A., Esposito, G., Callicott, J.H. *et al.* (2000b) Specific relationship between prefrontal neuronal N-acetylaspartate and activation of the working memory cortical network in schizophrenia. *American Journal of Psychiatry* **157**, 26–33.

Boos, H.B., Aleman, A., Cahn, W., Hulshoff Pol, H. & Kahn, R.S. (2007) Brain volumes in relatives of patients with schizophrenia: a meta-analysis. *Archives of General Psychiatry* **64**, 297–304.

Buchsbaum, M.S., Tang, C.Y., Peled, S. *et al.* (1998) MRI white matter diffusion anisotropy and PET metabolic rate in schizophrenia. *Neuroreport* **9**, 425–430.

Burns, J., Job, D., Bastin, M.E. *et al.* (2003) Structural disconnectivity in schizophrenia: a diffusion tensor magnetic resonance imaging study. *British Journal of Psychiatry* **182**, 439–443.

Cahn, W., Hulshoff Pol, H.E., Lems, E.B. *et al.* (2002) Brain volume changes in first-episode schizophrenia: a 1-year follow-up study. *Archives of General Psychiatry* **59**, 1002–1010.

Cannon, T.D., Thompson, P.M., van Erp, T.G. *et al.* (2002) Cortex mapping reveals regionally specific patterns of genetic and disease-specific gray-matter deficits in twins discordant for schizophrenia. *Proceedings of the National Academy of Science USA* **99**, 3228–3233.

Chakos, M.H., Lieberman, J.A., Bilder, R.M. *et al.* (1994) Increase in caudate nuclei volumes of first-episode schizophrenic patients taking antipsychotic drugs. *American Journal of Psychiatry* **151**, 1430–1436.

Chakos, M., Lieberman, J.A., Alvir, J. *et al.* (1995) Caudate nuclei volumes in schizophrenic patients treated with typical antipsychotics or clozapine. *Lancet* **345**, 456–457.

Csernansky, J.G., Joshi, S., Wang, L. *et al.* (1998) Hippocampal morphometry in schizophrenia by high dimensional brain mapping. *Proceedings of the National Academy of Science USA* **95**, 11406–11411.

Egan, M.F., Kojima, M., Callicott, J.H. *et al.* (2003) The BDNF val66met polymorphism affects activity-dependent secretion of BDNF and human memory and hippocampal function. *Cell* **112**, 257–269.

Ellison-Wright, I. & Bullmore, E. (2009) Meta-analysis of diffusion tensor imaging studies in schizophrenia. *Schizophrenia Research* **108**, 3–10.

Ellison-Wright, I., Glahn, D.C., Laird, A.R., Thelen, S.M. & Bullmore, E. (2008) The anatomy of first-episode and chronic schizophrenia: an anatomical likelihood estimation meta-analysis. *American Journal of Psychiatry* **165**, 1015–1023.

Foong, J., Maier, M., Clark, C.A., Barker, G.J., Miller, D.H. & Ron, M.A. (2000) Neuropathological abnormalities of the corpus callosum in schizophrenia: a diffusion tensor imaging study. *Journal of Neurology Neurosurgery and Psychiatry* **68**, 242–244.

Fornito, A., Whittle, S., Wood, S.J., Velakoulis, D., Pantelis, C. & Yucel, M. (2006) The influence of sulcal variability on morphometry of the human anterior cingulate and paracingulate cortex. *Neuroimage* **33**, 843–854.

Fornito, A., Yung, A.R., Wood, S.J. *et al.* (2008) Anatomic abnormalities of the anterior cingulate cortex before psychosis onset: an MRI study of ultra-high-risk individuals. *Biological Psychiatry* **64**, 758–765.

Fornito, A., Yucel, M. & Pantelis, C. (2009a) Reconciling neuroimaging and neuropathological findings in schizophrenia and bipolar disorder. *Current Opinion in Psychiatry* **22**, 312–319.

Fornito, A., Yucel, M., Patti, J., Wood, S.J. & Pantelis, C. (2009b) Mapping grey matter reductions in schizophrenia: an anatomical likelihood estimation analysis of voxel-based morphometry studies. *Schizophrenia Research* **108**, 104–113.

Friedman, J.I., Tang, C., Carpenter, D. *et al.* (2008) Diffusion tensor imaging findings in first-episode and chronic schizophrenia patients. *American Journal of Psychiatry* **165**, 1024–1032.

Garner, B., Pariante, C.M., Wood, S.J. *et al.* (2005) Pituitary volume predicts future transition to psychosis in individuals at ultra-high risk of developing psychosis. *Biological Psychiatry* **58**, 417–423.

Gaser, C., Volz, H.P., Kiebel, S., Riehemann, S. & Sauer, H. (1999) Detecting structural changes in whole brain based on nonlinear deformations-application to schizophrenia research. *Neuroimage* **10**, 107–113.

Glahn, D.C., Laird, A.R., Ellison-Wright, I. *et al.* (2008) Meta-analysis of gray matter anomalies in schizophrenia: application of anatomic likelihood estimation and network analysis. *Biological Psychiatry* **64**, 774–781.

Goldstein, J.M., Goodman, J.M., Seidman, L.J. (1999) Cortical abnormalities in schizophrenia identified by structural magnetic resonance imaging. *Archives of General Psychiatry* **56**, 537–547.

Gur, R.E., Cowell, P.E., Latshaw, A. *et al.* (2000) Reduced dorsal and orbital prefrontal gray matter volumes in schizophrenia. *Archives of General Psychiatry* **57**, 761–768 [erratum in **57**, 858].

Gur, R.E., Keshavan, M.S. & Lawrie, S.M. (2007) Deconstructing psychosis with human brain imaging. *Schizophrenia Bulletin* **33**, 921–931.

Harris, J.M., Moorhead, T.W., Miller, P. *et al.* (2007) Increased prefrontal gyrification in a large high-risk cohort characterizes those who develop schizophrenia and reflects abnormal prefrontal development. *Biological Psychiatry* **62**, 722–729.

Harrison, P.J. (1999) The neuropathology of schizophrenia. A critical review of the data and their interpretation. *Brain* **122**, 593–624.

Harrison, P.J., Freemantle, N. & Geddes, J.R. (2003) Meta-analysis of brain weight in schizophrenia. *Schizophrenia Research* **64**, 25–34.

Ho, B.C., Andreasen, N.C., Dawson, J.D. & Wassink, T.H. (2007) Association between brain-derived neurotrophic factor Val66Met gene polymorphism and progressive brain volume changes in schizophrenia. *American Journal of Psychiatry* **164**, 1890–1899.

Hulshoff Pol, H.E. & Kahn, R.S. (2008) What happens after the first episode? A review of progressive brain changes in chronically ill patients with schizophrenia. *Schizophrenia Bulletin* **34**, 354–366.

Jacobson, K.B. (1959) Studies on the role of N-acetylaspartic acid in mammalian brain. *Journal of General Physiology* **43**, 323–333.

Jessen, F., Scherk, H., Traber, F. *et al.* (2006) Proton magnetic resonance spectroscopy in subjects at risk for schizophrenia. *Schizophrenia Research* **87**, 81–88.

Job, D.E., Whalley, H.C., McConnell, S., Glabus, M., Johnstone, E.C. & Lawrie, S.M. (2002) Structural gray matter differences between first-episode schizophrenics and normal controls using voxel-based morphometry. *Neuroimage* **17**, 880–889.

Job, D.E., Whalley, H.C., Johnstone, E.C. & Lawrie, S.M. (2005) Grey matter changes over time in high risk subjects developing schizophrenia. *Neuroimage* **25**, 1023–1030.

Job, D.E., Whalley, H.C., McIntosh, A.M., Owens, D.G., Johnstone, E.C. & Lawrie, S.M. (2006) Grey matter changes can improve the prediction of schizophrenia in subjects at high risk. *BMC Medicine* **4**, 29.

Jones, D.K., Griffin, L.D., Alexander, D.C. *et al.* (2002) Spatial normalization and averaging of diffusion tensor MRI data sets. *Neuroimage* **17**, 592–617.

Johnstone, E.C. & Owens, D.G. (2004) Early studies of brain anatomy in schizophrenia. In: Lawrie, S.M., Johnstone, E.C. & Weinberger, D.R., eds. *Schizophrenia: from Neuroimaging to Neuroscience*. Oxford: Oxford University Press, pp. 1–19.

Johnstone, E.C., Crow, T.J., Frith, C.D., Husband, J. & Kreel, L. (1976) Cerebral ventricular size and cognitive impairment in chronic schizophrenia. *Lancet* **2**, 924–926.

Kanaan, R.A., Kim, J.S., Kaufmann, W.E., Pearlson, G.D., Barker, G.J. & McGuire, P.K. (2005) Diffusion tensor imaging in schizophrenia. *Biological Psychiatry* **58**, 921–929.

Kanaan, R., Barker, G., Brammer, M. *et al.* (2009) White matter microstructure in schizophrenia: effects of disorder, duration and medication. *British Journal of Psychiatry* **194**, 236–242.

Keshavan, M.S., Anderson, S. & Pettegrew, J.W. (1994) Is schizophrenia due to excessive synaptic pruning in the prefrontal cortex? The Feinberg hypothesis revisited. *Journal of Psychiatry Research* **28**, 239–265.

Keshavan, M.S., Montrose, D.M., Pierri, J.N. *et al.* (1997) Magnetic resonance imaging and spectroscopy in offspring at risk for schizophrenia: preliminary studies. *Progress in Neuropsychopharmacology and Biological Psychiatry* **21**, 1285–1295.

Keshavan, M.S., Stanley, J.A. & Pettegrew, J.W. (2000) Magnetic resonance spectroscopy in schizophrenia: methodological issues and findings—part II. *Biological Psychiatry* **48**, 369–380.

Klemm, S., Rzanny, R., Riehemann, S. *et al.* (2001) Cerebral phosphate metabolism in first-degree relatives of patients with schizophrenia. *American Journal of Psychiatry* **158**, 958–960.

Konick, L.C. & Friedman, L. (2001) Meta-analysis of thalamic size in schizophrenia. *Biological Psychiatry* **49**, 28–38.

Koutsouleris, N., Meisenzahl, E.M., Davatzikos, C. *et al.* (2009) Use of neuroanatomical pattern classification to identify subjects in at-risk mental states of psychosis and predict disease transition. *Archives of General Psychiatry* **66**, 700–712.

Kubicki, M., Westin, C.F., Maier, S.E. *et al.* (2002) Uncinate fasciculus findings in schizophrenia: a magnetic resonance diffusion tensor imaging study. *American Journal of Psychiatry* **159**, 813–820.

Kubicki, M., Westin, C.F., Nestor, P.G. *et al.* (2003) Cingulate fasciculus integrity disruption in schizophrenia: a magnetic resonance diffusion tensor imaging study. *Biological Psychiatry* **54**, 1171–1180.

Kubicki, M., Park, H., Westin, C.F. *et al.* (2005) DTI and MTR abnormalities in schizophrenia: analysis of white matter. *Neuroimage* **26,** 1109–1118.

Kuperberg, G.R., Broome, M.R, McGuire, P.K. *et al.* (2003) Regionally localized thinning of the cerebral cortex in schizophrenia. *Archives of General Psychiatry* **60**, 878–888.

Lawrie, S.M. & Abukmeil, S.S. (1998) Brain abnormality in schizophrenia. A systematic and quantitative review of volumetric magnetic resonance imaging studies. *British Journal of Psychiatry* **172**, 110–120.

Lawrie, S.M., Whalley, H.C., Abukmeil, S.S. *et al.* (2001) Brain structure, genetic liability, and psychotic symptoms in subjects at high risk of developing schizophrenia. *Biological Psychiatry* **49**, 811–823.

Lawrie, S.M., McIntosh, A.M., Hall, J., Owens, D.G. & Johnstone, E.C. (2008) Brain structure and function changes during the development of schizophrenia: the evidence from studies of subjects at increased genetic risk. *Schizophrenia Bulletin* **34**, 330–340.

Lewis, S. (1991) Computerised tomography in schizophrenia. *British Journal of Psychiatry* **159**, 158–159.

Lieberman, J., Chakos, M., Wu, H. *et al.* (2001) Longitudinal study of brain morphology in first episode schizophrenia. *Biological Psychiatry* **49**, 487–499.

Lieberman, J.A., Tollefson, G.D., Charles, C. *et al.* (2005) Antipsychotic drug effects on brain morphology in first-episode psychosis. *Archives of General Psychiatry* **62**, 361–370.

Lim, K.O., Hedehus, M., Moseley, M., de Crespigny, A., Sullivan, E.V. & Pfefferbaum, A. (1999) Compromised white matter tract integrity in schizophrenia inferred from diffusion tensor imaging. *Archives of General Psychiatry* **56**, 367–374.

Malhi, G.S., Valenzuela, M., Wen, W. & Sachdev, P. (2002) Magnetic resonance spectroscopy and its applications in psychiatry. *Australian and New Zealand Journal of Psychiatry* **36**, 31–43.

Marenco, S., Weinberger, D.R. & Bertolino, A. (2004) Magnetic resonance spectroscopy. In: Lawrie, S.M, Johnstone, E.C. & Weinberger, D.R., eds. *Schizophrenia: From Neuroimaging to Neuroscience*. Oxford: Oxford University Press, pp. 73–92.

Mathalon, D.H., Pfefferbaum, A., Lim, K.O., Rosenbloom, M.J. & Sullivan, E.V. (2003) Compounded brain volume deficits in schizophrenia-alcoholism comorbidity. *Archives of General Psychiatry* **60**, 245–252.

McIntosh, A.M & Lawrie, S.M. (2004) Structural magnetic resonance imaging. In: Lawrie, S.M., Johnstone, E.C. & Weinberger, D.R., eds. *Schizophrenia: From Neuroimaging to Neuroscience.* Oxford: Oxford University Press, pp. 21–57.

McIntosh, A.M., Baig, B.J., Hall, J. *et al.* (2007) Relationship of catechol-O-methyltransferase variants to brain structure and function in a population at high risk of psychosis. *Biological Psychiatry* **61**, 1127–1134.

McIntosh, A.M., Maniega, S.M., Lymer, G.K. *et al.* (2008) White matter tractography in bipolar disorder and schizophrenia. *Biological Psychiatry* **64**, 1088–1092.

McNeil, T.F., Cantor-Graae, E. & Weinberger, D.R. (2000) Relationship of obstetric complications and differences in size of brain structures in monozygotic twin pairs discordant for schizophrenia. *American Journal of Psychiatry* **157**, 203–212.

Moffett, J.R., Ross, B., Arun, P., Madhavarao, C.N. and Namboodiri, A.M. (2007) N-acetylaspartate in the CNS: from neurodiagnostics to neurobiology. *Progress in Neurobiology* **81**, 89–131.

Nakamura, M., Nestor, P.G., McCarley, R.W. *et al.* (2007) Altered orbitofrontal sulcogyral pattern in schizophrenia. *Brain* **130**, 693–707.

Nasrallah, H.A., Skinner, T.E., Schmalbrock, P. & Robitaille, P.M. (1994) Proton magnetic resonance spectroscopy (1H MRS) of the hippocampal formation in schizophrenia: a pilot study. *British Journal of Psychiatry* **165**, 481–485.

Pantelis, C., Velakoulis, D., McGorry, P.D. *et al.* (2003) Neuroanatomical abnormalities before and after onset of psychosis: a cross-sectional and longitudinal MRI comparison. *Lancet* **361**, 281–288.

Pantelis, C., Yücel, M., Wood, S.J. *et al.* (2005) Structural brain imaging evidence for multiple pathological processes at different stages of brain development in schizophrenia. *Schizophrenia Bulletin* **31**, 672–696.

Pariante, C.M., Dazzan, P., Danese, A. *et al.* (2005) Increased pituitary volume in antipsychotic-free and antipsychotic-treated patients of the AEsop first-onset psychosis study. *Neuropsychopharmacology* **30**, 1923–1931.

Rais, M., Cahn, W., Van Haren, N. *et al.* (2008) Excessive brain volume loss over time in cannabis-using first-episode schizophrenia patients. *American Journal of Psychiatry* **165**, 490–496.

Raz, S. & Raz, N. (1990) Structural brain abnormalities in the major psychoses: a quantitative review of the evidence from computerized imaging. *Psychological Bulletin* **108**, 93–108.

Renshaw, P.F., Yurgelun-Todd, D.A., Tohen, M., Gruber, S. & Cohen, B.M. (1995) Temporal lobe proton magnetic resonance spectroscopy of patients with first-episode psychosis. *American Journal of Psychiatry* **152**, 444–446.

Salisbury, D.F., Kuroki, N., Kasai, K., Shenton, M.E. & McCarley, R.W. (2007) Progressive and interrelated functional and structural evidence of post-onset brain reduction in schizophrenia. *Archives of General Psychiatry* **64**, 521–529.

Seal, M.L., Yücel, M., Fornito, A. *et al.* (2008) Abnormal white matter microstructure in schizophrenia: A voxelwise analysis of axial and radial diffusivity. *Schizophrenia Research* **101**, 106–110.

Shapleske, J., Rossell, S.L., Woodruff, P.W. & David, A.S. (1999) The planum temporale: a systematic, quantitative review of its structural, functional and clinical significance. *Brain Research and Brain Research Reviews* **29**, 26–49.

Smith, S.M., Jenkinson, M., Johansen-Berg, H. *et al.* (2006) Tract-based spatial statistics: voxelwise analysis of multi-subject diffusion data. *Neuroimage* **31**, 1487–1505.

Shenton, M.E., Kikinis, R., Jolesz, F.A. *et al.* (1992) Abnormalities of the left temporal lobe and thought disorder in schizophrenia. A quantitative magnetic resonance imaging study. *New England Journal of Medicine* **327**, 604–612.

Shenton, M.E., Dickey, C.C., Frumin, M. & McCarley, R.W. (2001) A review of MRI findings in schizophrenia. *Schizophrenia Research* **49**, 1–52.

Stanley, J.A., Williamson, P.C., Drost, D.J. *et al.* (1995) An *in vivo* study of the prefrontal cortex of schizophrenic patients at different stages of illness via phosphorus magnetic resonance spectroscopy. *Archives of General Psychiatry* **52**, 399–406.

Stanley, J.A., Pettegrew, J.W. & Keshavan, M.S. (2000) Magnetic resonance spectroscopy in schizophrenia: methodological issues and findings—part I. *Biological Psychiatry* **48**, 357–368.

Steen, R.G., Hamer, R.M. & Lieberman, J.A. (2005) Measurement of brain metabolites by 1H magnetic resonance spectroscopy in patients with schizophrenia: a systematic review and meta-analysis. *Neuropsychopharmacology* **30**, 1949–1962.

Steen, R.G., Mull, C., McClure, R., Hamer, R.M. & Lieberman, J.A. (2006) Brain volume in first-episode schizophrenia: systematic review and meta-analysis of magnetic resonance imaging studies. *British Journal of Psychiatry* **188**, 510–518.

Suddath, R.L., Christison, G.W., Torrey, E.F., Casanova, M.F. & Weinberger, D.R. (1990) Anatomical abnormalities in the brains of monozygotic twins discordant for schizophrenia. *New England Journal of Medicine* **322,** 789–794.

Sun, D., Stuart, G.W., Jenkinson, M. *et al.* (2009a) Brain surface contraction mapped in first-episode schizophrenia: a longitudinal magnetic resonance imaging study. *Molecular Psychiatry* **14**, 976–986.

Sun, D., Phillips, L., Velakoulis, D. *et al.* (2009b) Progressive brain structural changes mapped as psychosis develops in "at risk" individuals. *Schizophrenia Research* **108**, 85–92.

Takahashi, T., Yücel, M. & Yung, A.R. *et al.* (2008) Adhesio interthalamica in individuals at high-risk for developing psychosis and patients with psychotic disorders. *Progress in Neuropsychopharmacology and Biological Psychiatry* **32**, 1708–1714.

Takahashi, T., Wood, S.J., Yung, A.R. *et al.* (2009) Progressive gray matter reduction of the superior temporal gyrus during transition to psychosis. *Archives of General Psychiatry* **66**, 366–376.

Tanskanen, P., Ridler, K., Murray, G.K. *et al.* (2008) Morphometric brain abnormalities in schizophrenia in a population-based sample: Relationship to duration of illness. *Schizophrenia Bulletin* [Epub ahead of print].

Theberge, J., Bartha, R., Drost, D.J. *et al.* (2002) Glutamate and glutamine measured with 4.0 T proton MRS in never-treated patients with schizophrenia and healthy volunteers. *American Journal of Psychiatry* **159**, 1944–1946.

Thompson, P.M., Vidal, C., Giedd, J.N. *et al.* (2001) Mapping adolescent brain change reveals dynamic wave of accelerated gray matter loss in very early-onset schizophrenia. *Proceedings of the National Academy of Science USA* **98**, 11650–11655.

van Erp, T.G., Saleh, P.A., Rosso, I.M. *et al.* (2002) Contributions of genetic risk and fetal hypoxia to hippocampal volume in patients with schizophrenia or schizoaffective disorder, their unaffected siblings, and healthy unrelated volunteers. *American Journal of Psychiatry* **159**, 1514–1520.

van Horn, J.D. & McManus, I.C. (1992) Ventricular enlargement in schizophrenia. A meta-analysis of studies of the ventricle:brain ratio (VBR). *British Journal of Psychiatry* **160**, 687–697.

Velakoulis, D., Wood, S.J., Wong, M.T. *et al.* (2006) Hippocampal and amygdala volumes according to psychosis stage and diagnosis: a magnetic resonance imaging study of chronic schizophrenia, first-episode psychosis, and ultra-high-risk individuals. *Archives of General Psychiatry* **63**, 139–149.

Vita, A., De Peri, L., Silenzi, C. & Dieci, M. (2006) Brain morphology in first-episode schizophrenia: a meta-analysis of quantitative magnetic resonance imaging studies. *Schizophrenia Research* **82**, 75–88.

Weber-Fahr, W., Ende, G., Braus, D.F. *et al.* (2002) A fully automated method for tissue segmentation and CSF-correction of proton MRSI metabolites corroborates abnormal hippocampal NAA in schizophrenia. *Neuroimage* **16**, 49–60.

Weinberger, D.R. (1999) Cell biology of the hippocampal formation in schizophrenia. *Biological Psychiatry* **45**, 395–402.

Weinberger, D.R. & McClure, R.K. (2002) Neurotoxicity, neuroplasticity, and magnetic resonance imaging morphometry: what is happening in the schizophrenic brain? *Archives of General Psychiatry* **59**, 553–558.

Weinberger, D.R., Torrey, E.F., Neophytides, A.N. & Wyatt, R.J. (1979) Structural abnormalities in the cerebral cortex of chronic schizophrenic patients. *Archives of General Psychiatry* **36**, 935–939.

Weinberger, D.R., Egan, M.F., Bertolino, A. *et al.* (2001) Prefrontal neurons and the genetics of schizophrenia. *Biological Psychiatry* **50**, 825–844.

Wood, S.J., Berger, G., Velakoulis, D. *et al.* (2003) Proton magnetic resonance spectroscopy in first episode psychosis and ultra high-risk individuals. *Schizophrenia Bulletin* **29**, 831–843.

Wood, S.J., Berger, G.E., Lambert, M. *et al.* (2006) Prediction of functional outcome 18 months after a first psychotic episode: a proton magnetic resonance spectroscopy study. *Archives of General Psychiatry* **63**, 969–976.

Wood, S.J., Berger, G.E., Wellard, R.M. *et al.* (2008a) A (1)H-MRS investigation of the medial temporal lobe in antipsychotic-naive and early-treated first episode psychosis. *Schizophrenia Research* **102**, 163–170.

Wood, S.J., Pantelis, C., Velakoulis, D., Yücel, M., Fornito, A. & McGorry, P.D. (2008b) Progressive changes in the development toward schizophrenia: studies in subjects at increased symptomatic risk. *Schizophrenia Bulletin* **34**, 322–329.

Wood, S.J., Pantelis, C., Yung, A.R., Velakoulis, D. & McGorry, P.D. (2009) Brain changes during the onset of schizophrenia: implications for neurodevelopmental theories. *Medical Journal of Australia* **190**, S10–13.

Wright, I.C., Rabe-Hesketh, S., Woodruff, P.W., David, A.S., Murray, R.M. & Bullmore, E.T. (2000) Meta-analysis of regional brain volumes in schizophrenia. *American Journal of Psychiatry* **157**, 16–25.

Yildiz-Yesiloglu, A. & Ankerst, D.P. (2006a) Neurochemical alterations of the brain in bipolar disorder and their implications for pathophysiology: a systematic review of the in vivo proton magnetic resonance spectroscopy findings. *Progress in Neuropsychopharmacology and Biological Psychiatry* **30**, 969–995.

Yildiz-Yesiloglu, A. & Ankerst, D.P. (2006b) Review of 1H magnetic resonance spectroscopy findings in major depressive disorder: a meta-analysis. *Psychiatry Research* **147**, 1–25.

Yücel, M., Stuart, G.W., Maruff, P. *et al.* (2002) Paracingulate morphologic differences in males with established schizophrenia: a magnetic resonance imaging morphometric study. *Biological Psychiatry* **52**, 15–23.

Yücel, M., Wood, S.J., Phillips, L.J. *et al.* (2003) Morphology of the anterior cingulate cortex in young men at ultra-high risk of developing a psychotic illness. *British Journal of Psychiatry* **182**, 518–524.

Yücel, M., Solowij, N., Respondek, C., *et al.* (2008) Regional brain abnormalities associated with long-term heavy cannabis use. *Archives of General Psychiatry* **65**, 694–701.

Zhou, S.Y., Suzuki, M. & Hagino, H. *et al.* (2005) Volumetric analysis of sulci/gyri-defined in vivo frontal lobe regions in schizophrenia: Precentral gyrus, cingulate gyrus, and prefrontal region. *Psychiatry Research* **139**, 127–139.

CHAPTER 17

Functional brain imaging in schizophrenia

Andreas Meyer-Lindenberg[1] and Edward T. Bullmore[2]

[1]Central Institute of Mental Health, University of Heidelberg, Heidelberg, Germany
[2]University of Cambridge, Cambridge, UK

Introduction

Searching the PubMed database for "schizophrenia"[ti] and ("functional magnetic resonance imaging") (a fairly conservative search) in January 2010 yielded over 300 papers (*vs.* fewer than 100 for depression). Clearly, if schizophrenia used to be the graveyard of neuropathology (Chapter 18), it has now emerged as the fairground of functional neuroimaging. This largely reflects a success story since modern imaging techniques, such as magnetic resonance imaging (MRI) and positron emission tomography (PET), provide access to a systems-level description of relevant neurobiology to an unprecedented degree. This has been especially useful for schizophrenia research, which is challenged with understanding how genetic contributions of a highly heritable (group of) disorders are translated into clinical symptoms, course of illness, and response to therapy. In this translational enterprise, neuroimaging occupies a useful middle ground in that findings at the neural systems level can be related both back to the level of cells and genes, and "upwards" to the level of behavior. Neuroimaging research has contributed enormously to establish and anchor schizophrenia research firmly in the broader neuroscience community, and has resulted in reduced stigma for patients and their families. In this chapter, we will attempt to synthesize this information, mindful of the fact that consideration of every facet will be impossible and the result necessarily somewhat idiosyncratic.

In contradistinction to structural neuroimaging, functional brain data are dependent on what cognitive state the participants are in. What is more, the more commonly used modality of functional MRI (fMRI) does not provide a stable baseline estimate of brain function, which means that most imaging paradigms include two or more cognitive states that can be contrasted. Even in PET or perfusion MRI, which do provide data on blood flow *versus* a stable baseline, cognitive paradigms are commonly used. This situation requires experimental choices that have largely been taken from the broader field of cognitive neuroscience. For example, a well-established paradigm to study working memory in fMRI can be used in patients and their functional neuroimages compared to healthy controls. This approach is straightforward if one assumes, as the field to some degree did, that specific neurocognitive abnormalities might explain a large proportion of the clinical picture of schizophrenia, because neuroimaging would then provide the neurofunctional correlate of exactly those implicated cognitive system(s). However, recent data suggest that the cognitive deficit in schizophrenia is broad and not specific for individual neurocognitive domains (see Chapter 8). This requires a change of perspective in that cognitive activation paradigms are used not as an end in themselves but as "reflex hammers" to reliably elicit

Schizophrenia, 3rd edition. Edited by Daniel R. Weinberger and Paul J Harrison © 2011 Blackwell Publishing Ltd.

functional activation that can be related to the biology of schizophrenia. Instead of an account that interprets dorsolateral prefrontal activation abnormalities seen during a working memory fMRI paradigm as the neural mechanism by which working memory dysfunction contributes to schizophrenia, one would view a working memory task as a tool to elicit dysfunction in a region that is preferentially impacted by the biology of the illness, just as a Babinski reflex response is useful not because one believes that dorsiflexion of the great toe is relevant for the pathophysiology of spasticity but because it reliably indicates abnormalities in the motor systems which *are* relevant for the disease. A second important preliminary point about functional imaging data is their extraordinary richness. Usually, information on blood oxygen level-dependent (BOLD) response or blood flow are available in about 40000 voxels every 2 s for minutes. In a first pass, these data are analyzed to identify regional abnormalities (as voxels will behave differently in patients and controls). However, they can also be used to understand how different regions of the brain interact, i.e., to parse neural systems. This is an approach that deeply resonates with ideas in schizophrenia research that emphasize the importance of functional interactions over regional pathology and that go back at least to Carl Wernicke.

In this setting, several strategies can and have been pursued. Manifestly ill patients can be compared to controls using functional imaging data acquired at rest or during a number of cognitive challenge paradigms. This approach comprises the large majority of work summarized in this chapter. Data obtained in this way have been used to test hypotheses about a specific neurocognitive function in schizophrenia (e.g., are there abnormalities in working memory symptoms?), specific neural systems (is hippocampal activity or prefrontal–hippocampal interaction preferentially impacted in schizophrenia?), symptoms (neural correlates of positive or negative symptoms, or more specifically hallucinations or delusions), course of illness (differences between first-episode and later stages of the illness), and therapy (effects of drug or neurocognitive treatment). Despite its enduring popularity, this approach has problems because manifest illness is associated with a myriad of confounding factors (hospitalization history, drug treatment effects, neurocognitive impairments impacting on task performance in the scanner, to name just a few) that are difficult to control experimentally. One way out of this conundrum is to utilize the fact that the major causal contribution is genetic. One can therefore use imaging genetics (see Chapter 14) to investigate, in healthy controls, the effects of genetic variants implicated in schizophrenia. In addition, people with increased genetic risk who are not ill, e.g., siblings of patients, who carry 50% of their genes and have an approximately 10-fold increased risk for later illness, can be studied using cognitive chal-

lenge paradigms. Abnormalities found in this group of people are likely to be related to the neurogenetic substrate of the illness, a link that can be substantiated further using approaches from formal genetics, such as Risch's lambda for siblings. This approach is reviewed at the end of the chapter.

Imaging neurocognitive functions

Psychomotor function

Patients with schizophrenia frequently exhibit psychomotor disturbances. Manifestations range from involuntary motor acts, neurological soft signs (e.g., coordination deficits) to complex disorders of behavioral control and catatonic symptoms (Schroeder *et al.*, 1991; Vrtunski *et al.*, 1986). Although quite a lot of fMRI research was performed in this domain, the neurofunctional basis of the disturbances is still only incompletely known. Most studies employed simple repetitive motor activities (e.g., sequential finger opposition) alternating with resting conditions in a block-design approach. Early investigations, e.g., the work of Wenz *et al.* (1994) or Schröder *et al.* (1995), reported hypoactivation of primary sensori- and supplementary-motor cortices in schizophrenia, a finding not consistently replicated by subsequent studies (Wenz *et al.*, 1994; Schröder *et al.*, 1995, 1999; Buckley *et al.*, 1997; Braus *et al.*, 1999). In addition, data indicating altered functional asymmetry of the cortical hemispheres during motor tasks have been published, e.g., by the group of Yurgelun-Todd (Rogowska *et al.*, 2004; Bertolino *et al.*, 2004a; Mattay *et al.*, 1997).

One emerging finding is that patients with schizophrenia may be characterized by a reduced lateralization index during motor performance. In light of the usually pronounced lateralization of cortical activation during motor function, this indicates an abnormal situation in terms of reduced contralateral recruitment or deficient ipsilateral inhibition of motor areas, respectively. However, a substantial number of contradictory findings, as well as some empirical data (Bertolino *et al.*, 2004a; Braus *et al.*, 1999, 2000b), show that further studies in this areas will benefit from controlling for confounding factors, such as medication effects (see also Imaging treatment effects, below).

Visual information processing

Neuropsychological research has repeatedly confirmed the presence of visual information processing deficits in schizophrenia (Braff & Saccuzzo, 1981; 1985; Keri *et al.*, 2000; Moritz *et al.*, 2001). Among others, patients exhibit a significantly increased error rate during performance of so-called "backward masking" tasks, which employ contiguous distractor presentations to disturb the sensory processing of target stimuli (Braff & Saccuzzo, 1981, 1985). Another affected visual domain is deficient perceptual discrimination of target velocities, a research area extensively investigated by Holzman and coworkers (Chen et al., 1999a,b,c). Since some studies indicate that visual processing abnormalities may be observable in asymptomatic relatives of patients with schizophrenia (Green et al., 1997; Chen et al., 1999b), they may be valuable as a trait marker of disease vulnerability. Delineation of the underlying neural processing deficit may therefore be valuable as an endophenotype (see Chapter 14).

Consequently, much research has been directed to the characterization of visual information processing deficits in behavioral experiments (see Chapter 15). Here, high error rates during processing of stimuli of higher spatial frequency, or moving stimuli, suggest a pathophysiological involvement of the dorsal visual processing stream in patients with schizophrenia patients (Schwartz et al., 1999; Cadenhead et al., 1998; O'Donnell et al., 1996). The so-called magnocellular network comprises cortical areas specialized for the handling of motion and depth cues, e.g., the motion-sensitive field V5 (hMT), posterior parietal cortex (PPC), and frontal eye fields (FEF) (Ungerleider et al., 1998; Ungerleider & Mishkin, 1982). The exact location of the presumed dorsal stream dysfunction, however, cannot be identified using a behavioral approach. Prior empirical data were therefore interpreted in manifold ways, e.g., as a sign of a deficient prefrontal control of lower visual areas or a thalamic filter dysfunction (Keri et al., 2000; Levin, 1984a,b). Among others (Chen et al., 1999a; Tek et al., 2002; Stuve et al., 1997), the group surrounding Holzman (Chen et al., 1999a,b,c) assumes a deficiency in "bottom up" processing of motion signals in V5 as being responsible for visual processing dysfunctions and executive deficits observable in schizophrenic patients (e.g., eye tracking dysfunction, spatial working memory deficits).

Only relatively few research groups have used fMRI to study early visual information processing in schizophrenia to date. Braus et al. (2002) investigated visuo-acoustic integration in 12 neuroleptic-naïve patients with a passive stimulation paradigm involving the simultaneous presentation of a visual 6 Hz checkerboard and an auditory drum beat stimulus. Compared to healthy controls, the patient group displayed a significant activation decrease in both the thalamic geniculate body and higher order areas of the dorsal processing stream [PPC, FEF, and dorso-lateral prefrontal cortex (DLPFC)]. The results indicate a fundamental visual processing deficit of the dorsal stream network that is already noticeable at disease onset, even in the absence of marked cognitive demands (Braus et al., 2002). Subsequent fMRI studies examined the pathophysiological model supposed by Holzman and colleagues, proposing a circumscribed functional deficiency of V5 during visual motion perception. During the passive perception of moving visual

targets (Tost et al., 2003a), significantly enhanced activation of controls was found in posterior parietal areas, whereas activation differences in V5 were absent in patients.

The assumption of a deficient processing of motion signals in V5 is largely based on behavioral experiments indicating a significantly lower contrast sensitivity for the discrimination of small velocity differences in schizophrenia (Chen et al., 1999c). Studying this phenomenon in fMRI, Tost et al. (2003b, 2004) found significantly decreased activation of PPC and DLPFC in the patient group; activation differences in V5, however, could not be verified. These results point to a deficient processing of motion cues at a higher level of the dorsal visual network usually associated with executive functioning, the control of eye movements and the "top-down" control of lower visual cortices (Kastner et al., 1998, 1999; Ungerleider et al., 1998).

Selective attention

The neuropsychological term attention describes the selection and integration of relevant information units from the perceptual stream, requiring the complex interplay of different brain regions and functions. In schizophrenia research, scientific descriptions of attentional dysfunction can be traced back to the initial descriptions by Kraepelin and Bleuler. These disturbances are considered by some as promising cognitive endophenotypes of disease vulnerability since they precede disease onset, persist during remissions, and are also found in asymptomatic relatives (Gold & Thaker, 2002; Cornblatt & Malhotra, 2001; Egan et al., 2000).

The continuous performance test (CPT)—rather a terminological label than a standardized test device—is one of the most popular neuropsychological measures in schizophrenia research. The term encompasses a variety of tasks best summarized as requiring selective attention (typical task requirements: selective responses to certain targets, inhibition of inadequate reactions to non-targets, high rate of stimuli over a period of less than 10 min). Apart from simple choice reaction tasks (involving the selection of a certain target from an assortment of stimuli, CPT-X), more complex CPT versions with additional cognitive requirements can be distinguished. So-called "degraded CPTs" use blurred visual presentations to manipulate the perceptual requirements of the task (e.g., Siegel et al., 1995). Appropriate handling of contingent CPTs requires the additional monitoring of preceding task conditions. Due to their strong resemblance to 1-back tasks, these cognitive tests extend into the working memory domain (e.g., CPT-AX, CPT-IP, and CPT-double-T). Other CPT variants use interspersed distractors to assay impulse control; the resulting task demands are similar to classical cognitive interference tasks (e.g., Stroop). Thus, any assessment of functional imaging findings in this domain needs to carefully take the specific task arrangements into account.

So far, most functional imaging studies have used contingent CPTs to examine selective attention dysfunction in schizophrenia. Dorso-lateral prefrontal hypoactivation of the patient group is a widely replicated finding, likely due to the moderate working memory load of the tasks (MacDonald & Carter, 2003; Volz *et al.*, 1999). Barch *et al.* (2001) observed a comparable DLPFC dysfunction in neuroleptic-naïve patients as well, arguing against medication effects. Simple CPT choice-reaction tasks, however, were rarely investigated with fMRI. Only one study by Eyler *et al.* (2004) used a simple CPT paradigm, providing evidence for a right inferior frontal activation decrease in the patient group. The authors hypothesized that the unusual ventral lateral location of the group difference may be a consequence of the lower executive demands of their task (Eyler *et al.*, 2004).

An important neural interface of cognition, emotion, and behavioral control, the dorsal anterior cingulate gyrus (ACG), is prominently activated during the performance of cognitive interference tasks (Cohen *et al.*, 2000). Early PET studies already showed ACG hypoperfusion during interference in schizophrenia (Carter *et al.*, 1997). According to Yücel *et al.* (2002), the activation loss may coincide with the absence of a morphologically differentiated paracingulate gyrus in patients. Several studies conducted by Carter *et al.* (1999, 2001) demonstrated a comparatively specific (performance correlated) ACG dysfunction in schizophrenia. The authors extended their results into a framework encompassing computational models of prefrontal dopamine function (Braver *et al.*, 1999). An fMRI study conducted by Heckers *et al.* (2004) confirmed, even under comparable task performance conditions, an absence or abnormal localization of dorsal ACG activation in patients with schizophrenia. The described functional ACG results are supplemented by growing diffusion tensor imaging (DTI) evidence indicating disturbed integrity of the cingulate bundle (Sun *et al.*, 2003; Kubicki *et al.*, 2003). Although the total number of studies on this topic is still limited to date, current evidence for a structural and functional disturbance of the ACG in schizophrenia is convincing (Weiss *et al.*, 2003). Importantly, conflict monitoring of the anterior cingulate cortex (ACC) also extends to emotionally discordant stimuli, forming a bridge into the processing of emotion and social cognition (Park *et al.*, 2008).

Executive function (including working memory)

The institution and flexible adaptation of behavioral patterns depending on environmental demands is one of the main functions of the PFC. The high rate of so-called executive dysfunction, e.g., working memory abnormalities, thus argues for involvement of the prefrontal regions in the

pathogenesis of schizophrenia (Silver *et al.*, 2003; Glahn *et al.*, 2000; Gold *et al.*, 1997; Goldman-Rakic, 1994; see also Chapter 8). However, of course, executive function and working memory are not synonymous, nor is the PFC the only brain region implicated in these groups of cognitive faculties. Nevertheless, working memory paradigms have been among the first, and most studied, approaches that have consistently elicited abnormalities in schizophrenia. Unlike short-term memory, the working memory concept is aimed at the active storage of information necessary for the performance of cognitive operations, but not available from the environment. So-called "n-back" tasks are a popular neuropsychological instrument for the assessment of working memory dysfunction. Here, participants are required to constantly monitor a sequence of stimulus presentations and react to items that match the one presented n stimuli previously. These tasks are popular because working memory load can be increased parametrically by increasing the parameter "n" (1-back, 2-back, etc.) while keeping the stimulus and response conditions constant. Another popular measure of executive function is the Wisconsin Card Sorting Test (WCST), a complex task requiring abstract reasoning and cognitive flexibility in addition to working memory. Both instruments have been used extensively in imaging research to examine the neurobiological correlates of frontal lobe dysfunction in schizophrenia.

A recent review (Minzenberg *et al.*, 2009) surveyed 41 studies of "executive cognition", which primarily meant the delayed match-to-sample, n-back, AX-CPT, and Stroop tasks. Using activation likelihood estimation meta-analytic techniques, the authors concluded that the topography of the distributed network subserving executive function was not altered in patients who activated the DLPFC, ventro-lateral PFC (VLPFC), ACC, and thalamus similar to controls. However, patients showed quantitative abnormalities, namely hypoactivation, in the DLPFC, rostral ACC, left medio-dorsal nucleus thalamus, inferior parietal lobule, and occipital (mainly visual) areas. Since the DLPFC and ACC have been ascribed a critical role in top-down regulation during executive cognition, these findings are consistent with disrupted frontal-based top-down control, where the DLPFC performs executive "computations", including working memory maintenance and manipulation, while the ACC is involved in conflict monitoring present during information processing and modulates the level of DLPFC task-related engagement. Conversely, the left VLPFC and ventro-medial cortex, areas near the frontal pole, and supplementary and premotor areas showed relatively increased activation in patients. While there were differences between task types, the congruence both of the activation pattern and the abnormalities within it were more striking.

A variety of confounders that might provide alternative explanations for a disease-related abnormality in DLPFC function have been examined, but largely discounted.

Patients with schizophrenia display irregular activation patterns during working memory tasks regardless of performance level (Honey *et al.*, 2002), motivation (Berman *et al.*, 1988) or the particular stimulus material used (Tek *et al.*, 2002; Stevens *et al.*, 1998; Thermenos *et al.*, 2004; Spindler *et al.*, 1997). Importantly, comparable differences to those seen in patients with overt disease can also be observed in healthy siblings of patients with schizophrenia (Callicott *et al.*, 2004), indicating that DLPFC dysfunction has a place in the neurogenetic risk architecture of schizophrenia, and is an "intermediate" or "endo" phenotype, a concept discussed fully in Chapter 14. While both common and rare genetic variants certainly therefore contribute to the prefrontal functional deficit, the precise cellular- and systems-level steps leading to this point are still a matter of some debate. The great majority of early functional imaging studies, as well as the recent meta-analysis (Minzenberg *et al.*, 2009), indicated a DLPFC hypoactivation both at rest and during working memory performance (Paulman *et al.*, 1990; Andreasen *et al.*, 1997; Volz *et al.*, 1999). Nevertheless, discrepant results accumulated in the last several years, have made it necessary that the theory of a pure "hypofrontality" in schizophrenia had to be revised, or at least amended (Ramsey *et al.*, 2002; Manoach *et al.*, 1999, 2000), and should be replaced by a more nuanced model.

Several lines of evidence support the contention that the simple descriptive term of a hypo- or hyper-activation underestimates the real complexity of the issue (Callicott *et al.*, 2003). First, even in healthy subjects, for instance, DLPFC activation follows a complex and load-dependent course similar to an inverted-U function. According to this, prefrontal activation level increases with task demands until a capacity limit is reached, followed by DLPFC activation decrease concomitant with behavioral decompensation (as indicated by the corresponding increase of performance errors; Callicott *et al.*, 1999). A comparable relationship between working memory effort and amount of prefrontal neural discharge was observed in animal studies (Goldman-Rakic *et al.*, 2000). Second, some groups have observed an increase of activation as subjects exceed their capacity limit (Mattay *et al.*, 2003), arguing for an "(in)efficiency" concept where increased activation may be indicative of excessive and task-inadequate neuronal recruitment. A further complication is derived from the fact that neuroimaging data typically reflect a mapping of statistical significance levels representing composite measures of "signal" and "noise" (as measured by the mean shift in BOLD effect and the residual variance, respectively), which may correspond to differing neuronal phenomena in the context of working memory. Callicott and Manoach especially have attempted to reconcile discrepant findings in this domain in the context of more complex functional models (Callicott *et al.*, 2000; Manoach, 2003) that appear to be in good agreement with the currently available evidence.

Current pathophysiological theories therefore assume a deficient neural processing in patients with schizophrenia that may, depending on the current capacity reserve, manifest as prefrontal hyper- or hypo-activation, respectively. The course of the DLPFC activation level may thus correspond to a pathological left shift in the inverted-U load –response curve described above: patients may display a relatively enhanced prefrontal activation level under low cognitive load (hyperactivity subsequent to the inefficient use of neural resources), while the reverse may be found under increasing working memory demands (hypoactivity as a sign of neural capacity constraints) (Jansma *et al.*, 2004; Manoach *et al.*, 2000). A recent paper by Callicott *et al.* (2003) found group differences in DLPFC activation, supporting the pathophysiological model of a shifted inverted-U function in schizophrenia. However, findings not compatible with this model were noted, as well. The functional correlates of DLPFC dysfunction thus seem to manifest as a highly complex, capacity-dependent pattern of coincident hyper- and hypo-activity states. The main commonality of most studies seems to be less the directionality than the location of the abnormality, namely, the middle frontal gyrus and the corresponding Brodmann areas 46 and 9. More work will be necessary before a theoretical account can be reached that encompasses the current empirical data while remaining predictive enough to be potentially falsifiable.

An interesting strand of the literature confirmed by the recent meta-analysis (Minzenberg *et al.*, 2009) is that increased activation is observed in VLPFC in settings where impairment during executive cognition is signaled by DLPFC hypoactivation. Tan *et al.* (2007) have provided evidence indicating that this may reflect the compensatory recruitment of evolutionarily older, and computationally less sophisticated, ventro-lateral areas in a situation where the DLPFC signal-to-noise ratio is compromised. This clinical evidence is supported by cognitive neuroscience findings during memory tasks, which show a cognitive differentiation of VLPFC and DLPFC: activity in the VLPFC has been found to be increased in conditions that require the inhibition of irrelevant information and the selection of goal-relevant information, while DLPFC activation is increased when relationships must be processed amongst items that are active in memory.

Episodic memory

Together with executive dysfunction, impairments in episodic memory are among the most pronounced and studied neurocognitive deficits of schizophrenia. Basic cognitive neuroscience has identified a distributed neural system subserving episodic memory centered around the hippocampal formation (HF) and regions of the PFC. Abnormalities of the HF have been amply documented in schizophrenia (see Chapter 18), and a large body of work, starting with early lesion studies and underpinned by extensive imaging studies, has shown that the HF is necessary for successful episodic memory consolidation and retrieval, as well as for relational binding. Despite this compelling congruence, however, the episodic memory deficit in schizophrenia does not resemble the amnesia seen in pronounced medial temporal lobe damage. Rather, patients exhibit a pattern of difficulties reminiscent of deficient prefrontal contribution to episodic memory, such as reduced verbal fluency and ability to use semantic cues. A recent meta-analysis surveyed 18 studies of episodic memory in which patients and healthy controls were compared in a paradigm including a low-level baseline condition, with a combined sample of 123 patients with schizophrenia and 137 control subjects (Ragland *et al.*, 2009). An earlier meta-analysis used similar activation likelihood estimation meta-analytic techniques, but also included coordinates significant in region-of-interest (ROI) analyses (Achim & Lepage, 2005), leading to 18 studies being included in these surveys. The concordant results of these two studies primarily highlighted prefrontal abnormalities: reduced activation was found in both encoding and retrieval of episodic memory information in the DLPFC and VLPFC (and also in the frontal pole during encoding only). Hyperactivation in patients was found in some prefrontal regions in encoding and retrieval as well, notably in the left precentral and right medial frontal gyrus. While VLPFC abnormalities were related to task performance aspects, this was not the case for DLPFC, highlighting this region again as one where a core deficit in schizophrenia can be localized. The finding of "ventro-lateral sparing" is also in agreement with the theory, mentioned above in the context of executive function, that the VLPFC is able to perform some compensatory operations in the context of DLPFC compromise.

In contradistinction to the consistent prefrontal abnormalities, meta-analytic support for activation differences in the HF was inconsistent. While Ragland *et al.* (2009), including only coordinates reported from a whole-brain analysis, found no changes in the HF proper, the earlier meta-analysis (Achim & Lepage, 2005), which did include ROI analyses, did provide evidence for reduced HF activation in episodic memory tasks. In our estimation, this is likely because of the difficulty of achieving robust and reliable hippocampal activation in episodic memory tasks at a whole-brain level. However, there was consistent evidence in both analyses for relative increases in activation in the parahippocampal gyrus, on the left during encoding and the right during retrieval. This may reflect decreased deactivation relative to a resting baseline or an increased reliance on familiarity-based retrieval decisions, for which parahippocampal activity is thought to be decisive, over conscious recollection.

Emotional regulation

Emotional dysfunction has been regarded as a central feature of schizophrenia from the time of Kraeplin and Bleuler. Blunted affect is the typical clinical manifestation. It is strongly related to other negative symptoms as well as social dysfunction. After a period in which executive cognition stood at the center of interest in schizophrenia neuroimaging research, a large number of papers have examined the functional correlates of emotion processing in the disorder. Interest has focused on the amygdala, which has widely been regarded to be a key region of the emotional brain, which also includes the medial prefrontal and orbito-frontal cortex, anterior cingulate, and insula. Of 12 studies summarized in a recent review (Aleman & Kahn, 2005), a consistent picture emerges of reduced amygdala activation in patients with schizophrenia when emotional stimuli are compared to similar but neutral stimuli. This appears to be stable over time (Reske *et al.*, 2007). Similar conclusions were reached in a narrative review. While this reflects limbic hyporeactivity, the truth may be more complex. First, some studies reported normal findings when amygdala activation was examined relative to a low-level baseline. This suggests that amygdala activation to neutral stimuli might be abnormal in schizophrenia, in line with evidence that in normal controls, amygdala activation to neural faces is dependent on state anxiety. Intriguingly, a recent event-related study (Gur *et al.*, 2007), which also found reduced activation compared with controls, found that opposite to controls, greater limbic activation in patients predicted misidentifications of facial emotion and levels of flat affect. It would be of interest to investigate whether these findings are sensitive to medication or other state variables, since studies in healthy siblings of patients with schizophrenia indicate that amygdala dysfunction is not pronounced in this genetically high-risk group (Rasetti *et al.*, 2009).

Departing from these findings of regional dysfunction, recent interest has focused on the question of regulation of amygdala and the extended limbic system by the PFC, especially the medial PFC. A number of studies have demonstrated reduced functional connectivity between the medial PFC and amygdala in schizophrenia, suggesting a relative impairment of a key regulatory circuit for fear expression and extinction that has also been implicated in genetic mechanisms related to gene–environment interactions and might therefore contribute to the pathophysiology of peristatic stressors implicated in schizophrenia, such as expressed emotion. Fakra *et al.* (2008) found inverse functional connectivity between medial PFC and amygdala in healthy controls, but not in patients, and Das *et al.* (2007) reported multiple qualitative abnormalities in amygdala connectivity in patients.

Impaired emotional processing also extends into more complex social cognition, e.g., judgments of trustworthiness. Here, reduced neural activation in the right amygdala, fusiform face area, and left VLPFC was found in patients with chronic schizophrenia (Pinkham *et al.*, 2008), and similarly in the medial orbito-frontal cortex, amygdale, and the right insula in another study (Baas *et al.*, 2008).

Reward and salience processing and delusions

In an influential hypothesis paper, Kapur (2003) proposed that a dysregulated, hyperdopaminergic state, which leads to an aberrant assignment of salience to the elements of perception, is a mechanism leading from dopaminergic dysfunction to the clinical picture and antipsychotic treatment of schizophrenia. Antipsychotics supposedly "dampen the salience" of these abnormal experiences and by doing so permit the resolution of symptoms. Data from laboratory animals indicate that prediction errors are signaled by midbrain dopamine neurons (Schultz, 1998). These neurons send dense projections to the basal ganglia and PFC, forming the mesocortico-limbic dopamine system. From this work, the major locations of the salience/ error prediction signal are in the midbrain, ventral striatum, and right DLPFC (Corlett *et al.*, 2007). A dysregulation of the error prediction signal has in fact been demonstrated in a number of imaging studies in schizophrenia (Murray *et al.*, 2008; Corlett *et al.*, 2007), as well as under the psychotomimetic drug, ketamine. Their data provide support for associative models of delusion formation, in which dysfunction of the mesocorticolimbic dopamine system causes delusion formation via disrupted prediction-error signaling, establishing a link between dopaminergic dysfunction and symptomatology, whereby abnormally increased, possibly strongly stochastic or even chaotic activity of the prediction error signaling system may abnormally imbue percepts with salience/perceptual significance leading into a state of delusional beliefs. An interesting example is hyperactivation to neutral face expressions in schizophrenia (Seiferth *et al.*, 2008). Blackwood *et al.* (2004) found absence of anterior cingulate activation during self-referential statements in patients with schizophrenia and persecutory delusions, indicating deficiencies in cognitive control in this domain.

As opposed to perceptual salience, response to direct (e.g., monetary) rewards seems to be reduced in schizophrenia, associated with medication status (with typical antipsychotics dampening the response more than atypical) and negative symptoms. In the initial study of the phenomenon, Juckel *et al.* (2006b) observed reduced activation of the ventral striatum to monetary reward in unmedicated patients, a finding that correlated with negative symptoms. No group differences (but some correlations with psychopathology) were seen in a small medicated

patient sample by Simon *et al.* (2010). Schlagenhauf *et al.* (2009) studied avoidance of adverse consequences (monetary loss) and found reduced activation to successful *versus* unsuccessful avoidance of loss in the ventral striatum in patients. Increased severity of delusions in patients with schizophrenia was associated with a decrease in medial PFC activation elicited by successful *versus* unsuccessful avoidance of loss, and functional connectivity between the medial PFC and the ventral striatum was reduced, suggesting abnormalities of prefrontal regulation of the reward system in schizophrenia. Walter *et al.* (2009) also identified primarily prefrontal hypoactivation in patients in a monetary reward paradigm. Several studies provide a bridge from striatal incentive signaling to learning in schizophrenia. A hypoactivation in the putamen, dorsal cingulate, and superior frontal cortex was also observed in patients during reinforcement-based learning (Koch *et al.*, 2010). In a passive conditioning paradigm, Waltz *et al.* (2009) studied the temporal difference response and found reduced activation in the putamen to unexpected positive reinforcers.

Social cognition/theory of mind

There is now clear evidence that social cognition is impaired in schizophrenia (Couture *et al.*, 2006; Green & Leitman, 2008) and in people at risk for schizophrenia (Chung *et al.*, 2008), somewhat independently of other cognitive dysfunctions (van Hooren *et al.*, 2008). Social dysfunction is a major predictor of adjustment and quality of life in schizophrenia. The social brain hypothesis of schizophrenia has even put forward (Burns, 2005; Brune & Brune-Cohrs, 2006) that psychosis comes as a costly by-product of social brain evolution.

While several domains of social cognition have been distinguished, most imaging research has focused on mentalizing/theory of mind (ToM), e.g., in properly distinguishing the intention of others and one's own, or to "see" intentions where there are none, can explain characteristic symptoms of schizophrenia-like paranoid delusions (Frith, 1992; Harrington *et al.*, 2005). A recent formal meta-analysis of behavioral ToM studies in schizophrenia (29 studies, n = 1518) found a large overall effect size for mentalizing deficits (d = –1.255; p < 0.0001) with large effect sizes in each and every study (range –0.64–2.3) which was not significantly affected by sample characteristics (Sprong *et al.*, 2007).

The neural network active during mentalizing tasks is well known from neuroimaging studies in healthy controls and encompasses the medial (and lateral) PFC, the precuneus/posterior cingulate, the superior temporal sulcus/temporo-parietal junction, and the anterior temporal poles (Ciaramidaro *et al.*, 2007). Several studies in schizophrenia have investigated neural activation during ToM tasks (Brunet-Gouet & Decety, 2006; Marjoram *et al.*, 2006;

Brune *et al.*, 2008; Andreasen *et al.*, 2008; Walter, 2009). Mainly, these tasks have highlighted abnormalities in the medial PFC, temporo-parietal junction, and amygdala. While amygdala activation deficits mainly relate to emotional processing components of these tasks (Brunet-Gouet & Decety, 2006), discussed more fully above, abnormal activation of prefrontal and temporo-parietal structures are more likely related to mentalizing proper. Reduced activation in patients was found in either the right (Andreasen *et al.*, 2008) or left (Brunet *et al.*, 2003) inferior or bilateral (Marjoram *et al.*, 2006) PFC, or in a cortico-cerebellar circuit (left PFC, right cerebellum) (Russell *et al.*, 2000). In paranoid patients, two key regions of the ToM network were significantly less activated in the patient group, namely the dorso-medial PFC and the temporo-parietal cortex bilaterally (Walter, 2009). Links between social cognition and emotional processing are discussed above. The involvement of the PFC points to links with executive cognition and cognitive control as well; confirming this, a study comparing patients before and after recovery with a working memory task (WCST) found that social cognitive performance correlated with PFC activation (Lee *et al.*, 2006). Prefrontal activation during ToM was related to the presence or absence of positive symptoms (Marjoram *et al.*, 2006).

Hallucinations

The perception of voices in the absence of external stimuli (auditory hallucinations) is one of the cardinal symptoms of schizophrenia. Cognitive models first suggested underlying abnormalities in the processing of inner speech, a notion not supported by functional imaging studies. Instead, in the last 15 years, empirical evidence repeatedly indicated structural and functional disturbances of the superior temporal gyrus (STG), a crucial part of the network controlling the perception and production of speech. A close relationship between the severity of auditory hallucinations and the extent of STG volume reduction, for instance, was already found in 1990 by Bartha *et al.* Functional imaging results provided by the groups of Schnorr, Murray, and Woodruff (1995, 1997) demonstrated a pronounced activity enhancement of auditory and speech processing cortices during hallucinatory experiences (Heschl's gyrus, Broca and Wernicke area) (Silbersweig *et al.*, 1995; McGuire *et al.*, 1993, 1995; Woodruff *et al.*, 1995, 1997). A particularly convincing study was conducted by Dierks *et al.* (1999), demonstrating the potential of event-related fMRI study designs for psychiatric research. From a neuroscientific point of view, these results yield a plausible explanation for the fact that patients accept the internally generated voices as real.

Consistent with the proposal of a regional disconnection syndrome contributing to the symptomatology of schizo-phrenia, current fMRI, DTI, and morphometric imaging data indicate a correlation of hallucination severity with the extent of the functional and structural connectivity abnormalities of the STG (Lawrie *et al.*, 2002; Gaser *et al.*, 2004; Hubl *et al.*, 2004). Furthermore, these alterations have been shown to interfere with the cortical processing of regular auditory stimuli in schizophrenia, as well. An fMRI study of Wible *et al.* (2001), for example, provided evidence for a dysfunctional processing of mismatch stimuli (a descriptive term for the presentation of differing tones embedded in a series of standard tones) in the primary auditory cortex. Other fMRI studies point to a diminished response of the temporal lobes to external speech during hallucinatory experiences (Woodruff *et al.*, 1997; David *et al.*, 1996). This phenomenon is usually explained as the competition of physiological and pathological processes for limited neural processing capacity.

Imaging treatment effects

The psychopharmacology of schizophrenia has progressed in the last 10 years, focusing on the development of novel antipsychotic drugs with an atypical effect profile (e.g., clozapine, amisulpride, olanzapine). Some studies indicate that, compared to typical neuroleptic drugs (e.g., haloperidol), these substances may be superior with regard to the treatment of negative symptoms and cognitive deficits (Meltzer *et al.*, 1994; Meltzer & McGurk, 1999), although recent large-scale trials have largely not confirmed this (Lieberman *et al.*, 2005), but see Kahn *et al.* (2008), and Chapter 8. Even if differential efficacy is in doubt, the absence of substantial extrapyramidal side effects in second-generation antipsychotics (SGAs) is a definite improvement in patient quality of life in many cases. Until the mid-1990s, research on antipsychotic drug effects was mainly limited to behavioral experiments (Nestor *et al.*, 1991; Lieberman *et al.*, 1994; Zahn *et al.*, 1994). MRI studies examining structural, functional, and metabolic correlates of antipsychotic drug treatment emerged at the turn of the last century (Ende *et al.*, 2000; Heitmiller *et al.*, 2004; Arango *et al.*, 2003; Bertolino *et al.*, 2001; Braus *et al.*, 2001).

To date, the majority of fMRI studies in this field have been aimed at drug-induced changes of voluntary motor control, reward/salience tasks, and executive functioning. In this context, favorable effects of atypical antipsychotics on putative functional disturbances in schizophrenia have been repeatedly reported (Ramsey *et al.*, 2002).

In voluntary motor control (finger-tapping task), compared to drug-naïve patients, SGAs reduced activity in the supplementary motor area and first-generation antipsychotics (FGAs) additionally in the primary motor cortex (Braus *et al.*, 1999). In a longitudinal study, Stephan *et al.* (2001) found that olanzapine partially "normalized" (made more similar to a sample of healthy controls scanned with the same protocol) functional connectivity between the PFC and cerebellum in a small sample (n = 6) of patients. A recent study by Bertolino et al. (2004a) also showed a normalization of sensorimotor hypoactivation in the course of olanzapine treatment.

With regard to reward processing, since antipsychotics are expected to dampen the reward system through D_2 blockade, the observation is of interest that patients switched from typical neuroleptics to olanzapine showed an increase in their ventral striatal reward response (Schlagenhauf et al., 2008a), a finding similar to that obtained by Kirsch et al. (2007) and Juckel et al. (2006a) in a cross-sectional comparison of patients treated with typical or atypical drugs. That even atypical antipsychotics dampen the ventral striatal response somewhat is suggested by a study of single-dose olanzapine in healthy volunteers who demonstrated reduced reward-related brain activation in the ventral striatum, anterior cingulate, and inferior frontal cortex (Abler et al., 2007).

With regard to emotion processing, results on quetiapine by Fahim et al. (2005) and Stip et al. (2005) are difficult to interpret because of the passive viewing methodology used, but results, which the authors relate to blunted affect, were felt to be broadly consistent with increased lateral prefrontal activation after SGA treatment.

In executive functioning, several studies suggest at least partially beneficial treatment effects. Prefrontal functions especially showed some degree of normalization with atypical (but not typical) antipsychotic drug treatment (Braus et al., 1999, 2000a,b,c; Honey et al., 1999). An important study was provided by Honey et al. (1999), who studied two cohorts (n = 10 each) of patients with schizophrenia longitudinally with a verbal working memory task. One cohort was treated with an FGA throughout, while the other was switched to an SGA (risperidone) after baseline assessment. The results showed that the latter group of patients had increased functional activation in critical nodes of the executive cognition network: the right PFC, supplementary motor area, and PPC. In general agreement with these findings, a cross-sectional comparison of patients on long-acting risperidone compared to patients on a FGA and controls observed VLPFC underactivation only in the FGA group, making the SGA group "more normal" in lateral prefrontal activation (Surguladze et al., 2007). A similar directionality of effects, that did not however reach accepted levels of significance, was also observed in patients studied longitudinally with the n-back task before and after treatment with the SGA quetiapine (Meisenzahl et al., 2006). Using a verbal fluency task, Jones et al. (2004) also found that quetiapine increased lateral prefrontal activation compared to the drug-naïve state. In contrast, a longitudinal switch study to olanzapine found no effect on working memory-related activation in the PFC (Schlagenhauf et al., 2008b), but observed increased BOLD response during the attentional control (0-back) condition. In effective connectivity, a cross-sectional study using the n-back task indicated that the SGA olanzapine increased interhemispheric connectivity (Schlosser et al., 2003a).

A conclusive picture has not emerged from imaging results on antipsychotic drug effects conducted to date. The number of scientific publications on this topic is still small and methodologically required study designs (e.g., double-blind) are almost completely lacking. Given the cross-sectional design of the majority of the studies, the conclusion of a "normalizing" or "restoring" drug effect—drawn by some authors from reductions or absence of fMRI group differences—must remain tentative. However, it is fair to say that the localization of drug effects in the lateral PFC and ventral striatum does argue for dopaminergic effects at the level of the cortex that agree with current theorizing about the importance of that region in schizophrenia even when the directionality is not consistent. Consistent directionality is in any case difficult to expect when even the directionality of the main task activation effects, as reviewed above, is not consistent, and especially when SGAs form a pharmacologically very heterogeneous group. Furthermore, even in longitudinal study designs, a demonstration of functional recovery is conditional on the reliable and valid characterization of the underlying pathology. Future fMRI studies with more complex study designs will certainly be capable of dissolving this apparent heterogeneity (e.g., double-blind investigation of genetically-defined responder groups). The identification of moderating factors, especially genetic factors, promises progress in this area, e.g., data indicating an association of functional and clinical improvement with the catechol-O-methyl transferase (*COMT*) genotype are major steps in this future direction (Bertolino et al., 2004b).

Imaging systems: connectivity

Investigation of connectivity closely coincides with the perspective of schizophrenia as a disturbance of integration that has been discussed since Wernicke, and accords with neuropathological data showing a reduction in cortical neuropil and synaptic density (see Chapter 18), as well as with evidence from structural data such as DTI (Chapter 16). Even more so than in studies of regional activation, the study of connectivity in functional neuroimaging data use a wide array of methods that can be bewildering. At one end of the spectrum, correlation over time between two brain regions has emerged as a useful metric of functional coupling and has come to be called "functional connectivity". It is clear that functional connectivity between two brain regions or voxels does not imply that these regions are in fact anatomically connected, because the correlation observed could be due to both regions being driven by a third one (the thalamus, say). Even if two regions are in fact anatomically connected, the functional interaction need not be linear. Finally, correlation never implies causality or even directionality of the influence of one brain region over another. Nevertheless, functional connectivity has emerged as an eminently useful and computationally tractable metric of neural interactions measured using neuroimaging. Psychophysical interaction (PPI) analyses extend the logic of interregional functional connectivity to studying the effects of a moderating variable, such as task condition or the activity of a third brain region, on functional connectivity measures. Another important extension of functional connectivity is going from pairs of connected regions or voxels to a multivariate perspective that allows the extraction of systems of areas that are coupled functionally. A number of methods, such as principal components analysis (PCA), canonical variates analysis (CVA), independent component analysis (ICA), and others, are available and have been used in schizophrenia neuroimaging.

If connectivity measures are derived from methods that do allow a statement about directionality, they are called "effective connectivity". Two such methods are structural equation modeling (SEM) and dynamic causal modeling (DCM). Both of these require the investigator to prespecify a model of how the brain regions are hypothesized to be connected and then provide effective connectivity measures for the interactions (paths) in the model, provided the model is compatible with the data. The need to prespecify a model is a substantial drawback of these methods because currently available data usually do not constrain the range of possible models enough and "tinkering" with the model to improve fit with the data causes problems in statistical inference. However, it is possible to derive well-fitting models directly from the data, although this requires additional validation steps. While SEM is a widely used method in the social sciences as well, DCM is specific to neuroimaging in specifying the model at the level of neural interactions and then coupling it with a forward model that determines how neural activity is reflected in the neuroimaging modality used (for fMRI, this includes a balloon model of the generation of the BOLD response through neurovascular coupling). If images are acquired fast enough (TR is low), temporal precedence information can also be exploited to map effective connectivity using an approach called Granger causality. This does not require the user to specify a model. This method has, however, not been applied to schizophrenia at the time of writing.

Finally, methods from topology have begun to be applied to global connectivity properties of brain functional and structural networks (Bullmore & Sporns, 2009). One conclusion emerging from this work is that the human brain shares topological properties with other complex systems (such as the Internet) that support an efficient and robust transfer of information while keeping wiring between regions low. This so-called economical "small world"

property of functional brain networks derived from fMRI data may be altered in schizophrenia: for example, clustering of local connections was reduced in fMRI brain networks measured in patients with schizophrenia (Liu et al., 2008). Recent studies have also demonstrated abnormal network hierarchy, wiring cost, and cost-efficiency in anatomical networks derived from structural MRI data (Bassett et al., 2008), and functional networks derived from motor evoked response (MEG) data recorded during a working memory task (Bassett et al., 2009) in patients with schizophrenia. Abnormalities of adult brain network organization related to schizophrenia would be expected to follow aberrant early brain development (Ridler et al., 2006), but we currently know little about the normal development of brain functional networks or how this might be perturbed preclinically in individuals at high risk of meeting diagnostic criteria later in life.

Currently, no meta-analysis of connectivity in schizophrenia is available. The literature up to this point indicates that both abnormally increased and decreased connectivity is observed in schizophrenia, depending on the system studied and the cognitive state of the probands. Instead of the earlier hypothesis of a uniform disruption, or disconnectivity, in schizophrenia the picture that emerges from these studies is rather that of "disconnectivity": functional interactions between brain regions are disturbed in schizophrenia, but in a regionally and functionally differentiated manner that must be viewed against the functional status of the systems affected. We will therefore review this primary literature with a focus on some of the key cortical nodes and cortico-subcortical loops or circuits that are likely to be most disconnected in schizophrenia: the PFC, medial and lateral temporal cortex, anterior cingulate cortex, and cerebellar–thalamic–prefrontal circuits.

Prefrontal connectivity

The literature has focused on connectivity of the PFC, especially the DLPFC and anterior cingulate. Regarding the DLPFC, two systems have been studied most: the interaction with the medial temporal lobe, specifically the HF, and the interaction with the cerebellum and thalamus. The first system, interactions with the HF, is an attractive target for schizophrenia research since the HF provides important input to the DLPFC (Goldman-Rakic et al., 1984) and neonatal HF lesions in animals induce postpubertally-manifested changes in the PFC (Lipska & Weinberger, 2000), mimicking aspects of schizophrenic pathophysiology. It has been hypothesized that the interaction between these two regions might be particularly disturbed in the disorder (Weinberger et al., 1992, Honey et al., 2005). This so-called fronto-hippocampal "disconnection" hypothesis (Lawrie et al., 2002) is also attractive since the HF is selectively vulnerable to some obstetrical insults (Schmidt-Kastner & Freund, 1991) and a disturbed interaction with the DLPFC would, thus, offer an explanation for the epidemiological data linking schizophrenia to early neurodevelopmental disturbances (Weinberger, 1987). Similarly, the examination of connectivity with the cerebellum is suggested by the "cognitive dysmetria" hypothesis of Andreasen et al. (1998), which is characterized cognitively by a disruption in control and coordination processes, and functionally by abnormal interregional connectivity within the cortico–cerebellar–thalamo–cortical circuit (CCTCC). For the DLPFC, abnormal connectivity during working memory has been identified consistently in patients with schizophrenia and subjects at risk (Wolf et al., 2009; Crossley et al., 2009; Whitfield-Gabrieli et al., 2009; Spoletini et al., 2009; Ragland et al., 2007). One consistent finding here is impaired interhemispheric prefrontal connectivity in patients (Schlosser et al., 2003a,b), which agrees well with functional evidence for reduced transcallosal inhibition during transcranial magnetic stimulation (TMS) (Fitzgerald et al., 2002; Boroojerdi et al., 1999) and structural evidence (see Chapters 16 and 18).

Hippocampal connectivity

Interactions between the hippocampal formation and lateral PFC are essential for episodic memory retrieval, but may be deleterious in working memory, where it is advantageous *not* to encode the presented items in long-term memory in order to avoid potential interference effects. Therefore, disconnectivity of the hippocampal formation could be hypothesized with cognitive state during memory processing, a prediction that is in good agreement with the available data. Decreased connectivity of the HF during episodic memory encoding (Wolf et al., 2007) and at rest (Zhou et al., 2008) has in fact been observed in patients. Conversely, during working memory, using functional connectivity in PET data, Meyer-Lindenberg et al. (2005) observed a significant dysfunctional increase in the connectivity of the HF: patients and controls exhibited the same pattern of connectivity to the contralateral DLPFC during a sensorimotor control task, but the imposition of a working memory load led to a group difference: while HF–DLPFC connectivity was attenuated in healthy subjects, the functional linkage between these regions persisted undiminished in patients, compatible with a failure to modulate HF–DLPFC linkage and lack of HF/DLPFC compartmentalization. A similar finding using ICA and fMRI (Wolf et al., 2009) was that in patients, functional connectivity indices in the left DLPFC and the right hippocampal cortex were positively correlated with accuracy during the task, while the connectivity strengths in the right DLPFC were negatively correlated with measures of symptom severity, suggesting increased and persistent DLPFC and hippocampal connectivity during working memory performance. Extending these results to the beginning of manifest disease, a similar abnormal increase in

prefrontal–temporal connectivity was found in subjects with first-episode psychosis (Crossley et al., 2009). More broadly, reduced fronto-temporal connectivity was also found to be related to auditory hallucinations (Lawrie et al., 2002).

Cerebellar–thalamic–prefrontal connectivity

Honey et al. (2005) observed a reduction of a task-specific relationship between the medial superior frontal gyrus and both the anterior cingulate and cerebellum in patients. A similar decreased connectivity between the right medial prefrontal regions and the contralateral cerebellum was also observed in subjects at high risk for schizophrenia (Whalley et al., 2005). In another study, patients showed increases in thalamo-cortical connectivity, while prefrontal–cerebellar and the cerebellar–thalamic connectivity was reduced (Schlosser et al., 2003a). Thalamo-cortical connectivity in patients was also modulated by nicotine (Jacobsen et al., 2004), and cerebellar–prefrontal connectivity by treatment with olanzapine (Stephan et al., 2001). Cerebellar and prefrontal systems were abnormal in structural MRI data for patients in the Northern Finland Birth Cohort and this was related to prospectively assessed delays in early infant motor development (Ridler et al., 2006), suggesting that abnormal configuration of prefronto-cerebellar systems might be an imaging marker of slow motor skills acquisition and at-risk neurodevelopment for later psychosis.

Anterior cingulate

Given the relevance of the anterior cingulate for cognitive control and the activation differences found in this structure (see above), the connectivity of this region has been the subject of several studies. Functional disconnectivity of the anterior cingulate during cognitive challenge paradigms was observed by Honey et al. (2005) and others (Spence et al., 2000; Fletcher et al., 1999), and has also been found during the resting state (Zhou et al., 2008).

Multivariate characterizations of connectivity

Multivariate approaches are useful to investigate entire brain systems characterized by abnormal connectivity, avoiding *a priori* hypotheses about which regions to study. In an investigation using PET data acquired during a working memory paradigm analyzed using canonical variants, Meyer-Lindenberg et al. (2001) found that the difference in connectivity between patients and controls was largely accounted for by a single pattern showing inferotemporal, (para-)hippocampal, and cerebellar loadings for patients *versus* DLPFC and anterior cingulate activity for comparison subjects. Similarly, an array of abnormalities in prefrontal–temporal interactions were found by Friston et al. (1996). This result was validated prospectively by successfully classifying unrelated scans from the same patients and data from a new cohort. Multivariate analyses using

ICA have uncovered different spatial distributions of the connectivity-defined resting state network in schizophrenia, with abnormalities most notably in the frontal, anterior cingulate, and parahippocampal gyri (Garrity *et al.*, 2007; Zhou *et al.*, 2008). Interestingly, within the resting state network, the strength of correlations was recently found to be increased, but more variable relative to controls (Jafri *et al.*, 2008), a finding confirmed and extended to subjects at risk by Whitfield-Gabrieli *et al.* (2009).

Not all system specificity involves failure to function. A set of observations from different laboratories indicates increased connectivity of the VLPFC (Tan *et al.*, 2006). This may indicate a compensatory circuit for DLPFC dysfunction, since VLPFC, while evolutionarily older and less capable of complex executive functions, is nevertheless able to fulfil some of the operations usually assigned to DLPFC in the context of working memory, such as maintenance. Of interest, similar changes of connectivity are observed in healthy subjects carrying risk genes for schizophrenia. Also, it should be noted frankly that the key nodes and systems are discussed here separately for didactic reasons, but will interact extensively and in many different configurations, and that this dynamic interaction may be relevant for the pathophysiology of schizophrenia. For example, abnormal cingulate function has been found to modulate prefrontal–temporal interactions (Fletcher *et al.*, 1999).

Studies in relatives and high-risk populations

Neuroimaging studies in overt disease are open to objections that any abnormalities found might be confounded by disease-associated factors, such as impaired social and economic functioning, medication status, and hospitalization history. Furthermore, given that epidemiological evidence clearly shows that aspects of the schizophrenic pathophysiology predate the onset of manifest illness by years, the study of high-risk, but not (yet) manifestly ill, populations is an important strategy to uncover core, unconfounded aspects of schizophrenia susceptibility. Given that the majority of disease risk is genetic, a major approach here has been to study subjects known to have an enriched set of schizophrenia susceptibility genes, such as siblings or children of patients with schizophrenia. Positive findings in this group are relevant for genetic studies, because an imaging phenotype enriched in genetically high-risk subjects strengthens the status of that phenotype as intermediate between genetic risk and overt disease (see Chapter 14). In addition to this genetic approach, it is possible to clinically define a population at high risk (which will then again be largely due to genetic factors) which is composed of individuals with clinical features such as attenuated psychotic symptoms, brief limited

intermittent psychotic symptoms (BLIPS) or a recent decline in functioning, characteristics that significantly increase the risk for imminent onset of psychosis. This has been termed the "at risk mental state" (ARMS), a concept that overlaps with that of the schizophrenia prodrome (Yung *et al.*, 1998). The risk of progressing to overt disease is different in these populations: while the prevalence in the general population is around 1%, first-degree relatives of patients with schizophrenia have an approximately 10-fold increased risk and at-risk monozygotic twins a 40–50% increased risk, and in ARMS subjects the probability of developing psychosis is around 40% (see Chapter 6 for discussion of the prodrome).

A recent meta-analysis of fMRI studies in high-risk populations identified 24 papers up to 2007 (Fusar-Poli *et al.*, 2007). The majority of studies used working memory or other executive cognition paradigms. In fMRI studies, vulnerability to psychosis was associated with medium-to-large effect sizes when prefrontal activation (in the DLPFC, but also the VLPFC) was compared with that in controls. In general, the prefrontal response was intermediate to that seen in manifest illness. While studies in first-episode patients showed similar inconsistencies in the directionality of activation differences to those discussed above for working memory in general, presently available evidence using working memory tasks in healthy siblings shows concordant evidence of hyperactivation in DLPFC (Callicott *et al.*, 2003; Rasetti *et al.*, 2009; Thermenos *et al.*, 2004; Seidman *et al.*, 2006; Woodward *et al.*, 2009), the sole exception being the study of Keshavan *et al.* (2002), which however used a memory-guided saccade test. During episodic memory, increased prefrontal activation in siblings was observed (Bonner-Jackson *et al.*, 2007). Regarding basic emotion processing, a small group of relatives studied by Habel *et al.* (2004) showed reduced amygdala and cingulate activity, while no such finding emerged from a recent better-powered study (Rasetti *et al.*, 2009).

An increasing number of studies have addressed connectivity in subjects at risk. By and large, the findings obtained mirror those found in overt disease, strengthening the case for disturbed connectivity as an intermediate phenotype. Reduced interhemispheric connectivity has been shown in healthy relatives, pointing towards a genetic component of disturbed interhemispheric connectivity in schizophrenia, using TMS (Saka *et al.*, 2005) and during fMRI in a working memory/choice reaction paradigm (Woodward *et al.*, 2009). Abnormally increased connectivity between the PFC and hippocampus during working memory has been observed in subjects in the ARMS (Crossley *et al.*, 2009), again mirroring findings in overt disease (Meyer-Lindenberg *et al.*, 2005). Increased connectivity to the parietal lobe during a sentence completion paradigm was observed by Whalley *et al.* (2005), similar to findings in patients (Tan *et al.*, 2006). Disrupted functional connectivity between the PFC and the precuneus was observed in obligate carriers while performing a verbal fluency task (Spence *et al.*, 2000). Our own work indicates that abnormal connectivity between the amygdala and cingulate, implicated in emotional regulation, may not be present in healthy siblings (Rasetti *et al.*, 2009). However, Habel *et al.* (2004) found reduced amydgala activation in unaffected brothers of patients, although in a small sample (n = 13). Finally, abnormalities in the default mode network mirroring those found in patients with overt disease were found in their relatives: decreased task-related suppression of default mode areas, especially the medial PFC, and increased connectivity within the default mode network (Whitfield-Gabrieli *et al.*, 2009).

Conclusions

A large literature has identified definite neural processing abnormalities using functional neuroimaging in schizophrenia. Abnormalities in PFC activation, which were the first-described and remain the most studied process, have been reliably confirmed and linked to memory function and theory of mind, but the directionality of the effects are not consistent and compensatory mechanisms within the lateral PFC can be identified. The prefrontal response has also been linked to genetic and clinical risk for psychosis and responds, although inconsistently, to medication. In comparison, reliable abnormalities in the hippocampal formation have not been consistently shown. Emotional stimuli elicit reduced activation of amygdala in schizophrenia. Striatal and brainstem reactivity to perceptually salient stimuli may be increased, while response to rewarding stimuli is reduced. This salience system is also responsive to medication with antipsychotic drugs. Hallucinations have been linked to abnormal activity of the lateral temporal lobe. In addition to these localized abnormalities, increasing evidence points to the fact that distributed neural processing in schizophrenia is profoundly abnormal. In these circuits, the PFC again plays a prominent role, but now as a key node of large-scale complex networks that typically also include temporal and anterior cingulate cortex and prefronto–subcortical circuits.

References

Abler, B., Erk, S. & Walter, H. (2007) Human reward system activation is modulated by a single dose of olanzapine in healthy subjects in an event-related, double-blind, placebo-controlled fMRI study. *Psychopharmacology (Berlin)* **191**, 823–833.

Achim, A.M. & Lepage, M. (2005) Episodic memory-related activation in schizophrenia: meta-analysis. *British Journal of Psychiatry* **187**, 500–509.

Aleman, A. & Kahn, R.S. (2005) Strange feelings: do amygdala abnormalities dysregulate the emotional brain in schizophrenia. *Progress in Neurobiology* **77**, 283–298.

Andreasen, N.C., O'Leary, D.S., Flaum, M. *et al.* (1997) Hypofrontality in schizophrenia: distributed dysfunctional circuits in neuroleptic-naive patients. *Lancet* **349**, 1730–1734.

Andreasen, N.C., Paradiso, S. & O'Leary, D.S. (1998) "Cognitive dysmetria" as an integrative theory of schizophrenia: a dysfunction in cortical-subcortical-cerebellar circuitry? *Schizophrenia Bulletin* **24**, 203–218.

Andreasen, N.C., Calage, C.A. & O'Leary, D.S. (2008) Theory of mind and schizophrenia: a positron emission tomography study of medication-free patients. *Schizophrenia Bulletin* **34**, 708–719.

Arango, C., Breier, A., McMahon, R., Carpenter, W.T. & Buchanan, R.W. (2003) The relationship of clozapine and haloperidol treatment response to prefrontal, hippocampal and caudate brain volumes. *American Journal of Psychiatry* **160**, 1421–1427.

Baas, D., Aleman, A., Vink, M., Ramsey, N.F., De Haan, E.H. & Kahn, R.S. (2008) Evidence of altered cortical and amygdala activation during social decision-making in schizophrenia. *Neuroimage* **40**, 719–727.

Barch, D.M., Carter, C.S., Braver, T.S. *et al.* (2001) Selective deficits in prefrontal cortex function in medication-naive patients with schizophrenia. *Archives of General Psychiatry* **58**, 280–288.

Bassett, D.S., Bullmore, E., Verchinski, B.A., Mattay, V.S., Weinberger, D.R. & Meyer-Lindberg, A. (2008) Hierarchical organization of human cortical networks in health and schizophrenia. *Journal of Neuroscience* **28**, 9239–9248.

Bassett, D.S., Bullmore, E., Meyer-Lindenberg, A., Apud, J.A., Weinberger, D.R. & Coppola, R. (2009) Cognitive fitness of cost-efficient brain functional networks. *Proceedings of the National Academy of Science USA* **106**, 11747–11752.

Berman, K.F., Illowsky, B.P. & Weinberger, D.R. (1988) Physiological dysfunction of dorsolateral prefrontal cortex in schizophrenia. IV. Further evidence for regional and behavioral specificity. *Archives of General Psychiatry* **45**, 616–622.

Bertolino, A., Callicott, J.H., Mattay, V.S. *et al.* (2001) The effect of treatment with antipsychotic drugs on brain N-acetylaspartate measures in patients with schizophrenia. *Biological Psychiatry* **49**, 39–46.

Bertolino, A., Blasi, G., Caforio, G., *et al.* (2004a) Functional lateralization of the sensorimotor cortex in patients with schizophrenia: effects of treatment with olanzapine. *Biological Psychiatry* **56**, 190–197.

Bertolino, A., Caforio, G., Blasi, G. *et al.* (2004b) Interaction of COMT (Val(108/158)Met) genotype and olanzapine treatment on prefrontal cortical function in patients with schizophrenia. *American Journal of Psychiatry* **161**, 1798–1805.

Blackwood, N.J., Bentall, R.P., Ffytche, D.H., Simmons, A., Murray, R.M. & Howard, R.J. (2004) Persecutory delusions and the determination of self-relevance: an fMRI investigation. *Psychological Medicine* **34**, 591–596.

Bonner-Jackson, A., Csernansky, J.G. & Barch, D.M. (2007) Levels-of-processing effects in first-degree relatives of individuals with schizophrenia. *Biological Psychiatry* **61**, 1141–1147.

Boroojerdi, B., Topper, R., Foltys, H. & Meincke, U. (1999) Transcallosal inhibition and motor conduction studies in patients with schizophrenia using transcranial magnetic stimulation. *British Journal of Psychiatry* **175**, 375–379.

Braff, D.L. & Saccuzzo, D.P. (1981) Information processing dysfunction in paranoid schizophrenia: a two- factor deficit. *American Journal of Psychiatry* **138**, 1051–1056.

Braff, D.L. & Saccuzzo, D.P. (1985) The time course of information-processing deficits in schizophrenia. *American Journal of Psychiatry* **142**, 170–174.

Braus, D.F., Ende, G., Weber-Fahr, W. *et al.* (1999) Antipsychotic drug effects on motor activation measured by functional magnetic resonance imaging in schizophrenic patients. *Schizophrenia Research* **39**, 19–29.

Braus, D.F., Ende, G., Hubrich-Ungureanu, P. & Henn, F.A. (2000a) Cortical response to motor stimulation in neuroleptic-naive first episode schizophrenics. *Psychiatry Research* **98**, 145–154.

Braus, D.F., Ende, G., Tost, H. *et al.* (2000b) Funktionelle Kernspintomographie und Schizophrenie: Medikamenteneffekte, methodische Grenzen und Perspektiven. *Nervenheilkunde* **3**, 121–128.

Braus, D.F., Ende, G., Weber-Fahr, W. *et al.* (2000c) Neuroleptika und einfache Informationsverarbeitungsprozesse. *Psychology* **26**, 97–101.

Braus, D.F., Ende, G., Weber-Fahr, W., Demirakca, T. & Henn, F.A. (2001) Favorable effect on neuronal viability in the anterior cingulate gyrus due to long-term treatment with atypical antipsychotics: an MRSI study. *Pharmacopsychiatry* **34**, 251–253.

Braus, D.F., Weber-Fahr, W., Tost, H., Ruf, M. & Henn, F.A. (2002) Sensory information processing in neuroleptic-naive first-episode schizophrenic patients: a functional magnetic resonance imaging study. *Archives of General Psychiatry* **59**, 696–701.

Braver, T.S., Barch, D.M. & Cohen, J.D. (1999) Cognition and control in schizophrenia: a computational model of dopamine and prefrontal function. *Biological Psychiatry* **46**, 312–328.

Brune, M. & Brune-Cohrs, U. (2006) Theory of mind – evolution, ontogeny, brain mechanisms and psychopathology. *Neuroscience and Biobehaviour Reviews* **30**, 437–455.

Brune, M., Lissek, S., Fuchs, N. *et al.* (2008) An fMRI study of theory of mind in schizophrenic patients with "passivity" symptoms. *Neuropsychologia* **46**, 1992–2001.

Brunet-Gouet, E. & Decety, J. (2006) Social brain dysfunctions in schizophrenia: a review of neuroimaging studies. *Psychiatry Research* **148**, 75–92.

Brunet, E., Sarfati, Y., Hardy-Bayle, M.C. & Decety, J. (2003) Abnormalities of brain function during a nonverbal theory of mind task in schizophrenia. *Neuropsychologia* **41**, 1574–1582.

Buckley, P.F., Friedman, L., Wu, D. *et al.* (1997) Functional magnetic resonance imaging in schizophrenia: Initial methodology and evaluation of the motor cortex. *Psychiatry Research and Neuroimaging* **74**, 13–23.

Bullmore, E. & Sporns, O. (2009) Complex brain networks: graph theoretical analysis of structural and functional systems. *Nature Reviews Neuroscience* **10**, 186–198.

Burns, J.K. (2005) An evolutionary theory of schizophrenia: cortical connectivity, metarepresentation, and the social brain. *Behaviour and Brain Science* **27**, 831–855; discussion 855–885.

Cadenhead, K.S., Serper, Y. & Braff, D.L. (1998) Transient versus sustained visual channels in the visual backward masking deficits of schizophrenia patients. *Biological Psychiatry* **43**, 132–138.

Callicott, J.H., Mattay, V.S., Bertolino, A. *et al.* (1999) Physiological characteristics of capacity constraints in working memory as revealed by functional MRI. *Cerebral Cortex* **9**, 20–26.

Callicott, J.H., Bertolino, A., Mattay, V.S. *et al.* (2000) Physiological dysfunction of the dorsolateral prefrontal cortex in schizophrenia revisited. *Cerebral Cortex* **10**, 1078–1092.

Callicott, J., Mattay, V., Verchinski, B.A., Marenco, S., Egan, M.F. & Weinberger, D.R. (2003) Complexity of prefrontal cortical dysfunction in schizophrenia: more than up or down. *American Journal of Psychiatry* **160**, 2209–2215.

Callicott, J., Egan, M.F., Mattay, V. *et al.* (2004) Abnormal fMRI response of the dorsolateral prefrontal cortex in cognitively intact siblings of patients with schizophrenia. *American Journal of Psychiatry* **160**, 709–719.

Carter, C.S., Mintun, M., Nichols, T. & Cohen, J.D. (1997) Anterior cingulate gyrus dysfunction and selective attention deficits in schizophrenia: [15O]H2O PET study during single-trial Stroop task performance. *American Journal of Psychiatry* **154**, 1670–1675.

Carter, C.S., Botvinick, M.M. & Cohen, J.D. (1999) The contribution of the anterior cingulate cortex to executive processes in cognition. *Reviews in Neuroscience* **10**, 49–57.

Carter, C.S., Macdonald, A.W., 3rd, Ross, L.L. & Stenger, V.A. (2001) Anterior cingulate cortex activity and impaired self-monitoring of performance in patients with schizophrenia: an event-related fMRI study. *American Journal of Psychiatry* **158**, 1423–1428.

Chen, Y., Levy, D.L., Nakayama, K., Matthysse, S., Palafox, G. & Holozman, P.S. (1999a) Dependence of impaired eye tracking on deficient velocity discrimination in schizophrenia. *Archives of General Psychiatry* **56**, 155–161.

Chen, Y., Nakayama, K., Levy, D.L., Matthysse, S. & Holzman, P.S. (1999b) Psychophysical isolation of a motion-processing deficit in schizophrenics and their relatives and its association with impaired smooth pursuit. *Proceedings of the National Academy of Science USA* **96**, 4724–4729.

Chen, Y., Palafox, G.P., Nakayama, K., Levy, D.L., Matthysse, S. & Holzman, P.S. (1999c) Motion perception in schizophrenia. *Archives of General Psychiatry* **56**, 149–154.

Chung, Y.S., Kang, D.H., Shin, N.Y., Yoo, S.Y. & Kwon, J.S. (2008) Deficit of theory of mind in individuals at ultra-high-risk for schizophrenia. *Schizophrenia Research* **99**, 111–118.

Ciaramidaro, A., Adenzato, M., Enrici, I., *et al.* (2007) The intentional network: how the brain reads varieties of intentions. *Neuropsychologia* **45**, 3105–3113.

Cohen, J.D., Botvinick, M. & Carter, C.S. (2000) Anterior cingulate and prefrontal cortex: who's in control? *Nature Neuroscience* **3**, 421–423.

Corlett, P.R., Murray, G. K., Honey, G.D. *et al.* (2007) Disrupted prediction-error signal in psychosis: evidence for an associative account of delusions. *Brain* **130**, 2387–2400.

Cornblatt, B.A. & Malhorta, A.K. (2001) Impaired attention as an endophenotype for molecular genetic studies of schizophrenia. *American Journal Medical Genetics* **105**, 11–15.

Couture, S.M., Penn, D.L. & Roberts, D.L. (2006) The functional significance of social cognition in schizophrenia: a review. *Schizophrenia Bulletin* **32** (Suppl. 1), S44–63.

Crossley, N.A., Mechelli, A., Fusar-Poli, P. *et al.* (2009) Superior temporal lobe dysfunction and frontotemporal dysconnectivity in subjects at risk of psychosis and in first-episode psychosis. *Human Brain Mapping* **30**, 4129–4137.

Das, P., Kemp, A.H., Flynn, G. *et al.* (2007) Functional disconnections in the direct and indirect amygdala pathways for fear processing in schizophrenia. *Schizophrenia Research* **90**, 284–294.

David, A.S., Woodruff, P.W., Howard, R. *et al.* (1996) Auditory hallucinations inhibit exogenous activation of auditory association cortex. *Neuroreport* **7**, 932–936.

Dierks, T., Linden, D.E., Jandl, M., Formisano, E., Goebel, R., Lanfermann, H. & Singer, W. (1999) Activation of Heschl's gyrus during auditory hallucinations. *Neuron* **22**, 615–621.

Egan, M.F., Goldberg, T.E., Gscheidle, T., Weirich, M., Bigelow, L.B. & Weinberger, D.R. (2000) Relative risk of attention deficits in siblings of patients with schizophrenia. *American Journal of Psychiatry* **157**, 1309–1316.

Ende, G., Braus, D.F., Walter, S. *et al.* (2000) Effects of age, medication, and illness duration on the N-acetyl aspartate signal of the anterior cingulate region in schizophrenia. *Schizophrenia Research* **41**, 389–395.

Eyler, L.T., Olsne, R.K., Jeste, D.V. & Brown, G.G. (2004) Abnormal brain response of chronic schizophrenia patients despite normal performance during a visual vigilance task. *Psychiatry Research and Neuroimaging* **130**, 245–257.

Fahim, C., Stip, E., Mancini-Marie, A., Gendron, A., Mensour, B. & Beauregard, M. (2005) Differential hemodynamic brain activity in schizophrenia patients with blunted affect during quetiapine treatment. *Journal of Clinical Psychopharmacology* **25**, 367–371.

Fakra, E., Salgado-Pineda, P., Delaveau, P., Hariri, A.R. & Blin, O. (2008) Neural bases of different cognitive strategies for facial affect processing in schizophrenia. *Schizophrenia Research* **100**, 191–205.

Fitzgerald, P.B., Brown, T.L., Daskalakis, Z.J., Decastella, A. & Kulkarni, J. (2002) A study of transcallosal inhibition in schizophrenia using transcranial magnetic stimulation. *Schizophrenia Research* **56**, 199–209.

Fletcher, P., McKenna, P.J., Friston, K.J., Frith, C.D. & Dolan, R.J. (1999) Abnormal cingulate modulation of fronto-temporal connectivity in schizophrenia. *Neuroimage* **9**, 337–342.

Friston, K.J., Frith, C.D., Fletcher, P., Liddle, P.F. & Frackowiak, R.S. (1996) Functional topography: multidimensional scaling and functional connectivity in the brain. *Cerebral Cortex* **6**, 156–164.

Frith, C. (1992) *The Cognitive Neuropsycholgy of Schizophrenia.* Hove: Psychology Press.

Fusar-Poli, P., Perez, J., Broome, M. *et al.* (2007) Neurofunctional correlates of vulnerability to psychosis: a systematic review and meta-analysis. *Neuroscience and Biobehavior Reviews* **31**, 465–484.

Garrity, A.G., Pearlson, G.D., McKiernan, K., Lloyd, D., Kiehl, K.A. & Calhoun, V.D. (2007) Aberrant "default mode" functional connectivity in schizophrenia. *American Journal of Psychiatry* **164**, 450–457.

Gaser, C., Nenadic, I., Volz, H.P., Buchel, C. & Sauer, H. (2004) Neuroanatomy of "hearing voices": a frontotemporal brain structural abnormality associated with auditory hallucinations in schizophrenia. *Cerebral Cortex* **14**, 91–96.

Glahn, D.C., Cannon, T.D., Gur, R.E., Ragland, J.D. & Gur, R.C. (2000) Working memory constrains abstraction in schizophrenia. *Biological Psychiatry* **47**, 34–42.

Gold, J.M., Carpenter, C., Randolph, C., Goldberg, T.E. & Weinberger, D.R. (1997) Auditory working memory and Wisconsin Card Sorting Test performance in schizophrenia. *Archives of General Psychiatry* **54**, 159–165.

Gold, J.M. & Thaker, G.K. (2002) Current progress in schizophrenia research. Cognitive phenotypes of schizophrenia: attention. *Journal of Nervous and Mental Disease* **190**, 638–639.

Goldman-Rakic, P.S. (1994) Working memory dysfunction in schizophrenia. *Journal of Neuropsychiatry and Clinical Neuroscience* **6**, 348–357.

Goldman-Rakic, P.S, Selemon, L.D. & Schwartz, M.L. (1984) Dual pathways connecting the dorsolateral prefrontal cortex with the hippocampal formation and parahippocampal cortex in the rhesus monkey. *Neuroscience* **12**, 719–743.

Goldman-Rakic, P.S., Muly, E.C., 3rd & Williams, G.V. (2000) D(1) receptors in prefrontal cells and circuits. *Brain Research and Brain Research Review* **31**, 295–301.

Green, M.F. & Leitman, D.I. (2008) Social cognition in schizophrenia. *Schizophrenia Bulletin* **34**, 670–672.

Green, M.F., Nuechterlein, K.H. & Breitmeyer, B. (1997) Backward masking performance in unaffected siblings of schizophrenic patients. Evidence for a vulnerability indicator. *Archives of General Psychiatry* **54**, 465–472.

Gur, R.E., Loughead, J., Kohler, C.G. *et al.* (2007) Limbic activation associated with misidentification of fearful faces and flat affect in schizophrenia. *Archives of General Psychiatry* **64**, 1356–1366.

Habel, U., Klein, M., Shah, N.J. *et al.* (2004) Genetic load on amygdala hypofunction during sadness in nonaffected brothers of schizophrenia patients. *American Journal of Psychiatry* **161**, 1806–1813.

Harrington, L., Langdon, R., Siegert, R.J. & McClure, J. (2005) Schizophrenia, theory of mind, and persecutory delusions. *Cognitive Neuropsychiatry* **10**, 87–104.

Heckers, S., Weiss, A.P., Deckersbach, T., Goff, D.C., Morecraft, R.J. & Bush, G. (2004) Anterior cingulate cortex activation during cognitive interference in schizophrenia. *American Journal of Psychiatry* **161**, 707–715.

Heitmiller, D.R., Nopoulos, P.C. & Andreasen, N.C. (2004) Changes in caudate volume after exposure to atypical neuroleptics in patients with schizophrenia may be sex-dependent. *Schizophrenia Research* **66**, 137–142.

Honey, G.D., Bullmore, E.T., Soni, W., Varatheesan, M., Williams, S.C. & Sharma, T. (1999) Differences in frontal cortical activation by a working memory task after substitution of risperidone for typical antipsychotic drugs in patients with schizophrenia. *Proceedings of the National Academy of Science USA* **96**, 13432–13437.

Honey, G.D., Bullmore, E.T. & Sharma, T. (2002) De-coupling of cognitive performance and cerebral functional response during working memory in schizophrenia. *Schizophrenia Research* **53**, 45–56.

Honey, G.D., Pomarol-Clotet, E., Corlett, P.R. *et al.* (2005) Functional dysconnectivity in schizophrenia associated with attentional modulation of motor function. *Brain* **128**, 2597–2611.

Hubl, D., Koenig, T., Strik, W. *et al.* (2004) Pathways that make voices: white matter changes in auditory hallucinations. *Archives of General Psychiatry* **61**, 658–668.

Jacobsen, L.K., D'Souza, D.C., Mencl, W.E., Pugh, K.R., Skudlarski, P. & Krystal, J.H. (2004) Nicotine effects on brain function and functional connectivity in schizophrenia. *Biological Psychiatry* **55**, 850–858.

Jafri, M.J., Pearlson, G.D., Stevens, M. & Calhoun, V.D. (2008) A method for functional network connectivity among spatially independent resting-state components in schizophrenia. *Neuroimage* **39**, 1666–1681.

Jansma, J.M., Ramsey, N.F., van der Wee, N.J. & Kahn, R.S. (2004) Working memory constraints in schizoprenia: a parametric fMRI study. *Schizophrenia Research* **68**, 159–171.

Jones, H.M., Brammer, M.J., O'Toole, M. *et al.* (2004) Cortical effects of quetiapine in first-episode schizophrenia: a preliminary functional magnetic resonance imaging study. *Biological Psychiatry* **56**, 938–942.

Juckel, G., Schlagenhauf, F., Koslowski, M., *et al.* (2006a) Dysfunction of ventral striatal reward prediction in schizophrenic patients treated with typical, not atypical, neuroleptics. *Psychopharmacology (Berlin)* **187**, 222–228.

Juckel, G., Schlagenhauf, F., Koslowski, M. *et al.* (2006b) Dysfunction of ventral striatal reward prediction in schizophrenia. *Neuroimage* **29**, 409–416.

Kahn, R.S., Fleischhacker, W.W., Boter, H. *et al.* (2008) Effectiveness of antipsychotic drugs in first-episode schizophrenia and schizophreniform disorder: an open randomised clinical trial. *Lancet* **371**, 1085–1097.

Kapur, S. (2003) Psychosis as a state of aberrant salience: a framework linking biology, phenomenology, and pharmacology in schizophrenia. *American Journal of Psychiatry* **160**, 13–23.

Kastner, S., de Weerd, P., Desimone, R. & Ungerleider, L.G. (1998) Mechanisms of directed attention in the human extrastriate cortex as revealed by functional MRI. *Science* **282**, 108–111.

Kastner, S., Pinsk, M.A., de Weerd, P., Desimone, R. & Ungerleider, L.G. (1999) Increased activity in human visual cortex during directed attention in the absence of visual stimulation. *Neuron* **22**, 751–761.

Keri, S., Antal, A., Szekeres, G., Benedek, G. & Janka, Z. (2000) Visual information processing in patients with schizophrenia: evidence for the impairment of central mechanisms. *Neuroscience Letters* **293**, 69–71.

Keshavan, M.S., Diwadkar, V.A., Spencer, S.M., Harenski, K.A., Luna, B. & Sweeney, J.A. (2002) A preliminary functional magnetic resonance imaging study in offspring of schizophrenic parents. *Progress in Neuropsychopharmacology and Biological Psychiatry* **26**, 1143–1149.

Kirsch, P., Ronshausen, S., Mier, D. & Gallhofer, B. (2007) The influence of antipsychotic treatment on brain reward system reactivity in schizophrenia patients. *Pharmacopsychiatry* **40**, 196–198.

Koch, K., Schachtzabel, C., Wagner, G. *et al.* (2010) Altered activation in association with reward-related trial-and-error learning in patients with schizophrenia. *Neuroimage* **50**, 223–232.

Kubicki, M., Westin, C.F., Nestor, P.G. *et al.* (2003) Cingulate fasciculus integrity disruption in schizophrenia: a magnetic resonance diffusion tensor imaging study. *Biological Psychiatry* **54**, 1171–1180.

Lawrie, S.M., Buecjel, C., Whalley, H.C., Frith, C.D., Friston, K.J. & Johnstone, E.C. (2002) Reduced frontotemporal functional connectivity in schizophrenia associated with auditory hallucinations. *Biological Psychiatry* **51**, 1008–1011.

Lee, K.H., Brown, W.H., Egleston, P.N. *et al.* (2006) A functional magnetic resonance imaging study of social cognition in schizophrenia during an acute episode and after recovery. *American Journal of Psychiatry* **163**, 1926–1933.

Levin, S. (1984a) Frontal lobe dysfunctions in schizophrenia. I. Eye movement impairments. *Journal of Psychiatric Research* **18**, 27–55.

Levin, S. (1984b) Frontal lobe dysfunctions in schizophrenia – II. Impairments of psychological and brain functions. *Journal of Psychiatric Research* **18**, 57–72.

Lieberman, J.A., Safferman, A.Z., Pollack, S. *et al.* (1994) Clinical effects of clozapine in chronic schizophrenia: response to treatment and predictors of outcome. *American Journal of Psychiatry* **151**, 1744–1752.

Lieberman, J.A., Stroup, T.S., McEvoy, J.P. *et al.* (2005) Effectiveness of antipsychotic drugs in patients with chronic schizophrenia. *New England Journal of Medicine* **353**, 1209–1223.

Lipska, B.K. & Weinberger, D.R. (2000) To model a psychiatric disorder in animals: Schizophrenia as a reality test. *Neuropsychopharmacology* **23**, 223–239.

Liu, Y., Liang, M., Zhou, Y. *et al.* (2008) Disrupted small-world networks in schizophrenia. *Brain* **131**, 945–961.

Macdonald, A.W., 3rd & Carter, C.S. (2003) Event-related FMRI study of context processing in dorsolateral prefrontal cortex of patients with schizophrenia. *Journal of Abnormal Psychology* **112**, 689–697.

Manoach, D.S. (2003) Prefrontal cortex dysfunction during working memory performance in schizophrenia: reconciling discrepant findings. *Schizophrenia Research* **60**, 285–298.

Manoach, D.S., Press, D.Z., Thangaraj, V. *et al.* (1999) Schizophrenic subjects activate dorsolateral prefrontal cortex during a working memory task, as measured by fMRI. *Biological Psychiatry* **45**, 1128–1137.

Manoach, D.S., Gollub, R.L., Benson, E.S. *et al.* (2000) Schizophrenic subjects show aberrant fMRI activation of dorsolateral prefrontal cortex and basal ganglia during working memory performance. *Biological Psychiatry* **48**, 99–109.

Marjoram, D., Job, D.E., Whalley, H.C. *et al.* (2006) A visual joke fMRI investigation into Theory of Mind and enhanced risk of schizophrenia. *Neuroimage* **31**, 1850–1858.

Mattay, V.S., Callicott, J.H., Bertolino, A. *et al.* (1997) Abnormal functional lateralization of the sensorimotor cortex in patients with schizophrenia. *Neuroreport* **8**, 2977–2984.

Mattay, V.S., Goldberg, T.E., Fera, F. *et al.* (2003) Catechol O-methyltransferase val158-met genotype and individual variation in the brain response to amphetamine. *Proceedings of the National Academy of Science USA* **100**, 6186–6191.

McGuire, P.K., Shah, G.M. & Murray, R.M. (1993) Increased blood flow in Broca's area during auditory hallucinations in schizophrenia. *Lancet* **342**, 703–706.

McGuire, P.K., Silbersweig, D.A., Wright, I. *et al.* (1995) Abnormal monitoring of inner speech: a physiological basis for auditory hallucinations. *Lancet* **346**, 596–600.

Meisenzahl, E.M., Scheuerecker, J., Zipse, M. *et al.* (2006) Effects of treatment with the atypical neuroleptic quetiapine on working memory function: a functional MRI follow-up investigation. *European Archives of Psychiatry and Clinical Neuroscience* **256**, 522–531.

Meltzer, H.Y. & McGurk, S.R. (1999) The effects of clozapine, risperidone, and olanzapine on cognitive function in schizophrenia. *Schizophrenia Bulletin* **25**, 233–255.

Meltzer, H.Y., Lee, M.A. & Ranjan, R. (1994) Recent advances in the pharmacotherapy of schizophrenia. *Acta Psychiatrica Scandinavica* **384** (Suppl.), 95–101.

Meyer-Lindenberg, A., Poline, J.B., Kohn, P.D. *et al.* (2001) Evidence for abnormal cortical functional connectivity during working memory in schizophrenia. *American Journal of Psychiatry* **158**, 1809–1817.

Meyer-Lindenberg, A.S., Olsen, R.K., Kohn, P.D. *et al.* (2005) Regionally specific disturbance of dorsolateral prefrontal-hippocampal functional connectivity in schizophrenia. *Archives of General Psychiatry* **62**, 379–386.

Minzenberg, M.J., Laird, A.R., Thelen, S., Carter, C.S. & Glahn, D.C. (2009) Meta-analysis of 41 functional neuroimaging studies of executive function in schizophrenia. *Archives of General Psychiatry* **66**, 811–822.

Moritz, S., Ruff, C., Wilke, U., Andersen, B., Krausz, M. & Naber, D. (2001) Negative priming in schizophrenia: effects of masking and prime presentation time. *Schizophrenia Research* **48**, 291–299.

Murray, G.K., Corlett, P.R., Clark, L. *et al* (2008) Substantia nigra/ventral tegmental reward prediction error disruption in psychosis. *Molecular Psychiatry* **13**, 239, 267–276.

Nestor, P.G., Faux, S.F., McCarley, R.W., Sands, S.F., Horvath, T.B. & Peterson, A. (1991) Neuroleptics improve sustained attention in schizophrenia. A study using signal detection theory. *Neuropsychopharmacology* **4**, 145–149.

O'Donnell, B.F., Swearer, J.M., Smith, L.T., Nestor, P.G., Shenton, M.E. & McCarley, R.W. (1996) Selective deficits in visual perception and recognition in schizophrenia. *American Journal of Psychiatry* **153**, 687–692.

Park, I.H., Park, H.J., Chun, J.W., Kim, E.Y. & Kim, J.J. (2008) Dysfunctional modulation of emotional interference in the medial prefrontal cortex in patients with schizophrenia. *Neuroscience Letters* **440**, 119–124.

Paulman, R.G., Devous, M.D., Sr, Gregory, R.R. *et al.* (1990) Hypofrontality and cognitive impairment in schizophrenia: dynamic single-photon tomography and neuropsychological assessment of schizophrenic brain function. *Biological Psychiatry* **27**, 377–399.

Pinkham, A.E., Hopfinger, J.B., Pelphrey, K.A., Piven, J. & Penn, D. L. (2008) Neural bases for impaired social cognition in schizophrenia and autism spectrum disorders. *Schizophrenia Research* **99**, 164–175.

Ragland, J.D., Yoon, J., Minzenberg, M.J. & Carter, C.S. (2007) Neuroimaging of cognitive disability in schizophrenia: search for a pathophysiological mechanism. *International Review of Psychiatry* **19**, 417–427.

Ragland, J.D., Laird, A.R., Ranganath, C., Blumenfeld, R.S., Gonzales, S.M. & Glahn, D.C. (2009) Prefrontal activation deficits during episodic memory in schizophrenia. *American Journal of Psychiatry* **166**, 863–874.

Ramsey, N.F., Koning, H.A., Welles, P., Cahn, W., van der Linden, J.A. & Kahn, R.S. (2002) Excessive recruitment of neural systems subserving logical reasoning in schizophrenia. *Brain* **125**, 1793–1807.

Rasetti, R., Mattay, V.S., Wiedholz, L.M. *et al.* (2009) Evidence that altered amygdala activity in schizophrenia is related to clinical state and not genetic risk. *American Journal of Psychiatry* **166**, 216–225.

Reske, M., Kellerman, T., Habel, U. *et al.* (2007) Stablity of emotional functions? A long-term fMRI study in first-episode schizophrenia. *Journal of Psychiatric Research* **41**, 918–927.

Ridler, K., Veijola, J.M., Tanskanen, P. *et al.* (2006) Fronto-cerebellar systems are associated with infant motor and adult executive functions in healthy adults but not in schizophrenia. *Proceedings of the Nationall Academy of Science USA* **103**, 15651–15651.

Rogowska, J., Gruber, S.A. & Yurgelun-Todd, D.A. (2004) Functional magnetic resonance imaging in schizophrenia: cortical response to motor stimulation. *Psychiatry Research and Neuroimaging* **130**, 227–243.

Russell, T.A., Rubia, K., Bullmore, E.T. *et al.* (2000) Exploring the social brain in schizophrenia: left prefrontal underactivation during mental state attribution. *American Journal of Psychiatry* **157**, 2040–2042.

Saka, M.C., Atbasoglu, E.C., Ozguven, H.D., Sener, H.O. & Ozay, E. (2005) Cortical inhibition in first-degree relatives of schizophrenic patients assessed with transcranial magnetic stimulation. *International Journal of Neuropsychopharmacology* **8**, 595–599.

Schlagenhauf, F., Juckel, G., Koslowski, M. *et al.* (2008a) Reward system activation in schizophrenic patients switched from typical neuroleptics to olanzapine. *Psychopharmacology (Berlin)* **196**, 673–684.

Schlagenhauf, F., Wustenberg, T., Schmack, K. *et al.* (2008b) Switching schizophrenia patients from typical neuroleptics to olanzapine: effects on BOLD response during attention and working memory. *European Neuropsychopharmacology* **18**, 589–599.

Schlagenhauf, F., Sterzer, P., Schmack, K. *et al.* (2009) Reward feedback alterations in unmedicated schizophrenia patients: relevance for delusions. *Biological Psychiatry* **65**, 1032–1039.

Schlosser, R., Gesierich, T., Kaufmann, B. *et al.* (2003a) Altered effective connectivity during working memory performance in schizophrenia: a study with fMRI and structural equation modeling. *Neuroimage* **19**, 751–763.

Schlosser, R., Gesierich, T., Kaufmann, B., Vucurevic, G. & Stoeter, P. (2003b) Altered effective connectivity in drug free schizophrenic patients. *Neuroreport* **14**, 2233–2237.

Schmidt-Kastner, R. & Freund, T.F. (1991) Selective vulnerability of the hippocampus in brain ischemia. *Neuroscience* **40**, 599–636.

Schröder, J., Wenz, F., Schad, L.R., Baudendistel, K. & Knopp, M.V. (1995) Sensorimotor cortex and supplementary motor area changes in schizophrenia. A study with functional magnetic resonance imaging. *British Journal of Psychiatry* **167**, 197–201.

Schröder, J., Essig, M., Baudendistel, K. *et al.* (1999) Motor dysfunction and sensorimotor cortex activation changes in schizophrenia: A study with functional magnetic resonance imaging. *Neuroimage* **9**, 81–87.

Schroeder, J., Niethammer, R., Geider, F.J. *et al.* (1991) Neurological soft signs in schizophrenia. *Schizophrenia Research* **6**, 25–30.

Schultz, W. (1998) Predictive reward signal of dopamine neurons. *Journal of Neurophysiology* **80**, 1–27.

Schwartz, B.D., Maron, B.A., Evans, W.J. & Winstead, D.K. (1999) High velocity transient visual processing deficits diminish ability of patients with schizophrenia to recognize objects. *Neuropsychiatry, Neuropsychology and Behavioural Neurology* **12**, 170–177.

Seidman, L.J., Thermenos, H.W., Poldrack, R.A. *et al.* (2006) Altered brain activation in dorsolateral prefrontal cortex in adolescents and young adults at genetic risk for schizophrenia: an fMRI study of working memory. *Schizophrenia Research* **85**, 58–72.

Seiferth, N.Y., Pauly,. K., Habel, U. *et al.* (2008) Increased neural response related to neutral faces in individuals at risk for psychosis. *Neuroimage* **40**, 289–297.

Siegel, B.V., Jr., Nuechterlein, K.H., Abel, L., Wu, J.C. & Buschbaum, M.S. (1995) Glucose metabolic correlates of continuous performance test performance in adults with a history of infantile autism, schizophrenics, and controls. *Schizophrenia Research* **17**, 85–94.

Silbersweig, D.A., Stern, E., Frith, C. *et al.* (1995) A functional neuroanatomy of hallucinations in schizophrenia. *Nature* **378**, 176–179.

Silver, H., Feldman, P., Bilker, W. & Gur, R.C. (2003) Working memory deficit as a core neuropsychological dysfunction in schizophrenia. *American Journal of Psychiatry* **160**, 1809–1816.

Simon, J.J., Biller, A., Walther, S. *et al.* (2010) Neural correlates of reward processing in schizophrenia – Relationship to apathy and depression. *Schizophrenia Research* **118**, 154–161.

Spence, S.A., Liddle, P.F., Stefan, M.D. *et al.* (2000) Functional anatomy of verbal fluency in people with schizophrenia and those at genetic risk. Focal dysfunction and distributed disconnectivity reappraised. *British Journal of Psychiatry* **176**, 52–60.

Spindler, K.A., Sullivan, E.V., Menon, V., Lim, K.O. & Pfefferbaum, A. (1997) Deficits in multiple systems of working memory in schizophrenia. *Schizophrenia Research* **27**, 1–10.

Spoletini, I., Cherubini, A., Di Paola, M. *et al.* (2009) Reduced fronto-temporal connectivity is associated with frontal gray matter density reduction and neuropsychological deficit in schizophrenia. *Schizophrenia Research* **108**, 57–68.

Sprong, M., Schothorst, P., Vos, E., Hox, J. & van Engeland, H. (2007) Theory of mind in schizophrenia: meta-analysis. *British Journal of Psychiatry* **191**, 5–13.

Stephan, K.E., Magnotta, V.A., White, T. *et al.* (2001) Effects of olanzapine on cerebellar functional connectivity in schizophrenia measured by fMRI during a simple motor task. *Psychological Medicine* **31**, 1065–1078.

Stevens, A.A., Goldman-Rakic, P.S., Gore, J.C., Fulbright, R.K. & Wexler, B.E. (1998) Cortical dysfunction in schizophrenia during auditory word and tone working memory demonstrated by functional magnetic resonance imaging. *Archives of General Psychiatry* **55**, 1097–1103.

Stip, E., Fahim, C., Mancini-Marie, A. *et al.* (2005) Restoration of frontal activation during a treatment with quetiapine: an fMRI study of blunted affect in schizophrenia. *Progress in Neuropsychopharmacology and Biological Psychiatry* **29**, 21–26.

Stuve, T. A., Friedman, L., Jesberger, J.A., Gilmore, G.C., Strauss, M.E. & Meltzer, H.Y. (1997) The relationship between smooth pursuit performance, motion perception and sustained visual attention in patients with schizophrenia and normal controls. *Psychological Medicine* **27**, 143–152.

Sun, Z., Wang, F., Cui, L. J. *et al.* (2003) Abnormal anterior cingulum in patients with schizophrenia: a diffusion tensor imaging study. *Neuroreport* **14**, 1833–1836.

Surguladze, S.A., Chu, E.M., Evans, A. *et al.* (2007) The effect of long-acting risperidone on working memory in schizophrenia: a functional magnetic resonance imaging study. *Journal of Clinical Psychopharmacology* **27**, 560–570.

Tan, H.Y., Sust, S., Buckholtz, J.W. *et al.* (2006) Dysfunctional prefrontal regional specialization and compensation in schizophrenia. *American Journal of Psychiatry* **163**, 1969–1977.

Tan, H.Y., Callicott, J.H. & Weinberger, D.R. (2007) Dysfunctional and compensatory prefrontal cortical systems, genes and the pathogenesis of schizophrenia. *Cerebral Cortex* **17** (Suppl 1.), i171–181.

Tek, C., Gold, J., Blaxton, T., Wilk, C., McMahon, R.P. & Buchanan, R.W. (2002) Visual perceptual and working memory impairments in schizophrenia. *Archives of General Psychiatry* **59**, 146–153.

Thermenos, H.W., Seidman, L.J., Breiter, H. *et al.* (2004a) Functional magnetic resonance imaging during auditory verbal working memory in nonpsychotic relatives of persons with schizophrenia: a pilot study. *Biological Psychiatry* **55**, 490–500.

Tost, H., Brassen, S., Schmitt, A. *et al.* (2003a) Passive visual motion processing in schizophrenic patients: a fMRI study. *Neuroimage* **19**, 1584.

Tost, H., Schmitt, A., Brassen, S. *et al.* (2003b) Discrimination of large and small velocity differences in healthy subjects: an fMRI study. *Neuroimage* **19**, 1535.

Tost, H., Wolf, I., Brassen, S., Ruf, M., Schmitt, A. & Braus, D.F. (2004) Visual motion processing dysfunction in schizophrenia: a "bottom up" or "top down" deficit? *Neuroimage* **22**, TU 374.

Ungerleider, L.G. & Mishkin, M. (1982) Two cortical visual systems. In: Ingle, D.J., Goodale, M.A. & Mansfield, R.J., eds. *Analysis of Visual Behavior*. Cambridge, MA: MIT Press.

Ungerleider, L.G., Courtney, S.M. & Haxby, J.V. (1998) A neural system for human visual working memory. *Proceedings of the National Academy of Science USA* **95**, 883–890.

van Hooren, S., Versmissen, D., Janssen, I. *et al.* (2008) Social cognition and neurocognition as independent domains in psychosis. *Schizophrenia Research* **103**, 257–265.

Volz, H., Gaser, C., Hager, F. *et al.* (1999) Decreased frontal activation in schizophrenics during stimulation with the continuous performance test – a functional magnetic resonance imaging study. *European Psychiatry* **14**, 17–24.

Vrtunski, P.B., Simpson, D.M., Weiss, K.M. & Davis, G.C. (1986) Abnormalities of fine motor control in schizophrenia. *Psychiatry Research* **18**, 275–284.

Walter, H., Ciaramidaro, A., Adenzato, M. *et al.* (2009) Dysfunction of the social brain is modulated by intention type: an FMRI study. *Social, Cognitive and Affective Neuroscience* **4**, 166–176.

Walter, H., Kammerer, H., Frasch, K., Spitzer, M. & Abler, B. (2009) Altered reward functions in patients on atypical antipsychotic medication in line with the revised dopamine hypothesis of schizophrenia. *Psychopharmacology (Berlin)* **206**, 121–132.

Waltz, J.A., Schweitzer, J.B., Gold, J.M. *et al.* (2009) Patients with schizophrenia have a reduced neural response to both unpredictable and predictable primary reinforcers. *Neuropsychopharmacology* **34**, 1567–1577.

Weinberger, D.R. (1987) Implications of normal brain development for the pathogenesis of schizophrenia. *Archives of General Psychiatry* **44**, 660–669.

Weinberger, D.R., Berman, K.F., Suddath, R. & Torrey, E.F. (1992) Evidence of dysfunction of a prefrontal-limbic network in schizophrenia: a magnetic resonance imaging and regional cerebral blood flow study of discordant monozygotic twins. *American Journal of Psychiatry* **149**, 890–897.

Weiss, E.M., Golaszewski, S., Mottaghy, F.M. *et al.* (2003) Brain activtion patterns during a selective attention test – a functional MRI study in healthy volunteers and patients with schizophrenia. *Psychiatry Research* **123**, 1–15.

Wenz, F., Schad, L.R., Knopp, M.V. *et al.* (1994) Functional magnetic resonance imaging at 1.5 T: activation pattern in schizophrenic patients receiving neuroleptic medication. *Magnetic Resonance Imaging* **12**, 975–982.

Whalley, H.C., Simonotto, E., Marshall, I. *et al.* (2005) Functional disconnectivity in subjects at high genetic risk of schizophrenia. *Brain* **128**, 2097–2108.

Whitfield-Gabrieli, S., Thermenos, H.W., Milanovic, S.T. *et al.* (2009) Hyperactivity and hyperconnectivity of the default network in schizophrenia and in first-degree relatives of persons with schizophrenia. *Proceedings of the National Academy of Science USA* **106**, 1279–1284.

Wible, C.G., Kubicki, M., Yoo, S.S. *et al.* (2001) A functional magnetic resonance imaging study of auditory mismatch in schizophrenia. *American Journal of Psychiatry* **158**, 938–943.

Wolf, D.H., Gur, R.C., Valdez, J.N. *et al.* (2007) Alterations of fronto-temporal connectivity during word encoding in schizophrenia. *Psychiatry Research* **154**, 221–232.

Wolf, R.C., Vasic, N., Sambataro, F. *et al.* (2009) Temporally anticorrelated brain networks during working memory performance reveal aberrant prefrontal and hippocampal connectivity in patients with schizophrenia. *Progress in Neuropsychopharmacology and Biological Psychiatry* **33**, 1464–1473.

Woodruff, P., Brammer, M., Mellers, J., Wright, I., Bullmore, E. & Williams, S. (1995) Auditory hallucinations and perception of external speech. *Lancet* **346**, 1035.

Woodruff, P.W., Wright, I.C., Bullmore, E.T. *et al.* (1997) Auditory hallucinations and the temporal cortical response to speech in schizophrenia: a functional magnetic resonance imaging study. *American Journal of Psychiatry* **154**, 1676–1682.

Woodward, N.D., Waldie, B., Rogers, B., Tibbo, P., Seres, P. & Purdon, S.E. (2009) Abnormal prefrontal cortical activity and connectivity during response selection in first episode psychosis, chronic schizophrenia, and unaffected siblings of individuals with schizophrenia. *Schizophrenia Research* **109**, 182–190.

Yung, A.R., Phillips, L.J., McGorry, P.D. *et al.* (1998) Prediction of psychosis. A step towards indicated prevention of schizophrenia. *British Journal of Psychiatry* **172** (Suppl), 14–20.

Yücel, M., Pantelis, C., Stuart, G.W. *et al.* (2002) Anterior cingulate activation during Stroop task performance: a PET to MRI coregistration study of individual patients with schizophrenia. *American Journal of Psychiatry* **159**, 251–254.

Zahn, T.P., Pickar, D. & Haier, R.J. (1994) Effects of clozapine, fluphenazine, and placebo on reaction time measures of attention and sensory dominance in schizophrenia. *Schizophrenia Research* **13**, 133–144.

Zhou, Y., Shu, N., Liu, Y. *et al.* (2008) Altered resting-state functional connectivity and anatomical connectivity of hippocampus in schizophrenia. *Schizophrenia Research* **100**, 120–132.

CHAPTER 18

Neuropathology of schizophrenia

Paul J. Harrison[1], David A. Lewis[2], and Joel E. Kleinman[3]

[1]University of Oxford, Oxford, UK
[2]University of Pittsburgh, Pittsburgh, PA, USA
[3]National Institute of Mental Health, Bethesda, MD, USA

There is no neuropathology of schizophrenia in the sense that there is a neuropathology of Huntington's disease, leukodystrophy, or a glioma. However, this stark statement conceals the fact that significant progress has been made in discovering the existence and nature of histological correlates of schizophrenia, both by ruling out certain processes, as well as by providing some intriguing results concerning cytoarchitectural alterations which may represent, or at least contribute to, the structural substrate of the disorder. Moreover, advances have been made in the identification of the molecular pathways that may underpin these anatomical features, and that begin to link neuropathology to pathophysiology and etiology.

Soon after the (in)famous remark that schizophrenia was the "graveyard of neuropathologists" (Plum, 1972), the field experienced an upturn of fortunes that has persisted. The renaissance came about for several reasons. First,

beginning in the mid 1970s, accumulating evidence from computerized tomography (CT) and magnetic resonance imaging (MRI) studies has identified unequivocally that structural brain abnormalities are present in schizophrenia (see Chapter 16). One simple but key finding, shown by meta-analysis, is that brain volume is reduced by about 4% (Wright *et al.*, 2000), paralleled by a 3% reduction in brain weight (Harrison *et al.*, 2003). This result not only negates the null hypothesis that there is no neuropathology of schizophrenia, but begs the question as to its histological and molecular basis. Equally, a neuropathological explanation must be sought for the other robust MRI findings pointing to localized differences in the brain in schizophrenia. Second, lessons have been learned from the earlier generation of studies, which were inadequate by current standards of study design and statistical analysis. Third, the resurgence of neuropathological interest has coincided with the rapid progress made in neuroscience and molecular biology, which has increased the sophistication of contemporary studies, and has provided a more powerful range of tools with which to conduct them.

Schizophrenia, 3rd edition. Edited by Daniel R. Weinberger and Paul J Harrison © 2011 Blackwell Publishing Ltd.

This chapter summarizes the current understanding of the neuropathology of schizophrenia and its interpretation. We have not attempted a comprehensive review, but emphasize those aspects for which there is a convergence and consistency to the findings in order to highlight the key points and major themes; anatomically, we have focused on the hippocampal formation, dorso-lateral prefrontal cortex (DLPFC), and thalamus. For more detailed coverage, see Arnold and Trojanowski (1996), Harrison (1999a), Harrison & Roberts (2000) and Dorph-Petersen and Lewis (2010). For a review of the largely disregarded earlier literature, see David (1957).

Neurodegeneration in schizophrenia

A critical question concerns the neuropathological nature of schizophrenia. In the most basic (and grossly oversimplified) sense, brain disease processes are either neurodegenerative or neurodevelopmental. In the former, there are usually cytopathological inclusions (e.g., neurofibrillary tangles, Lewy bodies) and evidence for neuronal and synaptic loss, accompanied by gliosis (reactive astrocytosis). A degenerative process underlies most dementias, as well as the pathology seen after hypoxia, infection, and trauma. In the absence of any evidence for abnormalities of this kind, a neurodevelopmental process, in which something goes awry with normal brain maturation, is by default the likely form of pathology to explain a brain disorder. Because this distinction—despite its limitations—has such important implications for the nature of the disease, we first review the studies which have sought, and failed, to find consistent evidence for neurodegeneration in schizophrenia.

Gliosis

In a paper which heralded the start of the current phase of research, Stevens (1982) described reactive astrocytosis in around 70% of her series of cases with schizophrenia. The gliosis was usually located in periventricular and subependymal regions of the diencephalon or in adjacent basal forebrain structures. This finding supported etiopathogenic scenarios for schizophrenia involving infective, ischemic, autoimmune or neurodegenerative processes.

In contrast to Stevens' findings, many subsequent investigations of schizophrenia have not found gliosis (Arnold et al., 1996; Roberts & Harrison, 2000; Schmitt et al., 2009)—and, indeed, recent studies suggest instead there may actually be a glial deficit (see below). The study of Bruton et al. (1990) was illuminating, finding that gliosis in schizophrenia was only seen in cases exhibiting separate neuropathological abnormalities, such as focal lesions and infarcts, many of which clearly postdated the onset of psychosis. This suggested strongly that gliosis is not an intrinsic feature of the disease, but is a sign of coincidental or superimposed pathological changes (which occur in a significant

minority of cases; Riederer et al., 1995). This view, although now broadly accepted, is subject to qualifications. First, the recognition and definition of gliosis is not as straightforward as sometimes assumed (Stevens et al., 1992; Da Cunha et al., 1993). Second, most studies have focused on the cerebral cortex rather than on the diencephalon where the gliosis of Stevens (1982) was concentrated, although the study of Falkai et al. (1999) overcomes this limitation. Third, there could be pathological heterogeneity, with a proportion of cases being "neurodegenerative"; however, the cumulative data suggest that this proportion would have to be small.

The gliosis debate was stimulated by its implications for the neuropathological timing of schizophrenia. The gliotic response is said not to develop until the end of the second trimester *in utero* (Friede, 1989). Hence, an absence of gliosis, in the context of other pathological abnormalities, is considered strong evidence for an earlier neurodevelopmental origin of schizophrenia. However, the developmental onset of the glial response has not been well investigated and so absence of gliosis should not be used to time the pathology of schizophrenia with any certainty. Moreover, gliosis is not always permanent (Kalman et al., 1993), nor is it thought to accompany the normal maturational programmed cell death (apoptosis) of neurons, which has been hypothesized to be relevant to schizophrenia. Furthermore, it is a moot point whether the subtle kinds of morphometric disturbance to be described in schizophrenia, whenever and however they occurred, would be sufficient to trigger detectable gliosis. Thus, the lack of gliosis does not mean that schizophrenia must be a neurodevelopmental disorder of prenatal origin; it is merely one argument in favor of that conclusion. Certainly, an absence of gliosis does not negate models of schizophrenia which include aberrant plasticity and perhaps mild neurotoxic or other ongoing processes (Lieberman, 1999; DeLisi, 2008).

Alzheimer's disease

The other area of controversy regarding neurodegeneration in schizophrenia concerns the supposedly greater prevalence of Alzheimer's disease.

The belief that Alzheimer's disease is more frequent in schizophrenia apparently originated in the 1930s (see Corsellis, 1962) and was bolstered by a large, although uncontrolled, study (Prohovnik et al., 1993), and by data implying that antipsychotic drugs might promote Alzheimer-type changes (Wisniewski et al., 1994). However, a meta-analysis (Baldessarini et al., 1997) and several subsequent studies, which have used sophisticated staining techniques and careful experimental designs, show conclusively that Alzheimer's disease is not more common than expected in schizophrenia (Arnold et al., 1998; Murphy et al., 1998; Niizato et al. 1998; Purohit et al., 1998; Jellinger & Gabriel,

1999). This negative conclusion also applies, albeit based on limited data, to late-onset schizophrenia (Bozikas *et al.*, 2002; Casanova *et al.*, 2002). Moreover, the evidence does not support the view that antipsychotic drugs predispose to neurofibrillary or amyloid-related pathology (Baldessarini *et al.*, 1997; Harrison, 1999b). Neither is the incidence of other neurodegenerative pathological features increased in schizophrenia (Arnold *et al.*, 1998) and, in the case of Lewy body/α-synuclein lesions, may actually be reduced (Jellinger, 2009). The latter finding might relate to the inter-action between dopamine and α-synuclein aggregation (Leong *et al.*, (2009).

Of note, the absence of Alzheimer's disease and other neurodegenerative features in schizophrenia also applies to elderly patients who were unequivocally demented (Arnold *et al.*, 1996, 1998; Niizato *et al.*, 1998; Purohit *et al.*, 1998). The only known neuropathological correlate of dementia in schizophrenia is a small increase in the number of glial fibrillary acidic protein (GFAP)-positive astrocytes, with no change in other indices of gliosis (Arnold *et al.*, 1996). Apart from this equivocal finding, the dementia of schizophrenia—let alone the milder but nevertheless robust cognitive deficits that are a core feature of the syndrome (see Chapter 8)—remains unexplained. It may just be a more severe manifestation of whatever pathology under-lies the disorder itself, or perhaps the brain in schizophre-nia is rendered more vulnerable to cognitive impairment in response to a normal age-related amount of neurodegen-eration. A recent study is supportive of the latter possibility (Rapp *et al.*, 2010).

In the absence of overt degenerative changes, neu-ropathological attention has focused on alterations in the cytoarchitecture (the morphology and arrangement of cells in the brain), in tandem with studies of synapses and den-drites. The majority of these studies have been in the hip-pocampal formation and PFC, and the data in these two areas are considered in turn.

Hippocampal formation

The hippocampal formation (hippocampus and parahip-pocampal gyrus, including the entorhinal cortex) in the medial temporal lobe has been extensively studied in schiz-ophrenia for several reasons (Harrison, 2004; Tamminga *et al.*, 2010). First, when the current renaissance began 25 years ago, it was the hippocampal formation wherein several of the most striking initial findings were described, and this has continued to be the case (Arnold, 1997; Weinberger, 1999). The search for histological changes has been encouraged by the demonstration *in vivo* that hip-pocampal volume is decreased in first-episode (Velakoulis *et al.*, 1999) as well as chronic (Nelson *et al.*, 1998) cases. Hippocampal volume also distinguishes affected from unaffected monozygotic twins (Suddath *et al.*, 1990).

Furthermore, proton resonance spectroscopy shows a reduced hippocampal *N*-acetyl aspartate (NAA) signal, suggestive of a neuronal pathology (Bertolino *et al.*, 1998; Fannon *et al.*, 2003), including in first-episode cases, pro-viding encouragement that the morphometric findings described below, although made in chronic cases, may also have been present at this time. Second, a range of findings from functional imaging (Heckers, 2001), neuropsychology (Boyer *et al.*, 2007), animal models (see Chapter 22), and genetic considerations (Talbot *et al.*, 2004; Callicott *et al.*, 2005; Law *et al.*, 2006), all implicate the hippocampal forma-tion in schizophrenia. Finally, the relatively precise cir-cuitry of the hippocampal formation lends itself to studies seeking to investigate neural connectivity (Benes, 2000; Harrison & Eastwood, 2001), a concept which has become central to pathophysiological theories of schizophrenia (e.g., Friston, 1998; Harrison, 1999a; Stephan *et al.*, 2006; Konrad & Winterer, 2008).

Hippocampal morphometric findings

Several types of abnormality affecting hippocampal neurons have been reported. Some have also been found in other brain regions, but they are described here to exem-plify this type of neuropathological approach.

Hippocampal neuronal disarray
Normally, pyramidal neurons within the *cornu Ammonis* of the hippocampus are aligned, as in a pallisade, with the apical dendrite orientated towards the stratum radiatum. Kovelman and Scheibel (1984) reported that this orienta-tion was more variable and even reversed in schizophrenia, hence the term neuronal disarray. The disarray was present at the boundaries of CA1 with the adjacent subfields CA2 and subiculum. They suggested that a developmental migrational disturbance might be responsible. Qualified support for a greater variability of hippocampal neuronal orientation came in subsequent work from the same group (Altshuler *et al.*, 1987; Conrad *et al.*, 1991). However, other studies, using computerized image analysis-assisted meas-urements of neuronal orientation, have not replicated the observation (Christison *et al.*, 1989; Benes *et al.*, 1991b; Arnold *et al.*, 1995; Zaidel *et al.*, 1997b). It is therefore unlikely that hippocampal neuronal disarray is associated with schizophrenia.

Hippocampal neuronal position
The second oft-cited feature of the hippocampal formation in schizophrenia is that of misplaced and aberrantly clus-tered neurons in lamina II (pre-α cells) and lamina III of the entorhinal cortex (anterior parahippocampal gyrus), described by Jakob and Beckmann (1986). This finding was also interpreted as being developmental in origin and resulting from aberrant neuronal migration; certainly it is difficult to think of another plausible mechanism by which

a cell population could show this kind of abnormality. Many studies have sought to investigate this feature subsequently, using a range of methods. Several, with larger samples, better control groups, or methodologies which take into account the significant intrinsic and interindividual heterogeneity of the entorhinal cortex, did not find any differences (Heinsen *et al.*, 1996; Akil & Lewis, 1997; Krimer *et al.*, 1997; Bernstein *et al.*, 1998). On the other hand, there have been several replications and related positive findings (Arnold *et al.*, 1991a, 1997; Falkai *et al.*, 2000; Kovalenko *et al.*, 2003). The latter two studies, in particular, have revived the issue. Falkai *et al.* (2000) reported robust quantitative evidence of abnormally located and smaller sized clusters of entorhinal cortex neurons (using a different form of analysis in the same brain series as that of Bernstein *et al.*, 1998), and the same group then repeated this finding in a different series (Kovalenko *et al.*, 2003). Overall, the current evidence is suggestive, but not conclusive. Because a consistent alteration of neuronal location or clustering would constitute strong evidence for an early neurodevelopmental anomaly, further research is essential to confirm or eliminate such abnormalities as being a feature of schizophrenia.

Hippocampal neuronal density

A loss of hippocampal neurons is a third finding sometimes described as a feature of schizophrenia. In fact, only one substantive study has found reductions in neuronal density (Jeste & Lohr, 1989) and one reported a lower number of pyramidal neurons (Falkai & Bogerts, 1986). In contrast, several have found no change in neuronal density (Falkai & Bogerts, 1986; Benes *et al.*, 1991b; Arnold *et al.*, 1995) and one found a right-lateralized increase (Zaidel *et al.* 1997a). As well as being contradictory, none of these studies used stereological, three-dimensional counting methods, and so their value is limited by the inherent weaknesses and biases of neuronal counts not made in this way (see Guillery, 2002). The fact that the three stereological studies which have been carried out found no difference in neuronal number or density in any subfield (Heckers *et al.*, 1991; Walker *et al.*, 2002; Schmitt *et al.*, 2009) supports the view that there is no overall change in neuronal content of the hippocampus in schizophrenia. In this context, reports of altered neuronal density restricted to a specific neuronal type (Benes *et al.*, 1998), subfield or hemisphere (Zaidel *et al.*, 1997b) remain in need of replication.

Hippocampal neuronal size and shape

Three studies, each counting large numbers of neurons, identified a smaller cross-sectional area of hippocampal pyramidal neurons in schizophrenia (Benes *et al.*, 1991b; Arnold *et al.*, 1995; Zaidel *et al.*, 1997a). Although different individual subfields reached significance in the latter two studies, the same trend was present in all CA fields and

in the subiculum. The non-replications comprise Christison *et al.* (1989) and Benes *et al.* (1998), perhaps because their measurements were limited to a restricted subset of neurons. The above studies were all two-dimensional approaches and subject to the limitations noted above for neuronal counts. One three-dimensional estimate of hippocampal neuronal volume in schizophrenia has been made using stereological techniques, and it found no differences (Highley *et al.*, 2003b). Finally, Zaidel *et al.* (1997a) found that pyramidal neurons were more elongated (as well as being smaller) in some hippocampal subfields in schizophrenia, which might relate to the abnormalities in dendritic arborization described in the next section.

Hippocampal synaptic and dendritic abnormalities

Changes in neuronal cell body parameters (such as size, shape, and packing density) are likely to be a sign, and probably a consequence, of alterations in other neuronal compartments and the cytoarchitecture in which they are situated. For example, cell body size is related to axonal diameter and other parameters of axodendritic arborization (Pierce & Lewin, 1994; Hayes & Lewis, 1996; Esiri & Pearson, 2000), because the majority of a neuron's total volume is in its processes (especially axons, in the case of projection neurons), and the size of the soma reflects the cellular machinery necessary to support these processes. Somal size varies normally within as well as between neuronal populations; it also changes (in both directions) in response to altered afferent and efferent connectivity (e.g., shrinkage after retrograde degeneration).

Starting in the mid-1990s, molecular approaches became available to investigate synapses and dendrites in postmortem brain, and were first applied to schizophrenia in studies of the hippocampus, in part to test these notions.

Investigation of synapses in schizophrenia has mainly used various proteins, concentrated in presynaptic terminals, to serve as markers thereof (Honer *et al.*, 2000; Eastwood & Harrison, 2001). First applied to Alzheimer's disease, using the protein synaptophysin (an integral protein of synaptic vesicles), this approach has been validated in various neuropathological and experimental situations. Dendrites can also be investigated in an analogous fashion using post-synaptically located proteins, notably microtubule-associated protein-2 (MAP-2) and spinophilin. In addition, the rapid Golgi method can be used, despite limitations, to study dendritic parameters (e.g., spine density, shape analysis) in postmortem material.

Key synaptic and dendritic findings in the hippocampal formation in schizophrenia are as follows (Harrison & Eastwood, 2001). Decreased expression of several presynaptic proteins, including synaptophysin, SNAP-25, and the complexins, has been found in several studies (Eastwood

& Harrison, 1995, 1999; Sawada et al., 2005; for review see Honer et al., 2000). Data in degenerative disorders indicate that these decreases are likely to be a reflection of a lowered density of synapses; this interpretation is supported by the few electron microscopy data available in the hippocampus in schizophrenia (Kolomeets et al., 2007); however, altered synaptic morphology (Kolomeets et al., 2005), decreases in synaptic activity, synaptic plasticity (Eastwood & Harrison, 1998), or the turnover of these gene products, may also contribute to the observations. Some data suggest that excitatory hippocampal neurons and their synapses may be more affected than inhibitory ones (Harrison & Eastwood, 1998; Sawada et al., 2005), but other data indicate the reverse pattern (Benes et al., 1998; Benes, 2000) or a similar involvement of both (Eastwood & Harrison, 2000).

Complementing these presynaptic alterations are data showing hippocampal dendritic alterations in schizophrenia, with decreased immunoreactivity for MAP-2, a dendritic marker (Arnold et al., 1991b), and decreased expression of MAP-2 and spinophilin (Law et al., 2004), as well as reduced density of dendritic spines on subicular neurons (Rosoklija et al., 2000).

In summary, there is good evidence for synaptic pathology in the hippocampal formation, but the specific characteristics of the alterations—as well as their cause—remain to be established.

Dorso-lateral prefrontal cortex

Although studies by Alzheimer identified the DLPFC as a possible site of pathological alterations in schizophrenia, it did not become a major focus of postmortem studies until the early 1990s. Investigations have been motivated by observations that subjects with schizophrenia exhibit altered metabolism of the DLPFC, and impaired performance on cognitive tasks, such as those involving working memory, which are known to depend upon the integrity of DLPFC circuitry. Indeed, studies examining neural activity using functional MRI indicate that subjects with schizophrenia exhibit an altered relationship between working memory load, behavioral performance, and DLPFC activation (Van Snellenberg et al., 2006). The idea that this dysfunction might be attributable to structural abnormalities has been supported by MRI studies which have revealed subtle reductions in gray matter volume of the DLPFC (see Chapter 16). The failure to detect such abnormalities in all studies has been hypothesized to be a consequence of several factors, including volume reductions that approach the level of sensitivity of MRI and the restriction of volumetric changes to certain DLPFC regions or gyri. Consistent with this view, postmortem studies have frequently revealed a 5–10% decrease in DLPFC cortical thickness in subjects with schizophrenia (Pakkenberg, 1993; Daviss & Lewis, 1995; Selemon et al., 1995; Woo et al., 1997a), although these changes were not always statisti-

cally significant. In addition, some (Bertolino et al., 1996, 2000; Deicken et al., 1997), but not all (Stanley et al., 1996) in vivo proton spectroscopy studies indicate that subjects with schizophrenia have reduced concentrations of DLPFC NAA. Interestingly, the magnitude of these NAA reductions correlates with the degree of impaired activation in other brain regions during working memory tasks, raising the possibility that a neuronal abnormality in the DLPFC could account for distributed functional disturbances in the working memory network (Bertolino et al., 2000).

Cellular and synaptic alterations in the dorso-lateral prefrontal cortex in schizophrenia

Several lines of evidence suggest that these changes may reflect disturbances in the synaptic connectivity of the DLPFC. For example, DLPFC levels of synaptophysin have been reported to be reduced in schizophrenia in many (Perrone-Bizzozero et al., 1996; Glantz & Lewis, 1997; Davidsson et al., 1999; Honer et al., 1999; Karson et al., 1999), but not all (Gabriel et al., 1997; Eastwood et al., 2000) studies. Alterations in other synapse-related proteins have also been described, although these observations are fewer in number and less consistent across studies and prefrontal regions (Thompson et al., 1998; Davidsson et al., 1999; Karson et al., 1999). Finally, reports of increased cell packing density (Daviss & Lewis, 1995; Selemon et al., 1995, 1998) have been interpreted as evidence that the DLPFC neuropil, which is composed of the axon terminals and dendritic spines and shafts that form most cortical synapses, is reduced in schizophrenia. This "reduced neuropil" hypothesis has been influential (Selemon & Goldman-Rakic, 1999). However, the findings of increased DLPFC neuronal density have not been well replicated (Akbarian et al., 1995; Pierri et al., 2001; Cullen et al., 2006), and the total number of PFC neurons was unchanged in subjects with schizophrenia in a study that used an unbiased stereological approach (Thune et al., 2001). Overall, various lines of evidence support the hypothesis that schizophrenia is associated with a decrease in the synaptic connectivity of the DLPFC, without any apparent loss of neurons. However, these studies may have lacked adequate sensitivity to detect a reduction in small subpopulations of neurons [e.g., a decrement of small neurons in layer 2 (Benes et al., 1991a) or in a subset of GABA interneurons; see below].

If there is no major loss of neurons, the reduction in DLPFC gray matter in schizophrenia could instead be caused, at least in part, by smaller neuronal cell bodies. The somal volume of pyramidal cells in deep layer 3 of DLPFC area 9 has been reported in two studies to be decreased (Rajkowska et al., 1998; Pierri et al., 2001). As discussed in the section "Hippocampal formation", this reduction may be associated with dendritic changes, and there is evidence for a decrease in total length of the basilar dendrites of these neurons (Glantz & Lewis, 2000; Kalus et al., 2000;

see also Plate 21.1.), as well as with the decreased synaptophysin levels mentioned above. In contrast, the size of DLPFC GABA neurons does not appear to be reduced (Benes et al., 1986; Woo et al., 1997a). Attempts to identify the class of affected pyramidal neurons based on immunocytochemical markers, such as those that express high levels of non-phosphorylated epitopes of neurofilament proteins (NNFP) and provide long distance corticocortical projections (Hof et al., 1996), have not yet yielded fruit. For example, the somal size of NNFP-containing layer 3 neurons was reported to be unaltered in schizophrenia (Law & Harrison, 2003; Pierri et al., 2003), but the studies were subject to a methodological confounder that resulted in an over-estimation of somal volumes (Maldonado-Aviles et al., 2006). Furthermore, the ability to distinguish other subpopulations of pyramidal neurons based on their molecular phenotype still awaits the types of gene expression profiling studies that have been successfully utilized for characterizing subclasses of cortical interneurons (Sugino et al., 2006).

In summary, the subtle reduction in DLPFC gray matter in schizophrenia appears attributable to a combination of smaller neurons and a decrease in the axon terminals, distal dendrites, and dendritic spines (see below) that represent the principal components of cortical synapses. Interestingly, this disturbance appears not to be restricted to the DLPFC. For example, smaller volumes of pyramidal cell bodies (Sweet et al., 2003, 2004) and shorter basilar dendrites (Broadbelt et al., 2002; Black et al., 2004) have been reported in other cortical regions. The issue of the cortical localization of schizophrenia neuropathology is considered further below.

Synaptic abnormalities and the connections of the dorso-lateral prefrontal cortex

Alterations in DLPFC synaptic connectivity in schizophrenia may involve synapses formed by intrinsic axon terminals arising from neurons within the DLPFC and/or from extrinsic axon terminals projecting to the DLPFC from other cortical regions, the brainstem, or the thalamus.

The DLPFC layer 3 pyramidal cells that are smaller in schizophrenia give rise to a substantial number of intrinsic excitatory synapses (Levitt et al., 1993; Pucak et al., 1996), suggesting that the synapses furnished by the intrinsic axon collaterals of these neurons may be reduced in number in schizophrenia. Consistent with this interpretation, gene expression profiling in the DLPFC in schizophrenia revealed lower levels of transcripts encoding for proteins involved in the regulation of presynaptic neurotransmitter release (Mirnics et al., 2000). Although these findings likely indicate a general impairment of synaptic transmission within the DLPFC in schizophrenia, it remains to be determined whether they represent a "primary" abnormality intrinsic to the DLPFC or a "secondary" response to defi-

cient inputs from other brain regions. The latter possibility is supported by the findings that synaptophysin mRNA levels are not reduced in the DLPFC in schizophrenia (Karson et al., 1999; Eastwood et al., 2000; Glantz et al., 2000), suggesting that the reduced amount of synaptophysin protein noted earlier may have an extrinsic source. This interpretation is supported by the observations that reduced pyramidal cell somal volume in layer 3 of the primary auditory cortex correlated with reduced levels of synaptophysin-positive puncta, putative axon terminals, in the middle layers of the adjacent auditory association cortex, which represents the terminal zone of the projections arising from the smaller neurons (Sweet et al., 2007).

In addition to these clues that DLPFC dysfunction in schizophrenia might relate to synaptic connectivity, other studies suggest that it might also reflect alterations in neuronal metabolic capacity. For example, the expression levels of various metabolic genes, or the proteins they encode, is reported to be reduced in schizophrenia (Mulcrone et al., 1995; Prince et al., 1999; Maurer et al., 2001), perhaps as part of a mitochondrial involvement in the disease process (Prabakaran et al., 2004; Altar et al., 2005). In particular, Middleton et al. (2002) used microarrays to examine the expression profile of genes comprising major metabolic pathways in postmortem samples of DLPFC (Brodmann area 9) from matched pairs of subjects with schizophrenia and controls.. Of the 71 metabolic pathways assessed, only five showed consistent changes in expression; specifically, reduced expression levels were identified for the transcripts of genes involved in the regulation of ornithine and polyamine metabolism, the mitochondrial malate shuttle system, the transcarboxylic acid (TCA) cycle, aspartate and alanine metabolism, and ubiquitin metabolism. Parallel studies in macaque monkeys treated chronically with haloperidol in a manner that mimicked its clinical use did not reveal similar reductions, and the transcript encoding the cytosolic form of malate dehydrogenase displayed a marked treatment-associated *increase* in expression. These findings suggest that metabolic alterations in the DLPFC of subjects with schizophrenia reflect specific abnormalities, at least at the level of gene expression, and that the therapeutic effect of antipsychotic medications might, in part, be mediated by the normalization of some of these alterations. Although the cause of the altered levels of these transcripts remains to be determined, the high metabolic demands placed on neurons by the processes involved in synaptic communication suggests that these changes are related to the synaptic abnormalities present in the DLPFC in schizophrenia.

In terms of subcortical inputs to the DLPFC, the dopamine (DA) projections from the mesencephalon may be reduced in schizophrenia. The densities of axons immunoreactive for tyrosine hydroxylase (TH), the rate-limiting enzyme in catecholamine synthesis, and the DA transporter (DAT), are both decreased in DLPFC area 9 (Akil et al., 1999). These findings suggest that the cortical DA signal might be diminished in schizophrenia, due to a reduced content of TH per axon, to a reduced density of DA axons, or to both. However, schizophrenia does not seem to be associated with a substantial loss of midbrain DA neurons, although the neurons are smaller (Bogerts et al., 1983). It should be noted that even if these findings do represent a decrement in the DA innervation of the DLPFC, they could not alone account for the observed reductions in gray matter volume, or synaptophysin levels, in the DLPFC of subjects with schizophrenia since DA axons are estimated to contribute less than 1% of cortical synapses (Lewis & Sesack, 1997). Plate 18.1 shows one schema linking DA alterations with other aspects of DLPFC neuropathology in schizophrenia.

Thalamic projections to the prefrontal cortex and thalamic pathology in schizophrenia

Excitatory projections from the medio-dorsal nucleus of the thalamus (MDN), the principal source of thalamic inputs to the DLPFC (Giguere & Goldman-Rakic, 1988) synapse primarily on dendritic spines (Melchitzky et al., 1999). These axons densely arborize in DLPFC deep layers 3 and 4, but do not innervate the deep cortical layers (Erickson & Lewis, 2004). Since the basilar dendrites of DLPFC deep layer 3 pyramidal neurons are present in the same location, a reduction in the number or activity of these afferents could contribute to the decrement in spine density in schizophrenia (Garey et al., 1998; Glantz & Lewis, 2000), which appears to be more prominent on layer 3 pyramidal neurons than on those located in the deep layers (Kolluri et al., 2005). Consistent with this hypothesis, total thalamic volume is decreased in schizophrenia, as determined by a meta-analysis of MRI data (Konick & Friedman, 2001), including in never-medicated subjects (Buchsbaum et al., 1996; Gilbert et al., 2001; Ettinger et al., 2001). Furthermore, reduced thalamic volume may mark the genetic contribution to the illness in studies of twin pairs concordant or discordant for schizophrenia (Ettinger et al., 2007). Finally, thalamic volume correlates with prefrontal white matter volume in subjects with schizophrenia (Portas et al., 1998), suggesting that a reduction in thalamic volume may be associated with fewer axonal projections to the DLPFC. However, although several reports indicated that the total number of MDN neurons was markedly lower in schizophrenia (Pakkenberg, 1990; Young et al., 2000; Popken et al., 2000; Byne et al., 2002), later studies have been conspicuously negative (Cullen et al., 2003; Dorph-Petersen et al., 2004; Young et al., 2004).

Recent studies have focused attention on another thalamic nucleus, the pulvinar, an association nucleus involved in higher-order visual processing, and which also projects to the DLPFC (Giguere & Goldman-Rakic, 1988). Several postmortem studies have reported reduced pulvinar

volume and neuron number in subjects with schizophrenia (Byne et al., 2002, 2007; Danos et al., 2003; Highley et al., 2003a), and two earlier studies found a similar trend (Lesch & Bogerts, 1984; Bogerts et al., 1990). The pulvinar data, mostly from unbiased stereological approaches, represent what is currently one of the most consistent neuropathological findings in schizophrenia, especially since there are congruent MRI observations (Byne et al., 2001; Gilbert et al., 2001; Kemether et al., 2003). Moreover, a preliminary study reported that the volume of the primary visual cortex, which projects to the pulvinar (Grieve et al., 2000), is also reduced in schizophrenia (Dorph-Petersen et al., 2007), raising the possibility that a developmental failure in the parcelation of this cortical area could not only contribute to disturbances in early visual processing in schizophrenia, but also to impairments in the pulvinar and its projections to the DLPFC. Clearly, understanding the nature of, and the relationship between, cortical and thalamic abnormalities in schizophrenia requires further study. Also, despite the consistency of the pulvinar literature, there are still complexities; for example, Highley et al. (2003b) found the reductions in schizophrenia to be concentrated in the medial subnucleus, and to be limited to the right hemisphere, but the other pulvinar studies have not shown this specific combination of alterations. For review of the thalamus in schizophrenia, see Byne et al. (2009).

Dorso-lateral prefrontal cortex interneurons and their connections

Perhaps the mostly widely replicated alteration in postmortem studies of schizophrenia involves altered expression of gene products that regulate gamma-aminobutyric acid (GABA) neurotransmission from cortical interneurons. An analysis of all data reported using specimens from the Stanley Neuropathology Consortium revealed that genes expressed in GABA interneurons had the most abnormal transcript and protein levels (Torrey et al., 2005).

The initial studies found decreased glutamic acid decarboxylase (GAD) activity (Bird et al., 1977), decreased GABA reuptake (Simpson et al., 1989), and increased binding to $GABA_A$ receptors (Hanada et al., 1987; Benes et al., 1996). Later studies of the DLPFC in schizophrenia, using microarrays, real-time quantitative polymerase chain reaction (PCR), or in situ hybridization, have consistently found reduced levels of the transcript for the 67 kDa isoform of GAD (GAD_{67}), the principal synthesizing enzyme for GABA (Akbarian et al., 1995; Mirnics et al., 2000; Guidotti et al., 2000; Volk et al., 2000; Vawter et al., 2002; Hashimoto et al., 2005; Straub et al., 2007). Similar findings have been reported in other neocortical regions (Woo et al., 2004; Akbarian & Huang, 2006). Indeed, within the same subjects with schizophrenia, the pattern of GABA-related transcript expression is conserved across the DLPFC and anterior cingulate, primary motor and primary visual cortices (Hashimoto *et al.* 2008). At the cellular level, the expression of GAD_{67} mRNA was not detectable in around 25–35% of GABA neurons in layers 1–5 of the DLPFC, but the remaining GABA neurons exhibited normal levels of GAD_{67} mRNA (Akbarian *et al.*, 1995; Volk *et al.*, 2000). Furthermore, levels of the mRNA for the GABA membrane transporter (GAT1), a protein responsible for re-uptake of GABA back into nerve terminals, was also decreased (Ohnuma *et al.*, 1999) and this decrease was restricted to a similar minority of GABA neurons (Volk *et al.*, 2001). These findings suggest that both the synthesis and re-uptake of GABA are lower in a subset of DLPFC neurons in schizophrenia.

Cortical GABA neurons can be subdivided according to their immunoreactivity for different calcium-binding proteins, notably parvalbumin (PV), calretinin, and calbindin. The approximately 50% of GABA neurons that express calretinin appear unaffected in the frontal cortex in schizophrenia (Beasley & Reynolds, 1997; Beasley *et al.* 2002; Cotter *et al.*, 2002; Hashimoto *et al.*, 2003), and there is little evidence for changes in the calbindin population (Beasley *et al.*, 2002; Cotter *et al.*, 2002). It is the PV-positive neurons, which comprise approximately 25% of GABA neurons in the human neocortex, which seem most affected. The effects are not primarily on the total density or number of the cells—studies in DLPFC report no change (Woo *et al.*, 1997a), a decrease (Beasley & Reynolds, 1997) or a marginal result (Beasley *et al.*, 2002). Rather, the main alterations affect the molecular and synaptic profile of PV-positive neurons. In individuals with schizophrenia, the expression level of PV mRNA is reduced, and approximately half of PV mRNA-containing neurons lack detectable levels of GAD_{67} mRNA (Hashimoto *et al.*, 2003).

Further evidence for PV-positive neuronal abnormalities in schizophrenia becomes apparent when their heterogeneity and connectivity is taken into account. PV-positive GABA interneurons can be further subdivided on morphological grounds. In the DLPFC in schizophrenia, GAT1 immunoreactivity is selectively reduced in the characteristic axon terminals (cartridges) of the chandelier class of PV-containing neurons (Woo *et al.*, 1998). In the postsynaptic targets of these axon cartridges, the axon initial segments of pyramidal neurons, immunoreactivity for the $GABA_A$ receptor α_2 subunit is markedly increased in schizophrenia (Volk *et al.*, 2002). These changes are not found in subjects with other psychiatric disorders, or in monkeys exposed chronically to antipsychotic medications (Volk *et al.*, 2000, 2001, 2002; Hashimoto *et al.*, 2003). The other major subclass of PV-containing GABA neurons is comprised of basket cells whose axons target the cell body and proximal dendritic spines and shafts of pyramidal neurons. Although more difficult to assess directly, similar pre- and post-synaptic alterations may also be present in the inputs of PV-containing, basket neurons to the perisomatic region

of pyramidal neurons. For example, the density of PV-immunoreactive puncta, possibly the axon terminals of wide arbor neurons (Erickson & Lewis, 2002), is reduced in the middle layers, and not in the superficial layers, of the DLPFC of subjects with schizophrenia (Lewis *et al.*, 2001), paralleling the laminar pattern of decreased PV-mRNA expression (Hashimoto *et al.*, 2003). Furthermore, the increased density of $GABA_A$ receptors found in ligand-binding studies was most prominent at pyramidal neuron cell bodies (Benes *et al.*, 1996). Together, these data suggest that the perisomatic inhibitory inputs from PV-containing chandelier and basket neurons are both reduced in schizophrenia.

Although the findings reviewed above provide convergent evidence for alterations in PV-containing GABA neurons in schizophrenia, they also suggest that these neurons cannot account for all of the observed GABAergic alterations. For example, the levels of GAD_{67} and GAT1 mRNAs are reduced to comparable degrees in layers 2–5 (Volk *et al.*, 2000, 2001), even though the density of PV-positive neurons is much greater in layers 3 and 4 than in layers 2 and 5 (Condé *et al.*, 1994). In addition, PV-mRNA expression was reduced in layers 3 and 4, but not in layers 2 and 5, in subjects with schizophrenia (Hashimoto *et al.*, 2003). Together, these findings suggest that one or more populations of GABA neurons in layers 2 and 5, that express neither PV nor calretinin, is altered in schizophrenia. For example, the expression of the neuropeptide somatostatin (SST), which is present in GABA neurons in layers 2 and 5 that do not express PV or calretinin, is reduced in subjects with schizophrenia (Hashimoto *et al.*, 2008; Morris *et al.*, 2008).

These various molecular and cellular findings together suggest that there is an alteration in schizophrenia affecting the intrinsic GABAergic circuitry of the DLPFC, in addition to the changes in extrinsic connectivity implicated by the thalamic and DA innervation data (Plate 18.2 and Plate 21.2.).

Oligodendrocytes in schizophrenia

In addition to the evidence implicating neuronal and synaptic subpopulations in schizophrenia, recent evidence suggests that oligodendrocytes, a glial cell type critically involved in myelination and neuronal development and support (Nave & Trapp, 2008), may be affected, both in the DLPFC and other regions. Reductions in the density of oligodendrocytes have been reported using Nissl-stained material and immunoreactivity for the oligodendrocyte marker 2′, 3′-cyclic nucleotide 3′-phosphodiesterase (CNP) (Hof *et al.*, 2003; Uranova *et al.*, 2004; Vostrikov *et al.*, 2007; Schmitt *et al.*, 2009). Consistent with a decreased number and/or activity of these cells, mRNA and protein studies have found reduced expression of many oligodendrocyte-enriched genes, such as myelin-associated glycoprotein which supports the myelin–axonal interface and the structure of myelin sheaths (Hakak *et al.*, 2001; Tkachev *et al.*, 2003; Dracheva *et al.*, 2006; but see Mitkus *et al.*, 2008). Altered oligodendrocyte ultrastructure has also been reported (Uranova *et al.*, 2001). These morphometric and molecular findings complement evidence from imaging modalities which show alterations in the structure of white matter tracts, consistent with—though not proof of—a pathophysiological role for oligodendrocytes, and thence for altered myelination, in schizophrenia (Davis *et al.*, 2003; Karoutzou *et al.*, 2008).

Neuropathological interpretations

Having reviewed the major themes and findings regarding the neuropathology of schizophrenia (summarized in Table 18.1), we briefly consider some of the diverse interpretational issues raised by these data.

Where is the core neuropathology?

This basic question, posed by Shapiro (1993), is still impossible to answer; it is not even clear if it is best framed in terms of brain areas, cell types, subcellular compartments, or neural circuits. Neither is it known whether there is a single causal factor that, if identified, would explain the where (or the what) of the core neuropathology.

Regarding regional distribution, surprisingly few studies have directly compared one area with another, and no brain region has been investigated in multiple studies and con-

Table 18.1 Selected neuropathological findings in schizophrenia.

General

Decreased brain weight

Absence of gliosis

Absence of Alzheimer's disease or other degenerative pathologies

Findings in the hippocampal formation and dorso-lateral prefrontal cortex (DLPFC)

Smaller pyramidal neuron cell bodies

Decreased presynaptic protein markers

Lower density of dendritic spines

Decreased markers of parvalbumin (PV)-positive GABA neurons and their synaptic terminals

Decreased number and activity of oligodendrocytes

No overall loss of neurons

Findings in other regions

Smaller pulvinar and medio-dorsal thalamic nuclei with fewer neurons

For more detailed listings and citations, see text.

sistently found to be unchanged in whatever parameter has been measured. Certainly, despite the focus in this chapter on the hippocampal formation, DLPFC, and thalamus, there are notable neuropathological findings of one kind or another in many other brain regions, some of which have been mentioned (see also, for example, Cotter *et al.*, 2004; Katsel *et al.*, 2005; Roberts *et al.*, 2005; Kreczmanski *et al.*, 2007; Perez-Costas *et al.*, 2010). For example, the primary visual cortex would generally be considered an "unaffected" cortical region in schizophrenia, yet it is smaller in volume (Dorph-Petersen *et al.*, 2007) and has a neuronal and synaptic pathology not dissimilar to that of the DLPFC (Selemon *et al.*, 1995; Eastwood *et al.*, 2000). As to the cellular perspective, the situation is arguably less clear than it was 10 years ago, when at least one could limit the discussion to which neuronal populations were most affected. Now, as noted above, glia, particularly oligodendrocytes, are also implicated. Finally, the localization of neuropathology can also be addressed in terms of subcellular compartments. Again, the findings are diverse, and, as discussed in this chapter, include axons, presynaptic terminals, dendrites and dendritic spines, and mitochondria.

It would be a major advance if the neuropathology of schizophrenia could be pinned down in terms of any of these three perspectives—regional, cellular, or subcellular—although it may, of course, also be that it is not definable in any such way.

Is there a cerebral asymmetry of neuropathology?

A number of postmortem studies, notably of the temporal lobe (Crow *et al.*, 1989; Zaidel *et al.*, 1997a,b; McDonald *et al.*, 2000; Smiley *et al.*, 2009), but also in some other regions (Highley *et al*, 2003a; Cullen *et al*, 2006), have shown changes in schizophrenia lateralized to one or other hemisphere, as do some results from other research modalities (Sommer *et al.*, 2001). However, many other studies find bilateral alterations, or have not been designed to address the question—the latter includes most investigations of the DLPFC. Overall, it remains unclear whether the neuropathology of schizophrenia is fundamentally asymmetrical (or affects normal asymmetries) in some way and, if it is, what its origin and significance might be (Holinger *et al.*, 2000). As such, Crow's (1990, 2004) theory of schizophrenia that ascribes a critical role to altered cerebral asymmetry remains neuropathologically speculative.

How are the pathology and symptoms related?

The question of clinicopathological correlations is a basic but neglected issue in the literature. It has several facets.

A neural circuitry-based model of schizophrenia requires an appreciation of the mechanistic relationships between the various abnormalities observed in different components of the circuitry. Specifically, understanding the pathophysiology of schizophrenia depends ultimately on knowledge of how abnormalities in one brain region or circuitry component produce and/or result from disturbances in others, a task that involves a consideration of cause, consequence, and compensation (Lewis, 2000). Does a given abnormality represent a primary pathogenic event (cause), does it reflect a secondary deleterious event (consequence) or does it reveal an attempted homeostatic response (compensation)? Distinguishing among these three possibilities for each component of a neural network will be necessary for understanding the pathophysiology of the disease, as well as for developing novel therapies designed to correct causes and consequences and/or to augment compensatory responses.

Another issue concerns the correspondence between clinical symptoms and pathological findings. To date, the clinical information available and the sample sizes used in postmortem research have been inadequate to allow this issue to be addressed. However, it may be hypothesized that the nature, distribution, and stability of pathological changes suggest that they might be particularly related to trait-related features (e.g. cognitive deficits) than to fluctuating features (e.g., positive symptoms; Harrison, 1999a). Although there are few data that directly address this proposal, Sawada *et al.* (2005) found that hippocampal synaptic protein reductions were related to a patient's cognitive status. A related point is whether one or several pathological processes underlie schizophrenia. Based on the current data, it is parsimonious to postulate a single pathological process which varies in severity between patients with schizophrenia—as is the case with the structural imaging findings. Across subjects, there may also be different genetic, molecular pathways leading to a common final functional and structural disturbance in brain circuitry. This view does not preclude a different conclusion as new data emerge (e.g., the possibility of a different pathological phenotype in late-onset schizophrenia).

The temporal relationship between neuropathology and the onset of symptoms is unknown, because postmortem studies of first-episode patients are impossible in practice. It is only by extrapolation (e.g., from the decreased NAA seen in first-episode cases, and the lack of correlation of postmortem findings with duration of illness) that the suggestion can be made that the alterations, at least partly, are present at or before the onset of illness. Equally, even if some of the neuropathological changes do only arise (or become more severe) later in the illness, this does not negate their importance or imply that they are epiphenomenal. Rather, if this were the case, it might mean that their development was a factor contributing to the oft progressive course of the illness.

Do the neuropathological data support a neurodevelopmental origin of schizophrenia?

Although the idea that schizophrenia is a late consequence of an early developmental lesion has many merits (Lewis & Levitt, 2002; see Chapter 19), it has proven difficult to obtain direct *positive* neuropathological evidence for a brain abnormality that necessarily supports such a model (i.e., which can confidently be timed to the second trimester, perinatal period, adolescence, etc.). To date, it remains the lack of evidence *against* there being a progressive or degenerative disease process that, by default, is the strongest neuropathological pointer towards a neurodevelopmental origin.

The dearth of positive neuropathological support has already been mentioned with regard to the failure to confirm unequivocally the occurrence of entorhinal dysplasia or hippocampal neuron disarray, either of which would constitute strong evidence of this kind. The same inference would apply to an altered distribution and/or density of interstitial neurons in the white matter of the neocortex, initially described by Akbarian *et al.* (1993a,b). These neurons are thought to be the surviving remnant of subplate neurons, a transient cell population that pioneers cortical development and the formation of corticothalamic connections. As such, the alterations were plausibly interpreted as being indicative of a developmental anomaly (Bloom, 1993). Again, however, the observations have not consistently been replicated (e.g., Cotter *et al*, 2002; Eastwood & Harrison, 2003). Instead, the cytoarchitectural and molecular changes which are more robustly demonstrable in schizophrenia, e.g., loss of synaptic proteins, smaller neurons, reductions in GABAergic markers, affect parameters which are dynamically regulated and could arise at any time point and for various reasons, including neuronal activity and hypoxia (e.g., Masliah *et al.*, 1993; Marti *et al.*, 1998; Bravin *et al.*, 1999). Thus, any developmental interpretations of such alterations should be made with due caution.

On the other hand, one should not neglect the corroborative and circumstantial evidence which, complementing the lack of gliosis, supports a developmental basis for the pathological findings in schizophrenia. There are three aspects to consider. First, the demonstration that the neural pathways implicated in the pathology of schizophrenia show marked developmental changes at relevant time periods. One example is in the hippocampal formation (Benes *et al.*, 1994); another is the circuitry of the primate DLPFC. For example, after rising dramatically during the main phase of synaptogenesis in prenatal and early postnatal life, the number of excitatory, but not inhibitory, synapses in the DLPFC declines by 50% during adolescence in primates (Huttenlocher, 1979; Bourgeois *et al.*, 1994). During this time period, dendritic spine densities decrease

(Anderson *et al.*, 1995), but pyramidal neuron size and total dendritic length increase (Lambe *et al.*, 2000). These maturational changes differ according to the neuronal and synaptic population being considered. For example, there are substantial changes to excitatory, inhibitory, and modulatory inputs to pyramidal neurons in deep layer 3 of the DLPFC. The terminals of intrinsic axon collaterals from DLPFC layer 3 pyramidal cells may be more extensively pruned than associational cortical projections (Woo *et al.*, 1997b), while serotonergic synapses upon these neurons develop much more rapidly than catecholaminergic ones (Lambe *et al.*, 2000). The apparent laminar specificity of at least some of these changes supports the observations that circuits involving these pyramidal neurons may be preferentially affected in schizophrenia (Lewis, 1997). Knowing whether projections from the thalamus are particularly vulnerable to this process might provide critical information for hypotheses regarding the mechanisms underlying disturbances in thalamocortical circuitry in schizophrenia.

Second, there are studies in schizophrenia of molecules known to be important in one or other aspect of brain maturation (e.g., neuronal migration, synaptogenesis). Reported alterations of reelin, *Wnt*, semaphorin, and netrin expression in schizophrenia exemplify this approach, and there will no doubt be many more reports of this kind as other key developmental genes are investigated (Weickert & Weinberger, 1998; Guidotti *et al.*, 2000; Eastwood *et al.*, 2003). The assumption behind these studies is that the altered gene expression seen in schizophrenia is a persistent sign (or "smoking gun") of aberrant neurodevelopment. This interpretation may well be true, but the very fact that a gene continues to be expressed in the adult brain may also indicate that it has other, non-developmental, functions and therefore a similarly non-developmental implication for schizophrenia (Harrison, 2007). As with morphometric alterations, a convergence and consistency of results will be needed to allow confidence in the developmental explanation.

Third, neuropathological findings in known neurodevelopmental disorders, although far from conclusive in their own right, provide another form of circumstantial support for a developmental interpretation of the schizophrenia data. For example, dendritic arborizations, dendritic proteins, and dendritic spine densities are decreased in the cortex in Rett syndrome and Williams syndrome (Kaufmann & Moser, 2000), dendritic spines are abnormal in fragile X syndrome (Irwin *et al.*, 2000), and neuronal size is reduced in Rett syndrome and autism (Kemper & Bauman, 1998).

Are the changes specific to schizophrenia?

The overlap with the morphometric findings reported in several neurodevelopmental disorders raises the issue of diagnostic specificity. Most classical neuropathological studies of schizophrenia have not included a comparison group comprised of patients with other psychiatric disorders and so, with few exceptions, the specificity of many alterations is uncertain. On the other hand, facilitated by the Stanley Medical Research Institute, an increasing number of morphometric and molecular studies have simultaneously evaluated bipolar disorder (and sometimes major depressive disorder). Review of the data collected in these brains reveals a marked but not complete concordance between schizophrenia and bipolar disorder, and a much lesser overlap with major depression (Torrey *et al.*, 2005; see also Harrison, 2002; Shao & Vawter, 2008). It is possible that the common findings reflect shared confounding factors between schizophrenia and bipolar disorder, but more likely points to shared pathophysiological and/or etiological pathways. In this regard, the relatively few neuropathological studies that show schizophrenia- or bipolar disorder-specific changes (e.g. Eastwood & Harrison, 2010; Pantazopoulos *et al.*, 2010), are of interest as pointing to potential points of separation between the disorder. Overall, however, the existing neuropathological data are insufficient to contribute in any conclusive way to the debate as to whether schizophrenia and bipolar disorder are distinct disorders or on a continuum. A similar debate may emerge with regard to autism, as its neuropathology begins to be evaluated in detail (Schmitz & Rezaie, 2008).

Are the changes brought about by medication?

Antipsychotic drugs, and other treatments, are often suspected as contributing to, or even causing, the neuropathological features reported in schizophrenia. Certainly, given that few subjects in postmortem studies have been medication-free at death, and virtually none medication-naïve, it is a difficult possibility to eliminate entirely.

An absence of demonstrable antipsychotic effects on cortical cytoarchitecture is suggested by findings in the DLPFC and MDN. Globally, the increase in DLPFC cell packing density seen in subjects with schizophrenia was not found in monkeys treated for 6 months with a variety of antipsychotics (Selemon *et al.*, 1999). In addition, treatment of monkeys for 12 months with haloperidol and benztropine at blood levels known to be therapeutic in humans was not associated with a reduction in the size or total neuron number of the MDN (Pierri *et al.*, 1999). The decreased dendritic spine density also appears to be specific to schizophrenia, in that it was not observed in a psychiatric disorder control group who had received antipsychotics (Glantz & Lewis, 2000). Likewise, many of the gene expression changes observed in schizophrenia have not been found in rodents or monkeys exposed to antipsychotic medications. However, these studies cannot, of course, exclude the possibility of human-specific effects of these medications, or of disease–drug interactions.

In contrast to these findings, a recent study in chronically antipsychotic-treated monkeys shared smaller gray matter volume, lower glial cell number, and higher neuron density without a difference in total neuron number (Dorph-Petersen *et al.*, 2005; Konopaske *et al.*, 2007). These results parallel observations in schizophrenia described above and that raise the possibility that the latter might be due, at least in part, to antipsychotic medication effects. Conversely, it is also possible that medication partially reverses, and therefore masks, some neuropathological features, as has been suggested based upon MRI studies (Scherk & Falkai, 2006), and exemplified by the DLPFC microarray findings discussed earlier (Middleton *et al.*, 2002).

There are few data as to the pathological consequences of other treatments sometimes used in schizophrenia, such as antidepressants, mood stabilizers, and electroconvulsive therapy, but those that exist do not suggest that they are major confounders (Harrison, 1999b).

Is the neuropathology genetic in origin?

The neuroimaging literature shows that a proportion of the structural brain differences seen in schizophrenia are also seen in unaffected relatives and those who have yet to develop the illness (see Chapter 16). It is therefore likely related to the genetic predisposition to the disorder. The same inference may be drawn for the neuropathological findings, although this can only be speculation as there has never been a postmortem study of at-risk subjects or unaffected relatives. Nevertheless, support for this notion is provided by recent reports that variants in several schizophrenia susceptibility genes are associated with differences in brain structure and connectivity seen *in vivo* (e.g., Callicott *et al.*, 2005; Prasad *et al.*, 2005; McIntosh *et al.*, 2008), and affect gene expression (e.g., Law *et al.*, 2006; Straub *et al.*, 2007). The apparent convergence of putative susceptibility genes upon synaptic (Harrison & Weinberger, 2005; Harrison & West, 2006) and oligodendrocyte (Carter, 2006) functioning is also noteworthy. It will be of interest to relate neuropathological findings to genotype in future studies (Kleinman *et al.*, 2011), albeit that they will inevitably be of limited power. Initial examples are provided by a report linking a *DISC1* genetic variant with the morphology of glial centrosomes (Eastwood *et al.*, 2010), and a study relating genome-wide association data with cytoarchitectural findings (Kim & Webster, 2010).

Will schizophrenia ever be diagnosable down a microscope?

The existing neuropathological data mean that the answer is a clear "'no" at present, and it is unknown whether this will change in the future. Comparison with Alzheimer's disease is relevant for illustrating the kinds of conditions which would need to be met if it is ever to be answered in the affirmative. First, in Alzheimer's disease there are reliably identifiable lesions (neurofibrillary tangles, amyloid plaques) that are qualitatively different from normal cytological and histological parameters, and which have a quantitative relationship to the presence and severity of the clinical syndrome, and their distribution and effect on the cortical circuitry gives a convincing explanation for the features of the syndrome. Second, key aspects of Alzheimer's disease pathology can now be reproduced in transgenic mice, which develop cognitive impairment; moreover, reversal of the pathology leads to corresponding improvement in memory performance. Finally, the neuropathological picture of Alzheimer's disease is different from that of other dementias, and in this sense it is diagnostically specific (although this becomes a circular argument once a disorder is defined by its neuropathology and not by its clinical features).

Ultimately, schizophrenia might become, like Alzheimer's disease, a disorder—or disorders —in which neuropathological features are necessary and/or sufficient for diagnostic purposes. Like Alzheimer's disease, it may also become possible to link the pathology directly to the etiology, as illustrated by the mice carrying mutations in the causative genes. Alternatively, new approaches, such as gene expression profiling or proteomic strategies, may provide molecular signatures that are diagnostic of schizophrenia(s). However, the value of the next generation of postmortem studies of schizophrenia may not rest in the realm of a "gold standard" for diagnosis, but in the types of pathogenic or pathophysiological insights that clarify genetic mechanisms, or reveal novel targets for pharmacological interventions.

Conclusions

Neuropathological studies provide clues as to the cellular and molecular correlates of the structural differences in the brain in schizophrenia identified by neuroimaging. There is strong evidence against the presence of a neurodegenerative process, with an absence of gliosis and of Alzheimer disease. There is a range of morphometric and cytoarchitectural findings, affecting the distribution, density, size, and phenotypic properties of various neuronal and glial populations. These are accompanied by alterations in the expression of various molecules indexing synaptic and oligodendrocyte functioning. The changes are prominent in, but not restricted to, the hippocampal formation, DLPFC, and thalamus. The robustness of these findings varies, and their interpretation remains under debate. It is likely that the neuropathology reflects, at least partly, a difference in subtle aspects of the neural circuitry arising from the neurodevelopmental and genetic origins of the syndrome. Antipsychotic medication and other confounders cannot be excluded as contributing to some of the findings. The diagnostic specificity of the changes reported in schizophrenia has not been determined, and there are few established clinicopathological correlations. Overall, the neuropathology of schizophrenia has made significant advances as an integral part of the broader progress in understanding the core neurobiology of the disorder, but it remains poorly characterized and lacks diagnostic or clinical value.

References

Akbarian, S. & Huang, H. S. (2006) Molecular and cellular mechanisms of altered GAD1/GAD67 expression in schizophrenia and related disorders. *Brain Research Reviews* **52**, 293–304.

Akbarian, S., Bunney, W.E., Jr, Potkin, S.G. *et al.* (1993a) Altered distribution of nicotinamide-adenine dinucleotide phosphate-diaphorase cells in frontal lobe of schizophrenics implies disturbances of cortical development. *Archives of General Psychiatry* **50**, 169–177.

Akbarian, S., Viñuela, A., Kim, J.J. *et al.* (1993b) Distorted distribution of nicotinamide-adenine dinucleotilde phosphate-diaphorase neurons in temporal lose of schizophrenic implies anomalous cortical development. *Archives of General Psychiatry* **50**, 178–187.

Akbarian, S., Kim, J.J., Potkin, S.G. *et al.* (1995) Gene expression for glutamic acid decarboxylase is reduced without loss of neurons in prefrontal cortex of schizophrenics. *Archives of General Psychiatry* **52**, 258–266.

Akil, M. & Lewis, D.A. (1997) The cytoarchitecture of the entorhinal cortex in schizophrenia. *American Journal of Psychiatry* **154**, 1010–1012.

Akil, M., Pierri, J.N., Whitehead, R.E. *et al.* (1999) Lamina-specific alteration in the dopamine innervation of the prefrontal cortex in schizophrenic subjects. *American Journal of Psychiatry* **156**, 1580–1589.

Altar, C.A., Jurata, L.W., Charles, V. *et al.* (2005) Deficient hippocampal neuron expression of proteasome, ubiquitin, and mitochondrial genes in multiple schizophrenia cohorts, *Biological Psychiatry* **58**, 85–96.

Altshuler, L.L., Conrad, A., Kovelman, J.A. & Scheibel, A.B. (1987) Hippocampal pyramidal cell orientation in schizophrenia: a controlled neurohistologic study of the Yakovlev collection. *Archives of General Psychiatry* **44**, 1094–1098.

Anderson, S.A., Classey, J.D., Condé, F. *et al.* (1995) Synchronous development of pyramidal neuron dendritic spines and parvalbumin-immunoreactive chandelier neuron axon terminals in layer III of monkey prefrontal cortex. *Neuroscience* **67**, 7–22.

Arnold, S.E. (1997) The medial temporal lobe in schizophrenia. *Journal of Neuropsychiatry and Clinical Neuroscience* **9**, 460–470.

Arnold, S.E. & Trojanowski, J.Q. (1996) Recent advances in defining the neuropathology of schizophrenia. *Acta Neuropathologica* **92**, 217–231.

Arnold, S.E., Hyman, B.T., Van Hoesen, G.W. & Damasio, A.R. (1991a) Some cytoarchitectural abnormalities of the entorhinal cortex in schizophrenia. *Archives of General Psychiatry* **48**, 625–632.

Arnold, S.E., Lee, V.M.Y., Gur, R.E. & Trojanowski, J.Q. (1991b) Abnormal expression of two microtubule-associated proteins (MAP2 and MAP5) in specific subfields of the hippocampal formation in schizophrenia. *Proceedings of the National Academy of Sciences USA* **88**, 10850–10854.

Arnold, S.E., Franz, B.R., Gur, R.C. *et al.* (1995) Smaller neuron size in schizophrenia hippocampal subfields that mediate cortical–hippocampal interactions. *American Journal of Psychiatry* **152**, 738–748.

Arnold, S.E., Franz, B.R., Trojanowski, J.Q. *et al.* (1996) Glial fibrillary acidic protein-immunoreactive astrocytosis in elderly patients with schizophrenia and dementia. *Acta Neuropathologica* **91**, 269–277.

Arnold, S.E., Ruscheinsky, D.D. & Han, L.Y. (1997) Further evidence of abnormal cytoarchitecture of the entorhinal cortex in schizophrenia using spatial point pattern analyses. *Biological Psychiatry* **42**, 639–647.

Arnold, S.E., Trojanowski, J.Q., Gur, R.E. *et al.* (1998) Absence of neurodegeneration and neural injury in the cerebral cortex in a sample of elderly patients with schizophrenia. *Archives of General Psychiatry* **55**, 225–232.

Baldessarini, R.J., Hegarty, J., Bird, E.D. & Benes, F.M. (1997) Meta-analysis of postmortem studies of Alzheimer's disease-like neuropathology in schizophrenia. *American Journal of Psychiatry* **154**, 861–863.

Beasley, C.L. & Reynolds, G.P. (1997) Parvalbumin-immunoreactive neurons are reduced in the prefrontal cortex of schizophrenics. *Schizophrenia Research* **24**, 349–355.

Beasley, C.L., Zhang, Z.J., Patten, I. & Reynolds, G.P. (2002) Selective deficits in prefrontal cortical GABAergic neurons in schizophrenia defined by the presence of calcium-binding proteins. *Biological Psychiatry* **52**, 708–715.

Benes, F.M. (2000) Emerging principles of altered neural circuitry in schizophrenia. *Brain Research Reviews* **31**, 251–269.

Benes, F.M., Davidson, J. & Bird, E.D. (1986) Quantitative cytoarchitectural studies of the cerebral cortex of schizophrenics. *Archives of General Psychiatry* **43**, 31–35.

Benes, F.M., McSparren, J., Bird, E.D. *et al.* (1991a) Deficits in small interneurons in prefrontal and cingulate cortices of schizophrenic and schizoaffective patients. *Archives of General Psychiatry* **48**, 996–1001.

Benes, F.M., Sorensen, I. & Bird, E.D. (1991b) Reduced neuronal size in posterior hippocampus of schizophrenic patients. *Schizophrenia Bulletin* **17**, 597–608.

Benes, F.M., Turtle, M., Khan, Y. & Farol, P. (1994) Myelination of a key relay zone in the hippocampal formation occurs in the human brain during childhood, adolescence, and adulthood. *Archives of General Psychiatry* **51**, 477–484.

Benes, F.M., Vincent, S.L., Marie, A. & Khan, Y. (1996) Up-regulation of GABA-A receptor binding on neurons of the prefrontal cortex in schizophrenic subjects. *Neuroscience* **75**, 1021–1031.

Benes, F.M., Kwok, E.W., Vincent, S.L. & Todtenkopf, M.S. (1998) Reduction of non-pyramidal cells in section CA2 of schizophrenics and manic depressives. *Biological Psychiatry* **44**, 88–97.

Bernstein, H.-G., Krell, D., Baumann, B. *et al.* (1998) Morphometric studies of the entorhinal cortex in neuropsychiatric patients and controls: clusters of heterotopically displaced lamina II neurons are not indicative of schizophrenia. *Schizophrenia Research* 33, 125–132.

Bertolino, A., Nawroz, S., Mattay, V.S. *et al.* (1996) Regionally specific pattern of neurochemical pathology in schizophrenia as assessed by multislice proton magnetic resonance spectroscopic imaging. *American Journal of Psychiatry* 153, 1554–1563.

Bertolino, A., Callicott, J.H., Elman, I. *et al.* (1998) Regionally specific neural pathology in untreated patients with schizophrenia: a proton magnetic resonance spectroscopic imaging study. *Biological Psychiatry* 43, 641–648.

Bertolino, A., Esposito, G., Callicott, J.H. *et al.* (2000) Specific relationship between prefrontal neuronal *N*-acetylaspartate and activation of the working memory cortical network in schizophrenia. *American Journal of Psychiatry* 157, 26–33.

Bird, E., Barnes, J., Iversen, L. *et al.* (1977) Increased brain dopamine and reduced glutamic acid decarboxylase and choline acetyl transferase activity in schizophrenia and related psychoses. *The Lancet* 310, 1157–1159.

Black, J.E., Kodish, I.M., Grossman, A.W. *et al.* (2004). Pathology of layer V pyramidal neurons in the prefrontal cortex of patients with schizophrenia. *American Journal of Psychiatry* 161, 742–744.

Bloom, F.E. (1993) Advancing a neurodevelopmental origin for schizophrenia, *Archives of General Psychiatry* 50, 224–227.

Bogerts, B., Hantsch, J. & Herzer, M. (1983) A morphometric study of the dopamine-containing cell groups in the mesencephalon of normals, Parkinson patients, and schizophrenics. *Biological Psychiatry* 18, 951–969.

Bogerts, B., Falkai, P., Haupts, M. *et al.* (1990) Post-mortem volume measurements of limbic system and basal ganglia structures in chronic schizophrenics. Initial results from a new brain collection. *Schizophrenia Research* 3, 295–301.

Bourgeois, J.-P., Goldman-Rakic, P.S. & Rakic, P. (1994) Synaptogenesis in the prefrontal cortex of rhesus monkeys. *Cerebral Cortex* 4, 78–96.

Boyer, P., Phillips, J.L., Rousseau, F.L. & Ilivitsky, S. (2007) Hippocampal abnormalities and memory deficits: New evidence of a strong pathophysiological link in schizophrenia. *Brain Research Reviews* 54, 92–112.

Bozikas, V.P., Kövari, E., Bouras, C. & Karavatos, A. (2002) Neurofibrillary tangles in elderly patients with late onset schizophrenia. *Neuroscience Letters* 324, 109–112.

Bravin, M., Morando, L., Vercelli, A. Rossi, F. & Strata, P. (1999) Control of spine formation by electrical activity in the adult rat cerebellum. *Proceedings of the National Academy of Sciences USA* 96, 1704–1709.

Broadbelt, K., Byne, W. & Jones, L.B. (2002). Evidence for a decrease in basilar dendrites of pyramidal cells in schizophrenic medial prefrontal cortex. *Schizophrenia Research* 58, 75–81.

Bruton, C.J., Crow, T.J., Frith, C. *et al.* (1990) Schizophrenia and the brain: a prospective cliniconeuropathological study. *Psychological Medicine* 20, 285–304.

Buchsbaum, M.S., Someya, T., Teng, C.Y. *et al.* (1996) PET and MRI of the thalamus in never-medicated patients with schizophrenia. *American Journal of Psychiatry* 153, 191–199.

Byne, W., Buchsbaum, M.S., Kemether, E. *et al.* (2001) Magnetic resonance imaging of the thalamic mediodorsal nucles and pulvinar in schizophrenia and schizotypal personality disorder. *Archives of General Psychiatry* 58, 133–140.

Byne, W., Buchsbaum, M.S., Mattiace, L.A. *et al.* (2002) Postmortem assessment of thalamic nuclear volumes in subjects with schizophrenia. *American Journal of Psychiatry* 159, 59–65.

Byne, W., Fernandes, J., Haroutunian, V. *et al.* (2007) Reduction of right medial pulvinar volume and neuron number in schizophrenia. *Schizophrenia Research* 90, 71–75.

Byne, W., Hazlett, E.A., Buchsbaum, M.S., & Kemether, E. (2009) The thalamus and schizophrenia: current status of research. *Acta Neuropathologica* 117, 347–368.

Callicott, J.H., Straub, R.E., Pezawas, L *et al.* (2005) Variation in DISC1 affects hippocampal structure and function and increases risk for schizophrenia. *Proceedings of the National Academy of Sciences USA* 102, 8627–8632.

Carter, C.J. (2006) Schizophrenia susceptibility genes converge on interlinked pathways related to glutamatergic transmission and long-term potentiation, oxidative stress and oligodendrocyte viability. *Schizophrenia Research* 86, 1–14.

Casanova, M.F., Stevens, J.R., Brown, R., Royston, C. & Bruton, C. (2002) Disentangling the pathology of schizophrenia and paraphrenia. *Acta Neuropathologica* 103, 313–320.

Christison, G.W., Casanova, M.F., Weinberger, D.R. *et al.* (1989) A quantitative investigation of hippocampal pyramidal cell size, shape, and variability of orientation in schizophrenia. *Archives of General Psychiatry* 46, 1027–1032.

Condé, F., Lund, J.S. Jacobowitz, D.M. *et al.* (1994) Local circuit neurons immunoreactive for calretinin, calbindin D-28k, or parvalbumin in monkey prefrontal cortex: Distribution and morphology. *Journal of Comparative Neurology* 341, 95–116.

Conrad, A.J., Abebe, T., Austin, R. *et al.* (1991) Hippocampal pyramidal cell disarray in schizophrenia as a bilateral phenomenon. *Archives of General Psychiatry* 48, 413–417.

Corsellis, J.A.N. (1962) Mental illness and the ageing brain. *Institute of Psychiatry Maudsley Monographs No. 9*. London: Oxford University Press.

Cotter, D., Landau, S., Beasley, C. *et al.* (2002) The density and spatial distribution of GABAergic neurons, labelled using calcium binding proteins, in the anterior cingulate cortex in major depressive disorder, bipolar disorder, and schizophrenia. *Biological Psychiatry* 51, 377–386.

Cotter, D., MacKay, D. Frangou, S. *et al.* (2004) Cell density and cortical thickness in Heschl's gyrus in schizophrenia, major depression and bipolar disorder. *British Journal of Psychiatry* 185, 258–259.

Crow, T.J. (1990) Temporal lobe asymmetries as the key to the etiology of schizophrenia. *Schizophrenia Bulletin* 16, 433–443.

Crow, T.J. (2004) Cerebral asymmetry and the lateralization of language: core deficits in schizophrenia as pointers to the gene. *Current Opinion in Psychiatry* 17, 97–106.

Crow, T.J., Ball, J., Bloom, S. *et al.* (1989) Schizophrenia as an anomaly of development of cerebral asymmetry. *Archives of General Psychiatry* 46, 1145–1150.

Cullen, T.J., Walker, M.A., Parkinson, N. *et al.* (2003) A postmortem study of the mediodorsal nucleus of the thalamus in schizophrenia. *Schizophrenia Research* 60, 157–166.

Cullen, T.J., Walker, M.A., Eastwood, S.L. *et al.* (2006) Anomalies of asymmetry of pyramidal cell density and structure in dorsolateral prefrontal cortex in schizophrenia. *British Journal of Psychiatry* **188**, 26–31.

Da Cunha, A., Jeffereson, J.J., Tyor, W.R. *et al.* (1993) Gliosis in human brain: relationship to size but not other properties of astrocytes. *Brain Research* **600**, 161–165.

Danos, P., Baumann, B., Krämer, A. *et al.* (2003) Volumes of association thalamic nuclei in schizophrenia: a postmortem study. *Schizophrenia Research* **60**, 141–155.

David, G.B. (1957) The pathological anatomy of the schizophrenias. In: Richter, D., ed. *Schizophrenia: Somatic Aspects*. Oxford: Pergamon, pp. 93–130.

Davidsson, P., Gottfries, J., Bogdanovic, N. *et al.* (1999) The synaptic-vesicle-specific proteins rab3a and synaptophysin are reduced in thalamus and related cortical brain regions in schizophrenic brains. *Schizophrenia Research* **40**, 23–29.

Davis, K.L., Stewart, D.G., Friedman, J.I. *et al.* (2003) White matter changes in schizophrenia – Evidence for myelin-related dysfunction. *Archives of General Psychiatry* **60**, 443–456.

Daviss, S.R. & Lewis, D.A. (1995) Local circuit neurons of the prefrontal cortex in schizophrenia: selective increase in the density of calbindin-immunoreactive neurons. *Psychiatry Research* **59**, 81–96.

Deicken, R.F., Zhou, L., Corwin, F. *et al.* (1997) Decreased left frontal lobe *N*-acetylaspartate in schizophrenia. *American Journal of Psychiatry* **154**, 688–690.

DeLisi, L.E. (2008) The concept of progressive brain change in schizophrenia: Implications for understanding schizophrenia. *Schizophrenia Bulletin* **34**, 312–321.

Dorph-Petersen, K.-A., Lewis, D.A. (2010) Stereological approaches to identifying neuropathology in psychosis. *Biological Psychiatry* doi:10.1016/j.biopsych.2010.10.04.30.

Dorph-Petersen, K.-A. Pierri, J.N. Sun, Z. *et al.* (2004) Stereological analysis of the mediodorsal thalamic nucleus in schizophrenia: Volume, neuron number, and cell types. *Journal of Comparative Neurology* **472**, 449–462.

Dorph-Petersen, K.-A. Pierri, J.N. Perel, J.M. *et al.* (2005) The influence of chronic exposure to antipsychotic medications on brain size before and after tissue fixation: A comparison of haloperidol and olanzapine in macaque monkeys. *Neuropsychopharmacolgy* **30**, 1649–1661.

Dorph-Petersen, K.A. Pierri, J.N. Wu, Q. *et al.* (2007) Primary visual cortex volume and total neuron number are reduced in schizophrenia. *Journal of Comparative Neurology* **501**, 290–301.

Dracheva, S., Davis, K.L., Chin, B. *et al.* (2006) Myelin-associated mRNA and protein expression deficits in the anterior cingulate cortex and hippocampus in elderly schizophrenia patients. *Neurobiology of Disease* **21**, 531–540.

Eastwood, S.L. & Harrison, P.J. (1995) Decreased synaptophysin in the medial temporal lobe in schizophrenia demonstrated using immunoautoradiography. *Neuroscience* **69**, 339–343.

Eastwood, S.L. & Harrison, P.J. (1998) Hippocampal and cortical growth-associated protein-43 messenger RNA in schizophrenia. *Neuroscience* **86**, 437–448.

Eastwood, S.L. & Harrison, P.J. (1999) Detection and quantification of hippocampal synaptophysin messenger RNA in schizophrenia using autoclaved, formalin-fixed paraffin wax-embedded sections. *Neuroscience* **93**, 99–106.

Eastwood, S.L. & Harrison, P.J. (2000) Hippocampal synaptic pathol-ogy in schizophrenia bipolar disorder and major depression: a study of complexin mRNAs. *Molecular Psychiatry* **5**, 425–432.

Eastwood, S.L. & Harrison, P.J. (2001) Synaptic pathology in the anterior cingulate cortex in schizophrenia and mood disorders: an immunoblotting study of synaptophysin, gap-43 and the complexins and a review. *Brain Research Bulletin* **55**, 569–578.

Eastwood, S.L. & Harrison, P.J. (2003) Interstitial white matter neurons express less reelin and are abnormally distributed in schizophrenia: towards an integration of molecular and morphologic aspects of the neurodevelopmental hypothesis. *Molecular Psychiatry* **8**, 821–831.

Eastwood, S.L. & Harrison, P.J. (2010) Markers of glutamate synaptic transmission and plasticity are increased in the anterior cingulate cortex in bipolar disorder. *Biological Psychiatry* **67**, 1010–1016.

Eastwood, S.L. Cairns, N.J. & Harrison, P.J. (2000) Synaptophysin gene expression in schizophrenia: investigation of synaptic pathology in the cerebral cortex. *British Journal of Psychiatry* **176**, 236–242.

Eastwood, S.L. Law, A.J. Everall, I.P. & Harrison, P.J. (2003) The axonal chemorepellant semaphorin 3A is increased in the cerebellum in schizophrenia and may contribute to its synaptic pathology. *Molecular Psychiatry* **8**, 148–155.

Eastwood, S.L., Walker, M., Hyde, T.M., Kleinman, J.E. & Harrison, P.J. (2010) The DISC1 Ser704Cys substitution affects centrosomal localisation of its binding partner PCM1 in glia in human brain. *Human Molecular Genetics* **19**, 2487–2496.

Erickson, S.L. & Lewis, D.A. (2002) Postnatal development of parvalbumin- and GABA transporter-immunoreactive axon terminals in monkey prefrontal cortex. *Journal of Comparative Neurology* **448**, 186–202.

Erickson, S.L. & Lewis, D.A. (2004). Cortical connections of the lateral mediodorsal thalamus in cynomolgus monkeys. *Journal of Comparative Neurology* **473**, 107–127.

Esiri, M.M. & Pearson, R.C.A. (2000) Perspectives from other diseases and lesions. In: Harrison, P.J. & Roberts, G.W., eds. *The Neuropathology of Schizophrenia: Progress and Interpretation* (eds), Oxford: Oxford University Press, pp. 257–276.

Ettinger, U., Chitnis, X.A., Kumari, V. *et al.* (2001) Magnetic resonance imaging of the thalamus in first-episode psychosis. *American Journal of Psychiatry* **158**, 116–118.

Ettinger, U., Picchioni, M., Landau, S. *et al.* (2007) Magnetic resonance imaging of the thalamus and adhesio interthalamica in twins with schizophrenia. *Archives of General Psychiatry* **64**, 401–409.

Falkai, P. & Bogerts, B. (1986) Cell loss in the hippocampus of schizophrenics. *European Archives of Psychiatry and Neurological Science* **236**, 154–161.

Falkai, P., Honer, W.G., David, S. *et al.* (1999) No evidence for astrogliosis in brains of schizophrenic patients: a postmortem study. *Neuropathology and Applied Neurobiology* **25**, 48–53.

Falkai, P., Schneider-Axmann, T. & Honer, W.G. (2000) Entorhinal cortex pre-alpha cell cluster in schizophrenia: quantitative evidence of a developmental abnormality. *Biological Psychiatry* **47**, 937–943.

Fannon, D., Simmons, A., Tennakoon, L. *et al.* (2003) Selective deficit of hippocampal N-acetylaspartate in antipsychotic-naive patients with schizophrenia. *Biological Psychiatry* **54**, 587–598.

Friede, R.J. (1989) *Developmental Neuropathology*. Berlin: Springer Verlag.

Friston, K.J. (1998) The disconnection hypothesis. *Schizophrenia Research* **30**, 115–125.

Gabriel, S.M., Haroutunian, V., Powchik, P. *et al.* (1997) Increased concentrations of presynaptic proteins in the cingulate cortex of subjects with schizophrenia. *Archives of General Psychiatry* **54**, 559–566.

Garey, L.J., Ong, W.Y., Patel, T.S. *et al.* (1998) Reduced dendritic spine density on cerebral cortical pyramidal neurons in schizophrenia. *Journal of Neurology, Neurosurgery and Psychiatry* **65**, 446–453.

Giguere, M. & Goldman-Rakic, P.S. (1988) Mediodorsal nucleus: Areal, laminar, and tangential distribution of afferents and efferents in the frontal lobe of rhesus monkeys. *Journal of Comparative Neurology* **277**, 195–213.

Gilbert, A.R., Rosenberg, D.R., Harenski, K. *et al.* (2001) Thalamic volumes in patients with first-episode schizophrenia. *American Journal of Psychiatry* **158**, 618–624.

Glantz, L.A. & Lewis, D.A. (1997) Reduction of synaptophysin immunoreactivity in the prefrontal cortex of subjects with schizophrenia: regional and diagnostic specificity. *Archives of General Psychiatry* **54**, 943–952.

Glantz, L.A. & Lewis, D.A. (2000) Decreased dendritic spine density on prefrontal cortical pyramidal neurons in schizophrenia. *Archives of General Psychiatry* **57**, 65–73.

Glantz, L.A., Austin, M.C. & Lewis, D.A. (2000) Normal cellular levels of synaptophysin mRNA expression in the prefrontal cortex of subjects with schizophrenia. *Biological Psychiatry* **48**, 389–397.

Grieve, K.L., Acuña, C. & Cudeiro, J. (2000) The primate pulvinar nuclei: vision and action. *Trends in Neurosciences* **23**, 35–39.

Guidotti, A., Auta, J., Davis, J.M. *et al.* (2000) Decrease in reelin and glutamic acid decarboxylase67 (GAD67) expression in schizophrenia and bipolar disorder. *Archives of General Psychiatry* **57**, 1061–1069.

Guillery, R. (2002) On counting and counting errors. *Journal of Comparative Neurology* **447**, 1–7.

Hakak, Y., Walker, J.R., Li, C. *et al.* (2001) Genome-wide expression analysis reveals dysregulation of myelination-related genes in chronic schizophrenia. *Proceedings of the National Academy of Sciences USA* **98**, 4746–4751.

Hanada, S., Mita, T., Nishino, N. & Tanaka, C. (1987) [3H] Muscimol binding sites increased in autopsied brains of chronic schizophrenics. *Life Sciences* **40**, 239–266.

Harrison, P.J. (1999a) The neuropathology of schizophrenia: a critical review of the data and their interpretation. *Brain* **122**, 593–624.

Harrison, P.J. (1999b) The neuropathological effects of antipsychotic drugs. *Schizophrenia Research* **40**, 87–99.

Harrison, P.J. (2002) The neuropathology of primary mood disorder. *Brain* **125**, 1428–1449.

Harrison, P.J. (2004) The hippocampus in schizophrenia: a review of the neuropathological evidence and its path-ophysiological implications. *Psychopharmacology* **174**, 151–162.

Harrison, P.J. (2007) Schizophrenia susceptibility genes and neurodevelopment, *Biological Psychiatry* **61**, 1119–1120.

Harrison, P.J. & Eastwood, S.L. (1998) Preferential involvement of excitatory neurons in medial temporal lobe in schizophrenia. *Lancet* **352**, 1669–1673.

Harrison, P.J. & Eastwood, S.L. (2001) Neuropathological studies of synaptic connectivity in the hippocampal formation in schizophrenia. *Hippocampus* **11**, 508–519.

Harrison, P.J. & Roberts, G.W. (2000) *The Neuropathology of Schizophrenia: Progress and Interpretation*. Oxford: Oxford University Press.

Harrison, P.J. & Weinberger, D.R. (2005) Schizophrenia genes, gene expression, and neuropathology: on the matter of their convergence. *Molecular Psychiatry* **10**, 40–68.

Harrison, P.J. & West, V.A. (2006) Six degrees of separation: on the prior probability that schizophrenia susceptibility genes converge on synapses, glutamate and NMDA receptors, *Molecular Psychiatry*, **11**, 981–983.

Harrison, P.J., Freemantle, N. & Geddes, J.R. (2003) Meta-analysis of brain weight in schizophrenia. *Schizophrenia Research* **64**, 25–34.

Hashimoto, T., Volk, D.W., Eggan, S.M. *et al.* (2003) Gene expression deficits in a subclass of GABA neurons in the prefrontal cortex of subjects with schizophrenia. *Journal of Neuroscience* **23**, 6315–6326.

Hashimoto, T., Bergen, S.E., Nguyen, Q.L. *et al.* (2005) Relationship of brain-derived neurotrophic factor and its receptor TrkB to altered inhibitory prefrontal circuitry in schizophrenia. *Journal of Neuroscience* **25**, 372–383.

Hashimoto, T., Arion, D., Unger, T. *et al.* (2008) Alterations in GABA-related transcriptome in the dorsolateral prefrontal cortex of subjects with schizophrenia. *Molecular Psychiatry* **13**, 147–161.

Hayes, T.L. & Lewis, D.A. (1996) Magnopyramidal neurons in the anterior motor speech region: dendritic features and inter-hemispheric comparisons. *Archives of Neurology* **53**, 1277–1283.

Heckers, S. (2001) Neuroimaging studies of the hippocampus in schizophrenia. *Hippocampus* **11**, 520–528.

Heckers, S., Heinsen, H., Geiger, B. & Beckmann, H. (1991) Hippocampal neuron number in schizophrenia: a stereological study. *Archives of General Psychiatry* **48**, 1002–1008.

Heinsen, H., Gössmann, E., Rüb, U. *et al.* (1996) Variability in the human entorhinal region may confound neuropsychiatric diagnoses. *Acta Anatomica* **157**, 226–237.

Highley, J.R., Walker, M.A., Crow, T.J. *et al.* (2003a) Low medial and lateral right pulvinar volumes in schizophrenia: a postmortem study. *American Journal of Psychiatry* **160**, 1177–1179.

Highley, J.R., Walker, M.A., McDonald, B. *et al.* (2003b) Size of hippocampal pyramidal neurons in schizophrenia. *British Journal of Psychiatry* **183**, 414–417.

Hof, P.R. Ungerleider, L.G. Webster, M.J. *et al.* (1996) Neurofilament protein in differentially distributed in subpopulations of corticocortical projection neurons in the macaque monkey visual pathways. *Journal of Comparative Neurology* **376**, 112–127.

Hof, P.R. Haroutunian, V. Friedrich, V.L. Jr. *et al.* (2003) Loss and altered spatial distribution of oligodendrocytes in the superior frontal gyrus in schizophrenia, *Biological Psychiatry* **53**, 1075–1085.

Holinger, D. Galaburda, A.M. & Harrison, P.J. (2000) Cerebral asymmetry. In: Harrison, P.J. & Roberts, G.W., eds. *The Neuropathology of Schizophrenia: Progress and Interpretation.* Oxford: Oxford University Press, pp. 151–171.

Honer, W.G., Falkai, P., Chen, C. *et al.* (1999) Synaptic and plasticity-associated proteins in anterior frontal cortex in severe mental illness. *Neuroscience* **91**, 1247–1255.

Honer, W.G. Young, C. & Falkai, P. (2000) Synaptic pathology. In: Harrison, P.J. & Roberts, G.W., eds. *The Neuropathology of Schizophrenia: Progress and Interpretation.* Oxford: Oxford University Press, pp. 105–136.

Huttenlocher, P.R. (1979) Synaptic density in human frontal cortex: developmental changes and effects of aging. *Brain Research* **163**, 195–205.

Irwin, S.A., Galvez, R. & Greenough, W.T. (2000) Dendritic spine structural anomalies in fragile X mental retardation syndrome. *Cerebral Cortex* **10**, 1038–1044.

Jakob, H. & Beckmann, H. (1986) Prenatal developmental disturbances in the limbic allocortex in schizophrenics. *Journal of Neural Transactions* **65**, 303–326.

Jellinger, K.A. (2009) Lewy body/alpha-synucleinopathy in schizophrenia and depression: a preliminary neuropathological study. *Acta Neuropathologica* **117**, 423–427.

Jellinger, K.A. & Gabriel, E. (1999) No increased incidence of Alzheimer's disease in elderly schizophrenics. *Acta Neuropathologica* **97**, 165–169.

Jeste, D.V. & Lohr, J.B. (1989) Hippocampal pathologic findings in schizophrenia: a morphometric study. *Archives of General Psychiatry* **46**, 1019–1024.

Kalman, M., Csillag, A., Schleicher, A. *et al.* (1993) Long-term effects of anterograde degeneration on astroglial reaction in the rat geniculo-cortico system as revealed by computerized image analysis. *Anatomical Embryology* **187**, 1–7.

Kalus, P., Muller, T.J., Zuschratter, W. & Senitz, D. (2000) The dendritic architecture of prefrontal pyramidal neurons in schizophrenic patients. *Neuroreport* **11**, 3621–3625.

Karoutzou, G., Emrich, H.M. & Dietrich, D.E. (2008) The myelin-pathogenesis puzzle in schizophrenia: a literature review. *Molecular Psychiatry* **13**, 245–260.

Karson, C.N., Mrak, R.E., Schluterman, K.O. *et al.* (1999) Alterations in synaptic proteins and their encoding mRNAs in prefrontal cortex in schizophenia: a possible neurochemical basis for 'hypofrontality'. *Molecular Psychiatry* **4**, 39–45.

Katsel, P., Davis, K.L. & Haroutunian, V. (2005) Variations in myelin and oligodendrocyte-related gene expression across multiple brain regions in schizophrenia: A gene ontology study. *Schizophrenia Research* **79**, 157–173.

Kaufmann, W.E. & Moser, H.W. (2000) Dendritic anomalies in disorders associated with mental retardation. *Cerebral Cortex* **10**, 981–991.

Kemether, E.M., Buchsbaum, M.S., Byne, W. *et al.* (2003) Magnetic resonance imaging of mediodorsal, pulvinar, and centromedian nuclei of the thalamus in patients with schizophrenia. *Archives of General Psychiatry* **60**, 983–991.

Kemper, T.L. & Bauman, M. (1998) Neuropathology of infantile autism. *Journal of Neuropathology and Experimental Neurology* **57**, 645–652.

Kim, S. & Webster, M.J. (2010) Integrative genome-wide association analysis of cytoarchitectural abnormalities in the prefrontal cortex of psychiatric disorders. *Molecular Psychiatry* [Epub ahead of print].

Kleinman, J.E., Law, A.J., Lipska, B.K. *et al.* (2011) Genetic neuropathology of schizophrenia: new approaches to an old question, and new uses for post mortem human brains. *Biological Psychiatry* (in press).

Kolluri, N., Sun, Z., Sampson, A.R. & Lewis, D.A. (2005) Lamina-specific reductions in dendritic spine density in the prefrontal cortex of subjects with schizophrenia. *American Journal of Psychiatry* **162**, 1200–1202.

Kolomeets, N.S. Orlovskaya, D.D. Rachmanova, V.I. & Uranova, N.A. (2005) Ultrastructural alterations in hippocampal mossy fiber synapses in schizophrenia: A postmortem morphometric study. *Synapse* **57**, 47–55.

Kolomeets, N.S., Orlovskaya, D.D. & Uranova, N.A. (2007) Decreased numerical density of CA3 hippocampal mossy fiber synapses in schizophrenia. *Synapse* **61**, 615–621.

Konick, L.C. & Friedman, L. (2001) Meta-analysis of thalamic size in schizophrenia. *Biological Psychiatry* **49**, 28–38.

Konopaske, G.T., Dorph-Petersen, K.-A., Pierri, J.N. *et al.* (2007). Effect of chronic exposure to antipsychotic medication on cell numbers in the parietal cortex of macaque monkeys. *Neuropsychopharmacology* **32**, 1216–1223.

Konrad, A. & Winterer, G. (2008) Disturbed structural connectivity in schizophrenia - Primary factor in pathology or epiphenomenon? *Schizophrenia Bulletin* **34**, 72–92.

Kovalenko, S., Bergmann, A., Schneider-Axmann, T. *et al.* (2003) Regio entorhinalis in schizophrenia: More evidence for migrational disturbances and suggestions for a new biological hypothesis. *Pharmacopsychiatry* **36** (Suppl. 3), S158–S161.

Kovelman, J.A. & Scheibel, A.B. (1984) A neurohistological correlate of schizophrenia. *Biological Psychiatry* **19**, 1601–1621.

Kreczmanski, P., Heinsen, H., Mantua, V. *et al.* (2007) Volume, neuron density and total neuron number in five subcortical regions in schizophrenia. *Brain* **130**, 678–692.

Krimer, L.S., Herman, M.M., Saunders, R.C. *et al.* (1997) A qualitative and quantitative analysis of the entorhinal cortex in schizophrenia. *Cerebral Cortex* **7**, 732–739.

Lambe, E.K., Krimer, L.S. & Goldman-Rakic, P.S. (2000) Differential postnatal development of catecholamine and serotonin inputs to identified neurons in prefrontal cortex of rhesus monkey. *Journal of Neuroscience* **20**, 8780–8787.

Law, A.J. & Harrison, P.J. (2003) The distribution and morphology of prefrontal cortex pyramidal neurons identified using anti-neurofilament antibodies SMI32, N200 and FNP7. Normative data and a comparison in subjects with schizophrenia, bipolar disorder or major depression. *Journal of Psychiatric Research* **37**, 487–499.

Law, A.J., Weickert, C.S., Hyde, T.M. *et al.* (2004) Reduced spinophilin but not microtubule-associated protein 2 expression in the hippocampal formation in schizophrenia and mood disorders: Molecular evidence for a pathology of dendritic spines, *American Journal of Psychiatry* **161**, 1848–1855.

Law, A.J., Lipska, B.K., Weickert, C.S. *et al.* (2006) Neuregulin 1 transcripts are differentially expressed in schizophrenia and regulated by 5′ SNPs associated with the disease. *Proceedings of the National Academy of Sciences of the United States of America* **103**, 6747–6752.

Leong, S.L., Cappai, R., Barnham, K.J. & Pham, C.L. (2009) Modulation of alpha-synuclein aggregation by dopamine: a review. *Neurochemical Research* **34**, 1838–1846.

Lesch, A. & Bogerts, B. (1984) The diencephalon in schizophrenia: evidence for reduced thickness of the periventricular grey matter. *European Archives of Psychiatry & Neurological Sciences* **234**, 212–219.

Levitt, J.B. Lewis, D.A. Yoshioka, T. & Lund, J.S. (1993) Topography of pyramidal neuron intrinsic connections in macaque monkey prefrontal cortex (areas 9 and 46). *Journal of Comparative Neurology* **338**, 360–376.

Lewis, D.A. (1997) Development of the prefrontal cortex during adolescence: insights into vulnerable neural circuits in schizophrenia. *Neuropsychopharmacology* **16**, 385–398.

Lewis, D.A. (2000) Distributed disturbances in brain structure and function in schizophrenia. *American Journal of Psychiatry* **157**, 1–2.

Lewis, D.A. & Levitt, P. (2002) Schizophrenia as a disorder of neurodevelopment, *Annual Review of Neuroscience* **25**, 409–432.

Lewis, D.A. & Sesack, S.R. (1997) Dopamine systems in the primate brain. In: Bloom, F.E., Björklund, A. & Hökfelt, T., eds. *Handbook of Chemical Neuroanatomy.* Amsterdam: Elsevier Science, pp. 261–373.

Lewis, D.A. & Lieberman, J.A. (2000) Catching up on schizophrenia: Natural history and neurobiology. *Neuron* **28**, 325–334.

Lewis, D.A. & Gonzales-Burgos, G. (2008) Neuroplasticity and neocortical circuits in schizophrenia. *Neuropsychopharmacology* **33**, 141–165.

Lewis, D.A., Cruz, D.A., Melchitzky, D.S. & Pierri, J.N. (2001) Lamina-specific deficits in parvalbumin-immunoreactive varicosities in the prefrontal cortex of subjects with schizophrenia: Evidence for fewer projections from the thalamus. *American Journal of Psychiatry* **158**, 1411–1422.

Lieberman, J.A. (1999) Is schizophrenia a neurodegenerative disorder? A clinical and neurobiological perspective. *Biological Psychiatry* **46**, 729–739.

Maldonado-Aviles, J.G., Wu, Q., Sampson, A.R. & Lewis, D. A. (2006). Somal size of immunolabeled pyramidal cells in the prefrontal cortex of subjects with schizophrenia. *Biological Psychiatry* **60**, 226–234.

Marti, E., Ferrer, I., Ballabriga, J. & Blasi, J. (1998) Increase in SNAP-25 immunoreactivity in mossy fibers following transient forebrain ischemia in the gerbil. *Acta Neuropathologica* **95**, 254–260.

Masliah, E., Mallory, M. Hansen, L. *et al.* (1993) Quantitative synaptic alterations in the human neocortex during normal aging. *Neurology* **43**, 192–197.

Maurer, I., Zierz, S. & Moller, H. (2001). Evidence for a mitochondrial oxidative phosphorylation defect in brains from patients with schizophrenia. *Schizophrenia Research* **48**, 125–136.

McDonald, B., Highley, J.R., Walker, M.A. *et al.* (2000) Anomalous asymmetry of fusiform and parahippocampal gyrus gray matter in schizophrenia: A postmortem study. *American Journal of Psychiatry* **157**, 40–47.

McIntosh, A.M., Moorhead, T.W., Job, D. *et al.* (2008) The effects of a neuregulin 1 variant on white matter density and integrity. *Molecular Psychiatry* **13**, 1054–1059.

Melchitzky, D.S., Sesack, S.R. & Lewis, D.A. (1999) Parvalbumin-immunoreactive axon terminals in macaque monkey and human prefrontal cortex: Laminar, regional and target specificity of Type I and Type II synapses. *Journal of Comparative Neurology* **408**, 11–22.

Middleton, F.A., Mirnics, K., Pierri, J.N. *et al.* (2002) Gene expression profiling reveals alterations of specific metabolic pathways in schizophrenia. *Journal of Neuroscience* **22**, 2718–2729.

Mirnics, K., Middleton, F.A., Marquez, A. *et al.* (2000) Molecular characterization of schizophrenia viewed by microarray analysis of gene expression in prefrontal cortex. *Neuron* **28**, 53–67.

Mitkus, S.N., Hyde, T.M., Vakkalanka, R. *et al.* (2008) Expression of oligodendrocyte-associated genes in dorsolateral prefrontal cortex of patients with schizophrenia. *Schizophrenia Research* **98**, 129–138.

Morris, H.M., Hashimoto, T. & Lewis, D.A. (2008) Alterations in somatostatin mRNA expression in the dorsolateral prefrontal cortex of subjects with schizophrenia or schizoaffective disorder. *Cerebral Cortex* **18**, 1575–1587.

Mulcrone, J., Whatley, S.A., Ferrier, I.N. & Marchbanks, R.M. (1995) A study of altered gene expression in frontal cortex from schizophrenic patients using differential screening. *Schizophrenia Research* **14**, 203–213.

Murphy, G.M., Jr, Lim, K.O., Wieneke, M. *et al.* (1998) No neuropathologic evidence for an increased frequency of Alzheimer's disease among elderly schizophrenics. *Biological Psychiatry* **43**, 205–209.

Nave, K.-A. & Trapp, B.D. (2008) Axon-glial signaling and the glial support of axon function. *Annual Review of Neuroscience* **31**, 535–561.

Nelson, M.D., Saykin, A.J., Flashman, L.A. & Riordan, H.J. (1998) Hippocampal volume reduction in schizophrenia as assessed by magnetic resonance imaging: a meta-analytic study. *Archives of General Psychiatry* **55**, 433–440.

Niizato, K., Arai, T., Kuroki, N., Kase, K., Iritani, S. & Ikeda, K. (1998) Autopsy study of Alzheimer's disease brain pathology in schizophrenia, *Schizophrenia Research*, **31**, pp. 177–184.

Ohnuma, T., Augood, S.J., Arai, H. *et al.* (1999). Measurement of GABAergic parameters in the prefrontal cortex in schizophrenia: Focus on GABA content, GABAA receptor a-1 subunit messenger RNA and human GABA transporter-1 (HGAT-1) messenger RNA expression. *Neuroscience* **93**, 441–448.

Pakkenberg, B. (1990) Pronounced reduction of total neuron number in mediodorsal thalamic nucleus and nucleus accumbens in schizophrenics. *Archives of General Psychiatry* **47**, 1023–1028.

Pakkenberg, B. (1993) Total nerve cell number in neocortex in chronic schizophrenics and controls estimated using optical disectors. *Biological Psychiatry* **34**, 768–772.

Pantazopoulos, H., Woo, T.-U.W., Lim, M.P., Lange, N. & Berretta, S. (2010) Extracellular matrix-glial abnormalities in the amygdala and entorhinal cortex of subjects diagnosed with schizophrenia. *Archives of General Psychiatry* **67**, 155–166.

Perez-Costas, E, Melendez-Ferro, M., & Roberts, R.C. (2010) Basal ganglia pathology in schizophrenia: dopamine connections and anomalies. *Journal of Neurochemistry* **113**, 287–302.

Perrone-Bizzozero, N.I., Sower, A.C., Bird, E.D. *et al.* (1996) Levels of the growth-associated protein GAP-43 are selectively increased in association cortices in schizophrenia. *Proceedings of the National Academy of Sciences* **93**, 14182–14187.

Pierce, J.P. & Lewin, G.R. (1994) An ultrastructural size principle. *Neuroscience* **58**, 441–446.

Pierri, J.N., Melchitzky, D.S. & Lewis, D.A. (1999) Volume and neuronal number of the primate mediodorsal thalamic nucleus: effects of chronic haloperidol administration. *Society for Neuroscience Abstracts* **25**, 1833.

Pierri, J.N., Volk, C.L.E., Auh, S. *et al.* (2001). Decreased somal size of deep layer 3 pyramidal neurons in the prefrontal cortex of subjects with schizophrenia. *Archives of General Psychiatry* **58**, 466–473.

Pierri, J.N., Volk, C.L., Auh, S. *et al.* (2003). Somal size of prefrontal cortical pyramidal neurons in schizophrenia: Differential effects across neuronal subpopulations. *Biological Psychiatry* **54**, 111–120.

Plum, F. (1972) Prospects for research on schizophrenia. Neuropathological findings. *Neuroscience Research Program Bulletin* **10**, 384–388.

Popken, G.J., Bunney, W.E., Jr., Potkin, S.G. & Jones, E.G. (2000) Subnucleus-specific loss of neurons in medial thalamus of schizophrenics. *Proceedings of the National Academy of Sciences USA* **97**, 9276–9280.

Portas, C.M., Goldstein, J.M., Shenton, M.E. *et al.* (1998) Volumetric evaluation of the thalamus in schizophrenic male patients using magnetic resonance imaging. *Biological Psychiatry* **43**, 649–659.

Prabakaran, S., Swatton, J.E., Ryan, M.M. *et al.* (2004) Mitochondrial dysfunction in Schizophrenia: evidence for compromised brain metabolism and oxidative stress. *Molecular Psychiatry* **9**, 684–697.

Prasad, K.M.R., Chowdari, K.V., Nimgaonkar, V.L. *et al.* (2005) Genetic polymorphisms of the RGS4 and dorsolateral prefrontal coretx morphometry among first episode schizophrenia patients., *Molecular Psychiatry* **10**, 213–219.

Prince, J.A., Blennow, K., Gottfries, C.G. *et al.* (1999) Mitochondrial function is differentially altered in the basal ganglia of chronic schizophrenics. *Neuropsychopharmacology* **21**, 372–379.

Prohovnik, I., Dwork, A.J., Kaufman, M.A. & Wilson, N. (1993) Alzheimer-type neuropathology in elderly schizophrenia patients. *Schizophrenia Bulletin* **19**, 805–816.

Pucak, M.L., Levitt, J.B., Lund, J.S. & Lewis, D.A. (1996) Patterns of intrinsic and associational circuitry in monkey prefrontal cortex. *Journal of Comparative Neurology* **376**, 614–630.

Purohit, D.P., Peri, D.P., Haroutunian, V. *et al.* (1998) Alzheimer disease and related neurodegenerative diseases in elderly patients with schizophrenia: a portmortem neuropathologic study of 100 cases. *Archives of General Psychiatry* **55**, 205–211.

Rajkowska, G., Selemon, L.D. & Goldman-Rakic, P.S. (1998) Neuronal and glial somal size in the prefrontal cortex: a post-mortem morphometric study of schizophrenia and Huntington disease. *Archives of General Psychiatry* **55**, 215–224.

Rapp, M.A., Schnaider-Beeri, M., Purohit, D.P. *et al.* (2010) Cortical neuritic plaques and neurofibrillary tangles are related to dementia severity in elderly schizophrenia patients. *Schizophrenia Research* **116**, 90–96.

Riederer, P., Gsell, W., Calza, L. *et al.* (1995) Consensus on minimal criteria of clinical and neuropathological diagnosis of schizophrenia and affective disorders for post mortem research. Report from the European Dementia and Schizophrenia Network (BIOMED 1). *Journal of Neural Transmission* **102**, 255–264.

Roberts, G.W. & Harrison, P.J. (2000) Gliosis and its implications for the disease process. In: Harrison, P.J. & Roberts, G.W., eds. *The Neuropathology of Schizophrenia: Progress and Interpretation.* Oxford: Oxford University Press, pp. 137–150.

Roberts, R.C., Roche, J.K., & Conley, R.R. (2005) Synaptic differences in the postmortem striatum of subjects with schizophrenia: A stereological ultrastructural analysis. *Synapse* **56**, 185–197.

Rosoklija, G., Toomayan, G., Ellis, S.P. *et al.* (2000) Structural abnormalities of subicular dendrites in subjects with schizophrenia and mood disorders: preliminary findings. *Archives of General Psychiatry* **57**, 349–356.

Sawada, K., Barr, A.M., Nakamura, M. *et al.* (2005) Hippocampal complexin proteins and cognitive dysfunction in schizophrenia. *Archives of General Psychiatry* **62**, 263–272.

Scherk, H. & Falkai, P. (2006) Effects of antipsychotics on brain structure. *Current Opinion in Psychiatry* **19**, 145–150.

Schmitt, A., Steyskal, C., Bernstein, H.G., *et al.* (2009) Stereologic investigation of the posterior part of the hippocampus in schizophrenia. *Acta Neuropathologica* **117**, 395–407.

Schmitz, C. & Rezaie, P. (2008) The neuropathology of autism: where do we stand? *Neuropathology and Applied Neurobiology* **34**, 4–11.

Selemon, L.D. & Goldman-Rakic, P.S. (1999) The reduced neuropil hypothesis: a circuit based model of schizophrenia. *Biological Psychiatry* **45**, 17–25.

Selemon, L.D. Rajkowska, G. & Goldman-Rakic, P.S. (1995) Abnormally high neuronal density in the schizophrenic cortex: a morphometric analysis of prefrontal area 9 and occipital area 17. *Archives of General Psychiatry* **52**, 805–818.

Selemon, L.D., Rajkowska, G. & Goldman-Rakic, P.S. (1998) Elevated neuronal density in prefrontal area 46 in brains from schizophrenic patients: application of a three-dimensional, stereologic counting method. *Journal of Comparative Neurology* **392**, 402–412.

Selemon, L.D., Lidow, M.S. & Goldman-Rakic, P.S. (1999) Increased volume and glial density in primate prefrontal cortex associated with chronic antipsychotic drug exposure. *Biological Psychiatry* **46**, 161–172.

Shao, L. & Vawter, M.P. (2008) Shared gene expression alterations in schizophrenia and bipolar disorder. *Biological Psychiatry* **64**, 89–97.

Shapiro, R.M. (1993) Regional neuropathology in schizophrenia: Where are we? Where are we going, *Schizophrenia Research* **10**, 187–239.

Simpson, M.D.C., Slater, P., Deakin, J.F.W. *et al.* (1989) Reduced GABA uptake sites in the temporal lobe in schizophrenia. *Neuroscience Letters* **107**, 211–215.

Smiley, J.F., Rosoklija, G., Mancevski, B., Mann, J.J., Dwork, A.J., & Javitt, D.C. (2009) Altered volume and hemispheric asymmetry of the superficial cortical layers in the schizophrenia planum temporal. *European Journal of Neuroscience* **30**, 449–463.

Sommer, I., Aleman, A., Ramsey, N. *et al.* (2001) Handedness, language lateralisation and anatomical asymmetry in schizophrenia—Meta-analysis. *British Journal of Psychiatry* **178**, 344–351.

Stanley, J.A., Williamson, P.C., Drost, D.J. *et al.* (1996) An *in vivo* proton magnetic resonance spectroscopy study of schizophrenia patients. *Schizophrenia Bulletin* **22**, 597–609.

Stephan, K.E., Baldeweg, T. & Friston, K.J. (2006) Synaptic plasticity and dysconnection in schizophrenia. *Biological Psychiatry* **59**, 929–939.

Stevens, J.R. (1982) Neuropathology of schizophrenia. *Archives of General Psychiatry* **39**, 1131–1139.

Stevens, J.R., Casanova, M.F., Poltorak, M. & Buchan, G.C. (1992) Comparison of immunocytochemical and Holzer's methods for detection of acute and chronic glioses in human postmortem material. *Journal of Neuropsychiatry and Clinical Neuroscience* **4**, 168–173.

Straub, R.E., Lipska, B.K., Egan, M.F. *et al.* (2007) Allelic variation in GAD1 (GAD67) is associated with schizophrenia and influences cortical function and gene expression. *Molecular Psychiatry* **12**, 854–869.

Suddath, R.L., Christison, G.W., Torrey, E.F. *et al.* (1990) Anatomical abnormalities in the brains of monozygotic twins discordant for schizophrenia. *New England Journal of Medicine* **322**, 789–794.

Sugino, K., Hempel, C.M., Miller, M.N. *et al.* (2006). Molecular taxonomy of major neuronal classes in the adult mouse forebrain. *Nature Neuroscience* **9**, 99–107.

Sweet, R.A., Pierri, J.N., Auh, S. *et al.* (2003). Reduced pyramidal cell somal volume in auditory association cortex of subjects with schizophrenia. *Neuropsychopharmacology* **28**, 599–609.

Sweet, R.A., Bergen, S.E., Sun, Z. *et al.* (2004). Pyramidal cell size reduction in schizophrenia: Evidence for involvement of auditory feedforward circuits. *Biological Psychiatry* **55**, 1128–1137.

Sweet, R.A., Bergen, S.E., Sun, Z. *et al.* (2007). Anatomical evidence of impaired feedforward auditory processing in schizophrenia. *Biological Psychiatry* **61**, 854–864.

Talbot, K., Eidem, W.L., Tinsley, C.L. *et al.* (2004) Dysbindin-1 is reduced in intrinsic, glutamatergic terminals of the hippocampal formation in schizophrenia. *Journal of Clinical Investigation* **113**, 1353–1363.

Tamminga, C.A., Stan, A.D. & Wagner, A.D. (2010) The hippocampal formation in schizophrenia. *American Journal of Psychiatry* (Epub ahead of print).

Thompson, P.M., Sower, A.C. & Perrone-Bizzozero, N.I. (1998) Altered levels of the synaptosomal associated protein SNAP-25 in schizophrenia. *Biological Psychiatry* **43**, 239–243.

Thune, J.J., Uylings, H.B.M. & Pakkenberg, B. (2001). No deficit in total number of neurons in the prefrontal cortex in schizophrenics. *Journal of Psychiatric Research* **35**, 15–21.

Tkachev, D., Mimmack, M.L., Ryan, M.M. *et al.* (2003). Oligodendrocyte dysfunction in schizophrenia and bipolar disorder. *Lancet* **362**, 798–805.

Torrey, E.F., Barci, B.M., Webster, M.J. *et al.* (2005) Neurochemical markers for schizophrenia, bipolar disorder, and major depression in postmortem brains. *Biological Psychiatry* **57**, 252–260.

Uranova, N.A., Orlovskaya, D.D., Vikhreva, O. *et al.* (2001) Electron microscopy of oligodendroglia in severe mental illness. *Brain Research Bulletin* **55**, 597–610.

Uranova, N.A., Vostrikov, V.M., Orlovskaya, D.D. & Rachmanova, V.I. (2004) Oligodendroglial density in the prefrontal cortex in schizophrenia and mood disorders: a study from the Stanley Neuropathology Consortium. *Schizophrenia Research* **67**, 269–275.

Van Snellenberg, J.X., Torres, I.J. & Thornton, A.E. (2006) Functional neuroimaging of working memory in schizophrenia: task performance as a moderating variable. *Neuropsychology* **20**, 497–510.

Vawter, M.P., Crook, J.M., Hyde, T.M. *et al.* (2002). Microarray analysis of gene expression in the prefrontal cortex in schizophrenia: A preliminary study. *Schizophrenia Research* **58**, 11–20.

Velakoulis, D., Panetelis, C., McGorry, P.D. *et al.* (1999) Hippocampal volume in first-episode psychosis and chronic schizophrenia: a high-resolution magnetic resonance imaging study. *Archives of General Psychiatry* **56**, 133–141.

Volk, D.W., Austin, M.C., Pierri, J.N. *et al.* (2000) Decreased GAD67 mRNA expression in a subset of prefrontal cortical GABA neurons in subjects with schizophrenia. *Archives of General Psychiatry* **57**, 237–245.

Volk, D.W., Austin, M.C., Pierri, J.N. *et al.* (2001) GABA transporter-1 mRNA in the prefrontal cortex in schizophrenia: Decreased expression in a subset of neurons. *American Journal of Psychiatry* **158**, 256–265.

Volk, D.W., Pierri, J.N., Fritschy, J.M. *et al.* (2002) Reciprocal alterations in pre- and postsynaptic inhibitory markers at chandelier cell inputs to pyramidal neurons in schizophrenia. *Cerebral Cortex* **12**, 1063–1070.

Vostrikov, V.M., Uranova, N.A. & Orlovskaya, D.D. (2007) Deficit of perineuronal oligodendrocytes in the prefrontal cortex in schizophrenia and mood disorders. *Schizophrenia Research* **94**, 273–280.

Walker, M.A., Highley, J.R., Esiri, M.M. *et al.* (2002) Estimated neuronal populations and volumes of the hippocampus and its subfields in schizophrenia. *American Journal of Psychiatry* **159**, 821–828.

Weickert, C. & Weinberger, D.R. (1998) A candidate molecular approach to defining the developmental pathology in schizophrenia. *Schizophrenia Bulletin* **24**, 303–316.

Weinberger, D.R. (1999) Cell biology of the hippocampal formation in schizophrenia. *Biological Psychiatry* **45**, 395–402.

Wisniewski, H.M., Constantinidis, J., Wegiel, J. *et al.* (1994) Neurofibrillary pathology in brains of elderly schizophrenics treated with neuroleptics. *Alzheimer Disease and Associated Disorders* **8**, 211–227.

Woo, T.U., Miller, J.L. & Lewis, D.A. (1997a) Schizophrenia and the parvalbumin-containing class of cortical local circuit neurons. *American Journal of Psychiatry* **154**, 1013–1015.

Woo, T.-U., Pucak, M.L., Kye, C.H. *et al.* (1997b) Peripubertal refinement of the intrinsic and associational circuitry in monkey prefrontal cortex. *Neuroscience* **80**, 1149–1158.

Woo, T.-U., Whitehead, R.E., Melchitzky, D.S. & Lewis, D.A. (1998) A subclass of prefrontal gamma-aminobutyric acid axon terminals are selectively altered in schizophrenia. *Proceedings of the National Academy of Sciences USA* **95**, 5341–5346.

Woo, T.-U., Walsh, J.P. & Benes, F.M. (2004) Density of glutamic acid decarboxylase 67 messenger RNA-containing neurons that express the N-methyl-D-aspartate receptor subunit NR2A in the anterior cingulate cortex in schizophrenia and bipolar disorder. *Archives of General Psychiatry* **61**, 649–657.

Wright, I.C., Rabe-Hesketh, S., Woodruff, P.W.R., David, A.S. *et al.* (2000) Meta-analysis of regional brain volumes in schizophrenia, *American Journal of Psychiatry* **157**, 16–25.

Young, K.A., Manaye, K.F., Liang, C.-L. *et al.* (2000) Reduced number of mediodorsal and anterior thalamic neurons in schizophrenia. *Biological Psychiatry* **47**, 944–953.

Young, K.A., Holcomb, L.A., Yazdani, U. *et al.* (2004) Elevated neuron number in the limbic thalamus in major depression. *American Journal of Psychiatry* **161**, 1270–1277.

Zaidel, D.W., Esiri, M.M. & Harrison, P.J. (1997a) The hippocampus in schizophrenia: lateralized increase in neuronal density and altered cytoarchitectural asymmetry. *Psychological Medicine* **27**, 703–713.

Zaidel, D.W., Esiri, M.M. & Harrison, P.J. (1997b) Size, shape and orientation of neurons in the left and right hippocampus: investigation of normal asymmetries and alterations in schizophrenia. *American Journal of Psychiatry* **154**, 812–818.

CHAPTER 19

Neurodevelopmental origins of schizophrenia

Daniel R. Weinberger[1] and Pat Levitt[2]

[1]National Institute of Mental Health, NIH, Bethesda, MD, USA
[2]Keck School of Medicine of University of Southern California, Los Angeles, CA, USA

Introduction

The idea that schizophrenia has its origins in early development dates back at least to the modern classification of the syndrome by Emil Kraepelin and Eugen Bleuler, both of whom noted abnormal neurological and behavioral signs in the childhood histories of adult patients. Some of the neuropathological findings reported in the early part of the 20th century were interpreted as evidence of abnormal brain development (e.g., Southard, 1915). Bender (1947), in her landmark study of cases of childhood-onset schizophrenia, argued that the condition was likely a developmental encephalopathy. In studies of children of mothers with schizophrenia, Fish and Hagin (1972) described a constellation of apparent lags and disruptions in neurological development, which predicted the later emergence of schizophrenia spectrum symptoms; they also proposed abnormal brain development as the cause. Other investigators had emphasized the early childhood social abnormalities of individuals with adult-onset schizophrenia (Watt, 1972), also potentially implicating abnormal brain development. In spite of this diverse literature, the general view among psychiatrists and researchers during much of the 20th century was that schizophrenia occurs principally

because of something that happens around early adult life, and that clinical remission is related to reversal of this process, while progression of the clinical condition is an expression of continuing progression of the pathology. This view echoed aspects of Kraepelin's codification of schizophrenia as an early dementia ("dementia praecox") and seemed consistent with the clinical fact that many patients with schizophrenia do not have a clearly abnormal premorbid history. The biochemical hypotheses that emerged in the 1960s, principally the dopamine hypothesis, fit nicely into biochemical disruption models that served to explain the manifestations of psychosis.

Beginning in the mid 1980s, a broad conceptual shift about the pathogenesis of schizophrenia began to gather momentum, as the possibility of abnormal brain development again became a popular idea and neurodevelopmental hypotheses of schizophrenia were proposed and embraced by both the clinical and research communities. The so-called neurodevelopment hypothesis of schizophrenia emerged as an appealing alternative to the neurotransmitter hypotheses because it addressed more of the phenomenology of the syndrome and newer areas of neuroscience research that pointed to disturbances in specific brain circuits. In contrast to the popular dopamine hypothesis, which rested in its early versions primarily on the pharmacological mechanism of antipsychotic drugs, the neurodevelopmental hypothesis addressed the role of

Schizophrenia, 3rd edition. Edited by Daniel R. Weinberger and
Paul J Harrison © 2011 Blackwell Publishing Ltd.

cortical physiological and cognitive deficits increasingly implicated in the disorder; it emphasized epidemiological evidence of obstetric complications increasing risk for schizophrenia and of developmental delays being associated with later development of schizophrenia; it also offered an explanation for the early adult onset of the syndrome. The neurodevelopmental hypothesis also accommodated the role of dopamine in antipsychotic treatment and it made sense of the failure of almost a century of neuropathological studies to unearth evidence of neurotoxicity or neurodegeneration in the postmortem brains of patients with the disorder. This new hypothesis was of course not really new. It was a recapitulation in the context of modern developmental neuroscience of earlier observations that patients with schizophrenia often have abnormal developmental histories. Moreover, in a strict sense, the neurodevelopmental hypothesis is not a hypothesis in terms of it being falsifiable; rather, it is a model or framework for understanding diverse aspects of the pathogenesis and course of the illness.

Previous editions of this book detailed various aspects of this neurodevelopmental model, from a summary of major events in early brain development to a consideration of pathophysiological mechanisms that lead to the emergence of the diagnostic syndrome in early adulthood. This substantially new chapter will review some of the earlier evidence for the neurodevelopmental hypothesis and update our thinking about the role of brain development in the context of recent landmark findings about the genetic origins and mechanisms of this illness.

There is no single "neurodevelopmental hypothesis", because different versions have focused on different aspects of brain development that might be relevant to the causes or expression of the condition. All hold, however, that abnormalities of brain development are critical to the pathogenesis of the disorder; some stress early developmental antecedents, others focus on periadolescent developmental events. For example, Murray and Lewis (1987) emphasized that schizophrenia was related to obstetric complications or to disruptions of the intrauterine microenvironment related to viral epidemics. Feinberg (1982) focused on the adolescent period of synaptic refinement, arguing that schizophrenia involved a disruption of the pruning of synapses, either too little or too much pruning. Weinberger (1986, 1987) offered a more agnostic hypothesis in terms of causation, but tried to account for the importance of cortical pathophysiology, the role of dopamine, and the implications of developmental neurobiology for the changing pattern of the clinical manifestations. Because of the hierarchical nature of building the circuitry that mediates complex cognitive and emotional functions disrupted in schizophrenia, he suggested that there were likely to be multiple histogenic events that could disrupt the development of critical systems in the brain, particu-

larly those related to connections between the prefrontal and limbic cortices and the prefrontal cortical regulation of the brainstem dopamine system. He also argued that the critical issue in the emergence of the syndrome in late adolescence was not related to a new pathological event at that time, but to an interaction of the early developmental abnormalities with other risk factors and normal biological changes in the brain that occur in late adolescence. Brain maturation was seen as a permissive process that brought out a preclinical diathesis based on developmental factors.

These three theoretical pillars of the neurodevelopmental view of schizophrenia have been revised and elaborated in several more recent derivations, including emphasis on a continuum or trajectory of genetically regulated developmental processes that begin early in development but that continue through the various phases of illness (Rapoport et al., 2005), and quantitative molecular effects early in development that initiate cascades of biological changes through various subsequent developmental stages and environmental changes that mark the course of illness (Lewis & Levitt, 2002). The model has been further modified recently to invoke the concept of developmental allostasis (Thompson & Levitt, 2010), meaning that abnormal early brain ontogeny results in adaptive changes and an altered developmental trajectory that allows normal functioning of systems that are under duress. Over time, and with other risk factors emerging, this becomes unsustainable, leading to overt circuit dysfunction and frank clinical presentation. The role that specific genes might play in shaping the developmental abnormalities and adaptive changes associated with schizophrenia has also become the subject of much speculation (e.g., Jaaro-Peled et al., 2009).

All efforts to understand the basic pathogenesis of schizophrenia must now consider the role of specific genes in the etiological landscape. As appealing as creative hypotheses might be, and schizophrenia research, like other areas of academic psychiatry, has not suffered from a paucity of creative hypotheses, hypotheses are by definition speculative and uncertain. Over a century of research about schizophrenia, from early neuropathological investigations, to modern epidemiological and neuropharmacological studies, to ground-breaking neuroimaging studies and studies of the molecular biology of schizophrenic brain tissue, all represent phenomenological observations (i.e., describing differences between people with schizophrenia or biological specimens from such people and a control sample). These observations, as compelling as the data may be, are associative and not mechanistic. They cannot determine the basic causation of the disease. This is not true of genes. Genes are objective causative factors, not the only factors and certainly not necessarily the most important factors, but they are, if validated, the only absolutely objective, incontrovertible elements of the risk architecture of the disease. In this respect, the discovery of genes related to schizophrenia promises to profoundly impact on our understanding of this devastating human disorder, and will ultimately help in the discovery of novel therapies. Genes will also help us understand the role of brain development in the pathogenesis of schizophrenia and will lead to a more finely derived neurodevelopmental hypothesis.

What is the evidence that abnormal brain development increases risk?

Impact of abnormal gestational experience

A number of well-designed epidemiological studies of large populations indicate that obstetric complications (OCs) of various denominations are associated with a slight increase in risk for schizophrenia, in the range of a 1.5-fold change in relative risk (Cannon *et al.*, 2002; see Chapter 10). The interpretation of the OC literature is not straightforward, and one of its more perplexing aspects is the heterogeneity of the findings. There is no specific complication (e.g., nuchal cord, prolonged labor, placental abruption, prematurity) that stands out as key, though evidence of fetal hypoxia has been implicated as the most frequently observed complication (Cannon *et al.*, 2008). There is no identified single cause of the obstetric problems, nor is it clear whether something goes wrong at the time of delivery or whether there have been subtle problems during intrauterine development that alter the molecular signals sent from the fetus to initiate and sustain a healthy birth process.

The inconsistencies in the OC literature reflect at least in part the relative weakness of the effect size of OCs on risk for schizophrenia. Meta-analyses of this literature have found that in general OCs increase risk from 1.3- to 2-fold (Cannon *et al.*, 2002; see Chapter 10); thus, they account for a relatively small number of cases, analogous to estimates of risk attributable to a single genetic locus. Nevertheless, it is difficult to escape the conclusion that OCs, of various sorts, depending probably on cohort and record-keeping variations, do slightly increase risk for the emergence of schizophrenia in later life. This means that abnormalities of the intrauterine environment can affect fetal development in a manner that has implications for the expression of schizophrenia. However, this broad conclusion may be as far as the association with OCs will ultimately go in clarifying the specific developmental mechanisms related to schizophrenia. OCs also are not specific for schizophrenia, and have been associated with increased risk for bipolar disorder (Marcelis *et al.*, 1998), although probably less so than with schizophrenia (Bain *et al.*, 2000), autism (Bolton *et al.*, 1997), and various neurological developmental disorders (Eschenbach, 1997). It may well be that many

psychiatric disorders have this antecedent and that OCs are a generic risk factor for a spectrum of behavioral complications.

Another confusing aspect of the OC literature is that while a disruption in brain development at different times might be expected to result in different outcomes, associations with schizophrenia have spanned most of the gestational period. It is also unclear why OCs affect some individuals adversely and appear to have no observable impact in others, probably the majority of people, including the unaffected identical co-twins of patients with schizophrenia (McNeil *et al.*, 2000). Several earlier studies have considered the possibility that OCs interact with genetic risk factors. Cannon *et al.* (1993) reported that a relationship with computed tomography (CT) abnormalities and OCs was found only in patients with a family history of schizophrenia. In a study aimed at determining whether evidence of hypoxia at birth implicates effects on fetal development that differ in those who will manifest schizophrenia as adults compared to those who will not, Cannon *et al.* (2008) examined the relationship between hypoxic indices at birth (low Apgar scores) and levels of circulating brain-derived neurotrophic factor (BDNF) in cord blood in a cohort of births in Philadelphia derived from the USA National Collaborative Perinatal Study, a large prospective public health study of factors related to cerebral palsy. They found that while hypoxia was associated with increased BDNF levels in control samples, the levels were reduced in patients who eventually developed schizophrenia as adults. These differences were not in maternal blood, arguing that the effects reflected a differential molecular experience of the fetus, though whether blood BDNF reflects brain or peripheral BDNF production is uncertain.

A recent study explored a potential interaction between OCs and schizophrenia risk-associated genes also specifically implicated in the molecular biology of hypoxic–ischemic neuronal injury (e.g., *BDNF*, *AKT1*, *GRM3*). In a family-based association study, Nicodemus *et al.* (2008) determined the impact on schizophrenia risk of inheriting variants in these genes in the context of serious OCs likely to be associated with hypoxia, in comparison to offspring inheriting the same alleles but in the absence of a history of OCs. Though the samples with risk alleles and a history of OCs were small, in some instances including fewer than 30 subjects, the effects were large, with increases in odds ratios from 4- to 12-fold. These results speak to a potential gene–environment interaction related to genetic risk and OC events, a potential insight into mechanisms that contribute to heterogeneity and variable expression of early developmental adversity.

Finally, it is important to point out that in almost all the OC literature there is no consideration of environmental risk factors, such as smoking and drug/alcohol use, on pregnancy outcome. It is clear from many studies that tobacco and alcohol use affect the frequency of OCs and brain development. The possibility that an association of such behaviors in the mothers of offspring who develop schizophrenia would provide a potential causative mechanism for OCs needs to be considered in future studies. The implications for prevention are also apparent.

In conclusion, while the OC literature does not provide a mechanistic account of how OCs biologically translate into risk for schizophrenia, it does add substantial evidence for a role of a neurodevelopmental abnormality *per se*, and is consistent with other data (*vide infra*) that developmental risk factors for the eventual expression of schizophrenia are protean and non-specific.

Several large epidemiological studies also indicate that abnormalities of the intrauterine microenvironment relatively early in development, most often during the first two trimesters when neuron production and migration to their final locations occur, can increase the risk of adult onset of the disorder (see Chapter 10). These include potential exposure to viruses and other infectious agents (Brown & Derkits, 2010), Rhesus incompatibility (Palmer *et al.*, 2002), ABO incompatibility (Insel *et al.*, 2005), elevated maternal homocysteine levels (Brown *et al.*, 2007), maternal severe stress during pregnancy (Khashan *et al.*, 2008), and nutritional deficiency (Susser & Lin, 1992). The early epidemiological literature on intrauterine infection reviewed in the second edition of this book (and see Chapter 10) was based largely on population studies that examined illness rates during known epidemics, but did not determine whether actual fetal infection occurred. More recent studies have employed prospective public health samples from selected healthcare networks (e.g., Kaiser Permanente in California) in which stored maternal or umbilical cord blood could be assayed many years later for biomarkers related to infection or fetal stress. These studies have confirmed the evidence that influenza infection in the mother is associated with increased rates of schizophrenia later in life (Brown & Derkits, 2010).

The earlier evidence from a study of the Nazi occupation of the Netherlands that starvation during gestation increases the risk of schizophrenia (Susser & Lin, 1992) has been confirmed in two large population studies from China In the first study (St Clair *et al.*, 2005), the risk for schizophrenia was examined in a region of Anhui Province (population approximately 1.5 million) that had been exposed to the major famine of 1959–61. The relative risk for schizophrenia was determined for individuals born during the famine and in the years before and after this. Despite a drop in the birth rate and a rise in mortality during the famine years, the overall risk for developing schizophrenia later in life rose on average two-fold for individuals born during the famine years, quite analogous to the effect size observed during the Dutch Hunger Winter Study (Susser & Lin, 1992). A subsequent independent study of the relative

risk of schizophrenia for children born during the famine years in the Liuzhou prefecture of the Guangxi autonomous region of China was conducted and the results, at least for children from rural areas, were quite analogous (Xu *et al.*, 2009). Curiously, in this latter study, children born in cities during the famine actually had reduced rates of schizophrenia. The studies from China provide further epidemiological evidence that prenatal malnutrition impacts on risk for schizophrenia long after birth, presumably by adversely affecting the molecular biology of fetal development.

In summary, over the past two decades there has been a substantial accumulation of data that OCs and intrauterine adversity slightly but significantly increase risk for adult emergence of schizophrenia. Because these factors reflect phenomena linked to aspects of brain development, they represent the most substantial evidence that abnormal brain development increases risk for schizophrenia. However, it is also clear from this large literature that there is no specific or consistent developmental factor, nor does there appear to be a specific vulnerable time or stage in human intrauterine development. This makes it difficult to implicate a specific biological mechanism, or a specific developmental defect, at least across the general population of affected patients. Moreover, the same developmental causes that increase risk for schizophrenia may also increase risk for other disorders, including affective psychosis. These results invite reflection upon the notion of specificity of causation and pathogenesis with respect to schizophrenia (see below). It is reasonable to assume that such diverse environmental factors that disrupt the normal programs of early human brain development have individually varying clinical effects depending on other modifying and protecting factors, including genetic background and environmental aspects of postnatal development.

Association with maturational deficits and delays in childhood

Developmental circuit disruptions in individuals at risk to manifest schizophrenia might be expected to yield at least subtle, if not overt, abnormalities of nervous system function during their childhood, prior to clinical illness. Indeed, there is a large epidemiological literature of neurological and cognitive development that consistently indicates a relationship between individuals destined to manifest schizophrenia as adults and delays in certain motor and cognitive milestones during childhood, even as early as the first 6 months of life (see Chapter 10, and reviewed by Weinberger & Marenco, 2003). This evidence includes delayed motor and speech milestones during the first year of life, various deficits in motor and cognitive development throughout childhood, and social and school abnormalities. A recent study from the Copenhagen

Perinatal Project confirmed in another population sample the association of delays in multiple early motor milestones (e.g., standing, walking unsupported) with increased risk for schizophrenia, though adults hospitalized with other psychiatric diagnoses also had some early motor delays, albeit not as prominent (Sorensen *et al.*, 2010). The magnitude of the delays or deficits reported in the studies of motor and cognitive development are very modest, not of the order that would cause parent or physician concern. Further, it is clear that most individuals who are slightly delayed in attaining these milestones do not evince schizophrenia as adults. At the population level, however, the data indicate that problems in brain maturation are preclinical signs of individuals who are at increased risk of manifesting schizophrenia in their lifetime, and possibly reflections of a core pathogenic process at an earlier stage of development.

A recent finding of the association of schizophrenia during adulthood with early childhood developmental abnormalities was seen in a large study of the prevalence of childhood enuresis in adult individuals with schizophrenia. Hyde *et al.* (2008) found a three-fold increase in the frequency of childhood enuresis in adult patients with schizophrenia as compared with normal subjects (21% in the patient sample *vs.* 7% in controls). Because enuresis is a well-documented neurological sign of cortical developmental delay, the biological implications of the findings are somewhat less obscure than for general motor or speech delay. Hyde *et al.* (2008) also tested directly the possibility that the history of childhood enuresis reflected a cortical maturational abnormality by examining cortical volume with magnetic resonance imaging (MRI) in adult patients with schizophrenia having positive enuresis histories in comparison to patients without such histories. While all subjects were continent as adults, the investigators found volume reductions in the medial prefrontal cortex in patients with positive childhood enuresis histories. These findings directly implicate the cortical region responsible for voluntary micturition control. This study also found evidence of significantly increased frequency of childhood enuresis in the histories of the healthy siblings of patients with schizophrenia, suggesting the developmental problem underlying the manifestation of enuresis is in part related to the genetics of schizophrenia.

Perhaps the most studied developmental antecedent of schizophrenia is premorbid IQ. Early studies found evidence that within a family, patients with schizophrenia tended to have the lowest IQ in their sibship, even if their IQ was within the normal range. More recent studies have focused on large public health epidemiological samples studied prospectively from early childhood. In a large meta-analysis of 18 studies of premorbid IQ of individuals who manifest schizophrenia as adults, Woodberry *et al.* (2008) found that schizophrenia was associated with approximately a one-half standard deviation reduction in IQ long before the emergence of the clinical syndrome. Importantly, in examining studies that included multiple premorbid IQ assessments, they found no evidence that IQ declined further during the premorbid years, suggesting that the deficit was stable and not a reflection of a continuing deteriorating pathological process. Reichenberg *et al.* (2010) explored the question of the stability of premorbid IQ deficits in a detailed analysis of serial assessments of children studied as part of the Dunedin Child Development Study in New Zealand. Over 1000 children were followed from birth to 32 years of age and serial IQ tests were performed to age 13. A comparison of 35 subjects who developed schizophrenia as adults with 98 subjects who manifested depression and 101 normal controls, all carefully matched, revealed that the patients who eventually manifested schizophrenia had the overall lowest premorbid IQ scores by more than one-half standard deviation (seven points), and that the sample with depression and the normal sample differed by only three points. More importantly, Reichenberg *et al.* (2010) used the serial IQ tests to examine three specific hypotheses: (1) whether IQ deteriorates during the premorbid period; (2) whether IQ deficits are stable; and (3) whether IQ lags maturationally, meaning it advances as expected with age but at a slower pace than normal. They found no evidence to support the first hypothesis, and some evidence for each of the other two. Specifically, deficits in verbal reasoning and information storage subscales of the IQ test battery were stable, while measures of attention and working memory improved but seemed to fail to keep pace with normal age-associated enhancement. They interpreted their data to suggest that children growing up to develop schizophrenia enter primary school with deficits in verbal reasoning and fall farther behind in executive cognitive processing as they enter early adolescence. They also predicted from their data at age 13 that by age 23, patients with schizophrenia would have IQ deficits of approximately one standard deviation from normal, consistent with what has been typically reported in the clinical literature.

While the role of prenatal adversity and genetic risk factors has not been studied systematically in relation to premorbid IQ in individuals who later develop schizophrenia, a large epidemiological study of male conscripts in Norway found that prenatal exposure to the Hong Kong influenza pandemic of 1969–70 was significantly associated with lower IQ scores at conscription (Eriksen *et al.*, 2009). Similarly, another large epidemiological study (n > 33 000) from the Perinatal Birth Study in the US revealed that advanced paternal age, which has been correlated positively with a number of developmental syndromes, including autism and schizophrenia, also predicts relatively lower IQ during childhood (Saha *et al.*, 2009).

Clearly, schizophrenia, as it is currently defined and diagnosed, is a disorder of early adult life, but antecedent abnormalities of cognitive, psychological, and neurological function are part of the extended syndrome. Thus, it can be concluded that such antecedents reflect disruption of normal developmental processes involved in building certain brain systems from relatively early in life. It is tempting to further conclude that these disturbances, which do not manifest as a clinical syndrome during childhood, are expressions of the same biological mechanisms that eventually translate into the recognizable psychiatric syndrome in early adulthood. However, because social and psychological deprivations also can affect cognitive and social development, the specific etiology of these antecedents of schizophrenia cannot be specified from the population studies. It also cannot be concluded that these premorbid deficits necessarily reflect the identical developmental processes that lead to the emergence of the clinical syndrome, as it is conceivable that they are associated manifestations, but not true intermediate phenotypes in the sense of being on the same pathogenic trajectory from cause to clinical syndrome.

These caveats notwithstanding, the premorbid risk and association data are the most objective evidence that schizophrenia is related to early neurodevelopmental deviations, at least to some degree. There are many other findings connected to schizophrenia that have been interpreted as reflecting developmental anomalies, including putative facial dysmorphias, fingerprint deviations, anomalous cerebral lateralization, and disrupted cellular architecture in the brain. These are controversial and inconclusive, however, as reviewed in this chapter in the previous edition of this book and in Chapter 10. One of the popular theories about schizophrenia based on brain development has proposed that the programs that determine cerebral asymmetry are disrupted, but a recent large, carefully controlled study of handedness and cerebral asymmetry in patients with schizophrenia and their healthy siblings did not support this hypothesis (Deep-Soboslay et al., 2010). It also has been noted frequently that evidence of brain degeneration, as is seen with many neurological disorders of adult onset, is generally lacking in postmortem studies of schizophrenic brain tissue (see Chapter 18). This has been offered as further evidence that the brain pathology in schizophrenia likely involves more basic aspects of circuitry wiring, which are organized relatively early in life. This too, however, is speculative. While the most appealing candidate genes for schizophrenia are involved in neurodevelopmental processes (see below), definitive evidence of a developmental etiology of schizophrenia will require identification of a molecular mechanism explaining both the associated premorbid deficits and the later emergence of the familiar clinical manifestations.

Clues to a molecular mechanism of developmental deviation

Insights to the cellular and molecular origins of schizophrenia will likely follow from an understanding of the role of genetic risk factors. While genes are certainly not the only important clues to etiology, they are the most objective and bounded. Genes by definition represent mechanisms of cellular function, and inheritance of risk-associated variations in genes presumably translate into compromised cell function that impacts on brain development. Genes may also illuminate the affected developmental processes that increase risk, as genes are developmental risk factors *pari passu*; they are usually expressed from early in fetal life and influence relevant cellular aspects of neural circuitry, development, and function. Indeed, congenital chromosomal defects associated with the diagnosis of schizophrenia, e.g., Klinefelter syndrome (XXY) and the 22q11 hemideletion or velocardiofacial syndrome (VCFS) (*vide infra*), invariably involve diverse aspects of development with protean clinical manifestations present from early in life (e.g., learning disabilities, physical dysmorphias, autism). Recent discoveries of other rare chromosomal microdeletions that increase risk for schizophrenia [e.g., hemideletions on chromosomes 1p (Stefansson et al., 2008), 2p (Rujescu et al., 2009), 15q (Stefansson et al., 2008), and 16p (Ingason et al., 2009)] also are associated with increased risk of other developmental syndromes with early life manifestations, such as autism, epilepsy, facial and skeletal abnormalities, and mental retardation. The fact that multiple chromosomal defects, involving a myriad of genes, may each translate into a spectrum of behavioral phenotypes that includes schizophrenia, suggests that from a developmental perspective, there are diverse genetic pathways to these clinical syndromes, echoing the diversity of environmental factors such as obstetric complications and prenatal adversities that also increase risk.

Biological studies of specific genes that have been implicated as risk factors for schizophrenia further suggest that the molecular mechanisms of risk are diverse and heterogeneous. For many of these candidates, there is a common biological convergence on mediating histogenic processes involved in the assembly and maturation of circuits and neural systems. The heterogeneous and diverse functions, both central and peripheral, that may be impacted in subpopulations of individuals with schizophrenia are consistent with the pleiotrophic nature of the gene products. That is, these genes impact more than one biological process in more than one type of cell or tissue. For example, the neurotrophic factor, neuregulin-1 (*NRG1*) and its tyrosine kinase receptor *ERBB4*, have been extensively studied as potential schizophrenia susceptibility genes based on evidence from clinical association studies and from studies of copy number variations (CNVs; Harrison & Law 2006; see

Chapter 13). NRG1–ERBB4 signaling has been shown to play a role in many developmental processes that are critical for the construction of cortical circuitry and neuronal plasticity, processes that are prominently implicated in pathophysiological formulations of schizophrenia. These processes include cell proliferation, radial glia differentiation, neuronal migration (both radial and tangential), neurite outgrowth, synaptic maturation, dendritic spine development, and various aspects of neurotransmitter functions, such as N-methyl-D-aspartate (NMDA) signaling, dopamine neuronal activity, and gamma-aminobutyric acid (GABA) neuronal function (Jaaro-Peled *et al.*, 2009). NRG1–ERBB4 also has been shown to be important in myelin formation, at least in the periphery, though controversy exists about whether signaling through the receptor also plays a role in central nervous system (CNS) oligodendrocyte maturation and function. NRG1 is expressed at much higher levels in the fetal than adult brain, and one recent study has shown that a region of the *NRG1* gene implicated in genetic risk for schizophrenia is associated specifically with an isoform of NRG1 that is primarily expressed in fetal life (Law *et al.*, 2006; Tan *et al.*, 2007). This suggests that at least one mechanism of genetic risk for schizophrenia related to *NRG1* involves the early developmental actions of the gene.

DISC1 is another well-studied candidate susceptibility gene for schizophrenia, based on identification of a highly penetrant chromosomal translocation disrupting this gene and on multiple clinical association studies (Porteous *et al.*, 2006; see Chapter 13). DISC1 is implicated in diverse developmental processes potentially relevant to the pathogenesis of schizophrenia (Brandon *et al.*, 2009), and in fact has been shown in experiments in mice to disrupt cell autonomous and non-autonomous development of the neocortex that results in postpubertal onset of relevant behavioral dysfunction (Niwa *et al.*, 2010; Clapcote *et al.*, 2007; Ayhan *et al.*, 2010). DISC1 is expressed at much higher levels during fetal than adult life (Jaaro-Peled *et al.*, 2009) and, as with *NRG1*, genetic variants in *DISC1* associated with risk for schizophrenia appear to predict expression specifically of fetal forms of DISC1 in the human brain (Nakata *et al.*, 2009). This suggests that the mechanism of genetic risk for schizophrenia related to *DISC1* involves the early developmental actions of this gene.

Many of the other genes prominently associated with schizophrenia have been shown to impact on basic processes of early brain development, especially the sculpting of neuronal circuitry, and a story can be fashioned for each of them playing a role in schizophrenia risk based on these developmental effects. For example, dysbindin (*DTNBP1*), one of the first genes to be associated with schizophrenia based on linkage, like *NRG1* and *DISC1*, is expressed at higher levels in fetal than adult brain and is important in synapse formation and plasticity (Talbot,

2009), particularly involving glutamate and dopamine synapses (Iizuka *et al.*, 2007; Tang *et al.*, 2009). *Neurexin-1*, a gene implicated from a rare CNV associated with schizophrenia and other developmental phenotypes (e.g., autism, mental retardation), is critical for synapse formation and plasticity, as is *NRGN1*, a gene identified from a large genome-wide association (GWA) study of schizophrenia (Stefansson *et al.*, 2009). *TCF4*, another gene implicated from GWA studies (Stefansson *et al.*, 2009), plays multiple roles in cortical development and nonsense mutations in this gene are associated with profound mental retardation syndromes. Loci in the major histocompatibility (MHC) region show genome-wide corrected statistical association with schizophrenia (Stefansson *et al.*, 2009) and MHC genes have been shown in experimental models to modulate synapse development, elimination, and plasticity (Shatz, 1990). The possibility that human leukocyte antigen (HLA) region genes may be involved in the neurodevelopmental origins of schizophrenia may also have implications for potential molecular mechanisms related to the effects of intrauterine adversity such as infection (Brown & Derkits, 2010).

A recent report of an association of schizophrenia with a potassium channel gene critical to neuronal repolarization and excitability (*KCNH2*) was shown to be based on regulation of expression of a novel, brain- and primate-specific isoform of this gene which affects adaptive neuronal firing patterns essential for normal circuitry dynamics (Huffaker *et al.*, 2009). The isoform of the gene associated with schizophrenia, both genetically and in expression differences between brains of patients and controls, was expressed very highly in early development, and much less abundantly after birth. This again suggests that the genetic mechanism related to risk for schizophrenia involves early cellular physiology and excitability, a factor thought to be critical for the early development of cortical circuits (Shatz, 1990).

These diverse biological roles played by schizophrenia risk-associated genes converge on the conclusion that their role in the etiology of schizophrenia is to interfere with critical stages in the wiring of the brain. One of the problems with this conclusion is that it offers no clue to specificity either in terms of which if any developmental processes are critical or why some genes are implicated and not others. Most genes in the human genome are expressed in brain and most play some role in brain development, though most so far have not been implicated in schizophrenia. This last point may ultimately undergo revision as a recent study suggests that the genetic origins of schizophrenia may be exceedingly complex and heterogeneous, potentially implicating many thousands of genes in many different constellations and combinations (Purcell *et al.*, 2009; Mitchell & Porteous, 2010). In other words, the emerging picture of multiple genetic factors impacting on diverse aspects of the development and refinement of cortical circuitry argues that there is no specificity in the pathogenesis of schizophrenia because there are many paths to a similar phenotypic state of brain development and function. That multiple genes can impact on risk for the same behavioral phenotype and that multiple behavioral phenotypes can be associated with the same genes likely reflect a fundamental aspect of brain development linked to complex cognitive and social behavior: the development of the cortex and the forebrain—structures subserving these complex behaviors—is inherently redundant and degenerate, meaning that there are many diverse processes involved in their development, reflected in the hierarchical fashion of how the circuitry is built. Thus, there are many stations along the way at which noise can be introduced into the molecular program to affect the trajectory, and many molecular alternatives that can affect compensation or buffering. In order to elucidate this molecular complexity, we will need a much deeper understanding of how our transcriptome is regulated during brain development, with regard to both spatial and temporal specificity, as well as the spectrum of alternative splicing and editing that adds significantly to the already complex genome.

As noted, circuit development in the brain follows a complex program involving cell proliferation, cell fate determination, migration, axon pathfinding to detect relevant targets, dendritic growth and arborization, synaptogenesis, and synaptic refinement. Myelination is another critical element for defining accessible periods of plasticity and improved information processing. For the cascade of complex events to lead to an adaptive functional outcome, there must be buffering capability to deal with molecular disruptions that can be introduced at various levels, based on genetic and environmental factors. This buffering in managing the "allostatic" load is presumably possible because of the complexity of the program and the built in redundancy and degeneracy, which has been demonstrated in multiple animal models (Mitchell, 2007). Thus, a single genetic variation by itself is not likely to have much of an impact, because the system can adapt to small amounts of noise. Small effects, however, despite their lack of appreciable individual impact, might sensitize the system to other genetic (i.e., epistatic gene interactions) and environmental factors (e.g., OCs or intrauterine stress), and to stochastic effects that will increasingly challenge the adaptive capability and bias the developmental path that is followed.

In other words, the more complex the program, and the more possibilities for disruption (genetic, environmental, and stochastic) and adaptation, the more the relationship between genotype and phenotype is non-linear. A recent study of epistatic interactions of genes in the NRG1/ERBB4/AKT1 signaling pathway illustrated this point in predicting risk for schizophrenia. While neither *NRG1* or

ERBB4 by themselves had significant effects on risk for schizophrenia in the clinical case–control sample studied, in the context of *AKT1* variation, the pattern of association was dramatically altered. Individuals with risk-associated genotypes at all three genes had a 27-fold increase in risk (Nicodemus *et al.*, 2010). *AKT1* did not interact with *NRG1* alone or with *ERBB4* alone to increase risk; only when all three gene effects were combined did the leap in risk occur, seeming to echo the multidimensional biological program of AKT1 activation induced by NRG1 binding to ERBB4.

The concept of developmental disruption considered so far has focused on early developmental events, and many of the genes implicated in schizophrenia appear to have particularly robust effects in early developmental models. Most of these genes, however, also are expressed throughout life and may affect synaptic function and plasticity into adulthood. Thus, the biological perturbations related to these factors may be expressed across the lifespan and continue to exert effects on differing maturational trajectories that characterize different stages of life. This may have additional implications for the changing manifestations of schizophrenia from early childhood to advanced age (*vide infra*).

This line of thinking about how genes and environment can interact to vary the trajectory of brain development echoes the seminal work of Conrad Waddington, who coined the phrase "epigenetic landscape" to suggest that the biological landscape from inherited genetic risk to clinical phenotype was one with many hills and valleys, representing distinct trajectories to the same phenotypic endpoints influenced by different combinations of developmental factors, including genes, environment, and stochastic factors (Waddington, 1972; see also Lewis & Levitt, 2002). Waddington proposed that because noise can be introduced at many levels of the landscape, there are likely to be many genetic and environmental events that can be associated with a deviation of the developmental landscape that biases the trajectory towards one hill or valley and a particular endpoint. Many different factors along the way can bias the trajectory towards a common endpoint, and any given risk factor can have its effects diverted from an expected endpoint by other factors that perturb the trajectory. Obviously, if the disruption is extreme, the impact on cortical development and the endpoint would tend to be a more extreme deviation, for example, resulting in intellectual disability or a profound congenital syndrome. The genetic and environmental events associated with schizophrenia, however, tend not to be extreme. For example, the OCs associated with schizophrenia do not disrupt general fetal growth and overt wellbeing or the development of other organ systems; the intrauterine environmental stresses associated with schizophrenia (e.g., influenza exposure, nutritional deficiency) do not disrupt gestation or cause major developmental lesions in other organ systems; and most of the genetic variations identified so far do not result in protein function abnormalities. The potential exceptions are the CNVs recently associated with schizophrenia, which are hemimicrodeletions or microduplications likely resulting in gene dosage effects. When many genes are involved, the CNVs tend to include intellectual disability or epilepsy as an associated phenotype, likely because of the greater biological burden imposed by the multiple mutations.

The syndrome of schizophrenia might, thus, be considered as an endpoint state of brain developmental wiring that can reflect multiple and subtle disruptions of diverse elements of the developmental landscape, all leading to a common pattern of cortical dysfunction, which during childhood is most apparent as cognitive and social deficits, but then during early adulthood takes on a new form of expression. In a sense, schizophrenia appears to be on a developmental continuum with other behavioral disorders that appear in childhood, including autism, intellectual disability, and epilepsy, arising perhaps from overlapping biological risk factors that may each have distinct covariants, but schizophrenia reflects the relatively least noise burden of this group of developmental disturbances. The early manifestations (and the subtle neuropathology) of schizophrenia suggest much less disruption of the early trajectory for cortical development than do disturbances leading to intellectual disability, autism, and involvement of other ectodermally-derived organ systems. In autism, for example, in which the cellular elements in the relevant circuits appear to be modestly impacted structurally, the regulatory processes that control cortical development are more significantly challenged (Webb *et al.*, 2007; Courchesne *et al.*, 2003). Thus, the principle opined by Waddington might be broadened to suggest that as individuals on a particular developmental trajectory move forward, the subtle course corrections from early cell differentiation and circuit construction become increasingly amplified and compounded as the phenotypic endpoint becomes increasingly mature and the circuits involved take on increasingly complex functions.

Why do the clinical manifestations of schizophrenia change over time?

To the extent that the origins of schizophrenia begin in early brain development, its major manifestations do not remain static across the lifespan, as seen, for example, with other neurodevelopmental syndromes such as intellectual disability or cerebral palsy. The illness appears to have cognitive and social correlates during childhood and then the dramatic appearance of further cognitive and social deficits along with frank perceptual abnormalities and thought disturbances in early adult life, i.e., the diagnostic symptoms of psychosis and thought disorganization

emerge long after the childhood antecedents. Later in the course of illness, many patients appear to deteriorate and become dilapidated and treatment resistant. MRI measures suggest that there is a loss of cortical volume associated with advancing illness (*vide infra*), causing some investigators to suggest that the brain may undergo some form of atrophy. Cognitive deterioration over time also has been reported in some studies, though, interestingly, most studies find that cognitive function is relatively stable after onset of the diagnostic symptoms in early adult life, despite other signs of deterioration (Gochman *et al.*, 2005; Caspi *et al.*, 2003; Mesholam-Gately & Giuliano, 2009). This dramatic change in the clinical expression of the state of brain function during the first few decades of life of affected individuals raises a number of challenges for understanding the pathogenesis of the disorder and the role of developmental factors. Among these questions are: (1) Is it plausible that early childhood antecedents of schizophrenia and psychosis in young adulthood are reflections of the same developmental abnormalities?; (2) Does the emergence of psychosis in early adulthood signal a new developmental event or an additional pathological "hit" occurring around this time?; (3) Does deterioration over time implicate a neurodegenerative process?; and (4) What are the molecular mechanisms that covary with the changing phenotype to account for the emergence of psychosis in early adult life?

Plausibility of a common etiology for the changing clinical state

The principle of Ocam's Razor would argue for a simple formulation, and given the evidence of anomalous brain development associated with schizophrenia, the changing clinical course—particularly the delayed emergence of the dramatic diagnostic symptoms two decades after birth—might represent another manifestation of the early life etiology. From the perspective of Waddington's epigenetic landscape, this would mean that the early developmental disruptions, as subtle as they may be functionally, increase the probability that the brain is developmentally at risk for schizophrenia. This manifests phenotypically in childhood as cognitive and social deficits, but changes its phenotypic expression as it enters a new stage of postnatal brain organization. One of the early neurodevelopmental formulations of schizophrenia echoed this thinking by suggesting that the emergence of psychosis in early adult life reflected an interaction between early cortical maldevelopment and normal developmental processes that occurmuch later (Weinberger, 1986, 1987). This view makes several implicit assumptions: that the clinical implications of a developmental defect vary with the maturational state of the brain; that the neural systems disrupted by the defect in early brain development destined to manifest as psychosis are normally late maturing neural systems; and that a defect in the function of these neural systems may not be reliably apparent until their normal time of functional maturation. In other words, certain neural systems may be primed from early in development to have the capacity to malfunction in a manner that accounts for the psychosis, but until a certain state of postnatal brain development, they either do not malfunction to a clinically significant degree, or their malfunctioning can be compensated for by other systems. The first of these assumptions, i.e., that the clinical implications of a developmental defect vary with the maturational state of the brain, has been repeatedly validated in developmental neurobiology. Indeed, a fundamental principle of the clinical impact of developmental neuropathology, as exemplified by the landmark work of Margaret Kennard (1936), is that in general early brain damage is most apparent early and tends to become less so over time. The young brain has a greater capacity for functional compensation than does the old brain (Kolb & Whishaw, 1989), presumably because immature pathways and connections are highly plastic, or those that are normally transient can be recruited and maintained in order to subserve the functions lost by the damaged circuits (Huttenlocher, 1990; Rakic et al., 1994). It also is a fundamental principle of pediatric neurology that in some cases congenital brain damage can have delayed or varying clinical effects if the neural systems involved are neurologically immature at birth; e.g., athetosis in association with a perinatal infarct is not apparent until a few years after birth as the basal ganglia mature (Adams & Lyons, 1982).

In the case of at least the diagnostic symptoms of schizophrenia, the "Kennard principle" appears to be inverted, in that the impact of putative early damage is less apparent early and more apparent late. In this respect, the other two assumptions of this perspective are much more speculative. It is not known whether the principle of clinical effects being delayed until the affected neural systems reach functional maturity applies to those neural systems implicated in psychosis. More data are needed about the neural systems that develop abnormally in schizophrenia and about their normal course of functional maturation. It is also important to be careful in defining these epochs of development, as the terms "early" and "late" are relative in context. In the primate brain, for example, prenatal disturbances may be viewed as early, but synapse formation, a late event on the histogenic timeline, begins in the third trimester in humans.

There is provocative evidence from other clinical disorders in which psychosis is common, and from animal models based on early cortical disruptions, that late-emerging behavioral states analogous with psychosis are plausible sequelae of the early disruptions. Animal models based on a variety of neonatal and prenatal pertur-

bations in cortical connectivity, analogous to what is implicated in schizophrenia, have been created (see Lipska & Weinberger, 2000 and Chapter 22). These animal models, especially those with disconnections involving prefrontal–temporo–limbic circuits, manifest subtle cognitive and social abnormalities during the prepubertal period, but a number of behaviors, cognitive deficits, and pharmacological responses considered as animal models of psychosis do not appear until early adulthood is reached. These results in animals (including the *DISC1* studies noted above) support the biological plausibility of the notion that early developmental changes in cortical circuitry can have a delayed impact on complex behaviors linked to psychosis, some of which do not become manifest until early adult life.

Data from studies of cortical function in patients with schizophrenia, including neuropsychological testing results (see Chapter 8) and studies of cortical physiology using functional brain imaging techniques (see Chapter 17), indicate that cortical dysfunction is a prominent characteristic of the illness and that prefrontal–temporal functional connectivity is especially affected. Even if cortical maldevelopment is widespread, the functional neural systems that appear to be particularly relevant to the clinical characteristics of schizophrenia are those involved in prefrontal–temporal cortical connectivity (see Chapter 17). If the functional maturation of such connectivity is prolonged normally over years, as a number of lines of evidence in human and non-human primates suggest (Bachevalier & Mishkin, 1984; Chelune & Baer 1986; Supekar et al., 2009), then this might predict that some of the manifestations of dysfunction of cortical connectivity would show delayed onset.

Further support for the model that developmental pathology can be a primary event underlying secondary emergent psychotic phenomena related to adolescence and relatively late cortical development comes from studies of various neurological conditions involving subtle developmental abnormalities of intracortical connections. Psychosis is not uncommon in many such conditions, including developmental epilepsies, intellectual disabilities of various types, and cerebral malformations. The remarkable aspect regarding the link with psychosis and these conditions is that, despite the variable etiology and pathology, if psychosis occurs, it appears around the same age as psychosis in schizophrenia, i.e., late adolescence or early adult life (Weinberger, 1987). This again speaks to the differentially regulated maturation process of the most relevant circuits (see below).

Metachromatic leukodystrophy (MLD), a rare genetic disorder of aryl sulfatase deficiency, is an informative example of this age association and also of the potential importance of functional "disconnection" of cortical regions. Hyde et al. (1992) demonstrated that when MLD presents between the ages of 13 and 25, it does so in the majority of cases as a schizophrenia-like illness. Patients have disorganized thinking, act bizarrely, have complex delusions, and when hallucinating, invariably have complex, "Schneiderian-type" auditory hallucinations. The condition is often misdiagnosed as schizophrenia, sometimes for years, before neurological symptoms appear. Interestingly, MLD is a disconnectivity disorder in that the neuropathological changes principally involve white matter. In its early neuropathological stages when it is most likely to present with psychosis, the changes are especially prominent in subprefrontal white matter. This suggests that a neural dysfunction with a high valence for producing psychotic symptoms is failure of some aspects of prefrontal connectivity, analogous functionally to what has been implicated in schizophrenia (see Chapter 17).

In the case of MLD, however, this functional "disconnection" does not appear to be sufficient. When MLD presents before this critical age range, it tends to present with intellectual and social deficits followed by motor deficits, and it almost never presents with psychosis, even though the location of the neuropathology is not age-dependent. In other words, the involvement of a critical neural system is not by itself sufficient for the expression of psychosis. An age-related factor that appears to be independent of the illness is also required. Again, since this age association is seen in other diseases and thus transcends specific illness boundaries, it is probably a function of normal postnatal brain maturation.

A hemideletion of the long arm of chromosome 22, the so-called VCFS or the 22q11 hemideletion syndrome, has been the subject of much interest in relation to schizophrenia, because a large portion (perhaps as much as 50%) of such cases develop psychiatric disorders, including autism and psychosis (Bassett & Chow, 2009). In addition, several genes implicated in association studies of schizophrenia are within the obligatory deletion region (e.g., *COMT*, *PRODH*; Karayiorgou *et al.*, 2010). Cases of VCFSs have subtle craniocerebral malformations and mental retardation, and typically manifest learning difficulties, autistic behavior, and attentional problems during childhood (Eliez *et al.*, 2001). While changes in the brain are clearly present at birth, and have childhood phenotypic repercussions, psychotic symptoms, if they are manifest, do not emerge until adolescence (Arnold *et al.*, 2001; Gothelf *et al.*, 2005). Interestingly, around the time that the psychosis appears, there also is a drop in IQ, analogous to what is seen in patients with schizophrenia. The etiology of both the childhood phenotypes and the early adolescent behavioral changes (including psychosis) that are associated with VCFS are the same. The difference is the impact that this etiology has at different stages of brain maturation. Similar observations have been made related to

other rare genetic variants associated with the diagnosis of schizophrenia, such as a nonsense mutation in the gene *SHANK3*, which has been associated with mental deficiency in childhood and a schizophrenia syndrome beginning in early adult life in the same individuals (Gauthier *et al.*, 2010).

While the genes deleted in the 22q11 region and *SHANK3* mutations impact on early aspects of brain development, and may thus set the stage for later appearing phenotypes, the hypomorphic genes likely impact on later aspects of brain function as well. The changing course of clinical manifestations may reflect this continuing biology of the genetic defect from early life to early adulthood. It likely involves a common etiology for this changing clinical landscape and an interaction of the biological effect of this etiology and the changing state of brain maturation. The fact that many neurological and developmental syndromes show the same chronological pattern with respect to early childhood cognitive and social deficits followed by the onset of psychosis years later argues that the factors leading to the manifestation of psychosis are generic and not specific to a particular condition. If they are specific to anything, it appears to be to early adult life.

Is there a second pathological "hit"?

The apparently deteriorating course of many patients with schizophrenia, their increasing dilapidation, and evidence of brain shrinkage on MRI scans has prompted some to suggest that there is another pathological process occurring other than a developmental one, specifically involving neurodegeneration or atrophy (Jarskog *et al.*, 2005). The evidence for this is largely circumstantial and inconsistent; yet the hypothesis is still provocative. Importantly, in postmortem tissue of patients who have died after many years of illness, where such evidence should be most obvious, signs of neurodegeneration have not been observed (see Chapter 18). Thus, the possibility of neurodegeneration in schizophrenia is based largely on two phenomena. First is the apparent progression of clinical aspects of the syndrome in some patients, such as personality deterioration, dilapidation, and treatment resistance (Lieberman, 1999). While some patients do show such apparent deterioration, overall the clinical course of most patients with schizophrenia is not chronically deteriorating. Moreover, clinical lore is replete with examples of patients who have "awakening"-like responses to new medications, even from states of extreme clinical deterioration. In longitudinal studies of cognitive function, a relatively direct and objective measure of the integrity of cortical neuronal systems, while there are occasional positive studies, the weight of the data are against progression, at least during the first 20 or so years of illness (e.g., Heaton *et al.*, 2001; Ho *et al.*, 2007; Gochman *et al.*, 2005; see Chapter 8).

Another possibility for apparent progressive changes that has been proposed is that psychosis itself is neurotoxic. If this were so, it might be expected that the longer one goes untreated in a psychotic state, the more obvious would be the signs of such toxicity. Most studies examining whether the duration of untreated psychosis has an impact on outcome after treatment, including medication response, cognition, social function, psychopathology, and structural measurements on MRI scan do not find evidence to support this assumption (Hoff *et al.*, 2000; Verdoux *et al.*, 2001; Ho *et al.*, 2005).

The most often cited and consistent body of evidence for a progressive and potentially degenerative disease process is based on changes of measurements made on structural MRI studies. While the first generation of longitudinal brain imaging studies of patients with schizophrenia, performed mainly with the CT scan, suggested that any observed anatomical changes were relatively static, more recent work has shown that changes occur over time and tend to imply loss of cortical volume. This literature has been reviewed elsewhere (Hulshoff Pol & Kahn, 2008) and is discussed in Chapter 16. The number of studies showing progression of measures of cortical volume loss after the onset of illness, even in first-episode patients (e.g., Sun *et al.*, 2009), has become voluminous and early concerns about ascertainment or methodological questions are no longer tenable. The data are unequivocal that reductions in MRI measures of cortical volume occur after the first diagnosis of schizophrenia and may continue for many years. The question about this literature is what the MRI changes represent, i.e., are they manifestations of a progressive neuropathological condition related to or independent of the developmental factors or are they associated epiphenomena (Weinberger & McClure, 2002)? If the MRI changes reflect a progressive neuropathology of any sort, it might be expected that they would predict worsening of the clinical state, i.e., more cognitive impairment, dilapidation, treatment resistance. While this has been reported in occasional studies, most studies do not find that progressive changes on MRI in patients with schizophrenia predict cognitive change (Ho *et al.*, 2007; Brans *et al.*, 2008; Sporn *et al.*, 2003), raising the possibility that the findings are not related to the pathogenesis of the clinical state.

It has also become clear that many environmental factors secondarily associated with being ill change volume measurements on MRI even in normal subjects and in the same direction as those reported in schizophrenia. These include alcohol consumption and related metabolic effects (Pfefferbaum *et al.*, 2004), weight gain (Taki *et al.*, 2008), exercise (Pajonk *et al.*, 2010), smoking (Brody *et al.*, 2004), and treatment with antipsychotic drugs (McClure *et al.*, 2006; Ho *et al.*, 2007). The possibility that the MRI changes may reflect such epiphenomena is further suggested by studies of sibling samples discordant for schizo-

phrenia. Brans *et al.* (2008) in a unique longitudinal study of discordant monozygotic and dizygotic twin pairs with schizophrenia found that progressive changes were at least as great, and in fact greater, in the healthy twins of both groups and not in the ill twins. In a study of healthy siblings of patients with childhood-onset schizophrenia, a patient sample with pronounced progressive MRI changes reported during the adolescent years (Rapoport *et al.*, 1999), a similar pattern and magnitude of changes have been found (Gogtay *et al.*, 2007). These remarkable results in genetically at-risk but unaffected family members suggest that the MRI findings may be at least to a considerable degree manifestations of associated, possibly familial, behaviors or environmental factors and that ongoing psychosis is not responsible. Finally, studies in monkeys treated chronically with antipsychotic drugs also demonstrate cortical volume reductions very similar in magnitude to that reported in patients, without loss of neurons or evidence of degeneration (Dorph-Petersen *et al.*, 2005; Konopaske *et al.*, 2007).

If the MRI changes do not implicate progressive atrophic processes related to the clinical illness mechanism, it leaves unanswered the question of why some patients appear to deteriorate over time. Many unfortunate human circumstances and behaviors appear to get worse in some individuals during their lifetime (e.g. joblessness and homelessness), without necessarily implicating degeneration of brain tissue. While chronic stressors, such as unemployment, may in fact be associated with dynamic changes in synaptic architecture, just as learning new behaviors and habits may involve changes in the connections made between cells, these presumably are *plastic* modifications (i.e., potentially reversible), not toxic degenerations (which usually imply irreversibility). It has become increasingly clear from studies in experimental animals that numerous environmental factors have an impact on neuronal plasticity and can be associated with changes in synaptic architecture. These non-degenerative adaptations, however, are potentially reversible—part of how a brain performs "molecular business" with its environment—in contrast to the implications of changes that reflect neurodegeneration.

In summary, while the course of schizophrenia implicates progressive processes in some individuals, the evidence that such processes reflect irreversible degeneration of neuronal elements, analogous to a neurotoxic process, are circumstantial and improbable. The apparent progressive changes observed in MRI studies are very likely epiphenomena related to secondary environmental factors and not to a primary illness mechanism. In terms of cognitive function and the capacity for clinical recovery, and at the level of cellular and molecular analysis, there is virtually no objective evidence for irreversible neurodegeneration or brain atrophy in schizophrenia.

Relevant biological events in adolescent brain development

If schizophrenia is related to abnormalities of early brain development that may manifest as cognitive and social deficits early in life, why do the manifestations change and take on the pattern of psychosis in young adulthood that accounts for the diagnosis? Indeed, in some patients the evidence of cognitive and social deficits is slight or virtually absent prior to the onset of psychosis in late adolescence, when the clinical diagnosis is first made. What accounts for the dramatic emergence of psychosis typically in the third decade after birth? Speculation about the answers to these questions has come primarily from two perspectives: (1) the possibility of an additional and seemingly independent developmental disruption occurring around the time of onset of the clinical illness; and (2) an interaction between developmental defects from early in life and developmental programs or events that occur in early adult life.

As the foremost proponent of the first perspective, Feinberg (1982) focused on the age at onset of schizophrenia as a clue to neurodevelopmental abnormalities that might explain the illness. He posited that schizophrenia is caused by a defect in adolescent synaptic reorganization, because either "too many, too few, or the wrong synapses are eliminated". In effect, he argued for a second pathological process, a specific pathology of synaptic elimination not necessarily related to possible maldevelopment from earlier in life. It is unclear what this pathology might be, in the sense of what would be abnormal about the pruning process. Since pruning is presumed to reflect a negative state, i.e., the end result of an absence of sustaining molecular and physiological processes that are required to support a synapse, the pathology would not likely be in the pruning *per se*, but rather in the mechanisms of synaptic sustenance. Numerous electrophysiological and molecular factors, involving classical neurotransmitters and trophic molecules, participate in the process of synaptic survival and plasticity. The abnormal pruning hypothesis has become very popular over the past decade as an explanation for a variety of clinical phenomena, including cortical thinning on MRI scans (Rapoport *et al.*, 1999; Mathalon *et al.*, 2001), and psychotic psychopathology (McGlashan & Hoffman, 2000).

It is possible that abnormalities of pruning or of other processes related to the formation and maintenance of neuronal connections (including myelination) could be abnormal without implicating a "second hit" hypothesis. Early developmental disruptions may set the stage for secondary synaptic disorganization that has its greatest neurobiological and clinical impact in adolescence. Sustaining specific connections that normally can be maintained could be challenged in an allostatic load model, in which temporal and new organizational dimensions, on the background of early disruptions, converge to deflect normal developmental trajectories. This could be likened to early-onset hypertension, in which an early developmental hit in terms of greatly reduced nephron number can sustain kidney function by adaptation (increase structural volume) for a period of time, but then ultimately fails under increased demand for renal function and age-associated involutional changes (Keller *et al.*, 2003). Consistent with the notion of altering the developmental trajectory, early developmental noise in the program of cortical circuit organization, involving both genetic and environmental factors (*vide infra*), could initiate an altered developmental path to maturity, which leads to cascading aberrations as cortical maturation proceeds. By this scenario, the phenotypic expression of the state of cortical function at the end of this trajectory would be expected to be quite different from that at its early stages. Neuronal circuitry that is anomalous from early in development has been shown in gross lesion models to have particularly profound implications for eventual connectivity (Schwartz & Goldman-Rakic, 1990; Marín-Padilla, 1997).

Interestingly, while it has been popular in the psychiatric literature to emphasize synaptic pruning as a critical maturational event in adolescent brain development, progressive synaptic events, involved in dendritic elaboration and spine maturation, are probably at least, if not even more, prominent during adolescence. Synaptic pruning is a relatively circumscribed process in early adulthood in the primate, involving a subpopulation of so-called asymmetric synapses, which are presumably excitatory and glutamatergic. GABAergic inhibitory connections are not pruned at this time. In fact, certain GABA synaptic markers increase in abundance throughout adolescence (Hashimoto *et al.*, 2009). Moreover, overall growth of dendrites and dendritic spines of pyramidal neurons, which are the postsynaptic targets of excitatory, glutamatergic inputs, actually increase in size and density quite remarkably in early adult life (Lambe *et al.*, 2000). It is tempting to conclude that the processes of pruning and of synaptic elaboration, which are occurring in parallel during adolescence, dynamically shape the synaptic landscape into a more mature, efficient, and environmentally adapted system. This is consistent with the notion that it is the stabilization of dynamic processes involved in postnatal cortical differentiation that signals the functional maturation of the cortex (Rakic, *et al.*, 1986; Lidow & Rakic, 1992) and the dynamics of efficient cortical network function (Supekar *et al.*, 2009).

In addition to progressive events at the level of dendritic and spine maturation, cortical inputs from subcortical projection neuronal systems also undergo progressive changes during early adulthood. In the primate prefrontal cortex, dopamine inputs show a dramatic postnatal developmental elaboration culminating in early adult life (Lambe *et al.*, 2000). A similar developmental trajectory is not seen with serotonergic inputs, which appear to reach their adult density level much earlier in development. Catechol-O-methyl transferase (COMT), an enzyme important for cortical dopamine metabolism, shows a similar pattern of increasing expression and activity in the prefrontal cortex of the postnatal human brain until it levels off in early adulthood (Tunbridge *et al.*, 2007).

In a more psychological vein, prefrontal–temporal connectivity has been viewed as facilitating the use of past experience to guide purposeful behavior when environmental cues are inadequate or maladaptive (Goldman-Rakic, 1987). The stresses of independent adult living might be especially likely to place a premium on this manner of circuit function. If the neural systems that permit such highly evolved behaviors are developmentally compromised, their malfunction might be relatively occult until either they alone are meant to subserve such functions and other systems (e.g., striatal) can no longer compensate, or until the environmental demands for such behavior overwhelm their diminished capacity (such as in the early-onset hypertension model above). It is important to note that this view does not predict that illness is inevitable, simply because of the existence of early pathology and of the eventual maturation of relevant brain systems in early adulthood. Clearly, catalytic events may be critical for many individuals, including environment adversity, stress, or substance abuse (see Chapter 11).

Candidate maturational processes and psychosis onset

Finally, it is of interest to speculate about the late molecular maturational processes that might interact with the early brain developmental abnormalities implicated in schizophrenia. The foregoing discussion militates towards processes involving cortical circuit development and maturation, i.e., on synaptic plasticity during development and during postnatal life. While schizophrenia may involve genetic variations that impact on the biology of synaptic plasticity (Harrison & Weinberger, 2005), and developmental adversity may disrupt the formation of normal cortical circuitry, the convergence of these risk factors on the processes that hone cortical connectivity during early adulthood would seem to be the final common pathway for the emergence of the syndrome. We believe that genetic risk factors and environmental adversity during brain development bias the normal molecular processes of postnatal synaptic assembly and plasticity towards abnormal connectivity that has its most dramatic impact during the early adult years. This biasing effect has implications at the cellular and molecular level, e.g., connections that are anomalous do not process signals normally and may not form normal secondary and tertiary connectivities. At the level of neuronal experience, anomalous circuits experience (i.e., perceive and process) environmental stimuli abnormally, and develop and maintain connections that are normal in terms of their cellular and molecular machinery, but are based on abnormal perception and processing of environmental events. This latter possibility also suggests that interactions between circuits that develop abnormally and those that are developmentally intact may color the phenotypic expression of the core deficits.

An interesting example of this latter possibility is implicated by a recent study of the effect of a risk-associated gene on cortical–striatal circuitry. Meyer-Lindenberg *et al.*, (2007) found association of the gene *PPP1R1B*, which encodes DARPP-32, with risk for schizophrenia in a family study. DARPP-32 has been of major interest as a protein phosphatase that modulates dopamine and glutamate signaling in the cortex and striatum. A surprising result of this study was that the common risk-associated variation in DARRP-32 translated into more efficient prefrontal–striatal processing of information in normal subjects. This raised the question of whether a genetic advantage in normal subjects may translate into a disadvantage in the context of functional impairments that are associated with schizophrenia based on other risk factors. Information flow through the striatum is thought to contribute to the automatization of behavioral and cognitive routines. In the normal brain functional state, this may subserve increased flexibility, working memory capacity, and cognitive control capabilities. In schizophrenia, on the other hand, the same information-processing constellation could facilitate the persistence and inflexibility of disorganized cortical information leading to environmentally maladaptive routines and perceptions. Stated another way, the common *DARPP-32* risk-associated genetic variation appears to be related to optimized frontal–striatal function, regardless of the specific information being processed through the system.

The emergence of the dramatic diagnostic symptoms in early adult life suggests that something has changed in how sensory, cognitive, and emotional information is processed in the brain. While cognitive information is processed in well-characterized cortical and cortical–striatal circuits, the neural systems that mediate the expression of psychotic systems are not well understood. Animal models have stressed abnormal dopamine function in the basal ganglia (see Chapter 20), but electrostimulation studies that induce hallucinations and bizarre thinking in humans (Gloor *et al.*, 1982) and neuroimaging studies of patients experiencing hallucinations (Shergill *et al.*, 2000) implicate temporo-limbic and prefrontal cortices. Thus, it seems reasonable to assume that the experience of psychosis, like abnormal cognitive function in schizophrenia, is a manifestation of alterations in the function of canonical cortical systems that are repeatedly implicated as abnormal in this disorder. Current thinking about how these systems malfunction in relation to the symptoms of schizophrenia has centered on a disorder of excitatory and inhibitory balance that is essential for the tuning of cortical microcircuitry, involving regulation of GABA activity by glutamate and dopamine (Winterer & Weinberger, 2007; Lewis & Gonzalez-Burgos, 2008). Indeed, the development and function of the system of GABAergic interneurons that is critical for fine-tuning of cortical function, and responsible for regulating cortical plasticity during critical developmental periods (Hensch, 2005), is another illustrative example of developmental risk factors for schizophrenia impacting on a developmental process critical for adult information processing in the cortex.

GABA neurons that seed dorsal pallial structures in the human brain arise, in part, in the ganglionic eminences and migrate tangentially into the cerebral cortex where they settle, elaborate processes, form synapses, and transition by the end of the first postnatal year from excitatory to inhibitory. As noted above, many of the genes implicated in risk for schizophrenia participate in various stages of GABA circuitry maturation, including in the genesis of GABA neurons (e.g., *DISC1*, *NRG1*), in their migration and settling (*DISC1*, *NRG1*, *ERBB4* ;Fazzari *et al.*, 2010), in synapse formation (e.g., *NRXN1*, *DISC1*, *NRG1*, *TGF4*, *NRGN1*), in neurotransmitter synthesis (*GAD1*), and in GABA becoming an inhibitory neurotransmitter (*CHRNA7*, *NRG1*; Liu *et al.*, 2006). Any of these risk factors could conceivably introduce noise in the early development of GABA circuitry. According to the principle articulated by Waddington, this noise, which could be etiologically quite heterogeneous, might impact on the trajectory of GABA microcircuit function and have ripple effects downstream in interactions with other maturing cortical circuits. For example, the response of GABA neurons to stimuli is mediated by glutamatergic excitatory input, and most of the same schizophrenia-associated genes that impact on GABA synaptic development and plasticity also impact on the development and function of glutamate, especially NMDA, synapses. Bottlenecks in the function of these neuronal systems, if not too extreme, might be expected to influence the tuning and efficiency of cortical information processing, but not necessarily derail this processing to the extent that might be implicated in autism or intellectual disability.

The evidence reviewed above that early adult life is particularly prone to the expression of psychosis when it occurs in association with other neurological conditions suggests that the impact of these early developmental bottlenecks has unique implications on cortical function in early adult life. This could occur due to changes in cortical tuning dynamics by early adulthood, or because the information processing load becomes too burdensome for compromised circuits, or a combination of the two. The pattern of expression of cortical GABA receptors shifts dramatically in early adulthood, suggesting age-dependent changes in GABA signaling (Hashimoto *et al.*, 2009). The unique

activity patterns of fast-spiking parvalbumin-expressing GABA neurons, which are critical for generating gamma frequency oscillations in the cortex, are late emerging in mice and not prominent before early adulthood (Okaty *et al.*, 2009). Gamma oscillations are thought to underlie complex cognitive processing in human brain and to be abnormal in schizophrenia (see Chapter 21). The electrophysiological changes in the behavior of these neurons in adolescence correlate with dramatic changes in the expression of genes regulating their excitability, such as potassium channel genes (Okaty *et al.*, 2009). Dopamine is important for tuning the excitability of fast-spiking GABA neurons, and this effect is not seen in the rat before early adult life (Tseng& O'Donnell, 2007). COMT, an enzyme linked to synaptic cortical dopamine levels, also reaches peak expression and activity in early adult life (Tunbridge *et al.*, 2007). These examples focus on the maturation and activity of GABA neurons that mediate cortical inhibition; they reflect only a small fraction of the complex processes that can be affected early and, because of the shifting trajectory of postnatal brain development related to cortical function, have changing phenotypic effects later. A similar story can be fashioned related to glutamate neuronal maturation, dopamine maturation, and likely other systems implicated in schizophrenia. These developmental cellular and molecular processes converge on the tuning of cortical circuitry implicated in schizophrenia; this circuitry undergoes profound changes in its tuning dynamics during the adolescent and early adult years. It seems to us reasonable to assume that these circuits—though seemingly compromised from early in development—are likely to be impacted most profoundly when their functional characteristics are most complex and most environmentally challenged.

Conclusions

The neurodevelopmental model of schizophrenia offers a framework for investigation that prompts us to focus on early antecedents and in particular on biological events involved in early brain development, during pregnancy and during early adolescence. It has obvious public health implications in that prevention should start early and include interventions at multiple ages. A vast body of research data supports this contention, but evidence of a "smoking gun" is lacking and evidence of specificity for schizophrenia is limited. We note, however, that specificity may not be critical from an outcomes perspective, for the avoidance or reduction of clinical symptoms over a lifetime may reflect an adaptational success.

The most parsimonious reduction of the available evidence argues that early developmental abnormalities based on genetic, environmental, and probably stochastic processes subtly alter the establishment of brain circuits and connectivity, which bias postnatal development towards further abnormalities of synaptic maturation and organization in critical cortical circuits. This increases the probability that schizophrenia as we currently diagnose it will be manifest in early adult life. The neurodevelopmental perspective about schizophrenia also links the adult features of the disorder with developmental problems in childhood that, though relatively subtle, are potential harbingers of more serious disabilities to come. The genetic overlap between schizophrenia, autism, and intellectual disabilities, the fact that certain genetic developmental abnormalities [e.g., Klinefelter syndrome (XXY), VCFS, *SHANK3* missense mutations, *NRXN1* deletions] can appear first as autism or intellectual disability and then change into what clinicians diagnose as schizophrenia by early adulthood illustrates the biological overlap between these syndromes and the lawful age-dependent transitions in their phenotypic expression. These various observations raise a much more fundamental epistemological question about the disease approach to schizophrenia. Schizophrenia, of course, is not something someone has; it is a diagnosis someone is given. It is worth considering that the syndrome of schizophrenia is not a disease at all, but a state of brain function based on an altered developmental trajectory from early programming with changing repercussions throughout life, much like autism and intellectual disability. That there appear to be numerous genetic and environmental factors that can contribute in various combinations to this recognizable state of altered brain function further suggests that what we call schizophrenia may represent "not the result of a discrete event or illness process at all, but rather one end of the developmental spectrum that for genetic and other reasons approximately 0.5% of the population will fall into" (Weinberger, 1987).

Nevertheless, there are major mysteries about schizophrenia that are barely addressed by the existing research data, and not adequately explained by neurodevelopmental models. What mediates the transition from relative clinical compensation to dramatic decompensation? Why does decompensation become chronic for most patients? What are the molecular events that mediate symptom relief and why is it a protracted process? How fixed are the deficits associated with this syndrome? Basic research about other neurodevelopmental disorders on this wide clinical spectrum, e.g., Fragile X and Rett syndrome (Dőlen *et al.*, 2010), suggest that long-standing changes in synaptic architecture, even from early in development, are not fixed, and can still be reversed even in adulthood (Ehninger *et al.*, 2008). Schizophrenia, too, despite its neurodevelopmental origins, may be more reversible (i.e., curable) than previously thought.

References

Adams, R.D. & Lyons, G. (1982) *Neurology of Hereditary Metabolic Diseases of Children*. New York: McGraw-Hill.

Arnold, P.D., Siegel-Bartelt, J., Cytrynbaum, C., Teshima, I. & Schachar, R. (2001) Velo-cardio-facial syndrome: implications of microdeletion 22q11 for schizophrenia and mood disorders. *American Journal of Medical Genetics* **105**, 354–362.

Ayhan, Y., Abazyan, B., Nomura, J. *et al.* (2010) Differential effects of prenatal and postnatal expressions of mutant human DISC1 on neurobehavioral phenotypes in transgenic mice: evidence for neurodevelopmental origin of major psychiatric disorders. *Molecular Psychiatry* [Epub ahead of print].

Bachevalier, J. & Mishkin, M. (1984) An early and a late developing system for learning and retention in infant monkeys. *Behavioral Neuroscience* **98**, 770–778.

Bain, M., Juszczak, E., McInneny, K. & Kendell, R.E. (2000) Obstetric complications and affective psychoses. Two case-control studies based on structured obstetric records. *British Journal of Psychiatry* **176**, 523–526.

Bassett, A.S. & Chow, E.W. (2009) 22q11 deletion syndrome, a genetic subtype of schizophrenia. *Biological Psychiatry* **46**, 882–891.

Bender, L. (1947) Childhood schizophrenia; clinical study on one hundred schizophrenic children. *American Journal of Orthopsychiatry* **17**, 40–56.

Bolton, P.F., Murphy, M., Macdonald, H., Whitlock, B., Pickles, A. & Rutter, M. (1997) Obstetric complications in autism: consequences or causes of the condition? *Journal of the American Academy of Child & Adolescent Psychiatry* **36**, 272–281.

Brandon, N.J., Millar, J.K., Korth, C. *et al.* (2009) Understanding the role of DISC1 in psychiatric disease and during normal development. *Journal of Neuorscience* **29**, 12768–12775.

Brans, R.G., van Haren, N.E., van Baal, G.C. *et al.* (2008) Longitudinal MRI study in schizophrenia patients and their healthy siblings. *British Journal of Psychiatry* **193**, 422–423.

Brody, A.L., Mandelkern, M.A., Jarvik, M.E. *et al.* (2004) Differences between smokers and nonsmokers in regional gray matter volumes and densities. *Biological Psychiatry* **55**, 77–84.

Brown, A.S. & Derkits, E.J. (2010) Prenatal infection and schizophrenia: a review of epidemiologic and translational studies. *American J Psychiatry* **167**, 261–820.

Brown, A.S., Bottiglieri, T., Schaefer, C.A. *et al.* (2007) Elevated prenatal homocysteine levels as a risk factor for schizophrenia. *Archives of General Psychiatry* **64**, 980–981.

Cannon, T.D., Mednick, S.A., Parnas, J. *et al.* (1993) Developmental brain abnormalities in the offspring of schizophrenic mothers. I. Contributions of genetic and perinatal factors. *Archives of General Psychiatry* **50**, 551–564.

Cannon, M., Caspi, A., Moffitt, T.E. *et al.* (2002) Evidence of early-childhood, pan-development impairment specific to schizophreniform disorder, results from a longitudinal birth cohort. *Archives of General Psychiatry* **59**, 449–456.

Cannon, T.D., Yolken, R., Buka, S. & Fuller, T. (2008) Decreased neurotrophic response to birth hypoxia in the etiology of schizophrenia. *Biological Psychiatry* **64**, 797–802.

Caspi, A., Reichenberg, A., Weiser, M. *et al.* (2003) Cognitive performance in schizophrenia patients assessed before and following the first psychotic episode. *Schizophrenia Research* **65**, 87–94.

Chelune, G.J. & Baer, R.A. (1986) Developmental norms for Wisconsin Card Sorting test. *Journal of Clinical Experimental Neuropsychology* **8**, 219–228.

Clapcote, S.J., Lipina, T.V., Millar, J.K. *et al.* (2007) Behavioral phenotypes of *Disc1* missense mutations in mice. *Neuron* **54**, 387–402.

Courchesne, E., Carper, R. & Akshoomoff, N. (2003) Evidence of brain outgrowth in the first year of life in autism. *Journal of the American Medical Association* **290**, 337–344.

Deep-Soboslay, A., Hyde, T.M., Lener, M.S, Apud, J.A., Weinberger, D.R. & Elvevåg, B. (2010) Handedness, heritability and neurocognition in schizophrenia. *Brain*; doi: 10.1093/brain/awq160.

Dőlen, G., Carpenter, R.L., Ocain, T.D. & Bear, M.F. (2010) Mechanism-based approaches to treating fragile X. *Pharmacology & Therapeutics* **127**, 78–93.

Dorph-Petersen, K.A., Pierri, J.N., Perel, J.M. *et al.* (2005) The influence of chronic exposure to antipsychotic medications on brain size before and after tissue fixation: a comparison of haloperidol and olanzapine in macaque monkeys. *Neuropsychopharmacology* **30**, 1649–1661.

Eliez, S., Antonarakis, S.E., Morris, M.A., Dahoun, S.P. & Reiss, A.L. (2001) Parental origin of the deletion 22q11.2 and brain development in velocardiofacial syndrome: a preliminary study. *Archives of General Psychiatry* **58**, 64–68.

Ehninger, D. Li, W., Fox, K., Stryker, M.P. & Silva, A.J. (2008) Reversing neurodevelopmental disorders in adults. *Neuron* **60**, 950–960.

Eriksen, W., Sundet, J.M. & Tambs, K. (2009) Register data suggest lower intelligence in men born the year after flu pandemic. *Annals of Neurology* **66**, 284–289.

Eschenbach, D.A. (1997) Amniotic fluid infection and cerebral palsy. Focus on the fetus. *Journal of the American Medical Association* **278**, 247–248.

Fazzari, P., Paternain, A.V., Valiente, M. *et al.* (2010) Control of cortical GABA circuitry development by Nrg1 and ErbB4 signalling. *Nature* **464**, 1376–1382.

Feinberg, I. (1982) Schizophrenia, caused by a fault in programmed synaptic elimination during adolescence? *Journal of Psychiatric Research* **17**, 319–334.

Fish, B. & Hagin, R. (1972) Visual-motor disorders in infants at risk for schizophrenia. *Archives of General Psychiatry* **27**, 594–598.

Gauthier, J., ChAmericanpagne, N., Lafrenière, R.G. *et al.* (2010) De novo mutations in the gene encoding the synaptic scaffolding protein SHANK3 in patients ascertained for schizophrenia. *Proceeding of the National Academy of Sciences USA* **107**, 7863–868.

Gloor, P., Olivier, A., Quesney, L.F., Anderrnann, F. & Horowitz, S. (1982) The role of the limbic system in experiential phenomena of temporal lobe epilepsy. *Annals of Neurology* **12**, 129–144.

Gochman, P.A., Greenstein, D., Sporn, A. *et al.* (2005) IQ stabilization in childhood-onset schizophrenia. *Schizophrenia Research* **77**, 271–277.

Gogtay, N.D., Greenstein, D., Lenane, M. *et al.* (2007) Cortical brain development in nonpsychotic siblings of patients with childhood-onset schizophrenia. *Archives of General Psychiatry* **64**, 772–780.

Goldman-Rakic, P.S. (1987) Development of cortical circuitry and cognitive function. *Child Development* **58**, 601–22.

Gothelf, D., Eliez, S., Thompson, T. *et al.* (2005) COMT genotype predicts longitudinal cognitive decline and psychosis in 22q11.2 deletion syndrome. *Nature Neuroscience* **8**, 1500–1502.

Harrison, P.J. & Law, A.J. (2006) Neuregulin 1 and schizophrenia: genetics, gene expression, and neurobiology. *Biological Psychiatry* **60**, 132–140.

Harrison, P. & Weinberger, D.R. (2005) Schizophrenia genes, gene expression, and neuropathology: on the matter of their convergence. *Molecular Psychiatry* **10**, 40–68.

Hashimoto, T., Nguyen, Q.L., Rotaru, D. *et al.* (2009) Protracted developmental trajectories of GABAA receptor alpha1 and alpha2 subunit expression in primate prefrontal cortex. *Biological Psychiatry* **65**, 1015–1023.

Heaton, R.K., Gladsjo, J.A., Palmer, B.W., Kuck, J., Marcotte, T.D. & Jeste, D.V. (2001) Stability and course of neuropsychological deficits in schizophrenia. *Archives of General Psychiatry* **58**, 24–32.

Hensch, T.K. (2005) Critical period plasticity in local cortical circuits. *Nature Reviews in Neuroscience* **6**, 877–888.

Ho, B.C., Alicata, D., Mola, C. & Andreasen, N.C. (2005) Hippocampus volume and treatment delays in first-episode schizophrenia. *American Journal of Psychiatry* **162**, 1527–1529.

Ho, B.C., Andreasen, N.C., Dawson, J.D. & Wassink, T.H. (2007) Association between brain-derived neurotrophic factor val66met gene polymorphism brain volume changes in schizophrenia. *American Journal of Psychiatry* **164**, 1890–1899.

Hoff, A.L., Sakuma, M., Razi, K., Heydebrand, G., Csernansky, J.G. & DeLisi, L.E. (2000) Lack of association between duration of untreated illness and severity of cognitive and structural brain deficits at the first episode of schizophrenia. *American Journal of Psychiatry* **157**, 1824–1828.

Huffaker, S.J., Chen, J., Nicodemus, K.K. *et al.* (2009) A primate-specific, brain isoform of KCNH2 affects cortical physiology, cognition, neuronal repolarization and risk of schizophrenia. *Nature Medicine* **15**, 509–518.

Hulshoff Pol, H.E. & Kahn, R.S. (2008) What happens after the first episode? A review of progressive brain changes in chronically ill patients with schizophrenia. *Schizophrenia Bulletin* **34**, 354–366.

Huttenlocher, P.R. (1990) Morphometric study of human cerebral cortex development. *Neuropsychologia* **28**, 517–527.

Hyde, T.M., Ziegler, J.C. & Weinberger, D.R. (1992) Psychiatric disturbances in metachromatic leukodystrophy, insight into the neurobiology of psychosis. *Archives of Neurology* **49**, 401–406.

Hyde, T.M., Deep-Soboslay, A., Iglesias, B. *et al.* (2008) Enuresis as a premorbid developmental marker of schizophrenia. *Brain* **131**, 2489–2498.

Iizuka, Y., Sei, Y., Weinberger, D.R. & Straub R.E. (2007) Evidence that the BLOC-1 protein dysbindin modulates dopamine D2 receptor internalization and signaling but not D1 internalization. *Journal of Neuroscience* **27**, 12390–12395.

Ingason, A., Rujescu, D., Cichon, S. *et al.* (2009) Copy number variations of chromosome 16p13.1 region associated with schizophrenia. *Molecular Psychiatry* [Epub ahead of print].

Insel, B.J., Brown, A.S., Bresnahan, M.A. *et al.* (2005) Maternal-fetal blood incompatibility and the risk of schizophrenia in offspring. *Schizophrenia Research* **80**, 331–342.

Jaaro-Peled, H., Hayashi-Takagi, A., Saurav, S. *et al.* (2009) Neurodevelopmental mechanisms of schizophrenia: understanding disturbed postnatal brain maturation through neuregulin-1-ErbB4 and DISC1. *Trends in Neuroscience* **32**, 485–495.

Jarskog, L.F., Glantz, L.A., Gilmore J.H. & Lieberman J.A. (2005) Apoptotic mechanisms in the pathophysiology of schizophrenia. *Progress in Neuropsychopharmacology Biological Psychiatry* **29**, 846–858.

Keller, G., Zimmer, G., Mall, G. *et al.* (2003) Nephron number in patients with primary hypertension. *New England Journal of Medicine* **348**, 101–108.

Kennard, M.A. (1936) Age and other factors in motor recovery from precentral lesions in monkeys. *American Journal of Physiology* **115**, 138–146.

Khashan, A.S., Abel K.M., McNamee, R. *et al.* (2008) Higher risk of offspring schizophrenia following antenatal maternal exposure to severe adverse life events. *Archives of General Psychiatry* **65**, 146–152.

Kolb, B. & Whishaw, I.Q. (1989) Plasticity in the neocortex: mechanisms underlying recovery from early brain damage. *Progress in Neurology* **32**, 235–276.

Konopaske, G.T., Dorph-Petersen, K.A., Pierri, J.N. *et al.* (2007) Effect of chronic exposure to antipsychotic medication on cell numbers in the parietal cortex of macaque monkeys. *Neuropsychopharmacology* **32**, 1216–1223.

Lambe, E.K., Krimer, L.S. & Goldman-Rakic, P.S. (2000) Differential postnatal development of catecholine and serotonin inputs to identified neurons in prefrontal cortex of rhesus monkey. *Journal of Neuroscience* **20**, 8780–8787.

Law, A.J., Lipska, B.K., Weickert, C.S. *et al.* (2006) Neuregulin 1 transcripts are differentially expressed in schizophrenia and regulated by 5′ SNPs associated with the disease. *Proceeding of the National Academy of Sciences USA* **103**, 6747–6752.

Lewis, D.A. & Gonzalez-Burgos, G. (2008) Neuroplasticity of neocortical circuits in schizophrenia. *Neuropsychopharmacology* **33**, 141–165.

Lewis, D.A. & Levitt, P. (2002) Schizophrenia as a disorder of neurodevelopment. *Annual Review of Neuorscience* **25**, 409–432.

Lidow, M.S. & Rakic, P. (1992) Scheduling of monoaminergic neurotransmitter receptor expression in the primate neocortex during postnatal development. *Cerebral Cortex* **2**, 401–416.

Lieberman, J.A. (1999) Is schizophrenia a neurodegenerative disorder? A clinical and neurobiological perspective. *Biological Psychiatry* **46**, 729–739.

Lipska, B. & Weinberger D.R. (2000) To model a psychiatric disorder in animals: Schizophrenia as a reality test. *Neuropsychopharmacology* **23**, 223–239.

Liu Z., Neff R.A. & Berg D.K. (2006) Sequential interplay of nicotinic and GABAergic signaling guides neuronal development *Science* **314**, 1610–1613.

Marcelis, M., van Os, J., Sham, P. *et al.* (1998) Obstetric complications and familial morbid risk of psychiatric disorders. *American Journal of Medical Genetics* **81**, 29–36.

Marín-Padilla M. (1997) Developmental neuropathology and impact of perinatal brain damage. II: white matter lesions of the neocortex. *Journal of Neuropathology & Experimental Neurology* **56**, 219–235.

Mathalon, D.H., Sullivan, E.V., Lim, K.O. & Pfefferbaum, A. (2001) Progressive brain volume changes and the clinical course of schizophrenia in men: a longitudinal magnetic resonance imaging study. *Archives of General Psychiatry* **58**, 148–157.

McClure, R.K., Phillips, I., Jazayerli, R., Barnett, A., Coppola, R. & Weinberger D.R. (2006) Regional change in brain morphometry in schizophrenia associated with antipsychotic treatment. *Psychiatry Research* **148**, 121–132.

McGlashan, T.H. & Hoffman, R.E. (2000) Schizophrenia as a disorder of developmentally reduced synaptic connectivity. *Archives of General Psychiatry* **57**, 637–648.

McNeil, T.F., Cantor-Graae, E. & Weinberger, DR. (2000) Relationship of obstetric complications and differences in size of brain structures in monozygotic twin pairs discordant for schizophrenia. *American Journal of Psychiatry* **157**, 203–212.

Mednick *et al.* (2010)

Mesholam-Gately, R. & Giuliano, A.J. (2009) Neurocognition in first-episode schizophrenia: a meta-analytic review. *Neuropsychology* **23**, 315–336.

Meyer-Lindenberg, A., Straub, R.E., Lipska, B.K. *et al.* (2007) Genetic evidence implicating DARP-32 in human fronto-striatal structure, function and cognition. *Journal of Clinical Investigations* **117**, 672–682.

Mitchell, K.J. (2007) The genetics of brain wiring, from molecule to mind. *PLoS Biology* **5**, 690–692.

Mitchell, K.J. & Porteous, D.J. (2010) Rethinking the genetic architecture of schizophrenia. *Psychological Medicine* [Epub ahead of print].

Murray R.M. & Lewis S.W. (1987) Is schizophrenia a neurodevelopmental disorder? *British Medical Journal* **295**, 681–682.

Nakata, K., Lipska, B.K., Hyde, T.M. *et al.* (2009) DISC1 splice variants are upregulated in schizophrenia and associated with risk polymorphisms. *Proceedings of the National Academy of Sciences USA* **106**, 15873–15878.

Nicodemus, K.K., Marenco, S., Batten, A.J. *et al.* (2008) Serious obstetric complications interact with hypoxia-regulated/vascular-expression genes to influence schizophrenia risk. *Molecular Psychiatry* **13**, 873–877.

Nicodemus, K.K., Law, A.J., Radulescu, E. *et al.* (2010) NRG1, ERBB4 and AKT1 epistasis increases schizophrenia risk and it biologically validated via functional neuroimaging in healthy controls. *Archives of General Psychiatry*, in press.

Niwa, M., Kamiya, A., Murai, R. *et al.* (2010) Knockdown of DISC1 by in utero gene transfer disturbs postnatal dopaminergic maturation in the frontal cortex and leads to adult behavioral deficits. *Neuron* **65**, 480–489.

Okaty, B.W., Miller, M.N., Sugino, K. *et al.* (2009) Transcriptional and electrophysiological maturation of neocortical fast-spiking GABAergic interneurons. *Journal of Neuroscience* **29**, 7040–7052.

Pajonk, F.G., Wobrock, T., Gruber, O. *et al.* (2010) Hippocampal plasticity in response to exercise in schizophrenia. *Archives of General Psychiatry* **67**, 133–143.

Palmer, C.G., Turunen, J.A., Sinsheimer, J.S. *et al.* (2002) RHD maternal-fetal genotype incompatibility increases schizophrenia susceptibility. *American Journal of Human Genetics* **71**, 1312–1319.

Porteous, D.J, Thomson, P., Brandon, N.J. & Millar, J.K. (2006) The genetics and Biology of DISC1—an emerging role in psychosis and cognition. *Biological Psychiatry* **60**, 123–131.

Pfefferbaum, A., Rosenbloom, M.J., Serventi, K.L. & Sullivan, E.V. (2004) Brain volumes, RBC status, and hepatic function in alcoholics after 1 and 4 weeks of sobriety: predictors of outcome. *American Journal of Psychiatry* **161**, 1190–1196.

Purcell, S.M., Wray, N.R., Stone J.L. *et al.* (2009) Common polygenic variation contributes to risk of schizophrenia and bipolar disorder. International Schizophrenia Consortium. *Nature* **460**, 748–752.

Rakic, P., Bourgeois, J.P., Eckenhoff, M.F. *et al.* (1986) Concurrent overproduction of synapses in diverse regions of the primate cerebral cortex. *Science* **232**, 232–235.

Rakic, P., Bourgeois, J.P. & Goldman-Rakic P.S. (1994) Synaptic development of the cerebral cortex: implications for learning, memory, and mental illness. *Progress in Brain Research* **102**, 227–243.

Rapoport, J.L., Giedd, J.N., Blumenthal, J. *et al.* (1999) Progressive cortical change during adolescence in childhood-onset schizophrenia. A longitudinal magnetic resonance imaging study. *Archives of General Psychiatry* **56**, 649–654.

Rapoport, J.L, Addington, A.M., Frangou, S. *et al.* (2005) The neurodevelopmental model of schizophrenia, update 2005. *Molecular Psychiatry* **10**, 434–449.

Reichenberg, A., Caspi, A., Harrington, H. *et al.* (2010) Static and dynamic cognitive deficits in childhood preceding adult schizophrenia, a 30-year study. *American Journal of Psychiatry* **167**, 160–169.

Rujescu, D., Ingason, A., Cichon, S., Pietiläinen, O.P. & Barnes, M.R. (2009) Disruption of the neurexin 1 gene is associated with schizophrenia. *Human Molecular Genetics* **18**, 988–996.

Saha, S., Barnett, A.G., Foldi, C. *et al.* (2009) Advanced paternal age is associated with impaired neurocognitive outcomes during infancy and childhood. *PLoS Medicine* **6**, e40.

Schwartz, M.L. & Goldman-Rakic, P. (1990) Development and plasticity of the primate cerebral cortex. *Clinical Perinatology* **17**, 83–102.

Shatz, C.J. (1990) Impulse activity and the patterning of connections during CNS development. *Neuron* **5**, 745–756.

Shergill, S.S., Brammer, M.J., Williams, S.C., Murray, R.M. & McGuire, P.K. (2000) Mapping auditory hallucinations in schizophrenia using functional magnetic resonance imaging. *Archives of General Psychiatry* **57**, 1033–1038.

Sorensen, H.J., Mortensen, E.L., Schiffman, J., Reinisch, J.M., Maeda, J. & Mednick, S.A. (2010) Early developmental milestones and rish of schizophrenia: a 45-year follow-up of the Copenhagen Perinatal Cohort. *Schizophrenia Research* **118**, 41–47.

Southard, E.E. (1915) On the topographical distribution of cortex lesions and anomalies in dementia praecox, with some account of their functional significance. *American Journal of Insanity* **71**, 603–671.

Sporn, A.L., Greenstein, D.K., Gogtay N. *et al.* (2003) Progressive brain volume loss during adolescence in childhood-onset schizophrenia. *American Journal of Psychiatry* **160**, 2181–2189.

St Clair, D., Xu, M., Wang, P. *et al.* (2005) Rate of adult schizophrenia following prenatal exposure to the Chinese famine of 1959–1961. *Journal of the American Medical Association* **294**, 557–562.

Stefansson, H., Rujescu, D., Cichon, S. *et al.* (2008) Large recurrent microdeletions associated with schizophrenia. *Nature* **455**, 232–236.

Stefansson, H., Ophoff, R.A., Steinberg, S. *et al.* (2009) Common variants conferring risk of schizophrenia. *Nature* **460**, 744–747.

Sun, D., Stuart, G.W., Jenkinson, M. *et al.* (2009) Brain surface contraction mapped in first-episode schizophrenia: a longitudinal magnetic resonance imaging study. *Molecular Psychiatry* **14**, 976–986.

Supekar, K., Musen, M. & Menon, V. (2009) Development of large-scale functional brain networks in children. *PLoS Biology* **7**, 1–15.

Susser, E.S. & Lin, S.P. (1992) Schizophreniaenia after prenatal exposure to the Dutch Hunger Winter of 1944–1945. *Archives of General Psychiatry* **49**, 983–988.

Taki, Y., Kinomura, S., Sato, K. *et al.* (2008) Relationship between body mass index and gray matter volume in 1,428 healthy individuals. *Obesity* **16**, 119–124.

Talbot, K. (2009) The sandy (sdy) mouse: a dysbindin-1 mutant relevant to schizophrenia research. *Progess in Brain Research* **179**, 87–94.

Tan, W., Wang, Y., Gold, B. *et al.* (2007) Molecular cloning of a brain-specific, developmentally regulated Neuregulin 1 (NRG1) isoform and identification of a functional promoter variant associated with schizophrenia. *Journal of Biological Chemistry* **33**, 24343–24351.

Tang, T.T., Yang, F., Chen, B.S. *et al.* (2009) Dysbindin regulates hippocampal LTP by controlling NMDA receptor surface expression. *Proceedings of the National Academy of Sciences USA* **106**, 21395–21400.

Tseng, K.Y. & O'Donnell, P. (2007) Dopamine modulation of prefrontal cortical interneurons changes during adolescence. *Cerebral Cortex* **17**, 1235–1240.

Thompson, B.L. & Levitt, P. (2010) Now you see it, now you don't—Closing in on allostasis and developmental basis of psychiatric disorders. *Neuron* **65**, 437–439.

Tunbridge, E.M., Weickert, C.S., Kleinman, J.E. *et al.* (2007) Catechol-o-methyltransferase enzyme activity and protein expression in human prefrontal cortex across the postnatal lifespan. *Cerebral Cortex* **5**, 1206–1212.

Verdoux, H., Liraud, F., Gonzales, B., Assens, F., Abalan, F. & van Os, J. (2001) Predictors and outcome characteristics associated with suicidal behaviour in early psychosis, a two-year follow-up of first-admitted subjects. *Acta Psychiatrica Scandinvica* **103**, 347–354.

Waddington, C.H. (1972) *Towards a Theoretical Biology*, vol 4, Essays. Edinburgh: Edinburgh University Press.

Watt, N.F. (1972) Longitudinal changes in the social behavior of children hospitalized for schizophrenia as adults. *Journal of Nervous and Mental Disease* **155**, 42–54.

Webb, S.J., Nalty, T., Munson, J. *et al.* (2007) Rate of head dircum-ference growth as a function of autism diagnosis and history of autistic regression. *Journal of Child Neurology* **22**, 1182–1190.

Weinberger, D.R. (1986) The pathogensis of schizophrenia: a neurodevlopmental theory. In Nasrallah H. A. & Weinberger (eds) *The Neurology of Schizophrenia*. Amsterdam: Elsevier, pp. 397–406.

Weinberger, D.R. (1987) Implications of normal brain develop-ment for the pathogenesis of schizophrenia. *Archives of General Psychiatry* **44**, 660–669.

Weinberger, D.R. & Marenco, S. (2003) Schizophrenia as a neu-rodevelopmental disorder. In: Hirsh, S.R. & Weinberger, D.R., eds. *Schizophrenia*, 2nd edn. Blackwell, London, pp. 326–348.

Weinberger, D.R. & McClure, R.K. (2002) Neurotoxicity, neuro-plasticity, and magnetic resonance imaging morphometry: What is happening in the schizophrenic brain? *Archives of General Psychiatry* **59**, 553–558.

Winterer, G. & Weinberger, D.R. (2007) Genes, dopamine and cortical signal-to-noise in schizophrenia. *Trends in Neuroscience* **27**, 683–690.

Woodberry, K.A., Giuliano, A.J. & Seidman, L.J. (2008) Premorbid IQ in schizophrenia: a meta-analytic review. *American Journal of Psychiatry* **165**, 579–587.

Xu, M.Q., Sun, W.S., Liu, B.X. *et al.* (2009) Prenatal malnutrition and adult schizophrenia: further evidence from the 1959–1961 Chinese famine. *Schizophrenia Bulletin* **35**, 568–576.

Dopamine and schizophrenia

Anissa Abi-Dargham[1] and Anthony A. Grace[2]
[1]Columbia Univeristy and New York State Psychiatric Institute, New York, NY, USA
[2]University of Pittsburgh, Pittsburgh, PA, USA

Introduction

Schizophrenia presents with multiple clinical features, ranging from positive symptoms (hallucinations, delusions, and thought disorder) to negative symptoms (social withdrawal, poverty of speech and thought, flattening of affect and lack of motivation) and disturbances in cognitive processes (attention, working memory, verbal fluency and learning, social cognition, and executive function). Dopamine (DA) dysregulation plays a role within each of these dimensions. While excess striatal DA relates most directly to the positive symptoms of the illness and to magnitude as well as speed of their response to antipsychotic treatment, the neurobiology of cognitive and negative symptoms is more complex and diverse, including, but not limited to, a prefrontal dopaminergic deficit. Furthermore, as negative symptoms are multifactorial (Blanchard & Cohen, 2006), including a factor associated with cognitive deficit such as poverty of expression, and a factor related

to deficits in reward functions, such as anhedonia and amotivation, they may relate to cortical and ventrostriatal DA dysfunction, respectively, although no direct data are available in this regard. We will first describe the evidence for a dopaminergic dysfunction within striatal and cortical regions underlying specific clinical domains within the schizophrenia spectrum; evidence derived largely from imaging studies in humans. This will be followed by a discussion of the properties of the dopaminergic neurons in the midbrain and the complex regulatory influences that modulate their activity states. This modulation, both inhibitory and excitatory, can affect the proportion of DA neurons that are active, and the firing rate of these neurons, such that it allows a wide dynamic range of neuronal activity and resulting DA release in the terminal fields. Phasic release is determined by burst firing of DA neurons and can be measured in humans with imaging paradigms using binding competition between D$_2$ radiotracers and DA, while tonic release is determined by single spike firing of DA neurons and is not measureable by imaging paradigms. We will discuss the pathology within structures that regulate DA neuronal firing and release, and could lead to the alterations observed in schizophrenia, then attempt to

Schizophrenia, 3rd edition. Edited by Daniel R. Weinberger and
Paul J Harrison © 2011 Blackwell Publishing Ltd.

integrate these various elements in one overall scheme as a potential mechanism by which a complex dysregulation of DA may occur in schizophrenia.

Historical perspective

The DA hypothesis of schizophrenia was first formulated by Rossum (1966) based on the observation that antipsychotics may block DA receptors. Additional support derived from the findings that DA receptors are activated by psychostimulants, that non-reserpine neuroleptics are DA antagonists and that DA plays an important role in the extrapyramidal motor system (Carlsson & Lindqvist, 1963). Later, it was further strengthened by the discovery of the correlation between clinical doses of antipsychotic drugs and their potency to block DA D_2 receptors (Seeman et al., 1975; Creese et al., 1976), and by the studies confirming the psychotogenic effects of DA-enhancing drugs, (for review, see Lieberman et al., 1987; Angrist & van Kammen, 1984). These observations supported a role for excess DA transmission in schizophrenia. Subsequently, the increasing awareness of enduring negative and cognitive symptoms in this illness and of their resistance to D_2 receptor antagonism led to a reformulation of this classical DA hypothesis. Functional brain imaging studies suggested that these symptoms might arise from altered prefrontal cortex (PFC) functions (for review, see Knable & Weinberger, 1997). A wealth of preclinical studies emerged documenting the importance of prefrontal DA transmission at D_1 receptors (the main DA receptor in the neocortex) for optimal PFC performance (for review, see Goldman-Rakic et al., 2000). Together, these observations led to the hypothesis that a deficit in DA transmission at D_1 receptors in the PFC might be implicated in the cognitive impairments and negative symptoms of schizophrenia (Davis et al., 1991; Weinberger, 1987). Thus, the current predominant view is that DA systems in schizophrenia might be characterized by an imbalance between subcortical and cortical DA systems: subcortical meso-limbic DA projections might be hyperactive (resulting in hyperstimulation of D_2 receptors and positive symptoms), while meso-cortical DA projections to the PFC might be hypoactive (resulting in hypostimulation of D_1 receptors, negative symptoms, and cognitive impairment). Furthermore, since the seminal work of Pycock et al. (1980), many laboratories have described reciprocal and opposite regulations between cortical and subcortical DA systems (for review, see Tzschentke, 2001). An abundant literature suggests that prefrontal DA activity exerts an inhibitory influence on subcortical DA activity (Karreman & Moghaddam, 1996; Kolachana et al., 1995; Wilkinson, 1997; Deutch et al., 1990). From these observations, it has been proposed that, in schizophrenia, both arms of the DA imbalance model might be related, inasmuch as a deficiency in meso-cortical DA function might

translate into disinhibition of meso-limbic DA activity (Weinberger, 1987).

Postmortem studies

The first test of the DA hypothesis came from postmortem studies, which have provided only partial support, partly because of the confounding effects of antemortem antipsychotic treatment.

Tissue dopamine and homovanillic acid

Direct measures of tissue content of DA and its metabolites have failed to demonstrate consistent and reproducible abnormalities (for review, see Davis et al., 1991; Reynolds, 1989). It should be noted, however, that some studies have reported higher DA tissue levels in samples from patients with schizophrenia in subcortical regions such as the caudate (Owen et al., 1978), nucleus accumbens (Mackay et al., 1982) or amygdala (Reynolds, 1983).

D_2 receptors

Increased density of striatal D_2 receptors in patients with schizophrenia has been a consistent finding in a large number of postmortem studies using [^{3}H]spiperone (Owen et al., 1978; Mackay et al., 1982; Lee et al., 1978; Cross et al., 1983; Seeman et al., 1984, 1987, 1993; Hess et al., 1987; Reynolds et al., 1987; Joyce et al., 1988; Mita et al., 1986; Sumiyoshi et al., 1995; Ruiz et al., 1992; Dean et al., 1997; Marzella et al., 1997; Lahti et al., 1996; Knable et al., 1994). Because chronic neuroleptic administration up-regulates D_2 receptor density (Burt et al., 1977), it is likely that these postmortem findings are related to prior neuroleptic exposure rather than to the disease process per se. In light of these very consistent results with [^{3}H]spiperone, it is interesting to note that the striatal binding of [^{3}H]raclopride has been reported to be increased in many studies (Ruiz et al., 1992; Sumiyoshi et al., 1995; Dean et al., 1997; Marzella et al., 1997), but normal in several others (Seeman et al., 1993; Knable et al., 1994; Lahti et al., 1996), even in patients exposed to neuroleptic drugs prior to death. This observation suggests that the increase in [^{3}H]raclopride binding is of lower magnitude than the increase in [^{3}H]spiperone binding. This discrepancy might simply reflect the observation that, for reasons that are not currently understood, antipsychotic drugs up-regulate more [^{3}H]spiperone than [^{3}H]raclopride binding to D_2 receptors (Schoots et al., 1995; Tarazi et al., 1997).

D_3 receptors

A significant increase in D_3 receptor number in ventral striata (VST) samples from patients with schizophrenia who were off neuroleptics at the time of death has been reported in one study (Gurevich et al., 1997). In contrast, in patients who had been treated with neuroleptics up to the time of death, D_3 receptor levels did not differ significantly from those of controls (Gurevich *et al.*, 1997). These data were interpreted as evidence that antipsychotics down-regulate the D_3 receptor in patients with schizophrenia who otherwise have a higher density of this receptor in the VST. The D_3 receptor gene expression is under the control of a neutrophin, called brain-derived neurotrophic factor (BDNF), which is synthesized in the ventral tegmental area (VTA) and the PFC, and released in the VST, where it maintains the expression of the D_3 receptor (Guillin *et al.*, 2001). Studies have shown increased (Takahashi *et al.*, 2000) and decreased (Weickert *et al.*, 2003; Hashimoto *et al.*, 2005) BDNF levels in the brain of patients with schizophrenia. Furthermore, D_3 receptors are up-regulated in the presence of hyperdopaminergic tone (Guillin *et al.*, 2001; Fauchey *et al.*, 2000; Bordet *et al.*, 1997; Le Foll *et al.*, 2002), under the control of BDNF, whose synthesis is in turn under the control of the activity of neurons projecting from the PFC or the VTA in the VST.

D_4 receptors

Based on ligand subtraction techniques, several studies have reported increased D_4-like receptors in schizophrenia (Seeman *et al.*, 1993; Murray *et al.*, 1995; Sumiyoshi *et al.*, 1995; Marzella *et al.*, 1997). These findings were not confirmed by other studies using the same technique (Lahti *et al.*, 1996; Reynolds & Mason, 1994), nor by a study using [^{3}H]NGD 94-1, a selective D_4 ligand (Lahti *et al.*, 1998). Moreover, the hypothesis that clozapine might act by blocking the D_4 receptor was not supported by a clinical trial with the D_4 selective agent L745,870 (Kramer *et al.*, 1997).

D_1 receptors

Striatal D_1 receptors have generally been reported to be unaltered in schizophrenia (Seeman *et al.*, 1987; Joyce *et al.*, 1988; Pimoule *et al.*, 1985; Reynolds & Czudek, 1988), although one study reported decreased density (Hess *et al.*, 1987). In the PFC, one study reported no changes (Laruelle *et al.*, 1990), and one reported a non-significant increase (Knable *et al.*, 1996).

Dopamine transporters

A large number of studies have reported unaltered DA transporter (DAT) density in the striatum of patients with schizophrenia (Joyce *et al.*, 1988; Knable *et al.*, 1994; Hirai *et al.*, 1988; Czudek & Reynolds, 1989; Pearce *et al.*, 1990; Chinaglia *et al.*, 1992).

Tyrosine hydroxylase immunolabeling

An interesting postmortem finding regarding DA parameters in patients with schizophrenia is the observation of decreased tyrosine hydroxylase (TH)-labeled axons in layers 3 and 6 of the entorhinal cortex (EC) and in layer 6

of the PFC, suggesting that schizophrenia might be associated with a deficit in DA transmission in the EC and PFC (Akil *et al.*, 1999, 2000). This finding was clearly unrelated to premortem neuroleptic exposure. Benes *et al.* (1997) observed no significant changes in TH-positive varicosities in the dorso-lateral PFC (DLPFC). In the anterior cingulate region (layer 2), these authors observed a significant shift in the distribution of TH varicosities from large neurons to small neurons.

Summary

Postmortem measurements of indices of DA transmission have generated a number of consistent observations in the striatum: (1) the binding of radioligand to D_2-like receptors in the striatum of patients with schizophrenia is increased, but the magnitude of this increase varies with the type of radioligands used, and it is difficult to exclude the contribution of premortem antipsychotic exposure in this set of findings; and (2) Striatal DAT and D_1 receptors density is unaffected in schizophrenia. Several interesting observations, such as the increase in D_3 receptors in the VST and alteration in TH immunolabeling in several cortical regions, do not appear to be consequences of premortem neuroleptic exposure, but these findings have yet to be independently confirmed.

Dopamine and psychosis: increased striatal phasic dopamine release

The more definitive evidence supporting a striatal dopaminergic dysregulation has derived from use of *in vivo* imaging techniques in drug-free and drug-naïve patients with schizophrenia. These studies assessed various aspects of DA transmission, including measurement of receptors, transporters, enzyme activity, and most importantly transmitter release and occupancy. We summarize below the most relevant work that has provided clear evidence for increased striatal DA activity.

The decrease in *in vivo* binding of $D_{2/3}$ radiotracers such as [^{11}C]raclopride and [^{123}I]IBZM following acute amphetamine challenge is a well-validated measure of the pharmacologically stimulated phasic DA release, while the increase in *in vivo* binding of [^{11}C]raclopride or [^{123}I]IBZM to $D_{2/3}$ receptors after acute depletion of synaptic DA using alpha-methyl-para-tyrosine (α-MPT) is associated with an acute unmasking of D_2 receptors previously occupied by DA (for review, see Laruelle, 2000a). The increased binding is a measure of baseline, or non-stimulated, phasic DA release which determines the degree of baseline occupancy of D_2 receptors by DA. The reasons we believe the imaging measures of DA are measures of DA phasic release are as follows: (1) phasic burst firing affects intrasynaptic DA levels, while extrasynaptic levels are essentially influenced by tonic or single spike firing of DA cells in the midbrain (see Preclinical considerations, below); and (2) changes in D_2 radiotracer binding following a challenge drug that affects DA levels reflect changes in intrasynaptic DA. This latter finding is based on the lack of correlation between the magnitude of DA increase measured with microdialysis and the magnitude of displacement of D_2 radiotracers across different challenge drugs (Laruelle, 2000a). Drugs that block the DAT, such as amphetamine and GBR12909, increase microdialysis-measured DA more than those that do not block the DAT, such as ketanserin and nicotine, yet the range of D_2 radiotracer displacement is similar for all, suggesting that it is affected only by changes in intrasynaptic DA. Thus, the imaging measures of DA in the stimulated (obtained with the amphetamine challenge) or baseline condition (obtained with the α-MPT depletion paradigm) are assumed to reflect measures of intrasynaptic or phasic release of DA. More definitive evidence supporting the exact molecular equivalence of the imaging measures is needed to confirm these interpretations. This evidence can derive from combining *in vivo* imaging using the amphetamine or AMPT paradigms with *ex vivo* measurements in rodent models of altered DA activity.

Both of these measures of intrasynaptic dopaminergic release have been shown to be increased in schizophrenia (Breier *et al.*, 1997; Laruelle *et al.*, 1996; Abi-Dargham et al., 1998, 2000). Furthermore, these measures are significantly related, as observed in a small study of drug-naïve patients with schizophrenia who underwent both assessments: stimulated and baseline DA release, measured with the amphetamine and the AMPT paradigm (Abi-Dargham *et al.*, 2009). This is also consistent with the reports of increased rate of dopa-decarboxylase enzyme activity in the striatum (McGowan *et al.*, 2004). The striatal DA excess exists in the presence of very mild elevations of striatal D_2 receptors, estimated to be in the range of 10% from a meta-analysis (Weinberger & Laruelle, 2002) and normal levels of both DA transporters (Lavalaye *et al.*, 2001; Laakso *et al.*, 2000, 2001; Laruelle, 2000b; Schmitt *et al.*, 2005), as well as vesicular monoamine transporters (Taylor *et al.*, 2000).

We will next review the evidence linking this excess DA to the pathophysiology and treatment of psychosis, and discuss its specificity to psychosis.

Excess striatal dopamine underlying psychosis

Using [^{123}I]IBZM and the amphetamine challenge, we observed a significant relationship between the magnitude of DA release and a transient induction or worsening of positive symptoms (Laruelle *et al.*, 1999). The increase in amphetamine-induced DA release was larger in patients experiencing an episode of illness exacerbation compared to patients in remission at the time of the scan (Laruelle *et al.*, 1999). Using similar methods and the same camera as in the studies in patients with schizophrenia (Laruelle

et al., 1996, 1999; Abi-Dargham *et al.*, 1998), we assessed a group of patients with schizotypal personality disorder (SPD) (Abi-Dargham *et al.*, 2004). The reduction in [^{123}I] IBZM induced by amphetamine in SPD had a similar magnitude to that previously observed in remitted patients with schizophrenia (p = 0.72), but was significantly lower than that observed in patients with schizophrenia studied during episodes of illness exacerbation (p < 0.01). The similarity in DA dysregulation between subjects with SPD and remitted patients with schizophrenia suggests that a modest increase in DA release in these groups might represent a trait variable, while the larger increases observed in the acute episodes of illness exacerbation might represent a state-related variable. While the increase in psychosis in patients with schizophrenia was related to DA release, we did not observe a relationship between baseline psychotic symptoms measured with the Positive and Negative Syndrome Scale (PANSS) positive symptoms subscale and DA release. This is probably related to the fact that a change in positive symptoms measured within one single session, in a short timeframe, is a less noisy measurement than ratings obtained at baseline across subjects, where positive symptoms may be influenced by different factors. This would predict that a study in a larger sample of patients may be needed to show a relationship. Furthermore, it is possible that DA release in other brain regions, not currently measureable with the available tracers, is more predictive of psychosis at baseline or after psychostimulant challenge. This can be assessed in future by using higher sensitivity tracers such as [^{11}C]FLB457 or [^{18}F]Fallypride, which are also sensitive to acute fluctuations in DA levels, to assess DA release in extrastriatal regions either at baseline or after a challenge. That said, the relationship we describe between striatal amphetamine-induced DA release and worsening of psychosis does not establish a causative link between these two events, and we cannot rule out a more fundamental causative effect in a DA system that is not reliably measured at present. Another interesting point to note is the absence of psychosis in SPD despite the increase in DA release due to amphetamine. This observation may suggest that a larger magnitude of DA dysregulation is necessary for overt psychosis to manifest, and subjects with SPD remain below these levels of release for reasons that are unclear at this point.

Relationship to treatment response

In the study of baseline phasic release, we also observed that higher occupancy of D_2 receptors by DA in patients with schizophrenia was predictive of good therapeutic response of these symptoms following 6 weeks of treatment with various antipsychotic medications (Abi-Dargham *et al.*, 2000). The fact that high levels of synaptic DA at baseline predicted better or faster response to atypical antipsychotic drugs suggested that the D_2 receptor blockade induced by these drugs is a key component of their initial mode of action. In a subsequent study, we assessed the relationship between occupancy of D_2 receptors and treatment response using [18F]Fallypride in striatal and extrastriatal regions (Kegeles et al., 2008). Seven subjects were rated with the PANSS before and after aripiprazole treatment, and we evaluated the relationships between the changes in the subscales and aripiprazole occupancy. Treatment was optimized for each patient independently of the study and the scan was obtained shortly after initiation of treatment. As it has been reported that most of the therapeutic response is measured in the first 4 weeks of treatment (Kerwin et al., 2007), we predicted that the treatment response measured then is likely to be close to the optimal response. Positive-symptom subscale changes correlated positively with striatal subregional occupancy. No such correlation was found in extrastriatal regions, and the negative-symptom subscale changes showed no significant correlation with occupancy in striatal or extrastriatal regions.

Correlations of ratings of clinical improvement of positive symptoms with occupancy in striatal but not extrastriatal regions are in agreement with one previous finding (Agid et al., 2007). These observations should be considered with caution as the samples are small but they do suggest, if confirmed in larger studies, that antipsychotics benefit positive symptoms of schizophrenia through modulation of striatal but not cortical or other extrastriatal DA activity. These data also confirm the predominant involvement of limbic and associative striatum compared to sensorimotor striatum in the therapeutic effect of antipsychotics. The lack of relationship with improvement in negative symptoms suggests that treatment of negative symptoms is multifactorial and therapeutic effects may depend on other systems in other regions.

Overall, striatal phasic DA excess mediates severity of psychosis and is most likely directly relevant to its treatment.

Dopamine and cognition: suboptimal cortical dopamine transmission

Preclinical studies have documented the importance of prefrontal DA function for cognitive processes (for review, see Goldman-Rakic, 1994; Goldman-Rakic et al., 2000). This important role has been recently confirmed in humans, by the repeated observation that carriers of the high activity allele of catechol-O-methyltransferase (COMT), an enzyme involved in DA metabolism, display lower performance in various cognitive tasks compared to carriers of the allele that induces a lower concentration of DA in PFC (for review, see Goldberg & Weinberger, 2004). Clinical studies have suggested a relationship between low cerebrospinal fluid (CSF) homovanillic acid (HVA), a measure reflecting

low DA activity in the PFC, and poor performance at tasks involving working memory in schizophrenia (Weinberger et al., 1988; Kahn et al., 1994). Administration of DA agonists might have beneficial effects on the pattern of prefrontal activation measured with positron emission tomography (PET) during these tasks (Daniel et al., 1991; Dolan et al., 1995). While these observations are consistent with the hypothesis of a hypodopaminergic state in the PFC of patients with schizophrenia, they do not constitute direct evidence for it. The most direct evidence so far has derived from postmortem studies showing decreased TH-labeled axons in the EC and PFC, suggesting that schizophrenia might be associated with deficit in DA transmission in these cortical regions (Akil et al., 1999, 2000).

Prefrontal cortical D_1 receptors

The D_1 receptor is the main mediator of DA effects in the PFC and is present at levels that allow quantification with imaging. Three PET studies of prefrontal D_1 receptor availability in patients with schizophrenia have been published. Two were performed with the D_1 radiotracer [11C]SCH 23390. The first reported decreased [11C]SCH 23390 binding potential in the PFC (Okubo et al., 1997), and the other reported no change (Karlsson et al., 1997). The third study was performed with [11C]NNC 112 (Abi-Dargham et al., 2000b), and reported increased [11C]NNC 112 binding potential in the DLPFC, and no change in other regions of the PFC, such as the medial PFC (MPFC) or the orbitofrontal cortex. In patients with schizophrenia, increased [11C]NNC 112 binding in the DLPFC was predictive of poor performance on a working memory task (Abi-Dargham et al., 2002). Many potential factors, including patient heterogeneity and differences in the boundaries of the sampled regions, might account for these discrepancies. However, severity of deficits at tasks involving working memory were reported to be associated with both decreased PFC [11C]SCH 23390 binding potential in one study (Okubo et al., 1997) and increased PFC [11C]NNC 112 binding potential in another (Abi-Dargham et al., 2000b), suggesting both alterations might reflect a common underlying deficit.

In an effort to understand the reasons for the discrepant results, we assessed the impact of acute and subchronic DA depletion on the in vivo binding of [11C]SCH 23390 and [11C] NNC 112 (Guo et al., 2001). Acute DA depletion did not affect the in vivo binding of [11C]NNC 112, but resulted in decreased in vivo binding of [3H]SCH 23390, a paradoxical response that might be related to DA depletion-induced translocation of D_1 receptors from the cytoplasmic to the cell surface compartment (Dumartin et al., 2000; Scott et al., 2002; Laruelle, 2000a). In contrast, chronic DA depletion is associated with increased in vivo [11C]NNC 112 binding, presumably reflecting a compensatory up-regulation of D_1

receptors. Interestingly, chronic DA depletion did not result in enhanced *in vivo* binding of [^{3}H]SCH 23390, possibly as a result of the opposing effects of receptor up-regulation and externalization on the binding of these tracers.

Consistent with the interpretation that up-regulation of D$_1$ receptors measured with [^{11}C]NNC 112 reflects a dopaminergic deficit, we have observed a similar increase in human volunteers who abuse N-methyl-D-aspartate (NMDA) antagonists (Narendran et al., 2005). Preclinical studies suggest that chronic hypofunction of NMDA receptors is associated with dysregulated prefrontal DA function (for review, see Jentsch & Roth, 1999; Jentsch et al., 1997). Furthermore, in non-human primates, chronic, intermittent exposure to the NMDA antagonist MK801 resulted in decreased performance at prefrontal tasks, decreased extracellular levels of DA in the DLPFC, and increased [^{11}C] NNC 112 BP in the DLPFC (Kakiuchi et al., 2001; Tsukada et al., 2005). Together, these preclinical data suggest that NMDA dysfunction might lead to decreased prefrontal DA activity and increased D$_1$ receptor availability, all three dysregulations contributing to working memory deficits.

Finally, we recently compared [^{11}C]NNC 112 binding in healthy volunteers homozygous for the Val allele to Met carriers of *COMT* (Slifstein et al., 2008). Subjects were otherwise matched for parameters known to affect [^{11}C]NNC 112 binding. Subjects with Val/Val alleles had significantly higher cortical [^{11}C]NNC 112 binding compared to Met carriers but did not differ in striatal binding. These results confirm the prominent role of COMT in regulating DA transmission in the cortex but not the striatum, and the reliability of [^{11}C]NNC 112 as a marker for low DA tone, as previously suggested by studies in patients with schizophrenia.

Functional implications

Based on the differential effects of DA depletion on the different D$_1$ radiotracers, it is justifiable to examine results obtained in different conditions with one tracer. Doing so with [^{11}C]NNC 112, we detected a consistent pattern of up-regulation, modest in magnitude but statistically significant throughout conditions, showing increased cortical D$_1$ in schizophrenia, in a DA depletion rat model, and in the human ketamine users model of NMDA dysfunction. The functional meaning of this up-regulation is subject to speculation and has different therapeutic implications. A most likely interpretation, supported by the rat model of DA depletion, is that the D$_1$ increases represent a compensatory up-regulation in response to a chronic deficiency in DA and a chronic *hypostimulation* of D$_1$ receptors. This explanation is congruent with all the clinical data reviewed above. An added validation to this hypothesis is the observation that a deficit in prefrontal DA innervation in schizophrenia

could contribute to the disinhibition of subcortical DA observed in these patients, as DA activity in PFC exerts a negative feedback on VTA activity. It has been shown that selective lesions of DA neurons in the PFC are associated with increased striatal DA release in rats (Jaskiw et al., 1990; Pycock et al., 1980, Bubser & Koch, 1994; Deutch et al., 1990; Thompson & Moss, 1995) and primates (Roberts et al., 1994), while augmentation of DA or gamma-aminobutyric acid (GABA) activity in the PFC inhibits striatal DA release (Jaskiw et al., 1991; Kolachana et al., 1995; Karreman & Moghaddam, 1996; for review, see Tzschentke, 2001).

The hypothesis of D$_1$ hypostimulation suggests that the relationship described between D$_1$ up-regulation and poor performance on working memory, which is true for severity of negative symptoms (Abi-Dargham, unpublished observations), means that cognitive deficit and negative symptoms are mediated to some extent by a lack of cortical D$_1$ stimulation. This can be tested using D$_1$ agonists in conjunction with antipsychotic treatment as a therapeutic enhancement strategy. Many challenges exist in terms of implementing this strategy in the treatment of cognitive deficits in schizophrenia, as the availability of D$_1$ agonists is limited, and the level and mode of D$_1$ stimulation, and the corresponding D1 occupancy, are all unclear at this point. Recently, subcutaneous administration of an investigational drug, DAR100, with poor bioavailability, has been tested in patients with schizophrenia. Initial studies showed safety and absence of negative or side effects (George et al., 2007). Further testing is currently underway to show efficacy against cognitive impairment. Some preclinical studies suggested long-lasting effects after single administration of a D$_1$ agonist in antipsychotic-induced cognitive impairment in non-human primates (Castner et al., 2000; Castner & Goldman-Rakic, 2004). Furthermore, an additional benefit of D$_1$ stimulation is the potential enhancement of NMDA transmission in schizophrenia as these two systems facilitate each other's function through many well-described interactions (Flores-Hernandez et al., 2002; Scott et al., 2002; Dunah & Standaert, 2001).

As an alternative to D$_1$ hypostimulation, the data may suggest the curve for D$_1$ stimulation in schizophrenia is a narrow inverted-U shape, with D$_1$ stimulation oscillating between low levels at baseline and superstimulation under conditions of stress and DA release.

Preclinical considerations

As stated above, there is substantial evidence for DA dysregulation in schizophrenia. The evidence relates to amphetamine-induced DA release and baseline occupancy of D$_2$ by DA in the striatum, both of which are measures of intrasynaptic phasic release. No information on basal release is available, which relates to extrasynaptic DA levels in the extracellular milieu, a measure not accessible to imaging. As there is little evidence for pathology within the DA neuron itself, it has been proposed that the pathology lies with the manner by which the DA neuron is regulated. However, defining the pathophysiology that drives this dysregulation has escaped identification. By examining the properties of the DA system regulation, we can study the contributions of well-known pathological changes in the brain of a patient with schizophrenia to the abnormal excitability observed within the DA system.

Dopamine systems of the brain

Most monoamine systems exhibit broadly divergent collateralizations, in that single norepinephrinergic or serotonergic neurons innervate multiple targets. However, this is not the case with the DA system. The DA neurons consist of clusters of neurons with discreet projections. Within the midbrain, the meso-limbic DA system exhibits projections to multiple subcortical regions involved in emotional regulation and reward (Montague *et al.*, 2004), including the ventro-medial limbic striatum, the amygdala, the septum, and the hippocampus. The meso-cortical system projects from the midbrain to the neocortical mantle, with highest concentrations in frontal cortical regions. The nigrostriatal system has traditionally been associated with more motor functions, due to its degeneration in Parkinson disease (Hornykiewicz, 1962). However, more recent studies have demonstrated that this system also has a strong involvement in habit formation and associative learning processes (Berke, 2003; Yin *et al.*, 2008). Finally, the tuberoinfundibular DA system is involved in the regulation of prolactin release, and likely contributes to some of the endocrine side effects of antipsychotic medication (Compton & Miller, 2002).

Dopamine neuron firing properties: tonic and phasic activity

The population of DA neurons in the midbrain is known to be under complex regulatory influences that modulate their activity states. DA neurons themselves are known to exhibit unique electrophysiological properties that enable the system to exhibit distinct states of activity depending on afferent drive. Thus, numerous studies have shown that under baseline conditions, both in anesthetized (Bunney & Grace, 1978; Grace & Bunney, 1984b) and awake (Freeman *et al.*, 1985) animals, a large proportion of DA neurons are not firing spontaneously, but are instead held in a hyperpolarized state. Neurons in this state often exhibit constant, high-amplitude GABAergic inhibitory postsynaptic potentials (Grace & Bunney, 1985). Moreover, the proportion of DA neurons that are spontaneously firing is under potent regulatory control; thus, even during the loss of DA neurons during lesion states modeling Parkinson disease,

the proportion of the remaining DA neurons exhibiting spontaneous activity is tightly regulated (Hollerman & Grace, 1990), whereas drugs that increase the number of neurons firing are known to induce pathological states, such as L-DOPA-induced motor syndromes (Harden & Grace, 1995) or antipsychotic drug-induced acute and chronic extrapyramidal symptoms (Bunney & Grace, 1978; Grace *et al.*, 1997). It is proposed that, by controlling the number of active neurons, the DA system is organized to maintain not baseline DA levels, but instead the dynamic range of response, enabling the system to recruit the same proportion of previously "silent" neurons during times of behavioral demand (Onn *et al.*, 2000; Hollerman & Grace, 1990). When this dynamic range is disrupted, as may occur in a number of DA-related disorders, including schizophrenia, patholophysiological consequences ensue.

Studies suggest that the origin of this inhibitory clamp over DA neuron firing is the pallidum. Thus, with respect to the meso-limbic and meso-cortical DA neuron system, the ventral pallidum is proposed to supply a potent GABAergic inhibitory influence over DA neuron firing (Floresco *et al.*, 2003). This is consistent both with the continuous bombardment of DA neurons with GABAergic inhibitory postsynaptic potentials (IPSPs; Grace & Bunney, 1985), and the fast firing rate of ventral pallidal neurons (Mogenson *et al.*, 1993). Moreover, inactivation of the ventral pallidum was found to cause a selective increase in the proportion of DA neurons firing spontaneously (Floresco *et al.*, 2001). The pathway that appears to most effectively regulate the number of neurons firing originates within the hippocampal complex; specifically, the ventral subiculum (Floresco *et al.*, 2001, 2003). Thus, activity within the ventral subiculum would activate VST GABAergic neurons, which in turn inhibit the ventral pallidum and release DA neurons from inhibitory influence (Fig. 20.1). Once this GABAergic tone is removed, the pacemaker conductance of the DA neuron would then initiate spontaneous spike discharge (Grace & Bunney, 1984b; Grace & Onn, 1989).

In addition to showing potent regulation of population activity in terms of neurons firing, the spontaneously active DA neurons also exhibit two unique firing patterns: single-spike firing and burst firing (Grace & Bunney, 1984a,b). The baseline activity state of DA neurons is an irregular, single-spike firing pattern. This pattern is driven by the pacemaker afferent input, as modulated by local (Grace & Bunney, 1979, 1985) and long-loop (Grace & Bunney, 1985) GABAergic inputs. However, when an animal is exposed to a behaviorally activating stimulus, the neurons fire in bursts (Schultz, 1998). Burst firing consists of rapid high-frequency firing of sets of 3–10 spikes (Grace & Bunney, 1984a), and is believed to represent the behaviorally salient output of the DA system (Grace, 1991, 1995). Burst firing is controlled by the glutamatergic drive of DA neurons acting

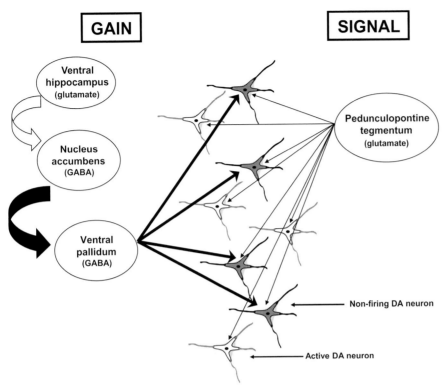

Fig. 20.1 Model of dopamine (DA) neuron regulation. Tonic DA neuron activity, defined as the proportion of DA neurons showing spontaneous spike discharge, is regulated by the ventral hippocampus. In baseline conditions, the ventral pallidum holds subsets of DA neurons inactive via powerful GABAergic inhibitory projections to the neurons. Activity within the ventral hippocampus produces a glutamate-mediated excitation of the nucleus accumbens, which in turn inhibits the ventral pallidum and releases DA neurons from inhibition. In contrast, a behaviorally relevant event causes the pedunculopontine tegmentum to elicit a rapid, phasic excitation of DA neurons causing them to burst fire. Only the DA neurons that the ventral subiculum causes to become active can respond to the phasic input from the pedunculopontine tegmentum. Therefore, the ventral subiculum determines the "gain", or how strong the phasic "signal" can be. In schizophrenia, it is proposed that hyperactivity within the hippocampus causes the "gain" to be too high, thereby causing a maximal DA "signal" to all stimuli independent of their behavioral salience.

on NMDA receptors (Grace & Bunney, 1984a; Overton & Clark, 1992; Chergui *et al.*, 1993). The glutamatergic input that drives meso-limbic DA neurons arises from the pedunculopontine tegmentum (PPT; Floresco *et al.*, 2001, 2003), and is dependent on another brainstem region, the laterodorsal tegmentum, that gates the ability of glutamate to drive burst firing (Lodge & Grace, 2006b).

Dopamine neuron activity and striatal dopamine dynamics

The state of activity of the DA neurons in turn determines the dynamics of DA release within the striatum. Thus, using microdialysis probes to sample the concentrations of DA in the extracellular milieu, it was found that tonic DA neuron firing was responsible for the tonic concentrations of DA present in the extrasynaptic space (Floresco *et al.*, 2003). This tonic DA is known to exist in low concentrations (i.e., nM range), which is sufficient to stimulate presynaptic DA receptors on cortical or DA terminals, but not postsynaptic sites (Grace, 1991). In contrast, when DA neurons elicit bursts of spikes, a rapid, high-amplitude phasic release of DA occurs within the synapse. This phasic release is much higher in amplitude (i.e., hundreds of micromolar), but is rapidly removed from the synapse by the DAT; thus, it fails to diffuse far from the release site (Floresco *et al.*, 2003). Activation of tonic and phasic DA release was found to have unique effects within the striatum; thus, increases in DA neuron population activity were found to act presynaptically on PFC glutamate afferents to the striatum (O'Donnell & Grace, 1994) to decrease cortical influence over the ventral striatum via actions on DA D_2 receptors (Goto & Grace, 2005), whereas increases in phasic DA release were found to selectively increase ventral hippocampal afferent drive via a D_1-dependent postsynaptic mechanism (Goto & Grace, 2005). Moreover, this was reflected in the behavior of the animal; thus, tonic DA release was found to interfere with behavioral flexibility in the face of changing task demands (which is consistent with interference with PFC drive; Ragozzino, 2007), whereas attenuation of phasic DA altered the animal's ability to acquire tasks (Goto & Grace, 2005).

Tonic single-spike firing and phasic burst firing, as illustrated above, are controlled by distinct afferent processes. However, these systems appear to function in a concerted manner. Thus, increases in tonic and phasic DA would shift the balance of prefrontal and limbic inputs in favor of limbic system drive (Goto & Grace, 2005; Goto et al., 2007). Moreover, the phasic DA response appears to depend on the amplitude of tonic DA neuron firing. Thus, pedunculopontine tegmental glutamatergic drive of DA neuron firing requires that the DA neuron be in an active state; otherwise, there is a magnesium blockade of hyperpolarized DA neurons that prevents NMDA-induced activation of burst firing (Floresco et al., 2003; Mayer et al., 1984). Thus, by controlling the number of DA neurons firing, the ventral hippocampus is positioned to control the "gain" of the phasic DA response (Lodge & Grace, 2006a). That is, when the ventral hippocampal drive is high, there are more DA neurons disinhibited and firing spontaneously; thus a signal that arrives via the PPT can cause a larger number of neurons to enter a burst firing mode, and lead to substantially greater phasic DA release.

Dopamine neuron activity and the pathophysiology of schizophrenia

The DA system is regulated by a number of systems. The PFC is known to provide an attenuation of subcortical DA systems, such that interference with prefrontal function leads to alteration in subcortical DA dynamics (Pycock et al., 1980; Jaskiw et al., 1990). Thus, by interfering with PFC function, an imbalance in tonic/phasic DA regulation in the subcortical systems can result (Grace, 1991; Weinberger et al., 1988). However, disruptions in PFC function can alter other subcortical systems as well; one region that is disrupted by pathology within the PFC is the hippocampus (Weinberger et al., 1992b, 1993). Indeed, one robust finding in patients with schizophrenia is altered hippocampal volume (Weinberger et al., 1992c; see Chapter 18). Indeed, rodent studies suggest a strong link between PFC function and hippocampal output systems, such as those affecting the ventral striatum (Belujon & Grace, 2008). Therefore, disruptions in either the hippocampus or in the PFC can disrupt the balance of regulation of the DA system in a manner that could contribute to the onset of schizophrenia.

An alternate potential disruption in hippocampal physiology has also been advanced as a means to understand the psychosis in schizophrenia. Thus, emerging evidence suggests that the hippocampus may exhibit hyperactivity in the patient with schizophrenia (Heckers et al., 1998; Medoff et al., 2001; Meyer-Lindenberg et al., 2005).

Moreover, the data are consistent with a role for hippocampal hyperactivity in psychosis in particular (Silbersweig et al., 1995). Indeed, it has been shown that temporal lobe epilepsy, that would activate the hippocampus, is associated with a psychosis not unlike that observed in patients with schizophrenia (Ounsted & Lindsay, 1981). Finally, studies in patients with schizophrenia have shown deficits in interneuron function in the hippocampus as well as the PFC (Heckers et al., 2002; Lewis et al., 2005; Benes et al., 2007; Zhang & Reynolds, 2002; Hashimoto et al., 2008; see Chapter 18). Indeed, developmental disruption rodent models of schizophrenia provide results that are consistent with this model. Thus, adult rats treated gestationally with a mitotoxin, methylazoxymethanol acetate (MAM), exhibit a number of features consistent with schizophrenia in humans, including decreased limbic cortical thickness, disruption of executive function, and hyper-responsivity to amphetamine (Grace & Moore, 1998, Moore et al., 2006). Moreover, these rats exhibit a selective loss of parvalbumin-containing interneurons within the ventral hippocampus and PFC that correlates with diminished gamma oscillations (Lodge et al., 2008), as observed in patients with schizophrenia (Herrmann & Demiralp, 2005; Lewis et al., 2001). Finally, VST neurons in MAM-treated rats do not show typical hippocampal gating, but instead appear to be in a continuous depolarized state (Moore et al., 2006).

Put together, these data suggest that in the MAM-treated rat, as may also be present in schizophrenia, there is hyperactivity within the ventral hippocampus. The results described above point to a model in which hyperactivity in the ventral hippocampus causes an abnormal increase in tonic DA neuron activity. Indeed, this is what was observed: MAM-treated rats exhibit nearly twice the number of DA neurons tonically firing as observed in control rats. Moreover, this increase is normalized by inactivation of the hippocampus. Finally, inactivation of the ventral hippocampus also normalizes the augmented behavioral responses to amphetamine observed in MAM-treated rats (Lodge & Grace, 2007). In summary, these data are consistent with a model whereby overdrive by the ventral hippocampus would cause the DA system to show abnormally augmented tonic activity; thus making it hyper-responsive to phasic activation by behaviorally relevant stimuli. In other words, under these conditions one would predict that rather benign stimuli would nonetheless cause hyperactivation of the phasic DA response, resulting in psychosis (Lodge & Grace, 2007; Grace et al., 2007).

These data are consistent with a hyperdopaminergic state that leads to over-release of DA in the ventral striatum of rats, which is proposed to be analogous to the augmented DA system response to amphetamine in patients with schizophrenia described above. However, in integrating the rodent and primate literature, caution must be observed in drawing comparisons. Many of the studies of DA system dynamics have been done in the rat, which is a species in which the caudate and frontal cortical system are much less differentiated than they are in humans. Thus, the ventro-medial striatal complex in both rat and humans receives inputs from MPFC and limbic structures, such as the hippocampus and the amygdala. However, in the human, these structures become more differentiated; thus, there is an expansion of the integrative striatal region that lies between the limbic and motor regions, and that receives inputs from the DLPFC (Haber et al., 2000). Indeed, this integrative striatal region has been shown in imaging studies to have the greatest amphetamine-induced DA release in subjects with schizophrenia (Kegeles et al., 2006). Nonetheless, anatomical studies demonstrate that the ventro-medial striatum in the primate, which receives limbic system inputs, will nonetheless affect the DA neurons that innervate the integrative striatal regions (Haber et al., 2000).

Antipsychotic drugs and their impact on tonic dopamine neuron firing

Given the evidence from both clinical and preclinical studies, how would antipsychotic drug treatment treat psychosis? One proposal is that long-term antipsychotic drug treatment would act in a manner opposite to that suggested to occur with ventral subicular activation. Thus, the effects of repeated antipsychotic drug treatment reported in rats is one of depolarization block (Grace et al., 1997; Bunney & Grace, 1978; Grace & Bunney, 1986). Depolarization block is the propensity of DA neurons to enter a state of inactivation of spike firing secondary to enhanced excitation. As a result, following 3 weeks of treatment with antipsychotic drugs, there is a decrease in the number of spontaneously firing DA neurons. The inactivation occurs with a delayed onset, which has been compared to the delayed maximal therapeutic action observed with antipsychotic drug treatment (Johnstone et al., 1978). Moreover, this induction of depolarization block corresponds with both the therapeutic potential and propensity for inducing extrapyramidal side effects. Thus, classical antipsychotic drugs induce depolarization block in both the nigrostriatal and meso-limbic DA neurons, whereas atypical agents only induce depolarization block in the meso-limbic DA system. It has been reported that individuals with schizophrenia exhibit variations in the onset of therapeutic actions, particularly when the DA system has been "sensitized" by prior therapeutic drug treatment regimens (Agid et al., 2006). Moreover, a compromised DA system, in which DA neurons are rendered hyper-responsive, more rapidly enters a state of depolarization block (Hollerman et al., 1992; Hollerman & Grace, 1989). Thus, in a state in which the DA system is already over-

driven, presumably via a hippocampal hyperactivation, one would predict that the DA neurons may be in a state that is more susceptible to rapid induction of depolarization block. However, this has not been tested as yet in animal models.

Dynamics of dopamine system regulation in the prefrontal cortex

The aforementioned description relates to DA actions within subcortical limbic systems, which are proposed to relate to the positive symptoms of schizophrenia (O'Donnell & Grace, 1998). However, patients with schizophrenia have substantial disruptions in cognitive function and present negative symptoms. Given the similarities in pathology observed in patients with frontal cortical damage with these cognitive/affective disturbances (O'Donnell & Grace, 1998), it is believed that the PFC has a substantial role in the pathophysiology of this disorder. The PFC exhibits a substantial DA innervation (Goldman-Rakic et al., 1992). The PFC is also believed to mediate many of the cognitive dysfunctions observed in schizophrenia, such as deficits in working memory function (Goldman-Rakic, 1995). Studies in primates have shown that visual working memory processes are strongly dependent on an intact DA innervation of the PFC, and that disruption of this DA innervation also disrupts working memory and other executive functions. Indeed, it has been proposed that deficiencies in PFC DA transmission may be a pathological factor in schizophrenia (Weinberger et al., 1992a). Moreover, PFC DA function has been implicated in the disruption of subcortical DA systems (Meyer-Lindenberg et al., 2002; Grace, 1991, 1993).

The dynamics of DA regulation in the PFC appear to be substantially different from those observed subcortically. Thus, in subcortical sites such as the striatum, DA is rapidly inactivated by reuptake into DA terminals. However, in the PFC, the dynamics are much different. Thus, it has been reported that DA terminals within the PFC do not have substantial levels of uptake sites (Sesack et al., 1998). As a result, DA released from terminals in the neocortex is free to diffuse from the release sites, and have actions at more distal locations. Inactivation of DA within the PFC is thus dependent on other processes, including: (1) diffusion from the site of release, which would have less impact in a dense terminal field; (2) inactivation by metabolizing enzymes; and (3) uptake into norepinephrine (NE) terminals (Yamamoto & Novotney, 1998). A primary means by which DA is inactivated in the PFC is proposed to be via the metabolizing enzyme COMT. Indeed, the primary metabolite of DA that is produced via an action of this enzyme is homovanillic acid (HVA), which is believed to be derived primarily from cortical DA turnover (Akil et al., 2003). This difference in DA dynamics between subcortical regions such as the striatum, where DA is inactivated primarily by reuptake, *versus* the PFC, where DA is inactivated primarily by metabolism, would therefore be impacted substantially differently by drugs that interfere with one or the other process. Thus, drugs of abuse that function as DA uptake blockers would preferentially increase DA levels within the striatum and other subcortical structures, whereas the increase in the PFC would not be as substantial. On the other hand, alterations of COMT will strongly impact synaptic transmission within the PFC. Indeed, it would appear that tonic and phasic DA transmission in these regions would be altered in substantially different manners by differences in COMT activity (Bilder *et al.*, 2004). As a result, an alteration in the cortical/subcortical balance of DA would occur.

COMT is known to exist in two different isoforms: one containing a valine allele (Val-COMT) and one containing a methionine allele at position 158 (Met-COMT) (see Tunbridge *et al.*, 2006). Studies show that COMT with the Val allele is more metabolically active than COMT with the Met allele (Weinshilboum *et al.*, 1999). Some clinical studies have shown that patients with schizophrenia have a higher predominance of the Val allele and diminished PFC function (Egan *et al.*, 2001). As a result, the time course of DA actions in the PFC, which is primarily controlled by COMT, would be limited, thereby potentially exacerbating the proposed DA deficit in the PFC via attenuation of the slower, phasic DA response in this region. However, since COMT would also preferentially metabolize DA that has escaped from the synaptic cleft, one model suggests that COMT would have a greater influence on the tonic DA system in the striatum (Bilder *et al.*, 2004). A decrease in tonic DA subcortically would be predicted to release the phasic DA system from autoinhibition at the level of the DA terminal (Grace, 1991; Bilder *et al.*, 2004). Therefore, the Val allele of COMT may potentially act to simultaneously exacerbate deficiencies in DA transmission in the PFC while potentially exacerbating the hyperdopaminergic state subcortically.

Once released from the synapse, DA can exert multiple and complex actions within the PFC. Direct application of DA tends to produce inhibitory effects *in vivo* (Lavin & Grace, 1997; Sesack & Bunney, 1989). However, the actions of this transmitter are much more complex when assessed on different DA receptor subtypes. Thus, DA can act on D_1 receptors on the principal neurons of the PFC, leading to an activation of their firing by increasing the duration of the plateau potential, and a decrease in slow potassium conductances, thereby increasing the duration of the "up" states (Yang *et al.*, 1999; Yang & Seamans, 1996). This could contribute to the observed facilitation of glutamate-driven "up" states by D_1 agonists *in vivo* (Moore *et al.*, 1998). Furthermore, D_1 agonists have been shown to affect pyramidal neurons differently depending on their state, in that only neurons in the "up" state show a D_1-mediated increase in excitability (Lavin & Grace, 2001). As such, D_1 agonists

can selectively potentiate excitatory inputs to the pyramidal neurons. In contrast, D_1 receptors will also activate the firing of GABAergic interneurons and in turn inhibit pyramidal output neurons (Gorelova *et al.*, 2002). This complex circuit of interactions may account in part for the finding that the level of D_1 receptor stimulation is critical in determining its actions, with pathologically low levels of D_1 stimulation producing similar functional deficits, as is observed with overstimulation of D_1 receptors (Zahrt *et al.*, 1997). DA acting on D_2 and D_4 receptors is reported to attenuate the activity of interneurons, and D_4 receptors and cannabinoids have been shown to disrupt normal emotional processing in this region (Laviolette *et al.*, 2005, 2006). Indeed, such an interaction could potentially account for the propensity of cannabis as a risk factor in schizophrenia (Arseneault *et al.*, 2004). Furthermore, the findings that cannabis use among individuals who express the COMT Val allele are at greater risk for schizophrenia (Caspi *et al.*, 2005), and that both DA and cannabis affect PFC and hippocampal interneurons (Lewis *et al.*, 2005), may point to a common pathophysiological mechanism involving interneuron dysfunction. The interactions between DA and the cellular components of the PFC have been synthesized into a model whereby DA input modifies the response of pyramidal neurons, causing them to respond preferentially to local circuit interactions that may subserve working memory (Yang *et al.*, 1999); however, a deficiency in DA would interfere with this function, and shift the PFC to a primarily externally-driven condition, interfering with its integrative function.

Animal models of schizophrenia based on developmental disruption also exhibit deficits within the PFC, particularly as it relates to the actions of DA in this system. Thus, after a neonatal ventral hippocampal lesion, MPFC neurons show alterations in their response to stimulation of the VTA, whereas in control rats such stimulation leads to a depolarization but inhibition of spike discharge; in the lesion adult rat the same type of stimulation now causes a depolarization and an increase in spike discharge (O'Donnell *et al.*, 2002). In MAM-treated rats, MPFC neurons lose their up/down state transitions (Moore *et al.*, 2006), and show a diminished sensitivity to DA (Lavin *et al.*, 2005). The loss of up/down states is also reflected in the absence of the slow, 1 Hz field potentials normally observed in this region, as well as a loss of the 40 Hz gamma rhythms (Goto & Grace, 2006); a characteristic also observed in patients with schizophrenia (Herrmann & Demiralp, 2005; Gallinat *et al.*, 2004). Given evidence that these oscillations may be critical for the processing of information in the MPFC (Engel *et al.*, 2001; Engel & Singer, 2001; Kaiser & Lutzenberger, 2003), such an alteration in network synchrony is likely to substantially impact cognitive processes. With respect to spike firing, there is an increase in regularity of firing and decrease in entropy, reflecting diminished information content in the outflow from this area (Goto & Grace, 2006). Moreover, synaptic plasticity in the hippocampal–MPFC pathway is also altered, and shows a much greater sensitivity to the disrupting effects of mild stressors (Goto & Grace, 2006).

Conclusions

We have reviewed above different sets of clinical and preclinical studies outlining a dopaminergic phenotype in schizophrenia, its potential mechanisms as well as its functional significance. From these studies an axis of pathology emerges that includes cortico-striatal DA and its modulation by hippocampal input. Increased striatal DA function is a well-established finding that appears most relevant to positive symptoms, as the severity of these correlates with the magnitude of DA release, and their response to treatment is also a function of the degree of dysregulation of striatal DA function. Indeed the most relevant site of therapeutic efficacy of antipsychotics is striatal, as measured by the strength of the relationship between D_2 occupancy in the striatum by antipsychotics and the response of positive symptoms. On the other hand, response of negative symptoms is unrelated to striatal occupancy, and the response of positive symptoms does not seem to be coupled to degree of extrastriatal occupancy. These observations need further confirmation in larger studies but indicate nevertheless that the striatal dopaminergic function determines severity and treatment response of psychosis.

Nonetheless, a striatal dopaminergic dysfunction can be reciprocally linked to a cortical dopaminergic dysfunction. Studies have documented that cortical DA affects subcortical DA dynamics, and more recently the reciprocal effect has been shown in a mouse model of striatal D_2 overexpression, showing cognitive impairment in tasks of working memory and behavioral flexibility, as well as altered PFC DA levels, rates of DA turnover, and activation of PFC D_1 receptors (Kellendonk et al., 2006). The mechanism by which this may occur is yet to be determined, but this finding suggests that flow of information in cortico-striato-thalamo-cortical loops can be impaired at the striatal level, producing a bottom-up impairment in cortical function.

The dopaminergic phenotype in the striatum can help explain and bring together many different elements of pathology that have been documented in schizophrenia, as the striatum represents an essential integrative station, by receiving input from the hippocampus and the cortex, two areas of pathology in schizophrenia, by modulating DA midbrain neurons, and by projecting indirectly back to the cortex. Pathological changes in hippocampal activity lead to dopaminergic dysregulation in animal models. Hippocampal pathology is also present in patients with schizophrenia (Heckers et al., 1998, Medoff et al., 2001,

Meyer-Lindenberg et al., 2005), suggesting that the hippocampus may play an essential role in the genesis of the dopaminergic pathology in schizophrenia. This could be mediated by a disinhibition of dopaminergic cells in the VTA via the pallidal projection, leading to an increased sensitivity to excitory inputs from the PPT and an increase in phasic firing. Testing in patients for an association between hippocampal hyperactivity and dopaminergic phasic dysregulation is needed to confirm the relevance of these preclinical observations to the pathophysiology of the disease in humans. The striatal DA dysregulation in turn may lead to an impairment of cortical inputs mediated by a D_2–glutamate interaction and a D_1-mediated potentiation of hippocampal inputs, thus imbalancing the cortico-limbic integration that takes place within the striatum and explaining the different domains of pathology that exist within the schizophrenia spectrum (Fig. 20.2).

In summary, we have illustrated how the different dynamics of DA system regulation within the PFC and subcortical structures and the receptors involved can lead to two very different states within these systems, with D_1 DA receptors mediating very different actions with respect to information integration and dynamics of regulation in the PFC, in contrast to the abnormally augmented stimulation of D_2.

Studies of cortical D_1 receptors have suggested alterations related to poor cognition and negative symptoms. A better classification of negative symptoms is needed to separate or distinguish those symptoms that may relate to cortical cognitive dysfunction *versus* those that may relate to limbic reward-related dysfunction. The role for DA release in the striatum in mediating some aspects of reward functions, and the alterations of reward processes in schizophrenia (Krystal et al., 2006) suggest that some components of negative symptoms may relate to alterations in ventrostriatal DA transmission. Future studies aimed at characterizing multidimensional factors within the negative symptoms domain as they relate to DA transmission in cortical *versus* striatal substructures are needed to test this conceptualization.

Finally, a more direct characterization of cortical DA as well as extrastriatal DA transmission in schizophrenia is needed, as the evidence for cortical deficit is largely by inference. These studies are now feasible with the development of high-affinity benzamide radiotracers which allow visualization of D_2 receptors in low-density areas of the brain and are sensitive to acute changes in DA tone. Thus, although the distinct pathophysiological aspects of schizophrenia have been examined independently in distinct brain structures, it is clear that the brain acts as an integrated whole, with a change in one system being reflected by alterations within a host of complex interrelated nuclei. As a consequence, a disorder as diverse as schizophrenia may encompass a number of sites of pathology, both corti-

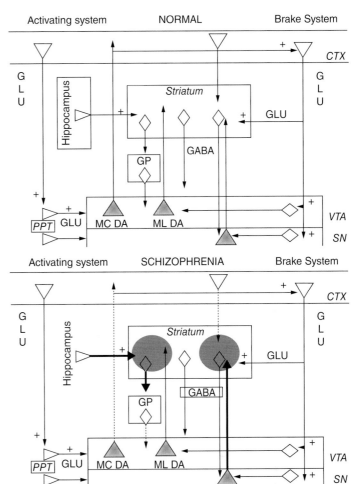

Fig. 20.2 Circuits and transmitters in the normal (upper panel) and in the schizophrenic brain (lower panel): dopamine (DA) activity in the ventral tegmental area/substantia nigra (VTA/SN) is stimulated by polysynaptic glutamatergic (Glu) tracks originating in the frontal cortex, perhaps involving relay in the pedunculopontine tegmentum (PPT), and inhibited via NMDA receptor-mediated stimulation of VTA GABAergic interneurons or striato-tegmental GABA neurons. In addition, the brake system regulating nigrostriatal/mesolimbic (NS/ML) DA activity is activated by MC DA projections. The striatum receives inputs from the cortex and hippocampus, and projects onto midbrain DA cells directly and via the pallidum (GP). In schizophrenia: DA is increased in the striatum, most predominantly in the associative substructure which receives dorso-lateral prefrontal cortex (DLPFC) input from the cortex (highlighted with shaded circle), this may weaken cortical input. Furthermore, hippocampal drive onto the striatum is increased (shaded circle), possibly contributing to DA dysregulation and to an altered processing at the level of the striatum of limbic *versus* cortical inputs. See text for details and references.

cally and subcortically, that could lead to common patho-physiological consequences across the integrated whole.

References

Abi-Dargham, A., Gil, R., Krystal, J. *et al.* (1998) Increased striatal dopamine transmission in schizophrenia: confirmation in a second cohort. *American Journal of Psychiatry* **155**, 761–767.

Abi-Dargham, A., Rodenhiser, J., Printz, D. *et al.* (2000a) Increased baseline occupancy of D2 receptors by dopamine in schizophrenia. *Proceedings of the National Academy of Science USA* **97**, 8104–8109.

Abi-Dargham, A., Martinez, D., Mawlawi, O. *et al.* (2000b) Measurement of striatal and extrastriatal dopamine D₁ receptor binding potential with [¹¹C]NNC 112 in humans: validation and reproducibility. *Journal of Cerebral Blood Flow Metabolism* **20**, 225–243.

Abi-Dargham, A., Mawlawi, O., Lombardo, I. *et al.* (2002) Prefrontal dopamine D1 receptors and working memory in schizophrenia. *Journal of Neuroscience* **22**, 3708–3719.

Abi-Dargham, A., Kegeles, L., Zea-Ponce, Y. *et al.* (2004) Striatal amphetamine-induced dopamine release in patients with schizotypal personality disorder studied with single photon emission computed tomography and [123I]iodobenzamide. *Biological Psychiatry* **55**, 1001–1006.

Abi-Dargham, A., Giessen, E.V., Slifstein, M., Kegeles, L.S. & Laruelle, M. (2009) Baseline and amphetamine-stimulated dopamine activity are related in drug-naive schizophrenic subjects. *Biologial Psychiatry* **65**, 1091–1093.

Agid, O., Seeman, P. & Kapur, S. (2006) The "delayed onset" of antipsychotic action—an idea whose time has come and gone. *Journal of Psychiatry and Neuroscience* **31**, 93–100.

Agid, O., Mamo, D., Ginovart, N. *et al.* (2007) Striatal vs extrastriatal dopamine D2 receptors in antipsychotic response—a double-blind PET study in schizophrenia. *Neuropsychopharmacology* **32**, 1209–1215.

Akil, M., Pierri, J.N., Whitehead, R.E. *et al.* (1999) Lamina-specific alterations in the dopamine innervation of the prefrontal cortex in schizophrenic subjects. *American Journal of Psychiatry* **156**, 1580–1589.

Akil, M., Edgar, C.L., Pierri, J.N., Casali, S. & Lewis, D.A. (2000) Decreased density of tyrosine hydroxylase-immunoreactive axons in the entorhinal cortex of schizophrenic subjects. *Biological Psychiatry* **47**, 361–370.

Akil, M., Kolanchana, B.S., Rothmond, D.A., Hyde, T.M., Weinberger, D.R. & Kleinman, J.E. (2003)

Catechol-O-methyltransferase genotype and dopamine regulation in the human brain. *Journal of Neuroscience* **23**, 2008–2013.

Angrist, B. & van Kammen, D.P. (1984) CNS stimulants as a tool in the study of schizophrenia. *Trends in Neuroscience* **7**, 388–390.

Arseneault, L., Cannon, M., Witton, J. & Murray, R.M. (2004) Causal association between cannabis and psychosis: examination of the evidence.[see comment]. *British Journal of Psychiatry* **184**, 110–117.

Belujon, P. & Grace, A.A. (2008) Critical role of the prefrontal cortex in the regulation of hippocampus-accumbens information flow. *Journal of Neuroscience* **28**, 9797–9805.

Benes, F.M., Todtenkopf, M.S. & Taylor, J.B. (1997) Differential distribution of tyrosine hydroxylase fibers on small and large neurons in layer II of anterior cingulated cortex of schizophrenic brain. *Synapse* **25**, 80–92.

Benes, F.M., Lim, B., Matzilevich, D., Walsh, J.P., Subburaju, S. & Minns, M. (2007) Regulation of the GABA cell phenotype in hippocampus of schizophrenics and bipolars. *Proceedings of the National Academy of Science USA* **104**, 10164–10169.

Berke, J.D. (2003) Learning and memory mechanisms involved in compulsive drug use and relapse. *Methods in Molecular Medicine* **79**, 75–101.

Bilder, R.M., Volavka, J., Lachman, H.M. & Grace, A.A. (2004) The catechol-O-methyltransferase polymorphism: relations to the tonic-phasic dopamine hypothesis and neuropsychiatric phenotypes. *Neuropsychopharmacology* **29**, 1943–1961.

Blanchard, J.J. & Cohen, A.S. (2006) The structure of negative symptoms within schizophrenia: implications for assessment. *Schizophrenia Bulletin* **32**, 238–245.

Bordet, R., Ridray, S., Carboni, S., Diaz, J., Sokoloff, P. & Schwartz, J.C. (1997) Induction of dopamine D3 receptor expression as a mechanism of behavioral sensitization to levodopa. *Proceedings of the National Academy of Science USA* **94**, 3363–3367.

Breier, A., Su, T.P., Saunders, R. *et al.* (1997) Schizophrenia is associated with elevated amphetamine-induced synaptic dopamine concentrations: evidence from a novel positron emission tomography method. *Proceedings of the National Academy of Science USA* **94**, 2569–2574.

Bubser, M. & Koch, M. (1994) Prepulse inhibition of the acoustic startle response of rats is reduced by 6-hydroxydopamine lesions of the medial prefrontal cortex. *Psychopharmacology (Berlin)* **113**, 487–492.

Bunney, B.S. & Grace, A.A. (1978) Acute and chronic haloperidol treatment: comparison of effects on nigral dopaminergic cell activity. *Life Sciences* **23**, 1715–1727.

Burt, D.R., Creese, I. & Snyder, S.H. (1977) Antischizophrenic drugs: chronic treatment elevates dopamine receptor binding in brain. *Science* **196**, 326–368.

Carlsson, A. & Lindqvist, M. (1963) Effect of chlorpromazine or haloperidol on formation of 3-methoxytyramine and normetanephrine in mouse brain. *Acta Pharmacologica Toxicologica* **20**, 140–144.

Caspi, A., Moffitt, T.E., Cannon, M. *et al.* (2005) Moderation of the effect of adolescent-onset cannabis use on adult psychosis by a functional polymorphism in the catechol-O-methyltransferase gene: longitudinal evidence of a gene X environment interaction. *Biological Psychiatry* **57**, 1117–1127.

Castner, S.A. & Goldman-Rakic, P.S. (2004) Enhancement of working memory in aged monkeys by a sensitizing regimen of dopamine D1 receptor stimulation. *Journal of Neuroscience* **24**, 1446–1450.

Castner, S.A., Williams, G.V. & Goldman-Rakic, P.S. (2000) Reversal of antipsychotic-induced working memory deficits by short-term dopamine D1 receptor stimulation. *Science* **287**, 2020–2022.

Chergui, K., Charlety, P.J., Akaoka, H. *et al.* (1993) Tonic activation of NMDA receptors causes spontaneous burst discharge of rat midbrain dopamine neurons in vivo. *European Journal of Neuroscience* **5**, 137–144.

Chinaglia, G., Alvarez, F.J., Probst, A. & Palacios, J.M. (1992) Mesostriatal and mesolimbic dopamine uptake binding sites are reduced in Parkinson's disease and progressive supranuclear palsy: a quantitative autoradiographic study using [3H] mazindol. *Neuroscience* **49**, 317–327.

Compton, M.T. & Miller, A.H. (2002) Antipsychotic-induced hyperprolactinemia and sexual dysfunction. *Psychopharmacology Bulletin* **36**, 143–164.

Creese, I., Burt, D.R. & Snyder, S.H. (1976) Dopamine receptor binding predicts clinical and pharmacological potencies of antischizophrenic drugs. *Science* **19**, 481–483.

Cross, A.J., Crow, T.J., Ferrier, I.N. *et al.* (1983) Dopamine receptor changes in schizophrenia in relation to the disease process and movement disorder. *Journal of Neural Transmission* **18** (Suppl.), 265–272.

Czudek, C. & Reynolds, G.P. (1989) [3H] GBR 12935 binding to the dopamine uptake site in post-mortem brain tissue in schizophrenia. *Journal of Neural Transmission* **77**, 227–230.

Daniel, D.G., Weinberger, D.R., Jones, D.W. *et al.* (1991) The effect of amphetamine on regional cerebral blood flow during cognitive activation in schizophrenia. *Journal of Neuroscience* **11**, 1907–1917.

Davis, K.L., Kahn, R.S., Ko, G. & Davidson, M. (1991) Dopamine in schizophrenia: a review and reconceptualization. *American Journal of Psychiatry* **148**, 1474–1486.

Dean, B., Pavey, G. & Opeskin, K. (1997) [3H]raclopride binding to brain tissue from subjects with schizophrenia: methodological aspects. *Neuropharmacology* **36**, 779–786.

Deutch, A., Clark, W.A. & Roth, R.H. (1990) Prefrontal cortical dopamine depletion enhances the responsiveness of the mesolimbic dopamine neurons to stress. *Brain Research* **521**, 311–315.

Dolan, R.J., Fletcher, P, Frith, C.D., Friston, K.J., Frackowiak, R.S. & Grasby, P.M. (1995) Dopaminergic modulation of impaired cognitive activation in the anterior cingulate cortex in schizophrenia. *Nature* **378**, 180–182.

Dumartin, B., Jaber, M., Gonon, F, Caron, M.G., Giros, B. & Bloch, B. (2000) Dopamine tone regulates D1 receptor trafficking and delivery in striatal neurons in dopamine transporter-deficient mice. *Proceedings of the National Academy of Sciences USA* **97**, 1879–1884.

Dunah, A.W. & Standaert, D.G. (2001) Dopamine D1 receptor-dependent trafficking of striatal NMDA glutamate receptors to the postsynaptic membrane. *Journal of Neuroscience* **21**, 5546–5558.

Egan, M.F., Goldberg, T.E., Kolachana, B.S. *et al.* (2001) Effect of COMT Val108/158 Met genotype on frontal lobe function and risk for schizophrenia. *Proceedings of the National Academy of Sciences USA* **98**, 6917–6922.

Engel, A.K. & Singer, W. (2001) Temporal binding and the neural correlates of sensory awareness. *Trends in Cognitive Science* **5**, 16–25.

Engel, A.K., Fries, P. & Singer, W. (2001) Dynamic predictions: Oscillations and synchrony in top-down processing. *Nature Reviews Neuroscience* **2**, 704–716.

Fauchey, V., Jaber, M., Caron, M.G., Bloch, B. & Le Moine, C. (2000) Differential regulation of the dopamine D1, D2 and D3 receptor gene expression and changes in the phenotype of the striatal neurons in mice lacking the dopamine transporter. *European Journal of Neuroscience* **12**, 19–26.

Flores-Hernandez, J., Cepeda, C., Hanandez-Echeagaray, E. *et al.* (2002) Dopamine enhancement of NMDA currents in dissociated medium-sized striatal neurons: role of D1 receptors and DARPP-32. *Journal Neurophysiology* **88**, 3010–3020.

Floresco, S.B., Todd, C.L. & Grace, A.A. (2001) Glutamatergic afferents from the hippocampus to the nucleus accumbens regulate activity of ventral tegmental area dopamine neurons. *Journal of Neuroscience* **21**, 4915–4922.

Floresco, S.B., West, A.R., Ash, B., Moore, H. & Grace, A.A. (2003) Afferent modulation of dopamine neuron firing differentially regulates tonic and phasic dopamine transmission. *Nature Neuroscience* **6**, 968–973.

Freeman, A.S., Meltzer, L.T. & Bunney, B.S. (1985) Firing properties of substantia nigra dopaminergic neurons in freely moving rats. *Life Science* **36**, 1983–1994.

Gallinat, J., Winterer, G., Herrman, C.S. & Senkowski, D. (2004) Reduced oscillatory gamma-band responses in unmedicated schizophrenic patients indicate impaired frontal network processing. *Clinical Neurophysiology* **115**, 1863–1874.

George, M.S., Molnar, C.E., Grenesko, E.L. *et al.* (2007) A single 20 mg dose of dihydrexidine (DAR-0100), a full dopamine D1 agonist, is safe and tolerated in patients with schizophrenia. *Schizophrenia Research* **93**, 42–50.

Goldberg, T.E. & Weinberger, D.R. (2004) Genes and the parsing of cognitive processes. *Trends in Cognitive Sciences* **8**, 325–335.

Goldman-Rakic, P.S. (1994) Working memory dysfunction in schizophrenia. *Journal of Neuropsychiatry Clinical Neuroscience* **6**, 348–357.

Goldman-Rakic, P.S. (1995) Cellular basis of working memory. *Neuron* **14**, 477–485.

Goldman-Rakic, P.S., Lidow, M.S., Smiley, J.F. & Williams, M.S. (1992) The anatomy of dopamine in monkeys and human prefrontal cortex. *Journal of Neural Transmission* **36** (Suppl.), 163–177.

Goldman-Rakic, P.S., Muly, E.C., 3rd & Williams, G.V. (2000) D(1) receptors in prefrontal cells and circuits. *Brain Research and Brain Research Reviews* **31**, 295–301.

Gorelova, N., Seamans, J.K. & Yang, C.R. (2002) Mechanisms of dopamine activation of fast-spiking interneurons that exert inhibition in rat prefrontal cortex. *Journal of Neurophysiology* **88**, 3150–3166.

Goto, Y. & Grace, A.A. (2005) Dopaminergic modulation of limbic and cortical drive of nucleus accumbens in goal-directed behavior. *Nature Neuroscience* **8**, 805–812.

Goto, Y. & Grace, A.A. (2006) Alterations in medial prefrontal cortical activity and plasticity in rats with disruption of cortical development. *Biological Psychiatry* **60**, 253–264.

Goto, Y., Otani, S. & Grace, A.A. (2007) The Yin and Yang of dopamine release: a new perspective. *Neuropharmacology* **53**, 583–587.

Grace, A.A. (1991) Phasic versus tonic dopamine release and the modulation of dopamine system responsivity: a hypothesis for the etiology of schizophrenia. *Neuroscience* **41**, 1–24.

Grace, A.A. (1993) Cortical regulation of subcortical dopamine systems and its possible relevance to schizophrenia. *Journal of Neural Transmission—General Section* **91**, 111–134.

Grace, A.A. (1995) The tonic/phasic model of dopamine system regulation: its relevance for understanding how stimulant abuse can alter basal ganglia function. *Drug & Alcohol Dependence* **37**, 111–129.

Grace, A.A. & Bunney, B.S. (1979) Paradoxical GABA excitation of nigral dopaminergic cells: indirect mediation through reticulata inhibitory neurons. *European Journal of Pharmacology* **59**, 211–218.

Grace, A.A. & Bunney, B.S. (1984a) The control of firing pattern in nigral dopamine neurons: burst firing. *Journal of Neuroscience* **4**, 2877–2890.

Grace, A.A. & Bunney, B. S. (1984b) The control of firing pattern in nigral dopamine neurons: single spike firing. *Journal of Neuroscience* **4**, 2866–2876.

Grace, A.A. & Bunney, B. S. (1985) Opposing effects of striatonigral feedback pathways on midbrain dopamine cell activity. *Brain Research* **333**, 271–284.

Grace, A.A. & Bunney, B.S. (1986) Induction of depolarization block in midbrain dopamine neurons by repeated administration of haloperidol: analysis using in vivo intracellular recording. *Journal of Pharmacology & Experimental Therapeutics* **238**, 1092–1100.

Grace, A.A. & Moore, H. (1998) Regulation of information flow in the nucleus accumbens: A model for the pathophysiology of schizophrenia. In: Lenzenweger, M.F. & Dworkin, R.H., eds. *Origins and Development of Schizophrenia: Advances in Experimental Psychopathology*. Washington D.C.: American Psychological Association Press.

Grace, A.A. & Onn, S.P. (1989) Morphology and electrophysiological properties of immunocytochemically identified rat dopamine neurons recorded in vitro. *Journal of Neuroscience* **9**, 3463–3481.

Grace, A.A., Bunney, B.S., Moore, H. & Todd, C.L. (1997) Dopamine-cell depolarization block as a model for the therapeutic actions of antipsychotic drugs. *Trends in Neurosciences* **20**, 31–37.

Grace, A.A., Floresco, S.B., Goto, Y. & Lodge, D.J. (2007) Regulation of firing of dopaminergic neurons and control of goal-directed behaviors. *Trends in Neuroscience* **30**, 220–227.

Guillin, O., Diaz, J., Carroll, P., Griffon, N., Schwartz, J.C. & Sokoloff, P. (2001) BDNF controls dopamine D3 receptor expression and triggers behavioural sensitization. *Nature* **411**, 86–89.

Guo, N., Hwang, D., Abdellhadi, S., Abi-Dargham, A., Zarahn, E. & Laruelle, M. (2001) The effect of chronic DA depletion on D1 ligand binding in rodent brain. *Society of Neurosciences Abstracts* **27**.

Gurevich, E.V., Bordelon, Y., Shapiro, R.M., Arnold, S.E., Gur R.E. & Joyce, J.N. (1997) Mesolimbic dopamine D3 receptors and use of antipsychotics in patients with schizophrenia. A postmortem study. *Archives of General Psychiatry* **54**, 225–232.

Haber, S.N., Fudge, J.L. & McFarland, N.R. (2000) Striatonigrostriatal pathways in primates form an ascending spiral from the shell to the dorsolateral striatum. *Journal of Neuroscience* **20**, 2369–2382.

Harden, D.G. & Grace, A.A. (1995) Activation of dopamine cell firing by repeated L-DOPA administration to dopamine-depleted rats: its potential role in mediating the therapeutic response to L-DOPA treatment. *Journal of Neuroscience* **15**, 6157–6166.

Hashimoto, T., Bergen, S.E., Nguyen, Q.L. *et al.* (2005) Relationship of brain-derived neurotrophic factor and its receptor TrkB to altered inhibitory prefrontal circuitry in schizophrenia. *Journal of Neuroscience* **25**, 372–383.

Hashimoto, T., Arion, D., Unger, T. *et al.* (2008) Alterations in GABA-related transcriptome in the dorsolateral prefrontal cortex of subjects with schizophrenia. *Molecular Psychiatry* **13**, 147–161.

Heckers, S., Rauch, S.L., Goff, D. *et al.* (1998) Impaired recruitment of the hippocampus during conscious recollection in schizophrenia. *Nature Neuroscience* **1**, 318–323.

Heckers, S., Stone, D., Walsh, J., Shick, J., Koul, P. & Benes, F.M. (2002) Differential hippocampal expression of glutamic acid decarboxylase 65 and 67 messenger RNA in bipolar disorder and schizophrenia. *Archives of General Psychiatry* **59**, 521–529.

Herrmann, C.S. & Demiralp, T. (2005) Human EEG gamma oscillations in neuropsychiatric disorders. *Clinical Neurophysiology* **116**, 2719–2733.

Hess, E.J., Bracha, H.S., Kleinman, J.E. & Creese, I. (1987) Dopamine receptor subtype imbalance in schizophrenia. *Life Science* **40**, 1487–1497.

Hirai, M., Kitamura, N., Hashimoto, T. *et al.* (1988) [3H]GBR-12935 binding sites in human striatal membranes: binding characteristics and changes in parkinsonians and schizophrenics. *Japanese Journal of Pharmacology* **47**, 237–243.

Hollerman, J.R. & Grace, A.A. (1989) Acute haloperidol administration induces depolarization block of nigral dopamine neurons in rats after partial dopamine lesions. *Neuroscience Letters* **96**, 82–88.

Hollerman, J.R. & Grace, A.A. (1990) The effects of dopamine-depleting brain lesions on the electrophysiological activity of rat substantia nigra dopamine neurons. *Brain Research* **533**, 203–212.

Hollerman, J.R., Abercrombie, E.D. & Grace, A.A. (1992) Electrophysiological, biochemical, and behavioral studies of acute haloperidol-induced depolarization block of nigral dopamine neurons. *Neuroscience* **47**, 589–601.

Hornykiewicz, O. (1962) [Dopamine (3-hydroxytyramine) in the central nervous system and its relation to the Parkinson syndrome in man.]. *Deutsch Medizin Wochenschrift* **87**, 1807–1810.

Jaskiw, G.E., Karoum, F., Freed, W.J., Phillips, I., Kleinman, J.E. & Weinberger, D.R. (1990) Effect of ibotenic acid lesions of the medial prefrontal cortex on amphetamine-induced locomotion and regional brain catecholamine concentrations in the rat. *Brain Research* **534**, 263–272.

Jaskiw, G.E., Weinberger, D.R. & Crawley, J.N. (1991) Microinjection of apomorphine into the prefrontal cortex of the rat reduces dopamine metabolite concentrations in microdialysate from the caudate nucleus. *Biological Psychiatry* **29**, 703–706.

Jentsch, J.D. & Roth, R.H. (1999) The neuropsychopharmacology of phencyclidine: from NMDA receptor hypofunction to the dopamine hypothesis of schizophrenia. *Neuropsychopharmacology* **20**, 201–225.

Jentsch, J.D., Elsworth, J.D., Redmond, D.E. Jr, Roth, R.H. (1997) Phencyclidine increases forebrain monoamine metabolism in rats and monkeys: modulation by the isomers of HA966, *Journal of Neuroscience* **17**, 1769–1775.

Johnstone, E.C., Crow, T.J., Frith, C.D., Carne, M.W.P. & Price, J.S. (1978) Mechanism of the antipsychotic effect in the treatment of acute schizophrenia. *Lancet* **1**, 848–851.

Joyce, J.N., Lexow, N., Bird, E. & Winokur, A. (1988) Organization of dopamine D1 and D2 receptors in human striatum: receptor autoradiographic studies in Huntington's disease and schizophrenia. *Synapse* **2**, 546–557.

Kakiuchi, T., Nishiyama, S., Sato, K., Ohba, H., Nakanishi, S. & Tsukada, H. (2001) Effect of MK801 on dopamine parameters in the monkey brain. *Neuroimage* **16**, 110.

Kahn, R.S., Harvey, P.D., Davidson, M. *et al.* (1994) Neuropsychological correlates of central monoamine function in chronic schizophrenia: relationship between CSF metabolites and cognitive function. *Schizophrenia Research* **11**, 217–224.

Kaiser, J. & Lutzenberger, W. (2003) Induced gamma-band activity and human brain function. *Neuroscientist* **9**, 475–585.

Karlsson, P., Farde, I., Hallidin, C. & Sedvall, G. (1997) D$_1$-dopamine receptors in schizophrenia examined by PET. *Schizophrenia Research* **24**, 179.

Karreman, M. & Moghaddam, B. (1996) The prefrontal cortex regulates the basal release of dopamine in the limbic striatum: an effect mediated by ventral tegmental area. *Journal of Neurochemistry* **66**, 589–598.

Kegeles, L., Frankle, W., Gil, R. *et al.* (2006) Schizophrenia is associated with increased synaptic dopamine in associative rather than limbic regions of the striatum: Implications for mechanisms of action of antipschotic drugs. *Journal of Nuclear Medicine* 139P.

Kegeles, L.S., Slifstein, M., Frankle, W.G *et al.* (2008) Dose-occupancy study of striatal and etrastriatal dopamine D(2) receptors by aripiprazole in schizophrenia with PET and [(18) F]fallypride. *Neuropsychopharmacology* **33**, 3111–3125.

Kellendonk, C., Simpson, E.H., Polan, H.J. *et al.* (2006) Transient and selective overexpression of dopamine D2 receptors in the striatum causes persistent abnormalities in prefrontal cortex functioning. *Neuron* **49**, 603–615.

Kerwin, R., Millet, B., Herman, E. *et al.* (2007) A multicentre, randomized, naturalistic, open-label study between aripiprazole and standard of care in the management of community-treated schizophrenic patients Schizophrenia Trial of Aripiprazole: (STAR) study. *European Psychiatry* **22**, 433–443.

Knable, M.B. & Weinberger, D.R. (1997) Dopamine, the prefrontal cortex and schizophrenia. *Journal of Psychopharmacology* **11**, 123–131.

Knable, M.B., Hyde, T.M., Herman, M.M., Carter, J.M., Bigelow, L. & Kleinman, J.E. (1994) Quantitative autoradiography of dopamine-D1 receptors, D2 receptors, and dopamine uptake sites in postmortem striatal specimens from schizophrenic patients. *Biological Psychiatry* **36**, 827–835.

Knable, M.B., Hyde, T.M., Murray, A.M., Herman, M.M. & Kleinman, J.E. (1996) A postmortem study of frontal cortical dopamine D1 receptors in schizophrenics, psychiatric controls, and normal controls. *Biological Psychiatry* **40**, 1191–1199.

Kolachana, B.S., Saunders, R. & Weinberger, D. (1995) Augmentation of prefrontal cortex monoaminergic activity inhibits dopamine release in the caudate nucleus: an *in vivo* neurochemical assessment in the rhesus monkey. *Neurosciences* **69**, 858–868.

Kramer, M.S., Last, B., Getson, A. & Reines, S.A. (1997) The effects of a selective D4 dopamine receptor antagonist (L-745,870) in acutely psychotic inpatients with schizophrenia. D4 Dopamine Antagonist Group. *Archives of General Psychiatry*, **54**, 567–572.

Krystal, J.H., D'Souza, D.C., Gallinat, J. *et al.* (2006) The vulnerability to alcohol and substance abuse in individuals diagnosed with schizophrenia. *Neurotoxicology Research* **10**, 235–252.

Laakso, A., Vilkman, H., Alakare, B. *et al.* (2000) Striatal dopamine transporter binding in neuroleptic-naive patients with schizophrenia studied with positron emission tomography. *American Journal of Psychiatry* **157**, 269–271.

Laakso, A., Bergman, J., Haaparanta, M. *et al.* (2001) Decreased striatal dopamine transporter binding in vivo in chronic schizophrenia. *Schizophrenia Research* **52**, 115–120.

Lahti, R.A., Roberts, R.C., Conley, R.R., Cochrane, E.V., Mutin, A. & Tamminga, C.A. (1996) D2-type dopamine receptors in postmortem human brain sections from normal and schizophrenic subjects. *Neuroreport* **7**, 1945–1948.

Lahti, R.A., Roberts, R.C., Cochrane, E.V. *et al.* (1998) Direct determination of dopamine D4 receptors in normal and schizophrenic postmortem brain tissue: a [3H]NGD-94-1 study. *Molecular Psychiatry* **3**, 528–533.

Laruelle, M. (2000a) Imaging synaptic neurotransmission with in vivo binding competition techniques: a critical review. *Journal of Cerebral Blood Flow and Metabolism* **20**, 423–451.

Laruelle, M. (2000b) The role of endogenous sensitization in the pathophysiology of schizophrenia: implications from recent brain imaging studies. *Brain Research and Brain Research Reviews* **31**, 371–384.

Laruelle, M., Casanova, M., Weinberger, D. & Kleinman, J. (1990) Postmortem study of the dopaminergic D1 receptors in the dorsolateral prefrontal cortex of schizophrenics and controls. *Schizophrenia Research* **3**, 30–31.

Laruelle, M., Abi-Dargham, A., van Dyck, C.H. *et al.* (1996) Single photon emission computerized tomography imaging of amphetamine-induced dopamine release in drug-free schizophrenic subjects. *Proceedings of the National Academy of Sciences USA* **93**, 9235–9240.

Laruelle, M., Abi-Dargham, A., Gil, R., Kegeles, L. & Innis, R. (1999) Increased dopamine transmission in schizophrenia: relationship to illness phases. *Biological Psychiatry* **46**, 56–72.

Lavalaye, J., Linszen, D.H., Booij, J. *et al.* (2001) Dopamine transporter density in young patients with schizophrenia assessed with [123]FP-CIT SPECT. *Schizophrenia Research* **47**, 59–67.

Lavin, A. & Grace, A.A. (1997) Effects of afferent stimulation and DA application on prefrontal cortical cells recorded intracellularly *in vivo*: Comparisons between intact rats and rats with pharmacologically-induced disruption of cortical development. *Society for Neuroscience Abstracts* **23**, 2080.

Lavin, A. & Grace, A.A. (2001) Stimulation of D1-type dopamine receptors enhances excitability in prefrontal cortical pyramidal neurons in a state-dependent manner. *Neuroscience* **104**, 335–346.

Lavin, A., Moore, H.M., Grace, A.A., Lavin, A., Moore, H.M. & Grace, A.A. (2005) Prenatal disruption of neocortical development alters prefrontal cortical neuron responses to dopamine in adult rats. *Neuropsychopharmacology* **30**, 1426–1435.

Laviolette, S.R., Lipski, W.J. & Grace, A.A. (2005) A subpopulation of neurons in the medial prefrontal cortex encodes emotional learning with burst and frequency codes through a dopamine D4 receptor-dependent basolateral amygdala input. *Journal of Neuroscience* **25**, 6066–6075.

Laviolette, S.R., Grace, A.A., Laviolette, S.R. & Grace, A.A. (2006) Cannabinoids P potentiate emotional learning plasticity in neurons of the medial prefrontal cortex through basolateral amygdala inputs. *Journal of Neuroscience* **26**, 6458–6468.

Lee, T., Seeman, P., Tourtellotte, W.W., Farley, I.J. & Hornykeiwicz, O. (1978) Binding of 3H-neuroleptics and 3H-apomorphine in schizophrenic brains. *Nature* **274**, 897–900.

Le Foll, B., Frances, H., Diaz, J., Schwartz, J.C. & Sokoloff, P. (2002) Role of the dopamine D3 receptor in reactivity to cocaine-associated cues in mice. *European Journal of Neuroscience* **15**, 2016–2026.

Lewis, D.A., Cruz, D.A., Melchitzky, D.S. & Pierri, J.N. (2001) Lamina-specific deficits in parvalbumin-immunoreactive varicosities in the prefrontal cortex of subjects with schizophrenia: evidence for fewer projections from the thalamus. *American Journal of Psychiatry* **158**, 1411–1414.

Lewis, D.A., Hashimoto, T. & Volk, D.W. (2005) Cortical inhibitory neurons and schizophrenia. *Nature Review Neuroscience* **6**, 312–324.

Lieberman, J.A., Kane, J.M. & Alvir, J. (1987) Provocative tests with psychostimulant drugs in schizophrenia. *Psychopharmacology* **91**, 415–433.

Lodge, D.J. & Grace, A.A. (2006a) The hippocampus modulates dopamine neuron responsivity by regulating the intensity of phasic neuron activation. *Neuopsychopharmacology* **31**, 1356–1361.

Lodge, D.J. & Grace, A.A. (2006b) The laterodorsal tegmentum is essential for burst firing of ventral tegmental area dopamine neurons. *Proceedings of the National Academy of Sciences USA* **103**, 5167–5172.

Lodge, D.J. & Grace, A.A. (2007) Aberrant hippocampal activity underlies the dopamine dysregulation in an animal model of schizophrenia. *Journal of Neuroscience* **27**, 11424–11430.

Lodge, D.J., Behrens, M.M. & Grace, A.A. (2008) A reduction in hippocampal and prefrontal cortical gamma oscillatory activity is associated with a decrease in parvalbumin interneurons in the MAM model of schizophrenia. *Program No. 657.2, 2008 Neuroscience Meeting Planner*. Washington, DC: Society for Neuroscience.

Mackay, A.V., Iversen, L.L., Rossor, M. *et al.* (1982) Increased brain dopamine and dopamine receptors in schizophrenia. *Archives of General Psychiatry* **39**, 991–997.

Marzella, P.L., Hill, C., Keks, N., Singh, B. & Copolov, D. (1997) The binding of both [3H]nemonapride and [3H]raclopride is increased in schizophrenia. *Biological Psychiatry* **42**, 648–654.

Mayer, M.L., Westbrook, G.L. & Guthrie, P.B. (1984) Voltage-dependent block by Mg2+ of NMDA responses in spinal cord neurones. *Nature* **309**, 261–263.

McGowan, S., Lawrence, A.D., Sales, T., Quested, D. & Grasby, P. (2004) Presynaptic dopaminergic dysfunction in schizophrenia: a positron emission tomographic [18F]fluorodopa study. *Archives of General Psychiatry* **61**, 134–142.

Medoff, D.R., Holcomb, H.H., Lahti, A.C. & Tamminga, C.A. (2001) Probing the human hippocampus using rCBF: contrasts in schizophrenia. *Hippocampus* **11**, 543–550.

Meyer-Lindenberg, A., Miletich, R.S., Kohn, P.D *et al.* (2002) Reduced prefrontal activity predicts exaggerated striatal dopaminergic function in schizophrenia. *Nature Neuroscience* **5**, 267–271.

Meyer-Lindenberg, A.S., Olsen, R.K., Kohn, P.D. *et al.* (2005) Regionally specific disturbance of dorsolateral prefrontal-hippocampal functional connectivity in schizophrenia. *Archives of General Psychiatry* **62**, 379–386.

Mita, T., Hanada, S., Nishino, N. *et al.* (1986) Decreased serotonin S2 and increased dopamine D2 receptors in chronic schizophrenics. *Biological Psychiatry* **21**, 1407–1414.

Mogenson, G.J., Brudzynski, S.M., Wu, M., Yang, C.R. & Yim, C.C.Y. (1993) From motivation to action: a review of dopaminergic regulation of limbic -> nucleus accumbens -> ventral pallidum -> pedunculopontine nucleus circuitries involved in limbic-motor integration. In: Kalivas, P.W. & Barnes, C.W., eds. *Limbic Motor Circuits and Neuropsychiatry*. Boca Raton, CRC.

Montague, P.R., Hyman, S.E. & Cohen, J.D. (2004) Computational roles for dopamine in behavioural control. *Nature* **431**, 760–767.

Moore, H., Lavin, A. & Grace, A.A. (1998) Interactions between dopamine and NMDA delivered locally by microdialysis during in vivo intracellular recording of rat prefrontal cortical neurons. *Society for Neuroscience Abstracts* **24**, 2061.

Moore, H., Jentsch, J.D., Ghajarnia, M., Geyer, M.A. & Grace, A.A. (2006) A neurobehavioral systems analysis of adult rats exposed to methylazoxymethanol acetate on E17: implications for the neuropathology of schizophrenia. *Biological Psychiatry* **60**, 253–264.

Murray, A.M., Hyde, T.M., Knable, M.B. *et al.* (1995) Distribution of putative D4 dopamine receptors in postmortem striatum from patients with schizophrenia. *Journal of Neuroscience* **15**, 2186–2191.

Narendran, R., Frankle, W.G., Keefe, R. *et al.* (2005) Altered prefrontal dopaminergic function in chronic recreational ketamine users. *American Journal of Psychiatry* **162**, 2352–2359.

O'Donnell, P. & Grace, A.A. (1994) Tonic D2-mediated attenuation of cortical excitation in nucleus accumbens neurons recorded in vitro. *Brain Research* **634**, 105–112.

O'Donnell, P. & Grace, A.A. (1998) Dysfunctions in multiple interrelated systems as the neurobiological bases of schizophrenia: Symptom clusters. *Schizophrenia Bulletin* **24**, 267–283.

O'Donnell, P., Lewis, B.L., Weinberger, D.R. & Lipska, B.K. (2002) Neonatal hippocampal damage alters electrophysiological properties of prefrontal cortical neurons in adult rats. *Cerebral Cortex* **12**, 975–982.

Okubo, Y., Suhara, T., Suzuki, K. *et al.* (1997) Decreased prefrontal dopamine D1 receptors in schizophrenia revealed by PET. *Nature* **385**, 634–636.

Onn, S.P., West, A.R. & Grace, A.A. (2000) Dopamine-mediated regulation of striatal neuronal and network interactions. *Trends in Neuroscience* **23**, S48–56.

Ounsted, C. & Lindsay, J. (1981) Epilepsy and psychiatry. In: Reynolds, E.H., & Trinble, M.R., eds. *A Textbook of Epilepsy*. Edinburgh: Churchill Livingstone.

Overton, P. & Clark, D. (1992) Iontophoretically administered drugs acting at the N-methyl-D-aspartate receptor modulate burst firing in A9 dopamine neurons in the rat. *Synapse* **10**, 131–140.

Owen, F., Cross, A.J., Crow, T.J., Longden, A., Poulter, M. & Riley, G.J. (1978) Increased dopamine-receptor sensitivity in schizophrenia. *Lancet* **2**, 223–226.

Pearce, R.K., Seeman, P., Jellinger, K. & Tourtellotte, W.W. (1990) Dopamine uptake sites and dopamine receptors in Parkinson's disease and schizophrenia. *European Neurology* **30** (Suppl. 1), 9–14.

Pimoule, C., Schoemaker, H., Reynolds, G.P. & Langer, S.Z. (1985) [3H]SCH 23390 labeled D1 dopamine receptors are unchanged in schizophrenia and Parkinson's disease. *European Journal of Pharmacology* **114**, 235–237.

Pycock, C.J., Kerwin, R.W. & Carter, C.J. (1980) Effect of lesion of cortical dopamine terminals on subcortical dopamine receptors in rats. *Nature* **286**, 74–77.

Ragozzino, M.E. (2007) The contribution of the medial prefrontal cortex, orbitofrontal cortex, and dorsomedial striatum to behavioral flexibility. *Annals of the New York Academy of Science* **1121**, 355–375.

Reynolds, G.P. (1983) Increased concentrations and lateral asymmetry of amygdala dopamine in schizophrenia. *Nature* **305**, 527–529.

Reynolds, G.P. (1989) Beyond the dopamine hypothesis. The neurochemical pathology of schizophrenia. *British Journal of Psychiatry* **155**, 305–316.

Reynolds, G.P. & Czudek, C. (1988) Status of the dopaminergic system in post-mortem brain in schizophrenia. *Psychopharmacology Bulletin* **24**, 345–347.

Reynolds, G.P. & Mason, S.L. (1994) Are striatal dopamine D4 receptors increased in schizophrenia? *Journal of Neurochemistry* **63**, 1576–1577.

Reynolds, G.P., Czudek, C., Bzowej, N. & Seeman, P. (1987) Dopamine receptor asymmetry in schizophrenia. *Lancet* **1**, 979.

Roberts, A.C., Desalvia, M.A., Wilkinson, L.S. *et al.* (1994) 6-hydroxydopamine lesions of the prefrontal cortex in monkeys enhance performance on an analog of the Wisconsin card sort test: possible interactions with subcortical dopamine. *Journal of Neuroscience* **14**, 2531–2544.

Rossum, V. (1966) The significance of dopamine receptor blockade for the mechanism of action of neuroleptic drugs. *Archives of International Pharmacodynamic Therapy* **160**, 492–494.

Ruiz, J., Gabilondo, A.M., Meana, J.J. & Garcia-Sevilla, J.A. (1992) Increased [3H] raclopride binding sites in postmortem brains from schizophrenic violent suicide victims. *Psychopharmacology (Berlin)* **109**, 410–414.

Schmitt, G.J., Meisenzahl, E.M., Frodl, T. *et al.* (2005) The striatal dopamine transporter in first-episode, drug-naive schizophrenic patients: evaluation by the new SPECT-ligand[99mTc] TRODAT-1. *Journal of Psychopharmacology* **19**, 488–493.

Schoots, O., Seeman, P., Guan, H.C., Paterson, A.D. & van Tol, H.H. (1995) Long-term haloperidol elevates dopamine D4 receptors by 2-fold in rats. *European Journal of Pharmacology* **289**, 67–72.

Schultz, W. (1998) The phasic reward signal of primate dopamine neurons. *Advances in Pharmacology* **42**, 686–690.

Scott, L., Kruse, M.S., Forssberg, H., Brismar, H., Greengard, P. & Aperia, A. (2002) Selective up-regulation of dopamine D1 receptors in dendritic spines by NMDA receptor activation. *Proceedings of the National Academy of Sciences, USA* **99**, 1661–1664.

Seeman, P., Guan, H.C. & van Tol, H.H. (1993) Dopamine D4 receptors elevated in schizophrenia. *Nature* **365**, 441–445.

Seeman, P., Chau-Wong, M., Tedesco, J. & Wong, K. (1975) Brain receptors for antipsychotic drugs and dopamine: direct binding assays. *Proceedings of the National Academy of Science USA* **72**, 4376–4380.

Seeman, P., Ulpian, C., Bergeron, C. *et al.* (1984) Bimodal distribution of dopamine receptor densities in brains of schizophrenics. *Science* **225**, 728–731.

Seeman, P., Bzowej, N.H., Guan, H.C. *et al.* (1987) Human brain D1 and D2 dopamine receptors in schizophrenia, Alzheimer's, Parkinson's, and Huntington's diseases. *Neuropsychopharmacology* **1**, 5–15.

Sesack, S.R. & Bunney, B.S. (1989) Pharmacological characterization of the receptor mediating electrophysiological responses to dopamine in the rat medial prefrontal cortex: a microiontophoretic study. *Journal of Pharmacology and Experimental Therapeutics* **248**, 1323–1333.

Sesack, S., Hawrylak, V., Matus, C., Guido, M. & Levey, A. (1998) Dopamine axon varicosities in the prelimbic division of the rat prefrontal cortex exhibit sparse immunoreactivity for the dopamine transporter. *Journal of Neuroscience* **18**, 2697–2708.

Silbersweig, D.A., Stern, E., Frith, C. *et al.* (1995) A functional neuroanatomy of hallucinations in schizophrenia. *Nature* **378**, 176–179.

Slifstein, M., Kolachana, B., Simpson, E.H. *et al.* (2008) COMT genotype predicts cortical-limbic D1 receptor availability measured with [(11)C]NNC112 and PET. *Molecular Psychiatry* **13**, 821–827.

Sumiyoshi, T., Stockmeier, C.A., Overholser, J.C., Thompson, P.A. & Meltzer, H.Y. (1995) Dopamine D4 receptors and effects of guanine nucleotides on [3H]raclopride binding in postmortem caudate nucleus of subjects with schizophrenia or major depression. *Brain Research* **681**, 109–116.

Takahashi, M., Shirakawa, O., Toyooka, K. *et al.* (2000) Abnormal expression of brain-derived neurotrophic factor and its receptor in the corticolimbic system of schizophrenic patients. *Molecular Psychiatry* **5**, 293–300.

Tarazi, F.I., Florijn, W.J. & Creese, I. (1997) Differential regulation of dopamine receptors after chronic typical and atypical antipsychotic drug treatment. *Neuroscience* **78**, 985–996.

Taylor, S.F., Koeppe, R.A., Tandon, R., Zubieta, J.K. & Frey, K.A. (2000) *In vivo* measurement of the vesicular monoamine transporter in schizophrenia. *Neuropsychopharmacology* **23**, 667–675.

Thompson, T.L. & Moss, R.L. (1995) In vivo stimulated dopamine release in the nucleus accumbens: modulation by the prefrontal cortex. *Brain Research* **686**, 93–98.

Tzschentke, T.M. (2001) Pharmacology and behavioral pharmacology of the mesocortical dopamine system. *Progress in Neurobiology* **63**, 241–320.

Tsukada, H., Miyasato, K., Nishiyama, S., Fukumoto, D., Kakiuchi, T. & Domino, E.F. (2005) Nicotine normalizes increased prefrontal cortical dopamine D1 receptor binding and decreased working memory performance produced by repeated pretreatment with MK-801: a PET study in conscious monkeys. *Neuropsychopharmacology* **30**, 2144–2153.

Tunbridge, E.M., Harrison, P.J. & Weinberger, D.R. (2006) Catechol-o-methyltransferase, cognition and psychosis: Val158Met and beyond. *Biological Psychiatry* **60**, 141–151.

Weickert, C.S., Hyde, T.M., Lipska, B.K., Herman, M.M., Weinberger, D.R. & Kleinman, J.E. (2003) Reduced brain-derived neurotrophic factor in prefrontal cortex of patients with schizophrenia. *Molecular Psychiatry* **8**, 592–610.

Weinberger, D.R. (1987) Implications of the normal brain development for the pathogenesis of schizophrenia. *Archives of General Psychiatry* **44**, 660–669.

Weinberger, D. & Laruelle, M. (2002) Neurochemical and neuropharmacological imaging in schizophrenia. In: *Neuropsychopharmacology: the Fifth Generation of Progress: An Official Publication of the American College of Neuropsychopharmacology.* Philadelphia: Lippincott/Williams & Wilkins.

Weinberger, D.R., Berman, K.F. & Illowsky, B.P. (1988) Physiological dysfunction of dorsolateral prefrontal cortex in schizophrenia. III. A new cohort and evidence for a monoaminergic mechanism. *Archives of General Psychiatry* **45**, 609–615.

Weinberger, D.R., Berman, K.F. & Daniel, D.G. (1992a) Mesoprefrontal cortical dopaminergic activity and prefrontal hypofunction in schizophrenia. *Clinical Neuropharmacology* **15**, 568A–569A.

Weinberger, D.R., Berman, K.F., Suddath, R. & Torrey, E.F. (1992b) Evidence of dysfunction of a prefrontal-limbic network in schizophrenia: a magnetic resonance imaging and regional cerebral blood flow study of discordant monozygotic twins. *American Journal of Psychiatry* **149**, 890–897.

Weinberger, D.R., Berman, K.F. & Torrey, E.F. (1992c) Correlations between abnormal hippocampal morphology and prefrontal physiology in schizophrenia. *Clinical Neuropharmacology* **15**, 393A–394A.

Weinberger, D.R., Berman, K.F., Ostrem, J.L., Abi-Dargham, A. & Torrey, E.F. (1993) Disorganization of prefrontal-hippocampal connectivity in schizophrenia: A PET study of discordant MZ twins. *Society for Neuroscience Abstracts* **19**, 7.

Weinshilboum, R.M., Otterness, D.M. & Szumlanski, C.L. (1999) Methylation pharmacogenetics: catechol O-methyltransferase, thiopurine methyltransferase, and histamine N-methyltransferase. *Annual Review of Pharmacology and Toxicology* **39**, 19–52.

Wilkinson, L.S. (1997) The nature of interactions involving prefrontal and striatal dopamine systems. *Journal of Psychopharmacology* **11**, 143–150.

Yamamoto, B.K. & Novotney, S. (1998) Regulation of extracellular dopamine by the norepinephrine transporter. *Journal of Neurochemistry* **71**, 274–280.

Yang, C.R. & Seamans, J.K. (1996) Dopamine D1 receptor actions in layers V-VI rat prefrontal cortex neurons *in vitro*: modulation of dendritic-somatic signal integration. *Journal of Neuroscience* **16**, 1922–1935.

Yang, C.R., Seamans, J.K. & Gorelova, N. (1999) Developing a neuronal model for the pathophysiology of schizophrenia based on the nature of electrophysiological actions of dopamine in the prefrontal cortex. *Neuropsychopharmacology* **21**, 161–194.

Yin, H.H., Ostlund, S.B. & Balleine, B.W. (2008) Reward-guided learning beyond dopamine in the nucleus accumbens: the integrative functions of cortico-basal ganglia networks. *European Journal of Neuroscience* **28**, 1437–1448.

Zahrt, J., Taylor, J.R., Mathew, R.G. & Arnsten, A.F. (1997) Supranormal stimulation of D1 dopamine receptors in the rodent prefrontal cortex impairs spatial working memory performance. *Journal of Neuroscience* **17**, 8528–8535.

Zhang, Z.J. & Reynolds, G.P. (2002) A selective decrease in the relative density of parvalbumin-immunoreactive neurons in the hippocampus in schizophrenia. *Schizophrenia Research* **55**, 1–10.

CHAPTER 21

Contributions of glutamate and GABA systems to the neurobiology and treatment of schizophrenia

John H. Krystal[1] and Bita Moghaddam[2]

[1]Yale University School of Medicine, New Haven, CT, USA
[2]University of Pittsburgh, Pittsburgh, PA, USA

Amino acid neurotransmission emerged in the forefront of schizophrenia research after languishing in the shadow of monoaminergic research for several decades. The demonstration of increased striatal dopamine release in a subgroup of patients with schizophrenia and the efficacy of dopamine-2 (D_2) receptor antagonist antipsychotic medications are core elements of our understanding of this disorder (Guillin *et al.*, 2007). Yet these medications are not particularly effective for treating negative symptoms or cognitive impairments associated with schizophrenia and there are large numbers of patients who fail to show adequate antipsychotic responses. As the dopamine "story" evolved, there was increasing focus on the interrelatedness of dopaminergic systems and amino acid neurotransmission. This shift is fitting because glutamate neurotransmission is the primary thoroughfare for excitatory communication in the brain and thus, all disturbances in monoaminergic neurotransmission must ultimately be expressed as an alteration in glutamatergic function. Similarly, as the primary system moderating and tuning the impact of glutamatergic activation, γ-aminobutyric acid (GABA) neurons are implicated in nearly all neural processes that engage glutamate systems. In this chapter

we will consider the contributions of glutamate and GABA systems to the neurobiology and treatment of schizophrenia. In doing so, we will consider the issue of how disturbances in the two most widely distributed neural systems in the brain might give rise to the neural and clinical features of schizophrenia. We will further consider how these systems might be targeted by treatments for this disorder.

Glutamatergic and GABAergic neuropathology in schizophrenia

Glutamatergic neuropathology in schizophrenia

Reduced glutamate neural connectivity
The integrity of the connectivity of cortical pyramidal neurons, neurons that use glutamate as their transmitter, appears to be compromised in schizophrenia. The breadth and severity of schizophrenia symptoms contrasts with the minimal evidence of gross tissue pathology, such as gliosis, in postmortem tissue from individuals with schizophrenia (Alzheimer, 1907; Damadzic *et al.*, 2001; Falkai *et al.*, 1999; Harrison, 1999). However, quantitative postmortem and structural neuroimaging studies readily identified a pattern of widespread reductions in cortical gray and white matter volume, most prominent in the frontal and temporal cortices, accompanied by increased ventricular volume

(Harrison, 1999). These structural deficits appeared to emerge as an exaggeration of normal trajectories for the development and pruning of cortical gray and white matter (Rapoport & Gogtay, 2008; Thompson *et al.*, 2001), and the divergence in the volume of cortical gray and white matter between people with schizophrenia and healthy individuals continues throughout adulthood (Mathalon *et al.*, 2001). In postmortem studies, reduced size of dendritic fields is suggested by smaller neuronal size and increased neuronal packing density (Plate 21.1; Rajkowska *et al.*, 1998; Selemon *et al.*, 1998). Direct measurement found reduction in the size and complexity of pyramidal neuronal dendritic fields, particularly basilar dendrites, and reduction in the density of dendritic spines in frontal cortical postmortem tissue from individuals with schizophrenia (Black *et al.*, 2004; Garey *et al.*, 1998; Glantz & Lewis, 2000; Kalus *et al.*, 2000). These findings are discussed in more detail in Chapter 18.

Although the technique is still being refined, diffusion tensor imaging (DTI) studies of individuals with schizophrenia also suggest reductions in the magnitude or organization of white matter tracks, particularly the long axonal pathways (Burns *et al.*, 2003; Jones *et al.*, 2006; Kubicki *et al.*, 2002; Szeszko *et al.*, 2007; see Chapter 16). In the hippocampus, schizophrenia was associated with reductions in the number of synapses and decreases in the expression of synaptophysin, a synaptic marker (Eastwood and Harrison, 1995; Kolomeets *et al.*, 2005; Webster *et al.*, 2001). In the cortex, gene expression levels for synaptophysin has been reported to be normal, but immunoreactivity levels for synaptophysin are reduced (Eastwood & Harrison, 2001; Glantz *et al.*, 2000; Glantz & Lewis, 1997a,b).

Alterations in glutamate receptors

The studies of glutamate-related synaptic proteins are marked by a high degree of heterogeneity in their findings. In evaluating the findings related to gene expression levels, protein levels, and ligand binding levels for glutamate synaptic proteins, a number of caveats apply. Under the best of conditions, studies of human postmortem tissue reflect the long-term adaptations to a pathophysiological process in response to the combined effects of abnormal development of a particular system and the impact of the abnormal function of that system. However, studies of postmortem tissue of schizophrenia face many additional challenges related to the heterogeneity of the diagnosis of schizophrenia, age and stage of illness-related expression of tissue pathology, and the impact of comorbid psychiatric and substance abuse diagnoses, and exposure to a wide range of pharmacotherapeutic agents from a large number of drug classes, in varying combinations and doses, and for inconsistent periods of time. These challenges are further complicated by the variable quality of the postmortem tissue that serves as the basis for these studies. Addressing the impact of all of these modifying characteristics is beyond the scope of this review, but is an important challenge to moving this field forward. The reader is referred to a number of reviews that have attempted to address aspects of the complexity of the postmortem literature and Chapter 18 (Harrison, 2004; Harrison & Weinberger, 2005; Kristiansen *et al.*, 2007; Meador-Woodruff & Healy, 2000).

There are two principal classes of glutamate receptors: the ionotropic receptors that, when stimulated by glutamate, permit the entry of cations into the cell; and the metabotropic receptors that are coupled by G-proteins to signal transduction mechanisms. There are three pharmacologically-based classes of ionotropic glutamate receptors: *N*-methyl-D-aspartate (NMDA), α-amino-3-hydroxy-5-methyl-4-isoxazole propionic acid (AMPA), and kainate receptors.

NMDA receptors

NMDA receptors are stimulated when two molecules of glutamate and two molecules of glycine bind to a receptor that is "activated" by membrane depolarization, which removes Mg^{2+} from its cation channel (reviewed in Kew & Kemp, 2005; Krystal *et al.*, 2003d). Because of the dual regulation of NMDA receptors by coincident presynaptic (glutamate release) and postsynaptic (membrane potential) state, these receptors play a distinctive role in signaling concurrent convergent excitatory inputs, events with particular significance for the integration of neural network functions and the induction of neuroplasticity (Tsien, 2000; Yuste *et al.*, 1999). NMDA receptors are tetramers comprised of two NR1 subunits and two NR2 subunits (NR2A–NR2D), encoded by separate genes. Of these NR2 subunits, the NR2B is the most common form *in utero*. With development, it is somewhat displaced within synapses by the NR2A subunit (Stocca & Vicini, 1998). The NR2C subunit is notable because of its relatively high density in the cerebellum compared to other brain regions. The NR2D subunit is distinctive in that NMDA receptors bearing it have properties that might make it more responsive to glutamate than receptors bearing the NR2A or NR2B subunits, including greater affinity for glutamate (Erreger *et al.*, 2007), a rapid unblocking of receptors by Mg^{2+} (Clarke & Johnson, 2006), and a shorter opening time (Cheffings & Colquhoun, 2000). Thus, recent data suggest that among synapses where NR2D, NR2B, and NR2A subunit-containing receptors are present together, modest levels of neuronal activation result in more NR2D receptors stimulated relative to the other two classes (Hires *et al.*, 2008). The NR3A and NR3B subunits substitute for the NR1 subunit. It is has a widespread distribution in the brain *in utero*, but its expression markedly declines with development (Bendel *et al.*, 2005; Fukaya *et al.*, 2005). It is distinctive in that receptors bearing this subunit do not flux cations when stimulated by glutamate, i.e., when it is expressed it reduces glutamate function at NMDA receptors, but may be stimulated by glycine (Chatterton *et al.*, 2002; Matsuda *et al.*, 2003; Nishi *et al.*, 2001). Consistent with the idea that NR3-containing receptors have consequences that resemble the pharmacological effects of blocking NMDA receptors, deletion of the *NR3B* gene in mice is associated with increased social behavior in a familiar environment and increased reactivity to novelty (Niemann *et al.*, 2007).

Postmortem data do not describe consistent alterations in NMDA receptor density or levels of subunit gene expression. Table 21.1 presents a brief selected summary of postmortem results related to NMDA receptors (for reviews giving additional regional detail, see Kristiansen *et al.*, 2007; Krystal *et al.*, 2000a; Meador-Woodruff & Healy, 2000). Reductions in NMDA receptor populations in the prefrontal cortex (PFC) might be expected on the basis of the reduction in the number of PFC dendritic spines and reductions in gene expression for the postsynaptic density-95 (PSD-95) protein (Table 21.1). NMDA receptors are preferentially located on dendritic spines (Conti *et al.*, 1997) and anchored to the neural membrane by PSD-95; thus, reductions in spines or PSD-95 might be expected to reduce NMDA receptors. However, a number of compensatory changes might explain the lack of NMDA receptor reductions. For example, there is some degree of

mobility of NMDA receptor subunits and the postsynaptic density (PSD-95), in and out of dendritic spines (Sharma *et al.*, 2006). The absence of gross reductions in NMDA receptor density in brain regions with clear reductions in dendritic spines may suggest that, in these regions, there are compensatory increases in extrasynaptic NMDA receptors.

NMDA receptor deficits in schizophrenia have been suggested by *in vivo* neuroimaging studies. These studies are made possible by the development of a single photon emission computed tomography (SPECT) radiotracer, [^{123}I] CNS1261, an uncompetitive NMDA receptor antagonist (Bressan *et al.*, 2004). Using this tracer, reductions in ligand binding in medication-free schizophrenic patients was observed in the hippocampus (Pilowsky *et al.*, 2006), a region where reductions in NR1 subunit gene expression have been reported (see Table 21.1). Antipsychotic treatment, particularly with clozapine, attenuated this deficit (Bressan *et al.*, 2005). Because this radiotracer produces a use-dependent blockade of the channel, results generated using this approach may reflect both the absolute number of receptors at the cell membrane as well as their activity state. However, studies have not yet resolved whether deficits in schizophrenia primarily reflect a reduction in receptor number or alterations in the activation state of the receptor.

Table 21.1 Summaries of glutamate receptor subunit and synaptic proteins in schizophrenia using postmortem brain samples.

Receptors/subunits	NMDA					AMPA			Kainate			Metabotropic			PSD	
Region	NR1	NR:2A	2B	2D	NR3A	GluR1	R2	R4	GluR5	R7	KA1/2	GrpI	II	III	PSD-95	PSD-93
DLPFC																
Gene expression	↑↓	–		–	↑* ↑	↑–	↓–	↓–		↑	↓	–	–		↓–	–
Protein levels	–	–		– –								↑a	↑a		–	–
Ligand binding	–					↑b–			↓b–							
Hippocampus																
Gene expression	↓–	–	↑–	–		↓	↓		↓–	↓–	↓–	–				–
Protein levels	–					↓a	↓a								↓a↓–	–
Ligand binding	–					↓b–			↓b–							
Striatum	–	–		– –											↓	–
Protein levels												–	–	–		
Ligand binding	↑b–					↑b↓b–	–		–							

Up and down arrows, and dash reflect, respectively, increases, decreases, and the absence of group differences. Black reflects gene expression, [a]reflects protein levels, and [b]reflects ligand binding.
*In one report there was a relative, but not absolute, increase in NR2D gene expression (Akbarian et al., 1996).
DLPFC, dorso-lateral prefrontal cortex; NMDA, N-methyl- D-aspartate; AMPA, α-amino-3-hydroxy-5-methyl-4-isoxazole propionic acid; PSD, postsynaptic density protein.
Findings were abstracted from reviews (Kristiansen et al., 2007; Krystal et al., 2000a; Meador-Woodruff & Healy, 2000) and supplemented by data from individual studies (Benes et al., 2001; Beneyto et al., 2007; Beneyto & Meador-Woodruff, 2006; Crook et al., 2002; Dracheva et al., 2005; Gao et al., 2000; Gupta et al., 2005; Meador-Woodruff et al., 2001; Noga et al., 2001; Noga & Wang, 2002; O'Connor et al., 2007; Ohnuma et al., 1998; Ohnuma et al., 2000; Porter et al., 1997; Vawter et al., 2002).

AMPA receptors

AMPA receptors are directly activated by glutamate, i.e., unlike NMDA receptors, they do not require coincident depolarization of the membrane in which they reside. This property suits their widespread role in mediating glutamate-related neural excitation. Further, long-term potentiation and long-term depression of excitatory synaptic function induced by the stimulation of NMDA receptors appears to effect change, in part, by introducing AMPA receptors to or removing them from the postsynaptic membrane, respectively (Malinow & Malenka, 2002; Takahashi et al., 2003). AMPA receptors are tetramers comprised of GluR1–GluR4 subunits, each encoded by a separate gene (Greger et al., 2007). Each of these subunits may be spliced in alternative ways (flip/flop). A critical distinction among AMPA receptors is that receptors bearing the GluR2 subunit do not flux Ca^{2+} and thus are relatively less liable to contribute to neurotoxicity and have a more limited role in the induction of neuroplasticity (Liu & Zukin, 2007).

Kainate receptors

Kainate receptors are the least understood ionotropic receptor due to historical absence of drugs that distinguished kainate and AMPA receptor function. Kainate receptors are tetramers including the GluR5–GluR7, KA1, and KA2 subunits, encoded by separate genes. Most kainate receptors are ionotropic and contribute to excitation in roles that parallel AMPA receptors and to mossy fiber long-term potentiation in the hippocampus (Bortolotto et al., 2005; Lerma, 2006). However, receptors bearing the KA2 subunit can be metabotropic and inhibitory, a role mediated by coupling via Gi to the regulation of the phosphoinositol signal transduction pathway (Mellor, 2006; Rodriguez-Moreno & Sihra, 2007). For example, kainate receptors play important roles inhibiting GABA and glutamate release that contribute to the emergence of cortical oscillations (Fisahn, 2005).

Metabotropic glutamate receptors (mGluR)

These are typical G-protein coupled receptors and they have a widespread distribution with region-, pathway-, and receptor-specific localizations to neurons and glia, presynaptic and postsynaptic elements, and excitatory or inhibitory neurons (Schoepp & Conn, 2002). The eight receptors in this class are encoded by separate genes and are pharmacologically clustered into group I (mGluR1, mGluR5), group II (mGluR2, mGluR3), and group III (mGluR4, mGluR6, mGluR7, mGluR8). Group I receptors are excitatory. They stimulate phospholipase C and activate the phosphoinositol signal transduction pathway. Group II and III receptors have inhibitory effects that are mediated by inhibition of adenyl cyclase activity. The Group II receptors, for example, appear to be located at the periphery of presynaptic glutamate terminals where they respond to the spillover of glutamate to the extrasynaptic space by providing feedback inhibition.

As noted in Table 21.1, postmortem studies have reported increases in the levels of mGluR1a and mGluR2/3 protein levels in the PFC in schizophrenia (Gupta et al., 2005). An allele of a polymorphism in the GRM3 gene has been associated with the risk for schizophrenia (Egan et al., 2004) and a meta-analysis was weakly positive (Albalushi et al., 2008). Variation in GRM3 was associated with impaired cortical activation and lower N-acetyl aspartate (NAA) levels in the PFC in healthy subjects (Egan et al., 2004; Marenco et al., 2006) and poorer negative symptom response to olanzapine treatment in patients (Bishop et al., 2005). The GRM3 polymorphism may alter mGluR3 receptor function by influencing RNA splicing (Sartorius et al., 2008) or altering the propensity of this receptor to dimerize (Corti et al., 2007). Although genetic studies would predict reductions in mGluR3 function in schizophrenia, this illness is also associated with elevated brain concentration of N-acetyl-aspartyl-glutamate (NAAG), a modified amino acid that has weak NMDA glutamate receptor antagonist and more potent mGluR3 agonist effects (Bergeron et al., 2007; Wroblewska et al., 1997). Increased NAAG levels in schizophrenia may arise from reduced function (Tsai et al., 1995), but not mRNA levels (Ghose et al., 2004), of its catabolic enzyme, carboxypeptidase II. Polymorphisms in the genes coding for two Group III glutamate receptors, mGluR7 (Ohtsuki et al., 2008) and mGluR8 (Takaki et al., 2004), have also been associated with schizophrenia.

Other proteins implicated in glutamatergic neurotransmission and in schizophrenia

The other implicated proteins are neuregulin, disrupted in schizophrenia-1 (DISC1), D-α-amino-oxidase (DAAO), D-serine racemase/G72, and dysbindin.

Neuregulin 1

Neuregulin 1 has diverse roles in regulating glutamatergic neural and glial development and function (Li et al., 2007). Interest in neuregulins emerged following a large Icelandic study and subsequent replications that implicated the gene coding for neuregulin 1 (NRG1) in the heritable risk for schizophrenia (Munafo et al., 2006; Stefansson et al., 2002). The exact nature of the neuregulin 1 alteration in schizophrenia is not yet clear. Postmortem studies have reported reduced expression of erbB3 (Corfas et al., 2004) or elevated levels of disease-related brain-specific splice variants of neuregulin 1 or erbB4 in schizophrenia (Law et al., 2006, 2007; Tan et al., 2007). These changes might decrease neuregulin levels or function and, in so doing, reduce NMDA receptor subunit expression and function (Bjarnadottir et al., 2007; Gu et al., 2005; Ozaki et al., 1997). One report found levels of neuregulin 1 and its receptor (erb4) to be unchanged in postmortem brain tissue from individuals with schizophrenia. However, in this study schizophrenia was associated with increased association of erbB4 with PSD-95, resulting in a reduction in NMDA receptor function (Hahn *et al.*, 2006). These studies suggest that alterations in neuregulin 1, erbB receptors, and their signaling pathways could contribute to NMDA receptor functional deficits associated with schizophrenia.

Disrupted in schizophrenia-1 (DISC1)

DISC1 has been implicated in the heritable risk for schizophrenia, bipolar disorder, depression, and autism. In one study where no change in DICS1 mRNA levels were found in postmortem brain tissue from individuals with schizophrenia, reduced levels of neurodevelopmental proteins that interact with DISC1, such as NUDEL, FEZ1, and LIS1, were found (Lipska *et al.*, 2006). No direct interactions between glutamate receptor proteins have been reported, but DISC1 is found in postsynaptic sites (Kirkpatrick *et al.*, 2006). Also indirect interactions between DISC1 and NMDA glutamate receptors have been hypothesized to be mediated by the AKAP9 protein (Millar *et al.*, 2003). DISC1 also interacts with phosphodiesterase 4B (PDE4B) and through this mechanism may influence cAMP-dependent signal transduction (Millar *et al.*, 2007).

D-α-amino-oxidase (DAAO), serine racemase, and D-amino-acid oxidase activator (DAOA; G72)

These are genes that code for proteins that influence the levels of D-serine, an endogenous co-agonist for the NMDA receptor that is released by glia in response to the synaptic release of glutamate (Schell *et al.*, 1997). DAAO oxidizes and inactivates D-serine, with DAOA/G72 interacting with and activating DAAO (Verrall *et al.*, 2010). The genes coding for these proteins have been implicated in "weakly" contributing to the heritable risk for schizophrenia (Chumakov *et al.*, 2002; Li & He 2007; Verrall *et al.*, 2010). The association may be linked to elevated brain DAAO expression and activity (Bendikov *et al.*, 2007; Burnet *et al.*, 2008; Madeira *et al.*, 2008), and to reduced cerebrospinal fluid and plasma D-serine levels, reported in schizophrenia (Bendikov *et al.*, 2007; Hashimoto *et al.*, 2003a). Serine racemase converts L-serine, the dominant form of this amino acid in humans, into D-serine, the form that facilitates NMDA receptor function. There is preliminary evidence of an association between a polymorphism in the serine racemase gene and schizophrenia (Morita *et al.*, 2007; Labrie *et al.*, 2009). Reduced serine racemase levels have been reported in postmortem brain tissue from individuals with schizophrenia, consistent with reduced ratios of D-serine/ L-serine in several brain regions from the tissue from this group (Bendikov *et al.*, 2007). However, other studies have reported increased protein and mRNA levels for serine racemase (Steffek *et al.*, 2006; Verrall *et al.*, 2007). D-serine

racemase also binds *PICK1*, a gene that has been preliminarily associated with schizophrenia (Hong *et al.*, 2004). Reductions in PICK1 function would reduce NMDA receptor function by impairing serine racemase function and reducing the phosphorylation of NMDA receptor subunits (Dev & Henley, 2006; Hikida *et al.*, 2008).

Dysbindin/dystrophin proteins

Originally studied in muscle in the context of Duchenne muscular dystrophy, these proteins play a role in the trafficking of glutamate vesicles and the branching of dendrites of glutamate neurons (Morris *et al.*, 2008a; Talbot *et al.*, 2006). The association of the dysbindin (*DTNB1*) gene with schizophrenia figured prominently when several large informative studies located this gene within a chromosomal region implicated in schizophrenia from linkage studies (Schwab *et al.*, 2003; Straub *et al.*, 2002; Vilella *et al.*, 2008). Further, several postmortem studies reported reductions in dysbindin levels in association with schizophrenia (Bray *et al.*, 2005; Talbot *et al.*, 2004; Weickert *et al.*, 2004). However, the exact single nucleotide repeats (SNPs) and haplotypes associated with schizophrenia across studies have been variable, leaving it unresolved exactly how *DTNB1* contributes to the risk for schizophrenia (Kendler, 2004; Mutsuddi *et al.*, 2006).

Glial pathology in schizophrenia

Glutamate metabolic roles of glia

Glia are integral partners with neurons in glutamatergic and GABAergic neurotransmission. Astrocytes and satellite oligodendroglia express the glutamate transporters that are primarily responsible for removal of glutamate from the synapse, the primary mode of inactivation. These glia express glutamine synthase, an enzyme that converts glutamate to glutamine. Glia then release glutamine into the extracellular space. Glutamatergic neurons avidly take up this glutamine and utilize it as the primary source for synaptic glutamate release. Impairment of these glial functions, might (1) overstimulate synaptic glutamate receptors and loss of the release of neurotrophic factors, producing neural atrophy and desensitization of AMPA receptors; (2) reduce cAMP response element-binding (CREB) levels, reducing gene expression for brain-derived neurotropic factor (BDNF) and other tropic factors; and (3) overstimulate mGluR2 receptors, resulting in reductions in synpatic glutamate release (Kendell *et al.*, 2005; Sanacora *et al.*, 2003).

There is evidence that schizophrenia is associated with reductions in the density, size, and/or functionality of astrocytes and oligodendroglia in a number of cortical regions (Benes *et al.*, 1986; Hof *et al.*, 2002; Rajkowska *et al.*, 2002; Stark *et al.*, 2004; Uranova *et al.*, 2004, 2007; Vostrikov *et al.*, 2007) and thalamus (Byne *et al.*, 2006; see Chapter 18. Also, reduced glutamine synthase immunoreactivity was found in the PFC in individuals with schizophrenia (Burbaeva *et al.*, 2003), accompanied by increased levels of glutamate dehydrogenase, a neuronal and glial enzyme that converts α-ketoglutarate to glutamate. This pattern might suggest a shift in the source of glutamate released in neurotransmission from the recycling of glutamate to newly synthesized glutamate. Generally, oligodendrocyte abnormalities were more prominent than astrocytes (Uranova *et al.*, 2007). However, the glial deficits are also prominent in mood disorders (Vostrikov *et al.*, 2007). Given current limitations in postmortem brain research, it is difficult to rule out the possibility that the findings reflect, in part, comorbid mood or substance abuse disorders (Sokolov, 2007). Another major potential confounder is the impact of antipsychotic treatment. Chronic administration of antipsychotics to non-human primates reduced cortical astrocyte numbers by approximately 20% and oligodendrocyte populations by half of this amount (Konopaske *et al.*, 2008). Chronic clozapine treatment in animals also reduced glial glutamate uptake (Vallejo-Illarramendi *et al.*, 2005). However, short-term NMDA antagonist administration also reduced the glial conversion of glutamate to glutamine (Kondziella *et al.*, 2006).

Myelination abnormalities

Oligodendrocyte abnormalities in schizophrenia are reflected in alterations in myelination that might influence glutamate neuronal structure and function (Davis *et al.*, 2003). For example, during development, the myelination of glutamatergic projections fosters the emergence of an adult pattern of cognitive capacities, particularly higher order reasoning and an enhanced working memory capacity (Nagy *et al.*, 2004). Postmortem studies provide evidence that schizophrenia is associated with reduced staining for myelin (Regenold *et al.*, 2007) and greater prevalence of atrophy of myelinated axons in the PFC (Uranova *et al.*, 2007). A large number of genes associated with the development of oligodendrocytes or their role in myelination show reduced expression levels in cortical regions in postmortem tissue from individuals with schizophrenia, including myelin-associated glycoprotein (*MAG*), mouse KH domain RNA-binding protein (*QK1*), myelin-associated lipoprotein (*MAL*), myelin-associated basic protein (*MBP*), transferrin (associated with myelination), myelin oligodendrocyte glycoprotein (*MOG*), tight and intercellular junction and peripheral myelin protein (*PMP22*), proteolipid protein 1 (*PLP1*), claudin (*CLD*), ankyrin 3, and tight junction protein (*TJP2/ZO2*) (Dracheva *et al.*, 2006; Hakak *et al.*, 2001; Haroutunian *et al.*, 2007; McCullumsmith *et al.*, 2007; Tkachev *et al.*, 2007). The expression of *SOX10*, a gene that influences the expression of MBP and PLP, may be regulated by methylation, suggesting that genetic and environmental factors might play a role in myelin-related alterations in schizophrenia (Iwamoto *et al.*, 2005). Although

the presence of antipsychotic medications was found to reduce the number of oligodendrocytes in monkey brain, antipsychotic treatment did not alter the pattern of expression of myelin-associated genes in schizophrenia (McCullumsmith *et al.*, 2007). However, there is some variability about the full range of myelin-associated gene expression alterations across studies (Byne *et al.*, 2008; Dracheva *et al.*, 2006; Mitkus *et al.*, 2008). In addition to gene expression findings, there is currently preliminary evidence that variation in genes coding for several myelination-associated proteins including *SOX10*, *MAG*, *MOG*, and *PLP1* are associated with the heritable risk for schizophrenia (Aberg *et al.*, 2006; Liu *et al.*, 2005b; Maeno *et al.*, 2007; Qin *et al.*, 2005; Yang *et al.*, 2005).

GABAergic neuropathology in schizophrenia

GABA neuronal populations

It remains unclear whether schizophrenia is associated with reduced numbers of GABA-releasing cortical interneurons (see Chapter 18). Reductions in the the density of non-pyramidal neurons were reported in layers II–VI of the anterior cingulate cortex and in layer II of the PFC (Beasley & Reynolds, 1997; Beasley *et al.*, 2002; Benes *et al.*, 1991; Reynolds *et al.*, 2001). Subsequent studies did not replicate these findings (Arnold *et al.*, 1995; Selemon *et al.*, 1995, 1998; Tooney & Chahl 2004; Woo *et al.*, 1997). It is possible that compensatory changes in GABA neuronal subpopulations mask changes within a particular subtype of GABA neurons. For example, increases in calretinin-containing neurons may occur in the context of reductions in parvalbumin-containing neuronal populations (Daviss & Lewis, 1995). It is also possible that reductions in GABA neuronal populations reflect the impact of clinical conditions that are commonly comorbid with schizophrenia. For example, reductions in GABA neuronal populations have been described in tissue from patients with schizoaffective disorder (Benes *et al.*, 1991), bipolar disorder (Benes *et al.*, 1997), and major depression (Rajkowska *et al.*, 1998).

It is also unclear whether disturbances in GABA neuronal migration contribute to deficits in cortical interneuron populations or to abnormal distribution of GABA neurons within the cortex. There are a few reports of abnormal distributions of schizophrenia-related GABA neurons across cortical layers or "nests" of GABA neurons in subcortical white matter (Akbarian *et al.*, 1993a,b; Kalus *et al.*, 1997), although there is also a negative finding (Akbarian *et al.*, 1995) and an attribution of maldistribution to bipolar disorder and not schizophrenia (Cotter *et al.*, 2002). Several cortical neuronal populations relevant to schizophrenia emerge from subregions of the ganglionic eminence that develops into the striatum (Wonders & Anderson, 2006). The GABA populations most affected in schizophrenia are the parvalbumin- and somatostatin-containing GABA neurons (Lewis & Gonzalez-Burgos, 2008). Parvalbumin-containing neurons appear to emerge from the ventral medial ganglionic emenince, while somatostatin-containing neurons migrate from the dorso-medial and caudal ganglionic eminence (Wonders *et al.*, 2008). The calretinin-containing GABA neurons, which are persevered in schizophrenia, emerge from the dorso-lateral ganglionic eminence (Wonders & Anderson, 2006). The genes that influence the migration abnormalities involving parvalbumin- and somatostatin-, but not calretinin-containing neurons, might distinctively play a role in migration abnormalities related to schizophrenia. These genes include the homeodomain-containing transcription factor, *Nkx2.1*, and a downstream transcription factor, *Lhx6* (Wonders & Anderson, 2006).

GABA neuronal abnormalities in development, distribution, and function also may be related to reductions in reelin gene expression arising through genetic or epigenetic mechanisms (Costa *et al.*, 2004; Eastwood & Harrison, 2003). Reelin is a lipoprotein implicated in neuronal migration and cortical development, particularly in the case of GABA neurons in superficial cortical layers, including Cajal–Retzius cells. In animal models, reelin deficits produce many GABA-related features of schizophrenia, including GABA neuronal migration deficits, reduced glutamic acid decarboxylase (GAD) expression, and reduced numbers of dendritic spines (Costa *et al.*, 2001). Animals that have reduced expression levels for reelin or its receptors also show impaired sensory gating and cognitive function (Barr *et al.*, 2007; Brigman *et al.*, 2006; Krueger *et al.*, 2006). Several studies of postmortem tissue from individuals with schizophrenia reported reduced levels of reelin gene expression, in association with other GABA-related abnormalities in the cortex and cerebellum (Eastwood & Harrison, 2003; Fatemi *et al.*, 2005; Guidotti *et al.*, 2000; Impagnatiello *et al.*, 1998; Torrey *et al.*, 2005). Building on these studies, polymorphisms in the reelin gene, particularly increasing numbers of trinucleotide repeats in the promotor region, that have been associated with reduced reelin expression (Persico *et al.*, 2006), were associated with the heritable vulnerability to schizophrenia in some (Goldberger *et al.*, 2005; Shifman *et al.*, 2008; Wedenoja *et al.*, 2008), but not all studies (Akahane *et al.*, 2002; Huang & Chen 2006). Other studies (Ruzicka *et al.*, 2007; Tochigi *et al.*, 2008), suggested that the function of the promotor region of the reelin gene in individuals with schizophrenia was functionally reduced by hypermethylation of CpG islands. Data are consistent with the hypothesis that the hypermethylation arises as a consequence of over-expression of DNA-methyltransferase 1 (DNMT1) (Noh *et al.*, 2005; Veldic *et al.*, 2004, 2005). This hypothesis would lead one to predict that drugs that prevent the methylation of the reelin gene, might play a role in the prevention of schizophrenia (Costa *et al.*, 2002). Drugs that reduce the acetylation of histone proteins, histone deactylases (HDACs), might also enhance GAD gene expression (Simonini *et al.*, 2006). The most commonly prescribed HDAC inhibitor, valproate, shows some efficacy in animal models (Tremolizzo *et al.*, 2005), though its clinical benefits are not obvious.

A number of other factors might influence GABA neuronal migration. NMDA glutamate receptors have been implicated in the radial migration of neurons to superficial cortical layers (Behar *et al.*, 1999; Komuro & Rakic, 1993). Also, D_1 receptor activation promotes and D_2 receptor activations inhibits GABA neuronal migration to the cortex (Crandall *et al.*, 2007). Thus, reductions in NMDA and D_1 receptor function and enhanced D_2 receptor function might contribution to impairments in GABA neuronal migration.

GABA neuronal functional integrity

Perhaps the most consistent finding arising from postmortem studies of schizophrenia is the reduction in GAD expression in many cortical regions in schizophrenia (Benes & Berretta, 2001; Benes *et al.*, 2007; Hashimoto *et al.*, 2008b; Lewis & Moghaddam, 2006). GAD is present in two forms, GAD_{65} and GAD_{67}, which are encoded by two genes, *GAD2* and *GAD1*, respectively (Erlander & Tobin, 1991; Soghomonian & Martin, 1998). Several studies report reductions in GAD_{67} mRNA and protein levels in studies of PFC and hippocampus tissue from patients with schizophrenia and bipolar disorder (Akbarian *et al.*, 1995; Guidotti *et al.*, 2000; Hashimoto & Lewis, 2006; Volk *et al.*, 2000). However, one study failed to replicate these findings within the hippocampus (Heckers *et al.*, 2002). Reduced methylation of the *GAD1* gene may have contributed to reduced GAD_{67} gene expression in schizophrenia (Huang & Akbarian, 2007). Consistent with this view, in the CA2/3 region of the hippocampus, reduced GAD_{67} gene expression is associated with increased expression of HDAC1 (Benes *et al.*, 2007). GAD alterations in schizophrenia may be influenced by comorbid mood disorders. In one study, GAD_{65} protein levels were reduced in the anterior cingulate cortex in tissue from patients who had been diagnosed with bipolar disorder or major depression, but not schizophrenia (Benes *et al.*, 2000; Todtenkopf & Benes, 1998). Consistent with reductions in GAD expression, schizophrenia is associated with reduced cortical GABA levels (Cross *et al.*, 1979; Perry *et al.*, 1979), although one study failed to find reduced cortical GAD activity (Bennett *et al.*, 1979).

Genetic and epigenetic regulation of *GAD* gene expression may contribute to GAD deficits in schizophrenia. Several studies indicated that schizophrenia is associated with functional polymorphisms in *GAD1* that are associated with reduced cortical GAD_{67} gene expression and altered cognitive activation of the PFC during functional magnetic resonance imaging (fMRI) (Straub *et al.*, 2007; Zhao *et al.*, 2007), although there are negative studies on this issue (Ikeda *et al.*, 2007; Lundorf *et al.*, 2005). In childhood-onset schizophrenia, the *GAD1* polymorphism also was associated with reduced frontal cortical gray matter volume (Addington *et al.*, 2005). Hypermethylation of the GAD_{67} promotor may reduce the expression of this gene in schizophrenia (Costa *et al.*, 2003; Ruzicka *et al.*, 2007). Two groups have suggested that epigenetic effects on GAD expression apply to schizophrenia but not bipolar disorder, where reductions in the level of transcription factors may contribute to GABA deficits (Benes *et al.*, 2007; Veldic *et al.*, 2007).

However, reduction in GAD expression associated with schizophrenia also may arise as a developmental consequence of abnormalities in glutamate synaptic function that reduce NMDA receptor function. This hypothesis was initially supported by evidence in non-human primates that loss of dendritic spines, the key postsynaptic structure at glutamate synapses, was associated with atrophy of the chandelier cell axon cartridges (Anderson *et al.*, 1995). Also, it is consistent with evidence that the deficit in neurons expressing GAD_{67} in schizophrenia is more pronounced among that subpopulation of interneurons that also express mRNA for the NR2A subunit of the NMDA glutamate receptor (Woo *et al.*, 2004). In intact animals and *in vitro* systems, blockade of NMDA receptors reduces GAD expression, particularly in NADPH oxidase- and parvalbumin-containing neurons (Abekawa *et al.*, 2007; Behrens *et al.*, 2007; Braun *et al.*, 2007; Paulson *et al.*, 2003).

GABA neuronal deficits have been reported in three subsets of interneurons, two groups of parvalbumin-containing neurons, chandelier cells and basket cells, and somatostatin/neuropeptide Y (NPY)-containing cells (Hashimoto *et al.*, 2008a; Lewis & Gonzalez-Burgos 2008; Morris *et al.*, 2008b) (Plate 21.2). Among the diverse types of interneurons (Freund 2003), schizophrenia is associated with abnormalities in neurons that stain for the calcium-binding proteins parvalbumin and calbindin, but not neurons that stain for calretinin (Beasley *et al.*, 2002; Hashimoto *et al.*, 2003b; Sakai *et al.*, 2008). Chandelier cells synapse on the initial axon segment of cortical pyramidal neurons (Lewis *et al.*, 2005). These cells show atrophy in schizophrenia, with reductions in the expression of calcium-binding proteins (parvalbumin, calbindin), reduced GAD expression, and reduced immunoreactivity for the GABA transporter (GAT1) in the terminal axon cartridges of these neurons (Konopaske *et al.*, 2006; Lewis & Gonzalez-Burgos, 2008; Pierri *et al.*, 1999; Woo *et al.*, 1998). Postsynaptic to the atrophied chandelier cells, increased expression is seen of $GABA_A$ receptors containing the α_2 subunit (Volk *et al.*, 2002).

Another population of dysfunctional parvalbumin-containing neurons are basket cells that synapse on the perisomatic region of cortical pyramidal neurons. Abnormalities in these cells in schizophrenia are the most likely explanation for reduced levels of cholecystokinin (CCK) gene expression (Hashimoto *et al.*, 2008a) and decreased ligand-binding to CCK receptors in some postmortem studies of cortical and hippocampal tissue (Bachus *et al.*, 1997; Farmery *et al.*, 1985; Kerwin *et al.*, 1992; Perry *et al.*, 1981). Basket cells possess cannabinoid-1 (CB1) receptors on their axon terminals (Freund, 2003), of interest to the field of schizophrenia research given the psychotigenic effects of tetra-hydrocannabinol in healthy humans and patients with schizophrenia (D'Souza *et al.*, 2004, 2005), the contributory effects of cannabis use to schizophrenia risk (Di Forti *et al.*, 2007), and the mixed preliminary findings associating genetic variation in the *CB1* receptor gene with vulnerability to schizophrenia (Hamdani *et al.*, 2008; Tsai *et al.*, 2000; Ujike *et al.*, 2002; Zammit *et al.*, 2007). One group has found reduced mRNA and protein levels in postmortem tissue from individuals with schizophrenia (Eggan *et al.*, 2010). However, other studies of schizophrenia described increased (Dean *et al.*, 2001b; Newell *et al.*, 2006) or no change (Deng *et al.*, 2007; Koethe *et al.*, 2007) rather than decreased ligand binding to the CB1 receptor in postmortem cortical tissue. This finding raises the possibility of an abnormal distribution of these receptors associated with schizophrenia. Another group of interneurons which express somatostatin (SST) and NPY also show reduced gene expression levels for these peptides associated with schizophrenia (Hashimoto *et al.*, 2008a; Kuromitsu *et al.*, 2001; Morris *et al.*, 2008b).

GABA receptors

Alterations in GABA receptor populations could reflect a heritable vulnerability to schizophrenia or a response to altered GABA synaptic function associated with the disorder. The family of GABA receptors includes $GABA_A$ receptors that contain a chloride channel (Mehta & Ticku, 1999; Whiting, 2003), $GABA_B$ receptors that are coupled by G-proteins to second messenger systems (Bettler *et al.*, 2004), and $GABA_C$ receptors that are neither blocked by bicuculline nor stimulated by baclofen (Chebib, 2004). $GABA_A$ receptors are pentamers that potentially contain combinations of 18 known subunits designated α_{1-6}, β_{1-3}, γ_{1-3}, δ, ε, θ_{1-3}, and π (Mehta & Ticku, 1999; Whiting, 2003).

$GABA_A$ receptors are typically found within the GABA synapse, i.e., "synaptic receptors", that mediate responses to benzodiazepine-like drugs (Krystal *et al.*, 2006; Mohler *et al.*, 2002; Whiting, 2003). Synaptic $GABA_A$ receptors typically include α, β and γ subunits in $\alpha_1\beta_2\gamma_2$, $\alpha_2\beta_3\gamma_2$, or $\alpha_3\beta_3\gamma_2$ subunit combinations. Synaptic $GABA_A$ receptors have lower affinity for GABA than receptor subclasses located at the periphery of GABA synapses, i.e., "extrasynaptic receptors" (Brickley *et al.*, 1999; Nusser *et al.*, 1998). However, synaptic receptors mediate a phasic, high chloride conductance GABA response by virtue of their exposure to brief pulses (10 ms) of near-saturating (≥ 1 mM) levels of GABA during GABA neuronal firing (Brickley et al., 1999; Farrant & Nusser, 2005; Nusser et al., 1998; Wallner et al., 2003). In contrast, extrasynaptic receptors typically do not respond to benzodiazepine agonist stimulation, although they respond to neurosteroids and benzodiazepine inverse agonists (Farrant & Nusser, 2005; Stell et al., 2003; Wohlfarth et al., 2002). In addition to the $\alpha_{1-3,5}$ subunits typical for synaptic receptors, extrasynaptic receptors on cerebellar granule cells also contain α_6 subunits, and extrasynaptic receptors in other regions may contain α_4 subunits. Extrasynaptic receptors also may contain a δ subunit instead of a γ subunit. Although these receptors have a higher affinity for GABA than the synaptic receptors, they are exposed to relatively low GABA levels associated with GABA spillover from the synapse into extracellular spaces ($<3\mu$M) (Borghese et al., 2006; Stell & Mody, 2002; Wei et al., 2003). These receptors comprise a small minority of GABA$_A$ receptors in the brain, but they play an important role in mediating the tonic component of GABAergic inhibition (Stell & Mody, 2002).

Molecular genetic studies have weakly implicated a number of GABA receptor or receptor subunits in the heritable risk for schizophrenia. Polymorphisms in genes coding for the α_1, α_6, and β_2 subunits have been associated with schizophrenia and reductions in gene expression levels for both the α_1 and α_6, subunits (Petryshen et al., 2005). However, these associations were not replicated in some small-to-moderately sized groups of subjects (Ikeda et al., 2005). The most widely studied and replicated finding links SNPs in the gene that codes for the β_2 subunit of the GABA$_A$ receptor (GABRAB2) and schizophrenia (Liu et al., 2005a; Lo et al., 2007a; Yu et al., 2006; Zhao et al., 2007). One study identified a haplotype of GABRB2 that was associated with schizophrenia (Lo et al., 2007b). Unlike most schizophrenia-related associations, this haplotype was associated with enhanced receptor function and it was positively selected for during evolution. Also, a preliminary association between the GABRB gene and schizophrenia was reported (Zai et al., 2005).

Ligand binding studies have produced a complicated picture of alterations in GABA$_A$ receptors in schizophrenia. Benes et al. (1992, 1996) described increases in GABA$_A$ receptor binding in superficial layers of the cingulate gyrus and PFC, where reductions in neuron number or levels of GAD gene expression were reported. However, in the hippocampus, schizophrenia was associated with regional increases in ligand binding to the GABA site of the GABA$_A$ receptor complex, while there were no parallel increases in the binding of a benzodiazepine agonist (Benes et al., 1997). Another study reported increases in [^{3}H]flumazenil binding, but not [^{3}H]muscimol binding, to be associated with schizophrenia (Dean et al., 2001a). These findings suggest that schizophrenia may be associated with dissociations of ligand binding to various sites of the GABA$_A$ receptor complex, possibly indicating that schizophrenia is associated with a shift in GABA$_A$ receptor subunit composition as well as receptor density. A relative increase in the benzodiazepine-insensitive subtypes of GABA receptors might be consistent with decreases in the levels of allopregnanolone in parietal cortex tissue from individuals with schizophrenia (Marx et al., 2006). Allopregnanolone is an endogenous agonist of the benzodiazepine-insensitive GABA$_A$ receptors (Smith et al., 2007).

Neurochemical brain imaging studies using radioligands for the benzodiazepine site of the GABA$_A$ receptor have not generated compelling findings, most likely, because SPECT and PET do not possess sufficient spatial resolution or GABA$_A$ receptor subtype selectivity. None of the published studies using [^{123}I]iomazenil or [^{11}C]Ro4513 (Abi-Dargham et al., 1999; Asai et al., 2008; Busatto et al., 1997; Verhoeff et al., 1999) has reported disease-related alterations.

Psychopharmacology and physiology of glutamate and GABA systems

Features of NMDA receptor antagonist psychosis

The study of the effects of NMDA glutamate receptor antagonists has proven to be enormously generative with respect to the development of hypotheses related to the role of glutamate and GABA in the pathophysiology of schizophrenia and in the development of novel pharmacotherapies for schizophrenia. Beginning in the late 1950s, 20 years before it was recognized that they bound to specific targets in the brain (Zukin & Zukin, 1979), investigators began to report that phencyclidine (PCP) and later, ketamine, produced effects in healthy human subjects that resembled the signs and symptoms of schizophrenia, including psychosis, withdrawal, and cognitive impairment (Cohen et al., 1962; Corssen & Domino 1966; Luby et al., 1959; Rosenbaum et al., 1959).

The best-studied NMDA receptor antagonist, ketamine, produced dose-related effects in healthy human subjects that resemble features of schizophrenia. At very low doses, it produces a mild euphoric effect that resembles one to two ethanol drinks (Krystal et al., 1994, 1998c). At higher doses, cognitive and perceptual deficits emerge. Most groups have studied ketamine at plasma levels in the 100–200 ng/ml range (Absalom et al., 2007; Krystal et al., 1998a; Malhotra et al., 1996; Morgan et al., 2004; Newcomer et al., 1999; Pomarol-Clotet et al., 2006; Vollenweider et al., 1997). At the higher end of this dose range, one may see many typical features of psychosis, including paranoia and grandiosity. One also sees perceptual distortions that may include hallucinations. These perceptual changes are influenced by the nature of the sensory environment where testing takes place. In a quiet, well-lit room, people predominately describe alterations in their experience of themselves (feelings of unreality, altered experiences of their body), time, and their testing environment. Commonly, during ketamine testing, subjects may experience the walls moving, a constricted range of attention (tunnel vision), and changes in the vividness or form of sensory stimuli. For example, quiet music from another room might be experienced as eminating from one's teeth or the sound of an MRI might be experienced as human speech. During ketamine administration, the form and content of thought are altered. Typically, thought becomes concrete and mildly to moderately idiosyncratic, loosely associated, and bizarre. Overall, the types of thought disorder produced by ketamine are not readily distinguishable from schizophrenia (Adler *et al.*, 1999; Krystal *et al.*, 1998b, 1999b). Ketamine produces "negative symptoms", including blunting of affect, withdrawal, and amotivational states. The extent to which ketamine produces negative symptoms is related to the degree to which it reduces ligand binding to the NMDA receptor *in vivo*. These negative symptoms are readily distinguished from sedation, in that they are not produced to the same degree by a similarly sedating dose of lorazepam

(Krystal *et al.*, 1998a) or haloperidol (Krystal *et al.*, 1999b). Ketamine also impairs many features of cognition, including the executive control of attention, working memory, the encoding and retrieval of declarative memory, planning, and abstract reasoning (Krystal *et al.*, 1994, 1998a, 1999b). However, ketamine does not produce a state of delerium, i.e., gross disorientation and global impairment of cognitive function (Krystal *et al.*, 1994). For example, ketamine impairs learning how to perform the Wisconsin Card Sorting Test (WCST), but once the task is learned, it does not appear to impair the execution of previously learned problem-solving strategies (Krystal *et al.*, 2000b).

The effects of ketamine are readily distinguished from the psychotigenic effects of amphetamine or the serotonergic hallucinogens, although there are many similarities between ketamine and cannabinoid effects (Table 21.2). Amphetamine produces a state of paranoid and grandiose ideation, irritability, and psychomotor activation (Krystal *et al.*, 2005c). Relative to amphetamine, ketamine produces more pronounced negative symptoms, cognitive impairments, and perceptual change. The serotonergic hallucinogens, such as mescaline, psilocybin, dimethyltryptamine (DMT), and lysergic acid diethylamide (LSD) are distinguished from ketamine or PCP by their relatively greater propensity to produce psychomotoric activation, a sense of

Table 21.2 Phenomenology of the model psychoses.

Sign/symptom	Ketamine	Amphetamine	THC	5-HT hallucinogen
Positive symptoms				
Delusion	+	++	+	+
Hallucinations	+	+/−	+	++
Other perceptual changes	++	0	+	++
Negative symptoms				
Blunted affect	++	0	++	+/−
Withdrawal	+	0	+	+
Anhedonia	+/−	0	+/−	0
Disorganization				
Thought disorder (overall)	++	+	+	+
Impaired abstraction	++	0	+	0
Impaired attention	+	+	+	+
Other effects				
Impaired working memory	++	+/−	+	?
Impaired declarative memory	++	+/−	++	?
Impaired planning/judgement	++	+/−	++	+

Modified from Krystal *et al.* (2003a), with the following additional papers considered: D'Souza *et al.* (2004), Krystal *et al.* (2005c), and Vollenweider & Geyer (2001).

5-HT, serotonin; THC, Δ9-tetrahydrocannabinol, 0, no effect; +/− inconsistent or minimal effect; +, mild-to-moderate effect; ++, moderate-to-large effect.

Based on the results of studies that have used these prototypical agents at doses sufficient to produce the array of effects relevant to this chapter. The 5HT hallucinogen effects are based primarily on studies of shorter-acting hallucinogens: mescaline, psilocybin, and dimethyltryptamine (DMT).

portentiousness (feeling that something important is happening), ego diffusion (sense of merging with the universe), and vivid psychedelic hallucinations (Cohen *et al.*, 1962; Hermle *et al.*, 1992; Strassman *et al.*, 1994; Vollenweider & Geyer, 2001).

PCP and ketamine have been administered to patients with schizophrenia, where they clearly worsen symptoms of this disorder (Itil *et al.*, 1967; Lahti *et al.*, 1995, 2001; Malhotra *et al.*, 1997b). Differences in the magnitude of the effects of ketamine on symptoms in patients and healthy individuals have not been clearly demonstrated. The lack of a group differences would question the existence of a systematic alteration in NMDA receptor function associated with schizophrenia. However, the sample sizes of the group comparisons have been small. Also, it is difficult to compare the magnitude of ketamine effects in patients and healthy subjects because the patients start at elevated baselines compared to healthy individuals on symptom rating scales, like the Brief Psychiatric Rating Scale (BPRS) or Positive and Negative Symptom Scale (PANSS), that do not have precise linear relationships with symptom severity (i.e., increasing scores reflect qualitative and quantitative changes).

Psychopharmacology of NMDA receptor antagonist psychosis

Dopamine

The inability of D_2 receptor antagonists to block the ketamine psychosis provides strong evidence that there are some forms of psychosis that are not dependent upon the activation of this type of receptors. This simple, but profound, observation is the single strongest justification for searching for antipsychotic medications that might work through other mechanisms.

While NMDA receptor antagonists increase cortical and limbic extracellular dopamine levels in animals (Moghaddam *et al.*, 1997; Takahata & Moghaddam, 1998) and increase the amphetamine-induced release of dopamine in humans (Kegeles *et al.*, 1999), the ketamine psychosis does not appear to be blocked by acute pretreatment with the D_2 receptor antagonist antipsychotics, haloperidol (Krystal *et al.*, 1999) or olanzapine (Lahti *et al.*, 1999). One report suggested that sertindole pretreatment reduced ketamine effects in healthy human subjects (Vollenweider *et al.*, 1999). In light of the prior antipsychotic studies, the sertindole effect, if replicable, is more likely to be attributable to action at a receptor other than the D_2 receptor. A small number of studies have evaluated the impact of chronic antipsychotic treatment in patients with schizophrenia. Chronic treatment with clozapine, but not haloperidol, appears to blunt the worsening of symptoms produced by ketamine administration in patients with schizophrenia (Lahti *et al.*, 1995; Malhotra *et al.*, 1997a).

These findings may be consistent with animal models suggesting that clozapine is more effective than haloperidol in reducing locomotor stimulatory effects, disruption of prepulse inhibition of the startle response, and cognitive impairments produced by NMDA receptor antagonists (Breese *et al.*, 2002). The differential efficacy of clozapine has been attributed to many actions, including $5HT_2$ receptor antagonism, D_4 receptor antagonism, α_2 noradrenergic receptor antagonism, and blockade of the glycine transporter (Meltzer *et al.*, 1989; Seeman 1992; Svensson 2003; Van Tol *et al.*, 1991; Williams *et al.*, 2004).

The interplay of the dopamine D_1 receptor and NMDA receptor may be important to the genesis and treatment of cognitive impairments associated with schizophrenia. Like NMDA receptors, alterations in D_1 receptors and their function in schizophrenia is suggested by findings from postmortem and *in vivo* neuroimaging studies (Abi-Dargham & Moore, 2003). In the PFC, D_1 receptors are located extrasynaptically on dendritic spines possessing NMDA receptors, where they are exposed to dopamine that overflows from the synapse (Smiley *et al.*, 1994). At a molecular level, there is interplay between these two receptors at the level of protein–protein interactions and via signal transduction pathways (Cepeda & Levine, 2006). This interplay has been best studied in the context of the neurobiology of working memory. In brain tissue slices and in awake behaving primates, both NMDA and D_1 receptors are involved in the preservation of persisting neural activity that seems necessary for the maintenance of information within working memory (Castner & Williams, 2007; Seamans & Yang 2004). This information seems applicable to schizophrenia because recent fMRI data indicate that PFC activation decays more rapidly during the maintenance of information in working memory in patients with schizophrenia relative to a healthy comparison group (Driesen *et al.*, 2008). These data raise the possibility that abnormalities in NMDA and D_1 receptors might contribute to PFC functional deficits in schizophrenia and that D_1-stimulating treatments might compensate for deficits in NMDA receptor function. This hypothesis is supported by human data suggesting that amphetamine reduces working memory impairments produced by ketamine (Krystal *et al.*, 2005b). It is also consistent with evidence that, in a dose-related fashion, D_1 receptor agonist administration may attenuate working memory deficits due to chronic antipsychotic exposure (Castner *et al.*, 2000) or aging (Cai & Arnsten, 1997). However, progress in this area has been slowed by the lack of an available D_1 receptor agonist for clinical trials.

GABA

Studying the interplay of glutamate and GABA systems in the NMDA glutamate receptor antagonist psychosis has provided new insights into the psychopharmacology of cognition and schizophrenia. When NMDA receptor antagonists are administered at subanesthetic doses, these drugs reduce GABA neuronal activation in the PFC (Homayoun & Moghaddam, 2007) and hippocampus (Grunze et al., 1996), decreasing GABA release and disinhibiting glutamate release by the "next" neuron in the feed-forward inhibition pathway (Plate 21.3). The resulting increase in glutamate release is reflected in animals by increased excitatory postsynaptic potentials and extracellular glutamate levels. In humans, ketamine activates resting cortical metabolism and perfusion in multiple brain regions. Thus, the NMDA receptor antagonist psychosis is an "activated' or "hyperglutamatergic" state even though these drugs block an excitatory receptor.

One obvious implication of this view of the NMDA receptor antagonist psychosis is that drugs that interfere with GABA action should increase psychosis risk, while drugs that stimulate GABA receptors should have antipsychotic effects. The anesthesiology literature suggested that hypnotic doses of benzodiazepines inhibited the perceptual effects of anesthetic doses of ketamine (Coppel et al., 1973; Lilburn et al., 1978). Thus, these studies had limited relevance to studying human cognition and behavior. At a subhypnotic dose, lorazepam tended to attenuate perceptual effects of subanesthetic ketamine, but this action was more prominent for "dissociative" rather than "psychotic" effects (Krystal et al., 1998b). Lorazepam also worsened cognitive impairments produced by ketamine. However, as will be reviewed in the next section, attempts to block ketamine effects with drugs that attenuate glutamate release have been productive.

Parvalbumin-containing or "fast-spiking" neurons, neurons sensitive to NMDA receptor antagonists and cell populations that are thought to be dysfunctional in schizophrenia, entrain cortical oscillations in the theta and gamma frequencies (Kawaguchi, 2001; Kawaguchi & Kubota, 1993; Klausberger et al., 2005; Traub et al., 1996; Tukker et al., 2007). Thus, deficits in cortical oscillations in these frequencies when individuals with schizophrenia perform cognitive and sensory tasks may reflect the underlying GABAergic pathology (Cho et al., 2006; Ford et al., 2008; Gallinat et al., 2004; Kwon et al., 1999; Spencer et al., 2004, 2008). Similarly, as is suggested by the simplified circuitry outlined in Plate 21.3, the ability of NMDA receptor antagonists to disrupt these types of cortical oscillations in vitro and in vivo may further reflect commonalities between neural circuit dysfunctions associated with schizophrenia and NMDA antagonist administration (Cunningham et al., 2006; D. Mathalon & J. Krystal, unpublished observation).

The role of GABA neurons in cortical oscillations raises the possibility that measurement of cortical oscillations in schizophrenia might serve as a biomarker to evaluate novel pharmacotherapies for schizophrenia aimed at compensating for deficits in GABA neuronal function. Examples of these types of treatments would be α_2 subunit-selective GABA$_A$ receptor agonists, that might compensate for reduced functionality of chandelier cells (Volk et al., 2002), or CB1 receptor antagonists, that might compensate for reduced basket cell function (Freund, 2003).

GABA deficits described in postmortem studies of schizophrenia might be expected to contribute to psychosis. A recent Cochrane review indicated that there was suggestive evidence that benzodiazepines reduced agitation and psychosis, but the overall data were inconclusive (Gillies et al., 2005). Further, these drugs generally have adverse effects on cognition and cortical information processing in patients with schizophrenia (Menzies et al., 2007; Murakami et al., 2002). To our knowledge, outside of the treatment of tardive dyskinesia, no other class of GABAergic agent (GABA transporter inhibitor, GABA transaminase inhibitor, subtype-selective GABA$_A$ receptor agonists or partial agonists, GABA$_B$ receptor agonists) has been studied in the treatment of schizophrenia. However, muscimol, a potent GABA$_A$ receptor agonist worsens behavioral disorganization and psychosis in patients with schizophrenia when administered at relatively high doses (Tamminga et al., 1978). Also, there have been some rare clinical reports of psychosis among individuals with epilepsy administered the potent GABA transaminase inhibitor, vigabatrin (Ferrie et al., 1996). However, it is not clear whether pre-existing psychiatric conditions led to these psychiatric "adverse events". The hypothesis that GABA deficits contribute to psychosis vulnerability is further supported by studies of benzodiazepine receptor inverse agonists. Studies of GABA$_A$ receptor full inverse agonists suggested that they were anxiogenic, but not psychotigenic (Dorow et al., 1983; Horowski & Dorrow, 2002). However, a subsequent study showed that administration of a GABA$_A$ receptor partial inverse agonist, iomazenil, created a vulnerability to psychosis produced by m-chlorophenylpiperazine (mCPP), a 5HT partial agonist that is psychotigenic in patients with schizophrenia but not healthy individuals (Abi-Saab et al., 2002; D'Souza et al., 2006; Krystal et al., 1993). Thus, GABA deficits might contribute to the observation that activation of monoaminergic (dopamine, serotonin) systems may worsen psychosis in patients with schizophrenia, but do not typically produce psychosis in healthy individuals. From this perspective, drugs that facilitate GABA function might have a prophylactic or protective role in muting the worsening of symptoms of schizophrenia produced by stress or other environmental situations associated with monoaminergic activation.

Glutamate

AMPAkines

There has been interest in the possibility that drugs that enhance glutamatergic activation could reduce symptoms and cognitive deficits associated with reductions in cortical metabolism. The principal pharmacological approaches pursued to address these deficits are the AMPAkines, agents that enhance AMPA receptor function (Arai & Kessler, 2007; Danysz, 2002). To date, only pilot studies of a few AMPAkines have been conducted in patients with schizophrenia and these have produced mixed results. In neuroleptic-free patients a small study did not report clinical efficacy, with some patients showing worsening of psychosis (Marenco et al., 2002). Two subsequent studies by another group reported conflicting results (Goff et al., 2001, 2008). The initial study found improvements in attention and working memory, but these benefits were not replicated in the follow-up study.

Glycine$_B$ receptor stimulation

The predominant strategy to treat deficits in NMDA receptor function has been to increase the stimulation of the glycine$_B$ receptor, the co-agonist site on the NMDA glutamate receptor (D'Souza et al., 1995). In animals and in humans, there is evidence that the administration of large doses of glycine or blockade of the glycine transporter can enter the central nervous system (CNS) and affect brain metabolism (D'Souza et al., 2000; Neumeister et al., 2006), more specifically, enhance NMDA receptor function and reduce the effects of uncompetitive NMDA receptor antagonists (Contreras 1990; D'Souza et al., 1997; Javitt et al., 1999; Linn et al., 2007; Nilsson et al., 1997; Toth & Lajtha, 1986). High levels of glycine are present in the extracellular fluid, raising questions as to whether glycine$_B$ receptors were saturated by glycine under physiological conditions. Subsequent studies showed that synaptic glycine levels were kept below the levels needed to saturate glycine$_B$ sites by a high activity transporter, GlyT1 (Supplisson & Bergman, 1997). Supporting this hypothesis, GlyT1 blockade enhanced NMDA receptor function (Bergeron et al., 1998).

Building on these advances, a series of small pilot clinical trials provided evidence that, at appropriate doses, glycine$_B$ receptor agonists or partial agonists, including glycine, D-alanine, and D-serine appeared to increase the effectiveness of antipsychotic treatment, particularly in the realms of negative symptoms and cognitive impairments (Heresco-Levy et al., 1996, 1999, 2004, 2005; Javitt et al., 1994, 2001; Tsai et al., 2004, 2006). The partial agonist, D-cycloserine, appears to be less effective than full agonists at the glycine site and, further, carries a risk of psychotic exacerbation at high doses (Cascella et al., 1994; Goff et al., 2005; Heresco-Levy & Javitt, 2004; van Berckel et al., 1999). One exception to this study is clozapine, a drug with antagonist activity at GlyT1 at clinical doses (Williams et al., 2004). When added to clozapine, full glycine$_B$ receptor agonists or glycine transporter antagonists are ineffective (Diaz et al., 2005; Lane et al., 2006) and the partial agonist,

D-cycloserine, worsens negative symptoms (Goff et al., 1999). In contrast to the generally encouraging results from the smaller studies, a multicenter study failed to find that either glycine or D-cycloserine was efficacious (Buchanan et al., 2007). These negative data highlighted important gaps in our understanding of the appropriate way to dose the amino acids during treatment. Thus, in the early studies, the positive result was the principal evidence supporting central activity of the amino acids administered to humans. It is unclear whether the negative data should be attributed to the mechanism or some aspects of the delivery (dose, timing) of the medications.

The most promising approach, to date, appears to be GlyT1 inhibition (Lane et al., 2005). These drugs robustly raise synaptic glycine levels and they are undergoing the type of industrial drug development necessary to determine dose-related efficacy in animals models and, eventually, humans. As a prelude to agents developed by the pharmaceutical industry, there are now preliminary data suggesting that GlyT1 inhibitors can increase the efficacy of antipsychotic treatment and perhaps even play a primary role in the treatment of symptoms in patients who are neuroleptic-naïve (Lane et al., 2008).

There are many unresolved issues relating to the role of glycine$_B$ receptor facilitation in schizophrenia (Krystal & D'Souza, 1998). One question is whether these drugs produce tolerance to their clinical benefit. This limitation has become evident in the use of D-cycloserine as an adjunct to exposure therapy in the treatment of anxiety disorders. It might be surprising that tolerance would develop to glycine-like agents since the glycine$_B$ receptor is tonically exposed to glycine. However, it is likely that the stimulation of the glycine$_B$ site of the NMDA receptor should be considered as having a tonic component, mediated by glycine, and a phasic component mediated by D-serine. D-serine is released by glia that are stimulated by synaptic glutamate release (Oliet & Mothet, 2006; Snyder & Kim, 2000). Thus, when adding a drug that raises glycine levels, one is converting a phasic activation of the glycine$_B$ receptor to a tonic activation.

The objective of facilitating NMDA receptor function could be compatible with glycine$_B$ receptor-facilitating treatments even if tolerance develops to continuous exposure to these agents. First, one could imagine that these treatments might facilitate network function within the context of cognitive function. However, it is not yet clear that drug exposure would be needed during sleep. Second, as has been previously suggested, glycine$_B$ receptor-facilitating treatment might play a more limited role in restoring a capacity for neuroplasticity that would be harnessed by rehabilitative therapies such as cognitive remediation or cognitive-behavioral therapy (Krystal, 2007; Krystal et al., 2003b). If so, then the role of glycine$_B$ receptor-facilitating treatments would be analogous to the role currently suggested for D-cycloserine, which is prescribed in combination with the extinction of fear conditioning (Ressler *et al.*, 2004). In this example, exposure to a glycine$_B$ receptor-facilitating agent is best limited to the period during which the cognitive therapy is delivered (Norberg *et al.*, 2008).

mGluR5 agonists

Alternatives to glycine$_B$ receptor facilitation are likely to be needed for schizophrenia to facilitate NMDA receptor function. In this regard, mGluR5 receptor agonism is a promising candidate mechanism. mGluR5 receptors are co-localized in many brain regions, particularly the hippocampus. In these regions, mGlur5 and NMDA receptors are functionally associated via the proteins, Homer and Shank (Ango *et al.*, 2000; Tu *et al.*, 1999). Recently, it has been shown that mGluR5 antagonists increase the effects of NMDA receptor antagonists upon PFC neuronal burst activity, working memory, locomotor activity, and pre-pulse inhibition of the startle response (Homayoun & Moghaddam, 2006; Homayoun *et al.*, 2004; Pietraszek *et al.*, 2005). Positive modulators of mGluR5 receptors reduce disruptive effects of NMDA receptor antagonists on PFC burst activity (Lecourtier *et al.*, 2007), learning, and pre-pulse inhibition (Chan *et al.*, 2008). Thus, mGluR5 agonism is a promising mechanism to explore for the treatment of schizophrenia.

mGluR2 agonists, glutamate release inhibitors, and AMPA receptor antagonists

In contrast to glutamate deficiency hypotheses that have lead to the study of AMPAkines, the "hyperglutamatergic" consequences of deficits in NMDA receptor function and GABA deficits predict that drugs that reduce glutamatergic excitation might play a role in the treatment of schizophrenia. The first approach to reduce glutamate release suggested by animal research was AMPA/kainate glutamate receptor antagonism. The first study to show that ketamine stimulated glutamate release in animals also showed that its dopaminergic and behavioral effects could be attenuated by administration of the AMPA/kainate receptor antagonist LY293558 (Moghaddam *et al.*, 1997). No selective AMPA/kainate receptor antagonist has ever been tested in patients with schizophrenia. However, topiramate, a drug that has some antagonist activity at these receptors, reduces mood symptoms, but it does not appear to enhance the efficacy of antipsychotics in treating positive or negative symptoms (Dursun & Deakin, 2001; Post, 1999; Tiihonen *et al.*, 2005).

Two approaches have been studied for reducing glutamate release: blocking voltage-gated cation channels and stimulating Group II mGlu receptors. The first approach is typified by studies of lamotrigine, a drug that blocks voltage-gated sodium channels and N- and P-type voltage-

gated calcium channels. Lamotrigine reduces glutamate release in several animal models, consistent with its anti-convulsant properties (Large *et al.*, 2005). In healthy humans, it attenuated the cognitive and perceptual effects of ketamine (Anand *et al.*, 2000). In animals, it reduced the neural injury, stimulation of cortical activation, disruption of pre-pulse inhibition of the startle response, and learning impairments produced by NMDA receptor antagonists (Brody *et al.*, 2003; Farber *et al.*, 1999; Gozzi *et al.*, 2008; Idris *et al.*, 2005). Several small clinical trials suggested that the addition of lamotrigine to ongoing antipsychotic treatment improved clinical outcomes (Dursun & Deakin 2001; Kremer *et al.*, 2004; Tiihonen *et al.*, 2003). However, this observation was not replicated in two large clinical trials (Goff *et al.*, 2007). Thus, while lamotrigine may produce clinical benefits in some patients, its effects are not likely to be sufficiently consistent to justify widespread clinical use based on current evidence.

The most promising glutamatergic treatment approach studied so far uses the Group II metabotropic glutamate receptor agonists. As noted earlier, mGluR3 receptors are implicated in the heritable risk for schizophrenia and in the actions of NAAG. Raising NAAG levels, through inhibition of its peptidase, attenuates the cognitive and behavioral effects of NMDA receptor antagonists in animals, presumably via stimulation of Group II mGluRs (Olszewski *et al.*, 2004, 2008). Although the agents tested to date stimulated both mGluR2 and mGluR3 receptors, some recent data implicate mGluR2 receptors more strongly than mGluR3 receptors in the therapeutic effects of these drugs (Woolley *et al.*, 2008). In animals, these drugs reduce the cortical excitatory effects of both serotonergic (LSD-like) hallucinogens (Marek *et al.*, 2000) and NMDA receptor antagonists (Gozzi *et al.*, 2008; Homayoun *et al.*, 2005; Moghaddam & Adams 1998). Further, the Group II metabotropic glutamate receptor agonist, LY354740, reduced the disruption of working memory, appearance of abnormal behaviors, and stimulation of locomotor activity produced by NMDA antagonist administration in animals (Cartmell *et al.*, 1999; Harich *et al.*, 2007; Moghaddam & Adams, 1998; Swanson & Schoepp, 2002). In humans, LY354740 reduced the disruption of working memory and there was a non-significant trend to reduce the psychotic symptoms produced by ketamine infusion (Krystal *et al.*, 2005a). In response to concerns about the central bioavailability of LY354740, another Group II metabotropic glutamate receptor agonist, LY2140023 (a prodrug of LY404039), was studied in patients with schizophrenia. A very promising initial study suggested that this drug, administered by itself, was as effective as olanzapine in treating schizophrenia (Patil *et al.*, 2007). If it proves to be effective, this drug will be the first non-D$_2$ blocking antipsychotic medication and the first to emerge from a hypothesis-driven translational neuroscience research effort.

Implications

Amino acid neurotransmission has emerged at the center of current efforts to understand the heritability, neuropathology, and pathophysiology of schizophrenia. All of these lines of research suggest that compromised glutamatergic synaptic function, particularly that component mediated by NMDA glutamate receptors, plays a major role in the collection of neurodevelopmental syndromes that we currently group under the diagnostic rubric of schizophrenia. There is already some evidence that the abnormalities in glutamatergic neuronal and synaptic function may be targeted by novel pharmacotherapeutic strategies for schizophrenia, exemplified by the efforts to enhance the stimulation of the glycine$_B$ site of the NMDA receptor complex.

This review highlights the inseparability of the glutamatergic and GABAergic pathophysiology of schizophrenia. There is evidence that the glutamatergic synaptic functional abnormalities contribute to the development of the GABAergic neuropathology associated with schizophrenia. Further, abnormalities in the activity of glutamatergic neuronal activity associated with schizophrenia, such as deficits in oscillatory activity, may be driven predominately by GABA neuronal functional deficits. These GABA deficits also serve to disinhibit cortical networks, resulting in hyperactivity or reduced efficiency.

This review has highlighted some inherent complexities of glutamatergic synaptic function that will challenge the development of medications for this disorder. For example, there appear to be reductions in cortical connectivity associated with schizophrenia, supporting the hypothesis that an AMPAkine would be helpful. Alternatively, the deficits in GABAergic function might yield a hyperglutamatergic state that would be exacerbated by an AMPAkine. We do not yet know whether these two dimensions of the pathophysiology of schizophrenia are in opposition, in which case both AMPA/kainate receptor-facilitating and drugs that reduce cortical excitability would need to be tested very cautiously to avoid symptom exacerbation. Alternatively, consistent with the high degree of variability in symptoms and deficits across patients, it may be possible to match patients to treatments that best suit their needs.

The most exciting aspect of research on amino acid neurotransmission in schizophrenia is its capacity to guide the development of fundamentally new treatments. Based on the convergence of many types of research within a translational neuroscience context, our field may have generated the first meaningful alternatives to the blockade of the dopamine D$_2$ receptor. The testing of the mGluR2 agonists for schizophrenia is just the tip of the iceberg as many more novel mechanisms have been identified and will be explored in upcoming years.

Acknowledgements

Dr Krystal acknowledges with gratitude the late Robert L. McNeil, Jr. His gift to Yale University School of Medicine has helped Dr Krystal to pursue many projects, such as the writing of this chapter.

The work outlined in this review was supported by the Department of Veterans Affairs through its support for the Schizophrenia Biological Research Center and Alcohol Research Center (J.K.), the National Institute of Mental Health [P50 MH068789-03 (JK), R37 MH4804, R21 MH065468 (BM)], the National Institute on Alcohol Abuse and Alcoholism (KO5 AA 14906-04, 2P50-AA012870-07), and NCRR for its support of the Yale Center for Clinical Investigation. The authors also acknowledge support from the Pittsburgh Life Sciences Greenhouse (BM).

The authors thank Dr David Lewis for sharing new data on CB1 receptor gene expression and insights on CB1 receptor alterations in schizophrenia.

Disclosure of Dr Krystal's industry-related financial interests are available at (http://journals.elsevierhealth.com/webfiles/images/journals/bps/Biological_Psychiatry_Editorial_Disclosures_02_22_08.pdf).

References

Abekawa, T., Ito, K., Nakagawa, S. & Koyama, T. (2007) Prenatal exposure to an NMDA receptor antagonist, MK-801 reduces density of parvalbumin-immunoreactive GABAergic neurons in the medial prefrontal cortex and enhances phencyclidine-induced hyperlocomotion but not behavioral sensitization to methamphetamine in postpubertal rats. *Psychopharmacology (Berlin)* **192**, 303–316.

Aberg, K., Saetre, P., Lindholm, E. *et al.* (2006) Human QKI, a new candidate gene for schizophrenia involved in myelination. *American Journal of Medical Genetics B Neuropsychiatric Genetics* **141**, 84–90.

Abi-Dargham, A. & Moore, H. (2003) Prefrontal DA transmission at D$_1$ receptors and the pathology of schizophrenia. *Neuroscientist* **9**, 404–416.

Abi-Dargham, A., Laruelle, M., Krystal, J. *et al.* (1999) No evidence of altered *in vivo* benzodiazepine receptor binding in schizophrenia. *Neuropsychopharmacology* **20**, 650–661.

Abi-Saab, W., Seibyl, J.P., D'Souza, D.C. *et al.* (2002) Ritanserin antagonism of m-chlorophenylpiperazine effects in neuroleptic-free schizophrenics patients: support for serotonin-2 receptor modulation of schizophrenia symptoms. *Psychopharmacology (Berlin)* **162**, 55–62.

Absalom, A.R., Lee, M, Menon, D.K. *et al.* (2007) Predictive performance of the Domino, Hijazi, and Clements models during low-dose target-controlled ketamine infusions in healthy volunteers. *British Journal of Anaesthesia* **98**, 615–623.

Addington, A.M., Gornick, M., Duckworth, J. *et al.* (2005) GAD1 (2q31.1), which encodes glutamic acid decarboxylase (GAD67), is associated with childhood-onset schizophrenia and cortical gray matter volume loss. *Molecular Psychiatry* **10**, 581–588.

Adler, C.M., Malhotra, A.K., Elman, I. *et al.* (1999) Comparison of ketamine-induced thought disorder in healthy volunteers and thought disorder in schizophrenia. *American Journal of Psychiatry* **156**, 1646–1649.

Akahane, A., Kunugi, H., Tanaka, H. & Nanko, S. (2002) Association analysis of polymorphic CGG repeat in 5′ UTR of the reelin and VLDLR genes with schizophrenia. *Schizophrenia Research* **58**, 37–41.

Akbarian, S., Bunney, W.E., Jr., Potkin, S.G. *et al.* (1993a) Altered distribution of nicotinamide-adenine dinucleotide phosphate-diaphorase cells in frontal lobe of schizophrenics implies disturbances of cortical development. *Archives of General Psychiatry* **50**, 169–177.

Akbarian, S., Vinuela, A., Kim, J.J., Potkin, S.G., Bunney, W.E., Jr. & Jones, E.G. (1993b) Distorted distribution of nicotinamide-adenine dinucleotide phosphate-diaphorase neurons in temporal lobe of schizophrenics implies anomalous cortical development. *Archives of General Psychiatry* **50**, 178–187.

Akbarian, S., Kim, J.J., Potkin, S.G. *et al.* (1995) Gene expression for glutamic acid decarboxylase is reduced without loss of neurons in prefrontal cortex of schizophrenics. *Archives of General Psychiatry* **52**, 258–266.

Akbarian, S., Sucher, N.J., Bradley, D. *et al.* (1996) Selective alterations in gene expression for NMDA receptor subunits in prefrontal cortex of schizophrenics. *Journal of Neuroscience* **16**, 19–30.

Albalushi, T., Horiuchi, Y., Ishiguro, H. *et al.* (2008) Replication study and meta-analysis of the genetic association of GRM3 gene polymorphisms with schizophrenia in a large Japanese case-control population. *American Journal of Medical Genetics B Neuropsychiatric Genetics* **147**, 392–396.

Alzheimer, A. (1907) Beiträge zur Pathologischen Anatomie der Hirnrinde und zur anatomiscen Grundlage der Psychozen. *Mschr Psychiat Neurol* **2**, 82–120.

Anand, A., Charney, D.S., Cappiello, A., Berman, R.M., Oren, D.A. & Krystal, J.H. (2000) Lamotrigine attenuates ketamine effects in humans: support for hyperglutamatergic effects of NMDA antagonists. *Archives of General Psychiatry* **57**, 270–276.

Anderson, S.A., Classey, J.D., Conde, F., Lund, J.S. & Lewis, D.A. (1995) Synchronous development of pyramidal neuron dendritic spines and parvalbumin-immunoreactive chandelier neuron axon terminals in layer III of monkey prefrontal cortex. *Neuroscience* **67**, 7–22.

Ango, F., Pin, J.P., Tu, J.C. *et al.* (2000) Dendritic and axonal targeting of type 5 metabotropic glutamate receptor is regulated by homer1 proteins and neuronal excitation. *Journal of Neuroscience* **20**, 8710–8716.

Arai, A.C. & Kessler, M. (2007) Pharmacology of ampakine modulators: from AMPA receptors to synapses and behavior. *Current Drug Targets* **8**, 583–602.

Arnold, S.E., Franz, B.R., Gur, R.C. *et al.* (1995) Smaller neuron size in schizophrenia in hippocampal subfields that mediate cortical-hippocampal interactions. *American Journal of Psychiatry* **152**, 738–748.

Asai, Y., Takano, A., Ito, H. *et al.* (2008) GABA(A)/Benzodiazepine receptor binding in patients with schizophrenia using [(11)C] Ro15-4513, a radioligand with relatively high affinity for alpha5 subunit. *Schizophrenia Research* **99**, 333–340.

Bachus, S.E., Hyde, T.M., Herman, M.M., Egan, M.F. & Kleinman, J.E. (1997) Abnormal cholecystokinin mRNA levels in entorhinal cortex of schizophrenics. *Journal of Psychiatric Research* **31**, 233–256.

Barr, A.M., Fish, K.N. & Markou, A. (2007) The reelin receptors VLDLR and ApoER2 regulate sensorimotor gating in mice. *Neuropharmacology* **52**, 1114–1123.

Beasley, C.L. & Reynolds, G.P. (1997) Parvalbumin-immunoreactive neurons are reduced in the prefrontal cortex of schizophrenics. *Schizophrenia Research* **24**, 349–355.

Beasley, C.L., Zhang, Z.J., Patten, I. & Reynolds, G.P. (2002) Selective deficits in prefrontal cortical GABAergic neurons in schizophrenia defined by the presence of calcium-binding proteins. *Biological Psychiatry* **52**, 708–715.

Behar, T.N., Scott, C.A., Greene, C.L. *et al.* (1999) Glutamate acting at NMDA receptors stimulates embryonic cortical neuronal migration. *Journal of Neuroscience* **19**, 4449–4461.

Behrens, M.M., Ali, S.S., Dao, D.N. *et al.* (2007) Ketamine-induced loss of phenotype of fast-spiking interneurons is mediated by NADPH-oxidase. *Science* **318**, 1645–1647.

Bendel, O., Meijer, B., Hurd, Y. & von Euler, G. (2005) Cloning and expression of the human NMDA receptor subunit NR3B in the adult human hippocampus. *Neuroscience Letters* **377**, 31–36.

Bendikov, I., Nadri, C., Amar, S. *et al.* (2007) A CSF and post-mortem brain study of D-serine metabolic parameters in schizophrenia. *Schizophrenia Research* **90**, 41–51.

Benes, F.M. & Berretta, S. (2001) GABAergic interneurons: implications for understanding schizophrenia and bipolar disorder. *Neuropsychopharmacology* **25**, 1–27.

Benes, F.M., Davidson, J. & Bird, E.D. (1986) Quantitative cytoarchitectural studies of the cerebral cortex of schizophrenics. *Archives of General Psychiatry* **43**, 31–35.

Benes, F.M., McSparren, J., Bird, E.D., SanGiovanni, J.P. & Vincent, S.L. (1991) Deficits in small interneurons in prefrontal and cingulate cortices of schizophrenic and schizoaffective patients. *Archives of General Psychiatry* **48**, 996–1001.

Benes, F.M., Vincent, S.L., Alsterberg, G., Bird, E.D. & SanGiovanni, J.P. (1992) Increased GABAA receptor binding in superficial layers of cingulate cortex in schizophrenics. *Journal of Neuroscience* **12**, 924–929.

Benes, F.M., Vincent, S.L., Marie, A. & Khan, Y. (1996) Upregulation of GABAA receptor binding on neurons of the prefrontal cortex in schizophrenic subjects. *Neuroscience* **75**, 1021–1031.

Benes, F.M., Wickramasinghe, R., Vincent, S.L., Khan, Y. & Todtenkopf, M. (1997) Uncoupling of GABA(A) and benzodiazepine receptor binding activity in the hippocampal formation of schizophrenic brain. *Brain Research* **755**, 121–129.

Benes, F.M., Todtenkopf, M.S., Logiotatos, P. & Williams, M. (2000) Glutamate decarboxylase(65)-immunoreactive terminals in cingulate and prefrontal cortices of schizophrenic and bipolar brain. *Journal of Chemical Neuroanatomy* **20**, 259–269.

Benes, F.M., Todtenkopf, M.S. & Kostoulakos, P. (2001) GluR5,6,7 subunit immunoreactivity on apical pyramidal cell dendrites in hippocampus of schizophrenics and manic depressives. *Hippocampus* **11**, 482–491.

Benes, F.M., Lim, B., Matzilevich, D., Walsh, J.P., Subburaju, S. & Minns, M. (2007) Regulation of the GABA cell phenotype in hippocampus of schizophrenics and bipolars. *Proceedings of the National Academy of Sciences USA* **104**, 10164–10166.

Beneyto, M., Kristiansen, L.V., Oni-Orisan, A., McCullumsmith, R.E. & Meador-Woodruff, J.H. (2007) Abnormal glutamate receptor expression in the medial temporal lobe in schizophrenia and mood disorders. *Neuropsychopharmacology* **32**, 1888–1902.

Beneyto, M. & Meador-Woodruff, J.H. (2006) Lamina-specific abnormalities of AMPA receptor trafficking and signaling molecule transcripts in the prefrontal cortex in schizophrenia. *Synapse* **60**, 585–598.

Bennett, J.P., Jr., Enna, S.J., Bylund, D.B., Gillin, J.C., Wyatt, R.J. & Snyder, S.H. (1979) Neurotransmitter receptors in frontal cortex of schizophrenics. *Archives of General Psychiatry* **36**, 927–934.

Bergeron, R., Meyer, T.M., Coyle, J.T. & Greene, R.W. (1998) Modulation of N-methyl-D-aspartate receptor function by glycine transport. *Proceedings of the National Academy of Sciences USA* **95**, 15730–15734.

Bergeron, R., Imamura, Y., Frangioni, J.V., Greene, R.W. & Coyle, J.T. (2007) Endogenous N-acetylaspartylglutamate reduced NMDA receptor-dependent current neurotransmission in the CA1 area of the hippocampus. *Journal of Neurochemistry* **100**, 346–357.

Bettler, B., Kaupmann, K., Mosbacher, J. & Gassmann, M. (2004) Molecular structure and physiological functions of GABA(B) receptors. *Physiology Reviews* **84**, 835–867.

Bishop, J.R., Ellingrod, V.L., Moline, J. & Miller, D. (2005) Association between the polymorphic GRM3 gene and negative symptom improvement during olanzapine treatment. *Schizophrenia Research* **77**, 253–260.

Bjarnadottir, M., Misner, D.L., Haverfield-Gross, S. *et al.* (2007) Neuregulin1 (NRG1) signaling through Fyn modulates NMDA receptor phosphorylation: differential synaptic function in NRG1+/− knock-outs compared with wild-type mice. *Journal of Neuroscience* **27**, 4519–4529.

Black, J.E., Kodish, I.M., Grossman, A.W., *et al.* (2004) Pathology of layer V pyramidal neurons in the prefrontal cortex of patients with schizophrenia. *American Journal of Psychiatry* **161**, 742–754.

Borghese, C.M., Stórustova, Sí., Ebert, B. *et al.* (2006) The delta subunit of γ-aminobutyric acid type A receptors does not confer sensitivity to low concentrations of ethanol. *Journal of Pharmacology & Experimental Therapeutics* **316**, 1360–1368.

Bortolotto, Z.A., Nistico, R., More, J.C., Jane, D.E. & Collingridge, G.L. (2005) Kainate receptors and mossy fiber LTP. *Neurotoxicology* **26**, 769–777.

Braun, I., Genius, J., Grunze, H., Bender, A., Moller, H.J. & Rujescu, D. (2007) Alterations of hippocampal and prefrontal GABAergic interneurons in an animal model of psychosis induced by NMDA receptor antagonism. *Schizophrenia Research* **97**, 254–263.

Bray, N.J., Preece, A., Williams, N.M. *et al.* (2005) Haplotypes at the dystrobrevin binding protein 1 (DTNBP1) gene locus mediate risk for schizophrenia through reduced DTNBP1 expression. *Human Molecular Genetics* **14**, 1947–1954.

Breese, G.R., Knapp, D.J. & Moy, S.S. (2002) Integrative role for serotonergic and glutamatergic receptor mechanisms in the action of NMDA antagonists: potential relationships to antipsychotic drug actions on NMDA antagonist responsiveness. *Neuroscience & Biobehavioral Reviews* **26**, 441–455.

Bressan, R.A., Erlandsson, K., Mulligan, R.S. *et al.* (2004) A bolus/infusion paradigm for the novel NMDA receptor SPET tracer [123I]CNS 1261. *Nuclear Medicine and Biology* **31**, 155–164.

Bressan, R.A., Erlandsson, K., Stone, J.M. *et al.* (2005) Impact of schizophrenia and chronic antipsychotic treatment on [123I]CNS-1261 binding to N-methyl-D-aspartate receptors *in vivo*. *Biological Psychiatry* **58**, 41–46.

Brickley S.G, Cull-Candy, S.G. & Farrant, M. (1999) Single-channel properties of synaptic and extrasynaptic GABAA receptors suggest differential targeting of receptor subtypes. *Journal of Neuroscience* **19**, 2960–2973.

Brigman, J.L., Padukiewicz, K.E., Sutherland, M.L. & Rothblat, L.A. (2006) Executive functions in the heterozygous reeler mouse model of schizophrenia. *Behavioral Neuroscience* **120**, 984–988.

Brody, S.A, Geyer, M.A. & Large, C.H. (2003) Lamotrigine prevents ketamine but not amphetamine-induced deficits in prepulse inhibition in mice. *Psychopharmacology (Berlin)* **169**, 240–246.

Buchanan, R.W, Javitt DC, Marder SR *et al.* (2007) The Cognitive and Negative Symptoms in Schizophrenia Trial (CONSIST): the efficacy of glutamatergic agents for negative symptoms and cognitive impairments. *American Journal of Psychiatry* **164**, 1593–1602.

Burbaeva, G., Boksha, I.S., Turishcheva, M.S., Vorobyeva, E.A., Savushkina, O.K. & Tereshkina, E.B. (2003) Glutamine synthetase and glutamate dehydrogenase in the prefrontal cortex of patients with schizophrenia. *Progress in Neuropsychopharmacology and Biological Psychiatry* **27**, 675–680.

Burnet, P.W.J., Eastwood, S.L., Bristow, G.C. *et al.* (2008) D-amino acid oxidase activity and expression are increased in schizophrenia. *Molecular Psychiatry* **13**, 658–660.

Burns, J., Job, D., Bastin, M.E. *et al.* (2003) Structural disconnectivity in schizophrenia: a diffusion tensor magnetic resonance imaging study. *British Journal of Psychiatry* **182**, 439–443.

Busatto, G.F., Pilowsky, L.S., Costa, D.C. *et al.* (1997) Correlation between reduced *in vivo* benzodiazepine receptor binding and severity of psychotic symptoms in schizophrenia. *American Journal of Psychiatry* **154**, 56–63.

Byne, W., Kidkardnee, S., Tatusov, A., Yiannoulos, G., Buchsbaum, M.S. & Haroutunian, V. (2006) Schizophrenia-associated reduction of neuronal and oligodendrocyte numbers in the anterior principal thalamic nucleus. *Schizophrenia Research* **85**, 245–253.

Byne, W., Dracheva, S., Chin, B., Schmeidler, J.M., Davis, K.L. & Haroutunian, V. (2008) Schizophrenia and sex associated differences in the expression of neuronal and oligodendrocyte-specific genes in individual thalamic nuclei. *Schizophrenia Research* **98**, 118–128.

Cai, J.X. & Arnsten, A.F. (1997) Dose-dependent effects of the dopamine D1 receptor agonists A77636 or SKF81297 on spatial working memory in aged monkeys. *Journal of Pharmacology & Experimental Therapeutics* **283**, 183–189.

Cartmell, J., Monn, J.A. & Schoepp, D.D. (1999) The metabotropic glutamate 2/3 receptor agonists LY354740 and LY379268 selectively attenuate phencyclidine versus d-amphetamine motor behaviors in rats. *Journal of Pharmacology & Experimental Therapeutics* **291**, 161–170.

Cascella, N.G., Macciardi, F., Cavallini, C. & Smeraldi, E. (1994) d-cycloserine adjuvant therapy to conventional neuroleptic treatment in schizophrenia: an open-label study. *Journal of Neural Transmission Genetics Section* **95**, 105–111.

Castner, S.A. & Williams, G.V. (2007) Tuning the engine of cognition: a focus on NMDA/D1 receptor interactions in prefrontal cortex. *Brain Cognition* **63**, 94–122.

Castner, S.A., Williams, G.V. & Goldman-Rakic, P.S. (2000) Reversal of antipsychotic-induced working memory deficits by short-term dopamine D1 receptor stimulation. *Science* **287**, 2020–2022.

Cepeda, C. & Levine, M.S. (2006) Where do you think you are going? The NMDA-D1 receptor trap. *Science STKE*, pe20.

Chan, M.H., Chiu, P.H., Sou, J.H. & Chen, H.H. (2008) Attenuation of ketamine-evoked behavioral responses by mGluR5 positive modulators in mice. *Psychopharmacology (Berlin)* **198**, 141–148.

Chatterton, J.E., Awobuluyi, M., Premkumar, L.S. *et al.* (2002) Excitatory glycine receptors containing the NR3 family of NMDA receptor subunits. *Nature* **415**, 793–798.

Chebib, M. (2004) GABAC receptor ion channels. *Clinical and Experimental Pharmacology and Physiology* **31**, 800–804.

Cheffings, C.M. & Colquhoun, D. (2000) Single channel analysis of a novel NMDA channel from Xenopus oocytes expressing recombinant NR1a, NR2A and NR2D subunits. *Journal of Physiology* **526**, 481–491.

Cho, R.Y., Konecky, R.O. & Carter, C.S. (2006) Impairments in frontal cortical gamma synchrony and cognitive control in schizophrenia. *Proceedings of the National Academy of Sciences USA* **103**, 19878–19883.

Chumakov, I., Blumenfeld, M., Guerassimenko, O. *et al.* (2002) Genetic and physiological data implicating the new human gene G72 and the gene for D-amino acid oxidase in schizophrenia. *Proceedings of the National Academy of Sciences USA* **99**, 13675–13680.

Clarke, R.J. & Johnson, J.W. (2006) NMDA receptor NR2 subunit dependence of the slow component of magnesium unblock. *Journal of Neuroscience* **26**, 5825–5834.

Cohen, B.D., Rosenbaum, G., Luby, E.D. & Gottlieb, J.S. (1962) Comparison of phencyclidine hydrochloride (sernyl) with other drugs: simulation of schizophrenic performance with phencyclidine hydrochloride (sernyl), lysergic acid diethylamide (LSD-25), amobarbital (amytal) sodium; II. symbolic and sequential thinking. *Archives of General Psychiatry* **6**, 79–85.

Conti, F., Minelli, A., DeBiasi, S. & Melone, M. (1997) Neuronal and glial localization of NMDA receptors in the cerebral cortex. *Molecular Neurobiology* **14**, 1–18.

Contreras, P.C. (1990) D-serine antagonized phencyclidine- and MK-801-induced stereotyped behavior and ataxia. *Neuropharmacology* **29**, 291–293.

Coppel, D.L., Bovill, J.G. & Dundee, J.W. (1973) The taming of ketamine. *Anaesthesia* **28**, 293–296.

Corfas, G., Roy, K. & Buxbaum, J.D. (2004) Neuregulin 1-erbB signaling and the molecular/cellular basis of schizophrenia. *Nature Neuroscience* **7**, 575–580.

Corssen, G. & Domino, E.F. (1966) Dissociative anesthesia: further pharmacologic studies and first clinical experience with the phencyclidine derivative CI-581. *Anesthesia & Analgesia* **45**, 29–40.

Corti, C., Crepaldi, L., Mion, S., Roth, A.L., Xuereb, J.H. & Ferraguti, F. (2007) Altered dimerization of metabotropic glutamate receptor 3 in schizophrenia. *Biological Psychiatry* **62**, 747–755.

Costa, E., Davis, J., Grayson, D.R., Guidotti, A., Pappas, G.D. & Pesold, C. (2001) Dendritic spine hypoplasticity and downregulation of reelin and GABAergic tone in schizophrenia vulnerability. *Neurobiological Disease* **8**, 723–742.

Costa, E., Chen, Y., Davis, J. *et al.* (2002) REELIN and schizophrenia: a disease at the interface of the genome and the epigenome. *Molecular Intervention* **2**, 47–57.

Costa, E., Grayson, D.R. & Guidotti, A. (2003) Epigenetic downregulation of GABAergic function in schizophrenia: potential for pharmacological intervention? *Molecular Intervention* **3**, 220–229.

Costa, E., Davis, J.M., Dong, E. *et al.* (2004) A GABAergic cortical deficit dominates schizophrenia pathophysiology. *Critical Reviews in Neurobiology* **16**, 1–23.

Cotter, D., Landau, S., Beasley, C. *et al.* (2002) The density and spatial distribution of GABAergic neurons, labelled using calcium binding proteins, in the anterior cingulate cortex in major depressive disorder, bipolar disorder, and schizophrenia. *Biological Psychiatry* **51**, 377–386.

Crandall, J.E., McCarthy, D.M., Araki, K.Y., Sims, J.R., Ren, J.Q. & Bhide, P.G. (2007) Dopamine receptor activation modulates GABA neuron migration from the basal forebrain to the cerebral cortex. *Journal of Neuroscience* **27**, 3813–3822.

Crook, J.M., Akil, M., Law, B.C., Hyde, T.M. & Kleinman, J.E. (2002) Comparative analysis of group II metabotropic glutamate receptor immunoreactivity in Brodmann's area 46 of the dorsolateral prefrontal cortex from patients with schizophrenia and normal subjects. *Molecular Psychiatry* **7**, 157–164.

Cross, A.J., Crow, T.J. & Owen, F. (1979) Gamma-aminobutyric acid in the brain in schizophrenia. *Lancet* **1**, 560–561.

Cunningham, M.O., Hunt, J., Middleton, S. *et al.* (2006) Region-specific reduction in entorhinal gamma oscillations and parvalbumin-immunoreactive neurons in animal models of psychiatric illness. *Journal of Neuroscience* **26**, 2767–2776.

Damadzic, R., Bigelow, L.B., Krimer, L.S. *et al.* (2001) A quantitative immunohistochemical study of astrocytes in the entorhinal cortex in schizophrenia, bipolar disorder and major depression: absence of significant astrocytosis. *Brain Research Bulletin* **55**, 611–618.

Danysz, W. (2002) CX-516 Cortex pharmaceuticals. *Current Opinion in Investigative Drugs* **3**, 1081–1088.

Davis, K.L., Stewart, D.G., Friedman, J.I. *et al.* (2003) White matter changes in schizophrenia: evidence for myelin-related dysfunction. *Archives of General Psychiatry* **60**, 443–456.

Daviss, S.R. & Lewis, D.A. (1995) Local circuit neurons of the prefrontal cortex in schizophrenia: selective increase in the density of calbindin-immunoreactive neurons. *Psychiatry Research* **59**, 81–96.

Dean, B., Pavey, G., McLeod, M., Opeskin, K., Keks, N. & Copolov, D. (2001a) A change in the density of [(3)H]flumazenil, but not [(3)H]muscimol binding, in Brodmann's Area 9 from subjects with bipolar disorder. *Journal of Affective Disorders* **66**, 147–158.

Dean, B., Sundram, S., Bradbury, R., Scarr, E. & Copolov, D. (2001b) Studies on [3H]CP-55940 binding in the human central nervous system: regional specific changes in density of cannabinoid-1 receptors associated with schizophrenia and cannabis use. *Neuroscience* **103**, 9–15.

Deng, C., Han, M. &, Huang, X.F. (2007) No changes in densities of cannabinoid receptors in the superior temporal gyrus in schizophrenia. *Neuroscience Bulletin* **23**, 341–347.

Dev, K.K. & Henley, J.M. (2006) The schizophrenic faces of PICK1. *Trends in Pharmacological Science* **27**, 57–49.

Di Forti, M., Morrison, P.D., Butt, A. & Murray, R.M. (2007) Cannabis use and psychiatric and cogitive disorders: the chicken or the egg? *Current Opinion in Psychiatry* **20**, 228–234.

Diaz, P., Bhaskara, S., Dursun, S.M. & Deakin, B. (2005) Double-blind, placebo-controlled, crossover trial of clozapine plus glycine in refractory schizophrenia negative results. *Journal of Clinical Psychopharmacology* **25**, 277–278.

Dorow, R., Horowski, R., Paschelke, G. & Amin, M. (1983) Severe anxiety induced by FG 7142, a beta-carboline ligand for benzodiazepine receptors. *Lancet* **2**, 98–99.

Dracheva, S., McGurk, S.R. & Haroutunian, V. (2005) mRNA expression of AMPA receptors and AMPA receptor binding proteins in the cerebral cortex of elderly schizophrenics. *Journal of Neuroscience Research* **79**, 868–878.

Dracheva, S., Davis, K.L., Chin, B., Woo, D.A., Schmeidler, J. & Haroutunian, V. (2006) Myelin-associated mRNA and protein expression deficits in the anterior cingulate cortex and hippocampus in elderly schizophrenia patients. *Neurobiological Diseases* **21**, 531–540.

Driesen, N.R., Leung, H.C., Calhoun, V.D. *et al.* (2008) Impairment of working memory maintenance and response in schizophrenia: functional magnetic resonance imaging evidence. *Biological Psychiatry* **64**, 1026–1034.

D'Souza, D.C., Charney, D.S. & Krystal, J.H. (1995) Glycine site agonists of the NMDA receptor: a review. *CNS Drug Reviews* **1**, 227–260.

D'Souza, D.C., Gil, R., Belger, A. *et al.* (1997) Glycine-ketamine interactions in healthy humans. 36th Annual Meeting, American College of Neuropsychopharmacology, Kona, HI, pp. 286.

D'Souza, D.C., Gil, R., Cassello, K. *et al.* (2000) IV glycine and oral D-cycloserine effects on plasma and CSF amino acids in healthy humans. *Biological Psychiatry* **47**, 450–462.

D'Souza, D.C., Perry, E., MacDougall, L. *et al.* (2004) The psychotomimetic effects of intravenous delta-9-tetrahydrocannabinol in healthy individuals: implications for psychosis. *Neuropsychopharmacology* **29**, 1558–1572.

D'Souza, D.C., Abi-Saab, W.M., Madonick, S. *et al.* (2005) Delta-9-tetrahydrocannabinol effects in schizophrenia: implications for cognition, psychosis, and addiction. *Biological Psychiatry* **57**, 594–608.

D'Souza, D.C., Gil, R., MacDougall, L. *et al.* (2006) Gamma-aminobutyric acid-serotonin interactions in healthy subjects:implications for psychosis and dissociation. *Biological Psychiatry* **59**, 128–137.

Dursun, S.M. & Deakin, J.F. (2001) Augmenting antipsychotic treatment with lamotrigine or topiramate in patients with treatment-resistant schizophrenia: a naturalistic case-series outcome study. *Journal of Psychopharmacology* **15**, 297–301.

Eastwood, S.L. & Harrison, P.J. (1995) Decreased synaptophysin in the medial temporal lobe in schizophrenia demonstrated using immunoautoradiography. *Neuroscience* **69**, 339–343.

Eastwood, S.L. & Harrison, P.J. (2001) Synaptic pathology in the anterior cingulate cortex in schizophrenia and mood disorders. A review and a Western blot study of synaptophysin, GAP-43 and the complexins. *Brain Research Bulletin* **55**, 569–578.

Eastwood, S.L. & Harrison, P.J. (2003) Interstitial white matter neurons express less reelin and are abnormally distributed in schizophrenia: towards an integration of molecular and morphologic aspects of the neurodevelopmental hypothesis. *Molecular Psychiatry* **8**, 769, 821–831.

Egan, M.F., Straub, R.E., Goldberg, T.E. *et al.* (2004) Variation in GRM3 affects cognition, prefrontal glutamate, and risk for schizophrenia. *Proceedings of the National Academy of Sciences USA* **101**, 12604–12609.

Eggan, S.M., Hashimoto, T. & Lewis, D.A. (2010) Reduced cortical cannabinoid 1 receptor mRNA and protein expression in schizophrenia. *Archives of General Psychiatry* (in press).

Erlander, M.G. & Tobin, A.J. (1991) The structural and functional heterogeneity of glutamic acid decarboxylase: a review. *Neurochemical Research* **16**, 215–226.

Erreger, K., Geballe, M.T., Kristensen, A. *et al.* (2007) Subunit-specific agonist activity at NR2A-, NR2B-, NR2C-, and NR2D-containing N-methyl-D-aspartate glutamate receptors. *Molecular Pharmacology* **72**, 907–920.

Falkai, P., Honer, W.G., David, S., Bogerts, B., Majtenyi, C. & Bayer, T.A. (1999) No evidence for astrogliosis in brains of schizophrenic patients. A post-mortem study. *Neuropathology and Applied Neurobiology* **25**, 48–53.

Farber, N.B., Newcomer, J.W. & Olney, J.W. (1999) Lamotrigine prevents NMDA antagonist neurotoxicity. *Schizophrenia Research* **36**, 308.

Farmery, S.M., Owen, F., Poulter, M. & Crow, T.J. (1985) Reduced high affinity cholecystokinin binding in hippocampus and frontal cortex of schizophrenic patients. *Life Science* **36**, 473–477.

Farrant, M. & Nusser, Z. (2005) Variations on an inhibitory theme: phasic and tonic activation of GABA(A) receptors. *Nature Reviews Neuroscience* **6**, 215–219.

Fatemi, S.H., Stary, J.M., Earle, J.A., Araghi-Niknam, M. & Eagan, E. (2005) GABAergic dysfunction in schizophrenia and mood disorders as reflected by decreased levels of glutamic acid decarboxylase 65 and 67 kDa and Reelin proteins in cerebellum. *Schizophrenia Research* **72**, 109–122.

Ferrie, C.D., Robinson, R.O. & Panayiotopoulos, C.P. (1996) Psychotic and severe behavioural reactions with vigabatrin: a review. *Acta Neurologica Scandinavica* **93**, 1–8.

Fisahn, A. (2005) Kainate receptors and rhythmic activity in neuronal networks: hippocampal gamma oscillations as a tool. *Journal of Physiology* **562**, 65–72.

Ford, J.M., Roach, B.J., Faustman, W.O. & Mathalon, D.H. (2008) Out-of-synch and out-of-sorts: dysfunction of motor-sensory communication in schizophrenia. *Biological Psychiatry* **63**, 736–743.

Freund, T.F. (2003) Interneuron Diversity series: Rhythm and mood in perisomatic inhibition. *Trends in Neuroscience* **26**, 489–495

Fukaya, M., Hayashi, Y. & Watanabe, M. (2005) NR2 to NR3B subunit switchover of NMDA receptors in early postnatal motoneurons. *European Journal of Neuroscience* **21**, 1432–1436.

Gallinat, J., Winterer, G., Herrmann, C.S. & Senkowski, D. (2004) Reduced oscillatory gamma-band responses in unmedicated schizophrenic patients indicate impaired frontal network processing. *Clinical Neurophysiology* **115**, 1863–1874.

Gao, X.M., Sakai, K., Roberts, R.C., Conley, R.R., Dean, B. & Tamminga, C.A. (2000) Ionotropic glutamate receptors and expression of N-methyl-D-aspartate receptor subunits in sub-regions of human hippocampus, effects of schizophrenia. *American Journal of Psychiatry* **157**, 1141–1149.

Garey, L.J., Ong, W.Y., Patel, T.S. *et al.* (1998) Reduced dendritic spine density on cerebral cortical pyramidal neurons in schiz-ophrenia. *Journal of Neurology, Neurosurgery & Psychiatry* **65**, 446–453.

Ghose, S., Weickert, C.S., Colvin, S.M. *et al.* (2004) Glutamate carboxypeptidase II gene expression in the human frontal and temporal lobe in schizophrenia. *Neuropsychopharmacology* **29**, 117–125.

Gillies, D., Beck, A., McCloud, A., Rathbone, J. & Gillies, D. (2005) Benzodiazepines alone or in combination with antipsy-chotic drugs for acute psychosis. *Cochrane Database Systematic Reviews*, CD003079.

Glantz, L.A & Lewis, D.A. (1997a) Reduction of synaptophysin immunoreactivity in the prefrontal cortex of subjects with schizophrenia. Regional and diagnostic specificity. *Archives of General Psychiatry* **54**, 943–952.

Glantz, L.A & Lewis, D.A. (1997b) Reduction of synaptophysin immunoreactivity in the prefrontal cortex of subjects with schizophrenia. Regional and diagnostic specificity. *Archives of General Psychiatry* **54**, 660–669.

Glantz, L.A & Lewis, D.A. (2000) Decreased dendritic spine density on prefrontal cortical pyramidal neurons in schizo-phrenia. *Archives of General Psychiatry* **57**, 65–73.

Glantz, L.A., Austin, M.C. & Lewis, D.A. (2000) Normal cellular levels of synaptophysin mRNA expression in the prefrontal cortex of subjects with schizophrenia. *Biological Psychiatry* **48**, 389–397.

Goff, D.C., Henderson, D.C., Evins, A.E. & Amico, E. (1999) A placebo-controlled crossover trial of D-cycloserine added to clozapine in patients with schizophrenia. *Biological Psychiatry* **45**, 512–514.

Goff, D.C., Leahy, L., Berman, I. *et al.* (2001) A placebo-controlled pilot study of the ampakine CX516 added to clozapine in schiz-ophrenia. *Journal of Clinical Psychopharmacology* **21**, 484–487.

Goff, D.C., Herz, L., Posever, T. *et al.* (2005) A six-month, placebo-controlled trial of D-cycloserine co-administered with conventional antipsychotics in schizophrenia patients. *Psychopharmacology (Berlin)* **179**, 144–150.

Goff, D.C., Keefe, R., Citrome, L. *et al.* (2007) Lamotrigine as add-on therapy in schizophrenia: Results of 2 placebo-controlled trials. *Journal of Clinical Psychopharmacology* **27**, 582–589.

Goff, D.C., Lamberti, J.S., Leon, A.C. *et al.* (2008) A placebo-controlled add-on trial of the ampakine, CX516, for cognitive deficits in schizophrenia. *Neuropsychopharmacology* **33**, 465–472.

Goldberger, C., Gourion, D., Leroy, S. *et al.* (2005) Population-based and family-based association study of 5'UTR polymor-phism of the reelin gene and schizophrenia. *American Journal of Medical Genetics B Neuropsychiatric Genetics* **137**, 5–15.

Gozzi, A., Large, C.H., Schwarz, A., Bertani, S., Crestan, V. & Bifone, A. (2008) Differential effects of antipsychotic and glutamatergic agents on the phMRI response to phencyclid-ine. *Neuropsychopharmacology* **33**, 1690–1703.

Greger, I.H., Ziff, E.B. & Penn, A.C. (2007) Molecular determi-nants of AMPA receptor subunit assembly. *Trends in Neuroscience* **30**, 407–416.

Grunze, H.C., Rainnie, D.G., Hasselmo, M.E. *et al.* (1996) NMDA-dependent modulation of CA1 local circuit inhibition. *Journal of Neuroscience* **16**, 2034–2043.

Gu, Z., Jiang, Q., Fu, A.K., Ip, N.Y. & Yan, Z. (2005) Regulation of NMDA receptors by neuregulin signaling in prefrontal cortex. *Journal of Neuroscience* **25**, 4974–4984.

Guidotti, A., Auta, J., Davis, J.M. *et al.* (2000) Decrease in reelin and glutamic acid decarboxylase67 (GAD67) expression in schizophrenia and bipolar disorder, a postmortem brain study. *Archives of General Psychiatry* **57**, 1061–1069.

Guillin, O., Abi-Dargham, A. & Laruelle, M. (2007) Neurobiology of dopamine in schizophrenia. *International Reviews in Neurobiology* **78**, 1–39.

Gupta, D.S., McCullumsmith, R.E., Beneyto, M., Haroutunian, V., Davis, K.L. & Meador-Woodruff, J.H. (2005) Metabotropic glutamate receptor protein expression in the prefrontal cortex and striatum in schizophrenia. *Synapse* **57**, 123–131.

Hahn, C.G., Wang, H.Y., Cho, D.S. *et al.* (2006) Altered neuregu-lin 1-erbB4 signaling contributes to NMDA receptor hypo-function in schizophrenia. *Nature Medicine* **12**, 824–828.

Hakak, Y., Walker, J.R., Li, C. *et al.* (2001) Genome-wide expres-sion analysis reveals dysregulation of myelination-related genes in chronic schizophrenia. *Proceedings of the National Academy of Sciences USA* **98**, 4746–4751.

Hamdani, N., Tabeze, J.P., Ramoz, N. *et al.* (2008) The CNR1 gene as a pharmacogenetic factor for antipsychotics rather than a susceptibility gene for schizophrenia. *European Neuropsychopharmacology* **18**, 34–40.

Harich, S., Gross, G. & Bespalov, A. (2007) Stimulation of the metabotropic glutamate 2/3 receptor attenuates social novelty discrimination deficits induced by neonatal phencyclidine treatment. *Psychopharmacology (Berlin)* **192**, 511–519.

Haroutunian, V., Katsel, P., Dracheva, S., Stewart, D.G. & Davis, K.L. (2007) Variations in oligodendrocyte-related gene expres-sion across multiple cortical regions: implications for the pathophysiology of schizophrenia. *International Journal of Neuropsychopharmacology* **10**, 565–573.

Harrison, P.J. (1999) The neuropathology of schizophrenia. A critical review of the data and their interpretation. *Brain* **122**, 593–624.

Harrison, P.J. (2004) The hippocampus in schizophrenia: a review of the neuropathological evidence and its pathophysi-ological implications. *Psychopharmacology (Berlin)* **174**, 151–162.

Harrison, P.J. & Weinberger, D.R. (2005) Schizophrenia genes, gene expression, and neuropathology: on the matter of their convergence. *Molecular Psychiatry* **10**, 40–68; image 5.

Hashimoto, T. & Lewis, D.A. (2006) BDNF Val66Met polymorphism and GAD67 mRNA expression in the prefrontal cortex of subjects with schizophrenia. *American Journal of Psychiatry* **163**, 534–537.

Hashimoto, K., Fukushima, T., Shimizu, E. *et al.* (2003a) Decreased serum levels of D-serine in patients with schizophrenia: evidence in support of the N-methyl-D-aspartate receptor hypofunction hypothesis of schizophrenia. *Archives of General Psychiatry* **60**, 572–576.

Hashimoto, T., Volk, D.W., Eggan, S.M. *et al.* (2003b) Gene expression deficits in a subclass of GABA neurons in the prefrontal cortex of subjects with schizophrenia. *Journal of Neuroscience* **23**, 6315–6326.

Hashimoto, T., Arion, D., Unger, T. *et al.* (2008a) Alterations in GABA-related transcriptome in the dorsolateral prefrontal cortex of subjects with schizophrenia. *Molecular Psychiatry* **13**, 147–161.

Hashimoto, T., Bazmi, H.H., Mirnics, K., Wu, Q., Sampson, A.R. & Lewis, D.A. (2008b) Conserved regional patterns of GABA-related transcript expression in the neocortex of subjects with schizophrenia. *American Journal of Psychiatry* **165**, 416–419.

Heckers, S., Stone, D., Walsh, J., Shick, J., Koul, P. & Benes, F.M. (2002) Differential hippocampal expression of glutamic acid decarboxylase 65 and 67 messenger RNA in bipolar disorder and schizophrenia. *Archives of General Psychiatry* **59**, 521–529.

Heresco-Levy, U. & Javitt, D.C. (2004) Comparative effects of glycine and D-cycloserine on persistent negative symptoms in schizophrenia: a retrospective analysis. *Schizophrenia Research* **66**, 89–96.

Heresco-Levy, U., Javitt, D.C., Ermilov, M., Mordel, C., Horowitz, A. & Kelly, D. (1996) Double-blind, placebo-controlled, crossover trial of glycine adjuvant therapy for treatment-resistant schizophrenia. *British Journal of Psychiatry* **169**, 610–617.

Heresco-Levy, U., Javitt, D.C., Ermilov, M., Mordel, C., Silipo, G. & Lichtenstein, M. (1999) Efficacy of high-dose glycine in the treatment of enduring negative symptoms of schizophrenia. *Archives of General Psychiatry* **56**, 29–36.

Heresco-Levy, U., Ermilov, M., Lichtenberg, P., Bar, G. & Javitt, D.C. (2004) High-dose glycine added to olanzapine and risperidone for the treatment of schizophrenia. *Biological Psychiatry* **55**, 165–171.

Heresco-Levy, U., Javitt, D.C., Ebstein, R. *et al.* (2005) D-serine efficacy as add-on pharmacotherapy to risperidone and olanzapine for treatment-refractory schizophrenia. *Biological Psychiatry* **57**, 577–585.

Hermle, L., Funfgeld, M., Oepen, G. *et al.* (1992) Mescaline-induced psychopathological, neuropsychological, and neurometabolic effects in normal subjects: experimental psychosis as a tool for psychiatric research. *Biological Psychiatry* **32**, 976–991.

Hikida, T., Mustafa, A.K., Maeda, K. *et al.* (2008) Modulation of D-serine levels in brains of mice lacking PICK1. *Biological Psychiatry* **63**, 997–1000.

Hires, S.A., Zhu, Y. & Tsien, R.Y. (2008) Optical measurement of synaptic glutamate spillover and reuptake by linker opti-mized glutamate-sensitive fluorescent reporters. *Proceedings of the National Academy of Sciences USA* **105**, 4411–4416.

Hof, P.R., Haroutunian, V., Copland, C., Davis, K.L. & Buxbaum, J.D. (2002) Molecular and cellular evidence for an oligodendrocyte abnormality in schizophrenia. *Neurochemical Research* **27**, 1193–1200.

Homayoun, H., Jackson, M.E. & Moghaddam, B. (2005) Activation of metabotropic glutamate 2/3 receptors reverses the effects of NMDA receptor hypofunction on prefrontal cortex unit activity in awake rats. *Journal of Neurophysiology* **93**, 1989–2001.

Homayoun, H. & Moghaddam, B. (2006) Bursting of prefrontal cortex neurons in awake rats is regulated by metabotropic glutamate 5 (mGlu5) receptors: rate-dependent influence and interaction with NMDA receptors. *Cerebral Cortex* **16**, 93–105.

Homayoun, H. & Moghaddam, B. (2007) NMDA receptor hypofunction produces opposite effects on prefrontal cortex interneurons and pyramidal neurons. *Journal of Neuroscience* **27**, 11496–11500.

Homayoun, H., Stefani, M.R., Adams, B.W., Tamagan, G.D. & Moghaddam, B. (2004) Functional interaction between NMDA and mGlu5 receptors: Effects on working memory, instrumental learning, motor behaviors, and dopamine release. *Neuropsychopharmacology* **29**, 1259–1269.

Hong, C.J., Liao, D.L., Shih, H.L. & Tsai, S.J. (2004) Association study of PICK1 rs3952 polymorphism and schizophrenia. *Neuroreport* **15**, 1965–1967.

Horowski, R. & Dorrow, R. (2002) Anxiogenic, not psychotogenic, properties of the partial inverse benzodiazepine receptor agonist FG 7142 in man. *Psychopharmacology (Berlin)* **162**, 223–224.

Huang, C.H. & Chen, C.H. (2006) Absence of association of a polymorphic GGC repeat at the 5' untranslated region of the reelin gene with schizophrenia. *Psychiatry Research* **142**, 89–92.

Huang, H.S. & Akbarian, S. (2007) GAD1 mRNA expression and DNA methylation in prefrontal cortex of subjects with schizophrenia. *PLoS ONE* **2**, e809.

Idris, N.F., Repeto, P., Neill, J.C. & Large, C.H. (2005) Investigation of the effects of lamotrigine and clozapine in improving reversal-learning impairments induced by acute phencyclidine and D-amphetamine in the rat. *Psychopharmacology (Berlin)* **179**, 336–348.

Ikeda, M., Iwata, N., Suzuki, T. *et al.* (2005) Association analysis of chromosome 5 GABAA receptor cluster in Japanese schizophrenia patients. *Biological Psychiatry* **58**, 440–445.

Ikeda, M., Ozaki, N., Yamanouchi, Y. *et al.* (2007) No association between the glutamate decarboxylase 67 gene (GAD1) and schizophrenia in the Japanese population. *Schizophrenia Research* **91**, 22–26.

Impagnatiello, F., Guidotti, A.R., Pesold, C. *et al.* (1998) A decrease of reelin expression as a putative vulnerability factor in schizophrenia. *Proceedings of the National Academy of Sciences USA* **95**, 15718–15723.

Itil, T., Keskiner, A., Kiremitci, N. & Holden, J.M.C. (1967) Effect of phencyclidine in chronic schizophrenics. *Canadian Psychiatric Association Journal* **12**, 209–212.

Iwamoto, K., Bundo, M., Yamada, K. *et al.* (2005) DNA methylation status of SOX10 correlates with its downregulation and oligodendrocyte dysfunction in schizophrenia. *Journal of Neuroscience* **25**, 5376–5381.

Javitt, D.C., Zylberman, I., Zukin, S.R., Heresco-Levy, U. & Lindenmayer, J.P. (1994) Amelioration of negative symptoms in schizophrenia by glycine. *American Journal of Psychiatry* **151**, 1234–1236.

Javitt, D.C., Balla, A., Sershen, H. & Lajtha, A. (1999) A.E. Bennett Research Award. Reversal of phencyclidine-induced effects by glycine and glycine transport inhibitors. *Biological Psychiatry* **45**, 668–679.

Javitt, D.C., Silipo, G., Cienfuegos, A. *et al.* (2001) Adjunctive high-dose glycine in the treatment of schizophrenia. *International Journal of Neuropsychopharmacology* **4**, 385–391.

Jones, D.K., Catani, M., Pierpaoli, C. *et al.* (2006) Age effects on diffusion tensor magnetic resonance imaging tractography measures of frontal cortex connections in schizophrenia. *Human Brain Mapping* **27**, 230–238.

Kalus, P., Senitz, D. & Beckmann, H. (1997) Altered distribution of parvalbumin-immunoreactive local circuit neurons in the anterior cingulate cortex of schizophrenic patients. *Psychiatry Research* **75**, 49–59.

Kalus, P., Muller, T.J., Zuschratter, W. & Senitz, D. (2000) The dendritic architecture of prefrontal pyramidal neurons in schizophrenic patients. *Neuroreport* **11**, 3621–3625.

Kawaguchi, Y. (2001) Distinct firing patterns of neuronal subtypes in cortical synchronized activities. *Journal of Neuroscience* **21**, 7261–7272.

Kawaguchi, Y. & Kubota, Y. (1993) Correlation of physiological subgroupings of nonpyramidal cells with parvalbumin- and calbindinD28k-immunoreactive neurons in layer V of rat frontal cortex. *Journal of Neurophysiology* **70**, 387–396.

Kegeles, L.S., Zea-Ponce, Y., Abi-Dargham, A., Mann, J.J. & Laruelle, M. (1999) Ketamine modulation of amphetamine-induced striatal dopamine release in humans. *Biological Psychiatry* **45**, 20S.

Kendell, S.F., Krystal, J.H. & Sanacora, G. (2005) GABA and glutamate systems as therapeutic targets in depression and mood disorders. *Expert Opinion in Therapeutic Targets* **9**, 153–168.

Kendler, K.S. (2004) Schizophrenia genetics and dysbindin: a corner turned? *American Journal of Psychiatry* **161**, 1533–1536.

Kerwin, R., Robinson, P. & Stephenson, J. (1992) Distribution of CCK binding sites in the human hippocampal formation and their alteration in schizophrenia: a post-mortem autoradiographic study. *Psychological Medicine* **22**, 37–43.

Kew, J.N. & Kemp, J.A. (2005) Ionotropic and metabotropic glutamate receptor structure and pharmacology. *Psychopharmacology (Berlin)* **179**, 4–29.

Kirkpatrick, B., Xu, L., Cascella, N., Ozeki, Y., Sawa, A. & Roberts, R.C. (2006) DISC1 immunoreactivity at the light and ultrastructural level in the human neocortex. *Journal of Comparative Neurology* **497**, 436–450.

Klausberger, T., Marton, L.F., O'Neill, J. *et al.* (2005) Complementary roles of cholecystokinin- and parvalbumin-expressing GABAergic neurons in hippocampal network oscillations. *Journal of Neuroscience* **25**, 9782–9793.

Koethe, D., Llenos, I.C., Dulay, J.R. *et al.* (2007) Expression of CB1 cannabinoid receptor in the anterior cingulate cortex in schizophrenia, bipolar disorder, and major depression. *Journal of Neural Transmission* **114**, 1055–1063.

Kolomeets, N.S., Orlovskaya, D.D., Rachmanova, V.I. & Uranova, N.A. (2005) Ultrastructural alterations in hippocampal mossy fiber synapses in schizophrenia: a postmortem morphometric study. *Synapse* **57**, 47–55.

Komuro, H. & Rakic, P. (1993) Modulation of neuronal migration by NMDA receptors. *Science* **260**, 95–97.

Kondziella, D., Brenner, E., Eyjolfsson, E.M., Markinhuhta, K.R., Carlsson, M.L. & Sonnewald, U. (2006) Glial-neuronal interactions are impaired in the schizophrenia model of repeated MK801 exposure. *Neuropsychopharmacology* **31**, 1880–1887.

Konopaske, G.T., Sweet, R.A., Wu, Q., Sampson, A. & Lewis, D.A. (2006) Regional specificity of chandelier neuron axon terminal alterations in schizophrenia. *Neuroscience* **138**, 189–196.

Konopaske, G.T., Dorph-Petersen, K.A., Sweet, R.A. *et al.* (2008) Effect of chronic antipsychotic exposure on astrocyte and oligodendrocyte numbers in macaque monkeys. *Biological Psychiatry* **63**, 759–765.

Kremer, I., Vass, A., Gorelik, I. *et al.* (2004) Placebo-controlled trial of lamotrigine added to conventional and atypical antipsychotics in schizophrenia. *Biological Psychiatry* **56**, 441–446.

Kristiansen, L.V., Huerta, I., Beneyto, M. & Meador-Woodruff, J.H. (2007) NMDA receptors and schizophrenia. *Current Opinion in Pharmacology* **7**, 48–55.

Krueger, D.D., Howell, J.L., Hebert, B.F., Olausson, P., Taylor, J.R. & Nairn, A.C. (2006) Assessment of cognitive function in the heterozygous reeler mouse. *Psychopharmacology (Berlin)* **189**, 95–104.

Krystal, J.H. (2007) Neuroplasticity as a target for the pharmacotherapy of psychiatric disorders: new opportunities for synergy with psychotherapy. *Biological Psychiatry* **62**, 833–834.

Krystal, J.H., Seibyl, J.P., Price, L.H. *et al.* (1993) m-Chlorophenylpiperazine effects in neuroleptic-free schizophrenic patients. Evidence implicating serotonergic systems in the positive symptoms of schizophrenia. *Archives of General Psychiatry* **50**, 624–635.

Krystal, J.H., Karper, L.P., Seibyl, J.P. *et al.* (1994) Subanesthetic effects of the noncompetitive NMDA antagonist, ketamine, in humans. Psychotomimetic, perceptual, cognitive, and neuroendocrine responses. *Archives of General Psychiatry* **51**, 199–214.

Krystal, J.H., Karper, L.P., Bennett, A. *et al.* (1998a) Interactive effects of subanesthetic ketamine and subhypnotic lorazepam in humans. *Psychopharmacology (Berlin)* **135**, 213–229.

Krystal, J.H., Karper, L.P., Bennett, A. *et al.* (1998b) Interactive effects of subanesthetic ketamine and subhypnotic lorazepam in humans. *Psychopharmacology* **135**, 213–229.

Krystal, J.H., Petrakis, I.L., Webb, E. *et al.* (1998c) Dose-related ethanol-like effects of the NMDA antagonist, ketamine, in recently detoxified alcoholics. *Archives of General Psychiatry* **55**, 354–360.

Krystal, J.H. & D'Souza, D.C. (1998) D-serine and the therapeutic challenge posed by the N-methyl-D-aspartate antagonist model of schizophrenia. *Biological Psychiatry* **44**, 1075–1076.

Krystal, J.H., D'Souza, D.C., Karper, L.P. *et al.* (1999b) Interactive effects of subanesthetic ketamine and haloperidol in healthy humans. *Psychopharmacology (Berlin)* **145**, 193–204.

Krystal, J.H., Belger, A., Abi-Saab, W. *et al.* (2000a) Glutamatergic contributions to cognitive dysfunction in schizophrenia. In: Harvey, P.D. & Sharma, T., eds. *Cognitive Functioning in Schizophrenia*. London: Oxford University Press, pp. 126–153.

Krystal, J.H., Bennett, A., Abi-Saab, D. *et al.* (2000b) Dissociation of ketamine effects on rule acquisition and rule implementation: possible relevance to NMDA receptor contributions to executive cognitive functions. *Biological Psychiatry* **47**, 137–143.

Krystal, J.H., Abi-Dargham, A., Laruelle, M. & Moghaddam, B. (2003a) Pharmacologic models of psychosis. In: Charney, D.S. & Nestler, E.J., eds. *Neurobiology of Mental Illness*. New York: Oxford University Press, pp. 287–298.

Krystal, J.H., D'Souza, D.C., Mathalon, D., Perry, E., Belger, A. & Hoffman, R. (2003b) NMDA receptor antagonist effects, cortical glutamatergic function, and schizophrenia: toward a paradigm shift in medication development. *Psychopharmacology (Berlin)* **169**, 215–233.

Krystal, J.H., Petrakis, I.L., Mason, G., Trevisan, L. & D'Souza, D.C. (2003c) N-methyl-D-aspartate glutamate receptors and alcoholism: reward, dependence, treatment, and vulnerability. *Pharmacology and Therapeutics* **99**, 79–94.

Krystal, J.H., Abi-Saab, W., Perry, E. *et al.* (2005a) Preliminary evidence of attenuation of the disruptive effects of the NMDA glutamate receptor antagonist, ketamine, on working memory by pretreatment with the group II metabotropic glutamate receptor (mGluR) agonist, LY354740, in healthy human subjects. *Psychopharmacology* **179**, 303–309.

Krystal, J.H., Perry, E., Gueorgueva, R. *et al.* (2005b) Comparative and interactive human psychopharmacologic effects of ketamine and amphetamine: implications for glutamatergic and dopaminergic model psychoses and cognitive function. *Archives of General Psychiatry* **62**, 985–994.

Krystal, J.H., Perry, E.B., Jr. & Gueorguieva, R. *et al.* (2005c) Comparative and interactive human psychopharmacologic effects of ketamine and amphetamine: implications for glutamatergic and dopaminergic model psychoses and cognitive function. *Archives of General Psychiatry* **62**, 985–994.

Krystal, J.H., Staley, J., Mason, G. *et al.* (2006) Gamma-aminobutyric acid type A receptors and alcoholism: intoxication, dependence, vulnerability, and treatment. *Archives of General Psychiatry* **63**, 957–968.

Kubicki, M., Westin, C.F., Maier, S.E. *et al.* (2002) Uncinate fasciculus findings in schizophrenia: a magnetic resonance diffusion tensor imaging study. *American Journal of Psychiatry* **159**, 813–820.

Kuromitsu, J., Yokoi, A., Kawai, T. *et al.* (2001) Reduced neuropeptide Y mRNA levels in the frontal cortex of people with schizophrenia and bipolar disorder. *Brain Research Gene Expression Patterns* **1**, 17–21.

Kwon, J.S., O'Donnell, B.F., Wallenstein, G.V. *et al.* (1999) Gamma frequency-range abnormalities to auditory stimulation in schizophrenia. *Archives of General Psychiatry* **56**, 1001–1015.

Labrie, V., Fukumura, R., Rastogi, A. *et al.* (2009) Serine racemase is associated with schizophrenia susceptibility in humans and in a mouse model. *Human Molecular Genetics* **18**, 3227–3243.

Lahti, A.C., Koffel, B., LaPorte, D. & Tamminga, C.A. (1995) Subanesthetic doses of ketamine stimulate psychosis in schizophrenia. *Neuropsychopharmacology* **13**, 9–19.

Lahti, A.C., Weiler, M.A., Parwani, A. *et al.* (1999) Blockade of ketamine-induced psychosis with olanzepine. *Schizophrenia Research* **36**, 310.

Lahti, A.C., Weiler, M.A., Tamara Michaelidis, B.A., Parwani, A. & Tamminga, C.A. (2001) Effects of ketamine in normal and schizophrenic volunteers. *Neuropsychopharmacology* **25**, 455–467.

Lane, H.Y., Chang, Y.C., Liu, Y.C., Chiu, C.C. & Tsai, G.E. (2005) Sarcosine or D-serine add-on treatment for acute exacerbation of schizophrenia: a randomized, double-blind, placebo-controlled study. *Archives of General Psychiatry* **62**, 1196–1204.

Lane, H.Y., Huang, C.L., Wu, P.L. *et al.* (2006) Glycine transporter I inhibitor, N-methylglycine (sarcosine), added to clozapine for the treatment of schizophrenia. *Biological Psychiatry* **60**, 645–649.

Lane, H.Y., Liu, Y.C., Huang, C.L. *et al.* (2008) Sarcosine (N-methylglycine) treatment for acute schizophrenia: a randomized, double-blind study. *Biological Psychiatry* **63**, 9–12.

Large, C.H., Webster, E.L. & Goff, D.C. (2005) The potential role of lamotrigine in schizophrenia. *Psychopharmacology (Berlin)* **181**, 415–436.

Law, A.J., Lipska, B.K., Weickert, C.S. *et al.* (2006) Neuregulin 1 transcripts are differentially expressed in schizophrenia and regulated by 5' SNPs associated with the disease. *Proceedings of the National Academy of Sciences USA* **103**, 674–752.

Law, A.J., Kleinman, J.E., Weinberger, D.R. & Weickert, C.S. (2007) Disease-associated intronic variants in the ErbB4 gene are related to altered ErbB4 splice-variant expression in the brain in schizophrenia. *Human Molecular Genetics* **16**, 129–141.

Lecourtier, L., Homayoun, H., Tamagnan, G. & Moghaddam, B. (2007) Positive allosteric modulation of metabotropic glutamate 5 (mGlu5) receptors reverses N-Methyl-D-aspartate antagonist-induced alteration of neuronal firing in prefrontal cortex. *Biological Psychiatry* **62**, 739–746.

Lerma, J. (2006) Kainate receptor physiology. *Current Opinion in Pharmacology* **6**, 89–97.

Lewis, D.A. & Gonzalez-Burgos, G. (2008) Neuroplasticity of neocortical circuits in schizophrenia. *Neuropsychopharmacology* **33**, 141–165.

Lewis, D.A. & Moghaddam, B. (2006) Cognitive dysfunction in schizophrenia: convergence of gamma-aminobutyric acid and glutamate alterations. *Archives of Neurology* **63**, 1372–1376.

Lewis, D.A., Hashimoto, T. & Volk, D.W. (2005) Cortical inhibitory neurons and schizophrenia. *Nature Review Neuroscience* **6**, 312–324.

Li, D. & He, L. (2007) G72/G30 genes and schizophrenia: a systematic meta-analysis of association studies. *Genetics* **175**, 917–922.

Li, B., Woo, R.S., Mei, L. & Malinow, R. (2007) The neuregulin-1 receptor erbB4 controls glutamatergic synapse maturation and plasticity. *Neuron* **54**, 583–597.

Lilburn, J.K., Dundee, J.W., Nair, S.G., Fee, J.P. & Johnston, H.M. (1978) Ketamine sequelae. Evaluation of the ability of various premedicants to attenuate its psychic actions. *Anaesthesia* **33**, 307–311.

Linn, G.S., O'Keeffe, R.T., Lifshitz, K., Schroeder, C. & Javitt, D.C. (2007) Behavioral effects of orally administered glycine in socially housed monkeys chronically treated with phencyclidine. *Psychopharmacology (Berlin)* **192**, 27–38.

Lipska, B.K., Mitkus, S.N., Mathew, S.V. *et al.* (2006) Functional genomics in postmortem human brain: abnormalities in a DISC1 molecular pathway in schizophrenia. *Dialogues in Clinical Neuroscience* **8**, 353–357.

Liu, S.J. & Zukin, R.S. (2007) Ca^{2+}-permeable AMPA receptors in synaptic plasticity and neuronal death. *Trends in Neuroscience* **30**, 126–134.

Liu, J., Shi, Y., Tang, W. *et al.* (2005a) Positive association of the human GABA-A-receptor beta 2 subunit gene haplotype with schizophrenia in the Chinese Han population. *Biochemical and Biophysical Research Communications* **334**, 817–823.

Liu, X., Qin, W., He, G. *et al.* (2005b) A family-based association study of the MOG gene with schizophrenia in the Chinese population. *Schizophrenia Research* **73**, 275–280.

Lo, W.S., Harano, M., Gawlik, M. *et al.* (2007a) GABRB2 association with schizophrenia: commonalities and differences between ethnic groups and clinical subtypes. *Biological Psychiatry* **61**, 653–660.

Lo, W.S., Xu, Z., Yu, Z. *et al.* (2007b) Positive selection within the Schizophrenia-associated GABA(A) receptor beta2 gene. *PLoS ONE* **2**, e462.

Luby, E.D., Cohen, B.D., Rosenbaum, G., Gottlieb, J.S. & Kelley, R. (1959) Study of a new schizophrenomimetic drug—sernyl. *Archives of Neurology Psychiatry* **81**, 363–369.

Lundorf, M.D., Buttenschon, H.N., Foldager, L. *et al.* (2005) Mutational screening and association study of glutamate decarboxylase 1 as a candidate susceptibility gene for bipolar affective disorder and schizophrenia. *American Journal of Medical Genetics B Neuropsychiatric Genetics* **135**, 94–101.

Madeira, C., Freitas, M.E., Vargas-Lopes, C., Wolosker, H. & Panizzutti, R. (2008) Increased brain D-amino acid oxidase (DAAO) activity in schizophrenia. *Schizophrenia Research* **101**, 76–83.

Maeno, N., Takahashi, N., Saito, S. *et al.* (2007) Association of SOX10 with schizophrenia in the Japanese population. *Psychiatric Genetics* **17**, 227–231.

Malhotra, A.K., Adler, C.M., Kennison, S.D., Elman, I., Pickar, D. & Breier, A. (1997a) Clozapine blunts N-methyl-D-aspartate antagonist-induced psychosis: a study with ketamine. *Biological Psychiatry* **42**, 664–668.

Malhotra, A.K., Pinals, D.A., Adler, C.M. *et al.* (1997b) Ketamine-induced exacerbation of psychotic symptoms and cognitive impairment in neuroleptic-free schizophrenics. *Neuropsychopharmacology* **17**, 141–150.

Malhotra, A.K., Pinals, D.A., Weingartner, H. *et al.* (1996) NMDA receptor function and human cognition: the effects of ketamine in healthy volunteers. *Neuropsychopharmacology* **14**, 301–307.

Malinow, R. & Malenka, R.C. (2002) AMPA receptor trafficking and synaptic plasticity. *Annual Review of Neuroscience* **25**, 103–126.

Marek, G.J., Wright, R.A., Schoepp, D.D. & Aghajanian, G.K. (2000) Physiological antagonism between 5-hydroxytryptamine(2A) and group II metabotropic glutamate receptors in prefrontal cortex. *Journal of Pharmacology & Experimental Therapeutics* **292**, 76–87.

Marenco, S., Egan, M.F., Goldberg, T.E. *et al.* (2002) Preliminary experience with an ampakine (CX516) as a single agent for the treatment of schizophrenia: a case series. *Schizophrenia Research* **57**, 221–226.

Marenco, S., Steele, S.U., Egan, M.F. *et al.* (2006) Effect of metabotropic glutamate receptor 3 genotype on N-acetylaspartate measures in the dorsolateral prefrontal cortex. *American Journal of Psychiatry* **163**, 740–742.

Marx, C.E., Stevens, R.D., Shampine, L.J. *et al.* (2006) Neuroactive steroids are altered in schizophrenia and bipolar disorder: relevance to pathophysiology and therapeutics. *Neuropsychopharmacology* **31**, 1249–1263.

Mathalon, D.H., Sullivan, E.V., Lim, K.O. & Pfefferbaum, A. (2001) Progressive brain volume changes and the clinical course of schizophrenia in men: a longitudinal magnetic resonance imaging study. *Archives of General Psychiatry* **58**, 148–157.

Matsuda, K., Fletcher, M., Kamiya, Y. & Yuzaki, M. (2003) Specific assembly with the NMDA receptor 3B subunit controls surface expression and calcium permeability of NMDA receptors. *Journal of Neuroscience* **23**, 10064–10073.

McCullumsmith, R.E., Gupta, D., Beneyto, M. *et al.* (2007) Expression of transcripts for myelination-related genes in the anterior cingulate cortex in schizophrenia. *Schizophrenia Research* **90**, 15–27.

Meador-Woodruff, J.H. & Healy, D.J. (2000) Glutamate receptor expression in schizophrenic brain. *Brain Research & Brain Research Reviews* **31**, 288–294.

Meador-Woodruff, J.H., Hogg, A.J., Jr. & Smith, R.E. (2001) Striatal ionotropic glutamate receptor expression in schizophrenia, bipolar disorder, and major depressive disorder. *Brain Research Bulletin* **55**, 631–640.

Mehta, A.K. & Ticku, M.K. (1999) An update on GABAA receptors. *Brain Research—Brain Research Reviews* **29**, 196–217.

Mellor, J.R. (2006) Synaptic plasticity of kainate receptors. *Biochemistry Society Transactions* **34**, 949–951.

Meltzer, H.Y., Matsubara, S. & Lee, J.C. (1989) Classification of typical and atypical antipsychotic drugs on the basis of dopamine D-1, D-2 and serotonin2 pKi values. *Journal of Pharmacology & Experimental Therapeutics* **251**, 238–246.

Menzies, L., Ooi, C., Kamath, S. *et al.* (2007) Effects of gamma-aminobutyric acid-modulating drugs on working memory and brain function in patients with schizophrenia. *Archives of General Psychiatry* **64**, 156–167.

Millar, J.K., Christie, S. & Porteous, D.J. (2003) Yeast two-hybrid screens implicate DISC1 in brain development and function. *Biochemical Biophysics Research Communications* **311**, 1019–1025.

Millar, J.K., Mackie, S., Clapcote, S.J. *et al.* (2007) Disrupted in schizophrenia 1 and phosphodiesterase 4B: towards an understanding of psychiatric illness. *Journal of Physiology* **584**, 401–405.

Mitkus, S.N., Hyde, T.M., Vakkalanka, R. *et al.* (2008) Expression of oligodendrocyte-associated genes in dorsolateral prefrontal cortex of patients with schizophrenia. *Schizophrenia Research* **98**, 129–138.

Moghaddam, B. & Adams, B.W. (1998) Reversal of phencyclidine effects by a group II metabotropic glutamate receptor agonist in rats. *Science* **281**, 1349–1352.

Moghaddam, B., Adams, B., Verma, A. & Daly, D. (1997) Activation of glutamatergic neurotransmission by ketamine: a novel step in the pathway from NMDA receptor blockade to dopaminergic and cognitive disruptions associated with the prefrontal cortex. *Journal of Neuroscience* **17**, 2921–2927.

Mohler, H., Fritschy, J.M. & Rudolph, U. (2002) A new benzodiazepine pharmacology. *Journal of Pharmacology & Experimental Therapeutics* **300**, 2–8.

Morgan, C.J., Mofeez, A., Brandner, B., Bromley, L. & Curran, H.V. (2004) Acute effects of ketamine on memory systems and psychotic symptoms in healthy volunteers. *Neuropsychopharmacology* **29**, 208–218.

Morita, Y., Ujike, H., Tanaka, Y. *et al.* (2007) A genetic variant of the serine racemase gene is associated with schizophrenia. *Biological Psychiatry* **61**, 1200–1203.

Morris, D.W., Murphy, K., Kenny, N. *et al.* (2008a) Dysbindin (DTNBP1) and the biogenesis of lysosome-related organelles complex 1 (BLOC-1): main and epistatic gene effects are potential contributors to schizophrenia susceptibility. *Biological Psychiatry* **63**, 24–31.

Morris, H.M., Hashimoto, T. & Lewis, D.A. (2008b) Alterations in somatostatin mRNA expression in the dorsolateral prefrontal cortex of subjects with schizophrenia or schizoaffective disorder. *Cerebral Cortex* **18**, 1575–1587.

Munafo, M.R., Thiselton, D.L., Clark, T.G. & Flint, J. (2006) Association of the NRG1 gene and schizophrenia: a meta-analysis. *Molecular Psychiatry* **11**, 539–546.

Murakami, T., Nakagome, K., Kamio, S. *et al.* (2002) The effects of benzodiazepines on event-related potential indices of automatic and controlled processing in schizophrenia: a preliminary report. *Progress in Neuropsychopharmacology and Biological Psychiatry* **26**, 651–661.

Mutsuddi, M., Morris, D.W., Waggoner, S.G., Daly, M.J., Scolnick, E.M. & Sklar, P. (2006) Analysis of high-resolution HapMap of DTNBP1 (Dysbindin) suggests no consistency between reported common variant associations and schizophrenia. *American Journal of Human Genetics* **79**, 903–909.

Nagy, Z., Westerberg, H. & Klingberg, T. (2004) Maturation of white matter is associated with the development of cognitive functions during childhood. *Journal of Cognitive Neuroscience* **16**, 1227–1233.

Neumeister, A., Carson, R., Henry, S. *et al.* (2006) Cerebral metabolic effects of intravenous glycine in healthy human subjects. *Journal of Clinical Psychopharmacology* **26**, 595–599.

Newcomer, J.W., Farber, N.B., Jevtovic-Todorovic, V. *et al.* (1999) Ketamine-induced NMDA receptor hypofunction as model of memory impairment and psychosis. *Neuropsychopharmacology* **20**, 106–118.

Newell, K.A., Deng, C. & Huang, X.F. (2006) Increased cannabinoid receptor density in the posterior cingulate cortex in schizophrenia. *Experimental Brain Research* **172**, 556–560.

Niemann, S., Kanki, H., Fukui, Y. *et al.* (2007) Genetic ablation of NMDA receptor subunit NR3B in mouse reveals motoneuronal and nonmotoneuronal phenotypes. *European Journal of Neuroscience* **26**, 1407–1420.

Nilsson, M., Carlsson, A. & Carlsson, M.L. (1997) Glycine and D-serine decrease MK-801-induced hyperactivity in mice. *Journal of Neural Transmission* **104**, 1195–1205.

Nishi, M., Hinds, H., Lu, H.P., Kawata, M. & Hayashi, Y. (2001) Motoneuron-specific expression of NR3B, a novel NMDA-type glutamate receptor subunit that works in a dominant-negative manner. *Journal of Neuroscience* **21**, RC185.

Noga, J.T., Hyde, T.M., Bachus, S.E., Herman, M.M. & Kleinman, J.E. (2001) AMPA receptor binding in the dorsolateral prefrontal cortex of schizophrenics and controls. *Schizophrenia Research* **48**, 361–363.

Noga, J.T. & Wang, H. (2002) Further postmortem autoradiographic studies of AMPA receptor binding in schizophrenia. *Synapse* **45**, 250–258.

Noh, J.S., Sharma, R.P., Veldic, M. *et al.* (2005) DNA methyltransferase 1 regulates reelin mRNA expression in mouse primary cortical cultures. *Proceedings of the National Academy of Sciences USA* **102**, 1749–1754.

Norberg, M.M., Krystal, J.H. & Tolin, D.F. (2008) A meta-snalysis of D-cycloserine and the facilitation of fear extinction and exposure therapy. *Biological Psychiatry* **63**, 1118–1126.

Nusser, Z., Sieghart, W. & Somogyi, P. (1998) Segregation of different GABAA receptors to synaptic and extrasynaptic membranes of cerebellar granule cells. *Journal of Neuroscience* **18**, 1693–1703.

O'Connor, J.A., Muly, E.C., Arnold, S.E. & Hemby, S.E. (2007) AMPA receptor subunit and splice variant expression in the DLPFC of schizophrenic subjects and rhesus monkeys chronically administered antipsychotic drugs. *Schizophrenia Research* **90**, 28–40.

Ohnuma, T., Augood, S.J., Arai, H., McKenna, P.J. & Emson, P.C. (1998) Expression of the human excitatory amino acid transporter 2 and metabotropic glutamate receptors 3 and 5 in the prefrontal cortex from normal individuals and patients with schizophrenia. *Brain Research Molecular Brain Research* **56**, 207–217.

Ohnuma, T., Tessler, S., Arai, H., Faull, R.L., McKenna, P.J. & Emson, P.C. (2000) Gene expression of metabotropic glutamate receptor 5 and excitatory amino acid transporter 2 in the schizophrenic hippocampus. *Brain Research Molecular Brain Research* **85**, 24–31.

Ohtsuki, T., Koga, M., Ishiguro, H. *et al.* (2008) A polymorphism of the metabotropic glutamate receptor mGluR7 (GRM7) gene is associated with schizophrenia. *Schizophrenia Research* **101**, 9–16.

Oliet, S.H. & Mothet, J.P. (2006) Molecular determinants of D-serine-mediated gliotransmission: from release to function. *Glia* **54**, 726–737.

Olszewski, R.T., Bukhari, N., Zhou, J. *et al.* (2004) NAAG peptidase inhibition reduces locomotor activity and some stereotypes in the PCP model of schizophrenia via group II mGluR. *Journal of Neurochemistry* **89**, 876–885.

Olszewski, R.T., Wegorzewska, M.M., Monteiro, A.C. *et al.* (2008) Phencyclidine and dizocilpine induced behaviors reduced by N-acetylaspartylglutamate peptidase inhibition via metabotropic glutamate receptors. *Biological Psychiatry* **63**, 86–91.

Ozaki, M., Sasner, M., Yano, R., Lu, H.S. & Buonanno, A. (1997) Neuregulin-beta induces expression of an NMDA-receptor subunit. *Nature* **390**, 691–694.

Patil, S.T., Zhang, L., Martenyi, F. *et al.* (2007) Activation of mGlu2/3 receptors as a new approach to treat schizophrenia: a randomized Phase 2 clinical trial. *Nature Medicine* **13**, 1102–1107.

Paulson, L., Martin, P., Persson, A. *et al.* (2003) Comparative genome- and proteome analysis of cerebral cortex from MK-801-treated rats. *Journal of Neuroscience Research* **71**, 526–533.

Perry, T.L., Kish, S.J., Buchanan, J. & Hansen, S. (1979) Gamma-aminobutyric-acid deficiency in brain of schizophrenic patients. *Lancet* **1**, 237–239.

Perry, R.H., Dockray, G.J., Dimaline, R., Perry, E.K., Blessed, G. & Tomlinson, B.E. (1981) Neuropeptides in Alzheimer's disease, depression and schizophrenia. A post mortem analysis of vasoactive intestinal peptide and cholecystokinin in cerebral cortex. *Journal of Neurological Science* **51**, 465–472.

Persico, A.M., Levitt, P. & Pimenta, A.F. (2006) Polymorphic GGC repeat differentially regulates human reelin gene expression levels. *Journal of Neural Transmission* **113**, 1373–1382.

Petryshen, T.L., Middleton, F.A., Tahl, A.R. *et al.* (2005) Genetic investigation of chromosome 5q GABAA receptor subunit genes in schizophrenia. *Molecular Psychiatry* **10**, 1074–1088, 1057.

Pierri, J.N., Chaudry, A.S., Woo, T.U. & Lewis, D.A. (1999) Alterations in chandelier neuron axon terminals in the prefrontal cortex of schizophrenic subjects. *American Journal of Psychiatry* **156**, 1709–1719.

Pietraszek, M., Gravius, A., Schafer, D., Weil, T., Trifanova, D. & Danysz, W. (2005) mGluR5, but not mGluR1, antagonist modifies MK-801-induced locomotor activity and deficit of prepulse inhibition. *Neuropharmacology* **49**, 73–85.

Pilowsky, L.S., Bressan, R.A., Stone, J.M. *et al.* (2006) First in vivo evidence of an NMDA receptor deficit in medication-free schizophrenic patients. *Molecular Psychiatry* **11**, 118–119.

Pomarol-Clotet. E., Honey, G.D., Murray, G.K. *et al.* (2006) Psychological effects of ketamine in healthy volunteers. Phenomenological study. *British Journal of Psychiatry* **189**, 173–179.

Porter, R.H., Eastwood, S.L. & Harrison, P.J. (1997) Distribution of kainate receptor subunit mRNAs in human hippocampus, neocortex and cerebellum, and bilateral reduction of hippocampal GluR6 and KA2 transcripts in schizophrenia. *Brain Research* **751**, 217–231.

Post, R.M. (1999) Comparative pharmacology of bipolar disorder and schizophrenia. *Schizophrenia Research* **39**, 153–158; discussion 163.

Qin, W., Gao, J., Xing, Q. *et al.* (2005) A family-based association study of PLP1 and schizophrenia. *Neuroscience Letters* **375**, 207–210.

Rajkowska, G., Selemon, L.D. & Goldman-Rakic, P.S. (1998) Neuronal and glial somal size in the prefrontal cortex: a postmortem morphometric study of schizophrenia and Huntington disease. *Archives of General Psychiatry* **55**, 215–224.

Rajkowska, G., Miguel-Hidalgo, J.J., Makkos, Z., Meltzer, H., Overholser, J. & Stockmeier, C. (2002) Layer-specific reductions in GFAP-reactive astroglia in the dorsolateral prefrontal cortex in schizophrenia. *Schizophrenia Research* **57**, 127–138.

Rapoport, J.L. & Gogtay, N. (2008) Brain neuroplasticity in healthy, hyperactive and psychotic children: insights from neuroimaging. *Neuropsychopharmacology* **33**, 181–197.

Regenold, W.T., Phatak, P., Marano, C.M., Gearhart, L., Viens, C.H. & Hisley, K.C. (2007) Myelin staining of deep white matter in the dorsolateral prefrontal cortex in schizophrenia, bipolar disorder, and unipolar major depression. *Psychiatry Research* **151**, 179–188.

Ressler, K.J., Rothbaum, B.O., Tannenbaum, L. *et al.* (2004) Cognitive enhancers as adjuncts to psychotherapy: use of D-cycloserine in phobic individuals to facilitate extinction of fear. *Archives of General Psychiatry* **61**, 1136–1144.

Reynolds, G.P., Zhang Z.J. & Beasley, C.L. (2001) Neurochemical correlates of cortical GABAergic deficits in schizophrenia: selective losses of calcium binding protein immunoreactivity. *Brain Research Bulletin* **55**, 579–584.

Rodriguez-Moreno, A. & Sihra, T.S. (2007) Metabotropic actions of kainate receptors in the CNS. *Journal of Neurochemistry* **103**, 2121–2135.

Rosenbaum, G., Cohen, B.D., Luby, E.D., Gottlieb, J.S. & Yelen, D. (1959) Comparison of sernyl with other drugs: simulation of schizophrenic performance with sernyl, LSD-25,and amobarbital (amytal) sodium; I. attention, motor function, and proprioception. *Archives of General Psychiatry* **1**, 651–656.

Ruzicka, W.B., Zhubi, A., Veldic, M., Grayson, D.R., Costa, E. & Guidotti, A. (2007) Selective epigenetic alteration of layer I GABAergic neurons isolated from prefrontal cortex of schizophrenia patients using laser-assisted microdissection. *Molecular Psychiatry* **12**, 385–397.

Sakai, T., Oshima, A., Nozaki, Y., Ida, I. *et al.* (2008) Changes in density of calcium-binding-protein-immunoreactive GABAergic neurons in prefrontal cortex in schizophrenia and bipolar disorder. *Neuropathology* **28**, 143–150.

Sanacora, G., Mason, G., Rothman, D.L. & Krystal, J.H. (2003) Clinical studies implementing glutamate neurotransmission in mood disorders. *Annals of the New York Academy of Sciences* **1003**, 292–308.

Sartorius, L.J., Weinberger, D.R., Hyde, T.M., Harrison, P.J., Kleinman, J.E. & Lipska, B.K. (2008) Expression of a GRM3 splice variant is increased in the dorsolateral prefrontal cortex of individuals carrying a schizophrenia risk SNP. *Neuropsychopharmacology* **33**, 2626–2634.

Schell, M.J., Brady, R.O., Jr., Molliver, M.E. & Snyder, S.H. (1997) D-serine as a neuromodulator: regional and developmental localizations in rat brain glia resemble NMDA receptors. *Journal of Neuroscience* **17**, 1604–1615.

Schoepp, D.D. & Conn, P.J. (2002) Metabotropic glutamate receptors. *Pharmacology and Biochemical Behaviour* **74**, 255–256.

Schwab, S.G., Knapp, M., Mondabon, S. *et al.* (2003) Support for association of schizophrenia with genetic variation in the 6p22.3 gene, dysbindin, in sib-pair families with linkage and in an additional sample of triad families. *American Journal of Human Genetics* **72**, 185–190.

Seamans, J.K. & Yang, C.R. (2004) The principal features and mechanisms of dopamine modulation in the prefrontal cortex. *Progress in Neurobiology* **74**, 1–58.

Seeman, P. (1992) Dopamine receptor sequences. Therapeutic levels of neuroleptics occupy D2 receptors, clozapine occupies D4. *Neuropsychopharmacology* **7**, 261–284.

Selemon, L.D., Rajkowska, G. & Goldman-Rakic, P.S. (1995) Abnormally high neuronal density in the schizophrenic cortex. A morphometric analysis of prefrontal area 9 and occipital area 17. *Archives of General Psychiatry* **52**, 805–818.

Selemon, L.D., Rajkowska, G. & Goldman-Rakic, P.S. (1998) Elevated neuronal density in prefrontal area 46 in brains from schizophrenic patients: application of a three-dimensional, stereologic counting method. *Journal of Comparative Neurology* **392**, 402–412.

Sharma, K., Fong, D.K. & Craig, A.M. (2006) Postsynaptic protein mobility in dendritic spines: long-term regulation by synaptic NMDA receptor activation. *Molecular and Cellular Neuroscience* **31**, 702–712.

Shifman, S., Johannesson, M., Bronstein, M. *et al.* (2008) Genome-wide association identifies a common variant in the reelin gene that increases the risk of schizophrenia only in women. *PLoS Genet* **4**, e28.

Simonini M.V., Camargo, L.M., Dong, E. *et al.* (2006) The benzamide MS-275 is a potent, long-lasting brain region-selective inhibitor of histone deacetylases. *Proceedings of the National Academy of Science USA* **103**, 1587–1592.

Smiley, J.F., Levey, A.I., Ciliax, B.J. & Goldman-Rakic, P.S. (1994) D1 dopamine receptor immunoreactivity in human and monkey cerebral cortex: predominant and extrasynaptic localization in dendritic spines. *Proceedings of the National Academy of Sciences USA* **91**, 5720–5724.

Smith, S.S., Shen, H., Gong, Q.H. & Zhou, X. (2007) Neurosteroid regulation of GABA(A) receptors: Focus on the alpha4 and delta subunits. *Pharmacology and Therapeutics* **116**, 58–76.

Snyder, S.H. & Kim, P.M. (2000) D-amino acids as putative neurotransmitters: focus on D-serine. *Neurochemical Research* **25**, 553–560.

Soghomonian, J.J. & Martin, D.L. (1998) Two isoforms of glutamate decarboxylase: why? *Trends in Pharmacological Sciences* **19**, 500–505.

Sokolov, B.P. (2007) Oligodendroglial abnormalities in schizophrenia, mood disorders and substance abuse. Comorbidity, shared traits, or molecular phenocopies? *International Journal of Neuropsychopharmacology* **10**, 547–555.

Spencer, K.M., Nestor, P.G., Perlmutter, R. *et al.* (2004) Neural synchrony indexes disordered perception and cognition in schizophrenia. *Proceedings of the National Academy of Sciences USA* **101**, 17288–17293.

Spencer, K.M., Niznikiewicz, M.A., Shenton, M.E. & McCarley, R.W. (2008) Sensory-evoked gamma oscillations in chronic schizophrenia. *Biological Psychiatry* **63**, 744–747.

Stark, A.K., Uylings, H.B., Sanz-Arigita, E. & Pakkenberg, B. (2004) Glial cell loss in the anterior cingulate cortex, a subregion of the prefrontal cortex, in subjects with schizophrenia. *American Journal of Psychiatry* **161**, 882–888.

Stefansson, H., Sigurdsson, E., Steinthorsdottir, V. *et al.* (2002) Neuregulin 1 and susceptibility to schizophrenia. *American Journal of Human Genetics* **71**, 877–892.

Steffek, A.E., Haroutunian, V. & Meador-Woodruff, J.H. (2006) Serine racemase protein expression in cortex and hippocampus in schizophrenia. *Neuroreport* **17**, 1181–1185.

Stell, B.M., Brickley, S.G., Tang, C.Y., Farrant, M. & Mody, I. (2003) Neuroactive steroids reduce neuronal excitability by selectively enhancing tonic inhibition mediated by delta subunit-containing GABAA receptors. *Proceedings of the National Academy of Sciences USA* **100**, 14439–14444.

Stell, B.M. & Mody, I. (2002) Receptors with different affinities mediate phasic and tonic GABA(A) conductances in hippocampal neurons. *Journal of Neuroscience* **22**, RC22.

Stocca, G. & Vicini, S. (1998) Increased contribution of NR2A subunit to synaptic NMDA receptors in developing rat cortical neurons. *Journal of Physiology* **507**, 13–24.

Strassman, R.J., Qualls, C.R., Uhlenhuth, E.H. & Kellner, R. (1994) Dose-response study of N,N-dimethyltryptamine in humans. II. Subjective effects and preliminary results of a new rating scale. *Archives of General Psychiatry* **51**, 98–108.

Straub, R.E., Jiang, Y., MacLean, C.J. *et al.* (2002) Genetic variation in the 6p22.3 gene DTNBP1, the human ortholog of the mouse dysbindin gene, is associated with schizophrenia. *American Journal of Human Genetics* **71**, 337–348.

Straub, R.E., Lipska, B.K., Egan, M.F. *et al.* (2007) Allelic variation in GAD1 (GAD67) is associated with schizophrenia and influences cortical function and gene expression. *Molecular Psychiatry* **12**, 854–869.

Supplisson, S. & Bergman, C. (1997) Control of NMDA receptor activation by a glycine transporter co-expressed in Xenopus oocytes. *Journal of Neuroscience* **17**, 4580–4590.

Svensson, T.H. (2003) Alpha-adrenoceptor modulation hypothesis of antipsychotic atypicality. *Progress in Neuropsychopharmacology and Biological Psychiatry* **27**, 1145–1158.

Swanson, C.J. & Schoepp, D.D. (2002) The group II metabotropic glutamate receptor agonist (-)-2-oxa-4-aminobicyclo[3.1.0.] hexane-4,6-dicarboxylate (LY379268) and clozapine reverse phencyclidine-induced behaviors in monoamine-depleted rats. *Journal of Pharmacology and Experimental Therapeutics* **303**, 919–927.

Szeszko, P.R., Robinson, D.G., Ashtari, M. *et al.* (2007) Clinical and neuropsychological correlates of white matter abnormalities in recent onset schizophrenia. *Neuropsychopharmacology* **33**, 976–984.

Takahashi, T., Svoboda, K. & Malinow, R. (2003) Experience strengthening transmission by driving AMPA receptors into synapses. *Science* **299**, 1585–1588.

Takahata, R. & Moghaddam, B. (1998) Glutamatergic regulation of basal and stimulus-activated dopamine release in the prefrontal cortex. *Journal of Neurochemistry* **71**, 1443–1449.

Takaki, H., Kikuta, R., Shibata, H., Ninomiya, H., Tashiro, N. & Fukumaki, Y. (2004) Positive associations of polymorphisms in the metabotropic glutamate receptor type 8 gene (GRM8) with schizophrenia. *American Journal of Medical Genetics B Neuropsychiatric Genetics* **128**, 6–14.

Talbot K, Eidem WL, Tinsley CL *et al.* (2004) Dysbindin-1 is reduced in intrinsic, glutamatergic terminals of the hippocampal formation in schizophrenia. *Journal of Clinical Investigation* **113**, 1353–1363.

Talbot, K., Cho, D.S., Ong, W.Y. *et al.* (2006) Dysbindin-1 is a synaptic and microtubular protein that binds brain snapin. *Human Molecular Genetics* **15**, 3041–3054.

Tamminga, C.A., Crayton, J.W. & Chase, T.N. (1978) Muscimol: GABA agonist therapy in schizophrenia. *American Journal of Psychiatry* **135**, 746–747.

Tan, W., Wang, Y., Gold, B. *et al.* (2007) Molecular cloning of a brain-specific, developmentally regulated neuregulin 1

(NRG1) isoform and identification of a functional promoter variant associated with schizophrenia. *Journal of Biological Chemistry* **282**, 24343–24351.

Thompson, P.M., Vidal, C., Giedd, J.N. *et al.* (2001) Mapping adolescent brain change reveals dynamic wave of accelerated gray matter loss in very early-onset schizophrenia. *Proceedings of the National Academy of Sciences USA* **98**, 11650–11655.

Tiihonen J, Hallikainen T, Ryynänen O-P *et al.* (2003) Lamotrigine in treatment-resistant schizophrenia: a randomized placebo-controlled crossover trial. *Biological Psychiatry* **54**, 1–6.

Tiihonen, J., Halonen, P., Wahlbeck, K. *et al.* (2005) Topiramate add-on in treatment-resistant schizophrenia: a randomized, double-blind, placebo-controlled, crossover trial. *Journal of Clinical Psychiatry* **66**, 1012–1015.

Tkachev, D., Mimmack, M.L., Huffaker, S.J., Ryan, M. & Bahn, S. (2007) Further evidence for altered myelin biosynthesis and glutamatergic dysfunction in schizophrenia. *International Journal of Neuropsychopharmacology* **10**, 557–563.

Tochigi, M., Iwamoto, K., Bundo, M. *et al.* (2008) Methylation status of the reelin promoter region in the brain of schizophrenic patients. *Biological Psychiatry* **63**, 530–533.

Todtenkopf, M.S. & Benes, F.M. (1998) Distribution of glutamate decarboxylase65 immunoreactive puncta on pyramidal and nonpyramidal neurons in hippocampus of schizophrenic brain. *Synapse* **29**, 323–332.

Tooney, P.A. & Chahl, L.A. (2004) Neurons expressing calcium-binding proteins in the prefrontal cortex in schizophrenia. *Progress in Neuropsychopharmacology and Biological Psychiatry* **28**, 273–278.

Torrey, E.F., Barci, B.M., Webster, M.J., Bartko, J.J., Meador-Woodruff, J.H. & Knable, M.B. (2005) Neurochemical markers for schizophrenia, bipolar disorder, and major depression in postmortem brains. *Biological Psychiatry* **57**, 252–260.

Toth, E. & Lajtha, A. (1986) Antagonism of phencyclidine-induced hyperactivity by glycine in mice. *Neurochemical Research* **11**, 393–400.

Traub, R.D., Whittington, M.A., Colling, S.B., Buzsaki, G. & Jefferys, J.G. (1996) Analysis of gamma rhythms in the rat hippocampus *in vitro* and *in vivo*. *Journal of Physiology* **493**, 471–484.

Tremolizzo, L., Doueiri, M.S., Dong, E. *et al.* (2005) Valproate corrects the schizophrenia-like epigenetic behavioral modifications induced by methionine in mice. *Biological Psychiatry* **57**, 500–509.

Tsai, G., Passani, L.A., Slusher, B.S. *et al.* (1995) Abnormal excitatory neurotransmitter metabolism in schizophrenic brains. *Archives of General Psychiatry* **52**, 829–836.

Tsai, S.J., Wang, Y.C. & Hong, C.J. (2000) Association study of a cannabinoid receptor gene (CNR1) polymorphism and schizophrenia. *Psychiatric Genetics* **10**, 149–151.

Tsai, G., Lane, H.Y., Yang, P., Chong, M.Y. & Lange, N. (2004) Glycine transporter I inhibitor, N-methylglycine (sarcosine), added to antipsychotics for the treatment of schizophrenia. *Biological Psychiatry* **55**, 452–456.

Tsai, G.E., Yang, P., Chang, Y.C. & Chong, M.Y. (2006) D-alanine added to antipsychotics for the treatment of schizophrenia. *Biological Psychiatry* **59**, 230–234.

Tsien, J.Z. (2000) Linking Hebb's coincidence-detection to memory formation. *Current Opinion in Neurobiology* **10**, 266–273.

Tu, J.C., Xiao, B., Naisbitt, S. *et al.* (1999) Coupling of mGluR/Homer and PSD-95 complexes by the Shank family of postsynaptic density proteins. *Neuron* **23**, 583–592.

Tukker, J.J., Fuentealba, P., Hartwich, K., Somogyi, P. & Klausberger, T. (2007) Cell type-specific tuning of hippocampal interneuron firing during gamma oscillations in vivo. *Journal of Neuroscience* **27**, 8184–8189.

Ujike, H., Takaki, M., Nakata, K. *et al.* (2002) CNR1, central cannabinoid receptor gene, associated with susceptibility to hebephrenic schizophrenia. *Molecular Psychiatry* **7**, 515–518.

Uranova, N.A., Vostrikov, V.M., Orlovskaya, D.D. & Rachmanova, V.I. (2004) Oligodendroglial density in the prefrontal cortex in schizophrenia and mood disorders: a study from the Stanley Neuropathology Consortium. *Schizophrenia Research* **67**, 269–275.

Uranova, N.A., Vostrikov, V.M., Vikhreva, O.V., Zimina, I.S., Kolomeets, N.S. & Orlovskaya, D.D. (2007) The role of oligodendrocyte pathology in schizophrenia. *International Journal of Neuropsychopharmacology* **10**, 537–545.

Vallejo-Illarramendi, A., Torres-Ramos, M., Melone, M., Conti, F. & Matute, C. (2005) Clozapine reduces GLT-1 expression and glutamate uptake in astrocyte cultures. *Glia* **50**, 276–279.

van Berckel, B.N., Evenblij, C.N., van Loon, B.J. *et al.* (1999) D-cycloserine increases positive symptoms in chronic schizophrenic patients when administered in addition to antipsychotics: a double-blind, parallel, placebo-controlled study. *Neuropsychopharmacology* **21**, 203–210.

Van Tol, H.H., Bunzow, J.R., Guan, H.C. *et al.* (1991) Cloning of the gene for a human dopamine D4 receptor with high affinity for the antipsychotic clozapine. *Nature* **350**, 610–614.

Vawter, M.P., Crook, J.M., Hyde, T.M. *et al.* (2002) Microarray analysis of gene expression in the prefrontal cortex in schizophrenia: a preliminary study. *Schizophrenia Research* **58**, 11–20.

Veldic, M., Caruncho, H.J., Liu, W.S. *et al.* (2004) DNA-methyltransferase 1 mRNA is selectively overexpressed in telencephalic GABAergic interneurons of schizophrenia brains. *Proceedings of the National Academy of Sciences USA* **101**, 348–353.

Veldic, M., Guidotti, A., Maloku, E., Davis, J.M. & Costa, E. (2005) In psychosis, cortical interneurons overexpress DNA-methyltransferase 1. *Proceedings of the National Academy of Sciences USA* **102**, 2152–2157.

Veldic, M., Kadriu, B., Maloku, E. *et al.* (2007) Epigenetic mechanisms expressed in basal ganglia GABAergic neurons differentiate schizophrenia from bipolar disorder. *Schizophrenia Research* **91**, 51–61.

Verhoeff, N.P.L.G., Soares, J.C., D'Souza, D.C. *et al.* (1999) [123I] iomazenil SPECT benzodiazepine receptor imaging in schizophrenia. *Psychiatry Research & Neuroimaging* **91**, 163–173.

Verrall, L., Walker, M., Rawlings, N. *et al.* (2007) d-Amino acid oxidase and serine racemase in human brain: normal distribution and altered expression in schizophrenia. *European Journal of Neuroscience* **26**, 1657–1669.

Verrall, L., Burnet, P.W.J., Betts, J.F. & Harrison, P.J. (2010) The neurobiology of D-amino acid oxidase and its involvement in schizophrenia. *Molecular Psychiatry* (in press).

Vilella, E., Costas, J., Sanjuan J. *et al.* (2008) Association of schizophrenia with DTNBP1 but not with DAO, DAOA, NRG1 and

RGS4 nor their genetic interaction. *Journal of Psychiatric Research* **42**, 278–288.

Volk, D.W., Austin, M.C., Pierri, J.N., Sampson, A.R. & Lewis, D.A. (2000) Decreased glutamic acid decarboxylase67 messenger RNA expression in a subset of prefrontal cortical gamma-aminobutyric acid neurons in subjects with schizophrenia. *Archives of General Psychiatry* **57**, 237–245.

Volk, D.W., Pierri, J.N., Fritschy, J.M., Auh, S., Sampson, A.R. & Lewis, D.A. (2002) Reciprocal alterations in pre- and postsynaptic inhibitory markers at chandelier cell inputs to pyramidal neurons in schizophrenia. *Cerebral Cortex* **12**, 1063–1070.

Vollenweider, F.X. & Geyer, M.A. (2001) A systems model of altered consciousness: integrating natural and drug-induced psychoses. *Brain Research Bulletin* **56**, 495–507.

Vollenweider, F.X., Leenders, K.L., Oye, I., Hell, D. & Angst, J. (1997) Differential psychopathology and patterns of cerebral glucose utilisation produced by (S)- and (R)-ketamine in healthy volunteers using positron emission tomography (PET). *European Neuropsychopharmacology* **7**, 25–38.

Vollenweider, F.X., Bachle, D., Umbricht, D., Geyer, M. & Hell, D. (1999) Sertindole reduces S-ketamine induced attentional deficits in healthy volunteers *Biological Psychiatry*, 100S.

Vostrikov, V.M., Uranova, N.A. & Orlovskaya, D.D. (2007) Deficit of perineuronal oligodendrocytes in the prefrontal cortex in schizophrenia and mood disorders. *Schizophrenia Research* **94**, 273–280.

Wallner, M., Hanchar, H.J. & Olsen, R.W. (2003) Ethanol enhances alpha 4 beta 3 delta and alpha 6 beta 3 delta gamma-aminobutyric acid type A receptors at low concentrations known to affect humans.[see comment]. *Proceedings of the National Academy of Sciences USA* **100**, 15218–15223.

Webster, M.J., Shannon Weickert, C., Herman, M.M., Hyde, T.M. & Kleinman, J.E. (2001) Synaptophysin and GAP-43 mRNA levels in the hippocampus of subjects with schizophrenia. *Schizophrenia Research* **49**, 89–98.

Wedenoja, J., Loukola, A., Tuulio-Henriksson, A. *et al.* (2008) Replication of linkage on chromosome 7q22 and association of the regional Reelin gene with working memory in schizophrenia families. *Molecular Psychiatry* **13**, 673–684.

Wei, W., Zhang, N., Peng, Z., Houser, C.R. & Mody, I. (2003) Perisynaptic localization of delta subunit-containing GABA(A) receptors and their activation by GABA spillover in the mouse dentate gyrus. *Journal of Neuroscience* **23**, 10650–10661.

Weickert, C.S., Straub, R.E., McClintock, B.W. *et al.* (2004) Human dysbindin (DTNBP1) gene expression in normal brain and in schizophrenic prefrontal cortex and midbrain. *Archives of General Psychiatry* **61**, 544–555.

Whiting, P.J. (2003) GABA-A receptor subtypes in the brain: a paradigm for CNS drug discovery? *Drug Discovery Today* **8**, 445–450.

Williams, J.B., Mallorga, P.J., Jeffrey Conn, P., Pettibone, D.J. & Sur, C. (2004) Effects of typical and atypical antipsychotics on human glycine transporters. *Schizophrenia Research* **71**, 103–112.

Wohlfarth KM, Bianchi MT, Macdonald RL (2002) Enhanced neurosteroid potentiation of ternary GABA(A) receptors containing the delta subunit. *Journal of Neuroscience* **22**, 1541–1549.

Wonders, C.P. & Anderson, S.A. (2006) The origin and specification of cortical interneurons. *Nature Review Neuroscience* **7**, 687–696.

Wonders, C.P., Taylor, L., Welagen, J., Mbata, I.C., Xiang, J.Z. & Anderson, S.A. (2008) A spatial bias for the origins of interneuron subgroups within the medial ganglionic eminence. *Developmental Biology* **314**, 127–136.

Woo, T.U., Whitehead, R.E., Melchitzky, D.S. & Lewis, D.A. (1998) A subclass of prefrontal gamma-aminobutyric acid axon terminals are selectively altered in schizophrenia. *Proceedings of the National Academy of Sciences USA* **95**, 5341–5346.

Woo, T.U., Miller, J.L. & Lewis, D.A. (1997) Schizophrenia and the parvalbumin-containing class of cortical local circuit neurons. *American Journal of Psychiatry* **154**, 1013–1015.

Woo, T.U., Walsh, J.P. & Benes, F.M. (2004) Density of glutamic acid decarboxylase 67 messenger RNA-containing neurons that express the N-methyl-D-aspartate receptor subunit NR2A in the anterior cingulate cortex in schizophrenia and bipolar disorder. *Archives of General Psychiatry* **61**, 649–657.

Woolley, M.L., Pemberton, D.J., Bate, S., Corti, C. & Jones, D.N. (2008) The mGlu2 but not the mGlu3 receptor mediates the actions of the mGluR2/3 agonist, LY379268, in mouse models predictive of antipsychotic activity. *Psychopharmacology (Berlin)* **196**, 431–440.

Wroblewska, B., Wroblewski, J.T., Pshenichkin, S., Surin, A., Sullivan, S.E. & Neale, J.H. (1997) N-acetylaspartylglutamate selectively activates mGluR3 receptors in transfected cells. *Journal of Neurochemistry* **69**, 174–181.

Yang, Y.F., Qin, W., Shugart, Y.Y. *et al.* (2005) Possible association of the MAG locus with schizophrenia in a Chinese Han cohort of family trios. *Schizophrenia Research* **75**, 11–19.

Yu, Z., Chen, J., Shi, H., Stoeber, G., Tsang, S.Y. & Xue, H. (2006) Analysis of GABRB2 association with schizophrenia in German population with DNA sequencing and one-label extension method for SNP genotyping. *Clinical Biochemistry* **39**, 210–218.

Yuste, R., Majewska, A., Cash, S.S. & Denk, W. (1999) Mechanisms of calcium influx into hippocampal spines: heterogeneity among spines, coincidence detection by NMDA receptors, and optical quantal analysis. *Journal of Neuroscience* **19**, 1976–1987.

Zai, G., King, N., Wong, G.W., Barr, C.L. & Kennedy, J.L. (2005) Possible association between the gamma-aminobutyric acid type B receptor 1 (GABBR1) gene and schizophrenia. *European Neuropsychopharmacology* **15**, 347–352.

Zammit, S., Spurlock, G., Williams, H. *et al.* (2007) Genotype effects of CHRNA7, CNR1 and COMT in schizophrenia: interactions with tobacco and cannabis use. *British Journal of Psychiatry* **191**, 402–407.

Zhao, X., Qin, S., Shi, Y. *et al.* (2007) Systematic study of association of four GABAergic genes: glutamic acid decarboxylase 1 gene, glutamic acid decarboxylase 2 gene, GABA(B) receptor 1 gene and GABA(A) receptor subunit beta2 gene, with schizophrenia using a universal DNA microarray. *Schizophrenia Research* **93**, 374–384.

Zukin, S.R. & Zukin, R.S. (1979) Specific [³H]phencyclidine binding in rat central nervous system. *Proceedings of the National Academy of Sciences USA* **76**, 5372–5376.

CHAPTER 22

Animal models of schizophrenia

Barbara K. Lipska[1] and Joseph A. Gogos[2]

[1]National Institute of Mental Health, Bethesda, MD, USA
[2]Columbia University Medical Center, New York, NY, USA

Pharmacological dopamine-based animal models

Traditionally, most animal models of schizophrenia have focused on phenomena linked to dopamine, because the dopaminergic system has been strongly implicated in this disorder, as all effective antipsychotic drugs are antagonists of dopamine receptors, and dopamine agonists induce symptoms that resemble psychosis (Table 22.1, and see Chapter 20). For instance, some dopamine-based models involve behavioral paradigms that were inspired by antipsychotic (i.e., antidopaminergic) pharmacology but bear no resemblance to schizophrenia (e.g., antagonism of apomorphine-induced emesis). Others reproduce phenomena isomorphic with selected characteristics of schizophrenia, such as motor behaviors (e.g., dopamimetic drug-induced stereotypies) and information processing deficits [e.g., apomorphine-induced prepulse inhibition of startle (PPI) abnormalities; Costall & Naylor, 1995]. These dopamine-linked behaviors, although not specific for or uniquely prominent in schizophrenia, can at least be detected and precisely quantified in non-human species and have been useful in screening drugs with a predicted mechanism of action (e.g., dopamine blockade). Thus, models based on perturbing dopamine have no construct validity, limited face validity, but relatively good predictive validity. The predictive validity is to be expected given that the models are based on changing dopamine function. However, as "dopamine-in, dopamine-out" models (i.e., models based on direct pharmacological manipulation of the dopaminergic system and tests of behavioral outcome related to dopamine function), they precluded exploring other than dopamine-based mechanisms of the disease and discovering novel antipsychotic therapies. Drugs that have emerged as a result of such models all exert antidopaminergic efficacy. Antidopaminergic drugs, however, although ameliorative of some of the symptoms of schizophrenia, do not cure the disease. It has become increasingly clear that models based on direct manipulations of the dopamine system may have exhausted their heuristic potential and that new strategies need to be developed to provide novel targets for the development of more effective therapeutic agents.

Novel approaches to modeling schizophrenia

In the context of our current knowledge about schizophrenia, innovative or heuristic models have several goals: (1) to test the plausibility of theories derived from the emerging research data about the disorder; (2) to probe the explanatory power of new biological findings about the disorder; (3) to uncover mechanisms of schizophrenia-like

Schizophrenia, 3rd edition. Edited by Daniel R. Weinberger and Paul J Harrison © 2011 Blackwell Publishing Ltd.

Table 22.1 Clinical aspects of schizophrenia and relevant behavioral changes in animals.

Schizophrenia: clinical phenomena	Animal models: behavioral changes
Psychotic symptoms	Behaviors related to increased dopaminergic transmission: Dopamimetic-induced hyperlocomotion Reduced haloperidol-induced catalepsy
Stereotypic behaviors symptoms by NMDA-antagonists	Dopamimetic-induced stereotypies Worsening of psychotic NMDA antagonists-induced locomotion
Vulnerability to stress	Stress-induced hyperlocomotion
Information processing deficits	Sensorimotor gating (PPI, P50) deficits
Attentional deficits	Deficits in latent inhibition
Cognitive deficits	Impaired performance in delayed alternation and spatial memory tests
Social withdrawal	Reduced contacts with unfamiliar partners

phenomena; and (4) to suggest potential new treatments. Thus, a heuristic model, in contrast to a traditional dopamine-based model, needs to evince other schizophrenia-like abnormalities besides the feature that it directly manipulates. For instance, a model based on hippocampal injury would be heuristic if it triggered behavioral and/or molecular changes outside the hippocampus that are associated with schizophrenia, enabled testing the mechanisms underlying the ensuing changes, and predicted novel therapies based on newly discovered mechanisms.

As interest in schizophrenia research has shifted from a principal focus on dopamine to theories of abnormal neurodevelopment, dysfunction of cortical glutamatergic neurons, and genetic susceptibility, animal models have followed a similar trend. The models considered below are either non-pharmacological or based on pharmacological manipulation of a neurotransmitter other than dopamine. Thus, they have ventured off the beaten path of "dopamine-in, dopamine-out" models, and offer the potential of elucidating non-dopamine mechanisms of disease and treatment. All animal models of schizophrenia, however, whether new or old, suffer from a generic problem–lack of a straightforward test of fidelity. This is because there is no valid genotype, cellular phenotype or other biological marker that is characteristic of the disorder, and no animal model can fully reproduce the perceptual, cognitive, and emotional features of the human illness. In the absence of a pathognomonic marker, a faithful model is expected to reproduce a constellation of behavioral and biological phenomena relevant to schizophrenia. If a model addresses a

cluster of relevant changes ranging from anatomical and neurochemical to behavioral and cognitive features, rather than a single or a few non-specific phenomena, then there is a higher probability that the model is heuristic and isomorphic with biological processes related to the human disorder. As new findings about the pathophysiology of schizophrenia emerge, new models increasingly focus on certain cell or tissue phenotypes and a variety of complex behavioral characteristics, in addition to time-honored effects on dopamine-related function (Tables 22.1 and 22.2); unfortunately, as shown in the examples below, rarely are multiple phenomena addressed in a single model.

In this chapter, we will examine three approaches to creating animal models related to schizophrenia: (1) neurodevelopmental models; (2) glutamatergic hypofunction models; and (3) genetic models. The first approach is based on experimentally-induced disruption of brain development that becomes evident in an adult animal in the form of altered brain neurochemistry and aberrant behavior (neurodevelopmental models). These models test hypotheses that schizophrenia is caused by a defect in cerebral development (Lillrank et al., 1995; Lipska & Weinberger, 2000; see Chapter 19), and in some instances, test whether the effects of early brain damage could remain inconspicuous until after a considerable delay, as appears to be the case in the human condition (Weinberger, 1986, 1987; Murray & Lewis, 1987; Bloom. 1993). Another popular modeling approach involves pharmacological disruption of brain function and behavior via N-methyl-D-aspartate (NMDA) antagonists. These models test the hypothesis that dysfunction of glutamate neurotransmission accounts for a variety of schizophrenic phenomena (Javitt & Zukin, 1991; see Chapter 21). Still another effort focuses on the search for susceptibility genes employing modern technologies of genetic engineering (genetic models; Arguello & Gogos, 2006). These models test the clinical evidence that susceptibility genes account for risk for illness and, together with epigenetic/environmental factors, for phenotypic variation (see Chapters 12 and 13). Characteristically, a majority of these new models, despite the diversity of their origins, target components of a common neural circuitry implicated in schizophrenia, i.e., the temporo-limbic cortices–nucleus accumbens/striatal complex–thalamus–prefrontal cortex. The involvement of this circuitry may account for the overlap in "schizophrenia-like" phenomena at the anatomical, neurochemical or behavioral level that is common to these various models.

Neurodevelopmental models

Models testing etiological theories

Many epidemiological and clinical correlational studies have been carried out in the search for early developmental

Table 22.2 Neonatal ventral hippocampal (VH) lesion model: schizophrenia-like phenomena.

	Neonatal VH lesion model	Schizophrenia
Behavioral changes	Hyperlocomotion to stress PPI deficits LI deficits Deficits in delayed alternation tests Reduced social contacts Social withdrawal	Stress vulnerability PPI deficits LI deficits Working memory deficits
Pharmacological responses	Amphetamine-induced hyperactivity ⎫ Apomorphine-induced stereotypies ⎬ Reduced catalepsy to haloperidol response to ketamine MK-801- and PCP-induced hyperactivity	Enhanced symptomatic response to dopamimetics Neuroleptic tolerance enhanced Symptomatic
Molecular changes in the PFC	NAA levels ↓ GAD$_{67}$ mRNA ↓ BDNF mRNA ↓	NAA levels ↓ GAD$_{67}$ mRNA ↓ BDNF mRNA ↓
Changes in synaptic morphology in the PFC	Spine density↓	Spine density ↓

BDNF, brain-derived neurotropic factor; GAD$_{67}$, glutamate decarboxylase-67; LI, latent inhibition; NAA, N-acetylaspartate; PCP, phencyclidine; PPI, prepulse inhibition of startle; PFC, prefrontal cortex; ↓,reduced *vs.* controls.

factors that may predispose to schizophrenia. There have been reports linking schizophrenia to obstetrical complications (Woerner *et al.*, 1973; DeLisi *et al.*, 1988; McNiel, 1988; Hultman *et al.*, 1997; Dalman *et al.*, 1999), *in utero* exposure to alcohol (Lohr & Bracha, 1989), and severe malnutrition (Susser & Lin, 1992). A number of animal models have been designed to test the plausibility that specific gestational factors play a role in the origin of this disorder. These "etiological" models, none of which directly manipulates dopamine, aspire to construct validity and heuristic value because they reproduce putative causes of the disease and theoretically model putative primary pathological mechanisms.

For instance, developmental malnutrition models (or more precisely, prenatal protein deprivation or gestational vitamin D deficiency) result in permanent changes in the development of the rat brain (Palmer *et al.*, 2004; Kesby *et al.*, 2006). Malnutrition affects neurogenesis, cell migration and differentiation, and leads to deviations in normal brain development, including disrupted formation of neural circuits and neurotransmitter systems, and debilitating effects on cognitive function and learning abilities (Lewis *et al.*, 1979; Cintra *et al.*, 1997). Thus, to some degree these models mimic certain "face" features of schizophrenia. In contrast to schizophrenia, however, morphological abnormalities are severe and widespread, and the behavioral consequences are varied and inconsistent, perhaps, at least in part, because the impact of malnutrition on brain development is likely to be quite variable and to depend

on many factors, which have only been explored to a small degree. As a test of the plausibility of the malnutrition theory of schizophrenia, this model has limited validity.

Prenatal exposure to influenza virus, another predisposing factor implicated in schizophrenia by several large epidemiological studies (Mednick *et al.*, 1988; Kendell & Kemp, 1989; O'Callaghan *et al.*, 1991; Adams *et al.*, 1993), has been shown to induce pyramidal cell disarray in a small subgroup of mice whose mothers were inoculated with the virus (Cotter *et al.*, 1995). This developmental defect is somewhat similar to that reported in two studies in the hippocampi of patients with schizophrenia (Conrad *et al.*, 1991; Scheibel & Kovelman, 1981). Other reports indicate that infection with human influenza of pregnant mice results in defective corticogenesis, as indicated by reduced thickness of the neocortex and hippocampus and behavioral changes (Fatemi *et al.*, 1999; Shi *et al.*, 2003). These are intriguing observations, but more conclusive data are required before conclusions about the relevance of this model for schizophrenia can be made.

The plausibility that other, less common, viruses may induce schizophrenia-like changes has also been investigated (Rott *et al.*, 1985; Waltrip *et al.*, 1995). *In utero* Borna disease virus (BDV), a neurotrophic virus with limbic selectivity, damages the hippocampus and prefrontal cortex (PFC), and results in complex changes in regional dopamine in rats and in behavioral hypersensitivity to psychostimulants (Solbrig *et al.*, 2000; Hornig *et al.*, 1999). While this model may invite further research into the mechanisms involved, notwithstanding convincing evidence of BDV infection in schizophrenia, its relevance to the pathophysiology of schizophrenia seems remote.

Another example of a viral model is neonatal infection with lymphocytic choriomeningitis virus (LCMV) which disrupts in adult rats the integrity of γ-aminobutyric acid (GABA)ergic neurons and excitatory amino acid systems, both of which are implicated in schizophrenia (reviewed by Pearce, 2001). The potential face validity of this model at a cellular level makes it particularly attractive because it addresses two theories about the pathophysiology of schizophrenia: vulnerability of GABAergic interneurons to developmental insult and adolescent vulnerability to excitotoxic injury (Benes et al., 1992; Olney & Farber, 1995). Although conceptually appealing, it has yet to address a broader spectrum of aspects of the disorder, and its basic construct, LCMV infection, is of dubious relevance to schizophrenia.

Prenatal exposure to infections represents a risk factor for the emergence of neuropsychiatric disorders, including schizophrenia. To test this, pregnant mice were exposed to the inflammatory agent polyriboinosinic–polyribocytidilic acid (PolyI:C). Their offspring showed a variety of dopamine- and glutamate-related pharmacological and neuroanatomical disturbances (Zuckerman et al., 2003). However, the adoption of prenatal control animals to immune-challenged surrogate mothers was also sufficient to induce specific pharmacological and neuroanatomical abnormalities in the fostered offspring (Meyer et al., 2008). These data suggest that immunological stress during pregnancy may affect the mothers in such a way that being reared by an immune-challenged mother can confer risk for some aspects of psychiatric illness in adult life.

The plausibility of obstetric and birth complications are difficult to explore in animals because their causes in schizophrenia are unknown. Nevertheless, studies of models of cesarean birth and of anoxia during birth in rats report changes in limbic dopamine function of adult animals consistent with hyper-responsiveness of the dopamine system to stimulants (reviewed by Boksa & El-Khodor, 2003). Surprisingly though, animals born by cesarian section and not subject to anoxia seem to be even more affected than anoxic rats (El-Khodor & Boksa, 1997). In humans, cesarian section is generally assumed to involve less stress to the fetus and has not been noted as one of the obstetric complications linked to schizophrenia.

Until a broader array of schizophrenia-related phenomena is assessed in each of these etiological models, it is premature to draw firm conclusions about whether any reproduces mechanisms underlying the human disorder. Moreover, the validity of these models is tempered by the lack of convincing evidence for the role of any of these various causative factors in schizophrenia, with the possible exception of influenza. These models illustrate, however, that certain early developmental insults may permanently disrupt brain function in ways that are similar to some of the phenomena reported in schizophrenia.

Models of disrupted neurogenesis

Several postmortem studies of schizophrenia have reported variations in cortical cytoarchitecture (Akbarian et al., 1993; Arnold et al., 1991; Kirkpatrick et al., 1999; see Harrison & Weinberger, 2005, and Chapter 18), possibly of a developmental nature. These reports have inspired models based on disrupted neurogenesis. Examples include cortical dysgenesis induced by gestational X-ray irradiation (Mintz et al., 1999; Selemon et al., 2005; Gelowitz et al., 2002), in-utero exposure to a mitotic toxin, methylazoxymethanol acetate (MAM), which destroys populations of rapidly dividing neurons, and systemic administration of nitric oxide synthase (NOS) inhibitors, which interfere with maturation of neurons and synaptogenesis. Animals that have undergone X-ray or MAM manipulations exhibit morphological changes in a broad array of brain structures implicated in schizophrenia, particularly the hippocampus, and frontal and entorhinal cortices, and a variety of behavioral alterations (Johnston et al., 1988; Talamini et al., 1998; Moore et al., 2006). Male rats exposed to an NOS inhibitor (L-nitroarginine) between 3 and 5 days of life show in adulthood locomotor hypersensitivity to amphetamine and deficits in PPI, but similarly treated females were not found to be affected on these measures (Black et al., 1999). These results are provocative and invite further research.

Models of aberrant neurogenesis, though the data are limited at this time, appear to have potential heuristic value in discovering mechanisms of specific neural circuit disruptions caused by elimination of maturing neurons.

Perinatal stress models

This group of models focuses on the long-lasting consequences of stress for brain development and for shaping adult behavioral responses. Stress has been postulated as a factor in so-called "two hit" models of schizophrenia in which two independent insults (e.g., aberrant genetic trait and stressful experience) are thought to be necessary for the occurrence of the disorder. In rodents, early life exposure to experiential stressors, such as maternal separation and social isolation, produce numerous hormonal, neurochemical, and behavioral changes, including locomotor hyperactivity in a novel environment, maze learning impairments, anxiety, latent inhibition, and sensorimotor gating deficits (reviewed by Sullivan et al., 2006). Of particular interest is that some of these alterations emerge in adult life and can be restored by a wide range of antipsychotics, including various typical and atypical drugs (Varty

& Higgins, 1995; Ellenbroek *et al.*, 1998; Bakshi *et al.*, 1998). Importantly, the effects of adverse early life events (e.g. maternal separation) on adult reactivity are strongly influenced by genetic as well as non-genomic factors (Zaharia *et al.*, 1996; Anisman *et al.*, 1998; Francis *et al.*, 1999).

Neonatal lesion models

Another series of studies has focused on neonatal damage of restricted brain regions in rats (Lipska *et al.*, 1993; Flores *et al.*, 1996a; Chambers *et al.*, 1996; Wan *et al.*, 1996, 1998; Wan & Corbett, 1997; Brake *et al.*, 1999; Black *et al.*, 1998; Becker *et al.*, 1999; Grecksch *et al.*, 1999; Schroeder *et al.*, 1999) and in monkeys (Beauregard & Bachevalier, 1996; Bertolino *et al.*, 1997; Saunders *et al.*, 1998; Bachevalier *et al.*, 1999). The main objective of many of these studies is to disrupt development of the hippocampus, a brain area consistently implicated in human schizophrenia (Falkai & Bogerts, 1986; Jeste & Lohr, 1989; Bogerts *et al.*, 1990; Suddath *et al.*, 1990; Eastwood *et al.*, 1995, 1997; Eastwood & Harrison 1995, 1998; Weinberger, 1999), and thus disrupts development of the widespread cortical and subcortical circuitry in which the hippocampus participates. The lesions were intended to involve regions of the hippocampus that directly project to the PFC, i.e., the ventral hippocampus and ventral subiculum (Jay *et al.*, 1989; Carr & Sesack, 1996), and that correspond to the anterior hippocampus in humans, a region that shows anatomical abnormalities in schizophrenia (Suddath *et al.*, 1990). Of all the recent studies of animal models based on developmental perturbations, the neonatal ventral hippocampal lesion model has been studied by far the most extensively (reviewed in Tseng *et al.*, 2009), and it will be discussed in some detail here.

Neonatal excitotoxic lesions of the rat ventral hippocampus (VH) lead in adolescence or early adulthood to the emergence of abnormalities in a number of dopamine-related behaviors, which bear close resemblance to behaviors seen in animals sensitized to psychostimulants. When tested as juveniles (postnatal day 35), rats with the neonatal VH lesions are less social than controls (Sams-Dodd *et al.*, 1997), but otherwise behave normally in motor tests involving exposure to stress and dopamine agonists. In adolescence and adulthood (postnatal day 56 and older), lesioned animals display markedly changed behaviors thought to be primarily linked to increased mesolimbic/nigrostriatal dopamine transmission (motor hyper-responsiveness to stress and stimulants, enhanced stereotypies). They also show enhanced sensitivity to glutamate antagonists (MK-801 and PCP), deficits in PPI and latent inhibition, impaired social behaviors, and working memory problems (Lipska & Weinberger, 1993, 1994a,b, 1995; Becker *et al.*, 1999; Grecksch *et al.*, 1999; Al-Amin *et al.*, 2000, 2001), phenomena showing many parallels with schizophrenia. Emergence

of the behavioral changes in adolescence appears not to be related to the surge of gonadal hormones during puberty because a similar temporal pattern of abnormalities is observed in animals depleted of gonadal hormones prior to puberty (Lipska & Weinberger, 1994b). Notably, removal of prefrontal neurons in adult animals with the earlier hippocampal lesion restores some of the behaviors (i.e., those modulated by but not critically dependent on the PFC, such as hyperlocomotion after amphetamine), suggesting that aberrant development of the PFC in the context of early damage to the hippocampus may be a critical factor in the expression of the syndrome (Lipska *et al.*, 1998a). In this context, it is important to emphasize that anatomical findings from postmortem studies and neuropsychological and neuroimaging studies of brain function in patients with schizophrenia have implicated PFC maldevelopment and a developmental "disconnection" of the temporo-limbic and prefrontal cortices (for review, see Weinberger & Lipska, 1995). Although the exact mechanisms of a seemingly similar "disconnection" and malfunction of the PFC in the VH-lesioned rats need to be elucidated, preliminary findings from molecular and electrophysiological studies [such as reduced cortical levels of *N*-acetylaspartate (NAA), attenuated stress-induced cortical dopamine release, attenuated cortical expression of a membrane glutamate transporter, EAAC1, and of a synthetic enzyme for GABA, glutamate decarboxylase-67 (GAD_{67}), reduced brain-derived neurotrophic factor (BDNF) expression, altered cortical expression of transcription factors, c-fos and ΔfosB, as well as altered firing pattern of cortical pyramidal neurons in response to ventral tegmental area (VTA) stimulation] suggest that aberrant cortical dopamine–glutamate–GABA interactions may underlie cortical dysfunction in the neonatally VH-lesioned rats (Lipska *et al.*, 1995; Bertolino *et al.*, 1999; Lee *et al.*, 1998; Ashe *et al.*, 2002; O'Donnell *et al.*, 2002; Powell *et al.*, 2006; Wong *et al.*, 2005). It has also been reported that excitotoxic PFC lesions in adult animals cause downstream striatal NAA losses and reduced GAD_{67} mRNA expression, and suggested that both changes might reflect trans-synaptic pathology (Roffman *et al.*, 2000). Electrophysiological studies provided further evidence that prefrontal dopamine and glutamatergic systems become altered after puberty in the neonatally lesioned rats (Tseng *et al.*, 2007) and that these alterations are mediated by changes in the GABAergic interneurons (Tseng & O'Donnell, 2004, 2007), reminiscent of the changes reported in schizophrenia.

It is interesting to note that many of these changes have been reported in stress- and psychostimulant-sensitization models (Vanderschuren *et al.*, 1999; Gambarana *et al.*, 1999; Feldpausch *et al.*, 1998), as well as in patients with schizophrenia (Akbarian *et al.*, 1995; Bertolino *et al.*, 1998). It is hypothesized that increased substance abuse disorder comorbidity in schizophrenia may reflect greater vulnerability to addictive processes because of inherent neurocircuit dysfunction in the schizophrenic brain. Indeed, using the neurodevelopmental hippocampal lesion model, it has been shown that altered patterns of behavioral sensitization, as a possible correlate of greater addiction vulnerability, can occur as a by-product of the neural system dysfunction that is responsible for major psychiatric syndromes. In particular, rats with neonatal lesions showed augmented locomotor effects and deficient learning of complex contingencies to guide an efficient reward approach when exposed to repeated cocaine (Chambers & Taylor, 2004; Chambers *et al.*, 2005). Subcortical function in the neonatally lesioned rats is also altered in a fashion consistent with at least some reports on behavioral sensitization, i.e., striatal dopamine release is attenuated in response to stress and amphetamine, midbrain expression of the membrane dopamine transporter (DAT) mRNA is reduced, striatal expression of dynorphin (an opioid peptide colocalized with D_1 receptors) and of ΔfosB (a transcription factor sensitive to persistent stimulation) are enhanced (Lipska *et al.*, 1998b; Powell *et al.*, 2006). It should be noted, however, that enhanced rather than attenuated striatal dopamine release has been observed in other paradigms of sensitization to psychostimulants (for review, see Spanagel & Weiss, 1999), as well as in a subgroup of individuals with schizophrenia, as evidenced by recent single photon emission computed tomography (SPECT) and positron emission tomography (PET) studies (Abi-Dargham *et al.*, 1998; Laruelle *et al.*, 1996; Breier *et al.*, 1997). Nevertheless, an array of behavioral and molecular changes associated with this model suggests that early developmental insult of the VH may facilitate sensitization of the dopamine system (Chambers & Taylor, 2004; Chambers *et al.*, 2005; Berg & Chambers 2008; Conroy *et al.*, 2007). Similar pathophysiological mechanisms have been hypothesized to underlie schizophrenia (Lieberman *et al.*, 1997; Meng *et al.*, 1998; Duncan *et al.*, 1999). It is of considerable heuristic interest to determine how the developmental lesion initiates the subsequent behavioral and molecular phenomena associated with sensitization.

In terms of the predictive validity of the neonatal VH lesion model, antipsychotic drugs normalize some lesion-induced behaviors (Lipska & Weinberger, 1994a; Sams-Dodd *et al.*, 1997; Becker & Grecksch 2000; Le Pen & Moreau, 2002; Rueter *et al.*, 2004; Richtand *et al.*, 2006). Drugs targeting the glutamate system may also prove beneficial; LY293558, an α-amino-3-hydroxy-5-methyl-4-isoxazole propionic acid (AMPA) antagonist, is highly efficient in blocking hyperlocomotion in neonatally lesioned rats at doses that do not affect locomotor activity in controls (Al-Amin *et al.*, 2000). Thus, this model may have predictive validity and heuristic potential to identify drugs with new mechanisms of action. The model also appears to mimic a spectrum of neurobiological and behav-

ioral features of schizophrenia, including functional pathology in presumably critical brain regions interconnected with the hippocampal formation and targeted by antipsychotic drugs—the striatum/nucleus accumbens and the PFC (see Table 22.2). It is noteworthy that in the nonhuman primate, early postnatal damage of the hippocampal region also alters development of the dorsal PFC and the mechanisms whereby the dorsal PFC regulates subcortical dopamine function, phenomena similar to those described in patients with schizophrenia (Saunders *et al.*, 1998; Bertolino *et al.*, 1997, 2000). Thus, neonatal damage to the hippocampus of the rat appears to reproduce a broad spectrum of schizophrenia-related phenomena, and establishes the neurobiological plausibility of early damage having a delayed impact on the neural functions implicated in schizophrenia.

Developmental lesions of other brain structures implicated in schizophrenia and components of a limbic–neocortical circuit (e.g., thalamus, PFC) also have been considered as models. For instance, thalamic excitotoxic lesions in PD7 rats result in adult expression of apomorphine- and amphetamine-induced hyperlocomotion (Rajakumar *et al.*, 1996), although other studies did not detect relevant changes after thalamic lesions in rats (Volk & Lewis, 2003; Lipska *et al.*, 2003). Intracerebroventricular infusions of kainic acid into neonatal (PD7) rats lead in adulthood to a reduction in neural numbers in the dorsal hippocampus, and are associated with changes in the expression of subpopulations of glutamate receptors and immediate early genes (Csernansky *et al.*, 1998, 2006; Montgomery *et al.*, 1999). Neonatal (PD7) excitotoxic damage of the medial PFC (MPFC) has been reported to produce delayed behavioral and neurochemical effects (Flores *et al.*, 1996b; Uehara *et al.*, 2007), although others have not confirmed these data (Lipska *et al.*, 1998a). The spectrum of behavioral and cellular parameters examined in these models is rather limited at this time.

Although developmental lesion models represent a rather crude technique to study the role of particular brain regions, transmitter systems or the connections between them (even when more functional techniques of "disconnection" are used; see Lipska *et al.*, 2002), they have confirmed the plausibility of neurodevelopmental damage having selected deleterious effects after a prolonged period of relative normality. In this respect, they appear to have face validity not just in terms of behavioral, cellular, and pharmacological phenomena, but also in terms of the temporal course of the clinical disorder. As models of developmental pathology, they certainly lack construct validity, as the schizophrenic brain does not manifest a "lesion" analogous to any of these models; but they may have heuristic value in discovering molecular consequences of early brain damage, and new treatment prospects.

Pharmacological models of glutamatergic antagonism

In addition to the non-pharmacological, non-dopaminergic approaches described above, pharmacological blockade of NMDA receptors in adult animals has gained popularity as a model of schizophrenia. Observations that non-competitive NMDA antagonists, such as phencyclidine (PCP) and ketamine, exacerbate some psychotic symptoms in patients with schizophrenia and have psychotomimetic effects in normal humans (Krystal et al., 1994; Lahti et al., 1995) have encouraged speculation that some aspects of schizophrenia may relate to abnormal glutamatergic function. This has been further supported by postmortem studies in schizophrenia showing a variety of changes in the glutamate system, including altered glutamate metabolism and expression of various glutamate receptors (Javitt & Zukin, 1991; Akbarian et al., 1996; Jentsch & Roth, 1999; Weinberger, 1999; see Chapter 21).

In rodents and monkeys, acute subanesthetic doses of NMDA antagonists produce a constellation of phenomena potentially relevant to schizophrenic symptomatology, including hyperlocomotion, enhanced stereotyped behaviors, cognitive and sensorimotor gating deficits, and impaired social interactions. PCP as well as other NMDA antagonists acutely increase extracellular levels of dopamine and glutamate (as well as norepinephrine and acetylcholine) in the PFC, and alter firing patterns of dopaminergic and nucleus accumbens neurons (Verma & Moghaddam, 1996; O'Donnell & Grace, 1998). Repeated administration of PCP can also induce robust behavioral and neurochemical changes, persisting after long-term withdrawal (Jentsch & Roth, 1999) even single doses of NMDA antagonists can have these effects (Harris et al., 2003). Of particular interest is differential dysregulation of the firing patterns of meso-limbic and meso-cortical dopaminergic neurons by low, behaviorally relevant doses of NMDA antagonists. These changes in dopamine cell firing may render them unresponsive or inappropriately responsive to salient environmental stimuli such as stress and reward (Murase et al., 1993; Mathe et al., 1998). If a similar process underlies psychotic symptoms and cognitive deficits in schizophrenia, the NMDA antagonist model may offer novel treatment strategies targeting glutamate rather than dopamine. Experimental approaches to reverse NMDA antagonist-induced abnormalities have included pharmacological enhancement of NMDA receptor activity, enhancement of metabotropic glutamate receptor (mGluR2) activity, and blockade of AMPA receptors (Moghaddam et al., 1997; Moghaddam & Adams, 1998), the latter approach shown to be also effective in the neonatal hippocampal lesion model (see above). Thus, a model based on a primary glutamatergic abnormality appears to show important heuristic properties in terms of identifying potential novel therapies. This model offers insight into molecular adaptations that follow chronic NMDA blockade, and has recently led to the identification of a new antipsychotic drug, LY404039, which is a selective agonist for metabotropic glutamate 2/3 (mGlu2/3) receptors (Patil et al., 2007). Notably, the repeated non-competitive NMDA blockade model, which had also been intensively investigated from the perspective of behavioral sensitization and its role in drug addiction and reward mechanisms (Wolf et al., 1993), shares certain behavioral and neurochemical similarities with the neonatal hippocampal lesion model, including cognitive deficits (in particular, in working memory tasks), reduced frontal dopamine transmission (Jentsch & Roth, 1999), reduced GABA activity, as indicated by reduced levels of GAD_{67} (Qin et al., 1994; Yonezawa et al., 1998), disrupted social behaviors, and augmented locomotor responses to stress and amphetamine. The similarities between the models may reflect a common disruption of cortical glutamate–GABA function which may converge towards a common underlying process of behavioral sensitization. Unlike the etiological or neonatal lesions models, the NMDA antagonist approach does not, however, address the developmental component of schizophrenia.

Genetic models

Schizophrenia is a highly heritable disorder that probably involves multiple genes with small effects across large populations (Kendler et al., 1996; see Chapter 12). Elucidating the roles of the susceptibility genes for this clinically diverse and probably genetically heterogeneous disorder will require considerable effort and is unlikely to be fully resolved soon. Modern technologies, involving targeted gene deletions or gene transfer techniques that have revolutionized experimental medicine, may provide a new generation of animal models for schizophrenia that may help in this daunting task.

Advantages, limitations, and challenges

Genetic factors play a prominent role in many psychiatric disorders and numerous putative candidate genes have been identified (Gogos & Gerber, 2006). Mouse models of "susceptibility genes" identified through human genetic studies hold tremendous promise and offer several unique advantages in understanding the function of a gene and its contribution to the pathophysiology of the disease or disease-related endophenotypes (Arguello & Gogos, 2006). They allow for a detailed analysis of the molecular and cellular pathways, neural circuits, and behaviors affected, including early mutational effects and their developmental progression. In addition, they allow for a thorough investigation of interactions among susceptibility genes and between genes and environmental factors. Despite these obvious advantages, interpreting results from even the most reliable genetic mouse models can be confounded by at least two factors (Arguello & Gogos, 2006). First, a gene-based model may not exhibit abnormalities in all schizophrenia-related endophenotypes. Second, genetic manipulations are the most upstream from the observed clinical psychopathology and, if efficient adaptive responses emerge (i.e., changes in activity and expression of other genes; Anholt *et al.*, 2003), they may require additional genetic, pharmacological or environmental manipulations to compromise the efficiency of this genomic buffering and become fully penetrant at the behavioral level. In that context, a mouse model for an individual candidate gene will not be representative of the entire disorder and at best it will reproduce either a subtype of the disorder or a particular aspect of an endophenotype.

Genetic architecture of complex psychiatric disorders

There are two predominating but not mutually exclusive hypotheses regarding the genetic architecture of complex psychiatric disorders such as schizophrenia (see Chapters 12 and 13). According to the common disease/common allele hypothesis (CD/CA; Pritchard & Cox, 2002), no single gene is necessary or sufficient to cause the disease, but instead, common (≥5%), low-penetrance genetic variants in more than one susceptibility gene, each contributing a small effect, act in combinations to increase the risk of illness. The alternative hypothesis (common disease/rare allele hypothesis, CD/RA) proposes that complex psychiatric disorders may instead result from the effects of rare, but highly penetrant, mutations (i.e., point mutations, copy number mutations, etc.) in single genes, with substantial allelic heterogeneity at disease-causing loci.

Within this human genetics context, the most important consideration in developing etiologically valid genetic mouse models has to do with the nature of the disease-associated genetic variants. Obviously, the minimum amount of information needed is whether the risk allele is a hypomorph or gain of function and therefore whether a mouse knockdown strategy or transgene-mediated over-expression, respectively, can model it accurately. A didactic example demonstrating the importance of modeling well-defined disease alleles rather than disease loci (using routine knockout or transgenic approaches) is provided by recent work by Sudhof and colleagues in developing genetic mouse models of autism spectrum disorders (ASDs). A small percentage of patients with an ASD carry mutations in genes encoding neuroligins (postsynaptic cell-adhesion molecules). Using a knockin approach, Tabuchi *et al.* (2007) introduced one of these mutations (R451C substitution in neuroligin-3) into mice. Mutant mice showed several autism-related behavioral changes, accompanied by an increase in inhibitory transmission. In sharp contrast, knockout of neuroligin-3 did not cause such changes, indicating that the R451C substitution represents a gain-of-function mutation that results in increased inhibitory transmission and that cannot be modeled by traditional knockout approaches.

With possibly few exceptions, results from studies based on the CD/CA hypothesis have not provided genetic variants with a *clear effect on gene function or expression* that unequivocally increase disease risk. One reason is that the associated variants usually have no obvious effect on protein structure (Rebbeck *et al.*, 2004) and in some cases may only serve as proxies for physically linked, true risk variant(s) residing within the identified gene or a nearby gene (linkage disequilibrium; Newton-Cheh & Hirschhorn, 2005). These uncertainties contribute to the challenging task of generating animal models based on CD/CA-based genetic findings. Nevertheless, the CD/CA hypothesis has generated several interesting leading "candidate" genes. Traditional knockout and other *in vivo* or *in vitro* approaches are used for follow-up gene function studies. Although they do not necessarily reproduce the risk alleles, such approaches are indispensable in deciphering the function of candidate genes and the genetic pathway(s) they participate in, as well as in generating hypotheses on how disruption of such genes could possibly contribute to disease risk.

Results from studies based on the CD/RA hypothesis have been more fruitful in identifying well-defined genetic lesions with clear effects on gene function or expression that unequivocally increase disease risk. Identification of such rare genetic lesions will definitely facilitate modeling efforts, especially when highly penetrant loss or gain-of-function alleles are involved that can be faithfully modeled by appropriate genetic engineering manipulations.

Two such examples exist to date and will be described in more detail below: *de novo* deletions on 22q11 and an inherited translocation in the disrupted-in-schizophrenia 1 (*DISC1*) gene. Considering that rare mutations may collectively account for a substantial portion of the genetic component of schizophrenia and other neuropsychiatric disorders (Karayiorgou *et al.*, 1995; Sebat *et al.*, 2007), animal model approaches based on such mutations are very likely to improve dramatically our knowledge of the genetic and biological basis of schizophrenia in the very near future.

Models based on the CD/CA hypothesis

For the most part, genetic mouse models based on the CD/CA hypothesis have been limited to constitutive or conditional knockouts or generation of dominant-negative transgenic mice. Some examples are outlined below and more detailed descriptions can be found in Chen *et al.* (2006) and O'Tuathaigh *et al.* (2007a).

Neuregulin 1 (NRG1), and to a lesser extent its receptor erbB4, are leading candidate susceptibility genes for schizophrenia (Stefansson *et al.*, 2002; Law *et al.*, 2007). Both genes have pleiotropic effects on neuronal migration, neurite outgrowth, synaptic transmission, glial cell proliferation, myelination, and various modes of cellular signaling (reviewed in Corfas *et al.*, 2004). *NRG1* hypomorphic mice, lacking various domains of the gene, have been extensively used to study the broad cellular deficits induced by impaired NRG1 function and their effects on behavior. These mice show deficits in several neurotransmitter systems, including decreased expression of NMDA receptors (Stefansson *et al.*, 2002) and increased levels of the serotonin 2A receptor and serotonin transporter. Behavioral analyses revealed deficits in PPI and latent inhibition (LI), alterations in locomotor motor activity, anxiety, and suites of spontaneous behaviors. *NRG1* mutants also showed disrupted social interactions, but, notably, cognitive assays showed that spatial learning and working memory processes appeared to be normal (Rimer *et al.*, 2005; Dean *et al.*, 2007; O'Tuathaigh *et al.*, 2006, 2007b,c; Karl *et al.*, 2007).

Based on prior evidence implicating NRG1–erbB signaling in oligodendrocyte (OL) development, Corfas and colleagues (Roy *et al.*, 2007) used transgenic mice in which erbB signaling is blocked in OLs *in vivo* (by the expression of a dominant-negative form of the gene) to test the hypothesis that NRG1–erbB signaling contributes to psychiatric disorders by regulating the structure or function of OLs. Loss of erbB signaling led to changes in OL number and morphology, reduced myelin thickness, and slower conduction velocity in central nervous system (CNS) axons. Interestingly, these transgenic mice showed increased levels of dopamine receptors and transporters as well as behavioral alterations, thus providing one potential mechanism by which NRG1 variants may increase the risk for schizophrenia.

It should be noted here that the functional implications of the *NRG1* genetic variation related to schizophrenia are unclear. A recent study on human postmortem tissue seems to indicate that NRG1 signaling may be *enhanced* in some individuals with schizophrenia (Hahn *et al.*, 2006). Another study has identified a unique brain-specific NRG1 isoform (Type IV) that is differentially expressed and processed during early development, and whose expression is regulated by a schizophrenia risk-associated functional promoter or single nucleotide polymorphism (SNP; Tan *et al.*, 2007; Law *et al.*, 2006). Thus, although the mouse studies summarized above provide initial insight into the basic function of *NRG1*, whether a knockout mutation can model the relevant clinical aspects of its genetic contribution is arguable and the subject of ongoing investigation.

In addition to the *NRG1* mouse models, another relevant example in the context of the CD/CA hypothesis is provided by a conditional knockout of the gene encoding for the calcineurin regulatory subunit. These mice demonstrate several schizophrenia-related phenotypes, such as

deficits in working memory and PPI (Miyakawa *et al.*, 2003). Although variants in this gene have not been shown to increase risk for schizophrenia, common variants in another gene in the pathway (*PPP3CC*) have identified it as a potential susceptibility gene (Gerber *et al.*, 2003). Mice deficient in another candidate gene, *AKT1* (Emamian *et al.*, 2004), provide an additional example. A greater sensitivity to the disrupting effects of AMPH on PPI was initially observed in an *AKT1*-deficient mouse model (Emamian *et al.*, 2004). Subsequent analysis using various genetic mouse models showed that AKT1 is a key signaling intermediate downstream of DRD2, the best-established target of antipsychotic drugs (Emamian *et al.*, 2004; Beaulieu *et al.*, 2005), and that it influences synaptic connectivity in the PFC and performance of working memory tests (Lai *et al.*, 2006).

Catechol-O-methyltransferase (COMT) is a major enzyme responsible for catecholamine catabolism and especially, for the catabolism of dopamine in the PFC, which has few dopamine transporters (Sesack *et al.*, 1998), and is encoded by a schizophrenia candidate gene. In humans, the *COMT* gene has a functional polymorphism (Val158Met) that affects enzyme activity and has been associated with schizophrenia and various cognitive domains (Egan *et al.*, 2001; Goldberg *et al.*, 2003; Glatt *et al.*, 2003; see Chapter 20). To test whether overexpression of human COMT Val affects cognitive function, transgenic mice overexpressing the human COMT Val variant (COMT Val-tg) were recently created (Papaleo *et al.*, 2008). COMT Val-tg mice have increased COMT enzyme activity compared to their control littermates, but are otherwise healthy in generalized tests of physical abilities. Tested in an attentional set-shifting test, modeled after the human version of the Wisconsin Card Sorting Test (WCST) and sensitive to PFC dopamine, the COMT Val-tg mice show selective impairments in their ability to shift an attentional-set, while their simple discrimination and reversal learning abilities are intact. Moreover, COMT Val-tg mice show working memory deficits and object recognition memory deficits, which can be reversed by amphetamine treatment. COMT knockout mice, on the other hand, show improved working memory, as demonstrated by their faster acquisition of the discrete paired-trial alternation T-maze task and more correct responses at different intra-trial delays (Papaleo *et al.*, 2008). Overall, these results demonstrate that life-long changes (either increases or reductions) in COMT activity markedly impact cognition. In particular, *COMT* gene modifications affect working memory processes and the abilities to shift an attentional set, perhaps because of COMT regulation of dopamine trafficking in the PFC.

Models based on the CD/RA hypothesis

A number of mouse models have been reported that are based on rare genetic lesions strongly linked to psychiatric disorders. Despite the fact that these models are based on rare genetic events, they nonetheless may help identify cellular pathways and neural circuits dysfunctional in schizophrenia in general.

Mouse models of the *DISC1* schizophrenia susceptibility locus

DISC1 was implicated as a susceptibility gene for major mental illness through a balanced chromosomal translocation, which truncates the *DISC1* gene and segregates with schizophrenia and affective disorders in a multigenerational Scottish pedigree (Millar *et al.*, 2000). A number of suggestive linkage and association studies indicate that common variation in *DISC1* may also play a role in schizophrenia, affective disorders, and related endophenotypes in karyotypically normal patient populations (Callicott *et al.*, 2005; Cannon *et al.*, 2005; Hennah *et al.*, 2003). In all, *DISC1* represents a potentially valuable tool for gaining insight into the pathogenesis of mental illnesses. Biochemical studies have provided initial evidence for a physical interaction between DISC1 and several cytoskeletal and centrosomal proteins as well as phosphodiesterase 4B (PDE4B), suggesting an involvement in cell migration, neurite outgrowth, and cAMP signaling (Millar *et al.*, 2005; Kamiya *et al.*, 2005; Morris *et al.*, 2003). How many of these interactions are relevant in understanding the contribution of the gene to psychiatric disorders is unknown and comprehensive analysis of genetic mouse models of this gene are instrumental towards this end.

Koike *et al.* (2006) used a knockin approach to generate mutant *DISC1* mice carrying a truncating lesion in the endogenous *DISC1* ortholog, genetically engineered to resemble the putative effects of the well-defined disease risk allele observed in the Scottish family (Millar *et al.*, 2000). Mutant *DISC1* mice demonstrated normal locomotor activity and PPI. Analysis of cognitive function in these mice revealed a specific pattern of cognitive deficits (Koike *et al.*, 2006; Kvajo *et al.*, 2008). Specifically, a battery of tests assessing cognitive processes, such as contextual fear association, object recognition, spatial reference memory, spatial short-term memory, and spatial working memory, revealed a highly specific deficit in working memory. This deficit was evident in both homozygous and heterozygous mice in two independent tasks requiring the robust and active maintenance of information online (Baddeley, 1992) and may relate to core deficits in working memory and executive function observed in patients with schizophrenia (Elvevag & Goldberg, 2000). These selective cognitive deficits were accompanied by specific neuronal pathology in the hippocampus and MPFC (Kvajo *et al.*, 2008). Analysis in the hippocampus showed normal gross morphology and volume, but revealed alterations in the distribution and organization of new and especially mature neurons of the dentate gyrus (DG), while no such deficits were observed in pyramidal cells in the CA1 area.

Additional mouse models overexpressing human truncated DISC1 protein *in vivo* have also been generated based on the assumption that a putative truncated form of DISC1 produced as a result of the translocation in the Scottish pedigree has dominant-negative properties. Pletnikov *et al.* (2007) used the αCaMKII promoter to generate transgenic mice with doxycycline-inducible expression of mutant human DISC1 (hDISC1) limited to the cerebral cortex, hippocampus, and striatum. Expression of mutant hDISC1 led to a mild enlargement of the lateral ventricles and attenuation of neurite outgrowth in primary cortical neurons, but was not associated with gross morphological abnormalities. Transgenic male mice exhibited spontaneous hyperactivity in the open field and alterations in social interaction, and transgenic female mice showed deficient spatial memory. Using a similar approach, Hikida *et al.* (2007) generated a transgenic mouse model where a dominant-negative form of DISC1 (DN-DISC1) is expressed under the αCaMKII promoter. Expression of mutant hDISC1 led to an enlargement of the lateral ventricles as well as a selective reduction in the immunoreactivity of parvalbumin in the cortex. Behavioral assessment revealed a number of abnormalities, including an increase in locomotor activity, a subtle disturbance in PPI, as well as deficits in olfactory-dependent and affective behavioral measures. The extent of phenotypic similarities between the knockin (Koike *et al.*, 2006; Kvajo *et al.*, 2008) and the transgenic mouse models are unknown due to methodological differences in their design and assessment. However, the levels and pattern of expression of the exogenous truncated protein in the latter may lead to neomorphic phenotypic features, especially at the neural circuit and behavior levels.

DISC1 is expressed at low levels in adult rodent and primate brain (Austin *et al.*, 2004a,b) and in human brain (Lipska *et al.* 2006) as compared with the fetal or early postnatal period. This pattern of expression suggests that the effect of the Scottish mutation may be, at least in part, developmental in origin. To test this hypothesis, Li *et al.* (2007) used an inducible and reversible transgenic system to induce expression of a C-terminal portion of DISC1 in mice. They found that early postnatal, but not adult, induction results in reduced hippocampal dendritic complexity in the DG, impaired synaptic transmission (but normal long-term plasticity), depressive-like traits, abnormal spatial working memory, and reduced sociability. These findings suggest that alterations in DISC1 function during brain development may contribute to schizophrenia pathogenesis.

Allelic heterogeneity at a given disease locus is often accompanied by phenotypic heterogeneity (Letts *et al.*,

2003). Although the Scottish translocation is the only *DISC1* mutation currently unequivocally associated with schizophrenia and affective disorders, the possibility exists that other mutations of the *DISC1* gene exist that may lead to related psychiatric phenotypes. Clapcote *et al.* (2007) addressed this issue by analyzing two independently derived ENU-induced mutations in exon 2 of mouse *DISC1*. Mice with mutation Q31L showed deficits in the forced swim test and other affective measures that were reversed by the antidepressant bupropion, but not by rolipram, a phosphodiesterase-4 (PDE4) inhibitor. In contrast, L100P mutant mice exhibited deficits in PPI and LI that were reversed by antipsychotic treatment. Although none of the assays used in this study is "diagnostic" of depression or schizophrenia in mice, the results clearly suggest that allelic heterogeneity at the *DISC1* locus may lead to phenotypic heterogeneity in the affected behavioral domains. By inference, *DISC1* allelic heterogeneity, if present in patient populations, may lead to distinct psychiatric phenotypes or symptoms.

In addition to the genetic mouse models described above, a number of studies have employed acute RNA interference approaches to interfere with the function of DISC1 in specific brain areas during development or in the adult brain. One such study (Duan *et al.*, 2007) employed acute shRNA-mediated downregulation of DISC1 in new DG cells to investigate the role of DISC1 in adult hippocampal neurogenesis. It was shown that downregulation of *DISC1* leads to a complex pattern of enhanced dendritic growth, appearance of ectopic apical and basal dendrites, accelerated spine formation, enhanced excitability, as well as mispositioning of new dentate granule cells. These findings led the authors to speculate that *DISC1* downregulation results in accelerated functional neuronal integration in the adult brain. A germline genetic lesion of *DISC1* also leads to mispositioning of young neurons in the DG. However, it also results in dendritic misorientation and reduced numbers of new neurons, in the absence of excessive dendritic growth and accelerated spine formation (Kvajo *et al.*, 2008). Thus, newly generated hippocampal neurons in mutant *DISC1* mice may be compromised and possibly unable to integrate into DG functional circuits. This possibility appears to be supported by the additional observation that in mutant *DISC1* mice, mature granule cells show impaired dendritic growth and reduced number of spines. These discrepant findings raise an important general issue pertaining to the information obtained by models based on shRNA-mediated approaches as opposed to models based on germline genetic lesions. They highlight several important differences between these approaches that have to do with the timing and the extent of the genetic disruption and the unique induction of compensatory responses that could be activated in germline genetic lesions to buffer against developmental insults.

Mouse models of the 22q11 schizophrenia susceptibility locus

Microdeletions of the 22q11.2 locus are among the most common chromosomal abnormalities and occur predominantly (~90%) *de novo* (McDonald-McGinn *et al.* 2001). Around 30% of children with the 22q11.2 microdeletion develop schizophrenia or schizoaffective disorder in adolescence or early adulthood (Chow *et al.*, 2006; Murphy *et al.*, 1999; Pulver *et al.*, 1994). Indeed, 22q11 microdeletions account for up to 1% of cases of schizophrenia in Caucasian populations (Horowitz *et al.*, 2005; Karayiorgou *et al.*, 1995; Wiehahn *et al.*, 2004) and represent the only known recurrent mutation responsible for introducing new (sporadic) cases of schizophrenia into the population. Individuals with the 22q11.2 microdeletion also exhibit a spectrum of deficits in cognitive tasks linked to activity in the hippocampus and PFC, such as measures of attention, working memory, executive function, and short-term verbal memory (Bearden *et al.*, 2001; Sobin *et al.*, 2005; Woodin *et al.*, 2001). This is notable given the recognition of similar cognitive dysfunction as an enduring core deficit of schizophrenia (Chow *et al.*, 2006; Elvevag & Goldberg, 2000). The majority of patients have a hemizygous 3-Mb deletion, while 7% have a nested 1.5-Mb deletion encompassing 27 known genes (Edelmann *et al.*, 1999). Most of these genes are expressed in the brain in a relatively wide pattern.

The syntenic region of the human 22q11 locus, which lies on mouse chromosome 16, includes nearly all human genes. This conserved arrangement of the mouse orthologs in the syntenic locus provides a unique opportunity to generate mouse models with strong etiological validity. Accordingly, the 22q11 microdeletion has been modeled in the mouse using chromosomal engineering approaches, and initial analysis of mice carrying deficiencies with variable overlap with the "schizophrenia critical region" (Karayiorgou *et al.*, 1995) indicated deficits in PPI, contextual and cued fear memory, as well as in the acquisition of a working-memory dependent task (Paylor *et al.*, 2006; Long *et al.*, 2006; Stark *et al.*, 2008). Stark *et al.* (2008) analyzed an engineered mouse strain carrying a hemizygous chromosomal deficiency, which spans a segment syntenic to the entire "schizophrenia critical region", and uncovered alterations in the biogenesis of brain microRNAs, a class of small non-coding RNAs that in animals regulates gene expression by inhibiting mRNA translation or stability. They showed that abnormal microRNA biogenesis is due to haploinsufficiency of the *DGCR8* gene, which encodes for an RNA-binding moiety of the microRNA "microprocessor" complex and contributes to the behavioral and neuronal deficits induced by this chromosomal deficiency. Heterozygous *DGCR8*-deficient mice showed deficits in a working memory-dependent learning task, as well as reductions in the size of dendritic spines and in dendritic complexity of hippocampal pyramidal neurons.

A number of additional single-gene models have been generated for candidate susceptibility genes from the 22q11 locus. Among them, *PRODH* is a leading candidate gene (Bender *et al.*, 2005; Jacquet *et al.*, 2005; Liu *et al.*, 2002), which encodes a mitochondrial enzyme that metabolizes L-proline, a putative neuromodulator of glutamatergic transmission (Renick *et al.*, 1999). A *PRODH* knockdown mouse strain (Gogos *et al.*, 1999; Paterlini *et al.*, 2005) showed abnormal PPI, deficits in fear memory, as well as hypersensitivity to the locomotor effects of the psychotogenic drug amphetamine (AMPH; Angrist & Gershon, 1970). The increased sensitivity to AMPH was also reflected in increased cortical dopamine efflux in the mutant mice following acute, systemic AMPH administration. Transcriptional profiling in the frontal cortex of *PRODH*-deficient mice revealed a highly reproducible increase in the levels of transcript and protein of COMT (Gothelf *et al.*, 2005), also located within the 22q11 microdeletion locus. There is strong evidence that COMT modulates clearance of extracellular dopamine in the PFC but not in the striatum (Yavich *et al.*, 2007). Consistent with this evidence, pharmacological inhibition of COMT activity by systemic administration of tolcapone potentiated the effect of AMPH on locomotor activity, exaggerated deficits in PPI, and induced deficits in a working memory-dependent task specifically in *PRODH*-deficient, but not wild-type, mice, suggesting that increase in COMT expression is engaged in a homeostatic response to buffer excessive dopamine signaling in the frontal cortex of *PRODH*-deficient mice (Paterlini *et al.*, 2005). Thus, this animal-model work revealed a genetic feedback loop, which involves two interacting 22q11 genes, affects dopamine transmission (a key feature of the disease; Davis *et al.*, 1991), and modulates the risk of schizophrenia associated with this locus, or the severity of the clinical symptoms. Notably, these animal-model-based predictions found support in recent studies of individuals with 22q11 microdeletions (Raux *et al.*, 2007).

Other genetic mouse models of candidate susceptibility genes from this locus have been reported. These include knockout mice for *COMT*, which have been used extensively to analyze the effect of COMT deficiency on dopamine metabolism and transmission (Huotari *et al.*, 2002, 2004; Yavich *et al.* 2007), as well as knockout mice for *Zdhhc8*, a palmitoyltransferase that plays a key role in the assembly of excitatory synapses and dendritic growth (Mukai *et al.*, 2004). Additional studies in animal models have focused on abnormalities of PPI and have identified several genes from the 22q11 region that exert both positive (Kimber *et al.*, 1999) and negative influences on PPI, such as *Tbx1*, a transcription factor, and *Gnbl1*, a gene of unknown function (Paylor *et al.*, 2006).

Overall, genetic studies in humans, augmented by analysis of reliable animal models, have identified a small subset of the deleted genes and their interactions as potentially contributing to the dramatic increase in schizophrenia risk by resulting in neuronal disconnectivity as well as aberrant neuromodulation.

Conclusions

The approach to studying the etiology and pathophysiology of schizophrenia at the level of animal neurobiology has become much more sophisticated. In light of mounting evidence linking schizophrenia to certain neuropathological processes in the brain, heuristic animal models may prove to be important tools in testing new theories about the origin and mechanisms of this disorder. In particular, some models have confirmed the plausibility of neurodevelopmental insults having prolonged effects on the dopamine system and behaviors relevant to schizophrenia, and supported the notion that disruption of glutamatergic neurotransmission may lead to new approaches to treatment. Modeling psychiatric disorders in mice is an evolving process that has reached a turning point, where accurate mouse models of candidate susceptibility genes are now becoming feasible and are likely to appear in abundance in the next few years. At the end, realization of the promise offered by the new generation of genetic models for understanding the pathophysiology of the disease and developing new treatments (Scolnick, 2006) will depend on (1) the careful interpretation of the accumulating genetic findings and their integration of large volumes of data obtained over many years of clinical research and work on models of pathophysiology and pathogenesis, and (2) the broadening and refining of our analytical tools for animal models, especially towards system and circuit level approaches.

References

Abi-Dargham, A., Gil, R., Krystal, J. *et al.* (1998) Increased striatal dopamine transmission in schizophrenia: confirmation in a second cohort. *American Journal of Psychiatry* **155**, 761–767.

Adams, W., Kendell, R.E., Hare, E.H. & Munk-Jorgensen, P. (1993) Epidemiological evidence that maternal influenza contributes to the aetiology of schizophrenia: an analysis of Scottish, English and Danish data. *British Journal of Psychiatry* **163**, 522–534.

Akbarian, S., Bunney, W.E. Jr., Potkin, S.G. *et al.* (1993) Altered distribution of nicotinamide-adenine dinucleotide phosphate-diaphorase cells in frontal lobe of schizophrenics implies disturbances of cortical development. *Archives of General Psychiatry* **50**, 169–177.

Akbarian, S., Kim, J.J., Potkin, S.G. *et al.* (1995) Gene expression for glutamic acid decarboxylase is reduced without loss of neurons in prefrontal cortex of schizophrenics. *Archives of General Psychiatry* **52**, 258–266.

Akbarian, S., Sucher, N.J., Bradley, D. *et al.* (1996) Selective alterations in gene expression for NMDA receptor subunits in prefrontal cortex of schizophrenics. *Journal of Neuroscience* **16**, 19–30.

Al-Amin, H.A., Weinberger, D.R. & Lipska, B.K. (2000) Exaggerated MK-801-induced motor hyperactivity in rats with the neonatal lesion of the ventral hippocampus. *Behavioural Pharmacology* **11**, 269–278.

Al-Amin, H.A., Weickert, C.S., Lillrank, S.M., Weinberger, D.R. & Lipska, B.K. (2001) Delayed onset of enhanced MK-801-induced motor hyperactivity after neonatal lesions of the rat ventral hippocampus. *Biological Psychiatry* **49**, 528–539.

Angrist, B.M. & Gershon, S. (1970) The phenomenology of experimentally induced amphetamine psychosis—preliminary observations. *Biological Psychiatry* **2**, 95–107.

Anholt, R.R., Dilda, C.L., Chang, S. *et al.* (2003) The genetic architecture of odor-guided behavior in Drosophila: epistasis and the transcriptome. *Nature Genetics* **35**, 180–184.

Anisman, H., Zaharia, M.D., Meaney, M.J. & Merali, Z. (1998) Do early-life events permanently alter behavioral and hormonal responses to stressors? *International Journal of Developmental Neuroscience* **16**, 149–164.

Arguello, P.A. & Gogos, J.A. (2006) Modeling madness in mice: one piece at a time. *Neuron* **52**, 179–196.

Arnold, S.E., Hyman, B.T., van Hoesen, G.W. & Damasio, A.R. (1991) Some cytoarchitectural abnormalities of the entorhinal cortex in schizophrenia. *Archives of General Psychiatry* **48**, 625–632.

Ashe, P.C., Chlan-Fourney, J., Juorio, A.V. & Li, X.M. (2002) Brain-derived neurotrophic factor (BDNF) mRNA in rats with neonatal ibotenic acid lesions of the ventral hippocampus. *Brain Research* **956**, 126–135.

Austin, C.P., Ky, B., Ma, L., Morris, J.A. & Shughrue, P.J. (2004a) DISC1 (Disrupted in Schizophrenia-1) is expressed in limbic regions of the primate brain. *Neuroreport* **14**, 951–954.

Austin, C.P., Ky, B., Ma, L., Morris, J.A. & Shughrue, P.J. (2004b) Expression of Disrupted-In-Schizophrenia-1, a schizophrenia-associated gene, is prominent in the mouse hippocampus throughout brain development. *Neuroscience* **124**, 3–10.

Bachevalier, J., Alvarado, M.C. & Malkova, L. (1999) Memory and socioemotional behavior in monkeys after hippocampal damage incurred in infancy or in adulthood. *Biological Psychiatry* **46**, 329–339.

Baddeley, A. (1992) Working memory. *Science* **255**, 556–559.

Bakshi, V.P., Swerdlow, N.R., Braff, D.L. & Geyer, M.A. (1998) Reversal of isolation rearing-induced deficits in prepulse inhibition by Seroquel and olanzapine. *Biological Psychiatry* **43**, 436–445.

Bearden, C.E., Woodin, M.F., Wang, P.P. *et al.* (2001) The neurocognitive phenotype of the 22q11.2 deletion syndrome: selective deficit in visual-spatial memory. *Journal of Clinical and Experimental Neuropsychology* **23**, 447–464.

Beaulieu, J.M., Sotnikova, T.D., Marion, S., Lefkowitz, R.J., Gainetdinov, R.R. & Caron, M.G. (2005) An Akt/beta-arrestin 2/PP2A signaling complex mediates dopaminergic neurotransmission and behavior. *Cell* **122**, 261–273.

Beauregard, M. & Bachevalier, J. (1996) Neonatal insult to the hippocampal region and schizophrenia: a review and a putative animal model. *Canadian Journal of Psychiatry* **41**, 446–445.

Becker, A., Grecksch, G., Bernsteinn, H.G., Hollt, V. & Bogerts, B. (1999) Social behavior in rats lesioned with ibotenic acid in the hippocampus: quantitative and qualitative analysis. *Psychopharmacology* **144**, 333–338.

Becker, A. & Grecksch, G. (2000) Social memory is impaired in neonatally ibotenic acid lesioned rats. *Behavioural Brain Research* **109**, 137–140.

Bender, H.U., Almashanu, S., Steel, G. *et al.* (2005) Functional consequences of PRODH missense mutations. *American Journal of Human Genetics* **76**, 409–420.

Benes, F.M., Vincent, S.L., Alsterberg, G., Bird, E.D. & san Giovanni, J.P. (1992) Increased GABA-A receptor binding in superficial laminae in cingulate cortex of schizophrenic brain. *Journal of Neuroscience* **12**, 924–929.

Berg, S.A. & Chambers, R.A. (2008) Accentuated behavioral sensitization to nicotine in the neonatal ventral hippocampal lesion model of schizophrenia. *Neuropharmacology* **54**, 1201–1207.

Bertolino, A., Saunders, R.C., Mattay, V.S., Bachevalier, J., Frank, J.A. & Weinberger, D.R. (1997) Altered development of prefrontal neurons in rhesus monkeys with neonatal mesial temporo-limbic lesions: A proton magnetic resonance spectroscopic imaging study. *Cerebral Cortex* **7**, 740–748.

Bertolino, A., Callicott, J.H., Elman, I. *et al.* (1998) Regionally specific neuronal pathology in untreated patients with schizophrenia: a proton magnetic resonance spectroscopic imaging study. *Biological Psychiatry* **43**, 641–648.

Bertolino, A., Roffman, J.L., Lipska, B.K., Van Gelderen, P., Olson, A., & Weinberger, D.R. (1999) Postpubertal emergence of prefrontal neuronal deficits and altered dopaminergic behaviors in rats with neonatal hippocampal lesions. *Social Neuroscience Abstract* **520**, 8.

Bertolino, A., Breier, A., Callicott, J.H. *et al.* (2000) The relationship between dorsolateral prefrontal neuronal N-acetylaspartate and evoked release of striatal dopamine in schizophrenia. *Neuropsychopharmacology* **22**, 125–132.

Black, M.D., Lister, S., Hitchcock, J.M., Giersbergen, P. & Sorensen, S.M. (1998) Neonatal hippocampal lesion model of schizophrenia in rats: sex differences and persistence of effects into maturity. *Drugs and Developmental Research* **43**, 206–213.

Black, M.D., Selk, D.E., Hitchcock, J.M., Wetttstein, J.G. & Sorensen, S.M. (1999) On the effect of neonatal nitric oxide synthase inhibition in rats: a potential neurodevelopmental model of schizophrenia. *Neuropharmacology* **38**, 1299–1306.

Bloom, F.E. (1993) Advancing a neurodevelopmental origin of schizophrenia. *Archives of General Psychiatry* **50**, 224–227.

Bogerts, B., Ashtar, M., Degreef, G., Alvir, J.M.J., Bilder, R.M. & Lieberman, J.A. (1990) Reduced temporal limbic structure volumes on magnetic resonance images in first-episode schizophrenia. *Psychiatric Research Neuroimaging* **35**, 1–13.

Boksa, P. & El-Khodor, B.F. (2003) Birth insult interacts with stress at adulthood to alter dopaminergic function in animal models: possible implications for schizophrenia and other disorders. *Neuroscience and Biobehavioral Review* **27**, 91–101.

Brake, W.G., Sullivan, R.M., Flores, G., Srivastava, L. & Gratton, A. (1999) Neonatal ventral hippocampal lesions attenuate the nucleus accumbens dopamine response to stress: an electrochemical study in the rat. *Brain Research* **831**, 25–32.

Breier, A., Su, T.P., Saunders, R. *et al.* (1997) Schizophrenia is associated with elevated amphetamine-induced synaptic dopamine concentrations: evidence from a novel positron emission tomography method. *Proceedings of the National Academy of Sciencs USA* **94**, 2569–2574.

Callicott, J.H., Straub, R.E., Pezawas, L. *et al.* (2005) Variation in DISC1 affects hippocampal structure and function and increases risk for schizophrenia. *Proceedings of the National Academy of Sciencs USA* **102**, 8627–8632.

Cannon, T.D., Hennah, W., van Erp, T.G. *et al.* (2005) Association of DISC1/TRAX haplotypes with schizophrenia, reduced prefrontal gray matter, and impaired short- and long-term memory. *Archives of General Psychiatry* **62**, 1205–1213.

Carr, D.B. & Sesack, S.R. (1996) Hippocampal afferents to the rat prefrontal cortex: Synaptic targets and relation to dopaminergic terminals. *Journal of Comparative Neurology* **369**, 1–15.

Chambers, R.A. & Taylor, J.R. (2004) Animal modeling dual diagnosis schizophrenia: sensitization to cocaine in rats with neonatal ventral hippocampal lesions. *Biological Psychiatry* **56**, 308–316.

Chambers, R.A., Moore, J., McEvoy, J.P. & Levin, E.D. (1996) Cognitive effects of neonatal hippocampal lesions in a rat model of schizophrenia. *Neuropsychopharmacology* **15**, 587–594.

Chambers, R.A., Jones, R.M., Brown, S. & Taylor, J.R. (2005) Natural reward-related learning in rats with neonatal ventral hippocampal lesions and prior cocaine exposure. *Psychopharmacology (Berlin)* **179**, 470–478.

Chen, J., Lipska, B.K. & Weinberger, D.R. (2006) Genetic mouse models of schizophrenia: from hypothesis-based to susceptibility gene-based models. *Biological Psychiatry* **59**, 1180–1188.

Chow, E.W., Watson, M., Young, D.A. & Bassett, A.S. (2006) Neurocognitive profile in 22q11 deletion syndrome and schizophrenia. *Schizophrenia Research* **87**, 270–278.

Cintra, L., Granados, L., Aguilar, A. *et al.* (1997) Effects of prenatal protein malnutrition on mossy fibers of the hippocampal formation in rats of four age groups. *Hippocampus* **7**, 184–191.

Clapcote, S.J., Lipina, T.V., Millar, J.K. *et al.* (2007) Behavioral phenotypes of Disc1 missense mutations in mice. *Neuron* **54**, 387–402.

Conrad, A.J., Abebe, T., Ron, A., Forsythe, S. & Scheibel, B. (1991) Hippocampal pyramidal cell disarray in schizophrenia as a bilateral phenomenon. *Archives of General Psychiatry* **48**, 413–417.

Conroy, S.K., Rodd, Z. & Chambers, R.A. (2007) Ethanol sensitization in a neurodevelopmental lesion model of schizophrenia in rats. *Pharmacology, Biochemistry & Behavior* **86**, 386–394.

Corfas, G., Roy, K. & Buxbaum, J.D. (2004) Neuregulin 1-erbB signaling and the molecular/cellular basis of schizophrenia. *Nature Neuroscience* **7**, 575–580.

Costall, B. & Naylor, R.J. (1995) Animal neuropharmacology and its prediction of clinical response. In: Hirsch S.R. & Weinberger, D.R., eds. *Schizophrenia*. Oxford: Blackwell Science, pp. 401–424.

Cotter, D., Takei, N., Farrell, M. *et al.* (1995) Does prenatal exposure to influenza in mice induce pyramidal cell disarray in the dorsal hippocampus? *Schizophrenia Research* **16**, 233–241.

Csernansky, J.G., Csernansky, C.A., Kogelman, L., Montgomery, E.M. & Bardgett, M.E. (1998) Progressive neurodegeneration after intracerebroventricular kainic acid administration in rats: implications for schizophrenia? *Biological Psychiatry* **44**, 1143–1150.

Csernansky, J.G., Martin, M.V., Czeisler, B., Meltzer, M.A., Ali, Z. & Dong, H. (2006) Neuroprotective effects of olanzapine in a rat model of neurodevelopmental injury. *Pharmacology, Biochemistry & Behavior* **83**, 208–213.

Dalman, C., Allebeck, P., Cullberg, J., Grunewald, C. & Koster, M. (1999) Obstetric complications and the risk of schizophrenia: a longitudinal study of a national birth cohort. *Archives of General Psychiatry* **56**, 234–240.

Davis, K.L., Kahn, R.S., Ko, G. & Davidson, M. (1991) Dopamine in schizophrenia: a review and reconceptualization. *American Journal of Psychiatry* **148**, 1474–1486.

Dean, B., Karl, T., Pavey, G., Boer, S., Duffy, L. & Scarr, E. (2007) Increased levels of serotonin 2A receptors and serotonin transporter in the CNS of neuregulin 1 hypomorphic/mutant mice. *Schizophrenia Research* **99**, 341–349.

DeLisi, L.E., Dauphinais, I.D. & Gershon, E.S. (1988) Perinatal complications and reduced size of brain limbic structures in familial schizophrenia. *Schizophrenia Bulletin* **14**, 185–191.

Duan, X., Chang, J.H., Ge, S. *et al.* (2007) Disrupted-In-Schizophrenia 1 regulates integration of newly generated neurons in the adult brain. *Cell* **130**, 1146–1158.

Duncan, G.E., Sheitman, B.B. & Lieberman, J.A. (1999) An integrated view of pathophysiological models of schizophrenia. *Brain Research Brain Research Review* **29**, 250–264.

Eastwood, S.L. & Harrison, P.J. (1995) Decreased synaptophysin in the medial temporal lobe in schizophrenia demonstrated using immunoautoradiography. *Neuroscience* **69**, 339–343.

Eastwood, S.L. & Harrison, P.J. (1998) Hippocampal and cortical growth-associated protein-43 messenger RNA in schizophrenia. *Neuroscience* **86**, 437–448.

Eastwood, S.L., McDonald, B., Burnet, P.W., Beckwith, J.P., Kerwin, R.W. & Harrison, P.J. (1995) Decreased expression of mRNAs encoding non-NMDA glutamate receptors GluR1 and GluR2 in medial temporal lobe neurons in schizophrenia. *Brain Research Molecular Brain Research* **29**, 211–223.

Eastwood, S.L., Burnet, P.W. & Harrison, P.J. (1997) GluR2 glutamate receptor subunit flip and flop isoforms are decreased in the hippocampal formation in schizophrenia: a reverse transcriptase-polymerase chain reaction (RT-PCR) study. *Brain Research Molecular Brain Research* **44**, 92–98.

Edelmann, L., Pandita, R.K. & Morrow, B.E. (1999) Low-copy repeats mediate the common 3-Mb deletion in patients with velo-cardio-facial syndrome. *American Journal of Human Genetics* **64**, 1076–1086.

Egan, M.F., Goldberg, T.E., Kolachana, B.S. *et al.* (2001) Effect of COMT Val108/158 Met genotype on frontal lobe function and risk for schizophrenia. *Proceedings of the National Academy of Sciences USA* **98**, 6917–6922.

El-Khodor, B.F. & Boksa, P. (1997) Long-term reciprocal changes in dopamine levels in prefrontal cortex versus nucleus accumbens in rats born by Cesarean section compared to vaginal birth. *Experimental Neurology* **145**, 118–129.

Ellenbroek, B.A., van den Kroonenberg, P.T. & Cools, A.R. (1998) The effects of an early stressful life event on sensorimotor gating in adult rats. *Schizophrenia Research* **30**, 251–260.

Elvevag, B. & Goldberg, T.E. (2000) Cognitive impairment in schizophrenia is the core of the disorder. *Critical Review of Neurobiology* **14**, 1–21.

Emamian, E.S., Hall, D., Birnbaum, M.J., Karayiorgou, M. & Gogos, J.A. (2004) Convergent evidence for impaired AKT1-GSK3beta signaling in schizophrenia. *Nature Genetics* **36**, 131–137.

Falkai, P. & Bogerts, B. (1986) Cell loss in the hippocampus of schizophrenics. *European Archives of Psychiatry & Neurological Sciences* **236**, 154–161.

Fatemi, S.H., Emamian, E.S., Kist, D. *et al.* (1999) Defective corticogenesis and reduction in Reelin immunoreactivity in cortex and hippocampus of prenatally infected neonatal mice. *Molecular Psychiatry* **4**, 145–154.

Feldpausch, D.L., Needham, L.M., Stone, M.P. *et al.* (1998) The role of dopamine D4 receptor in the induction of behavioral sensitization to amphetamine and accompanying biochemical and molecular adaptations. *Journal of Pharmacological & Experimental Therapeutics* **286**, 497–508.

Flores, G., Barbeau, D., Quirion, R. & Srivastava, L.K. (1996a) Decreased binding of dopamine D3 receptors in limbic subregions after neonatal bilateral lesion of rat hippocampus. *Journal of Neuroscience* **16**, 2020–2026.

Flores, G., Wood, G.K., Liang, J.J., Quirion, R. & Srivastava, L.K. (1996b) Enhanced amphetamine sensitivity and increased expression of dopamine D2 receptors in postpubertal rats after neonatal excitotoxic lesions of the medial prefrontal cortex. *Journal of Neuroscience* **16**, 7366–7375.

Francis, D., Diorio, J., Liu, D. & Meaney, M.J. (1999) Nongenomic transmission across generations of maternal behavior and stress responses in the rat. *Science* **286**, 1155–1158.

Gambarana, C., Masi, F., Tagliamonte, A., Scheggi, S., Ghiglieri, O. & De Montis, M.G. (1999) A chronic stress that impairs reactivity in rats also decreases dopaminergic transmission in the nucleus accumbens: a microdialysis study. *Journal of Neurochemistry* **72**, 2039–2046.

Gelowitz, D.L., Rakic, P., Goldman-Rakic, P.S. & Selemon, L.D. (2002) Craniofacial dysmorphogenesis in fetally irradiated nonhuman primates: implications for the neurodevelopmental hypothesis of schizophrenia. *Biological Psychiatry* **52**, 716–720.

Gerber, D.J., Hall, D., Miyakawa, T. *et al.* (2003) Evidence for association of schizophrenia with genetic variation in the 8p21.3 gene, PPP3CC, encoding the calcineurin gamma subunit. *Proceedings of the National Academy of Sciencs USA* **100**, 8993–8998.

Glatt, S.J., Faraone, S.V. & Tsuang, M.T. (2003) Association between a functional catechol *O*-methyltransferase gene polymorphism and schizophrenia: Meta-analysis of case-control and family-based studies. *American Journal of Psychiatry* **160**, 469–476.

Gogos, J.A. & Gerber, D.J. (2006) Schizophrenia susceptibility genes: emergence of positional candidates and future directions. *Trends in Pharmacological Sciences* **27**, 226–233.

Gogos, J.A., Santha, M., Takacs, Z. *et al.* (1999) The gene encoding proline dehydrogenase modulates sensorimotor gating in mice. *Nature Genetics* **21**, 434–439.

Goldberg, T.E., Egan, M.F., Gscheidle, T. *et al.* (2003) Executive subprocesses in working memory: relationship to catechol-O-methyltransferase Val158Met genotype and schizophrenia. *Archives of General Psychiatry* **60**, 889–896.

Gothelf, D., Eliez, S., Thompson, T. *et al.* (2005) COMT genotype predicts longitudinal cognitive decline and psycho-

sis in 22q11.2 deletion syndrome. *Nature Neuroscience* **8**, 1500–1502.

Grecksch, G., Bernstein, H.G., Becker, A., Hollt, V. & Bogerts, B. (1999) Disruption of latent inhibition in rats with postnatal hippocampal lesions. *Neuropsychopharmacology* **20**, 525–532.

Hahn, C.G., Wang, H.Y., Cho, D.S. *et al.* (2006) Altered neuregulin 1-erbB4 signaling contributes to NMDA receptor hypofunction in schizophrenia. *Nature Medicine* **12**, 824–828.

Harris, L.W., Sharp, T., Gartlon, J. *et al.* (2003) Long-term behavioural, molecular and morphological effects of neonatal NMDA receptor antagonism. *European Journal of Neuroscience* **18**, 1706–1710.

Harrison, P.J. & Weinberger, D.R. (2005) Schizophrenia genes, gene expression, and neuropathology: on the matter of their convergence. *Molecular Psychiatry* **10**, 40–68.

Hennah, W., Varilo, T., Kestilä, M. *et al.* (2003) Haplotype transmission analysis provides evidence of association for DISC1 to schizophrenia and suggests sex-dependent effects. *Human Molecular Genetics* **12**, 3151–3159.

Hikida, T., Jaaro-Peled, H., Seshadri, S. *et al.* (2007) Dominant-negative DISC1 transgenic mice display schizophrenia-associated phenotypes detected by measures translatable to humans. *Proceedings of the National Academy of Sciencs USA* **104**, 14501–14506.

Hornig, M., Weissenbock, H., Horscroft, N. & Lipkin, W.I. (1999) An infection-based model of neurodevelopmental damage. *Proceedings of the National Academy of Sciencs USA* **96**, 12102–12107.

Horowitz, A., Shifman, S., Rivlin, N., Pisante, A. & Darvasi, A. (2005) A survey of the 22q11 microdeletion in a large cohort of schizophrenia patients. *Schizophrenia Research* **73**, 263–267.

Hultman, C.M., Ohman, A., Cnattingius, S., Wieselgren, I.M. & Lindstrom, L.H. (1997) Prenatal and neonatal risk factors for schizophrenia. *British Journal of Psychiatry* **170**, 128–133.

Huotari, M., Gogos, J.A., Karayiorgou, M. *et al.* (2002) Brain catecholamine metabolism in catechol-O-methyltransferase (COMT)-deficient mice. *European Journal of Neuroscience* **15**, 246–256.

Huotari, M., Garcia-Horsman, J.A., Karayiorgou, M., Gogos, J.A. & Mannisto, P.T. (2004) D-amphetamine responses in catechol-O-methyltransferase (COMT) disrupted mice. *Psychopharmacology (Berlin)* **172**, 1–10.

Jacquet, H., Demily, C., Houy, E. *et al.* (2005) Hyperprolinemia is a risk factor for schizoaffective disorder. *Molecular Psychiatry* **10**, 479–485.

Javitt, D.C. & Zukin, S.R. (1991) Recent advances in the phencyclidine model of schizophrenia. *American Journal of Psychiatry* **148**, 1301–1308.

Jay, T.M., Glowinski, J. & Thierry, A.M. (1989) Selectivity of the hippocampal projection to the prelimbic area of the prefrontal cortex in the rat. *Brain Research* **505**, 337–340.

Jentsch, J.D. & Roth, R.H. (1999) The neuropsychopharmacology of phencyclidine: from NMDA receptor hypofunction to the dopamine hypothesis of schizophrenia. *Neuropsychopharmacology* **20**, 201–225.

Jeste, D.V. & Lohr, J.B. (1989) Hippocampal pathologic findings in schizophrenia: a morphometric study. *Archives of General Psychiatry* **46**, 1019–1024.

Johnston, M.V., Barks, J., Greenmyre, T. & Silverstein, F. (1988) Use of toxins to disrupt neurotransmitter circuitry in the developing brain. *Progress in Brain Research* **73**, 425–446.

Kamiya, A., Kubo, K., Tomoda, T. *et al.* (2005) A schizophrenia-associated mutation of DISC1 perturbs cerebral cortex development. *Nature Cellular Biology* **7**, 1067–1078.

Karayiorgou, M., Morris, M.A., Morrow, B. *et al.* (1995) Schizophrenia susceptibility associated with interstitial deletions of chromosome 22q11. *Proceedings of the National Academy of Sciencs USA* **92**, 7612–7616.

Karl, T., Duffy, L., Scimone, A., Harvey, R.P. & Schofield, P.R. (2007) Altered motor activity, exploration and anxiety in heterozygous neuregulin 1 mutant mice: implications for understanding schizophrenia. *Genes Brain Behavior* **6**, 677–687.

Kendell, R.E. & Kemp, I.W. (1989) Maternal influenza in the etiology of schizophrenia. *Archives of General Psychiatry* **46**, 878–882.

Kendler, K.S., MacLean, C.J., O'Neill *et al.* (1996) Evidence for a schizophrenia vulnerability locus on chromosome 8p in the Irish study of high-density schizophrenia families. *American Journal of Psychiatry* **153**, 1534–1540.

Kesby, J.P., Burne, T.H., McGrath, J.J. & Eyles, D.W. (2006) Developmental vitamin D deficiency alters MK 801-induced hyperlocomotion in the adult rat: An animal model of schizophrenia. *Biological Psychiatry* **60**, 591–596.

Kimber, W.L., Hsieh, P., Hirotsune, S. *et al.* (1999) Deletion of 150 kb in the minimal DiGeorge/velocardiofacial syndrome critical region in mouse. *Human Molecular Genetics* **8**, 2229–2237.

Kirkpatrick, B., Conley, R.C., Kakoyannis, A., Reep, R.L. & Roberts, R.C. (1999) Interstitial cells of the white matter in the inferior parietal cortex in schizophrenia: An unbiased cell-counting study. *Synapse* **34**, 95–102.

Koike, H., Arguello, P.A., Kvajo, M., Karayiorgou, M. & Gogos, J.A. (2006) Disc1 is mutated in the 129S6/SvEv strain and modulates working memory in mice. *Proceedings of the National Academy of Sciencs USA* **103**, 3693–3697.

Krystal, J.H., Karper, L.P., Seibyl, J.P. *et al.* (1994) Subanesthetic effects of the noncompetitive NMDA antagonist, ketamine, in humans Psychotomimetic, perceptual, cognitive, and neuroendocrine responses. *Archives of General Psychiatry* **51**, 199–214.

Kvajo, M., McKellar, H., Arguello, P.A. *et al.* (2008) A mutation in mouse *Disc1* that models a schizophrenia risk allele leads to specific alterations in neuronal architecture and cognition. *Proceedings of the National Academy of Sciencs USA* **105**, 7076–7081.

Lahti, A.C., Koffel, B., LaPorte, D. & Tamminga, C.A. (1995) Subanesthetic doses of ketamine stimulate psychosis in schizophrenia. *Neuropsychopharmacology* **13**, 9–19.

Lai, W.S., Xu, B. & Westphal, K.G. (2006) Akt1 deficiency affects neuronal morphology and predisposes to abnormalities in prefrontal cortex functioning. *Proceedings of the National Academy of Sciencs USA* **103**, 16906–16911.

Laruelle, M., Abi-Dargham, A., van Dyck, C.H. *et al.* (1996) Single photon emission computerized tomography imaging of amphetamine-induced dopamine release in drug-free schizophrenic subjects. *Proceedings of the National Academy of Sciences USA* **93**, 9235–9240.

Law, A.J., Lipska, B.K., Weickert, C.S. *et al.* (2006) Neuregulin 1 transcripts are differentially expressed in schizophrenia and regulated by 5' SNPs associated with the disease. *Proceedings of the National Academy of Sciencs USA* **103**, 6747–6752.

Law, A.J., Kleinman, J.E., Weinberger, D.R. & Weickert, C.S. (2007) Disease-associated intronic variants in the ErbB4 gene are related to altered ErbB4 splice-variant expression in the brain in schizophrenia. *Human Molecular Genetics* **16**, 129–141.

Le Pen, G. & Moreau, J.L. (2002) Disruption of prepulse inhibition of startle reflex in a neurodevelopmental model of schizophrenia: reversal by clozapine, olanzapine and risperidone but not by haloperidol. *Neuropsychopharmacology* **27**, 1–11.

Lee, C.J., Binder, T., Lipska, B.K. *et al.* (1998) Neonatal ventral hippocampal lesions produce an elevation of Δ-FosB-like protein(s) in the rodent neocortex. *Social Neuroscience Abstracts* **24**, 489.

Letts, V.A., Kang, M.G., Mahaffey, C.L. *et al.* (2003) Phenotypic heterogeneity in the stargazin allelic series. *Mammalian Genome* **14**, 506–513.

Lewis, P., Patel, A. & Balazs, R. (1979) Effect of undernutrition on cell generation in the adult rat brain. *Brain Research* **168**, 186–189.

Li, W., Zhou, Y., Jentsch, J.D. *et al.* (2007) Specific developmental disruption of disrupted-in-schizophrenia-1 function results in schizophrenia-related phenotypes in mice. *Proceedings of the National Academy of Sciencs USA* **104**, 18280–18285.

Lieberman, J.A., Sheitman, B.B. & Kinon, B.J. (1997) Neurochemical sensitization in the pathophysiology of schizophrenia: deficits and dysfunction in neuronal regulation and plasticity. *Neuropsychopharmacology* **17**, 205–229.

Lillrank, S.M., Lipska, B.K. & Weinberger, D.R. (1995) Neurodevelopmental animal models of schizophrenia. *Clinical Neuroscience* **3**, 98–104.

Lipska, B.K., Jaskiw, G.E. & Weinberger, D.R. (1993) Postpubertal emergence of hyperresponsiveness to stress and to amphetamine after neonatal hippocampal damage: A potential animal model of schizophrenia. *Neuropsychopharmacology* **9**, 67–75.

Lipska, B.K. & Weinberger, D.R. (1993) Delayed effects of neonatal hippocampal damage on haloperidol-induced catalepsy and apomorphine-induced stereotypic behaviors in the rat. *Developmental Brain Research* **75**, 13–22.

Lipska, B.K. & Weinberger, D.R. (1994a) Subchronic treatment with haloperidol or clozapine in rats with neonatal excitotoxic hippocampal damage. *Neuropsychopharmacology* **10**, 199–205.

Lipska, B.K. & Weinberger, D.R. (1994b) Gonadectomy does not prevent novelty- or drug-induced hyperresponsiveness in rats with neonatal excitototxic hippocampal damage. *Developmental Brain Research* **78**, 253–258.

Lipska, B.K. & Weinberger, D.R. (1995) Genetic variation in vulnerability to the behavioral effects of neonatal hippocampal damage in rats. *Proceedings of the National Academy of Sciencs USA* **92**, 8906–8910.

Lipska, B.K. & Weinberger, D.R. (2000) To model a psychiatric disorder in animals: Schizophrenia as a reality test. *Neuropsychopharmacology* **23**, 223–239.

Lipska, B.K., Chrapusta, S.J., Egan, M.F. & Weinberger, D.R. (1995) Neonatal excitotoxic ventral hippocampal damage alters dopamine response to mild chronic stress and haloperidol treatment. *Synapse* **20**, 125–130.

Lipska, B.K., Al-Amin, H.A. & Weinberger, D.R. (1998a) Excitotoxic lesions of the rat medial prefrontal cortex: effects on abnormal behaviors associated with neonatal hippocampal damage. *Neuropsychopharmacology* **19**, 451–464.

Lipska, B.K., Khaing, Z.Z., Lerman, D.N. & Weinberger, D.R. (1998b) Neonatal damage of the rat ventral hippocampus reduces expression of a dopamine transporter. *Social Neurosciences Abstracts* **24**, 365.

Lipska, B.K., Halim, N.D., Segal, P.N. & Weinberger, D.R. (2002) Effects of reversible inactivation of the neonatal ventral hippocampus on behavior in the adult rat. *Journal of Neuroscience* **22**, 2835–2842.

Lipska, B.K., Luu, S., Halim, N.D. & Weinberger, D.R. (2003) Behavioral effects of neonatal and adult excitotoxic lesions of the mediodorsal thalamus in the adult rat. *Behavioural Brain Research* **141**, 105–111.

Lipska, B.K., Peters, T., Halim, N. *et al.* (2006) Expression of DISC1 binding partners is reduced in schizophrenia and associated with DISC1 SNPs. *Human Molecular Genetics* **15**, 1245–1258.

Liu, H., Heath, S.C., Sobin, C. *et al.* (2002) Genetic variation at the 22q11 PRODH2/DGCR6 locus presents an unusual pattern and increases susceptibility to schizophrenia. *Proceedings of the National Academy of Sciencs USA* **99**, 3717–3722.

Lohr, J.B. & Bracha, S. (1989) Can schizophrenia be related to prenatal exposure to alcohol? Some speculations. *Schizophrenia Bulletin* **15**, 595–603.

Long, J.M., LaPorte, P., Merscher, S. *et al.* (2006) Behavior of mice with mutations in the conserved region deleted in velocardiofacial/DiGeorge syndrome. *Neurogenetics* **7**, 247–257.

Mathe, J.M., Nomikos, G.G., Schilstrom, B. & Svensson, T.H. (1998) Non-NMDA excitatory amino acid receptors in the ventral tegmental area mediate systemic dizocilpine (MK-801) induced hyperlocomotion and dopamine release in the nucleus accumbens. *Journal of Neuroscience Research* **51**, 583–592.

McDonald-McGinn, D.M., Tonnesen, M.K., Laufer-Cahana *et al.* (2001) Phenotype of the 22q11.2 deletion in individuals identified through an affected relative: cast a wide FISHing net! *Genetics in Medicine* **3**, 23–29.

McNiel, T.F. (1988) Obstetric factors and perinatal injuries. In; Tsuang, M.T. & Simpson, J.C., eds. *Handbook of Schizophrenia, 3. Nosology, Epidemiology and Genetic*. Amsterdam: Elsevier, pp. 319–344.

Mednick, S.A., Machon, R.A., Huttunen, M.O. & Bonett, D. (1988) Adult schizophrenia following prenatal exposure to influenza epidemic. *Archives of General Psychiatry* **45**, 189–192.

Meng, Z.H., Feldpaush, D.L. & Merchant, K.M. (1998) Clozapine and haloperidol block the induction of behavioral sensitization to amphetamine and associated genomic responses in rats. *Brain Research Molecular Brain Research* **61**, 39–50.

Meyer, U., Nyffeler, M., Schwendener, S., Knuesel, I., Yee, B.K. & Feldon, J. (2008) Relative prenatal and postnatal maternal contributions to schizophrenia-related neurochemical dysfunction after *in utero* immune challenge. *Neuropsychopharmacology* **33**, 441–456.

Millar, J.K., Wilson-Annan, J.C., Anderson, S. *et al.* (2000) Disruption of two novel genes by a translocation co-segregating with schizophrenia. *Human Molecular Genetics* **9**, 1415–1423.

Millar, J.K., Pickard, B.S., Mackie, S. *et al.* (2005) DISC1 and PDE4B are interacting genetic factors in schizophrenia that regulate cAMP signaling. *Science* **310**, 1187–1191.

Mintz, M., Gigi, A., Shohami, D. & Myslobodsky, M.S. (1999) Effects of prenatal exposure to gamma rays on circling and activity behavior in prepubertal and postpubertal rats. *Behavioural Brain Research* **98**, 45–51.

Miyakawa, T., Leiter, L.M., Gerber, D.J. *et al.* (2003) Conditional calcineurin knockout mice exhibit multiple abnormal behaviors related to schizophrenia. *Proceedings of the National Academy of Sciencs USA* **100**, 8987–8992.

Moghaddam, B., Adams, B., Verma, A. & Daly, D. (1997) Activation of glutamatergic neurotransmission by ketamine: a novel step in pathway from NMDA receptor blockade to dopaminergic and cognitive disruptions associated with the prefrontal cortex. *Journal of Neuroscience* **17**, 2921–2927.

Moghaddam, B. & Adams, B. (1998) Reversal of phencyclidine effects by group II metabotropic glutamate receptor agonist in rats. *Science* **281**, 1349–1352.

Montgomery, E.M., Bardgett, M.E., Lall, B., Csernansky, C.A. & Csernansky, J.G. (1999) Delayed neuronal loss after administration of intracerebroventricular kainic acid to preweanling rats. *Brain Research Developmental Brain Research* **112**, 107–116.

Moore, H., Jentsch, J.D., Ghajarnia, M., Geyer, M.A. & Grace, A.A. (2006) A neurobehavioral systems analysis of adult rats exposed to methylazoxymethanol acetate on E17: implications for the neuropathology of schizophrenia. *Biological Psychiatry* **60**, 253–264.

Morris, JA, Kandpal, G, Ma, L, & Austin, CP (2003) DISC1 (Disrupted-In-Schizophrenia 1) is a centrosome-associated protein that interacts with MAP1A, MIPT3, ATF4/5 and NUDEL: regulation and loss of interaction with mutation. *Human Molecular Genetics* **12**, 1591–1608.

Mukai, J., Liu, H., Burt, R.A. *et al.* (2004) Evidence that the gene encoding ZDHHC8 contributes to the risk of schizophrenia. *Nature Genetics* **36**, 725–731.

Murase, S., Mathe, J.M., Grenhoff, J. & Svensson, T.H. (1993) Effects of dizocilpine (MK-801) on rat midbrain dopamine cell activity: differential actions on firing pattern related to anatomical localization. *Journal of Neural Transmission Genetics Section* **91**, 13–25.

Murphy, K.C., Jones, L.A. & Owen, M.J. (1999) High rates of schizophrenia in adults with velo-cardio-facial syndrome. *Archives of General Psychiatry* **56**, 940–945.

Murray, R.M. & Lewis, S.W. (1987) Is schizophrenia a neurodevelopmental disorder? *British Medical Journal* **295**, 681–682.

Newton-Cheh, C. & Hirschhorn, J.N. (2005) Genetic association studies of complex traits: design and analysis issues. *Mutation Research* **573**, 54–69.

O'Callaghan, E., Sham, P., Takei, N., Glover, G. & Murray, R.M. (1991) Schizophrenia after prenatal exposure to 1957 A2 influenza epidemic. *Lancet* **337**, 248–1250.

O'Donnell, P. & Grace, A.A. (1998) Phencyclidine interferes with the hippocampal gating of nucleus accumbens neuronal activity *in vivo*. *Neuroscience* **87**, 823–830.

O'Donnell, P., Lewis, B.L., Weinberger, D.R. & Lipska, B.K. (2002) Neonatal hippocampal damage alters electrophysiological properties of prefrontal cortical neurons. *Cerebral Cortex* **12**, 975–982.

Olney, J.W. & Farber, N.B. (1995) Glutamate receptor dysfunction and schizophrenia. *Archives of General Psychiatry* **52**, 998–1007.

O'Tuathaigh, C.M., O'Sullivan, G.J., Kinsella, A. *et al.* (2006) Sexually dimorphic changes in the exploratory and habituation profiles of heterozygous neuregulin-1 knockout mice. *Neuroreport* **17**, 79–83.

O'Tuathaigh, C.M., Babovic, D., O'Meara, G., Clifford, J.J., Croke, D.T. & Waddington, JL (2007a) Susceptibility genes for schizophrenia: characterisation of mutant mouse models at the level of phenotypic behaviour. *Neuroscience Biobehavioral Review* **31**, 60–78.

O'Tuathaigh, C.M., Babovic, D., O'Sullivan, G.J. *et al.* (2007b) Phenotypic characterization of spatial cognition and social behavior in mice with "knockout" of the schizophrenia risk gene neuregulin 1. *Neuroscience* **147**, 18–27.

O'Tuathaigh, C.M., O'Connor, A.M., O'Sullivan, G.J. *et al.* (2007c) Disruption to social dyadic interactions but not emotional/anxiety-related behaviour in mice with heterozygous "knockout" of the schizophrenia risk gene neuregulin-1. *Progress in Neuropsychopharmacology and Biological Psychiatry* **32**, 462–466.

Palmer, A.A., Printz, D.J., Butler, P.D., Dulawa, S.C. & Printz, M.P. (2004) Prenatal protein deprivation in rats induces changes in prepulse inhibition and NMDA receptor binding. *Brain Research* **996**, 193–201.

Papaleo, F., Crawley, J.N., Song, J. *et al.* (2008) Genetic dissection of the role of catechol-O-methyltransferase in cognition and stress reactivity in mice. *Journal of Neuroscience* **28**, 8709–8723.

Paterlini, M., Zakharenko, S.S., Lai, W.S. *et al.* (2005) Transcriptional and behavioral interaction between 22q11.2 orthologs modulates schizophrenia-related phenotypes in mice. *Nature Neuroscience* **8**, 1586–1594.

Patil, S.T., Zhang, L., Martenyi, F. *et al.* (2007) Activation of mGlu2/3 receptors as a new approach to treat schizophrenia: a randomized Phase 2 clinical trial. *Nature Medicine* **13**, 1102–1107.

Paylor, R., Glaser, B., Mupo, A. *et al.* (2006) Tbx1 haploinsufficiency is linked to behavioral disorders in mice and humans: implications for 22q11 deletion syndrome. *Proceedings of the National Academy of Sciencs USA* **103**, 7729–7734.

Pearce, B.D. (2001) Schizophrenia and viral infection during neurodevelopment: a focus on mechanisms. *Molecular Psychiatry* **6**, 634–646.

Pletnikov, M.V., Ayhan, Y., Nikolskaia, O. *et al.* (2007) Inducible expression of mutant human DISC1 in mice is associated with brain and behavioral abnormalities reminiscent of schizophrenia. *Molecular Psychiatry* **13**, 173–186.

Powell, K.J., Binder, T.L., Hori, S. *et al.* (2006) Neonatal ventral hippocampal lesions produce an elevation of ?FosB-like protein(s) in the rodent neocortex. *Neuropsychopharmacology* **31**, 700–711.

Pritchard, J.K. & Cox, N.J. (2002) The allelic architecture of human disease genes: common disease-common variant…or not? *Human Molecular Genetics* **11**, 2417–2423.

Pulver, A.E., Nestadt, G., Goldberg, R. *et al.* (1994) Psychotic illness in patients diagnosed with velo-cardio-facial syndrome and their relatives. *Journal of Nervous and Mental Diseases* **182**, 476–478.

Qin, Z.H., Zhang, S.P. & Weiss, B. (1994) Dopaminergic and glutamatergic blocking drugs differentially regulate glutamic acid decarboxylase mRNA in mouse brain. *Brain Research and Molecular Brain Research* **21**, 293–302.

Rajakumar, N., Williamson, P.C., Stoessl, J.A. & Flumerfelt, B.A. (1996) Neurodevelopmental pathogenesis of schizophrenia. *Social Neuroscience Abstracts* **22**, 1187.

Raux, G., Bumsel, E., Hecketsweiler, B. *et al.* (2007) Involvement of hyperprolinemia in cognitive and psychiatric features of the 22q11 deletion syndrome. *Human Molecular Genetics* **16**, 83–91.

Rebbeck, T.R., Spitz, M. & Wu, X. (2004) Assessing the function of genetic variants in candidate gene association studies. *Nature Review Genetics* **5**, 589–597.

Renick, S.E., Kleven, D.T., Chan, J. *et al.* (1999) The mammalian brain high-affinity L-proline transporter is enriched preferentially in synaptic vesicles in a subpopulation of excitatory nerve terminals in rat forebrain. *Journal of Neuroscience* **19**, 21–33.

Richtand, N.M., Taylor, B., Welge, J.A. *et al.* (2006) Risperidone pretreatment prevents elevated locomotor activity following neonatal hippocampal lesions. *Neuropsychopharmacology* **31**, 77–89.

Rimer, M., Barrett, D.W., Maldonado, M.A., Vock, V.M. & Gonzalez-Lima, F. (2005) Neuregulin-1 immunoglobulin-like domain mutant mice: clozapine sensitivity and impaired latent inhibition. *Neuroreport* **16**, 271–275.

Roffman, J.L., Lipska, B.K., Bertolino, A. *et al.* (2000) Local and downstream effects of excitotoxic lesions in the rat medial prefrontal cortex on *in vivo* ^{1}H-MRS signals. *Neuropsychopharmacology* **22**, 430–439.

Rott, R., Herzog, S., Fleischer, B. *et al.* (1985) Detection of serum antibodies to Borna disease virus in patients with psychiatric disorders. *Science* **228**, 755–756.

Roy, K., Murtie, J.C., El-Khodor, B.F. *et al.* (2007) Loss of erbB signaling in oligodendrocytes alters myelin and dopaminergic function, a potential mechanism for neuropsychiatric disorders. *Proceedings of the National Academy of Sciencs USA* **104**, 8131–8136.

Rueter, L.E., Ballard, M.E., Gallagher, K.B., Basso, A.M., Curzon, P. & Kohlhaas, K.L. (2004) Chronic low dose risperidone and clozapine alleviate positive but not negative symptoms in the rat neonatal ventral hippocampal lesion model of schizophrenia. *Psychopharmacology (Berlin)* **176**, 312–319.

Sams-Dodd, F., Lipska, B.K. & Weinberger, D.R. (1997) Neonatal lesions of the rat ventral hippocampus result in hyperlocomotion and deficits in social behaviour in adulthood. *Psychopharmacology* **132**, 303–310.

Saunders, R.C., Kolachana, B.S., Bachevalier, J. & Weinberger, D.R. (1998) Neonatal lesions of the temporal lobe disrupt prefrontal cortical regulation of striatal dopamine. *Nature* **393**, 169–171.

Scheibel, A.B. & Kovelman, J.A. (1981) Disorientation of the hippocampal pyramidal cell and its processes in the schizophrenic patient. *Biological Psychiatry* **16**, 101–102.

Schroeder, H., Grecksch, G., Becker, A., Bogerts, B. & Höllt, V. (1999) Alterations of the dopaminergic and glutamatergic neurotransmission in adult rats with postnatal ibotenic acid hippocampal lesion. *Psychopharmacology* **145**, 61–66.

Scolnick, E.M. (2006) Mechanisms of action of medicines for schizophrenia and bipolar illness: status and limitations. *Biological Psychiatry* **59**, 1039–1045.

Sebat, J., Lakshmi, B., Malhotra, D. *et al.* (2007) Strong association of *de novo* copy number mutations with autism. *Science* **316**, 445–449.

Selemon, L.D., Wang, L., Nebel, M.B., Csernansky, J.G., Goldman-Rakic, P.S. & Rakic, P. (2005) Direct and indirect effects of fetal irradiation on cortical gray and white matter volume in the macaque. *Biological Psychiatry* **57**, 83–90.

Sesack, S.R., Hawrylak, V.A., Matus, C., Guido, M.A. & Levey, A.I. (1998) Dopamine axon varicosities in the prelimbic division of the rat prefrontal cortex exhibit sparse immunoreactivity for the dopamine transporter. *Journal of Neuroscience* **18**, 2697–2708.

Shi, L., Fatemi, S.H., Sidwell, R.W. & Patterson, P.H. (2003) Maternal influenza infection causes marked behavioral and pharmacological changes in the offspring. *Journal of Neuro_science* **23**, 297–302.

Sobin, C., Kiley-Brabeck, K., Daniels, S. *et al.* (2005) Neuropsychological characteristics of children with the 22q11 Deletion Syndrome: a descriptive analysis. *Child Neuropsychology* **11**, 39–53.

Solbrig, M.V., Koob, G.F. & Parsons, L.H. *et al.* (2000) Neurotrophic factor expression after CNS viral injury produces enhanced sensitivity to psychostimulants: potential mechanism for addiction vulnerability. *Journal of Neuroscience* **20**, RC104.

Spanagel, R. & Weiss, F. (1999) The dopamine hypothesis of reward: past and current status. *Trends in Neuroscience* **22**, 521–527.

Stark, K.L., Xu, B., Bagchi, A. *et al.* (2008) Altered brain microRNA biogenesis in mice deficient for the 22q11 region contributes to behavioral and neuronal deficits. *Nature Genetics* **40**, 751–760.

Stefansson, H., Sigurdsson, E., Steinthorsdottir, V. *et al.* (2002) Neuregulin 1 and susceptibility to schizophrenia. *American Journal of Human Genetics* **71**, 877–892.

Suddath, R.L., Christisin, G.W., Torrey, E.F., Casanova, M. & Weinberger, D.R. (1990) Anatomical abnormalities in the brains of monozygotic twins discordant for schizophrenia. *New England Journal of Medicine* **322**, 789–794.

Sullivan, R., Wilson, D.A., Feldon, J. *et al.* (2006) The International Society for Developmental Psychobiology annual meeting symposium: Impact of early life experiences on brain and behavioral development. *Developmental Psychobiology* **48**, 583–602.

Susser, E.S. & Lin, S.P. (1992) Schizophrenia after prenatal exposure to the Dutch Hunger Winter of 1944–1945. *Archives of General Psychiatry* **49**, 983–988.

Tabuchi, K., Blundell, J., Etherton, M.R. *et al.* (2007) A neuroligin-3 mutation implicated in autism increases inhibitory synaptic transmission in mice. *Science* **318**, 71–76.

Talamini, L.M., Koch, T., Ter Horst, G.J. & Korf, J. (1998) Methylazoxymethanol acetate-induced abnormalities in the entorhinal cortex of the rat; parallels with morphological findings in schizophrenia. *Brain Research* **789**, 293–306.

Tan, W., Wang, Y., Gold, B. *et al.* (2007) Molecular cloning of a brain-specific, developmentally regulated neuregulin 1 (NRG1) isoform and identification of a functional promoter variant associated with schizophrenia. *Journal of Biological Chemistry* **282**, 24343–24351.

Tseng, K.Y. & O'Donnell, P. (2004) Dopamine-glutamate interactions controlling prefrontal cortical pyramidal cell excitability involve multiple signaling mechanisms. *Journal of Neuroscience* **24**, 5131–5139.

Tseng K.Y. & O'Donnell, P. (2007) D2 dopamine receptors recruit a GABA component for their attenuation of excitatory synaptic transmission in the adult rat prefrontal cortex. *Synapse* **61**, 843–850.

Tseng, K.Y., Lewis, B.L., Lipska, B.K., O'Donnell, P. (2007) Postpubertal disruption of medial prefrontal cortical dopamine-glutamate interactions in a developmental animal model of schizophrenia. *Biological Psychiatry* **62**, 730–738.

Tseng, K.Y., Chambers, R.A. & Lipska, B.K. (2009) The neonatal ventral hippocampal lesion as a heuristic neurodevelopmental model of schizophrenia. *Behavioural Brain Research* **204**, 295–305.

Uehara, T., Sumiyoshi, T., Matsuoka, T., Itoh, H. & Kurachi, M. (2007) Effect of prefrontal cortex inactivation on behavioral and neurochemical abnormalities in rats with excitotoxic lesions of the entorhinal cortex. *Synapse* **61**, 391–400.

Vanderschuren, L.J., Schmidt, E.D., De Vries, T.J., Van Moorsel, C.A., Tilders, F.J. & Schoffelmeer, A.N. (1999) A single exposure to amphetamine is sufficient to induce long-term behavioral, neuroendocrine, and neurochemical sensitization in rats. *Journal of Neuroscience* **19**, 9579–9586.

Varty, G.B. & Higgins, G.A. (1995) Examination of drug-induced and isolation-induced disruptions of prepulse inhibition as models to screen antipsychotic drugs. *Psychopharmacology* **122**, 15–26.

Verma, A. & Moghaddam, B. (1996) NMDA receptor antagonists impair prefrontal cortex function as assessed via spatial delayed alternation performance in rats: modulation by dopamine. *Journal of Neuroscience* **16**, 373–379.

Volk, D.W. & Lewis, D.A. (2003) Effects of a mediodorsal thalamus lesion on prefrontal inhibitory circuitry: implications for schizophrenia. *Biological Psychiatry* **53**, 385–389.

Waltrip, R.W. 2nd, Buchanan, R.W., Summerfeld, A. *et al.* (1995) Borna disease virus and schizophrenia. *Psychiatric Research* **56**, 33–44.

Wan, R.-Q., Giovanni, A., Kafka, S.H. & Corbett, R. (1996) Neonatal hippocampal lesions induced hyperresponsiveness to amphetamine: behavioral and in vivo microdialysis studies. *Behavioural Brain Research* **78**, 211–223.

Wan, R.Q. & Corbett, R. (1997) Enhancement of postsynaptic sensitivity to dopaminergic agonists induced by neonatal hippocampal lesions. *Neuropsychopharmacology* **16**, 259–268.

Wan, R.Q., Hartman, H. & Corbett, R. (1998) Alteration of dopamine metabolites in CSF and behavioral impairments induced by neonatal hippocampal lesions. *Physiological Behavior* **65**, 429–436.

Weinberger, D.R. (1986) The pathogenesis of schizophrenia: a neurodevelopmental theory. In: Nasrallah, H.A. & Weinberger, D.R., eds. *The Neurology of Schizophrenia*. Amsterdam: Elsevier, pp. 397–406.

Weinberger, D.R. (1987) Implications of normal brain development for the pathogenesis of schizophrenia. *Archives of General Psychiatry* **44**, 660–669.

Weinberger, D.R. (1999) Cell biology of the hippocampal formation in schizophrenia. *Biological Psychiatry* **45**, 395–402.

Weinberger, D.R. & Lipska, B.K. (1995) Corticol maldevelopment anti-psychotic drugs, and schizophrenia: in search of common ground. *Schizophrenia Research* **16**, 87–110.

Wiehahn, G.J., Bosch, G.P., du Preez, R.R., Pretorius, H.W., Karayiorgou, M. & Roos, J.L. (2004) Assessment of the frequency of the 22q11 deletion in Afrikaner schizophrenic patients. *American Journal of Medical Genetics B Neuropsychiatric Genetics* **129**, 20–22.

Woerner, M.G., Pollack, M. & Klein, D.F. (1973) Pregnancy and birth complications in psychiatric patients: a comparison of schizophrenic and personality disorder patients with their siblings. *Acta Psychiatrica Scandinavica* **49**, 712–721.

Wolf, M.E., White, F.J. & Hu, X.-T. (1993) Behavioral sensitization to MK-801 (dizocilpine): neurochemical and electrophysiological correlates in the mesoaccumbens dopamine system. *Behavioral Pharmacolgy* **4**, 429–442.

Wong, H.A.C., Lipska, B.K., Likhodi, O. *et al.* (2005) Cortical gene expression in the neonatal ventral-hippocampal lesion model of schizophrenia. *Schizophrenia Research* **77**, 261–270.

Woodin, M., Wang, P.P., Aleman, D., McDonald-McGinn, D., Zackai, E. & Moss, E. (2001) Neuropsychological profile of children and adolescents with the 22q11.2 microdeletion. *Genetic Medicine* **3**, 34–39.

Yavich, L., Forsberg, M.M., Karayiorgou, M., Gogos, J.A. & Männistö, P.T. (2007) Site-specific role of catechol-O-methyltransferase in dopamine overflow within prefrontal cortex and dorsal striatum. *Journal of Neuroscience* **27**, 10196–10209.

Yonezawa, Y., Kuroki, T., Kawahara, T., Tashiro, N. & Uchimura, H. (1998) Involvement of gamma-aminobutyric acid neurotransmission in phencyclidine-induced dopamine release in the medial prefrontal cortex. *European Journal of Pharmacology* **341**, 45–56.

Zaharia, M.D., Kulczycki, J., Shanks, N., Meaney, M.J. & Anisman, H. (1996) The effects of early postnatal stimulation on Morris water-maze acquisition in adult mice: genetic and maternal factors. *Psychopharmacology* **128**, 227–239.

Zuckerman, L., Rehavi, M., Nachman, R. & Weiner, I. (2003) Immune activation during pregnancy in rats leads to a postpubertal emergence of disrupted latent inhibition, dopaminergic hyperfunction, and altered limbic morphology in the offspring: a novel neurodevelopmental model of schizophrenia. *Neuropsychopharmacology* **28**, 1778–1789.

PART 3

Physical Treatments

CHAPTER 23

Pharmacology and neuroscience of antipsychotic drugs

John L. Waddington[1], Colm M.P. O'Tuathaigh[1], and Gary J. Remington[2]

[1]Royal College of Surgeons in Ireland, Dublin, Ireland
[2]Centre for Addiction and Mental Health, Toronto, Canada

Schizophrenia, 3rd edition. Edited by Daniel R. Weinberger and
Paul J Harrison © 2011 Blackwell Publishing Ltd.

Origins of contemporary concepts and challenges

Increasing knowledge in most domains of scientific enquiry usually leads, over time, to practical advantage. Yet, while the serendipitous discovery and introduction of neuroleptic drugs in the 1950s has been of profound significance (for a uniquely personal memoir of these early events, see Deniker, 1983), neuroscience and therapeutics are now traversing the sixth decade of an incremental search for (1) the basis of their antipsychotic effect and (2) the pathobiology of psychosis. Encouragingly, over recent years we have been witnessing perhaps a greater rate of progress than occurred during preceding decades due to two complementary developments: advances in basic neuroscience that continually replenish the knowledge base from which we can generate new hypotheses; and the emergence of deeper insights into human brain function fostered by new investigatory tools, including molecular, cellular, and neuroimaging techniques that increasingly allow the direct exploration of drug action and functional effects in living subjects (Ross *et al.*, 2006; Waddington, 2007).

While the tranche of new antipsychotic agents continues to evolve, the extent to which the clinical profiles of second-generation ("atypical") antipsychotics might be superior to those of their first-generation ("typical") counterparts (see Geddes *et al.*, 2000; Davis *et al.*, 2003; Leucht *et al.*, 2003; see Chapter 25) is currently the topic of considerable empirical scrutiny (Rosenheck *et al.*, 2003; Lieberman *et al.*, 2005; Jones *et al.*, 2006; Tiihonen *et al.*, 2006) and editorial analysis (Freedman, 2005; Rosenheck. 2006; Tandon & Nasrallah, 2006). This is not without pharmacological import, as assumed superiority of second-generation agents leads readily to a search for the mechanistic basis of that advantage; however, were this to have been overstated materially, resources may have been applied injudiciously in relation to a clinically less advantageous group of agents than has been appreciated previously.

Since recent reviews of antipsychotic drug action (Waddington & Casey, 2000; Waddington *et al.*, 2003; Miyamoto *et al.*, 2005), it has been suggested that putative superiority of second-generation over first-generation antipsychotics may *inter alia* reflect: (1) artifacts of trial methodology (Leucht *et al.*, 2007); (2) the nature of trial sponsorship (Jorgensen *et al.*, 2006); and (3) differences in evidence base *vis-à-vis* regulatory procedures across diverse cultures (Adams *et al.*, 2006). As the field engages in this essential debate, there are additional challenges of mechanistic import: where, if they exist at all, are the boundaries of antipsychotic activity, e.g., in relation to the treatment of bipolar disorder (Johnstone *et al.*, 1988; Cousins & Young, 2007; Scherk *et al.*, 2007) and unipolar psychotic depression (Wijkstra *et al.*, 2006)? Additionally, the boundaries of adverse effects, especially for newer antipsychotics,

extend to an increasing number of critical areas, particularly physical morbidity in terms of weight gain/glucose dysregulation/risk for diabetes during the treatment of psychosis at large (Basu & Meltzer, 2006; see Chapter 28) and increased mortality during the treatment of behavioral disturbances in dementia (Schneider *et al.*, 2005; Wang *et al.*, 2005; Kales *et al.*, 2007; see Chapter 27). Furthermore, there may be mechanistic import in renewed evidence for therapeutic advantage from combining antipsychotic therapy with psychosocial interventions (Petersen *et al.*, 2005; Penn *et al.*, 2005; Byrne, 2007).

Here, the nomenclature of first- and second-generation antipsychotics is retained, not in prejudgment of ongoing debates, but as pragmatic recognition of the temporal emergence of these agents and of a nomenclature that may prove difficult to shift; though widely utilized, the terminology "atypical" is avoided because of lack of clarity as to meaning and definition. This chapter seeks to document advances and controversies in relation to mechanisms of antipsychotic drug action. It focuses on findings for second-generation agents; yet it is mindful of what we have learned and have still to learn from their first-generation counterparts. Thereafter, it considers putative "third-generation" agents and then considers novel mechanisms and possible future developments.

Evolution of the D₂ receptor blockade hypothesis

Dopamine receptor antagonism

It should be recognized that the extent of interrogation of second-generation antipsychotics during their development and subsequent introduction into clinical practice has generated an unprecedented wealth of studies, many of which make unprecedented use of new molecular, cellular, and human imaging techniques. Yet enthusiasm engendered by these events must be tempered by recognition that the concept which still underpins much contemporary theorizing, namely the dopamine (DA) receptor blockade hypothesis, is now over 45 years old. It remains a chastening fact that *all* known antipsychotic drugs evidencing clinical efficacy in appropriately controlled clinical trials exert *inter alia* at least some competitive antagonism of brain DA receptors. However, only recently has this notion been given material pathophysiological relevance by neuroimaging findings in living patients that indicate increased subcortical release of DA in schizophrenia, primarily during phases of exacerbation of positive psychotic symptoms; conversely, cognitive impairment and possibly aspects of the negative symptom domain may reflect reduced release of DA in the prefrontal cortex (PFC; Waddington & Morgan, 2001; Guillin *et al.*, 2007; see also Chapter 20).

The common action of first-generation antipsychotic drugs to block brain DA receptors was posited initially from neurochemical observations (Carlsson & Lindqvist, 1963) that were subsequently elaborated by a wealth of behavioral (Niemegeers & Janssen, 1978) and clinical (Johnstone *et al.*, 1978) findings. The relationship of these properties to therapeutic efficacy in schizophrenia received strong, though indirect, support from data indicating the *in vitro* affinities of a wide range of antipsychotic drugs for brain DA antagonist binding sites to correlate highly with their clinical potencies to control psychotic symptoms (Seeman, 1980).

Dopamine receptor typology

In conceptual terms, these now classical (though at the time radical and heuristic) notions endure, but have required material modification in their detail as our knowledge base in the neurosciences has expanded. In particular, our concepts of DA receptor typology and function have undergone substantial revision. Specifically, it was recognized subsequently that DA receptors existed as two major subtypes, D_1 and D_2 (Kebabian & Calne, 1979). Re-evaluation of the above relationship in terms of this D_1/D_2 schema indicated the clinical potencies of antipsychotics to be correlated highly with their affinities for the D_2 but not for the D_1 receptor; furthermore, this relationship held not just for rat striatal but also for postmortem human putamen tissue and, importantly, no differences were apparent between the affinities of such drugs for D_2 receptors in caudate or putamen [the meso-striatal DAergic system, presumed to mediate extrapyramidal side effects (EPS)] versus nucleus accumbens (the meso-cortico-limbic system, presumed to mediate antipsychotic efficacy) of human postmortem brain (see Waddington, 1993; Lidsky, 1995). Similarly, selective or preferential D_2 antagonists, such as the substituted benzamide sulpiride or the butyrophenone haloperidol, respectively, appeared to reproduce the essential clinical activity of non-selective antipsychotics, such as the phenothiazines (e.g., fluphenazine) and thioxanthenes (e.g., flupenthixol), that block both D_1 and D_2 receptors (Ehman et al. 1987). On this basis, D_2 receptor blockade was ascribed a prepotent or even exclusive role in mediating antipsychotic activity (Seeman, 1980, 1992).

Molecular biological/gene cloning techniques subsequently indicated the number of DA receptor subtypes to be yet larger than envisaged originally. Until very recently, theory has encompassed six DA receptor protein sequences which, on the basis of structural and pharmacological characteristics, are best subsumed under the umbrella of two families of D_1-like (D_1 and D_5) and D_2-like ($D_{2long/short}$, D_3, and D_4) receptors (Missale et al., 1998; Waddington et al., 2005). Within the D_1-like family, the D_1 receptor evidences a general meso-striatal–cortico-limbic localization, while its D_5 counterpart evidences primarily a characteristic, low-density localization within particular cortico-limbic areas (Niznik et al., 2002). Conversely, within the D_2-like family, the D_2 receptor, having a general meso-striatal–limbic localization, exists in both "long" and "short" isoforms generated by alternative splicing; the D_3 and D_4 receptors evidence low density localizations within distinct striatal subregions and cortico-limbic areas (Levant, 1997; Tarazi & Baldessarini. 1999; Waddington et al., 2005).

A putative, variant D_2-like receptor, $D_{2longer}$, has a unique TG splice site that has been identified in some (but not all) postmortem brains both from control subjects and from patients with schizophrenia (Seeman *et al.*, 2000; Liu *et al.*, 2000). However, given its variable prevalence in human brain, occurrence at about 2–3% of the total population of D_2 transcripts therein, unknown regional distribution or functional characteristics other than high affinity for antipsychotics and linkage to inhibition of adenylyl cyclase, and no known selective agonists or antagonists for more incisive studies, any relevance for antipsychotic drug action remains to be clarified.

Current status of selective D_2 antagonism

On this basis, previous studies of the correlation between clinical antipsychotic potencies and affinities for the "D_2" receptor actually reflected generic affinities for all members of the D_2-like family (i.e., D_2, D_3, and D_4) due to the inability of the ligands utilized to distinguish between them. However, subsequent studies using cloned cell lines have indicated both clinical antipsychotic potencies and the free concentrations of antipsychotics in patient plasma to correlate generally with their affinities for the D_2 receptor when expressed independently of its D_3 and D_4 siblings (Seeman, 1992). The primacy of D_2 antagonism in antipsychotic activity is nourished by the established therapeutic efficacy of amisulpride, a selective D_2 antagonist having negligible affinity for essentially any known receptor other than its D_3 sibling (Mota *et al.*, 2002; Moller, 2003; McKeage & Plosker, 2004).

More recently, focus on the D_2 receptor has shifted to its high- and low-affinity states. D_2^{High} represents the functional physiological state and it has been hypothesized that numbers of D_2^{High} receptors may be increased in conditions such as schizophrenia, i.e., DA supersensitivity (Seeman *et al.*, 2005, 2006). In support of this model are data indicating that drugs with psychotomimetic properties increase the high-affinity state of D_2 receptors, while antipsychotics, both first- and second-generation, block such an effect (Seeman *et al.*, 2006). This distinction serves to reconcile, at least in part, the contradictory evidence regarding D_2 receptor density in individuals with schizophrenia (Guillin *et al.*, 2007). Moreover, evidence that multiple and diverse non-dopaminergic strategies can alter this supersensitive state is in line with the notion that DA can be modulated through numerous pathways and systems (Guillin *et al.*, 2007). Thus, DA remains the final common pathway in psychosis, although mechanisms by which it can be altered are diverse. Perhaps the greatest challenge to this model at present is specificity in measurement of the D_2^{High} state (McCormick *et al.*, 2008).

Current status of selective D_3 antagonism

A high affinity for most antipsychotics and predominantly "peristriatal", limbic localization initially generated much interest in the D_3 receptor as a potentially novel therapeutic target for antipsychotic activity (Sokoloff *et al.*, 1992). However, no known antipsychotic shows more than modest preference for D_3 over D_2 receptors, and clinical antipsychotic potencies correlate less strongly with affinities for the D_3 than for the D_2 receptor (Seeman, 1992). On the basis of the most recent preclinical studies with new preferential/selective D_3 antagonists or partial agonists, and in D_3 "knockout" mice, the role of D_3 antagonism in antipsychotic activity remains uncertain (Joyce & Millan, 2005; Waddington *et al.*, 2005). Thus, only controlled clinical trials with selective D_3 antagonists will ultimately clarify this long-standing conundrum.

Current status of selective D_4 antagonism

Similarly, the D_4 receptor has long been considered as a potential novel therapeutic target on the basis of its high affinity for many antipsychotics and its predominantly cortico-limbic localization (Van Tol *et al.*, 1991; Tarazi & Baldessarini, 1999). However, no known antipsychotic shows more than modest preference for D_4 over D_2 receptors, and clinical antipsychotic potencies appear to correlate less strongly with affinities for the D_4 than for the D_2 receptor (Seeman, 1992). On the basis of the most recent preclinical studies with new selective D_4 antagonists, and in D_4 "knockout" mice, the role of D_4 antagonism in antipsychotic activity remains uncertain (Wong & Van Tol, 2003; Waddington *et al.*, 2005).

Nevertheless, on the basis of the above profiles and inconsistent evidence suggesting *inter alia* abnormalities of the D_4 receptor in schizophrenia (Tarazi & Baldessarini, 1999; Hrib, 2000), clinical trials with selective D_4 antagonists have proceded. In the first such study (Kramer *et al.*, 1997), the selective D_4 antagonist L745,870 was found to be without either antipsychotic activity or EPS in schizophrenia; indeed, it was associated with some worsening of psychotic symptoms relative to placebo. However, subsequent studies have indicated L745,870, like some other first- and second-generation antipsychotics and putative "third-generation" agents to be considered below, to evidence partial agonist activity at the D_4 receptor (Gazi *et al.*, 1999;

Newman-Tancredi *et al.*, 2008); thus, their capacity to reveal antipsychotic activity for D_4 antagonists may be compromised. In subsequent studies, the mixed D_4–5-HT$_{2A}$ antagonist fananserin (Truffinet *et al.*, 1999) and the selective D_4 antagonist sonepiprazole (Corrigan *et al.*, 2004) were also found to be without antipsychotic activity.

Such evidence indicates that selective D_4 antagonists are unlikely to prove effective as primary treatments for psychotic symptoms in schizophrenia. However, they serve an important purpose in focusing attention on how we evaluate findings in individual preclinical models of antipsychotic activity in which some such drugs are active and still under investigation; e.g., the actions of FAUC 213 to reduce amphetamine-induced hyperactivity and restore apomorphine-induced disruption of prepulse inhibition in the absence of catalepsy (Boeckler *et al.*, 2004). Furthermore, the D_4 receptor may not be without therapeutic potential; the selective D_4 antagonist PNU-101387 has been reported to prevent stress-induced cognitive deficits (Arnsten *et al.*, 2000), while the selective D_4 agonists A-412997, CP226269, and PD168077 show some cognitive enhancing properties, particularly in relation to social recognition memory (Browman *et al.*, 2005); furthermore, the selective D_4 agonist ABT-670 may have efficacy for the treatment of erectile dysfunction (Patel *et al.*, 2006).

Current status of selective D_1-like antagonism

Given the above weight of evidence indicating a primary role for D_2 receptor antagonism in antipsychotic drug action, it engendered some initial surprise that studies with selective D_1-like antagonists indicated them to be active in many traditional functional models held to predict antipsychotic activity (Waddington, 1993); however, this unexpected profile might have a basis in D_1-like–D_2-like interactions, which play a critical role in regulating the totality of DAergic neurotransmission (Waddington *et al.*, 1994). Though subsequent clinical trials have indicated each of the selective D_1-like antagonists ecopipam (also designated SCH 39166; de Beaurepaire *et al.*, 1995; Den Boer *et al.*, 1995; Karlsson *et al.*, 1995; Labelle *et al.*, 1998) and NNC 01-0687 (Karle *et al.*, 1995) to be without either antipsychotic activity or major adverse effects, these limited trials have been conducted generally in small numbers of patients with varying degrees of experimental rigor; unexpectedly, two of these (Den Boer *et al.*, 1995; Karle *et al.*, 1995) have suggested some modest activity to ameliorate negative symptoms.

While this area has subsequently experienced some considerable neglect, it should be noted that cortical D_1-like receptor-mediated processes may play an important role in regulating aspects of cognitive function known to be impaired in schizophrenia; neuroimaging findings in living patients indicate cognitive impairment, and aspects of the negative symptom domain may possibly reflect reduced release of DA in the PFC (Seamans & Yang, 2004; Guillin *et al.* 2007; see Chapter 20). Such findings raise the possibility of D$_1$-like receptor-mediated therapeutic effects at the level of cognition and suggest a putative role for D$_1$-like agonists rather than antagonists, as considered further below.

As no known agonists or antagonists are able to distinguish meaningfully between D$_1$ and D$_5$ receptors (Niznik *et al.*, 2002), there is currently little evidence on which to evaluate any differential involvement in processes related to psychosis and its treatment.

Reappraisal of the D$_2$ receptor blockade hypothesis by PET and SPECT

In the course of their evolution, the above notions of receptor action have proved heuristic over several decades. However, it must be emphasized that, in the main, they derive from indirect lines of investigation. One of the major subsequent advances has been the emergence of functional neuroimaging techniques for the direct visualization and quantization of drug–receptor interactions in living patients, namely positron emission tomography (PET) and single photon emission computed tomography (SPECT). These techniques cannot yet address directly all of the issues raised by indirect approaches, but they are a powerful new approach to determining both their validity and, critically, their specific relationship to clinical phenomena on an individual patient as well as a population basis.

Concepts of striatal D$_2$ receptor occupancy threshold

With techniques such as PET and SPECT now available, there has arisen the opportunity to generate *in vivo* evidence to better delineate parameters of brain receptor occupancy in relation both to clinical efficacy and to adverse effects. In general, PET and SPECT radioligands, like the majority of antipsychotics, are unable to distinguish materially within members of either the D$_1$-like or the D$_2$-like families of DA receptor. Henceforth, D$_1$ is used as convenient shorthand for D$_1$-like, i.e., D$_1$ and D$_5$ receptors, and D$_2$ is used as convenient shorthand for D$_2$-like, i.e., D$_2$, D$_3$, and D$_4$ receptors, unless specifically indicated otherwise.

Critical to our understanding regarding the relationship between D$_2$ occupancy and antipsychotic efficacy has been the proposal that there is a "threshold", in the range of 65–70% (Farde *et al.*, 1992; Nordstrom *et al.*, 1993; Kapur *et al.*, 2000a). This is not absolute, that is, individuals can respond below this threshold and, conversely, lack of response can be seen in individuals with D$_2$ blockade exceeding this threshold (Wolkin *et al.*, 1989; Coppens *et al.*, 1991; Kapur *et al.*, 2000a). However, administering an antipsychotic dose that exceeds this threshold appears to optimize the chance of clinical response. This has been given real clinical meaning in a study where low-dose haloperidol, i.e., 1 or 2.5 mg daily, was administered to 22 patients with first-episode schizophrenia (Kapur *et al.*, 2000a). A threshold of 65% occupancy optimally separated responders and non-responders: 80% of responders were above this threshold, while 67% of non-responders were below it. Of the 11 non-responders, all could tolerate a dose increase to 5 mg/day. Six of seven individuals with previous D$_2$ occupancies below 65% demonstrated clinical improvement, in contrast to only one of four individuals who had previous D$_2$ occupancies above 65%. This latter finding is thus in keeping with other reports indicating that, while response may be optimized by exceeding a threshold of 65–70%, non-response exists in the face of adequate D$_2$ blockade.

Added to this information have been data indicating that exceeding a threshold of 80% striatal D$_2$ occupancy markedly increases the risk of EPS (Farde *et al.*, 1992; Nordstrom *et al.*, 1993; Kapur *et al.*, 2000a) and depressive symptoms (Bressan *et al.*, 2002). This also indicates that there is a relatively narrow therapeutic window, as defined by D$_2$ occupancy: the optimal chance of clinical response occurs with D$_2$ blockade above 65% but EPS risk is greatest with 80% or greater occupancy (Kapur *et al.*, 2000a). How does this translate into actual clinical doses? Using haloperidol as the reference, 2 mg daily has been reported to result in a mean D$_2$ occupancy of 67% (Kapur *et al.*, 1996); therefore, it represents the minimal dose that would be associated with the best chance of clinical efficacy. Haloperidol in the range of 5 mg results in D$_2$ occupancy in the range of 80% (Nyberg *et al.*, 1996), and one would expect a substantial increase in risk for EPS with doses at or above this level. Saturation of D$_2$ receptors is approached at 10–20 mg haloperidol (Coppens *et al.*, 1991). These data dovetail with clinical evidence, including several large reviews and meta-analyses, indicating that optimal dosing is in the range of 2–12 mg haloperidol equivalents daily (Baldessarini *et al.*, 1988; Bollini *et al.*, 1994). Findings with haloperidol decanoate, administered monthly, indicate that antipsychotic efficacy can be maintained when mean D$_2$ occupancy decreases from 73% (60–82%) at week 1 to 52% (20–74%) at week 4 (Nyberg *et al.*, 1995).

It is necessary to acknowledge that optimal dosage may vary as a function both of phase (acute *vs.* stabilized) and of stage (first or early episode *vs.* chronic) of illness. It has been suggested, for example, that first-episode patients may require lower doses of antipsychotic medication and clinical studies suggest that patients who have been previously treated may need higher doses than first-episode patients (Remington *et al.*, 1998). Subsequent PET data offer indirect support for this, reporting a 34% increase in D$_2$ receptors after long-term antipsychotic exposure (Silvestri et al., 1999); theoretically, up-regulation in D_2 receptors could require increments in dose to obtain the same effect on DAergic transmission (Kapur, 2000). That said, such a finding is unlikely to account for or justify the megadoses which have been documented in relation to antipsychotic use, and do not factor in the receptor changes seen as a function of age that likely contribute to the lower doses required in geriatric populations (Fitzgerald & Seeman, 1999).

Striatal D_2 receptor occupancy in relation to 5-HT$_2$ receptor occupancy

A pharmacological feature held to characterize all second-generation antipsychotics identified to date, with the notable exception of amisulpride, is greater 5-HT$_2$ (actually 5-HT$_{2A/C}$) versus D_2 blockade, and this has long been an influential postulate for the putative advantageous profiles of these compounds (Meltzer et al., 1989), particularly diminished risk for EPS. This line of thinking is based on evidence that 5-HT can modulate DAergic function, particularly at the level of the nigro-striatal and meso-cortical DAergic pathways, as well as reports indicating that administration of selective 5-HT$_2$ antagonists can diminish antipsychotic-induced EPS (Kapur & Remington, 1996; Meltzer et al., 2003). The net result is a wider therapeutic window between those doses that maximize chance of clinical response and those that induce EPS. This proposition, amenable to examination by PET and SPECT in terms of the relationship between D_2 and 5-HT$_2$ occupancies, is not without limitations, as will be considered further below in relation to individual second-generation agents; for example, it should be noted that the first-generation antipsychotic chlorpromazine is associated with almost complete occupancy of both D_2 and 5-HT$_2$ receptors, while the second-generation antipsychotic amisulpride is associated with occupancy of D_2 but not 5-HT$_2$ receptors (Trichard et al., 1998).

A second adverse event that has been linked to D_2 blockade, and one that certainly characterizes all first-generation antipsychotics, is hyperprolactinemia. As with other D_2-related processes, neuroimaging has been able to illuminate the nature of this relationship. For example, D_2 occupancy significantly predicted risk for elevated prolactin: the likelihood was 15% with D_2 occupancy below 72% but this rose to 86% with higher D_2 occupancies (Kapur et al., 2000a). A second report, in this case using raclopride, reported a lower threshold for hyperprolactinemia of 50% (Nordstrom & Farde, 1998). This difference may be accounted for, at least in part, by pharmacodynamic differences between blood–brain barrier permeability; in addition, a number of factors are known to influence prolactin levels (Molitch, 1995). Both reports, though, suggest that a threshold for hyperprolactinemia exists but, as with other

D_2 thresholds discussed, this is not an all-or-none phenomenon.

Finally, some comment is warranted regarding reported D_2 occupancy values. Various factors may influence these, including the scanner itself, the ligands employed, time at scanning in relation to last administered dose, and other technical variables. Differences between reports may be partly explained thereby and in comparing results it is important to consider such factors. It should be noted also that the values reported here reflect striatal D_2 occupancy levels. However, antipsychotic response has been linked to extrastriatal, meso-cortico-limbic D_2 blockade (Davis et al., 1991; see Evolution of the D_2 receptor blockade hypothesis above), while prolactin levels are mediated through D_2 blockade in the pituitary.

Extrastriatal D_2 receptor occupancy

Though it was held originally that PET findings on striatal D_2 occupancy could be extrapolated to reflect D_2 occupancy in extrastriatal regions, such as areas of the limbic system and cortex, some initial SPECT studies with both first- and second-generation agents indicated the contrary (Farde et al., 1997; Pilowsky et al., 1997a; Bigliani et al., 1999, 2000; Talvic et al., 2001; Xiberas et al., 2001). While there remain a number of technical concerns relating to this issue (Olsson & Farde, 2001; Erlandsson et al., 2003), with the introduction of new radioligands and advances in PET and SPECT technologies there is now a considerable body of evidence for differential D_2 occupancy in the temporal cortex, insular cortex, and thalamus vis-à-vis the striatum (Jones & Pilowsky, 2002). These findings will be considered further below in relation to individual second-generation agents.

Clozapine as the prototype second-generation antipsychotic

Evolving concepts of the antipsychotic action of clozapine

We have recently traversed the 20th anniversary of the pivotal trial (Kane et al., 1988) that established the antipsychotic efficacy of clozapine in a material minority of patients refractory to conventional antipsychotics, in the essential absence of EPS (see Chapter 26). However, it should be emphasized that clozapine, even at that time, was not a new drug; rather; it had been synthesized and investigated pharmacologically in the early 1960s and enjoyed long appreciation in Europe for its high therapeutic efficacy with low EPS liability before diminishing utilization due to concern over its propensity to induce potentially fatal agranulocytosis (for a personal memoir of these early events, see Hippius 1989).

Nevertheless, such historical completeness cannot detract from the status of clozapine as an agent that has, over the past two decades, influenced materially our perspectives on antipsychotic drug action. Meta-analysis has sustained the superior clinical efficacy and EPS profile of clozapine, though the extent to which this might relate particularly to negative symptoms, aspects of the deficit syndrome and cognitive impairment, or refractoriness *per se*, and might be reflected in levels of functioning, may have been overstated initially (Wahlbeck *et al.*, 1999; Leucht *et al.*, 2003; McEvoy *et al.*, 2006; Murphy *et al.*, 2006). However, its agranulocytosis liability and associated mandatory blood-count monitoring program, together with its propensity to induce weight gain/glucose dysregulation, seizures, sedation, hypotension, hypersalivation, and myocarditis mean that this important agent does not attract widespread use as a "front-line" antipsychotic, though it still appears underutilized for patients unresponsive to or intolerant of other agents (McEvoy *et al.*, 2006). Uniquely, however, it indicates that our clinical expectations for new antipsychotics can be revised upwards and suggests that pharmacological efforts be directed towards identifying the basis of its advantageous therapeutic profile and resolving the mechanisms of its numerous non-motoric side effect liabilities with a view to identifying more utilitarian agents.

Yet this mission is far from straightforward. Clozapine is a highly non-selective agent that demonstrates an extensive range of actions at multiple levels of neuronal function associated with numerous neurotransmitter systems (Waddington & Casey, 2000; Miyamoto *et al.*, 2005). Indeed, in seriously confounding any such goal, the breadth of these actions means that clozapine can be considered either as a rich reservoir for theorizing on or, alternatively, extremely muddy waters in which to fish for the substrate of a new generation of improved antipsychotic agents.

While clozapine shows modest *in vitro* affinity both for D_2-like ($D_4 > D_2 = D_3$) and D_1-like ($D_1 = D_5$) receptors, particular attention has focused on a purported selectivity for the D_4 receptor (Van Tol *et al.*, 1991; Seeman *et al.*, 1997), which might be better described as a limited preference of uncertain functional significance (Waddington & Casey, 2000). The importance of its D_4 antagonist affinity has been revised downwards by a major proponent in favor of mechanisms based on the nature of its actions at the D_2 receptor (Seeman & Tallerico, 1998; Seeman *et al.* 2006). More specifically, it has been argued that the ability of clozapine (a drug with a high dissociation constant, i.e., "loose" binding) to occupy D_2 receptors appears reduced using a ligand of lower dissociation constant (i.e., "tight" binding), particularly in the presence of higher levels of endogenous DA in competition therewith.

Thus, on taking into account the characteristics of the ligand used, competition from endogenous DA, and antipsychotic cerebrospinal fluid concentrations of free drug, including active metabolites, it may be possible to sustain the relationship between affinity for the D_2 receptor and clinical antipsychotic potency (Seeman *et al.*, 1997, 2006; Seeman & Tallerico, 1998). There are also clinical implications to this complex but heuristic pharmacodynamic analysis, in that "loose"-binding antipsychotics such as clozapine should, in competition with endogenous DA in basal ganglia *versus* cortico-limbic regions: (1) induce less EPS than "tight"-binding antipsychotics such as haloperidol; and (2) may lead to more rapid relapse after discontinuation, due to rapid dissociation from D_2 receptors; indeed, essentially "all" aspects of the pathobiology of psychosis and of antipsychotic efficacy and EPS liability for clozapine are purported to be explicable in terms of D_2 receptor-mediated effects (Seeman & Tallerico, 1999; Seeman *et al.*, 2006). It will be important to clarify through further preclinical and clinical experimentation the extent to which these putative pharmacodynamic effects and their predictions can be sustained.

Variant mechanisms

Clozapine shows considerably higher *in vitro* antagonist affinity for multiple non-DAergic than for DA receptor subtypes, particularly α ($\alpha_1 > \alpha_2$), H ($H_1 > H_3$), M ($M_1 > M_5 > M_{4(agonist)} > M_3 > M_2$) and 5-HT (5-HT$_{2A}$ = 5-HT$_6$ > 5-HT$_{2C}$ > 5-HT$_7$ > 5-HT$_3$ > 5-HT$_{1A[partial agonist]}$), together with actions at other levels of synaptic transmission (Waddington & Casey, 2000; Miyamoto *et al.*, 2005). These diverse non-DAergic effects of clozapine have engendered many alternative formulations for its clinical profile in terms of antipsychotic efficacy with low EPS liability but propensity for numerous other adverse effects.

Its profile of high 5-HT$_{2A}$ affinity with D_2 antagonism has been posited to result in enhanced release of DA to mitigate EPS due to D_2 blockade in the basal ganglia, and to ameliorate negative symptoms and cognitive dysfunction due to putative DAergic deficits in the PFC (Meltzer *et al.*, 2003; but see Carpenter *et al.*, 2000); however, while clozapine, but not haloperidol, has been shown to preferentially augment DA release in the PFC relative to the striatum in both rodents and non-human primates (Youngren *et al.*, 1999; Meltzer *et al.*, 2003), some anomalies are evident (Seeman *et al.*, 1997). Nevertheless, this proposition has proven influential and heuristic to the field. The high affinity of clozapine for 5-HT$_6$ and 5-HT$_7$ receptors has prompted consideration of these sites also as contributing to an advantageous antipsychotic profile (Meltzer *et al.*, 2003; Semenova *et al.*, 2008); however, these have received less systematic evaluation. Another influential variant emphasizes 5-HT$_{1A}$ partial agonist activity; when occurring in combination with D_2 antagonist activity, this may contribute not only to mitigation of EPS but additionally to enhancement of prefrontal DA release and putative therapeutic advantage (Meltzer *et al.*, 2003; Bardin *et al.*, 2007;

Lawrence, 2007). A further variant posits α_0-antagonist activity to also augment prefrontal DA release, perhaps via interactions with D_1/N-methyl-D-aspartate (NMDA)-mediated mechanisms (Sokoloff, 2005; Wadenberg *et al.* 2007).

Though heterogeneous, each of these formulations encompasses, in addition to D_2 antagonism, an action associated putatively with enhancement of DA release in the PFC, in accordance with contemporary perspectives on the pathophysiology of schizophrenia (Waddington & Morgan, 2001; Guillin *et al.*, 2007; see Chapter 20).

N-desmethylclozapine

In humans, clozapine has a major metabolite, *N*-desmethylclozapine (also designated ACP-104) with *in vitro* antagonist affinities that include: $H_1 > 5\text{-}HT_{2A/C/6/7} > D_{2[\text{partial agonist}]} = D_{3[\text{partial agonist}]} = D_4 = \alpha_{1A/B} = M_{1[\text{partial agonist}]} > 5\text{-}HT_{1A[\text{partial agonist}]}$ (Bursten *et al.*, 2005; Lameh *et al.*, 2007). Thus, this metabolite shows both similarities and differences *vis-à-vis* its parent compound. The extent to which *N*-desmethylclozapine may contribute to the overall clinical profile of clozapine, or indeed constitute a novel antipsychotic in its own right, is rendered uncertain by conflicting data as to its effects in preclinical models held to predict antipsychotic activity (Lameh *et al.*, 2007; Natesan *et al.*, 2007).

Continuing appraisal of clozapine by PET and SPECT

Data in patients with schizophrenia have confirmed low D_2 occupancy for clozapine, even at the highest therapeutic dose of 900 mg; in contrast, $5\text{-}HT_2$ blockade is consistently higher, with occupancy approaching saturation (Farde *et al.*, 1992, 1994; Kapur *et al.*, 1999); while there is appreciable occupancy of $5\text{-}HT_{1A}$ receptors in non-human primates (Chou *et al.*, 2003), no such occupancy was observed in patients (Bantick *et al.*, 2004a). Clozapine shows appreciable occupancy of muscarinic receptors; this may contribute both to anticholinergic side effects and to low liability for EPS (Raedler *et al.*, 2003; Raedler, 2007).

These *in vivo* D_2 occupancy data for clozapine constitute a fundamental finding. As discussed above, neuroimaging studies have led to the notion that optimal clinical response is achieved when D_2 blockade exceeds a 65–70% threshold (Farde *et al.*, 1992; Nordstrom *et al.*, 1993; Kapur *et al.*, 1999); yet data now indicate clozapine, an agent with at least comparable and likely greater efficacy than all other antipsychotics, achieves that efficacy at D_2 occupancies below this proposed threshold. How can this apparent anomaly be reconciled? One explanation is that the model of a 65–70% threshold is incorrect. However, this finding has been confirmed at several centers, using different antipsychot-

ics. An alternative explanation is that antipsychotic efficacy can be achieved through mechanisms that are not exclusively dependent on D_2 activity. Indeed, in the case of clozapine, might D_2 activity be a "red herring", without material relation to its antipsychotic effect and distinguishing it from a class of antipsychotics that are dependent on D_2 antagonism to effect antipsychotic activity?

An answer to this conundrum appears to evolve through an integration of both *in vitro* and *in vivo* evidence. Based on the *in vitro* work described above, suggesting that antipsychotic compounds may differ in the nature of their binding to the D_2 receptor, first-generation antipsychotics such as haloperidol bind "tightly" and dissociate slowly, while clozapine binds "loosely" and dissociates rapidly (Seeman & Tallerico, 1999; Kapur & Seeman, 2000). More recent *in vivo* data involving PET complements this line of thinking. It appears that clozapine is characterized by transient D_2 occupancy, such that levels measured 12–24 h after the last administered dose are markedly lower than those evident within the first several hours (Kapur *et al.*, 2000b,c). Thus, the apparently low striatal D_2 occupancy of antipsychotic agents such as clozapine can be accounted for, at least in part, by transient D_2 blockade, and their clinical efficacy does not contradict a model predicated on D_2 antagonism. The question remains, though, as to how long an antipsychotic must bind to the D_2 receptor in order to optimize the likelihood of clinical response while minimizing risk of D_2-related adverse events.

It is increasingly apparent that while D_2 occupancy represents the *sine qua non* of antipsychotic activity, sustained blockade may not be necessary (Kapur & Seeman, 2001; Tauscher *et al.*, 2002; Uchida *et al.*, 2008). Indeed, clinical advantages that may be ascribed to other pharmacological features of the second-generation antipsychotics, characterized in general by heterogeneous receptor binding profiles, may relate to their relative "sparing" of DA. More specifically, D_2 blockade is associated with numerous side effects beyond EPS and hyperprolactinemia, including motivational deficits and dysphoria (de Visser *et al.*, 2001; de Haan *et al.*, 2004; Voruganti & Awad, 2004; Saeedi *et al.*, 2006). Clinical benefits in each of these areas may be achieved through avoiding continuous D_2 occupancy. Furthermore, there is at least theoretical evidence to suggest that transient exposure may enhance response by avoiding DA supersensitivity, as reflected by D_2 receptors in the high-affinity state (Samaha *et al.*, 2008).

Another factor is evidence that clozapine exerts greater occupancy of extrastriatal than of striatal D_2 receptors, with the following rank order: temporal cortex > thalamus = amygdala > striatum > substantia nigra; occupancy in the temporal cortex approaches the threshold of 60%, though such selectivity may be lost at very high plasma concentrations (Grunder *et al.*, 2006; Kessler *et al.*, 2006); within the striatum, occupancy has been reported to be greater in limbic-related ventral striatum/caudate than in putamen in one study (Grunder *et al.*, 2006) but not in another (Kessler *et al.*, 2006).

There is consistent evidence that clozapine exerts greater occupancy of striatal D_1-like receptors than does any other antipsychotic, to a level similar to its occupancy of striatal D_2 receptors (Nordstom *et al.*, 1995; Tauscher *et al.*, 2004) and possibly to a level greater than its occupancy of D_2 receptors in the frontal cortex (Chou *et al.*, 2006). Given the uncertain role of D_1-like antagonism in antipsychotic activity (see Current status of selective D_1-like antagonism, above), this action of clozapine is of similarly uncertain import but may have been underestimated.

Subsequent second-generation antipsychotics

Given the evolving controversy over the extent to which the clinical profiles of second-generation ("atypical") antipsychotics might be superior to those of their first-generation ("typical") counterparts (see Origins of contemporary concepts and challenges, above), it is important to evaluate the pharmacological actions of each second-generation agent individually and then consider unity *versus* heterogeneity in their profiles *vis-à-vis* their first-generation counterparts. Essentially, all second-generation agents show generally similar (though not identical) psychopharmacological profiles in behavioral and other functional models held to predict therapeutic efficacy *vis-à-vis* side effect liability, particularly in relation to EPS; these effects have been considered exhaustively elsewhere (Arnt & Skarsfeldt, 1998; Waddington & Casey, 2000; Geyer & Ellenbroek, 2003; Waddington *et al.*, 2003; Kapur *et al.*, 2005). Similarly, their clinical profiles have received exhaustive review and meta-analysis (Davis *et al.*, 2003; Leucht *et al.*, 2003; see Chapter 25). The focus here is on (1) their relative actions at the levels of transmitter receptors and selected aspects of cellular function, and (2) the extent to which PET and SPECT can inform directly on these processes in living patients in relation to clinical and adverse effects.

Amisulpride and the enigma of sulpiride

Amisulpride

This substituted benzamide is *in vitro* a low affinity, selective antagonist of D_2-like ($D_2 > D_3 \gg D_4$) with little or no affinity for D_1-like or non-DAergic receptors (Coukell *et al.*, 1996; Schoemaker *et al.*, 1997; Waddington & Casey, 2000; Miyamoto *et al.*, 2005). It has been argued on the basis of preclinical studies that (1) lower doses of amisulpride preferentially block presynaptic D_2-like autoreceptors to give a relative enhancement of DAergic function, which may subserve clinical effectiveness against negative symptoms (Leucht *et al.*, 2002), and (2) higher doses antagonize certain

postsynaptic DA receptor-mediated functions, particularly in cortico-limbic regions and the pituitary, to exert antipsychotic efficacy with low EPS liability but prominent elevation of prolactin secretion (Perrault *et al.*, 1997; Schoemaker *et al.*, 1997; Mota *et al.*, 2002; McKeage & Plosker, 2004). There is evidence for only transient occupancy of D_2 receptors ("loose" binding) due to rapid dissociation (Seeman, 2002).

In patients with schizophrenia, PET studies indicate lower doses of amisulpride (50–100 mg] to occupy only 4–26% of striatal D_2 receptors, while higher doses (200–800 mg) occupy 38–76% thereof (Martinot *et al.*, 1996); a recent study has indicated such doses to give occupancies of 43–85% in the putamen and 67–90% in the caudate (Vernaleken *et al.*, 2004). It has been confirmed that such occupancy of D_2 receptors by 200–1200 mg amisulpride occurs in the absence of cortical 5-HT_2 receptor occupancy (Trichard *et al.*, 1998). Amisulpride occupies extrastriatal D_2 receptors with a rank order of temporal cortex > thalamus > striatum (Xiberas *et al.*, 2001; Bressan *et al.*, 2003a) and occupancy of limbic-related ventral striatum/caudate may exceed that in the putamen (Stone *et al.*, 2005). Hyperprolactinemia induced by amisulpride appears uncoupled from brain D_2 receptor occupancy, reflecting poor blood–brain barrier penetration and accounting for high levels of prolactin with low EPS (Bressan *et al.*, 2004).

As a selective D_2-like antagonist without meaningful interactions at any other known receptor site, amisulpride constitutes a fundamental challenge for any generalized mechanism(s) of antipsychotic activity for first- or second-generation agents that invoke activity at other DA or non-DA receptor subtypes.

Sulpiride

The ongoing debate on the extent to which the superiority of second-generation antipsychotics over their first-generation counterparts may have been overstated (see Origins of contemporary concepts and challenges, above) presents a number of mechanistic as well as clinical challenges. In one influential study, the most frequently administered first-generation agent was sulpiride and the least frequently administered second-generation agent was amisulpride (Jones *et al.*, 2006). Thus, to interpret fully the clinical finding of no advantage for second-generation agents, whether in terms of symptomatology, quality of life or associated costs of care, it is necessary to evaluate carefully the pharmacology of sulpiride *vis-à-vis* that of amisulpride; in particular, it is instructive to revisit these authors' opinion that for sulpiride "… its pharmacological features have little in common with amisulpride" (Jones *et al.*, 2006, p. 1086). Because sulpiride was developed in the 1960s, the database thereon is substantially from a different era and lacks the contemporary breadth, depth, and rigor of that on amisulpride. Nevertheless, the comparison is important.

Like amisulpride, sulpiride is a substituted benzamide that exerts *in vitro* low affinity, selective antagonism of D_2-like receptors ($D_2 > D_3 \gg D_4$) with little or no affinity for D_1-like or non-DAergic receptors (Jenner *et al.*, 1982; O'Connor & Brown, 1982; Caley & Weber, 1995; Waddington *et al.*, 1997; Miyamoto *et al.*, 2005). Similarly, as for amisulpride, it has been argued on the basis of preclinical studies that (1) lower doses of sulpiride preferentially block presynaptic D_2-like autoreceptors to give a relative enhancement of DAergic function, which may subserve clinical effectiveness against negative symptoms, while (2) higher doses antagonize certain postsynaptic DA receptor-mediated functions, particularly in cortico-limbic regions and the pituitary, to exert antipsychotic efficacy with low EPS liability but prominent elevation of prolactin secretion (Caley & Weber, 1995; Mauri *et al.*, 1996; Schoemaker *et al.*, 1997); in this context, the available clinical data (Caley & Weber, 1995; Mauri *et al.*, 1996; Soares *et al.*, 2000) are insufficient to clarify (but do not disprove) any particular efficacy of sulpiride against negative symptoms *vis-à-vis* that indicated for amisulpride. Furthermore, as for amisulpride, there is evidence for only transient occupancy of D_2 receptors ("loose" binding) due to rapid dissociation (Seeman & Tallerico, 1998).

In normal subjects, PET studies indicate low doses of sulpiride (200–400 mg) occupy 17–28% of striatal D_2 receptors (Mehta *et al.*, 2008), while higher doses (200–800 mg) give D_2 occupancies of 25–68% in extrastriatal regions (temporal cortex, PFC, and thalamus; Takano *et al.* 2006); these occupancy values are comparable to those achieved by amisulpride in patients with schizophrenia. There are few PET or SPECT studies on sulpiride in schizophrenia, with one systematic study (Farde *et al.*, 1992) indicating striatal D_2 receptor occupancies similar to those reported for amisulpride. There are no systematic studies in extrastriatal regions.

In overview, the pharmacological profile of sulpiride has much in common with that of amisulpride and the extent to which the clinical profile of sulpiride is similar to or differs from that of amisulpride is not clear. As a selective D_2-like antagonist without meaningful interactions at any other known receptor site, sulpiride joins amisulpride in constituting a joint challenge for any generalized mechanism(s) of antipsychotic activity for first- or second-generation agents that invoke activity at other DA or non-DA receptor subtypes.

Olanzapine

This thienobenzodiazepine *in vitro* is a high-affinity antagonist of 5-HT ($5\text{-}HT_{2A/C} > 5\text{-}HT_6 > 5\text{-}HT_3) = M_{1-4} = H_1 > D_2$-like ($D_2 = D_3 = D_4$) > D_1-like = α ($\alpha_1 > \alpha_2$)(Bymaster *et al.*,

1996; Schotte *et al.*, 1996; Waddington & Casey, 2000; Miyamoto *et al.*, 2005).

Initial PET and SPECT studies in patients with schizophrenia have demonstrated that at therapeutic doses, striatal D_2 occupancy appears greater than for clozapine but less than for risperidone (Pilowsky *et al.*, 1996; Kapur *et al.*, 1998, 1999). At currently recommended therapeutic doses, i.e., 5–20 mg daily, a profile of greater $5\text{-}HT_2$ *versus* D_2 occupancy can be shown; however, as dosage is increased, $5\text{-}HT_2$ occupancy approaches saturation while D_2 occupancy continues to rise, with diminution in the $5\text{-}HT_2$:D_2 ratio purported to account for features such as increased EPS (Kapur *et al.*, 1998, 1999).

Nevertheless, this agent appears to have a wider than expected therapeutic dose range before EPS are evident clinically. One additional explanation for this may be the inherent muscarinic activity that has been identified for olanzapine, both *in vitro* (Bymaster *et al.*, 1996) and *in vivo* by SPECT (Raedler *et al.*, 2000; Raedler, 2007); however, this is less than is evident for clozapine (Raedler *et al.*, 2003; Raedler, 2007). Additionally, among second-generation antipsychotics, olanzapine exerts the highest occupancy of striatal D_1 receptors other than clozapine (Tauscher *et al.*, 2004).

While some studies have reported olanzapine to preferentially occupy extrastriatal sites with a rank order of temporal cortex > thalamus > striatum (Bigliani *et al.*, 2000; Xiberas *et al.*, 2001), there are also contradictory data (Kessler *et al.*, 2005). Occupancy of D_2 receptors in the striatum is predictive of amelioration of positive but not negative symptoms by olanzapine, while occupancy in extrastriatal regions does not predict responsivity (Agid *et al.*, 2007); D_2 occupancy in each of ventral and dorsal striatum and temporal and insular cortex is predictive of negative subjective experience during treatment with olanzapine (Mizrahi *et al.*, 2007).

Recently, olanzapine has been examined in patients with bipolar disorder (Attarbaschi *et al.*, 2007); as in schizophrenia, the therapeutic dose range of 5–20 mg daily was associated with striatal D_2 occupancy of 28–68% in the absence of EPS.

Long-acting injectable olanzapine

Olanzapine has also been developed in a long-acting, injectable preparation, as a pamoate derivative that is administered intramuscularly at intervals of 2–4 weeks (Mamo *et al.*, 2008a).

PET data in schizophrenia indicate a therapeutic dose of 300 mg given every 4 weeks to occupy 53–62% of striatal D_2 receptors over 3–6 months of repeated administration, when assessed before the administration of the next injection; there were no consistent changes in psychiatric status, EPS or other adverse effects from baseline at discontinuation of oral medication (Mamo *et al.*, 2008a).

Quetiapine

This dibenzothiazepine *in vitro* is a low-affinity antagonist of $H_1 > 5\text{-HT}$ ($5\text{-HT}_{2A} > 5\text{-HT}_7$) $= \alpha_{1/2} > D_2$-like ($D_2 = D_3 > D_4$) $> D_1$-like $=$ M receptors (Fulton & Goa, 1995; Schotte *et al.*, 1996; Waddington & Casey, 2000; Miyamoto *et al.*, 2005).

PET and SPECT data in patients with schizophrenia are particularly interesting on several levels. Like clozapine, striatal D_2 occupancy is quite low (Tauscher *et al.*, 2004); while 5-HT_2 occupancy is consistently higher, it does not approach saturation across the recommended therapeutic dose range up to 750 mg daily (Kapur *et al.*, 2000c; Tauscher-Wisniewski *et al.*, 2002). An important additional finding is its transient D_2 occupancy; it is like clozapine in this respect and, in fact, shows yet "looser" binding (Kapur *et al.*, 2000c). Furthermore, while *in vivo* data indicate high 5-HT_2 blockade with clozapine, even at the lowest therapeutic doses, this is not the case for quetiapine, where doses of 300–600 mg have been associated with occupancy of 5-HT_2 receptors of up to 78% (Kapur *et al.*, 2000c), and 450–750 mg with 57–74% occupancy thereof (Gefvert *et al.*, 2001).

Quetiapine preferentially occupies extrastriatal D_2 receptors with a rank order of temporal cortex > thalamus > striatum, with similar occupancies in the ventral striatum, putamen, and substantia nigra (Stephenson *et al.*, 2000; Kessler *et al.*, 2006), but exerts yet higher occupancy of 5-HT_2 receptors in the frontal cortex (Jones *et al.*, 2001).

Extended-release quetiapine

Quetiapine has also been developed in an extended-release formulation of film-coated quetiapine fumarate for once-daily oral administration (Kahn *et al.*, 2007). Initial PET studies indicate that once-daily dosing of 300–800 mg extended-release quetiapine fumarate results in striatal D_2 occupancies comparable to twice-daily administration of quetiapine (Mamo *et al.*, 2008b)

Risperidone and related antipsychotic preparations

This benzisoxazole has very high *in vitro* affinity for 5-HT ($5\text{-HT}_{2A} > 5\text{-HT}_7 \gg 5\text{-HT}_{1A/2C/3/6}$) and high affinity for D_2-like ($D_2 > D_3 = D_4$), α ($\alpha_1 > \alpha_2$) and H_1 receptors (Schotte *et al.*, 1996; Waddington & Casey, 2000; Miyamoto *et al.*, 2005); an active metabolite, 9-OH-risperidone (see below), has a pharmacological profile very similar to that of the parent compound and contributes substantively to its overall clinical activity.

PET data in schizophrenia have confirmed that at the recommended therapeutic dose range, 2–6 mg daily, a profile of greater striatal 5-HT_2 *versus* D_2 blockade is evident; however, as dosage is increased, 5-HT_2 occupancy approaches saturation while D_2 occupancy continues to rise such that, ultimately, the $5\text{-HT}_2{:}D_2$ ratio purported to account for features such as reduced EPS is lost, and from this standpoint risperidone begins to look like a first-generation antipsychotic (Kapur & Remington, 1996; Kapur *et al.*, 1995; 1999; Reimold *et al.*, 2007). At such therapeutic doses, substantive occupancy of striatal D_2 receptors is associated with only low occupancy of their D_1 counterparts (Tauscher *et al.*, 2004; Reimold *et al.* 2007).

Risperidone preferentially occupies extrastriatal sites with a rank order of temporal cortex > thalamus > striatum (Xiberas *et al.*, 2001; Bressan *et al.*, 2003b). Occupancy of D_2 receptors in the striatum is predictive of amelioration of positive but not negative symptoms by risperidone, while occupancy in extrastriatal regions does not predict responsivity (Agid *et al.*, 2007). As D_2 occupancy in ventral striatum/caudate may exceed that in the putamen (Stone *et al.*, 2005), the limbic-related ventral striatum may be an important mediator of antipsychotic activity. Conversely, D_2 occupancy in each of the ventral and dorsal striatum and temporal and insular cortex is predictive of negative subjective experience during treatment with risperidone (Mizrahi *et al.*, 2007).

Long-acting injectable risperidone

Risperidone has also been developed in a long-acting, injectable preparation, using a microsphere formulation that is administered intramuscularly in aqueous solution at intervals of 2–3 weeks (Moller, 2007).

PET data in schizophrenia have indicated therapeutic doses of 25 and 50 mg given every 2 weeks to stabilization, to occupy 25–48% and 59–83% of striatal D_2 receptors, respectively (Gefvert *et al.*, 2005). A subsequent study utilizing these same doses has indicated mean occupancies of 71–74% shortly after injection and 54–65% shortly before the following injection (Remington *et al.*, 2006).

Extended-release paliperidone

This active 9-OH metabolite of risperidone, like the parent compound, shows very high *in vitro* affinity for 5-HT ($5\text{-HT}_{2A} > 5\text{-HT}_7 \gg 5\text{-HT}_{1A/2C/3/6}$) and high affinity for D_2-like ($D_2 > D_3 = D_4$), α ($\alpha_1 > \alpha_2$) and H_1 receptors (Schotte *et al.*, 1996).

Paliperidone has been developed primarily in an extended-release, osmotic membrane-based tablet formulation to effect controlled delivery of this active metabolite of risperidone during once-daily oral administration (Kane *et al.*, 2007; Marder *et al.*, 2007; Yang & Plosker, 2007). Initial PET studies in schizophrenia during sustained administration of 3–15 mg daily (Arakawa *et al.*, 2008) indicate D_2 receptor occupancy of 54–86% in the striatum and 35–87% in the temporal cortex, with therapeutic doses of 6–9 mg associated with 70–80% occupancy of D_2 receptors in both striatal and extrastriatal regions.

Sertindole

This phenylindole *in vitro* is a high-affinity antagonist of 5-HT ($5\text{-HT}_{2A/C} > 5\text{-HT}_7$) > α_1 > D_2-like ($D_2 = D_3 = D_4$) receptors (Dunn & Fitton, 1996; Schotte *et al.*, 1996; Waddington & Casey, 2000; Miyamoto *et al.*, 2005). Following its launch in 1996, sertindole was in 1998 the subject of a voluntary product withdrawal in European Union countries by the manufacturers due to concerns about cardiac arrhythmias associated with prolongation of QTc interval. It was re-introduced in 2002 under strict regulatory conditions and oversight (Lewis *et al.*, 2005; Murdoch & Keating, 2006) and continues to receive experimental as well as clinical interrogation (Lindstrom *et al.*, 2005; Hertel, 2006; Peuskens *et al.*, 2007).

PET and SPECT data in schizophrenia indicate that 20–24 mg sertindole shows high occupancy both of striatal D_2 and of cortical 5-HT_2 receptors (Pilowsky *et al.*, 1997b; Travis *et al.*, 1997). More recently, quantitative SPECT studies have indicated 8–24 mg sertindole to occupy 47–74% of striatal D_2 receptors and suggest that previous higher estimates may have been influenced by prior treatment with depot antipsychotics (Kasper *et al.*, 1998; Bigliani *et al.*, 2000). In the face of conflicting data, whether sertindole exerts preferential occupancy of extrastriatal *versus* striatal D_2 receptors remains unresolved (Bigliani *et al.*, 2000; Nyberg *et al.*, 2002).

Because of concerns over the cardiac safety of sertindole, this aspect of its pharmacology has continued to receive investigation. An initial observation of high-affinity antagonism of the human cardiac potassium channel HERG as a basis for prolongation of QTc interval (Rampe *et al.*, 1998), particularly in relation to the effects of sertindole on other cardiac functions and its affinity for D_2 and 5-HT_2 receptors (Kongsamut *et al.*, 2002; Crumb *et al.*, 2006), has generated continuing interest in cardiac parameters (Lindstrom *et al.*, 2005).

Ziprasidone

This indolone derivative *in vitro* is a high-affinity antagonist of 5-HT ($5\text{-HT}_{2A} = 5\text{-HT}_{1D/7} > 5\text{-HT}_{1A[agonist]/2C}$) > D_2-like ($D_2 = D_3 > D_4$) > α ($\alpha_1 > \alpha_2$) > H_1 receptors; in addition, it inhibits reuptake of both norepinephrine and 5-HT (Seeger *et al.*, 1995; Schotte *et al.*, 1996; Waddington & Casey, 2000; Miyamoto *et al.*, 2005).

Initial PET data in healthy volunteers confirmed a profile of greater striatal 5-HT_2 *versus* D_2 occupancy at doses of 20–40 mg (Bench *et al.*, 1996; Fischman *et al.*, 1996), with little occupancy of 5-HT_{1A} receptors (Bantick *et al.*, 2004b). Subsequent studies in schizophrenia at therapeutic doses of 40–120 mg daily indicate striatal D_2 occupancy of 10–73% *versus* frontal cortical 5-HT_2 occupancy of 52–99% (Mamo *et al.*, 2004). While ziprasidone appears to be associated with both lower occupancy of striatal D_2 receptors and fewer EPS (Swainston *et al.*, 2006) than haloperidol, D_2 receptor occupancy during treatment of acute psychotic exacerbations with 80–120 mg daily is predictive of clinical efficacy and EPS (Corripio *et al.*, 2005). Although the issue of transience of binding to D_2 receptors has yet to be formally assessed, initial time–activity curves, in conjunction with evidence indicating only short-term prolactin elevation, would suggest that its occupancy may be more transient than would be seen with first-generation antipsychotics (Bench *et al.*, 1996). Similarly, the issue of any preferential occupancy of extrastriatal *versus* striatal D_2 receptors has yet to receive systematic study.

While many antipsychotics have been associated with prolongation of QTc interval, ziprasidone has attracted perhaps the greatest attention other than sertindole (Haddad & Sharma, 2007). In comparison with sertindole, the affinity of ziprasidone for the human cardiac potassium channel HERG is both lower and less selective *vis-à-vis* its affinity for D_2 and 5-HT_2 receptors (Kongsamut *et al.*, 2002). Thus, residual concerns should be evaluated in context (Taylor, 2003; Haddad & Sharma, 2007).

Zotepine

This dibenzothiazepine *in vitro* is a high-affinity antagonist of 5-HT ($5\text{-HT}_{2A/C} = 5\text{-HT}_{6/7}$) = α_1 = H_1 > D_2-like ($D_2 = D_3 = D_4$) > D_1-like receptors, which also inhibits reuptake of norepinephrine (Schotte *et al.*, 1996; Prakash & Lamb, 1998; Waddington & Casey, 2000; Miyamoto *et al.*, 2005).

Zotepine has not received extensive investigation using either PET or SPECT. Initial SPECT studies in schizophrenia using 150 and 300 mg daily were associated with mean striatal D_2 occupancies of 66% and 78%, respectively, in the absence of any clinically relevant EPS (Barnas *et al.*, 2001). There are as yet no studies of any preferential occupancy of extrastriatal *versus* striatal D_2 receptors or occupancy of 5-HT_2 receptors.

Putative "third-generation" antipsychotics

The second-generation agents considered above have generated both an unprecedented research database on antipsychotic drug action and a search for yet safer and more effective medications. Perhaps inevitably, as newer antipsychotics have been developed, some of which are already available for clinical use while others remain in clinical development or traverse regulatory processes, these have been held by some to constitute a "third-generation". For individual agents, novel mechanisms have been proposed, while others appear to act through variants of existing mechanisms. In considering these agents, this terminology is noted here only in its temporal sense. The debate *vis-à-vis* first- *versus* second-generation agents (see Origins of contemporary concepts and challenges, above) behoves us to be highly circumspect in interpreting "third-generation" in terms of relative safety and efficacy.

Aripiprazole

This quinolinone derivative (previously designated OPC-14597) *in vitro* has high affinity for D_2-like ($D_2 > D_3 > D_4$) and 5-HT (5-HT$_{c/6/7}$ > 5-HT$_{1A[partial agonist]}$ > 5-HT$_{2C/67}$) receptors, with modest affinities for $\alpha_{1/2}$ and H_1 receptors; at D_2 and 5-HT$_{1A}$ receptors this affinity is manifest as partial agonist activity (Lawler *et al.*, 1999; Shapiro *et al.*, 2003; Tadori *et al.*, 2005). Evidence as to whether it increases release of DA in the PFC is equivocal (Assie *et al.*, 2005; Li *et al.*, 2004). Aripiprazole may be metabolized differentially in humans and rodents, with an active metabolite in humans retaining partial agonist activity at D_2 receptors but an active metabolite in rodents acting as a D_2 antagonist (Wood *et al.*, 2006); this may complicate extrapolation from rodent studies to those in humans (Natesan *et al.*, 2006a).

It has been proposed that in schizophrenia, partial agonist activity at D_2 receptors results in attenuation of DAergic function, particularly phasic DAergic *hyper*function in subcortical brain regions, but only down to the tonic level of its modest intrinsic activity, thus retaining residual activity through subcortical D_2 receptors and reducing the likelihood of EPS (Grunder *et al.*, 2003; Hamamura & Harada, 2007); more speculatively, partial agonist activity at D_2 receptors might also result in reversal of phasic DAergic *hypo*function in cortical brain regions, but only up to the tonic level of its modest intrinsic activity, thus promoting residual activity through cortical D_2 receptors to perhaps exert some therapeutic effect on the domains of cognitive impairment and negative symptoms (see Waddington & Morgan, 2001; Guillin *et al.*, 2007; Chapter 20). The actions of aripiprazole to induce transient nausea and small decreases in prolactin levels in patients with schizophrenia (El-Sayeh *et al.*, 2006; Bhattacharjee & El-Sayeh, 2008) would be consistent with low but functionally relevant D_2 receptor partial agonism, respectively, in the chemoreceptive trigger zone and pituitary.

Initial PET data in healthy volunteers indicated that while low doses of aripiprazole (0.5–2 mg) occupy <80% of striatal D_2 receptors, higher doses (10–30 mg) occupy up to 95% thereof without EPS or elevated levels of prolactin (Yokoi *et al.*, 2002). Subsequent PET data in schizophrenia have reported therapeutic doses (10–30 mg) to result in mean D_2 receptor occupancies of 87% in the putamen, 93% in the caudate, and 91% in the ventral striatum, with 10 mg occupying 81–88% and 30 mg occupying 90–94% of D_2 receptors in the putamen, in the absence of any material EPS; there was modest (mean, 54%; range, 31–79%) occu-

pancy of 5-HT$_2$ receptors, with minimal (mean, 17%; range, 0–44%) occupancy of 5-HT$_{1A}$ receptors, in temporal and frontal cortices (Mamo *et al.*, 2007). These data are consistent with the modest D_2 partial agonist activity of aripiprazole attenuating DAergic hyperfunction while preserving tonic activity through D_2 receptors to reduce the likelihood of EPS. However, as for findings with amisulpride, they question any substantive involvement of 5-HT$_2$ antagonist and particularly of 5-HT$_{1A}$ partial agonist activity.

Asenapine

This dibenzoxepinopyrrole derivative (previously designated ORG 5222) *in vitro* is a high-affinity antagonist of 5-HT (5-HT$_{2A/C/7}$ > 5-HT$_{1A}$) > D_2-like ($D_2 = D_3 = D_4 > D_1$) = $H_1 = \alpha_{1/2}$ >> M receptors (Schotte *et al.*, 1996; Richelson & Souder, 2000). Asenapine is active in a range of preclinical models predictive of antipsychotic activity with low EPS liability, and additionally, like clozapine, it increases the efflux of DA and potentiates NMDA-induced responses in the PFC (Franberg *et al.*, 2008). The extent to which the receptor and pharmacological profiles of asenapine may relate to initial evidence suggesting efficacy against negative symptoms and cognitive dysfunction in the absence of material EPS, weight gain, and changes in clinical laboratory values or cardiovascular parameters (Alphs *et al.*, 2007; Potkin *et al.*, 2007) remains to be determined.

Initial PET data in healthy volunteers indicated a low dose of asenapine (0.1 mg) to occupy 15–30% of frontal cortical 5-HT$_{2A}$ receptors and 12–23% of striatal D_2 receptors (Andree *et al.*, 1997). As these doses are considerably below those that are clinically effective (10 mg; Potkin *et al.*, 2007), systematic PET and SPECT studies using doses in the therapeutic range are required. The issue of any preferential occupancy of extrastriatal *versus* striatal D_2 receptors remains to be investigated.

Bifeprunox

This benzoxazolone derivative (previously designated DU 127090) has high *in vitro* affinity for D_2-like ($D_2 > D_{3/4}$) > 5-HT$_{1A}$ > 5-HT$_{2A/7}$ receptors; at D_2-like receptors these affinities manifest as D_2 and D_4 partial agonist and D_3 agonist activities, while at 5-HT receptors these affinities manifest as 5-HT$_{1A}$ agonist, 5-HT$_{2A}$ antagonist, and 5-HT$_7$ partial agonist activities (Feenstra *et al.*, 2001; Cuisiat *et al.*, 2007; Newman-Tancredi *et al.*, 2007a). Bifeprunox is active in a range of preclinical models predictive of antipsychotic activity with low EPS liability, but does not appear to increase release of DA in the PFC (Assie *et al.*, 2005; Newman-Tancredi *et al.*, 2007). The extent to which the receptor and pharmacological profiles of bifeprunox may relate to preliminary evidence suggesting therapeutic efficacy in the absence of material EPS, weight gain, and changes in clinical laboratory values or cardiovascular parameters remains to be determined.

There is as yet little information in the scientific literature on its effects in patients, whether in clinical trials or using PET/SPECT.

Iloperidone

This benzisoxazole (previously designated HP 873) *in vitro* has very high affinity for 5-HT ($5-HT_{2A} > 5-HT_{1A/2C/6/7}$) = α ($\alpha_1 > \alpha_2$), high affinity for D_2-like ($D_2 = D_3 > D_4 >> D_1$) > H_1, and low affinity for M receptors (Richelson & Souder, 2000; Kalkman *et al.*, 2001).

Iloperidone is active in a range of preclinical models predictive of antipsychotic activity with low EPS liability, and appears to increase release of DA in the PFC (Szewczak *et al.*, 1995; Ichikawa *et al.*, 2002; Barr *et al.*, 2006). The extent to which the receptor and pharmacological profiles of iloperidone may relate to preliminary evidence (Cucchiaro *et al.*, 2001; Albers *et al.*, 2008) suggesting therapeutic efficacy in the absence of material EPS, weight gain, and changes in clinical laboratory values or cardiovascular parameters, but with liability for hypotension, remains to be determined. Iloperidone is being developed in two additional contexts: in an extended-release, injectable formulation that is administered at intervals of up to 4 weeks; and, more speculatively, in association with pharmacogenetic evaluation.

There is as yet little information in the scientific literature on its effects in patients, whether in clinical trials or using PET/SPECT.

Interim synthesis

Biological mechanisms of antipsychotic activity

Despite over 50 years of research, the only action known to be common to all clinically effective antipsychotic drugs remains varying affinities to block brain DA receptors, primarily those of the D_2 subtype (Kapur & Remington, 2001; Kapur & Mamo, 2003). Current uncertainty regarding the extent to which the clinical profiles of second-generation antipsychotics might be superior to those of their first-generation counterparts confounds putative explanations for the "superiority" of second-generation agents.

Recognizing this uncertainty, the three main variants of D_2 antagonism offered as the substrate of such "superiority" are "loose" binding to D_2 receptors (Kapur & Seeman, 2001) and combined interactions with D_2 and 5-HT receptors; these combination effects are posited to take the form of high-affinity $5-HT_{2A}$ antagonism and/or $5-HT_{1A}$ partial agonism, which are held to mitigate risk for EPS and enhance efficacy via increased cortical DA release (Meltzer *et al.*, 2003; Bardin *et al.*, 2007). Embedded in these proposi-

tions are uncertainties as to the optimal ratio of affinities for distinct receptors and the optimal extent of intrinsic (i.e., partial agonist or inverse agonist) activity, if any, at those receptors. However, while many newer (and indeed some older) antipsychotics do appear to exert such actions, none has yet been shown to have the universality of D_2 antagonism. Furthermore, the pharmacological and human PET/SPECT profiles of amisulpride, and to some extent of aripiprazole, pose specific challenges. Interactions with $5-HT_{2C}$, $5-HT_6$, $5-HT_7$, and α_2 receptors (Meltzer *et al.*, 2003; Sokoloff, 2005; Bardin *et al.*, 2007; Lawrence, 2007; Richtand *et al.*, 2007; Wadenberg *et al.*, 2007; Semenova *et al.*, 2008) have yet to receive the same breadth and depth of investigation but remain heuristic.

Psychological mechanisms of antipsychotic activity

The analysis above has concentrated on mechanistic issues at the level of receptors and related aspects of cellular function. However, there is a clear and substantive explanatory gap between this level of effect and how it translates to the level of psychological processes and associated behavior at which the disorder is manifest and therapeutic benefit assessed. Recent theoretical accounts have sought to elaborate the relationship between pharmacological–neurobiological data and the phenomenological experience of psychosis with respect to its course and treatment.

Kapur and colleagues have postulated a role for DA in psychosis and the action of antipsychotic medication based upon existing findings concerning the role of DA in emotion and behavior (Kapur 2003, 2004; Kapur *et al.* 2005, 2006). In an attempt to reconcile apparently contradictory experimental data indicating dopaminergic involvement in behavioral responses to appetitive and aversive stimuli, contemporary theorists have posited a complementary role for DA in reward prediction (Schultz, 2002, 2007) and motivational salience (Berridge & Robinson, 1998; Kapur *et al.*, 2005). Therefore, it is now established that DA appears to be crucially involved in detecting and encoding the motivational valence of external stimuli and their relationships, which in turn facilitates goal-directed behavior.

Kapur and colleagues hypothesize that in schizophrenia, the interplay of genetic vulnerability and environmental factors act to produce an imbalance in DA neurotransmission. Inappropriate firing and release of DA in a cue- and context-independent manner results in the misattribution of salience to irrelevant events in the external environment. This process, at a neurobiological and psychological level, is hypothesized to proceed for months (a "prodromal" period) prior to the onset of the florid "positive" symptoms of psychosis, such as delusions and hallucinations. In essence, this progressive alteration in perception of novelty and salience attribution, accompanied by the disturbance in DA function, results in the misinterpretation of internally generated percepts and memories as externally driven input. Within this framework, delusions comprise a top-down driven, cognitive explanation on behalf of the patient to rationalize the experience of disturbed novelty perception and salience.

Antipsychotics, by blocking DA function, act to normalize these novelty/salience-based processes. Pharmacological intervention via antipsychotic treatment progressively reduces the formation of new inappropriate associations associated with disturbed salience, and existing faulty associations start to extinguish gradually. With respect to existing delusional formations and hallucinations, Kapur suggests that antipsychotic treatment does not relieve or abolish these symptoms. Rather, it is posited that antipsychotics *lessen their behavioral impact* on the patient. Hence, the process of remission, which is triggered by the salience-attenuating effect of antipsychotic drugs, is attributable to a reduction in the distressing and intrusive effect of psychotic symptoms, allowing the patient to achieve a form of psychological "quiescence". Discontinuation of antipsychotic treatment results in renewed DAergic imbalance, recurrence of abnormal salience processes, and the re-emergence of hitherto suppressed delusions and hallucinations. A number of recent clinical studies in patients with schizophrenia support the notion that the action of antipsychotics may consist of a reduction in the subjective impact of psychotic symptoms rather than their reduction or elimination *per se* (Mizrahi *et al.*, 2005, 2006).

The proposed function of antipsychotics to dampen salience processing also explains the reporting of dysphoria-like symptoms in patients taking antipsychotic medication; chronic blockade of DA neurotransmission attenuates aberrant perceptual and attentional processes, but also disrupts normal functioning in these domains, thereby impacting upon motivational behavior.

Movement disorders

As noted at the outset (see Origins of contemporary concepts and challenges, above), the numerous clinical advantages claimed by second-generation antipsychotics since their inception have been called into question. This even holds true for EPS, the lack of which has been touted as the essence of atypicality (Meltzer, 1995). The challenge has been driven by several lines of thinking. It has been argued that routinely using haloperidol as the comparator, a high-potency first-generation agent with a marked liability of EPS, favors second-generation antipsychotics on this dimension. Also, dosing of haloperidol has often been excessive according to current guidelines, further biasing results in the direction of newer drugs (Geddes *et al.*, 2000). In fact, data involving lower haloperidol doses, as well as less potent conventional agents, support these arguments

(Geddes *et al.*, 2000; Leucht *et al.*, 2003). In addition, it has become increasingly clear that second-generation antipsychotics differ in risk of EPS, with compounds like risperidone and ziprasidone demonstrating a dose-dependent increase in EPS liability (Daniel *et al.*, 1999; Kapur *et al.*, 1995), in contrast to agents such as aripiprazole, clozapine, and quetiapine where this is not observed (Kane *et al.*, 2002; Kapur *et al.*, 2000a; Nordstrom *et al.*, 1995).

While mechanistic explanations can account for these differences between different second-generation antipsychotics (Kapur *et al.* 1999, 2000a), what remains to be answered is how this translates to risk of tardive dyskinesia (TD). Implicit in the assumption of diminished EPS is reduced TD liability, as EPS has been identified as a risk factor in TD (Andrew, 1994; Chouinard *et al.*, 1988; O'Hara *et al.*, 1993; Tenback *et al.*, 2006). Evidence to date, albeit preliminary, suggests that second-generation antipsychotics have a lower risk of TD (Correll *et al.*, 2004; Tarsy & Baldessarini, 2006); however, it is not yet clear whether this will be sustained by longer-term data and whether there are material differences between second-generation antipsychotics based on their diverse mechanisms of action. As an aside, there is also at least theoretical evidence to suggest that advantages in this regard may be influenced by formulation, e.g., oral *versus* depot formulation (Turrone *et al.*, 2002, 2005).

The advantage of reduced TD, given its potential irreversibility and poor response to treatment, cannot be ignored. Whether the newer antipsychotics bestow a benefit in this regard represents a critical but as yet unanswered question, as the purported differences between first- and second-generation antipsychotics shrink and concerns grow around metabolic and weight gain issues (see below).

Weight gain and metabolic dysregulation

One aspect of the increasing scrutiny directed towards second-generation antipsychotic drugs is concern over their variable liabilities, and in some instances marked propensities, to cause weight gain and glucose/lipid dysregulation, and to predispose to diabetes (Meltzer, 2007); indeed this metabolic syndrome, with associated morbidity and mortality, has been considered the "new TD" of second-generation antipsychotics (see Chapter 28).

The wide range of neurotransmitter receptors and related cellular processes targeted by antipsychotic drugs constitutes a rich pharmacology for seeking the biological basis of these effects (Nasrallah, 2008). Recently, second-generation antipsychotics have been shown to potently and selectively exert H_1-receptor-mediated activation of arcuate and paraventricular hypothalamic AMP-kinase, previously associated with the regulation of food intake, in proportion with their orexigenic liability (Kim *et al.*, 2007). If this effect is sustained, it may constitute an essential step in the holistic improvement of antipsychotic treatment.

Of note, there has been a shift in thinking regarding the increased risk of glucose dysregulation associated with second-generation antipsychotics as a class. At least initially, it seemed reasonable to assume that this was simply a secondary effect of the marked weight gain observed with treatment. However, various lines of investigation suggest that there may also be an immediate effect that can occur independent of weight gain (Chintoh *et al.*, 2008; Houseknecht *et al.*, 2006). This would be in line with diabetic ketoacidosis being observed soon after treatment with second-generation antipsychotics in the absence of notable weight gain (Ramankutty, 2002; Nihalani *et al.*, 2007; Ramaswamy *et al.*, 2007).

Pharmacogenetics, pharmacokinetics, and pharmaceutics

The molecular biology era has facilitated understanding not only of the genetics of schizophrenia (Gogos, 2007; Waddington *et al.*, 2007a,b; see Chapters 13 and 19), but also of the genetic prediction of drug pharmacokinetics, therapeutic response, and adverse effects. Consideration of these issues is beyond the scope of this article but has been the subject of recent, authoritative review (Arranz & de Leon, 2007).

In relation to other aspects of pharmacokinetics, both first- and second-generation antipsychotics show material dissociation between brain and plasma levels; they persist at higher concentrations in the brain, in a region-specific manner, relative to decline in plasma concentration, whether using PET imaging in living subjects (Tauscher *et al.*, 2002) or direct measurement in postmortem tissue (Kornhuber *et al.*, 2006). Such effects may be overlooked in interpreting fully the therapeutic and adverse effects of antipsychotic drugs.

New pharmaceutical preparations are available for (1) controlled delivery of antipsychotics during once-daily oral administration, using osmotic membrane and film-coated derivatives, and (2) delivering sustained levels of antipsychotics during periods of 2–4 weeks, using oil-based decanoate/pamoate derivatives and aqueous suspension of microspheres (see Subsequent second-generation antipsychotics, above). As yet longer-acting preparations could be of advantage in certain clinical situations, formulations such as an implantable, biodegradable polylactide-co-glycolide polymer have been shown in proof-of-concept studies in rodents and rabbits to effect antipsychotic delivery over periods of up to 1 year after implantation (Metzger *et al.*, 2007). However, such preparations present practical, clinical, and ethical challenges that may limit their widespread applicability.

Reconceptualizing schizophrenia and its target symptoms

This chapter has as it focus "antipsychotic" drugs, with the identified limitations of even the newer agents demanding an ongoing search for medications that are more effective and/or tolerable. That said, there has been a shift in the direction of drug development for schizophrenia that frames its progressive reconceptualization. The historical primacy of positive symptoms has given way to a broader definition that incorporates various other symptom domains, including cognition (both neurocognition and social cognition) as well as negative/deficit symptoms (Green & Nuechterlein, 1999, 2004; Green *et al.*, 2008; Harvey *et al.*, 2006; Marder & Fenton, 2004; Sergi *et al.*, 2007). Paralleling this has been a shift from clinical to functional measures of outcome, driven in part by "recovery" models and diminishing healthcare resources (Bellack, 2006; Davidson *et al.*, 2008; Goeree *et al.*, 2005; Lester & Gask, 2006). Evidence that it is cognitive and negative, not positive, symptoms that represent the rate-limiting step in functional recovery (Brekke *et al.*, 2007; Dickinson *et al.*, 2007; Greenwood *et al.*, 2005; Harvey *et al.*, 2006), in combination with data indicating that second-generation antipsychotics are not substantially better in the treatment of these domains than first-generation agents (Buckley & Stahl, 2007; Marder, 2006a), has tempered our enthusiasm for the "magic bullet" approach that holds to a single drug effectively managing all features of the illness. Instead, there is a growing interest in the development of symptom-specific pharmacological treatments that can be used individually and in combinations tailored to meet a patient's specific symptom profile.

The practical implications of this shift in thinking can already be observed. First, more and more trials are investigating compounds that are circumscribed in their clinical actions (Alphs, 2007; Gray & Roth, 2007; Marder, 2006a,b). Second, regulatory agencies are now acknowledging this conceptual shift and indicating their willingness to move from the idea of a "one size fits all" antischizophrenia drug to a multifaceted model that builds upon effective antipsychotic treatment with add-on strategies addressing these other symptom domains (Laughren & Levin, 2006).

Experimental approaches

As the above second- and "third"-generation antipsychotics are perhaps at best conceptualized as more an incremental advance than any radical shift in our therapeutic armamentarium, they reinforce the necessity of continuing to search for yet more effective and benign treatment modalities. One approach to this challenge seeks to identify improved agents within our current understanding (or presumption) of putative mechanisms and most of these experimental approaches thus involve variant effects on DA-mediated transmission. A more intellectually satisfying approach seeks to identify and target alternative, non-DAergic systems based on increased understanding of the pathophysiology of schizophrenia (Lewis & Gonzales-Burgos, 2006), some of which may interact with DAergic function. Yet another approach is to improve treatment with existing agents, in terms of pharmacogenetic prediction of optimal responsivity to individual agents; this strategy, now generic to clinical pharmacology in all medical specialities, is a developing area in antipsychotic therapy (Arranz & de Leon, 2007).

New dopamine-related mechanisms

D_2-like receptor "stabilization"

Dopaminergic "stabilizers" have been defined as drugs that inhibit dopaminergic function when it is elevated, and stimulate dopaminergic function when it is reduced (Carlsson et al., 2004). Conceptually and in terms of their therapeutic potential, these agents bear some similarity to D_2-like partial agonists (see Aripiprazole, above). However, unlike aripiprazole, the evidence base for therapeutic efficacy of the prototype agent OSU6162 in schizophrenia remains sparse and anecdotal (Gefvert et al., 2000) and proposals for the mechanism of action of OSU6162 and the related agent ACR16 remain in a state of flux.

These agents were proposed initially to be D_2-like partial agonists but this proposition has metamorphosed through preferential autoreceptor antagonist and partial antagonist activity to effects on extrastriatal D_2-like receptors; most recently, it has been proposed that such agents inhibit elevated dopaminergic function through low-affinity binding to the orthostatic site of D_2-like receptors, but stimulate reduced dopaminergic function through high-affinity binding to an allosteric site of D_2-like receptors (Carlsson & Carlsson, 2006; Lahti et al., 2007). In the face of such mechanistic diversity, the preclinical pharmacology of these intriguing agents (Rung et al., 2005; Natesan et al., 2006b; Seeman & Guan, 2007) is in urgent need of sustenance through clinical data from controlled trials.

More generally, it has been suggested that antipsychotic drugs may be distinguished by their relative positions along a continuum ranging from partial agonism, through antagonism to inverse agonism at D_2 receptors (Heusler et al., 2007).

D_2-like antagonism in combination with serotonergic actions

Arguments based on combining D_2-like antagonism with 5-HT$_{2A/C}$ antagonism and/or 5-HT$_{1A}$ agonism have been influential stimuli for the investigation of numerous addi-

tional compounds having various permutations and combinations of these and related properties.

Commonly, the underlying premise is that a specific balance between two or more of these properties will confer particular advantage in terms of efficacy and/or adverse effects (Lawrence, 2007), as typified by the following investigatory agents: the $D_2/D_3/5$-HT$_{2A}$ antagonist AD-5423 (blonanserin; Nagai et al., 2003); the D_2/D_3 antagonist/5-HT$_{1A}$ agonists SSR181507 (Claustre et al., 2003), and SLV313 (McCreary et al., 2007); the $D_3/5$-HT$_{1A}$ antagonist KKHA-761 (Park et al., 2005); the D_2/D_3 antagonist, D_4 partial agonist, and 5-HT$_{1A}$ agonist F15063 (Newman-Tancredi et al., 2007b); the $D_3/5$-HT$_{2/7}/\alpha_{2C}$ antagonist S33138 (Millan et al., 2008); the D_4 antagonist/5-HT reuptake inhibitor Lu 35-138 (Hertel et al., 2007). An elaboration of this approach involves seeking to duplicate the yet broader, multitarget interactions of clozapine in a novel chemical structure (QF2004B; Brea et al., 2006). However, only data from controlled clinical trials will inform on the validity of these underlying premises.

Selective D_1-like agonists

While selective D_1-like antagonists appear to be without material antipsychotic activity, there may be a putative role for selective D_1-like agonists in relation to cognitive impairment and possibly negative symptoms mediated via reduced DAergic activity through D_1-like receptors in the PFC (see Current status of selective D_1-like antagonism, above). However, studies with the D_1-like agonist dihydrexidine (also designated DAR-0100) in patients with schizophrenia indicate a single subcutaneous dose to be safe and tolerated but without material clinical or cognitive effects, despite an increase in both prefrontal and non-prefrontal perfusion on functional magnetic resonance imaging (fMRI; George et al., 2007; Mu et al., 2007).

While this lack of acute effect might indicate a requirement for more sustained administration, it may reflect the non-selective affinity of dihydrexidine for D_2-like as well as D_1-like receptors (Deveney & Waddington, 1997; Niznik et al., 2002). Preclinical studies with selective D_1-like agonists indicate facilitation of social cognition with enhancement of acetylcholine levels in the hippocampus and PFC (Di Cara et al., 2007), where there are prominent interactions between D_1 and NMDA-glutamate receptors (Castner & Williams, 2007). Thus, further clinical studies with selective D_1-like agonists are warranted.

New non-dopamine-related mechanisms

Selective serotonergic approaches

Arguments based on combining D_2-like antagonism with 5-HT$_{2A/C}$ antagonism and/or 5-HT$_{1A}$ agonism have generated renewed interest in the therapeutic potential of interactions with 5-HT receptor subtypes in the absence of D_2-like antagonism, as typified by the following investigatory agents: the 5-HT$_{2A/C}$ antagonists SR46349B (Meltzer et al., 2004) and ACP-103 (Gardell et al., 2007), which may have inverse agonist activity at 5-HT$_{2A}$ receptors (Nordstrom et al., 2008); the 5-HT$_{2C}$ agonist WAY-163909 (Marquis et al., 2007). The very early phase of investigation of such compounds necessitates studies in a broader range of preclinical models and, ultimately, in controlled clinical trials to clarify the status of such compounds as novel antipsychotics or adjuncts to existing antipsychotic agents.

Neurokinin 3 and other peptide antagonists

On the basis of preclinical studies (Spooren et al., 2005), the neurokinin 3 antagonists osanetant (also designated SR142801) and talnetant (also designated SB-223412) have been the subject of initial clinical trials; in particular, osanetant was associated with modest improvement in psychopathology, to an extent less than that associated with haloperidol, while the cannabinoid 1 antagonist rimonabant (also designated SR141716) and the neurotensin 1 antagonist SR48692 were without effect (Meltzer at al., 2004). Only further studies will clarify the status of such compounds as novel antipsychotics or adjuncts to existing antipsychotic agents.

α7 nicotinic agonists

On the basis of convergent evidence from neurobiological and genetic studies implicating the α7 nicotinic receptor as a possible pathological mechanism in schizophrenia, particularly in relation to cognitive impairment, the partial α7 nicotinic receptor agonists DMXB-A and tropisetron have been the subject of initial clinical trials; these indicated some improvement in cognitive function, particularly in terms of sensory gating (Koike et al., 2005; Olincy et al., 2006). α7 Nicotinic receptor agonists such as NS1738 (Timmermann et al., 2007), PNU-282987 (Hansen et al., 2007), and SSR180711 (Pichat et al., 2007) are the subject of continuing investigations in this heuristic area of therapy.

Glutamatergic approaches

Perhaps the most enduring and, until recently, unfulfilled non-dopaminergic approach to antipsychotic treatment is based on evidence for hypoglutamatergic function in schizophrenia (see Chapter 21). Fuelled by the more homologous psychotomimetic activity of the non-competitive NMDA antagonist phencyclidine (PCP) and evidence for NMDA deficits in postmortem brain in schizophrenia (Coyle, 2006; Stone et al., 2007; see Chapter 21), this proposition has been reinforced by recent SPECT evidence for an NMDA receptor deficit in living patients (Pilowsky et al.,

2006); it may connect to aspects of previous pathobiological and pharmacological schemas through prominent interactions between NMDA and D_1 receptors in the PFC (Castner & Williams, 2007).

An important element of this evolving research front has been a series of clinical trials involving agents such as glycine, D-serine, and D-cycloserine that promote the actions of glycine at an accessory site necessary for NMDA receptor function and thus enhance NMDA-mediated transmission. Meta-analysis of 18 short-term trials indicates some effect of glycine and D-serine, but not D-cycloserine, to attenuate negative but not positive symptoms with little effect on cognition; limited data from studies with the related non-NMDA glutamatergic ampakine CX516 did not allow conclusions to be drawn (Tuominen et al., 2005). The most recent and extensive, placebo-controlled study of glycine and D-cycloserine indicates that neither agent is a generally effective therapeutic option for the treatment of negative symptoms or cognitive impairment in schizophrenia (Buchanan et al., 2007).

A related but alternative therapeutic approach is the promotion of glycine action, and hence facilitation of NMDA transmission, via inhibition of the glycine transporter (Javitt, 2008). The naturally occurring glycine transporter inhibitor sarcosine has received initial study both as adjunctive (Lane et al., 2005) and as monotherapy (Lane et al., 2008); however, these preliminary studies do not yet allow conclusions to be drawn. Preclinical and clinical studies with the glycine transporter inhibitors ORG24461, ORG24598, and SSR504734 (Javitt, 2008) may inform further on the therapeutic potential of this approach.

More provocatively, a recent placebo-controlled clinical trial with the metabotropic glutamate 2/3 receptor agonist LY404039 (Rorick-Kehn et al., 2007), administered for 4 weeks via the prodrug LY2140023, was as effective as olanzapine in reducing both positive and negative symptoms in the absence of prolactin elevation, EPS or weight gain; any effects on cognitive function remain to be determined (Patil et al., 2007). If this finding can be replicated and elaborated with related agents, subsequent recourse to the "retrospectoscope" may recognize it as the progenitor of a new generation of safe and effective non-dopaminergic antipsychotic agents and thus a landmark study in the pharmacotherapy of schizophrenia.

Neuroprotection and related cellular processes as targets for "fourth-generation" antipsychotics

A "one size fits all" medication precludes the possibility of shaping treatment to the specific features that predominate in a given individual at a given stage in their illness. A more sophisticated pharmacological approach would be to define the different dimensions (Tamminga & Davis, 2007), develop targeted treatments for each, and combine these drugs in a flexible manner that addresses each patient's unique requirements along those diverse dimensions. This, of course, requires that we better understand the pathobiologies that appear to underlie different symptom clusters. While most theorizing on and empirical research into the pathobiology and treatment of schizophrenia focuses on neurotransmitter receptor mechanisms, understanding more fundamental levels of cellular dysfunction (see Chapter 18) during evolution of psychotic illness may favor this approach.

Developmental and, more controversially, "neuroprogressive" aspects of the pathobiology of schizophrenia, often considered separately but best subsumed within a lifetime trajectory perspective for the disorder (Baldwin et al., 2004; Waddington et al., 2007a ; see also Chapters 18 and 19), offer related targets for pharmacological intervention. Molecular genetics and putative biomarkers are not yet able to identify on an individual basis those infants and children "at risk" for the disorder in young adulthood (Waddington, 2007). However, the evolving literature on identification of "at-risk" mental state in young adults before the emergence of psychosis has resulted in a series of heuristic studies exploring the potential of early intervention with second-generation antipsychotic drugs to attenuate conversion to psychosis (McGorry et al., 2002; McGlashan et al., 2006). These studies open up the possibility of alternative treatment modalities for neuroprotection. While such actions are predicated on understanding the pathobiology of the underlying cellular process(es) through which psychosis emerges, some tantalizing preliminary findings are emerging; these include the use of antidepressants, omega-3 fatty acids, and anti-inflammatory agents such as COX-2 inhibitors (Akhondzadeh et al., 2007; Berger et al., 2007).

At a more mechanistic level, the tetracycline antimicrobial minocycline has activity to inhibit production of nitric oxide and expression of caspase-1, and caspase-3 expression and exerts neuroprotective effects in preclinical models of ischemic injury and neurodegenerative disease; it is notable that minocycline also protects against the emergence of neurochemical abnormalities and behavioral deficits in the NMDA antagonist model of schizophrenia (Levkovitz et al., 2007; Zhang et al., 2007). The importance of a recent description of sustained benefit from minocycline administration in two patients with catatonic schizophrenia, one near to illness onset and another experiencing an acute exacerbation (Miyaoka et al., 2007), remains to be determined.

Though evidence for a neuroprogressive process over the course of schizophrenia is growing (Waddington & Morgan, 2001; Waddington et al., 2007a), its cellular basis is also poorly understood. Descriptively, active psychosis may mediate clinical deterioration and progressive brain changes via as yet unknown mechanisms that may include disruption of normal processes of synaptic plasticity (McGlashan, 2006). In this regard, it is notable that DA has been reported to exert both toxic and protective effects on neurons in various situations, with D_2 receptors being particularly implicated (Bozzi & Borrelli, 2006). Among several possibilities, apoptosis, a form of programmed cell death, is regulated by a complex cascade of pro- and anti-apoptotic proteins that may be altered in schizophrenia and might mediate subtle, progressive disruption to, and ultimately loss of, cerebral gray matter, particularly over the early course of illness, in the absence of evidence for any neurodegenerative process as currently conceptualized (Glantz et al., 2006; Catts et al., 2006; Waddington, 2007; Waddington et al., 2007a; Tandon et al., 2008).

MRI studies (see Chapter 16) have indicated that exposure to first-generation antipsychotics may be associated with increase in volume of the basal ganglia and pituitary with reduction in cortical gray matter (Lieberman et al., 2005; Pariante et al., 2005), while exposure to second-generation antipsychotics may be associated with increase in cortical gray matter (Dazzan et al., 2005; Garver et al., 2005; Molina et al., 2005); furthermore, there is now a substantial body of evidence for white matter pathology in schizophrenia (Walterfang et al., 2006) and these changes may be modulated by exposure to second-generation antipsychotics (Molina et al., 2005; Garver et al., 2008). While the mechanism(s) underlying these effects are unknown, roles for neurogenesis, forebrain neural stem cell proliferation, neurotrophins, and orexins/hypocretins, the extent to which these cellular processes may be regulated by DA and NMDA, and how they might be influenced by antipsychotic drugs (Kippin et al., 2005; Reif et al., 2007; Buckley et al., 2007; Deutch & Bubser, 2007), remain conjectural but heuristic.

By way of example, the microtubule stabilizer epothilone D elaborates the action of antipsychotics to ameliorate the morphological, physiological, and behavioral phenotype associated with disruption to the murine gene encoding the microtubule-associated protein STOP (Andrieux et al., 2006). Similarly, a putative effect of the orexin/hypocretin modulator modafinil to enhance cognition in schizophrenia (Morein-Zamir et al., 2007) may involve its action to enhance deficient thalamocortical activity (Lambe et al., 2007; Urbano et al., 2007); interestingly, we have shown recently that deletion of the murine gene *Sema6A*, which *inter alia* regulates connectivity in the thalamocortical pathway, is associated with a schizophrenia-like phenotype that is sensitive to very low doses of clozapine (Mitchell et al., 2008). Thus, further understanding of these cellular and morphological mechanisms, both in clinical studies and in mutant models (O'Tuathaigh et al., 2007; Waddington et al., 2007b) holds out the prospect of identifying targets for antipsychotic drugs capable of influencing fundamental neuronal processes to mitigate pathological changes associated with the disease process of schizophrenia at various stages over its lifetime trajectory.

Acknowledgements

The authors' studies are supported by Science Foundation Ireland (07/IN.1/B960) and the Health Research Board of Ireland (PD/2007/20).

References

Adams, C.E., Tharyan, P., Coutinho, E.S. *et al.* (2006) The schizophrenia drug-treatment paradox. *British Journal of Psychiatry* **189**, 391–392.

Agid, O., Mamo, D., Ginovart, N. *et al.* (2007) Striatal vs extrastriatal dopamine D2 receptors in antipsychotic response. *Neuropsychopharmacology* **32**, 1209–1215.

Andrew, H.G. (1994) Clinical relationship of extrapyramidal symptoms and tardive dyskinesia. *Canadian Journal of Psychiatry* **39**, S76–S80

Akhondzadeh, S., Tabatabee, M. & Behnam B. (2007) Celecoxib as adjunctive therapy in schizophrenia. *Schizophrenia Research* **90**, 179–185

Albers, L.J., Musenga A. & Raggi, A. (2008) Iloperidone: a new benzisoxazole atypical antipsychotic drug. *Expert Opinion on Investigational Drugs* **17**, 61–75.

Alphs, L. (2006) An industry perspective on the NIMH consensus statement on negative symptoms. *Schizophrenia Bulletin* **32**, 225–230.

Alphs, L., Panagides J., & Lancaster, S. (2007) Asenapine in the treatment of negative symptoms of schizophrenia. *Psychopharmacology Bulletin* **40**, 41–53.

Andree, B., Halldin, C., Vrijmoed-deVries, M. *et al.* (1997) Central 5-HT2A and D2 dopamine receptor occupancy after sublingual administration of ORG 5222 in healthy men. *Psychopharmacology* **131**, 339–345.

Andrieux, A., Salin, P., Schweitzer, A. *et al.* (2006) Microtubule stabilizer ameliorates synaptic function and behavior in a mouse model for schizophrenia. *Biological Psychiatry* **60**, 1224–1230.

Arakawa, R., Ito, H., Takano, A. *et al.* (2008) Dose-finding study of paliperidone ER based on striatal and extrastriatal dopamine D(2) receptor occupancy in patients with schizophrenia. *Psychopharmacology* **197**, 229–335.

Arnsten, A.F.T., Murphy, B. & Merchant, K. (2000) The selective dopamine D4 receptor antagonist, PNU-101387G, prevents stress-induced cognitive deficits in monkeys. *Neuropsychopharmacology* **23**, 405–410.

Arnt, J. & Skarsfeldt, T. (1998) Do novel antipsychotics have similar pharmacological characteristics? *Neuropsychopharmacology* **18**, 63–101.

Arranz, M.J. & de Leon, J. (2007) Pharmacogenetics and pharmacogenomics of schizophrenia: a review of last decade of research. *Molecular Psychiatry* **12**, 707–747.

Assie, M.B., Ravailhe, V., Faucillon, V. *et al.* (2005) Contrasting contribution of 5-hydroxytryptamine1A receptor activation to neurochemical profile of novel antipsychotics. *Journal of Pharmacology and Experimental Therapeutics* **315**, 265–272.

Attarbaschi, T., Sacher, J., Geiss-Granadia, T. *et al.* (2007) Striatal D(2) receptor occupancy in bipolar patients treated with olanzapine. *European Neuropsychopharmacology* **17**, 102–107.

Baldwin, P.A., Hennessy, R.J., Morgan, M.G. *et al.* (2004) Controversies in schizophrenia research. In: Gattaz, W. & Hafner, H. eds. *Search for the Causes of Schizophrenia.* Darmstadt: Steinkopff, pp. 394–409.

Baldessarini, R.J., Cohen, B.M. & Teicher M.H. (1988) Significance of neuroleptic dose and plasma level in the pharmacological treatment of psychoses. *Archives of General Psychiatry* **45**, 79–91

Bantick, R.A., Montgomery, A.J., Bench, C.J. *et al.* (2004a) A positron emission tomography study of the 5-HT1A receptor in schizophrenia and during clozapine treatment. *Journal of Psychopharmacology* **18**, 346–354.

Bantick, R.A., Rabiner, E.A., Hirani, E. *et al.* (2004b) Occupancy of agonist drugs at the 5-HT1A receptor. *Neuropsychopharmacology* **29**, 847–859.

Bardin, L., Auclair, A., Kleven, M.S. *et al.* (2007) Pharmacological profiles in rats of novel antipsychotics with combined dopamine D2/serotonin 5-HT1A activity. *Behavioural Pharmacology* **18**, 103–118.

Barnas, C., Quiner, S., Tauscher, J. *et al.* (2001) In vivo (123)I IBZM SPECT imaging of striatal dopamine 2 receptor occupancy in schizophrenic patients. *Psychopharmacology* **157**, 236–242.

Barr, A.M., Powell, S.B., Markou, A. *et al.* (2006) Iloperidone reduces sensorimotor gating deficits in pharmacological models, but not a developmental model, of disrupted prepulse inhibition in rats. *Neuropharmacology* **51**, 457–465.

Basu, A. & Meltzer, H.Y. (2006) Differential trends in prevalence of diabetes and unrelated general medical illness for schizophrenia patients before and after the atypical antipsychotic era. *Schizophrenia Research* **86**, 99–109.

Bellack, A.S. (2006) Scientific and consumer models of recovery in schizophrenia. *Schizophrenia Bulletin* **32**, 432–442.

Bench, C.J., Lammertsma, A.A., Grasby, P.M. *et al.* (1996) The time course of binding to striatal dopamine D2 receptors by the neuroleptic ziprasidone (CP-88,059-01) determined by positron emission tomography. *Psychopharmacology* **124**, 141–147.

Berger, G.E., Proffitt, T.M., McConchie M. *et al.* (2007) Ethyl-eicosapentaenoic acid in first-episode psychosis. *Journal of Clinical Psychiatry* **68**, 1867–1875

Berridge, K.C., & Robinson, T.E. (1998) What is the role of dopamine in reward? *Brain Research Reviews* **28**, 309–369.

Bhattacharjee, J. & El-Sayeh, H.G. (2008) Aripiprazole versus typicals for schizophrenia. *Cochrane Database Systematic Review*, CD006617.

Bigliani, V., Mulligan, R.S., Acton, P.D. *et al.* (1999) In vivo occupancy of striatal and temporal cortical D2/D3 dopamine receptors by typical antipsychotic drugs. *British Journal of Psychiatry* **175**, 231–238

Bigliani, V., Mulligan, R.S., Acton, P.D. *et al.* (2000) Striatal and temporal cortical D2/D3 receptor occupancy by olanzapine and sertindole in vivo. *Psychopharmacology* **150**, 132–140.

Boeckler, F., Russig, H., Zhang, W. *et al.* (2004) FAUC 213, a highly selective dopamine D4 receptor full antagonist, exhibits atypical antipsychotic properties in behavioural and neurochemical models of schizophrenia. *Psychopharmacology* **175**, 7–17.

Bollini, P., Pampaliona, S., Orza, M.J. *et al.* (1994) Antipsychotic drugs: is more worse? *Psychological Medicine* **24**, 307–316.

Bozzi, Y. & Borrelli, E. (2006) Dopamine in neurotoxicity and neuroprotection. *Trends in Neuroscience* **29**, 167–174.

Brea, J., Castro, M., Loza, M. I. *et al.* (2006) QF2004B, a potential antipsychotic butyrophenone derivative with similar pharmacological properties to clozapine. *Neuropharmacology* **51**, 251–262.

Brekke, J.S., Hoe, M., Long, J. *et al.* (2007) How neurocognition and social cognition influence functional change during community-based psychosocial rehabilitation for individuals with schizophrenia. *Schizophrenia Bulletin* **33**, 1247–1256.

Bressan, R.A., Costa, D.C., Jones, H.M. *et al.* (2002) Typical antipsychotic drugs: D(2) receptor occupancy and depressive symptoms in schizophrenia. *Schizophrenia Research* **56**, 31–36.

Bressan, R.A., Erlandsson, K., Spencer, E.P. *et al.* (2004) Prolactinemia is uncoupled from central D2/D3 dopamine receptor occupancy in amisulpride treated patients. *Psychopharmacology* **175**, 367–373.

Bressan, R.A., Erlandsson, K., Jones, H.M. *et al.* (2003a) Is regionally selective D2/D3 dopamine occupancy sufficient for atypical antipsychotic effect? An in vivo quantitative [123I] epidepride SPET study of amisulpride-treated patients. *American Journal of Psychiatry* **160**, 1413–1420.

Bressan, R.A., Erlandsson, K., Jones, H.M. *et al.* (2003b) Optimizing limbic selective D2/D3 receptor occupancy by risperidone. *Journal of Clinical Psychopharmacoogyl* **23**, 5–14.

Browman, K.E., Curzon, P., Pan, J.B. *et al.* (2005) A-412997, a selective dopamine D4 agonist, improves cognitive performance in rats. *Pharmacology, Biochemistry & Behavior* **82**, 148–155.

Buchanan, R.W., Javitt, D.C., Marder, S.R. *et al.* (2007) The Cognitive and Negative Symptoms in Schizophrenia Trial (CONSIST): the efficacy of glutamatergic agents for negative symptoms and cognitive impairments. *American Journal of Psychiatry* **164**, 1593–1602.

Buckley, P.F. & Stahl, S.M. (2007) Pharmacological treatment of negative symptoms of schizophrenia. *Acta Psychiatrica Scandinavica* **115**, 93–100.

Buckley, P.F., Mahadik, S., Pillai, A. *et al.* (2007) Neurotrophins and schizophrenia. *Schizophrenia Research* **94**, 1–11.

Burstein, E.S., Ma, J., Wong, S. *et al.* (2005) Intrinsic efficacy of antipsychotics at human D2, D3, and D4 dopamine receptors: identification of the clozapine metabolite N-desmethylclozapine as a D2/D3 partial agonist. *Journal of Pharmacology and Experimental Therapeutics* **315**, 1278–1287.

Bymaster, F.P., Calligaro, D.O., Falcone, J.F. *et al.* (1996) Radioreceptor binding profile of the atypical antipsychotic olanzapine. *Neuropsychopharmacology* **14**, 87–96.

Byrne, P. (2007) Managing the acute psychotic episode. *British Medical Journal* **334**, 686–692.

Caley, C.F. & Weber, S.S. (1995) Sulpiride: an antipsychotic with selective dopaminergic antagonist properties. *Annals of Pharmacotherapy* **29**, 152–160.

Carlsson, A. & Lindqvist, A. (1963) Effect of chlorpromazine or haloperidol on formation of 3-methoxytyramine in mouse brain. *Acta Pharmacologica et Toxicologica* **20**, 140–144.

Carlsson, A. & Carlsson, M.L. (2006) A dopaminergic deficit hypothesis of schizophrenia. *Dialogues in Clinical Neuroscience* **8**, 137–142.

Carlsson, M. L., Carlsson A., & Nilsson, M. (2004) Schizophrenia: from dopamine to glutamate and back. *Current Medicinal Chemistry* **11**, 267–277.

Carpenter, W.T., Conley, R. & Kirkpatrick, B. (2000) On Schizophrenia and new generation drugs. *Neuropsychopharmacology* **22**, 660–661.

Castner, S.A. & Williams, G.V. (2007) Tuning the engine of cognition: a focus on NMDA/D1 receptor interactions in prefrontal cortex. *Brain and Cognition* **63**, 94–122.

Catts, V.S., Catts, S.V., McGrath, J.J. *et al.* (2006) Apoptosis and schizophrenia. *Schizophrenia Research* **84**, 20–28.

Chintoh, A.F., Mann, S.W., Lam, L. *et al.* (2008) Insulin resistance and decreased glucose-stimulated insulin secretion after acute olanzapine administration. *Journal of Clinical Psychopharmacology* **28**, 494–499.

Chou, Y.H., Halldin C., & Farde, L. (2003) Occupancy of 5-HT1A receptors by clozapine in the primate brain: a PET study. *Psychopharmacology* **166**, 234–240.

Chou, Y.H., Halldin C., & Farde, L. (2006) Clozapine binds preferentially to cortical D1-like dopamine receptors in the primate brain: a PET study. *Psychopharmacology* **185**, 29–35.

Chouinard, G., Annable, L., Ross-Chouinard, A. *et al.* (1988) A 5-year prospective longitudinal study of tardive dyskinesia. *Journal of Clinical Psychopharmacology* **8**, 21S–26S.

Claustre, Y., Peretti, D.D., Brun, P. *et al.* (2003) SSR181507, a dopamine D(2) receptor antagonist and 5-HT(1A) receptor agonist. *Neuropsychopharmacology* **28**, 2064–2076.

Coppens, H.J., Slooff, C.J., Paans, A.M., *et al.* (1991) High central D2-dopamine receptor occupancy as assessed with positron emission tomography in medicated but therapy-resistant schizophrenic patients. *Biological Psychiatry* **29**, 629–634.

Correll, C.U., Leucht, S., & Kane, J.M. (2004) Lower risk for tardive dyskinesia associated with second-generation antipsychotics. *American Journal of Psychiatry* **161**, 414–425.

Corrigan, M.H., Gallen, C.C., Bonura, M.L. *et al.* (2004) Effectiveness of the selective D4 antagonist sonepiprazole in schizophrenia. *Biological Psychiatry* **55**, 445–451.

Corripio, I., Catafau, A.M., Perez, V. *et al.* (2005) Striatal dopaminergic D2 receptor occupancy and clinical efficacy in psychosis exacerbation: a 123I-IBZM study with ziprasidone and haloperidol. *Progress in Neuropsychopharmacology and Biological Psychiatry* **29**, 91–96.

Coukell, A.J., Spencer, C.M. & Benfield, P. (1996) Amisulpride: a review of its pharmacodynamic and pharmacokinetic properties and therapeutic efficacy in the management of schizophrenia. *CNS Drugs* **6**, 237–256.

Cousins, D.A. & Young, A.H. (2007) The armamentarium of treatments for bipolar disorder. *International Journal of Neuropsychopharmacology* **10**, 411–431.

Coyle, J.T. (2006) Glutamate and schizophrenia: beyond the dopamine hypothesis. *Cellular and Molecular Neurobiology* **26**, 365–384.

Crumb, W.J., Ekins, S. Sarazan, R.D. *et al.* (2006) Effects of antipsychotic drugs on I(to), I (Na), I (sus), I (K1), and hERG. *Pharmacological Research* **23**, 1133–1143.

Cucchiaro, J., Nann-Vernotica, R., Lasser, T. *et al.* (2001) A randomised, double-blind multicenter phase III study of iloperidone versus haloperidol and placebo in patients with schizophrenia or schizoaffective disorder. *Schizophrenia Research* **49**, 223–224.

Cuisiat, S., Bourdiol, N., Lacharme, V. *et al.* (2007) Towards a new generation of potential antipsychotic agents combing D2 and 5-HT1A receptor activities. *Journal of Medicinal Chemistry* **22**, 865–876

Daniel, D.G., Zimbroff, D.L., Potkin, S.G., *et al.* (1999) Ziprasidone 80 mg/day and 160 mg/day in the acute exacerbation of schizophrenia and schizoaffective disorder. *Neuropsychopharmacology* **20**, 491–505.

Davidson, L., Schmutte, T., Dinzeo, T. *et al.* (2008) Remission and recovery in schizophrenia. *Schizophrenia Bulletin* **34**, 5–8.

Davis, K.L., Kahn, R.S., Ko, G. *et al.* (1991) Dopamine in schizophrenia. *American Journal of Psychiatry* **148**, 1474–1486.

Davis, J.M., Chen, N. & Glick I.D. (2003) A meta-analysis of the efficacy of second-generation antipsychotics. *Archives of General Psychiatry* **63**, 553–564.

Dazzan, P., Morgan, K.D., Orr, K. *et al.* (2005) Different effects of typical and atypical antipsychotics on grey matter in first episode psychosis. *Neuropsychopharmacology* **30**, 765–774.

De Beaurepaire, R., Labelle., Naber, D. *et al.* (1995) An open trial of the D_1 antagonist SCH 39166 in six cases of acute psychotic states. *Psychopharmacology* **121**, 323–327.

De Haan, L., Lavalaye, J., van Bruggen, M. *et al.* (2004) Subjective experience and dopamine D_2 receptor occupancy in patients treated with antipsychotics. *Canadian Journal of Psychiatry* **49**, 290–296.

De Visser, S.J., van der Post, J., Pieters, M.S.M., *et al.* (2001) Biomarkers for the effects of antipsychotic drugs in healthy volunteers. *British Journal of Clinical Pharmacology* **51**, 119–132.

Den Boer, J.A., van Megen, H.J.G.M., Fleischhacker, W. W. *et al.* (1995) Differential effects of the D1-DA receptor antagonist SCH 39166 on positive and negative symptoms of schizophrenia. *Psychopharmacology* **121**, 317–322.

Deniker, P. (1983) Discovery of the clinical uses of neuroleptics. In: Parnham, M.J. & Bruinvels, J., eds. *Discoveries in Pharmacology*, Vol. **1**. Amsterdam: Elsevier, pp. 163–180.

Deutch, A.Y. & Bubser, M. (2007) The orexins/hypocretins and schizophrenia. *Schizophrenia Bulletin* **33**, 1277–1283.

Deveney, A.M. & Waddington, J.L. (1997) Psychopharmacological distinction between novel full-efficacy "D1-like" dopamine receptor agonists. *Pharmacology, Biochemstry & Behavior* **58**, 551–558.

Di Cara, B., Panayi, F., Gobert, A. *et al.* (2007). Activation of dopamine D1 receptors enhances cholinergic transmission and social cognition. *International Journal of Neuropsychopharmacology* **10**, 383–399.

Dickinson, D., Bellack, A.S., & Gold, J.M. (2007) Social/communication skills, cognition, and vocational functioning in schizophrenia. *Schizophrenia Bulletin* **33**, 1213–1220.

Dunn, C.J. & Fitton, A. (1996) Sertindole. *CNS Drugs* **5**, 224–230.

Ehmann, T.S., Delva, J.J. & Beninger. R.J. (1987) Flupenthixol in chronic schizophrenic inpatients. *Journal of Clinical Psychopharmacology* **3**, 173–175.

El-Sayeh, H.G., Morganti C. & Adams, C.E. (2006) Aripiprazole for schizophrenia. *British Journal of Psychiatry* **189**, 102–108.

Erlandsson, K., Bressan, R. A., Mulligan, R.S. *et al.* (2003). Analysis of D2 dopamine receptor occupancy with quantitative SPET using the high-affinity ligand [123I]epidepride. *Neuroimage* **19**, 1205–1214.

Farde, L., Nordstrom, A.L., Wiesel, F.A. *et al.* (1992) Positron emission tomographic analysis of central D1 and D2 dopamine receptor occupancy in patients treated with classical neuroleptics and clozapine. *Archives of General Psychiatry* **49**, 538–544.

Farde, L., Nordstrom, A.L., Nyberg, S. *et al.* (1994) D1-, D2-, and 5-HT2-receptor occupancy in clozapine-treated patients. *Journal of Clinical Psychiatry* **55** (Suppl B), 67–69.

Farde, L., Suhara, T., Nyberg, S. *et al.* (1997) A PET-study of [11C]FLB 457 binding to extrastriatal D2-dopamine receptors in healthy subjects and antipsychotic drug-treated patients. *Psychopharmacology* **133**, 396–404.

Feenstra, R.W., de Moes, J., Hofma, J.J. *et al.* (2001) New 1-aryl-4-(biarylmethylene)piperazines as potential atypical antipsychotics sharing dopamine D(2)-receptor and serotonin 5-HT(1A)-receptor affinities. *Bioorganic and Medicinal Chemistry Letters* **11**, 2345–2349.

Fischman, A.J., Bonab, A.A., Babich, J.W. *et al.* (1996) Positron emission tomographic analysis of central 5-hydroxytryptamine2 receptor occupancy in healthy volunteers treated with the novel antipsychotic agent, ziprasidone. *Journal of Pharmacology & Experimental Therapeutics* **279**, 939–947.

Fitzgerald, P, & Seeman, P. (1999) Neuroreceptor studies in the elderly. In: Howard, R. & Castle, D., eds. *Late-onset Schizophrenia*. Philadelphia: Wrightson Biomedical Publishing, pp. 205–216.

Franberg, O., Wiker, C., Marcus, M.M. *et al.* (2008) Asenapine, a novel psychopharmacologic agent. *Psychopharmacology* **196**, 417–429.

Freedman, R., (2005) The choice of antipsychotic drugs for schizophrenia. *New England Journal of Medicine* **353**, 1286–1288.

Fulton, B. & Goa, K.L. (1995) ICI-204,636: an initial appraisal of its pharmacological properties and clinical potential in the treatment of schizophrenia. *CNS Drugs* **4**, 68–78.

Gardell, L.R., Vanover, K., E. Pounds, L. *et al.* (2007) ACP-103, a 5-hydroxytryptamine 2A receptor inverse agonist, improves the antipsychotic efficacy and side-effect profile of haloperidol and risperidone in experimental models. *Journal of Pharmacology and Experimental Therapeutics* **322**, 862–870.

Garver, D.L., Holcomb J.A. & Christensen, J.D. (2005) Cerebral cortical gray expansion associated with two second-generation antipsychotics. *Biological Psychiatry* **58**, 62–66.

Garver, D.L., Holcomb J.A. & Christensen, J.D. (2008) Compromised myelin integrity during psychosis with repair during remission in drug-responding schizophrenia. *International Journal of Neuropsychopharmacology* **11**, 49–61.

Gazi, L., Bobirnac, I., Danzeisen, M. *et al.* (1999) Receptor density as a factor governing the efficacy of the dopamine D4 receptor ligands, L-745,870 and U-101958 at human recombinant D4,4 receptors expressed in CHO cells. *British Journal of Pharmacology* **128**, 613–620.

Geddes, J., Freemantle, N., Harrison, P. *et al*. (2000) Atypical antipsychotics in the treatment of schizophrenia. *British Medical Journal* **321**, 1371–1376.

Gefvert, O., Lindstrom, L.H., Dahlback, O. *et al*. (2000) (-)-OSU6162 induces a rapid onset of antipsychotic effect after a single dose. In: von Knorring, L., ed. *Scandinavian Society for Psychopharmacology*. Stockholm: Scandinavian Society for Psychopharmacology, pp. 93–94.

Gefvert, O., Eriksson, B., Persson, P. *et al*. (2005) Pharmacokinetics and D2 receptor occupancy of long-acting injectable risperidone (Risperdal Consta) in patients with schizophrenia. *International Journal of Neuropsychopharmacology* **8**, 27–36.

Gefvert, O., Lundberg, T., Wieselgren, I.M. *et al*. (2001) D(2) and 5HT(2A) receptor occupancy of different doses of quetiapine in schizophrenia: a PET study. *European Neuropsychopharmacology* **11**, 105–110.

George, M.S., Molnar, C.E., Grenesko, E.L. *et al*. (2007) A single 20 mg dose of dihydrexidine (DAR-0100), a full dopamine D1 agonist, is safe and tolerated in patients with schizophrenia. *Schizophrenia Research* **93**, 42–50.

Geyer, M.A. & Ellenbroek, B. (2003) Animal behavior models of the mechanisms underlying antipsychotic atypicality. *Progress in Neuropsychopharmacology & Biological Psychiatry* **27**, 1071–1079.

Glantz, L.A., Gilmore, J.E., Lieberman, J.A. *et al*. (2006) Apoptotic mechanisms and the synaptic pathology of schizophrenia. *Schizophrenia Research* **81**, 47–63.

Goeree, R., Farahati, F., Burke, N. *et al*. (2005) The economic burden of schizophrenia in Canada in 2004. *Current Medical Research and Opinion* **21**, 2017–2028.

Gogos, J.A. (2007) Schizophrenia susceptibility genes. *International Review of Neurobiology* **78**, 397–422.

Gray, J.A. & Roth, B.L. (2007) Molecular targets for treating cognitive dysfunction in schizophrenia. *Schizophrenia Bulletin* **33**, 1100–1119.

Green, M.F. & Nuechterlein, K.H. (1999) Should schizophrenia be treated as a neurocognitive disorder? *Schizophrenia Bulletin* **25**, 309–319.

Green, M.F. & Nuechterlein, K.H. (2004) The MATRICS initiative: developing a consensus cognitive battery for clinical trials. *Schizophrenia Research* **72**, 1–3.

Green, M.F., Penn, D.L., Bentall, R. *et al*. (2008) Social cognition in schizophrenia. *Schizophrenia Bulletin* **34**, 1211–1220.

Greenwood, K.E., Landau, S. & Wykes, T. (2005) Negative symptoms and specific cognitive impairments as combined targets for improved functional outcome within cognitive remediation therapy. *Schizophrenia Bulletin* **31**, 910–921.

Grunder, G., Carlsson A. & Wong, D.F. (2003) Mechanism of new antipsychotic medications. *Archives of General Psychiatry* **60**, 974–977.

Grunder, G., Landvogt, C., Vernaleken, I. *et al*. (2006) The striatal and extrastriatal D2/D3 receptor-binding profile of clozapine in patients with schizophrenia. *Neuropsychopharmacology* **31**, 1027–1035.

Guillin, O., Abi-Dargham, A. & Laruelle, M. (2007) Neurobiology of dopamine in schizophrenia. *International Review of Neurobiology* **78**, 1–39.

Haddad, P.M. & Sharma, S.G. (2007) Adverse effects of atypical antipsychotics. *CNS Drugs* **21**, 911–936.

Hamamura, T. & Harada, T. (2007) Unique pharmacological profile of aripiprazole as the phasic component buster. *Psychopharmacology* **191**, 741–743.

Hansen, H.H., Timmermann, D.B., Peters, D. *et al*. (2007) Alpha-7 nicotinic acetylcholine receptor agonists selectively activate limbic regions of the rat forebrain. *Journal of Neuroscience Research* **85**, 1810–1818.

Harvey, P.D., Koren, D., Reichenberg, A. *et al*. (2006) Negative symptoms and cognitive deficits. *Schizophrenia Bulletin* **32**, 250–258.

Hertel, P. (2006) Comparing sertindole to other new generation antipsychotics on preferential dopamine output in limbic versus striatal projection regions: mechanism of action. *Synapse* **60**, 543–552.

Hertel, P., Didriksen, M., Pouzet, B. *et al*. (2007) Lu 35-138 ((+)-(S)-3-{1-[2-(1-acetyl-2,3-dihydro-1H-indol-3-yl)ethyl]-3,6-dihydro-2H -pyridin-4-yl}-6-chloro-1H-indole), a dopamine D4 receptor antagonist and serotonin reuptake inhibitor. *European Journal of Pharmacology* **573**, 148–160.

Heusler, P., Newman-Tancredi, A., Castro-Fernandez, A. *et al*. (2007) Differential agonist and inverse agonist profile of antipsychotics at D_{2L} receptors coupled to GIRK potassium channels. *Neuropharmacology* **52**, 1106–1113.

Hippius, H. (1989) The history of clozapine. *Psychopharmacology* **99**, S3–S5.

Houseknecht, K.L., Robertson, A.S., Zavadoski, W. *et al*. (2006) Acute effects of atypical antipsychotics on whole-body insulin resistance in rats. *Neuropsychopharmacology* **32**, 289–297.

Hrib, N.J. (2000) The dopamine D_4 receptor. *Drugs of the Future* **25**, 587–611.

Ichikawa, J., Li, Z., Dai, J. *et al*. (2002) Atypical antipsychotic drugs, quetiapine, iloperidone, and melperone, preferentially increase dopamine and acetylcholine release in rat medial prefrontal cortex: role of 5-HT1A receptor agonism. *Brain Research* **956**, 349–357.

Javitt, D. C. (2008) Glycine transport inhibitors and the treatment of schizophrenia. *Biological Psychiatry* **63**, 6–8.

Jenner, P., Theodorou A. & Marsden, C.D. (1982) Specific receptors for substituted benzamide drugs in brain. *Advances in Biochemical Psychopharmacology* **35**, 109–141.

Johnstone, E.C., Crow, T.J., Frith, C.D. *et al*. (1978) Mechanism of antipsychotic effect in the treatment of acute schizophrenia. *Lancet* **1**, 848–851.

Johnstone, E.C., Crow, T.J., Frith, C.D. *et al*. (1988) The Northwick park 'functional' psychosis study. *Lancet* **2**, 119–125.

Jones, H.M. & Pilowsky, L.S. (2002) Dopamine and antipsychotic drug action revisited. *British Journal of Psychiatry* **181**, 271–275.

Jones, H.M., Travis, M.J., Mulligan, R. *et al*. (2001) In vivo 5-HT2A receptor blockade by quetiapine. *Psychopharmacology* **157**, 60–66.

Jones, P.B., Barnes, T.R., Davies, L. *et al*. (2006) Randomized controlled trial of the effect on Quality of Life of second- vs first-generation antipsychotic drugs in schizophrenia. *Archives of General Psychiatry* **63**, 1079–1087.

Jorgensen, A.W., Hilden J. & Gotzsche, P.C. (2006) Cochrane reviews compared with industry supported meta-analyses and other meta-analyses of the same drugs. *British Medical Journal* **333**, 782.

Joyce, J.N. & Millan, M.J. (2005) Dopamine D3 receptor antagonists as therapeutic agents. *Drug Discovery Today* **10**, 917–925.

Kahn, R.S., Schulz, S.C., Palazov, V.D. *et al.* (2007) Efficacy and tolerability of once-daily extended release quetiapine fumarate in acute schizophrenia. *Journal of Clinical Psychiatry* **68**, 832–842.

Kales, H.C., Valenstein, M., Kim, H.M. *et al.*(2007) Mortality risk in patients with dementia treated with antipsychotics versus other psychiatric medications. *American Journal of Psychiatry* **164**, 1568–1576

Kalkman, H.O., Subramanian N. & Hoyer, D. (2001) Extended radioligand binding profile of iloperidone. *Neuropsychopharmacology* **25**, 904–914.

Kane, J.M., Carson, W.H., Saha, A.R. *et al.* (2002) Efficacy and safety of aripiprazole and haloperidol versus placebo in patients with schizophrenia and schizoaffective disorder. *Journal of Clinical Psychiatry* **63**, 763–771.

Kane, J., Canas, F., Kramer, M. *et al.* (2007) Treatment of schizophrenia with paliperidone extended-release tablets. *Schizophrenia Research* **90**, 147–161.

Kane, J., Honigfield, G., Singer, J., *et al.* (1988) Clozapine for the treatment-resistant schizophrenic. *Archives of General Psychiatry* **45**, 789–796.

Kapur, S. & Remington, G. (1996) Serotonin-dopamine interaction and its relevance to schizophrenia. *American Journal of Psychiatry* **153**, 466–476.

Kapur, S. & Seeman, P. (2000) Antipsychotic agents differ in how fast they come off the dopamine D2 receptors. *Journal of Psychiatry and Neuroscience* **25**, 161–166.

Kapur, S. (2000) Receptor occupancy by antipsychotics. In: Lidow, M.S., ed. *Neurotransmitter Receptors in Actions of Antipsychotics.* London: CRC Press, pp. 163–176.

Kapur, S. (2003) Psychosis as a state of aberrant salience. *American Journal of Psychiatry* **160**, 13–23.

Kapur, S. (2004) How antipsychotics become anti-"psychotic". *Trends in Pharmacological Science* **25**, 402–406.

Kapur, S. & Mamo, D. (2003) Half a century of antipsychotics and still a central role for dopamine D2 receptors. *Progress in Neuropsychopharmacology and Biological Psychiatry* **27**, 1081–1090.

Kapur, S. & Remington, G. (2001) Dopamine D(2) receptors and their role in atypical antipsychotic action. *Biological Psychiatry* **50**, 873–883.

Kapur, S., & Seeman, P. (2001) Does fast dissociation from the dopamine D₂ receptor explain the action of atypical antipsychotics? *American Journal of Psychiatry* **158**, 360–369.

Kapur, S., Agid, O., Mizrahi, R. *et al.* (2006) How antipsychotics work. *NeuroReceptor* **3**, 10–21.

Kapur, S., Mizrahi, R. & Li, M. (2005) From dopamine to salience to psychosis-linking biology, pharmacology and phenomenology of psychosis. *Schizophrenia Research* **79**, 59–68.

Kapur, S., Remington, G., Jones, C. *et al.* (1996) High levels of dopamine D2 receptor occupancy with low-dose haloperidol treatment. *American Journal of Psychiatry* **153**, 948–950.

Kapur, S., Remington, G., Zipursky, R.B. *et al.* (1995) The D2 dopamine receptor occupancy of risperidone and its relationship to extrapyramidal symptoms. *Life Sciences* **57**, 103–107.

Kapur, S., Zipursky, R.B. & Remington, G. (1999) Clinical and theoretical implications of 5-HT₂ and D₂ receptor occupancy of clozapine, risperidone, and olanzapine in schizophrenia. *American Journal of Psychiatry* **156**, 286–293.

Kapur, S., Zipursky, R., Jones, C. *et al.* (2000a) Relationship between dopamine D(2) occupancy, clinical response, and side effects. *American Journal of Psychiatry* **157**, 514–520.

Kapur, S., Zipursky, R., Jones, C. *et al.* (2000c) A positron emission tomography study of quetiapine in schizophrenia. *Archives of General Psychiatry* **57**, 553–559.

Kapur, S., Zipursky, R., Remington, G. *et al.* (2000b) Fast Koff at the dopamine D2 receptor (not high affinity at other receptors) is the key to clozapine's uniqueness and atypical antipsychotic activity. *International Journal of Neuropsychopharmacology* **3** (Suppl 1), S95.

Kapur, S., Zipursky, R.B., Remington, G. *et al.* (1998) 5-HT2 and D2 receptor occupancy of olanzapine in schizophrenia. *American Journal of Psychiatry* **55**, 921–928.

Karle, J., Clemmesen, L., Hansen, L. *et al.* (1995) NNC 01-0687, a selective dopamine D1 receptor antagonist, in the treatment of schizophrenia. *Psychopharmacology* **121**, 328–329.

Karlsson, P., Smith, L., Farde, L. *et al.* (1995) Lack of apparent antipsychotic effect of the D₁-dopamine receptor antagonist SCH 39166 in acutely ill schizophrenic patients. *Psychopharmacology* **121**, 309–316.

Kasper, S., Tauscher, J., Kufferle, B. *et al.* (1998) Sertindole and dopamine D2 receptor occupancy in comparison to risperidone, clozapine and haloperidol. *Psychopharmacology* **136**, 367–373.

Kebabian, J.W. & Calne, D.B. (1979) Multiple receptors for dopamine. *Nature* **277**, 93–96.

Kessler, R.M., Ansari, M.S., Riccardi, P. *et al.* (2005) Occupancy of striatal and extrastriatal dopamine D2/D3 receptors by olanzapine and haloperidol. *Neuropsychopharmacology* **30**, 2283–2289.

Kessler, R.M., Ansari, M. S., Riccardi, P. *et al.* (2006) Occupancy of striatal and extrastriatal dopamine D2 receptors by clozapine and quetiapine. *Neuropsychopharmacology* **31**, 1991–2001.

Kim, S.F., Huang, A.S., Snowman, A.M. *et al.* (2007) Antipsychotic drug-induced weight gain mediated by histamine H1 receptor-linked activation of hypothalamic AMP-kinase. *Proceedings of the National Acadamy of Sciences USA* **104**, 3456–3459.

Kippin, T.E., Kapur S. & van der Kooy, D. (2005) Dopamine specifically inhibits forebrain neural stem cell proliferation, suggesting a novel effect of antipsychotic drugs. *Journal of Neuroscience* **25**, 5815–5823.

Koike, K., Hashimoto, K., Takai, N. *et al.* (2005) Tropisetron improves deficits in auditory P50 suppression in schizophrenia. *Schizophrenia Research* **76**, 67–72.

Kongsamut, S., Kang, J., Chen, X.L. *et al.* (2002) A comparison of the receptor binding and HERG channel affinities for a series of antipsychotic drugs. *European Journal of Pharmacology* **450**, 37–41.

Kornhuber, J., Wiltfang, J., Riederer, P. *et al.* (2006). Neuroleptic drugs in the human brain: clinical impact of persistence and region-specific distribution. *European Archives of Psychiatry & Clinical Neuroscience* **256**, 274–280.

Kramer, M.S., Last, B., Getson, A. *et al.* (1997) The effects of a selective D₄ dopamine receptor antagonist (L-745,870) in acutely psychotic inpatients with schizophrenia. *Archives of General Psychiatry* **54**, 567–572.

Labelle, A., de Beaurepaire, R., Boulay, L.J. *et al.* (1998) A pilot study of the safety and tolerance of SCH 39166 in patients with schizophrenia. *Journal of Psychiatry & Neuroscience* **23**, 93–94.

Lahti, R.A., Tamminga C.A. & Carlsson, A. (2007) Stimulating and inhibitory effects of the dopamine "stabilizer" (-)-OSU6162 on dopamine D(2) receptor function in vitro. *Journal of Neural Transmission* **114**, 1143–1146.

Lambe, E.K., Liu R.J. & Aghajanian, G.K. (2007) Schizophrenia, hypocretin (orexin), and the thalamocortical activating system. *Schizophrenia Bulletin* **33**, 1284–1290.

Lameh, J., Burstein, E.S., Taylor, E. *et al.* (2007) Pharmacology of N-desmethylclozapine. *Pharmacology and Therapeutics* **115**, 223–231.

Lane, H.Y., Chang, Y.C., Liu, Y.C. *et al.* (2005) Sarcosine or D-serine add-on treatment for acute exacerbation of schizophrenia. *Archives of General Psychiatry* **62**, 1196–1204.

Lane, H.Y., Liu, Y.C., Huang, C.L. *et al.* (2008) Sarcosine (N-methylglycine) treatment for acute schizophrenia. *Biological Psychiatry* **63**, 9–12.

Laughren, T. & Levin, R. (2006) Food and Drug Administration perspective on negative symptoms in schizophrenia as a target for a drug treatment claim. *Schizophrenia Bulletin* **32**, 220–222.

Lawler, C.P., Prioleau, C., Lewis, M.M. *et al.* (1999) Interactions of the novel antipsychotic aripiprazole (OPC-14597) with dopamine and serotonin receptor subtypes. *Neuropsychopharmacology* **20**, 612–627.

Lawrence, A.J. (2007) Optimisation of anti-psychotic therapeutics. *British Journal of Pharmacology* **151**, 161–162.

Lester, H. & Gask, L. (2006) Delivering medical care for patients with serious mental illness or promoting a collaborative model of recovery? *British Journal of Psychiatry* **188**, 465–471.

Leucht, S., Pitschel-Walz, G., Engel, R.R. *et al.* (2002) Amisulpride, an unusual "atypical" antipsychotic. *American Journal of Psychiatry* **159**, 180–190.

Leucht, S., Engel, R.R., Bauml, J. *et al.* (2007) Is the superior efficacy of new generation antipsychotics an artifact of LOCF? *Schizophrenia Bulletin* **33**, 183–191.

Leucht, S., Wahlbeck, K., Hamann, J. *et al.* (2003) New generation antipsychotics versus low-potency conventional antipsychotics. *Lancet* **361**, 1581–1589.

Levant, B. (1997) The D3 dopamine receptor. *Pharmacological Reviews* **49**, 231–252

Levkovitz, Y., Levi, U., Braw, Y. *et al.* (2007) Minocycline, a second-generation tetracycline, as a neuroprotective agent in an animal model of schizophrenia. *Brain Research* **1154**, 154–162.

Lewis, D.A. & Gonzalez-Burgos, G. (2006) Pathophysiologically based treatment interventions in schizophrenia. *Nature Medicine* **12**, 1016–1022.

Lewis, R., Bagnall A. M. & Leitner, M. (2005) Sertindole for schizophrenia. *Cochrane Database Systematic Reviews* CD001715.

Li, Z., Ichikawa, J., Dai, J. *et al.* (2004) Aripiprazole, a novel antipsychotic drug, preferentially increases dopamine release in the prefrontal cortex and hippocampus in rat brain. *European Journal of Pharmacology* **493**, 75–83.

Lidsky, T.I. (1995) Reevaluation of the mesolimbic hypothesis of antipsychotic drug action. *Schizophrenia Bulletin* **21**, 67–74.

Lieberman, J.A., Stroup, T.S., McEvoy, J.P. *et al.* (2005) Effectiveness of antipsychotic drugs in patients with chronic schizophrenia. *New England Journal of Medicine* **353**, 1209–1223.

Lindstrom, E., Farde, L., Eberhard, J. *et al.* (2005) QTc interval prolongation and antipsychotic drug treatments. *International Journal of Neuropsychopharmacology* **8**, 615–629.

Liu, I.S.C., George, S.R. & Seeman, P. (2000) The human D2$_{Longer}$ receptor has a high-affinity state and inhibits adenylyl cyclase. *Molecular Brain Research* **77**, 281–284.

Mamo, D., Graff, A., Mizrahi, R. *et al.* (2007) Differential effects of aripiprazole on D(2), 5-HT(2), and 5-HT(1A) receptor occupancy in patients with schizophrenia. *American Journal of Psychiatry* **164**, 1411–1417.

Mamo, D., Kapur, S., Shammi, C.M. *et al.* (2004) A PET study of dopamine D2 and serotonin 5-HT2 receptor occupancy in patients with schizophrenia treated with therapeutic doses of ziprasidone. *American Journal of Psychiatry* **161**, 818–825.

Mamo, D., Kapur, S., Keshavan, M. *et al.* (2008a) D2 receptor occupancy of olanzapine pamoate depot using positron emission tomography. *Neuropsychopharmacology* **33**, 298–304.

Mamo, D.C., Uchida, H., Vitcu, I. *et al.* (2008b) Quetiapine extended-release versus immediate-release formulation. *Journal of Clinical Psychiatry* **69**, 81–86.

Marder, S.R. & Fenton, W. (2004) Measurement And Treatment Research to Improve Cognition in Schizophrenia. *Schizophrenia Research* **72**, 5–9.

Marder, S.R. (2006a) Drug initiatives to improve cognitive function. *Journal of Clinical Psychiatry* **67** (Suppl. 9), 31–35.

Marder, S.R. (2006b) Initiatives to promote the discovery of drugs to improve cognitive function in severe mental illness. *Journal of Clinical Psychiatry* **67**, e03.

Marder, S.R., Kramer, M., Ford, L. *et al.* (2007) Efficacy and safety of paliperidone extended-release tablets. *Biological Psychiatry* **62**, 1363–1370.

Marquis, K.L., Sabb, A.L., Logue, S.F. *et al.* (2007) WAY-163909 [(7bR,10aR)-1,2,3,4,8,9,10,10a-octahydro-7bH-cyclopenta-[b][1,4]diazepino[6,7,1hi]indole]: A novel 5-hydroxytryptamine 2C receptor-selective agonist with preclinical antipsychotic-like activity. *Journal of Pharmacology and Experimental Therapeutics* **320**, 486–496.

Martinot, J.L., Pailliere-Martinot, M.L., Poirier, M.F. *et al.* (1996) *In vivo* characteristics of dopamine D2 receptor occupancy by amisulpride in schizophrenia. *Psychopharmacology* **124**, 154–158.

Mauri, M.C., Bravin, S., Bitetto, A. *et al.* (1996) A risk-benefit assessment of sulpiride in the treatment of schizophrenia. *Drug Safety* **14**, 288–298.

McCormick, P.N., Kapur, S., Seeman, P. *et al.* (2008) Dopamine D2 receptor radiotracers [^{11}C](+)-PHNO and [^{3}H] raclopride are indistinguishably inhibited by D$_2$ agonists and antagonists *ex vivo*. *Nuclear Medicine and Biology* **35**, 11–17.

McCreary, A.C., Glennon, J.C., Ashby, C.R. *et al.* (2007) SLV313 (1-(2,3-dihydro-benzo[1,4]dioxin-5-yl)-4- [5-(4-fluoro-phenyl)-pyridin-3-ylmethyl]-piperazine monohydrochloride): a novel dopamine D2 receptor antagonist and 5-HT1A receptor agonist potential antipsychotic drug. *Neuropsychopharmacology* **32**, 78–94.

McEvoy, J.P., Lieberman, J.A., Stroup, T.S. *et al.* (2006) Effectiveness of clozapine versus olanzapine, quetiapine, and risperidone in patients with chronic schizophrenia who did not respond to prior atypical antipsychotic treatment. *American Journal of Psychiatry* **163**, 600–610.

McGlashan, T.H., (2006) Is active psychosis neurotoxic? *Schizophrenia Bulletin* **32**, 609–613.

McGlashan, T.H., Zipursky, R.B., Perkins, D. *et al.* (2006) Randomized, double-blind trial of olanzapine versus placebo in patients prodromally symptomatic for psychosis. *American Journal of Psychiatry* **163**, 790–799.

McGorry, P.D., Yung, A.R., Philips, L.J. *et al.* (2002) Randomized controlled trial of interventions designed to reduce the risk of progression to first-episode psychosis in a clinical sample with subthreshold symptoms. *Archives of General Psychiatry* **59**, 921–928.

McKeage, K. & Plosker, G.L. (2004) Amisulpride: a review of its use in the management of schizophrenia. *CNS Drugs* **18**, 933–956.

Mehta, M.A., Montgomery, A.J., Kitamura, Y. *et al.* (2008) Dopamine D2 receptor occupancy levels of acute sulpiride challenges that produce working memory and learning impairments in healthy volunteers. *Psychopharmacology* **196**, 157–165.

Meltzer, H. (1995) Atypical antipsychotic drugs. In: Kupfer, D. & Bloom, F.E., eds. *Psychopharmacology: The Fourth Generation of Progress.* New York: Raven Press, pp. 1277–1286.

Meltzer, H.Y. (2007) Iluminating the molecular basis for some antipsychotic drug-induced metabolic burden. *Proceedings of the National Acadamy of Sciences USA* **104**, 3019–3020.

Meltzer, H.Y., Arvanitis, L., Bauer, D. *et al.* (2004) Placebo-controlled evaluation of four novel compounds for the treatment of schizophrenia and schizoaffective disorder. *American Journal of Psychiatry* **161**, 975–984.

Meltzer, H.Y., Li, Z., Kaneda, Y. *et al.* (2003) Serotonin receptors: their key role in drugs to treat schizophrenia. *Progress in Neuropsychopharmacology and Biological Psychiatry* **27**, 1159–1172.

Meltzer, H.Y., Matsubara, S. & Lee, J-C. (1989) Classification of typical and atypical antipsychotic drugs on the basis of dopamine D-1, D-2 and serotonin2 pKi values. *Journal of Pharmacology and Experimental Therapeutics* **251**, 238–246.

Metzger, K.L., Shoemaker, J.M., Kahn, J.B. *et al.* (2007) Pharmacokinetic and behavioral characterization of a long-term antipsychotic delivery system in rodents and rabbits. *Psychopharmacology* **190**, 201–211.

Millan, M.J., Svenningsson, P., Ashby, C.R. *et al.* (2008) S33138 [N-[4-[2-[(3aS,9bR)-8-cyano-1,3a,4,9b-tetrahydro[1]-benzopyrano[3,4-c]pyrr ol-2(3H)-yl)-ethyl]phenylacetamide], a preferential dopamine D3 versus D2 receptor antagonist and potential antipsychotic agent. *Journal of Pharmacology and Experimental Therapeutics* **324**, 600–611.

Missale, C., Nash, S.R., Robinson, S.W. *et al.* (1998) Dopamine receptors: from structure to function. *Physiological Reviews* **78**, 189–225.

Mitchell, K., Runker, A., Little, G. *et al.* (2008) Semaphorin and plexin genes specify limbic and cortical connectivity and are implicated in the etiology of schizophrenia. *Schizophrenia Research* **102** (Suppl. 2), 26–27.

Miyamoto, S., Duncan, G.E., Marx, C.E. *et al.* (2005) Treatments for schizophrenia: a critical review of pharmacology and mechanisms of action of antipsychotic drugs. *Molecular Psychiatry* **10**, 79–104.

Miyaoka, T., Yasukawa, R., Yasuda, H. *et al.* (2007) Possible antipsychotic effects of minocycline in patients with schizophrenia. *Progress in Neuropsychopharmacology and Biological Psychiatry* **31**, 304–307.

Mizrahi, R., Bagby, R.M., Zipursky, R.B. *et al.* (2005) How antipsychotics work. *Progress in Neuropsychopharmacology and Biological Psychiatry* **29**, 859–864.

Mizrahi, R., Kiang, M., Mamo, D.C., *et al.* (2006) The selective effect of antipsychotics on the different dimensions of the experience of psychosis in schizophrenia spectrum disorders. *Schizophrenia Research* **88**, 111–118.

Mizrahi, R., Rusjan, P., Agid, O. *et al.* (2007) Adverse subjective experience with antipsychotics and its relationship to striatal and extrastriatal D2 receptors. *American Journal of Psychiatry* **164**, 630–637.

Molina, V., Reig, S., Sanz, J. *et al.* (2005) Increase in gray matter and decrease in white matter volumes in the cortex during treatment with atypical neuroleptics in schizophrenia. *Schizophrenia Research* **80**, 61–71.

Molitch, M. (1995) Prolactin. In: Molitch, M., ed. *The Pituitary.* pp 136-183. Oxford: Blackwell, pp. 136–183.

Moller, H.J., (2003) Amisulpride: limbic specificity and the mechanism of antipsychotic atypicality. *Progress in Neuropsychopharmacology and Biological Psychiatry* **27**, 1101–1111.

Moller, H.J., (2007) Long-acting injectable risperidone for the treatment of schizophrenia: clinical perspectives. *Drugs* **67**, 1541–1566.

Morein-Zamir, S., Turner D.C. & Sahakian, B.J. (2007) A review of the effects of modafinil on cognition in schizophrenia. *Schizophrenia Bulletin* **33**, 1298–1306.

Mota, N.E., Lima M.S. & Soares, B.G. (2002) Amisulpride for schizophrenia. *Cochrane Database Systematic Reviews* CD001357.

Mu, Q., Johnson, K., Morgan, P.S. *et al.* (2007) A single 20 mg dose of the full D1 dopamine agonist dihydrexidine (DAR-0100) increases prefrontal perfusion in schizophrenia. *Schizophrenia Research* **94**, 332–341.

Murdoch, D. & Keating, G.M. (2006) Sertindole. *CNS Drugs* **20**, 233–255.

Murphy, B.P., Chung, Y.C., Park, T.W. *et al.* (2006) Pharmacological treatment of primary negative symptoms in schizophrenia. *Schizophrenia Research* **88**, 5–25.

Nagai, T., Noda, Y., Une, T. *et al.* (2003) Effect of AD-5423 on animal models of schizophrenia. *Neuroreport* **14**, 269–272.

Nasrallah, H.A., (2008) Atypical antipsychotic-induced metabolic side effects. *Molecular Psychiatry* **13**, 27–35.

Natesan, S., Reckless, G.E., Nobrega, J.N. *et al.* (2006a) Dissociation between in vivo occupancy and functional antagonism of dopamine D2 receptors: comparing aripiprazole to other antipsychotics in animal models. *Neuropsychopharmacology* **31**, 1854–1863.

Natesan, S., Svensson, K. A., Reckless, G. E. *et al.* (2006b) The dopamine stabilizers (S)-(-)-(3-methanesulfonyl-phenyl)-

1-propyl-piperidine [(-)-OSU6162] and 4-(3-methanesulfonyl phenyl)-1-propyl-piperidine (ACR16) show high in vivo D2 receptor occupancy, antipsychotic-like efficacy, and low potential for motor side effects in the rat. *Journal of Pharmacology and Experimental Therapeutics* **318**, 810–818.

Natesan, S., Reckless, G. E., Barlow, K. B. *et al.* (2007) Evaluation of N-desmethylclozapine as a potential antipsychotic-preclinical studies. *Neuropsychopharmacology* **32**, 1540–1549.

Newman-Tancredi, A., Cussac D. & Depoortere, R. (2007a) Neuropharmacological profile of bifeprunox. *Current Opinion on Investigational Drugs* **8**, 539–554.

Newman-Tancredi, A., Assie, M.B., Martel, J.C. *et al.* (2007b) F15063, a potential antipsychotic with D2/D3 antagonist, 5-HT 1A agonist and D4 partial agonist properties. *British Journal of Pharmacology* **151**, 237–252.

Newman-Tancredi, A., Heusler, P., Martel, J.C. *et al.* (2008) Agonist and antagonist properties of antipsychotics at human dopamine D4.4 receptors. *International Journal of Neuropsychopharmacolgy* **11**, 293–307.

Niemegeers, C.J.E. & Janssen, P.A.J. (1978) A systematic study of the pharmacological activities of dopamine antagonists. *Life Sciences* **24**, 2201–2216.

Nihalani, N.D., Tu, X., Lamberti, J.S., *et al.* (2007) Diabetic ketoacidosis among patients receiving clozapine. *Annals of Clinical Psychiatry* **19**, 105–112.

Niznik, H.B., Sugamori, K.S., Clifford, J.J. *et al.* (2002) D$_1$-like dopamine receptors. In: Di Chiara, G., ed. *Handbook of Experimental Pharmacology: Dopamine in the CNS*. Heidelberg, Springer, pp. 121–158.

Nordstrom, A.L., Farde, L., Nyberg, S. *et al.* (1995) D$_1$, D$_2$, and 5-HT$_2$ receptor occupancy in relation to clozapine serum concentration. *American Journal of Psychiatry* **152**, 1444–1449.

Nordstrom, A.L. & Farde, L. (1998) Plasma prolactin and central D2 receptor occupancy in antipsychotic drug-treated patients. *Journal of Clinical Psychopharmacology* **18**, 305–310.

Nordstrom, A.L., Farde, L., Wiesel, F.A. *et al.* (1993) Central D2-dopamine receptor occupancy in relation to antipsychotic drug effects. *Biological Psychiatry* **33**, 227–235.

Nordstrom, A.L., Mansson, M., Jovanovic, H. *et al* (2008) PET analysis of the 5HT$_{2A}$ receptor inverse agonist ACP-103 in human brain. *International Journal of Neuropsychopharmacology* **11**, 163–171.

Nyberg, S., Farde, L., Halldin, C., *et al.* (1995) D2 dopamine receptor occupancy during low-dose treatment with haloperidol decanoate. *American Journal of Psychiatry* **152**, 173–178.

Nyberg, S., Olsson, H., Nilsson, U. *et al.* (2002) Low striatal and extra-striatal D2 receptor occupancy during treatment with the atypical antipsychotic sertindole. *Psychopharmacology* **162**, 37–41.

Nyberg, S., Nakashima, Y., Nordstrom, A.L. *et al.* (1996) Positron emission tomography of *in-vivo* binding characteristics of atypical antipsychotic drugs. *British Journal of Psychiatry* **168** (Suppl. 29), 40–44.

O'Connor, S.E. & Brown, R.A. (1982) The pharmacology of sulpiride. *General Pharmacology* **13**, 185–193.

O'Hara, P., Brugha, T.S., Lesage, A. *et al.* (1993) New findings on tardive dyskinesia in a community sample. *Psychological Medicine* **23**, 453–465.

O'Tuathaigh, C.M.P., Babovic, D., O'Meara, G. *et al.* (2007) Susceptibility genes for schizophrenia: phenotypic characterisation of mutant models. *Neuroscience & Biobehavioural Reviews* **31**, 60–78.

Olincy, A., Harris, J.G., Johnson, L.L. *et al.* (2006) Proof-of-concept trial of an alpha7 nicotinic agonist in schizophrenia. *Archives of General Psychiatry* **63**, 630–638.

Olsson, H. & Farde, L. (2001) Potentials and pitfalls using high affinity radioligands in PET and SPET determinations on regional drug induced D2 receptor occupancy. *NeuroImage* **14**, 936–945.

Pariante, C.M., Dazzan, P., Danese, A., *et al.* (2005) Increased pituitary volume in antipsychotic-free and antipsychotic-treated patients of the AESOP first-onset psychosis study. *Neuropsychopharmacology* **30**, 1923–1931

Park, W.K., Jeong, D., Cho, H. *et al.* (2005) KKHA-761, a potent D3 receptor antagonist with high 5-HT1A receptor affinity, exhibits antipsychotic properties in animal models of schizophrenia. *Pharmacology, Biochemistry & Behavior* **82**, 361–372.

Patel, M.V., Kolasa, T., Mortell, K. *et al.* (2006) Discovery of 3-methyl-N-(1-oxy-3',4',5',6'-tetrahydro-2'H-[2,4'-bipyridine]-1'-ylmethyl)benzamide (ABT-670), an orally bioavailable dopamine D4 agonist for the treatment of erectile dysfunction. *Journal of Medicinal Chemistry* **49**, 7450–7465.

Patil, S.T., Zhang, L., Martenyi, F. *et al.* (2007) Activation of mGlu2/3 receptors as a new approach to treat schizophrenia. *Nature Medicine* **13**, 1102–1107.

Penn, D.L., Waldheter, E.J., Perkins, D.O. *et al.* (2005) Psychosocial treatment for first-episode psychosis. *American Journal of Psychiatry* **162**, 2220–2232.

Perrault, G.H., Depoortere, R., Morel, E. *et al.* (1997) Psychopharmacological profile of amisulpride. *Journal of Pharmacology and Experimental Therapeutics* **280**, 73–82.

Petersen, L., Jeppesen, P., Thorup, A. *et al.* (2005) A randomised multicentre trial of integrated versus standard treatment for patients with a first episode of psychotic illness. *British Medical Journal* **331**, 602.

Peuskens, J., Moore, N., Azorin, J.M. *et al.* (2007) The European sertindole safety and exposure survey. *Pharmacoepidemiology of Drug Safety* **16**, 804–811.

Pichat, P., Bergis, O.E., Terranova, J.P. *et al.* (2007) SSR180711, a novel selective alpha7 nicotinic receptor partial agonist. *Neuropsychopharmacology* **32**, 17–34

Pilowsky, L. S., Bressan, R. A., Stone, J. M. *et al.* (2006) First in vivo evidence of an NMDA receptor deficit in medication-free schizophrenic patients. *Molecular Psychiatry* **11**, 118–119.

Pilowsky, L.S., Busatto, G.F., Taylor, M. *et al.* (1996) Dopamine D2 receptor occupancy in vivo by the novel atypical antipsychotic olanzapine. *Psychopharmacology* **124**, 148–153.

Pilowsky, L.S., Mulligan, R.S., Acton, P.D. *et al.* (1997a) Limbic selectivity of clozapine. *Lancet* **350**, 490–491.

Pilowsky, L.S., O'Connell, P., Davies, N. *et al.* (1997b) In vivo effects on striatal dopamine D$_2$ receptor binding by the novel atypical antipsychotic drug sertindole. *Psychopharmacology* **130**, 152–158.

Potkin, S. G., Cohen M. & Panagides, J. (2007) Efficacy and tolerability of asenapine in acute schizophrenia. *Journal of Clinical Psychiatry* **68**, 1492–1500.

Prakash, A. & Lamb, H.M. (1998) Zotepine. *CNS Drugs* **9**, 153–175.

Raedler, T.J., Knable, M.B., Jones, D.W. *et al.* (2000) In vivo olanzapine occupancy of muscarinic acetylcholine receptors in patients with schizophrenia. *Neuropsychopharmacology* **23**, 56–68.

Raedler, T.J., Knable, M.B., Jones, D.W. *et al.* (2003) Central muscarinic acethylcholine receptor availability in patients treated with clozapine. *Neuropsychopharmacology* **28**, 1531–1537.

Raedler, T. J. (2007) Comparison of the in-vivo muscarinic cholinergic receptor availability in patients treated with clozapine and olanzapine. *International Journal of Neuropsychopharmacology* **10**, 275–280.

Ramankutty, G. (2002) Olanzapine-induced destabilization of diabetes in the absence of weight gain. *Acta Psychiatrica Scandinavica* **105**, 237–236.

Ramaswamy, K., Kozma, C. M. & Nasrallah, H. (2007) Risk of diabetic ketoacidosis after exposure to risperidone or olanzapine. *Drug Safety* **30**, 589–599.

Rampe, D., Murawsky, M.K., Grau, J. *et al.* (1998) The antipsychotic agent sertindole is a high affinity antagonist of the human cardiac potassium channel HERG. *Journal of Pharmacology and Experimental Therapeutics* **286**, 788–793.

Reif, A., Schmitt, A., Fritzen, S. *et al.* (2007) Neurogenesis and schizophrenia. *European Archives of Psychiatry and Clinical Neuroscience* **257**, 290–299.

Reimold, M., Solbach, C., Noda, S. *et al.* (2007) Occupancy of dopamine D(1), D (2) and serotonin (2A) receptors in schizophrenic patients treated with flupentixol in comparison with risperidone and haloperidol. *Psychopharmacology* **190**, 241–249.

Remington, G., Mamo, D., Labelle, A. *et al.* (2006) A PET study evaluating dopamine D2 receptor occupancy for long-acting injectable risperidone. *American Journal of Psychiatry* **163**, 396–401.

Remington, G., Kapur, S. & Zipursky, R.B. (1998) Pharmacotherapy of first-episode schizophrenia. *British Journal of Psychiatry* **172** (Suppl.), 66–70.

Richelson, E. & T. Souder, (2000) Binding of antipsychotic drugs to human brain receptors focus on newer generation compounds. *Life Science* **68**, 29–39.

Richtand, N.M., Welge, J.A., Logue, A.D. *et al.* (2007) Dopamine and serotonin receptor binding and antipsychotic efficacy. *Neuropsychopharmacology* **32**, 1715–1726.

Rorick-Kehn, L.M., Johnson, B.G., Knitowski, K.M., *et al.* (2007) In vivo pharmacological characterization of the structurally novel, potent, selective mGlu2/3 receptor agonist LY404039 in animal models of psychiatric disorders. *Psychopharmacology* **193**, 121–136.

Rosenheck, R.A. (2006) Outcomes, costs, and policy caution. *Archives of General Psychiatry* **63**, 1074–1076.

Rosenheck, R., Perlick, D., Bingham, S. *et al.* (2003) Effectiveness and cost of olanzapine and haloperidol in the treatment of schizophrenia. *Journal of the American Medical Association* **290**, 2693–2702.

Ross, C.A., Margolis, R.L., Reading, S.A. *et al.* (2006) Neurobiology of schizophrenia. *Neuron* **52**, 139–153.

Rung, J.P., Carlsson, A., Markinhuhta, K.R. *et al.* (2005) The dopaminergic stabilizers (-)-OSU6162 and ACR16 reverse (+)-MK-801-induced social withdrawal in rats. *Progress in Neuropsychopharmacology and Biological Psychiatry* **29**, 833–839.

Saeedi, H., Remington, G. & Christensen, B.K. (2006) Impact of haloperidol, a dopamine D2 antagonist, on cognition and mood. *Schizophrenia Research* **85**, 222–231.

Samaha, A.N., Reckless, G.E., Seeman, P. *et al.* (2008) Less is more: antipsychotic drug effects are greater with transient rather than continuous delivery. *Biological Psychiatry* **64**, 145–152.

Seamans, J.K. & Yang, C.R. (2004) The principle features and mechanisms of dopamine modulation in the prefrontal cortex. *Progress in Neurobiology* **74**, 1–58.

Scherk, H., Pajonk F.G. & Leucht, S. (2007) Second-generation antipsychotic agents in the treatment of acute mania. *Archives of General Psychiatry* **64**, 442–455.

Schneider, L.S., Dagerman K.S. & Insel, P. (2005) Risk of death with atypical antipsychotic drug treatment for dementia. *Journal of the American Medical Association* **294**, 1934–1943.

Schoemaker, H., Claustre, Y., Fage, D. *et al.* (1997) Neurochemical characteristics of amisulpride, an atypical dopamine D_2/D_3 receptor antagonist with both presynaptic and limbic selectivity. *Journal of Pharmacology and Experimental Therapeutics* **280**, 83–97.

Schotte, A., Janssen, P.F., Gommeren, W. *et al.* (1996) Risperidone compared with new and reference antipsychotic drugs. *Psychopharmacology* **124**, 57–73.

Schultz, W. (2002). Getting formal with dopamine and reward. *Neuron* **36**, 241–263.

Schultz, W. (2007) Multiple dopamine functions at different time courses. *Annual Review of Neuroscience* **30**, 259–288.

Seeger, T.F., Seymour, P.A., Schmidt, A.W. *et al.* (1995) Ziprasidone (CP-88,059): a new antipsychotic with combined dopamine and serotonin receptor antagonist activity. *Journal of Pharmacology & Experimental Therapeutics* **275**, 101–113.

Seeman, P. & Tallerico, T. (1998) Antipsychotic drugs which elicit little or no Parkinsonism bind more loosely than dopamine to brain D2 receptors, yet occupy high levels of these receptors. *Molecular Psychiatry* **3**, 123–134.

Seeman, P. & Tallerico, T. (1999) Rapid release of antipsychotic drugs from dopamine D_2 receptors. *American Journal of Psychiatry* **156**, 876–884.

Seeman, P. (1980) Brain dopamine receptors. *Pharmacological Reviews* **32**, 229–313.

Seeman, P. (1992) Dopamine receptor sequences: therapeutic levels of neuroleptics occupy D_2 receptors, clozapine occupies D_4. *Neuropsychopharmacology* **7**, 261–284.

Seeman, P. & Guan, H. C. (2007) Dopamine partial agonist action of (-)OSU6162 is consistent with dopamine hyperactivity in psychosis. *European Journal of Pharmacology* **557**, 151–153.

Seeman, P. (2002) Atypical antipsychotics. *Canadian Journal of Psychiatry* **47**, 27–38.

Seeman, P., Corbett, R. & Van Tol, H.H.M. (1997) Atypical neuroleptics have low affinity for dopamine D_2 receptors or are selective for D_4 receptors. *Neuropsychopharmacology* **16**, 93–110.

Seeman, P., Nam, D., Ulpian, C. *et al.* (2000) New dopamine receptor, $D2_{Longer}$, with unique TG splice site, in human brain. *Molecular Brain Research* **76**, 132–141.

Seeman, P., Schwarz, J., Chen, J. F. *et al.* (2006) Psychosis pathways converge via D_2^{High} dopamine receptors. *Synapse* **60**, 319–346.

Seeman, P., Weinshenker, D., Quirion, R. *et al.* (2005) Dopamine supersensitivity correlates with D_2^{High} states, implying many paths to psychosis. *Proceedings of the National Academy of Sciences USA* **102**, 3513–3518.

Semenova, S., Geyer, M.A., Sutcliffe, J.G. *et al.* (2008) Inactivation of the 5-HT(7) receptor partially blocks phencyclidine-induced disruption of prepulse inhibition. *Biological Psychiatry* **63**, 98–105.

Sergi, M.J., Rassovsky, Y., Widmark, C., *et al.* (2007) Social cognition in schizophrenia. *Schizophrenia Research* **90**, 316–324.

Shapiro, D.A., Renck, S., Arrington, E. *et al.* (2003) Aripiprazole, a novel atypical antipsychotic drug with a unique and robust pharmacology. *Neuropsychopharmacology* **28**, 1400–1411.

Silvestri, S., Seeman, J.C., Negrte, S. *et al.* (1999) Dopamine D2 upregulation and 5HT2 downregulation measured after neuroleptic withdrawal using PET. *Schizophrenia Research* **36**, 247.

Soares, B.G., Fenton M. & Chue, P. (2000) Sulpiride for schizophrenia. *Cochrane Database Systemtic Reviews*, CD001162.

Sokoloff, P. (2005) Focus on clozapine: a new explanation for its atypical character. *International Journal of Neuropsychopharmacology* **8**, 311–313.

Sokoloff, P., Martres, M.-P., Giros, B. *et al.* (1992) The third dopamine receptor (D_3) as a novel target for antipsychotics. *Biochemical Pharmacology* **43**, 659–666.

Spooren, W., Riemer, C. & Meltzer, H.Y. (2005) NK3 receptor antagonists: the next generation of antipsychotics? *Nature Reviews in Drug Discovery* **4**, 967–975.

Stephenson, C.M., Bigliani, V., Jones, H.M. *et al.* (2000) Striatal and extra-striatal D(2)/D(3) dopamine receptor occupancy by quetiapine in vivo. *British Journal of Psychiatry* **177**, 408–415.

Stone, J.M., Morrison P.D. & Pilowsky, L.S. (2007) Glutamate and dopamine dysregulation in schizophrenia. *Journal of Psychopharmacology* **21**, 440–452.

Stone, J.M., Bressan, R.A., Erlandsson, K. *et al.* (2005) Non-uniform blockade of intrastriatal D2/D3 receptors by risperidone and amisulpride. *Psychopharmacology* **180**, 664–669.

Swainston-Harrison, T. & Scott, L. J. (2006) Ziprasidone. *CNS Drugs* **20**, 1027–1052.

Szewczak, M.R., Corbett, R., Rush, D.K. *et al.* (1995) The pharmacological profile of iloperidone, a novel atypical antipsychotic agent. *Journal of Pharmacology and Experimental Therapeutics* **274**, 1404–1413.

Tadori, Y., Miwa, T., Tottori, K. *et al.* (2005) Aripiprazole's low intrinsic activities at human dopamine D2L and D2S receptors render it a unique antipsychotic. *European Journal of Pharmacology* **515**, 10–19.

Takano, A., Suhara, T., Yasuno, F. *et al.* (2006) The antipsychotic sultopride is overdosed. *International Journal of Neuropsychopharmacology* **9**, 539–545.

Talvik, M., Nordstrom, A.L., Nyberg, S. *et al.* (2002) No support for regional selectivity in clozapine-treated patients: a PET study with [(11)C]raclopride and [(11)C]FLB 457. *American Journal of Psychiatry* **158**, 926–930.

Tamminga, C.A. & Davis, J.M. (2007) The neuropharmacology of psychosis. *Schizophrenia Bulletin* **33**, 937–946.

Tandon, R. & Nasrallah, H.A. (2006) Subjecting meta-analyses to closer scrutiny: Little support for differential efficacy among second-generation antipsychotics at equivalent doses. *Archives of General Psychiatry* **63**, 935–937.

Tandon, R., Keshaven, M.S. & Nasrallah, H.A. (2008) Schizophrenia, "Just the Facts": What we know in 2008 Part 1: Overview. *Schizophrenia Research* **100**, 4–19.

Tarazi, F.I. & Baldessarini, R.J. (1999) Dopamine D_4 receptors. *Molecular Psychiatry* **4**, 529–538.

Tarsy, D. & Baldessarini, R.J. (2006) Epidemiology of tardive dyskinesia. *Movement Disorders* **21**, 589–598.

Tauscher, J., Jones, C., Remington, G. *et al.* (2002) Significant dissociation of brain and plasma kinetics with antipsychotics. *Molecular Psychiatry* **7**, 317–321.

Tauscher, J., Hussain, T., Agid, O. *et al.* (2004) Equivalent occupancy of dopamine D1 and D2 receptors with clozapine. *American Journal of Psychiatry* **161**, 1620–1625.

Tauscher-Wisniewski, S., Kapur, S., Tauscher, J. *et al.* (2002) Quetiapine: an effective antipsychotic in first-episode schizophrenia despite only transiently high dopamine-2 receptor blockade. *Journal of Clinical Psychiatry* **63**, 992–997.

Taylor, D. (2003) Ziprasidone in the management of schizophrenia. *CNS Drugs* **17**, 423–430.

Tenback, D.E., van Harten, P.N., Slooff, C.J. *et al.* (2006) Evidence that early extrapyramidal symptoms predict later tardive dyskinesia. *American Journal of Psychiatry* **163**, 1438–1440.

Tiihonen, J., Walhbeck, K., Lonnqvist, J. *et al.* (2006) Effectiveness of antipsychotic treatments in a nationwide cohort of patients in community care after first hospitalisation due to schizophrenia and schizoaffective disorder. *British Medical Journal* **333**, 224.

Timmermann, D.B., Gronlien, J.H., Kohlhaas, K.L. *et al.* (2007) An allosteric modulator of the alpha7 nicotinic acetylcholine receptor possessing cognition-enhancing properties in vivo. *Journal of Pharmacology and Experimental Therapeutics* **323**, 294–307.

Travis, M.J., Busatto, G.F., Pilowsky, L.S. *et al.* (1997) Serotonin: 5-HT2A receptor occupancy in vivo and response to the new antipsychotics olanzapine and sertindole. *British Journal of Psychiatry* **171**, 290–291.

Trichard, C., Paillere-Martinot, M.L., Attar-Levy, D, *et al.* (1998) Binding of antipsychotic drugs to cortical 5-HT$_{2A}$ receptors. *American Journal of Psychiatry* **155**, 505–508.

Truffinet, P., Tamminga, C.A., Fabre, L.F. *et al.* (1999) Placebo-controlled study of the D$_4$/5-HT$_{2A}$ antagonist fananserin in the treatment of schizophrenia. *American Journal of Psychiatry* **156**, 419–425.

Tuominen, H.J., Tiihonen J. & Wahlbeck, K. (2005) Glutamatergic drugs for schizophrenia. *Schizophrenia Research* **72**, 225–234.

Turrone, P., Remington, G. & Nobrega, J.N. (2002) The vacuous chewing movement (VCM) model of tardive dyskinesia revisited. Is there a relationship to dopamine D_2 receptor occupancy? *Neuroscience and Biobehavioral Reviews* **26**, 361–380.

Turrone, P., Remington, G., Kapur, S. *et al.* (2005) Continuous but not intermittent olanzapine infusion induces vacuous chewing movements in rats. *Biological Psychiatry* **57**, 406–411.

Uchida, H., Mamo, D.C., Kapur, S. *et al.* (2008) Monthly administration of long-acting injectable risperidone and striatal dopamine D$_2$ receptor occupancy. *Journal of Clinical Psychiatry* **69**, 1281–1286.

Urbano, F.J., Leznik E. & Llinas, R.R. (2007) Modafinil enhances thalamocortical activity by increasing neuronal electrotonic coupling. *Proceedings of the National Acadamy of Sciences USA* **104**, 12554–12559.

Van Tol, H.H.M., Bunzow, J.R., Guan, H.-C. *et al.* (1991) Cloning of the gene for a human dopamine D$_4$ receptor with high affinity for the antipsychotic clozapine. *Nature* **350**, 610–614.

Vernaleken, I., Siessmeier, T., Buchholz, H.G. *et al.* (2004) High striatal occupancy of D2-like dopamine receptors by amisulpride in the brain of patients with schizophrenia. *International Journal of Neuropsychopharmacology* **7**, 421–430.

Voruganti, L., & Awad, A.G. (2004) Neuroleptic dysphoria. *Psychopharmacology* **171**, 121–132.

Waddington, J.L., Scully, P.J. & O'Callaghan, E. (1997) The new antipsychotics, and their potential for early intervention in schizophrenia. *Schizophrenia Research* **28**, 207–222.

Waddington, J.L., Kapur, S. & Remmington, G.J. (2003) The neuroscience and clinical psychopharmacology of first- and second-generation antipsychotics drugs. In: Hirsh, S.R. & Weinbergery, D.R., eds. *Schizophrenia*. Oxford: Blackwell, pp. 421–441.

Waddington, J.L., Daly, S.A., McCauley, P.G. *et al.* (1994) Levels of functional interaction between 'D-1-like' and 'D-2-like' dopamine receptor systems. In: Niznik, H.B., eds. *Dopamine Receptors*. New York: Marcel Dekker, pp. 511–537.

Waddington, J.L. & Casey. D.E. (2000) Comparative pharmacology of classical and novel [second-generation] antipsychotics. In: Buckley, P.F. & Waddington, J.L., eds. *Schizophrenia and Mood Disorders: The New Drug Therapies in Clinical Practice*. Oxford: Butterworth Heinemann, pp. 3–13.

Waddington, J.L. & Morgan, M.G. (2001) Pathobiology of schizophrenia. In: Lieberman, J.A. & Murray, R.M., eds. *Comprehensive Care of Schizophrenia: A Textbook of Clinical Management*. London: Martin Dunitz, pp. 27–35.

Waddington, J.L. (1993) Pre- and postsynaptic D-1 to D-5 dopamine receptor mechanisms in relation to antipsychotic activity. In: Barnes, T.R.E., ed. *Antipsychotic Drugs and their Side Effects*. London: Academic Press, pp. 65–85.

Waddington, J.L. (2007) Neuroimaging and other neurobiological indices in schizophrenia. *British Journal of Psychiatry* **50** (Suppl.), s52–s57.

Waddington, J.L., Kingston, T. & O'Tuathaigh, C.M.P. (2007a) Longitudinal studies on course of illness in schizophrenia. A lifetime trajectory perspective. In: Carpenter, W.T. & Thaker, G., ed. *The Year in Schizophrenia*, Vol. **1**. Oxford: Oxford Clinical Publishing, pp. 77–99.

Waddington, J.L., Corvin, A.P., Donohue, G. *et al.* (2007b) Functional genomics and schizophrenia. Endophenotypes and mutant models. *Psychiatric Clinics of North America* **30**, 365–399.

Waddington, J.L., O'Tuathaigh, C., O'Sullivan, G. *et al.* (2005) Phenotypic studies on dopamine receptor subtype and associated signal transduction mutants. *Psychopharmacology* **181**, 611–638.

Wadenberg, M.L., Wiker, C. & Svensson, T.H. (2007) Enhanced efficacy of both typical and atypical antipsychotic drugs by adjunctive alpha2 adrenoceptor blockade. *International Journal of Neuropsychopharmacology* **10**, 191–202.

Wahlbeck, K., Cheine, M., Essali, A. *et al.* (1999) Evidence of clozapine's effectiveness in schizophrenia. *American Journal of Psychiatry* **156**, 990–999.

Walterfang, M., Wood, S.J., Velakoulis, D. *et al.* (2006) Neuropathological, neurogenetic and neuroimaging evidence for white matter pathology in schizophrenia. *Neuroscience & Biobehavioural Reviews* **30**, 918–948.

Wang, P.S., Schneeweiss, S., Avorn, J. *et al* (2005) Risk of death in elderly users of conventional vs. atypical antipsychotic medications. *New England Journal of Medicine* **353**, 2335–2341.

Wijkstra, J., Lijmer, J., Balk, F.J. *et al.* (2006) Pharmacological treatment for unipolar psychotic depression. *British Journal of Psychiatry* **188**, 410–415.

Wolkin, A., Barouche, F., Wolf, A.P. *et al.* (1989) Dopamine blockade and clinical response: evidence for two biological subgroups of schizophrenia. *American Journal of Psychiatry* **146**, 905–908.

Wong, A.H. & Van Tol, H.H. (2003) The dopamine D4 receptors and mechanisms of antipsychotic atypicality. *Progress in Neuropsychopharmacology and Biological Psychiatry* **27**, 1091–1099.

Wood, M.D., Scott, C., Clarke, K. *et al.* (2006) Aripiprazole and its human metabolite are partial agonists at the human dopamine D2 receptor, but the rodent metabolite displays antagonist properties. *European Journal of Pharmacology* **546**, 88–94.

Xiberas, X., Martinot, J.L., Mallet, L. *et al.* (2001) Extrastriatal and striatal D(2) dopamine receptor blockade with haloperidol or new antipsychotic drugs in patients with schizophrenia. *British Journal of Psychiatry* **179**, 503–508.

Yang, L.P. & Plosker, G.L. (2007) Paliperidone extended release. *CNS Drugs* **21**, 417–425.

Yokoi, F., Grunder, G., Biziere, K. *et al.* (2002) Dopamine D2 and D3 receptor occupancy in normal humans treated with the antipsychotic drug aripiprazole (OPC 14597). *Neuropsychopharmacology* **27**, 248–259.

Youngren, K.D., Inglis, F.M., Pivirotto, P.J. *et al.* (1999) Clozapine preferentially increases dopamine release in the Rhesus monkey prefrontal cortex compared with the caudate nucleus. *Neuropsychopharmacology* **20**, 403–412.

Zhang, L., Shirayama, Y., Iyo, M. *et al.* (2007) Minocycline attenuates hyperlocomotion and prepulse inhibition deficits in mice after administration of the NMDA receptor antagonist dizocilpine. *Neuropsychopharmacology* **32**, 2004–2010.

Principles of pharmacological treatment in schizophrenia

Thomas R.E. Barnes[1] and Stephen R. Marder[2]

[1]Imperial College, London, UK
[2]Semel Institute for Neuroscience at UCLA, Los Angeles, CA, USA

Who benefits from these medications?

The important effect of antipsychotic medications in schizophrenia is their ability to reduce and sometimes eliminate psychotic thought processes. As a result, there is less misinterpretation of information in the person's environment or generated from memories, and delusions are less likely to emerge and are often eliminated. Similarly, the tendency to misinterpret internally generated information is reduced as auditory or other sensations are decreased. In other words, hallucinations are reduced. Some individuals describe antipsychotics as improving their ability to "filter" extraneous or irrelevant information. Individuals who experience psychomotor agitation will usually experience a calming effect from an antipsychotic. Finally, antipsychotics are effective in reducing the risk of psychotic relapse in stable patients with illnesses that tend to recur. These benefits are experienced by individuals with schizophrenia as well as those with other conditions associated with psychosis: schizoaffective illness, bipolar mania or mixed states, depression with psychosis, psychoses secondary to drugs, and psychoses from medical conditions.

It is important to note that antipsychotic medications are not antischizophrenia medications. Other symptom dimen-

sions of schizophrenia are often unaffected by these drugs. Negative symptoms of schizophrenia, including restricted affect, avolition, apathy, and anhedonia, may be unchanged by antipsychotics or improved to only a minimal degree. The same is true for the impairments in cognition, including deficits in memory, attention, and executive functioning. Patients with schizophrenia often perform 1.5–2 standard deviations below the mean on neuropsychological tests (see Chapter 8). First- or second-generation antipsychotics (FGAs and SGAs) may improve cognitive performance but only correct a small percentage of this deficit (Harvey & Keefe, 2001). This limitation is important since the functional outcome of schizophrenia, that is, the ability of patients to work, carry out family responsibilities, engage in education, and to socialize, is more related to their negative and cognitive symptoms than to their psychosis (Green, 1996; Kirkpatrick et al., 2006).

These limited but important effects of available antipsychotics support the treatment of nearly all patients with schizophrenia with an antipsychotic medication. The effects are clearest for patients who are burdened by psychotic symptoms. Antipsychotics reduce the discomfort and the behavioral consequences from psychosis. Even when symptoms persist with an antipsychotic, they tend to persist in a milder form than if untreated. Patients who are free of psychotic symptoms will often question whether they are deriving any benefit from drug treatment and ask to have it discontinued. These individuals are correct in

---

Schizophrenia, 3rd edition. Edited by Daniel R. Weinberger and Paul J Harrison © 2011 Blackwell Publishing Ltd.

asserting that antipsychotics probably have little effect on their immediate subjective state or their behavior. However, in these individuals, antipsychotics are effective in preventing recurrences of psychotic symptoms. The impact of reducing psychosis and preventing recurrences can have other secondary effects. Antipsychotic treatment, particularly treatment with clozapine, reduces the risk of suicide in schizophrenia (Meltzer *et al.*, 2003). Also, as will be noted below, patients who are stabilized on antipsychotic medications derive greater benefit from psychosocial treatment and rehabilitation (Marder, 2000). Patients who relapse when they are not being treated with an antipsychotic also tend to have more severe relapses that are more often associated with involuntary hospitalization (Johnson *et al.*, 1983).

The benefits from antipsychotic medications should be balanced against their side effects, which are probably a burden to nearly every patient treated with these drugs (see Chapters 27 and 28). This raises the question as to whether there are any patients for whom the benefits derived from these medications do not justify the burden from adverse effects. In our experience these individuals are very uncommon. Some have very mild psychotic symptoms and are able to manage through self-monitoring. Others can be managed without antipsychotic medications between episodes because they are able to identify early warning signs of an unfolding psychotic episode and resume treatment before the episode fully emerges.

Prescribing principles

Titration of dose

Each new prescription should constitute an individual clinical trial, with explicit expectations of what will represent a satisfactory response, how long treatment will be required to achieve such a response, and the criteria for discontinuation. If an adequate trial is ensured in terms of dosage, duration, and adherence, the nature and degree of the clinical response can more reliably inform any longer-term medication treatment strategy for that individual.

Optimizing dosage can be complex, as there is commonly a need to balance clinical response against the emergence of side effects, and reduction of dosage to tackle unwanted effects runs the risk of compromising the control of symptoms or increasing the risk of relapse. For each patient, the dose should be titrated to the lowest known to be effective, with increases in dosage of oral medication generally only warranted after 2 weeks of assessment, during which the patient has shown little or no evidence of a therapeutic response. When treating an acute psychotic episode, any decision to titrate the dosage against efficacy should be taken in the light of the likely timeframe and evolution of clinical response. Following a review of rele-

vant trials of antipsychotic response, Agid *et al.* (2003, 2006) concluded that there is little delay in the onset of antipsychotic action. Improvement occurs most rapidly in the first 2 weeks and then slowly reaches a plateau, with more improvement observed in the first month than in the rest of the subsequent year. In those first few weeks of treatment, the various dimensions of psychosis may be differentially affected. While rapid reduction of the behavioral impact of key psychotic symptoms may occur, along with a decrease in cognitive and emotional preoccupation, a patient's degree of conviction about psychotic experiences may take longer to respond (Mizrahi *et al.*, 2006).

When initiating medication in those presenting with their first episode, clinicians should start at the lowest recommended dosage for the antipsychotic being used (Lehman *et al.*, 2004), given the evidence that first-episode subjects respond to lower doses of antipsychotics than those with established schizophrenia, even when stringent criteria for response are applied (Robinson *et al.*, 1999; Rummel *et al.*, 2003; Schooler *et al.*, 2005). When treating an acute episode, little is to be gained by a high initial "loading" dose, the so-called "rapid neuroleptization" strategy (Barnes *et al.*, 2006), compared with doses in the recommended range. With advancing age, changes in the metabolism and physiology of the gastrointestinal, hepatic, renal, and cardiovascular systems substantially alter drug distribution and render older people more sensitive to side effects. Therefore, any antipsychotic drug used in the elderly should be started at the lowest possible dose, and subsequently monitored and titrated carefully with regular reviews (Howard *et al.*, 2000; Saltz *et al.*, 2000, 2004).

In line with such principles, UK recommendations for the drug treatment of schizophrenia are that the dose of an individual antipsychotic should be within its Summary of Product Characteristics (SPC)/British National Formulary (BNF) limits, that individuals receive only one antipsychotic at a time (National Institute for Clinical Excellence, 2002a), and that FGAs and SGAs are not prescribed concurrently (National Institute for Clinical Excellence, 2002b). Despite this guidance, and a lack of any convincing evidence for any benefit with either high-dose (Barnes *et al.*, 2006) or, with the exception of clozapine augmentation, combined antipsychotics, such prescribing is common in clinical practice. For example, UK audit data suggest that about a third of acute adult inpatients and forensic inpatients are prescribed a high dose, over 40% are prescribed combined antipsychotics, and around 30% are prescribed an FGA and SGA together, which presumably compromises any tolerability advantage of the latter (Prescribing Observatory for Mental Health, 2007a, 2007b). However, the use of PRN ("as required") antipsychotic medication makes a major contribution to these figures (Paton *et al.*, 2008).

With depot medication, achievement of peak plasma levels, therapeutic effect, and steady-state plasma levels takes considerably longer, so titration against response is a protracted process (Barnes & Curson, 1994; Kane *et al.*, 1998). For example, any increase in risk of relapse after a reduction in depot dosage or extension of the injection interval may take months or years to be evident.

Switching antipsychotic

The advent of SGAs raised expectations among clinicians and patients for beneficial outcomes with antipsychotic medication, leading to more switching of antipsychotic medication in pursuit of an optimal balance of efficacy and tolerability. However, the evidence base for such a strategy is relatively limited (Kinon et al., 1993; Weiden, 2006). The main reasons for switching from one antipsychotic to another are a disappointing therapeutic response, or intolerable side effects, or both. A poor response may prompt a switch, most commonly, perhaps, to try and achieve better control of positive symptoms that are persistent despite an adequate trial of monotherapy, but problems with recurrent relapse, or poor response in other domains, such as negative symptoms or affective disturbance, may also provoke a change in drug. A switch may also be warranted by adverse effects that are distressing, disabling or intolerable, or that may compromise the patient's physical health in the short or long term.

The risks of switching are destabilization of the illness and the provocation of switch-emergent adverse effects, problems that are potentially attributable to the discontinuation of the first antipsychotic, and/or a response to the second, and/or differences in pharmacological profile between the first and second (Lambert, 2007). To minimize such problems, an abrupt switch should be avoided. A gradual cross-tapering approach is usually recommended, whereby the first antipsychotic agent is either maintained at a therapeutic dose as the dose of the new antipsychotic is slowly titrated up, or gradually discontinued over the same period that the dose of the new drug is gradually titrated up (Weiden, 2006, Lambert, 2007).

Assessment of side effects

Antipsychotics have a broad range of side effects, with both FGAs and SGAs sharing, for example, the capacity to produce endocrine and metabolic disturbance, sexual dysfunction, cardiovascular abnormalities, hepatic effects, sedation, and a reduced seizure threshold (Barnes & McPhillips, 1999; see also Chapters 27 and 28). A clinician's choice of an antipsychotic will often be largely determined by its known relative liability for particular side effects matched to the perceived susceptibility, impact, and acceptability of such side effects in the person to be treated.

Effective evaluation of side effects requires more than one approach, combining physical health screening, investigation, and examination with careful enquiry informed by the recognized side effect profile of the particular antipsychotic prescribed. The full extent of side effect burden can only be ascertained by systematic inquiry (Weiden & Miller, 2001; Jordan *et al.*, 2002; Byerly *et al.*, 2006; Yusufi *et al.*, 2007). Many patients will fail to attribute certain side effects to the medication, or be embarrassed about mentioning them. Thus, some problems, such as sexual side effects and menstrual irregularities, are only likely to be elicited by direct but sensitive questioning (Yusufi *et al.*, 2007). Careful enquiry will be required to establish the clinical relevance of any particular side effect, that is, the level of associated distress as well as any impact on social, occupational or interpersonal functioning. Similarly, only systematic interview with a patient will yield reliable information about the presence and severity of possible subjective side effects. Not only is the clinician faced with the challenge of distinguishing between reported experiences that may have shared elements, such as daytime sleepiness, lethargy and lassitude, loss of energy, problems with concentration, and a sense of emotional numbness, but also deciding whether these phenomena are predominantly a manifestation of the illness or a consequence of its treatment.

The potential overlap between side effects and the signs and symptoms of illness occur in a range of domains, including extrapyramidal side effects (EPS). For example, some of the manifestations of bradykinesia, a sign of drug-induced parkinsonism, resemble features of retarded depression or negative symptoms such as flattened affect, and the feelings of restlessness and inner tension that characterize akathisia may be mistaken for psychomotor agitation associated with the psychotic illness.

Provision of information to patients about possible side effects, and the regular, comprehensive assessment of such problems is good practice, although there is no widely accepted minimum assessment standard in terms of frequency or the use of a formal side effect checklist or rating scale. Most of the general side effect assessment tools that are available were introduced some years ago, and address the presence and severity of those adverse effects commonly seen with FGAs rather than both FGAs and SGAs. Further, they often fail to cover the detailed assessment of important common adverse reactions such as dysphoric subjective experiences, glucose and lipid dysregulation, and sexual and urinary dysfunction. These scales were essentially designed for research purposes and many would be too time-consuming or limited in range to have much clinical utility (Jordan *et al.*, 2004), particularly as screening instruments. More specific rating scales are available for particular problems, such as EPS (parkinsonism, akathisia, and tardive dyskinesia; Gervin & Barnes, 2000) and sexual side effects (Byerly *et al.*, 2006), as well as treatment tolerability. Such scales can be useful clinically for both the identification and monitoring of these problems.

In addition to side effect assessment by systematic enquiry and the use of rating scales (Ohlsen *et al.*, 2008), there is also a need for routine physical investigations. For example, plasma prolactin should be monitored where there is a risk of persistently elevated levels, which are associated with several adverse consequences such as sexual dysfunction, reduction in bone mineral density, and menstrual disturbance (Montejo, 2008). Screening and monitoring are also required in relation to the cluster of features (hypertension, central obesity, glucose intolerance/ insulin resistance, dyslipidemia) that constitute the metabolic syndrome. This is commonly manifest in people with psychotic disorder who are receiving antipsychotic medication (Holt *et al.*, 2004; Mackin *et al.*, 2005), and is predictive of both Type 2 diabetes and cardiovascular disease (Grundy *et al.*, 2004). Reviews of the association between psychotic illness, the metabolic syndrome, and antipsychotic medication have led to recommendations for routine physical health screening for all people prescribed antipsychotic drugs (American Diabetes Association *et al.*, 2004; De Nayer *et al.*, 2005; Newcomer, 2007), although there is evidence that screening for the metabolic syndrome falls short of the optimum in routine practice (Barnes *et al.*, 2007). The Mount Sinai Guidelines suggest that clinicians should intervene when a patient shows a weight increase of 1 body mass index (BMI) unit. The intervention may include closer monitoring, recommendations for diet and exercise, and switching to an antipsychotic with a lower liability for metabolic effects. Changing antipsychotics for patients who gain weight or show other metabolic disturbances is supported by the findings from Phase 2 of the NIMH Clinical Antipsychotic Trials of Intervention Effectiveness (CATIE) study. In that trial, patients who had gained weight in Phase 1 were likely to lose weight and have improvements in their metabolic parameters when switched to ziprasidone or risperidone (see Chapter 28).

Choice of antipsychotic

Key considerations when choosing an antipsychotic drug are its likely efficacy and tolerability, and the likely adherence to the regimen by the particular individual for whom the drug will be prescribed. Evidence of past response, or lack of it, to specific antipsychotic drugs is useful, as is information on the patient's history of side effects with particular antipsychotics, general attitudes to medication, and record of adherence. It is recommended that such a choice is made jointly between the prescriber and the service user (and/or carer in some situations), based on an informed discussion of the relative benefits of the drugs and their known side-effect profiles (National Institute for Clinical Excellence, 2009). There is some expectation that patients who have the chance to express their preference in this way will show better adherence (Hamann *et al.*, 2003).

Leaving aside clozapine, which has a particular claim for effectiveness in treatment-resistant schizophrenia (Lewis *et al.*, 2006), the other available SGAs have been considered to be at least as effective as FGAs. However, none has been consistently or conclusively shown to be superior in terms of symptom response. (For a detailed discussion, see Chapter 25). So when considering the risk–benefit balance of a particular antipsychotic for a patient, a clinician will tend to turn to the evidence for the relative liability of antipsychotics for the common and potentially distressing and disabling side effects, such as metabolic effects and EPS (Shirdazi & Ghaemi, 2006).

Extrapyramidal side effects

The defining advantage of the SGAs when they were introduced was a lower liability for EPS than FGAs, although this benefit has not proved immune to challenge. It has been pointed out that interpretation of the randomized controlled trial evidence for the superiority of SGAs over FGAs in respect of acute EPS should take into account the dose and choice of FGA comparator, most commonly haloperidol, which is considered a high potency dopamine D_2 receptor antagonist with a relatively high liability for EPS (Geddes *et al.*, 2000). Even in studies where low doses of haloperidol have been used, e.g., in a first-episode study in comparison with a low-dose SGA, risperidone (Schooler *et al.*, 2005), the latter still showed a significant advantage with regard to EPS. But the situation may not be so clear where the comparator is a non-haloperidol, so-called low-potency FGA. A systematic review and meta-analysis of relevant trials by Leucht *et al.* (2003b) concluded that optimum doses of low-potency FGAs might not induce more EPS than SGAs. Further, the incidence of acute EPS reported in clinical trials may not be very generalizable, as it tends to relate to the short-term and antipsychotic monotherapy in standard dosage. In routine clinical practice, an additional issue is the common prescription of combined antipsychotics and high dosage, which are potential risk factors for EPS (Carnahan *et al.*, 2006).

Two major effectiveness studies have compared SGAs and FGAs: the CATIE study (Lieberman *et al.*, 2005) and the Cost Utility of the Latest Antipsychotics in Schizophrenia Study (CUtLASS1; Jones *et al.*, 2006). The FGA tested in CATIE was a low-potency drug, perphenazine, while in the CUtLASS1 various FGAs were chosen by the participating clinicians, the most common being sulpiride, which is also considered to be a low-potency agent. The findings of these studies are commonly cited as evidence for a lack of any major differences in risk of acute EPS between SGAs and

FGAs. But it is also noted that in the CATIE study a proxy measure of EPS liability, treatment discontinuation due to EPS, was significantly higher in the group receiving perphenazine. Of course, individual SGAs differ in their propensity to cause EPS: for some SGAs (e.g., clozapine and quetiapine) acute EPS liability does not differ from placebo across their full dose range, while for others (e.g., amisulpride, risperidone) the risk is dose dependent. These differences may reflect individual drug profiles in relation to properties such as selective dopamine D_2-like receptor antagonism, potent 5-HT_{2A} antagonism, and rapid dissociation from the D_2 receptor, and for aripiprazole, partial agonism at D_2 and 5-HT_{1A} receptors (see Chapter 23).

In relation to tardive dyskinesia (TD), the findings of a systematic review of 1-year studies (Correll *et al.*, 2004) suggested that people treated with SGAs had a markedly lower rate of TD over such a period. The estimated annualized incidence of TD in adults receiving SGAs was 0.8%, compared with 5.4% for those treated with FGAs, although haloperidol was the FGA comparator and was used in relatively high doses. Nevertheless, the results of a 3-year prospective study of the treatment of schizophrenia provided further evidence that SGAs have a genuine advantage in terms of a lower incidence and persistence of TD in clinical practice (Tenback *et al.*, 2005).

Several conclusions may be tentatively drawn. The evidence suggests that SGAs have a lower liability for acute EPS and TD than haloperidol, even at low dosage. The evidence for a lower liability for EPS with SGAs in comparison with low-dose, low-potency FGAs is less convincing. The common use of high-dose or combined SGAs, or combined SGAs and FGAs in clinical practice may compromise any advantage in relation to EPS. Certainly parkinsonism and akathisia remain major problems despite the widespread use of SGAs (Shirdazi & Ghaemi, 2006). In relation to TD specifically, preliminary evidence suggests a lower risk with SGAs, but this remains to be confirmed. For further discussion of the evidence base regarding antipsychotic effectiveness, see Chapter 25.

Long-term treatment

Relapse prevention

As mentioned above, antipsychotic medications are effective for decreasing the risk of psychotic relapse in schizophrenia. Studies of patients stabilized on an antipsychotic have randomized them to either changing to a placebo or continuing on an antipsychotic. The results differ depending on the population and the study design, but there is some consistency in the results. Approximately 70% of patients changed to placebo will relapse during the first year compared to only 30% of patients who remain on an antipsychotic (Davis, 1985). The differences between active

drug and placebo are likely to be larger when drug delivery is assured with a long-acting depot antipsychotic (Kane, 1984).

It is unclear if SGAs differ from FGAs with regard to relapse prevention in stable patients. A meta-analysis of clinical trials by Leucht *et al.* (2003a) found a modest but statistically significant difference favoring the SGAs tested. However, the use of haloperidol as the comparator FGA in many of these trials, an issue already mentioned above, should be taken into account when interpreting these findings. For example, because haloperidol has a greater liability for discomforting EPS, it is possible that patients assigned to this drug were less adherent. This contrast was demonstrated in a comparison of haloperidol and risperidone in which patients were followed for 2 years (Marder *et al.*, 2003). Even at low doses of both agents, patients on risperidone experienced less anxiety and depression. This appeared to be related to increased EPS, particularly akathisia, with haloperidol.

Duration of antipsychotic treatment for relapse prevention

Patients whose illnesses have been stable on an antipsychotic for years will often believe that the stability protects them against the risk of relapse, and that they are well despite rather than because of the continued medication. As a result, these patients will often challenge the need for continued medication, and pressure their clinician to stop it. Others will merely stop seeing their provider and/or stop refilling prescriptions. However, studies indicate that long periods of stability do not necessarily protect patients from relapse if their medications are discontinued. Rather, their relapse rates are similar to those of patients who have had recent relapses (Hogarty *et al.*, 1976). One can also make the case that those patients who have been in full remission for a prolonged period of time are deriving the most benefit from an antipsychotic. However, what has not been adequately tested is whether individuals who benefit from non-pharmacological treatments such as cognitive–behavioral therapy (CBT) for psychosis may be better candidates for drug discontinuation since they may be better able to detect impending relapse and resume medication.

Given the absence of reliable predictors of prognosis or long-term drug response, pharmacological relapse prevention is generally recommended for every patient diagnosed with schizophrenia for at least 1–2 years (Lehman *et al.*, 2004; National Institute for Clinical Excellence, 2009). Bosveld-van Haandel *et al.* (2001) considered this an arbitrary recommendation based on medium-term studies of therapeutic efficacy lasting less than 3 years. Given that rehabilitation programs aimed at improving social function, stable social integration, and subjective wellbeing take a long time, their view was that antipsychotic treatment should be maintained for longer, despite the lack of robust evidence.

Other goals

There is a growing consensus among clinicians, patients, and family members that the goal of long-term treatment should be more ambitious than merely preventing psychotic relapse. This has led to the designation of recovery as a treatment goal. Although definitions of "recovery" vary, for the purposes of this chapter we use the term to refer to a process whereby patients establish their own personal goals. Goals may include functioning more independently, improving social relationships, achieving educational goals, or finding a satisfying job. For the great majority of patients, "recovery" does not mean being cured of schizophrenia. Instead, it means being able to live a more satisfying life despite the burden of a chronic illness.

Pharmacological treatment plays an essential role in a treatment plan that is focused on recovery. There is substantial evidence indicating that patients who are receiving optimal long-term pharmacotherapy are more likely to benefit from psychosocial treatments and rehabilitation programs. Early National Institute of Mental Health (NIMH) studies showed that patients who were not treated with medications could demonstrate a clinical deterioration when they were stressed with psychosocial treatments. Hogarty et al. (1979) found that patients who received guaranteed drug delivery with a long-acting depot antipsychotic derived greater benefit from psychosocial treatments. An interesting study by Rosenheck et al. (1998) focused on the use of psychosocial treatments and rehabilitation in patients assigned to a comparison of clozapine or haloperidol. Although the psychosocial treatment was not a component of the study, patients receiving clozapine were more likely to utilize higher levels of psychosocial treatment. Moreover, use of these higher levels was associated with greater improvements in quality of life. This suggests that patients who experience more improvement in symptoms on a better pharmacotherapy have a greater potential to benefit from psychosocial interventions. It also suggests that one of the long-term goals of pharmacotherapy is to facilitate participation in psychosocial treatments.

Drug selection

Selecting the optimal regimen for long-term treatment requires a number of considerations. Since the most common reason for relapse among stable patients with schizophrenia is non-adherence with an antipsychotic, finding a drug and a treatment regimen that a patient will continue to accept is an important aim. Since the subjective experience of a medication is usually related to side effects, tolerability is likely to be the major consideration in drug selection. Moreover, tolerability can be related to a side effect that causes discomfort for the patient or to something that affects a patient's health, such as weight gain or an endocrine effect. Taking akathisia as an example, even mild to moderate symptoms can be difficult to live with if a patient experiences restlessness during every waking hour. Also, patients will differ in how they accommodate to different side effects. Some patients appreciate the mild sedation that is associated with antipsychotics such as olanzapine or quetiapine. Others may find that mild sedation interferes with their ability to perform at work or elsewhere. Patients who experience these discomforts are less likely to continue taking their medications regularly. These considerations suggest that clinicians should be aware of an individual's experience on an antipsychotic. In contrast to acute treatment, when side effects may be tolerated and clinical response is the priority, patients may be less likely to accept side effects that impair the quality of their lives.

There are other considerations in selecting an antipsychotic for long-term treatment. Patients who have a history of unreliable pill taking may benefit from a long-acting injectable antipsychotic. The key advantage for depot preparations over oral antipsychotics is the avoidance of the covert non-adherence possible with tablets. Non-adherence with depot is evident to the clinical team because of the failure of the patient to attend for, or refuse to accept, the injection. Nevertheless, it should not be assumed that depot preparations guarantee good adherence. During a follow-up period of 7 years, Curson et al., (1985) found adherence problems at some time in up 40% of patients established on FGA depot preparations. Other potential advantages of depot preparations include being more convenient and easier to remember than regular tablet taking for some patients, more predictable and stable serum drug levels, a reduced variability between patients in steady-state blood levels for a given dose, and a reduced risk of inadvertent or deliberate overdose (Barnes & Curson, 1994; Patel & David, 2005). Further, if a patient suffers a relapse despite the guaranteed medication delivery with depot, then non-adherence can be safely excluded as the cause. Clinical disadvantages include the lack of acceptability of regular intramuscular injections by a proportion of patients who see them as potentially painful, intrusive or ignominious, and some reduced flexibility in dosage.

Patients who receive long-acting depot agents are at least as likely to remain in a stable remission as those on maintenance oral medication (Adams et al., 2001, Nadeem et al., 2004). The studies comparing relapse rates on oral and depot preparations over the relatively short term show only a modest advantage for the latter (Adams et al., 2001), but they may underestimate the advantage of the latter in clinical practice for a couple of reasons: the superiority of depot treatment may require a longer period to be more clearly manifest, and those patients consenting to participate in such trials will tend to be those who would adhere well to oral medication regimens.

Management of non-adherence

The most common cause of relapse in patients with schizophrenia is non-adherence with prescribed medication (Weiden, 2007). Moreover, there is evidence that poor adherence is also associated with poorer long-term functioning (Ascher-Svanum *et al.*, 2006). Non-adherence among patients with schizophrenia is relatively common (Bebbington, 1995). For example, Valenstein *et al.* (2006) found that 61% of the patients they studied had problems with adherence at some time during a 4-year period. Even with first-episode patients, around half will be non-adherent or poorly adherent to their medication regimen in the first year of treatment (Bebbington, 1995; Coldham *et al.*, 2002). The high prevalence of medication non-adherence and its consequences indicate that assessing and managing adherence should be an important component of everyday outpatient management.

Certain patient factors should alert clinicians that there is an increased likelihood of non-adherence. In patients with a recent onset of schizophrenia, a lack of insight into their illness, substance abuse, and depression are indicators that medication adherence should be a concern (Mutsatsa *et al.*, 2003; Perkins *et al.*, 2008). Other factors that are commonly associated with non-adherence are medication side effects and a lack of antipsychotic effectiveness (Byerly *et al.*, 2007). However, while people with psychosis commonly identify side effects as a reason for not taking medication, there are other important influences on medication adherence, such as a complex drug regimen (Diaz *et al.*, 2004), negative attitudes toward medication, and a relative lack of insight (Mutstasta *et al.*, 2006; Cooper *et al.*, 2007). Choosing a drug with a good tolerability and safety profile does not obviate the need to consider how to tackle these other factors. A good therapeutic relationship is central (Bebbington, 1995), allowing frank discussion about medication, with the clinician expressing a commitment to provide a considered response to reports of side effects.

Blackwell (1976) has recommended an approach to evaluating the level of adherence. Merely asking a patient whether they are taking their medication is likely to lead to defensive over-reporting of their level of adherence. Blackwell suggests asking questions in a manner that will lead to an open discussion of adherence. For example, the clinician can note that individuals often find that it is a burden to remember to take medications daily, twice daily, or more often. This may lead patients to reveal more about their ambivalence about taking their pills, their difficulties remembering, or their tendencies to intentionally miss doses.

Patients who are agreeable to an antipsychotic, but are unreliable pill takers, may be candidates for a long-acting medication. As mentioned earlier, there is some evidence to suggest that patients who receive a long-acting antipsychotic preparation have a lower risk for psychotic relapse.

Strategies to educate patients and their families about schizophrenia may improve treatment adherence. A specific adherence (or compliance) therapy was developed to improve patients' cooperation with recommended treatments. It is based on motivational interviewing and uses CBT to assist patients in making their own decisions when they consider treatment options. However, recent studies of this intervention in people with schizophrenia have yielded inconsistent results (O'Donnell *et al.*, 2003) and to date there is inadequate evidence to support its effectiveness (Gray *et al.*, 2006; McIntosh *et al.*, 2006).

Drug discontinuation

Gradual withdrawal of antipsychotic medication is less likely to be associated with relapse, at least in the subsequent 6 months, compared with stopping medication rapidly (Viguera *et al.*, 1997; Jeste *et al.*, 1999). Clinicians should warn patients of this, and of the other risks of abrupt discontinuation, which include symptoms attributable to cholinergic rebound, such as sweating, diarrhea, nausea and vomiting, and insomnia (Borison *et al.*, 1996). Cholinergic rebound is a consequence of an antipsychotic with intrinsic anticholinergic activity, or an anticholinergic antiparkinsonian agent, being stopped too rapidly, leading to rebound cholinergic hypersensitivity. A similar mechanism is also hypothesized for dopamine receptor supersensitivity on abrupt withdrawal of an antipsychotic, provoking both EPS and symptoms of a "supersensitivity psychosis". This seems a reasonable explanation for EPS such as dystonia, akathisia, parkinsonism, and "withdrawal dyskinesia" resembling TD, occurring as recognized discontinuation problems. The status of psychotic symptoms appearing after stopping antipsychotic medication remains less clear. For example, there has been particular concern that abrupt discontinuation of clozapine can be associated with rapid relapse (Goudie, 2000) characterized by relatively transient symptoms such as delusions, hallucinations, hostility, and paranoid reactions (Tollefson *et al.*, 1999). However, clozapine treatment in recommended dosage is not associated with increased dopamine D_2 binding or D_2 receptor supersensitivity (Verghese *et al.*, 1996). While some have adduced evidence in support of the dopamine supersensitivity/rebound psychosis notion (Chouinard & Jones, 1980; Moncrieff, 2006), it is also plausible that in some cases the symptoms represent a relapse of the underlying illness, or, as Haddad *et al.* (2000) suggest, a combination of the two, that is, sudden drug termination altering the natural course of the illness.

References

Adams, C.E., Fenton, M.K., Quraishi, S. & David, A.S. (2001) Systematic meta-review of depot antipsychotic drugs for people with schizophrenia. *British Journal of Psychiatry* **179**, 290–299.

Agid, O., Kapur, S., Arenovich, T. & Zipursky, R.B. (2003) Delayed-onset hypothesis of antipsychotic action: a hypothesis tested and rejected. *Archives of General Psychiatry* **60**, 1228–1235.

Agid, O., Seeman, P. & Kapur, S. (2006) The "delayed onset" of antipsychotic action – an idea whose time has come and gone. *Journal of Psychiatry and Neuroscience* **31**, 93–100.

American Diabetes Association, American Psychiatric Association; American Association of Clinical Endocrinologists; North American Association for the Study of Obesity (2004) Consensus development conference on antipsychotics and obesity and diabetes. *Diabetes Care* **27**, 596–601.

Ascher-Svanum, H., Faries, D.E., Zhu, B., Ernst, F.R., Swartz, M.S. & Swanson, J.W. (2006) Medication adherence and long-term functional outcomes in the treatment of schizophrenia in usual care. *Journal of Clinical Psychiatry* **67**, 453–460.

Barnes, T.R.E. & Curson, D.A. (1994) Long-acting depot antipsychotics: a risk-benefit assessment. *Drug Safety* **10**, 464–479.

Barnes, T.R.E. & McPhillips, M.A. (1999) Critical analysis and comparison of the side-effect and safety profiles of the new antipsychotics. *British Journal of Psychiatry* **173** (Suppl. 38), 34–43.

Barnes, T.R.E., Davison, S., Ferrier, I.N. et al. (2006) *Consensus Statement on High-Dose Antipsychotic Medication.* CR138. London: Royal College of Psychiatrists.

Barnes, T.R.E., Paton, C., Cavanagh, M.-R., Hancock, E., Taylor, D.M., on behalf of the UK Prescribing Observatory for Mental Health (2007) A UK audit of screening for the metabolic side effects of antipsychotics in community patients. *Schizophrenia Bulletin* **33**, 1397–1401.

Bebbington, P.E. (1995) The content and context of compliance. *International Clinical Psychopharmacology* **9** (Suppl. 5), 41–50.

Blackwell, B. (1976) Treatment adherence. *British Journal of Psychiatry* **129**, 513–531.

Borison, R.L. and Consensus Study Group on Risperidone Dosing (1996) Changing antipsychotic medication: guidelines on the transition to treatment with risperidone. *Clinical Therapeutics* **18**, 592–607.

Bosveld-van Haandel, L.J., Sloof, C.J. & van den Bosch, R.J. (2001) Reasoning about the optimal duration of prophylactic antipsychotic medication in schizophrenia: evidence and arguments. *Acta Psychiatrica Scandinavica* **103**, 335–346.

Byerly, M.J., Nakonezny, P.A., Fisher, R., Magouirk, B. & Rush, A.J. (2006) An empirical evaluation of the Arizona sexual experience scale and a simple one-item screening test for assessing antipsychotic-related sexual dysfunction in outpatients with schizophrenia and schizoaffective disorder. *Schizophrenia Research* **81**, 311–316.

Byerly, M.J., Nakonezny, P.A. & Lescouflair, E. (2007) Antipsychotic medication adherence in schizophrenia. *Psychiatric Clinics of North America* **30**, 437–452.

Carnahan, R.M., Lund, B.C., Perry, P.J. & Chrischilles, E.A. (2006) Increased risk of extrapyramidal side-effect treatment associated with atypical antipsychotic polytherapy. *Acta Psychiatrica Scandinavica* **113**, 135–141.

Chouinard, G. & Jones, B.D. (1980) Neuroleptic-induced supersensitivity psychosis: clinical and pharmacologic characteristics. *American Journal of Psychiatry* **137**, 16–21.

Coldham, E.L., Addington, J. & Addington, D. (2002) Medication adherence of individuals with a first episode of psychosis. *Acta Psychiatrica Scandinavica* **106**, 286–290.

Cooper, C., Bebbington, P., King, M. et al. (2007) Why people do not take their psychotropic drugs as prescribed: results of the 2000 National Psychiatric Morbidity Survey. *Acta Psychiatrica Scandinavica* **116**, 47–53.

Correll, C.U., Leucht, S. & Kane, J.M. (2004) Lower risk for tardive dyskinesia associated with second-generation antipsychotics: a systematic review of 1-year studies. *American Journal of Psychiatry* **161**, 414–425.

Curson, D.A., Barnes, T.R.E., Bamber, R.W.K., Platt, S.D., Hirsch, S.R. & Duffy, J.C. (1985) Long-term depot maintenance of chronic schizophrenic outpatients: the seven year follow-up of the Medical Research Council fluphenazine/placebo trial. *British Journal of Psychiatry* **146**, 464–480.

Davis, J.M. (1985) Maintenance therapy and the natural course of schizophrenia. *Journal of Clinical Psychiatry* **46**, 18–21.

De Nayer, A., De Hert, M., Scheen, A., Van Gaab, L., Peuskens, J., on behalf of the Consensus Group (2005) Conference report: Belgian consensus on metabolic problems associated with second-generation antipsychotics. *International Journal of Psychiatric Clinical Practice* **9**, 130–137.

Diaz, E., Neuse, E., Sullivan, M.C., Pearsall, H.R. & Woods, S.W. (2004) Adherence to conventional and atypical antipsychotics after hospital discharge. *Journal of Clinical Psychiatry* **65**, 354–360.

Geddes, J., Freemantle, N., Harrison, P. & Bebbington, P. (2000) Atypical antipsychotics in the treatment of schizophrenia: systematic overview and meta-regression analysis. *BMJ* **321**, 1371–1376.

Gervin, M. & Barnes, T.R.E. (2000) Assessment of drug-related movement disorders in schizophrenia. *Advances in Psychiatric Treatment* **6**, 332–343.

Goudie, A.J. (2000) What is the clinical significance of the discontinuation syndrome seen with clozapine? *Journal of Psychopharmacology* **14**, 188–190.

Gray, R., Leese, M., Bindman, J. et al. (2006) Adherence therapy for people with schizophrenia. European multicentre randomised controlled trial. *British Journal of Psychiatry* **189**, 508–514.

Green, M.F. (1996) What are the functional consequences of neurocognitive deficits in schizophrenia? *American Journal of Psychiatry* **153**, 321–330.

Grundy, S.M., Brewer, H.B. Jr, Cleeman, J.I., Smith, S.C. Jr, Lenfant, C; American Heart Association; National Heart, Lung, and Blood Institute (2004) Definition of metabolic syndrome: Report of the National Heart, Lung, and Blood Institute/American Heart Association conference on scientific issues related to definition. *Circulation* **109**, 433–438.

Haddad, P., Hellewell, J. & Young, A. (2000) Reply to A.J. Goudie—What is the clinical significance of the discontinuation syndrome seen with clozapine? *Journal of Psychopharmacology* **14**, 191–192.

Hamann, J., Leucht, S. & Kissling, W. (2003) Shared decision making in psychiatry. *Acta Psychiatrica Scandinavica* **107**, 403–409.

Harvey, P.D. & Keefe, R.S.E. (2001) Studies of the cognitive change in patients with schizophrenia following novel antipsychotic treatment. *American Journal of Psychiatry* **158**, 176–184.

Hogarty, G.E., Schooler, N.R., Ulrich, R., Mussare, F., Ferro, P. & Herron, E. (1979) Fluphenazine and social therapy in the aftercare of schizophrenic patients: relapse analysis of two year controlled study of fluphenazine decanoate and fluphenazine hydrochloride. *Archives of General Psychiatry* **36**, 1283–1294.

Hogarty, G.E., Ulrich, R.F., Mussare, F. & Aristigueta, N. (1976) Drug discontinuation among long-term successfully maintained schizophrenic outpatients. *Diseases of the Nervous System* **37**, 494500.

Holt, R.I.G., Peveler, R.C. & Byrne, C.D. (2004) Schizophrenia, the metabolic syndrome and diabetes. *Diabetic Medicine* **21**, 515–523.

Howard, R., Rabins, P.V., Seeman, M.V., Jeste, D.V., and the International Late-Onset Schizophrenia Group (2000) Late-onset schizophrenia and very-late-onset schizophrenia-like psychosis: an international consensus. *American Journal of Psychiatry* **157**, 172–178.

Jeste, D.V., Palmer, B.W. & Harris, M.J. (1999) Neuroleptic discontinuation in clinical and research settings: scientific issues and ethical dilemmas. *Biological Psychiatry* **46**, 1050–1059.

Johnson, D.A.W., Pasterski, J.M., Ludlow, J.M., Street, K. & Taylor, R.D. (1983) The discontinuance of maintenance neuroleptic therapy in chronic schizophrenic patients: drug and social consequences. *Acta Psychiatrica Scandinavica* **67**, 339–352.

Jones, P.B., Barnes, T.R., Davies L. *et al.* (2006) Randomized controlled trial of the effect on Quality of Life of second- vs first-generation antipsychotic drugs in schizophrenia: Cost Utility of the Latest Antipsychotic Drugs in Schizophrenia Study (CUtLASS 1). *Archives of General Psychiatry* **63**, 1079–1087.

Jordan, S., Tunnicliffe, C. & Sykes, A. (2002) Minimizing side-effects: the clinical impact of nurse-administered 'side-effect' checklists. *Journal of Advances in Nursing* **37**, 155–165.

Jordan, S., Knight, J. & Pointon, D. (2004) Monitoring adverse drug reactions: Scales, profiles, and checklists. *International Nursing Review* **51**, 208–221.

Kane, J.M. (1984) The use of depot neuroleptics: clinical experience in the United States. *Journal of Clinical Psychiatry* **45**, 5–12.

Kane, J.M., Aguglia, E., Altamura, A.C. *et al.* (1998) Guidelines for depot antipsychotic treatment in schizophrenia. *European Neuropsychopharmacology* **8**, 55–66.

Kinon, B.J., Kane, J.M., Johns, C. *et al.* (1993) Treatment of neuroleptic-resistant schizophrenic relapse. *Psychopharmacology Bulletin* **29**, 309–314.

Kirkpatrick, B., Fenton, W.S., Carpenter, W.T., Jr & Marder, S.R. (2006) The NIMH-MATRICS consensus statement on negative symptoms. *Schizophrenia Bulletin* **32**, 214–219.

Lambert, T.J. (2007) Switching antipsychotic therapy: What to expect and clinical strategies for improving therapeutic outcomes. *Journal of Clinical Psychiatry* **68** (Suppl. 6), 10–13.

Lehman, A.F., Kreyenbuhl, J., Buchanan, R.W. *et al.* (2004) The Schizophrenia Patient Outcomes Research Team (PORT): Updated Treatment Recommendations 2003. *Schizophrenia Bulletin* **30**, 193–217.

Leucht, S., Barnes, T.R.E., Kissling, W., Engel, R.R., Correll, C. & Kane, J.M. (2003a) Relapse prevention in schizophrenia with new generation antipsychotics: A systematic review and explorative meta-analysis of randomized controlled trials. *American Journal of Psychiatry* **160**, 1209–1222.

Leucht, S., Wahlbeck, K., Hamann, J. & Kissling, W. (2003b) New generation antipsychotics versus low-potency conventional antipsychotics: a systematic review and meta-analysis. *Lancet* **361**, 1581–1589.

Lewis, S.W., Barnes, T.R.E. & Davies, L. *et al.* Randomised controlled trial of effect of prescription of clozapine versus other second generation antipsychotic drugs in resistant schizophrenia. *Schizophrenia Bulletin* **32**, 715–723.

Lieberman, J.A., Stroup, T.S., McEvoy, J.P. *et al.* (2005) Effectiveness of Antipsychotic Drugs in Patients with Chronic Schizophrenia. *New England Journal of Medicine* **353**, 1209–1223.

Mackin, P., Watkinson, H.M. & Young, A.H. (2005) Prevalence of obesity, glucose homeostasis disorders and metabolic syndrome in psychiatric patients taking typical or atypical antipsychotic drugs: a cross-sectional study. *Diabetalogia* **48**, 215–221.

Marder, S.R. (2000) Integrating pharmacological and psychosocial treatments for schizophrenia. *Acta Psychiatrica Scandinavica* **102**, 87–90.

Marder, S.R., Glynn, S.M., Wirshing, W.C. *et al.* (2003) Maintenance treatment of schizophrenia with risperidone or haloperidol: 2-year outcomes. *American Journal of Psychiatry* **160**, 1405–1412.

McIntosh, A.M., Conlon, L., Lawrie, S.M. & Stanfield, A.C. (2006) Compliance therapy for schizophrenia. *Cochrane Database of Systematic Reviews* Issue 3, CD003442.

Meltzer, H.Y., Alphs, L., Green, A.I. *et al.*; International Suicide Prevention Trial Study Group (2003) Clozapine treatment for suicidality in schizophrenia: International Suicide Prevention Trial (InterSePT). *Archives of General Psychiatry* **60**, 82–91.

Mizrahi, R., Kiang, M., Mamo, D.C. *et al.* (2006) The selective effect of antipsychotics on the different dimensions of the experience of psychosis in schizophrenia spectrum disorders. *Schizophrenia Research* **88**, 111–118.

Moncrieff, J. (2006) Does antipsychotic withdrawal provoke psychosis? Review of the literature on rapid onset psychosis (supersensitivity psychosis) and withdrawal-related relapse. *Acta Psychiatrica Scandinavica* **114**, 3–13.

Montejo, A.L. (2008) Prolactin awareness: An essential consideration for physical health in schizophrenia. *European Neuropsychopharmacology* **18**, S108–S114.

Mutsatsa, S., Joyce, E.M., Hutton, S. *et al.* (2003) Clinical correlates of early medication compliance: the west London first episode schizophrenia study. *Acta Psychiatrica Scandinavica* **108**, 439–446.

Mutsatsa, S., Joyce, E.M., Hutton, S. & Barnes, T.R.E. (2006) Relationship between insight, cognitive function, social function and symptomatology in schizophrenia. *European Archives of Psychiatry and Clinical Neuroscience* **256**, 356–363.

National Institute for Health and Clinical Excellence (2009) *Schizophrenia: Core Interventions in the Treatment and Management of Schizophrenia in Primary and Secondary Care (update)*. NICE clinical guideline 82. London: NICE.

Nadeem, H., Bhanjia, N.H., Chouinard, G. & Margolese, H.C. (2004) A review of compliance, depot intramuscular antipsychotics and the new long-acting injectable atypical antipsychotic risperidone in schizophrenia. *European Neuropsychopharmacology* **14**, 87–92.

National Institute for Clinical Excellence (2002a) Core interventions in the treatment and management of schizophrenia in primary and secondary care. Clinical Guideline 1. www.nice.org.uk

National Institute for Clinical Excellence (2002b) Guidance on the use of newer (atypical) antipsychotic drugs for the treatment of schizophrenia. NICE Health Technology Appraisal Guidance Number 43. www.nice.org.uk

Newcomer, J.W. (2007) Antipsychotic medications: metabolic and cardiovascular risk. *Journal of Clinical Psychiatry* **68** (Suppl. 4), 8–13.

O'Donnell, C., Donohoe, G., Sharkey, L. *et al.* (2003) Compliance therapy: a randomised controlled trial in schizophrenia. *BMJ* **327**, 834–837.

Ohlsen, R.I., Williamson, R.J., Yusufi, B. *et al.* (2008) Interrater reliability of the Antipsychotic Non-Neurological Side-Effects Rating Scale (ANNSERS). *Journal of Psychopharmacology* **22**, 323–329.

Patel, M.X. & David, A.S. (2005) Why aren't depot antipsychotics prescribed more often and what can be done about it? *Advances in Psychiatric Treatment* **11**, 203–213.

Paton, C., Barnes, T.R., Cavanagh, M.R., Taylor, D., on behalf of the POMH-UK Project Team (2008) High-dose and combination antipsychotic prescribing in acute adult wards in the UK; the challenges posed by PRN. *British Journal of Psychiatry* **192**, 435–439.

Perkins, D.O., Gu, H., Weiden, P.J., McEvoy, J.P., Hamer, R.M., Lieberman, J.A.; Comparison of Atypicals in First Episode Study Group (2008) Predictors of treatment discontinuation and medication nonadherence in patients recovering from a first episode of schizophrenia, schizophreniform disorder, or schizoaffective disorder: a randomized, double-blind, flexible-dose, multicenter study. *Journal of Clinical Psychiatry* **69**, 106–113.

Prescribing Observatory for Mental Health (2007a) Topic 1 report 1b. Prescribing of high-dose and combination antipsychotics on adult acute and intensive care wards: 12-month re-audit. Prescribing Observatory for Mental Health.

Prescribing Observatory for Mental Health (2007b) Topic 3 report 3a. Prescribing of high-dose and combination antipsychotics on forensic wards: baseline audit. Prescribing Observatory for Mental Health.

Robinson, D., Woerner, M.G., Alvir, J.M. *et al.* (1999) Predictors of relapse following response from a first episode of schizophrenia or schizoaffective disorder. *Archives of General Psychiatry* **56**, 241–247.

Rosenheck, R., Tekell, J., Peters, J. *et al.* (1998) Does participation in psychosocial treatment augment the benefit of clozapine? *Archives of General Psychiatry* **55**, 618–625.

Rummel, C., Hamann, J., Kissling, W. & Leucht, S. (2003) New generation antipsychotics for first episode schizophrenia. *Cochrane Database of Systematic Reviews* Issue 4, CD004410.

Saltz, B.L., Woerner, M.G., Robinson, D.G. & Kane, J.M. (2000) Side effects of antipsychotic drugs: avoiding and minimizing their impact in elderly patients. *Postgraduate Medicine* **107**, 169–178.

Saltz, B.L., Robinson, D.G. & Woerner, M.G. (2004) Recognizing and managing antipsychotic drug treatment side effects in the elderly. *Primary Care Companion Journal of Clinical Psychiatry* **6** (Suppl. 2), 14–19.

Schooler, N., Rabinowitz, J., Davidson, M. *et al.*; Early Psychosis Global Working Group (2005) Risperidone and haloperidol in first-episode psychosis: A long-term randomized trial. *American Journal of Psychiatry* **162**, 947–953.

Shirzadi, A.A. & Ghaemi, S.N. (2006) Side effects of atypical antipsychotics: extrapyramidal symptoms and the metabolic syndrome. *Harvard Review of Psychiatry* **14**, 152–164.

Tenback, D.E., van Harten, P.N., Slooff, C.J., Belger, M.A., van Os, J.; SOHO Study Group (2005) Effects of antipsychotic treatment on tardive dyskinesia: a 6-month evaluation of patients from the European Schizophrenia Outpatient Health Outcomes (SOHO) study. *Journal of Clinical Psychiatry* **66**, 1130–1133.

Tollefson, G.D., Dellva, M.A., Mattler, C.A., Kane, J.M., Wirshing, D.A. & Kinon, B.J. (1999) Controlled, double-blind investigation of the clozapine discontinuation symptoms with conversion to either olanzapine or placebo: The Collaborative Crossover Study Group. *Journal of Clinical Psychopharmacology* **19**, 435–443.

Valenstein, M., Ganoczy, D., McCarthy, J.F., Myra Kim, H., Lee, T.A. & Blow, F.C. (2006) Antipsychotic adherence over time among patients receiving treatment for schizophrenia: a retrospective review. *Journal of Clinical Psychiatry* **67**, 1542–1550.

Verghese, C., DeLeon, J., Nair, C. & Simpson, G.M. (1996) Clozapine withdrawal effects and receptor profiles of typical and atypical neuroleptics. *Biological Psychiatry* **39**, 135–138.

Viguera, A.C., Baldessarini, R.J., Hegarty, J.D., van Kammen, D.P. & Tohen, M. (1997) Clinical risk following abrupt and gradual withdrawal of maintenance neuroleptic treatment. *Archives of General Psychiatry* **54**, 49–55.

Weiden, P.J. (2006) Switching in the era of atypical antipsychotics. An updated review. *Postgradraduate Medicine* Spec No, 27–44.

Weiden, P.J. (2007) Understanding and addressing adherence issues in schizophrenia: from theory to practice. *Journal of Clinical Psychiatry* **68** (Suppl. 14), 14–19.

Weiden, P.J. & Miller, A.L. (2001) Which side effects really matter? Screening for common and distressing side effects of antipsychotic medications. *Journal of Psychiatric Practice* **7**, 41.

Yusufi, B., Mukherjee, S., Flanagan, R. *et al.* (2007) Prevalence and nature of side effects during clozapine maintenance treatment and the relationship with clozapine dose and plasma concentration. *International Clinical Psychopharmacology* **22**, 238–243.

25

Comparative efficacy and effectiveness in the drug treatment of schizophrenia

John R. Geddes[1], T. Scott Stroup[2], and Jeffrey A. Lieberman[2]

[1]University of Oxford, Oxford, UK
[2]Columbia University College of Physicians and Surgeons and the New York State Psychiatric Institute, New York, NY, USA

Introduction

Until the introduction of effective pharmacological treatment, the plight of many individuals with schizophrenia was long-term institutional care. Effective drug treatment became available in the 1950s and led to a revolution in care allowing many patients to return to the community and remain well for extended periods. Despite the undeniable benefits of the first generation of antipsychotic drugs (FGAs), they caused a number of troublesome adverse effects which were considered to be a largely unavoidable consequence of the therapeutic effect (see Chapter 27). Moreover, the early drugs only alleviated the positive symptoms of the disorder, such as hallucinations, and hallucinations and did little to help—and probably even

worsened—the negative, cognitive, and mood symptoms, which cause a substantial part of the disability attributable to the disorder. There was great hope that the second generation of drugs (SGAs) would more comprehensively help patients and be more tolerable. In this chapter we summarize the clinical effects of the FGAs and SGAs and outline their comparative efficacy and tolerability in the treatment of schizophrenia (see also Chapters 24 and 28). We will focus particularly on the clinical evidence and explore the factors that led to the premature conclusion that the SGAs were more effective and better tolerated that the FGAs. Finally, we will summarize the current status of the drug treatment of schizophrenia.

First-generation antipsychotics

Chlorpromazine, introduced in 1953, was the first modern antipsychotic drug. Randomized, placebo-controlled trials

Schizophrenia, 3rd edition. Edited by Daniel R. Weinberger and Paul J Harrison © 2011 Blackwell Publishing Ltd.

(RCTs) demonstrated efficacy (Adams *et al.*, 2007) and in the absence of other effective drug treatments for schizophrenia, chlorpromazine was heralded as a breakthrough and widely prescribed worldwide. Other antipsychotic drugs followed during the 1950s and 1960s, notably haloperidol (Joy *et al.*, 2001) and trifluoperazine (Marques *et al.*, 2004).

Mechanism of action

Carlsson and Lindqvist (1963) measured dopamine metabolites in the brains of mice treated with chlorpromazine or haloperidol and reported increases in dopamine turnover. This observation led to the "dopamine hypothesis" of schizophrenia that proposed that elevations in dopamine caused the characteristic psychotic symptoms. More directly, it provided a potential mechanism of action of antipsychotic drugs and led to the development of a number of animal models that could be used for the initial development of new agents (see Chapter 23). Until the introduction of clozapine (see below), dopamine blockade was considered to be necessary and probably sufficient for a candidate drug to be an effective antipsychotic. Despite the centrality of dopamine blockade, the individual FGAs vary substantially in their affinity for the dopamine receptor as measured by blockade of stereo-specific binding of [^{3}H]haloperidol in calf caudate in the pioneering work by Seeman *et al.* (1976).

The pharmacological profiles of the FGAs are also heterogeneous with respect to their effects on other neurotransmitter systems. Some, such as haloperidol, are highly potent and relatively selective antagonists of dopamine receptors. Others such as chlorpromazine, also block cholinergic, histaminergic, serotonergic, and adrenergic transmission. These varying pharmacological profiles account for the heterogeneous adverse effect profiles of the individual agents.

Until the advent of the SGAs, non-dopamine actions were not usually considered to be related to antipsychotic efficacy, although some, such as the anticholinergic activity of drugs like thioridazine, were considered to be potentially helpful in reducing the risk of extrapyramidal side effects (EPS) (see below).

Efficacy and tolerability

FGAs are highly effective in the acute phase of schizophrenia with rapid onset of action (Agid *et al.*, 2003). There is no reliable evidence that one or other FGA is superior in efficacy to another and most attempts to differentiate them have been based on their dissimilar adverse event profiles. FGAs have been demonstrated to reduce the risk of relapse (Gilbert *et al.*, 1995).

Adverse effects

Short-term

The main short-term problem with FGAs is their propensity to cause EPS, including parkinsonism (muscle rigidity, tremor, and bradykinesia), acute dystonic reactions (including oculogyric crises), and akathisia (see Chapter 27). FGAs with high potency for D_2 receptors (haloperidol) are more likely to produce EPS than low-potency drugs (such as chlorpromazine). In the case of high-potency drugs such as haloperidol, the EPS commonly occur at clinically effective doses.

Long-term

In the longer term, FGAs produce weight gain but their propensity to cause tardive dyskinesia at an annual incidence of about 5% per year (Chakos *et al.*, 1996) was the factor usually considered to be the most serious long-term complication. The practices of preferentially using high-potency FGAs and doses that may have been higher than the minimum effective dose may have contributed to the generally accepted incident rates.

Several additional FGAs were introduced throughout the 1970s and 1980s. Dopamine receptor blockade remained the common mechanism of action, although the drugs differed in both their potency on dopamine receptors and their actions on other neurotransmitters, which produced varying profiles of adverse effects. Despite their undoubted efficacy, it was recognized that the efficacy and acceptability of all FGAs was limited by the occurrence of EPS.

Clozapine and atypicality

Early experience with clozapine

Clozapine, a dibenzodiazepine derivative (Fig. 25.1), was initially identified and used clinically in Europe in the early 1960s (Hippius, 1989). Initial enthusiasm was limited *because* of the absence of EPS which were believed to be a prerequisite of an effective antipsychotic. Early trials in the early 1970s confirmed its efficacy. The drug was beginning to be more widely used when reports from Finland of 16 cases of agranulocytosis, including eight fatalities, in patients treated with clozapine led to its withdrawal from the market (Hippius, 1989). The absence of EPS and the failure of clozapine to induce catalepsy in animal models led to clozapine being recognized as "atypical" of drugs with antipsychotic efficacy.

Reintroduction of clozapine

The withdrawal of clozapine meant that a potentially effective treatment was no longer available for patients. Equally important was the possibility that clozapine offered a new approach to treating schizophrenia which could be used to

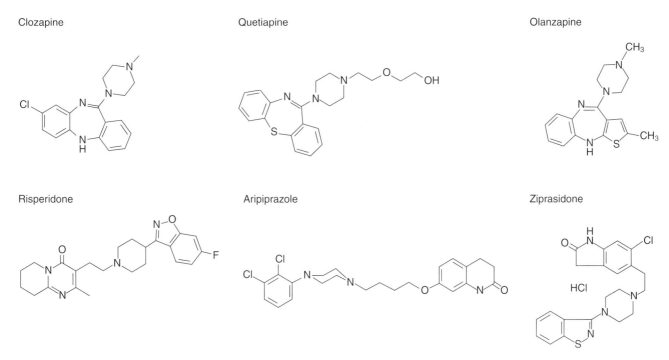

Fig. 25.1 Structure of atypical, second-generation, antipsychotic drugs.

develop new agents that did not share the propensity of clozapine to cause agranulocytosis. For these reasons, by the 1980s it was considered essential to establish reliably if clozapine was more effective than conventional agents, at least in some patients. The key patient subgroup for further trials was those whose illness was not helped by existing conventional dopamine-blocking agents. These patients had no available treatment option and carefully controlled treatment with clozapine in a trial was therefore ethical because the benefits might outweigh the risks. An important and carefully designed RCT was conducted in multiple US sites to investigate the efficacy of clozapine efficacy in the treatment of patients who had not responded to conventional antipsychotics (Kane *et al.*, 1988). Patients with schizophrenia who had failed to respond to at least three different neuroleptics were treated with haloperidol (mean dose, 61 mg/day) for 6 weeks in a single blind active run-in phase. Patients whose illness did not respond were then randomly assigned to double-blind treatment with clozapine (up to 900 mg/day) or chlorpromazine (up to 1800 mg/day) for 6 weeks. Of the 268 participants in the randomized phase, 30% treated with clozapine responded compared to 4% treated with chlorpromazine. This is a very substantial difference, although it is worth noting that just under a third of patients responded to clozapine. The authors noted that improvements in negative as well as positive symptoms were observed.

The trial had a major impact on clinical practice. Clozapine was subsequently reintroduced for the treat-

ment of patients who had failed to respond to conventional agents and the search for agents that replicated the efficacy of clozapine without the risk of blood dyscrasias accelerated. With the intensive hematological monitoring required in the marketing authorization, a very low incidence of serious adverse events was observed (Alvir *et al.*, 1993).

Subsequent trials confirmed the superiority of clozapine in treatment-resistant cases (Essali *et al.*, 2009; see Chapter 26). This replicated superiority is less apparent in treatment-responsive patients and first-episode cases (Lieberman *et al.*, 2003), perhaps indicating the presence of heterogeneity of response according to clinical subgroup. There is reasonable evidence that clozapine is superior to other SGAs in treatment-resistant schizophrenia, both in terms of symptoms (McEvoy *et al.*, 2006) and suicidal behavior (Meltzer *et al.*, 2003).

Second-generation (atypical) antipsychotics

The so-called atypical or second-generation antipsychotics (SGAs) are a heterogeneous group of compounds (Fig. 25.1). Their common, or atypical, feature is that they are less likely to induce EPS than FGAs. As described above, the development of SGAs was spurred by the demonstration that clozapine was both effective in patients who had failed to respond to FGAs and was less likely to induce EPS (Kane *et al.*, 1988). The starting point for the search for new clozapine-like agents was the chemical structure of clozapine itself. Olanzapine, for example, is a thienobenzo-diazepine, closely related to clozapine, and the member of a family of molecules that proved to be both antipsy-chotic and free from the hematological adverse effects of clozapine.

Mechanism of action

In general, the SGAs are more potent antagonists at 5-HT$_{2A}$ receptors than at D$_2$ receptors. The exception is aripipra-zole, which is a partial D$_2$ antagonist. The relative lower level of dopamine activity led to the formulation of the hypothesis that the mechanism of action of SGAs was not direct D$_2$ antagonism, but perhaps a balance between 5-HT$_{2A}$ and D$_2$ activity. To date, no mechanism of therapeu-tic action other than D$_2$ blockade has been convincingly demonstrated. It has been proposed that SGAs may dis-sociate from the dopamine receptors more rapidly than FGAs, explaining their efficacy and lower propensity to cause EPS (Kapur & Seeman, 2000). It has also been proposed that the 5-HT$_{2A}$ blocking actions on midbrain dopamine signaling mitigated its EPS effects, thus con-tributing to its greater tolerability but not therapeutic effi-cacy (Lieberman et al., 1998). For further discussion, see Chapter 23.

Efficacy and tolerability

Efficacy compared to placebo

All currently marketed SGAs have been evaluated in double-blind, placebo-controlled trials and shown to be efficacious (Leucht et al., 1999a). Placebo-controlled trials are challenging to conduct in acute psychosis and are mainly conducted for regulatory purposes. More clinically relevant evidence is perhaps provided by trials with an active FGA comparator.

Efficacy compared to first-generation antipsychotics

Although poor tolerability of FGAs was one of the main drivers for the development of the SGAs, the demonstra-tion that clozapine is efficacious in patients who fail to respond to FGAs also raised the intriguing possibility that SGAs would show superior efficacy across a range of symptom domains. Initial interest focused principally on negative symptoms, but as the importance of mood symp-toms and cognitive impairment as contributions to overall disability was increasingly recognized, these too became a focus.

We will describe the comparative evaluation of SGAs and FGAs in three phases: industry sponsored trials, sys-tematic reviews, and meta-analyses of the initial trials and independent trials.

Industry-sponsored Phase III trials

Compared to placebo-controlled trials, the pivotal Phase III trials comparing SGAs and FGAs were less challenging in terms of patient recruitment and retention, and established new methodological standards in psychiatry, especially in terms of size (Tollefson et al., 1997). Nonetheless, perhaps inevitably in view of their pioneering status, these trials were also fraught with methodological difficulties, includ-ing the selection of patients, choice and dose of FGA, dura-tion, patient retention, and analysis.

Patient selection: most trials recruited patients who had already been exposed to treatment with FGAs. Clearly, there would have been a selection of patients who had not responded completely to, or were unable to tolerate, FGAs (see below). While this was perfectly ethical and clinically reasonable at the time, trials randomizing such selected patients could not provide a fair comparison of FGAs and SGAs. Rather, trials conducted in such patients could dem-onstrate only that treatment with the new agents was not inferior and may be superior to re-exposure to an FGA.

Choice and dose of comparator: the standard comparator used in the trials was haloperidol which was seen as a rela-tively pure D$_2$ antagonist and, therefore, the most typical conventional agent. However, haloperidol is a high-potency FGA and is known to have a higher propensity to cause EPS. Futhermore, it was already known that the dose of haloperidol required to produce optimal blockade of D$_2$ receptors and clinical response was lower than had previ-ously been thought (van Putten et al., 1985, 1987, 1990, 1992). Consequently, higher doses may be counterproduc-tive in that they produce little additional benefit, but increase the risk of EPS (van Putten et al., 1992).

Duration: most of these trials were of around 6 weeks' duration. While this may be a reasonable length of time to assess initial treatment response in an acute episode, it is clearly difficult to extrapolate the results of such trials to the decades of treatment which the patient with schizo-phrenia typically receives in the course of their illness.

Patient retention: notwithstanding the short duration of the trials, they also had very low rates of retention (often <50%), and the rates of withdrawal differed between the treatment arms. Higher drop-out rates in the compara-tor arms meant that these patients had shorter exposure to study treatment and less time to experience symptom reduction.

Analysis: conducting the required intent-to-treat analysis in the presence of substantial drop-out is a well recognized but difficult problem (Streiner, 2002). The analysis method of last observation carried forward is prone to bias, espe-cially if it is possible to manipulate drop-out by using a supraoptimal dose of comparator drug, as in the case of the FGA *versus* SGA comparisons. In such cases, this analysis method would use outcome ratings that were higher in the treatment group which had the greater drop-out rate.

These methodological issues limited the confidence in the results of these trials, especially in view of the tendency to be more enthusiastic about the advantages of SGAs than the evidence supported (Huston & Moher, 1996; Cipriani & Geddes, 2003).

Systematic reviews and meta-analyses

Systematic reviews differ from conventional narrative reviews in that they use clearly stated methods to identify, appraise, and synthesize the primary trials. Systematic reviews are less susceptible to bias because the conclusion is made after data synthesis rather than the data being sought in order to bolster a prior conclusion or position. This was clearly shown in the classic comparison between systematic and narrative reviews by Antman *et al.* (1992), which was replicated in the specific area of reviews of the comparative efficacy of FGAs and SGAs (Cipriani & Geddes, 2003).

There have been several systematic reviews of the comparative efficacy of FGAs and SGAs, including reviews of specific agents and more general reviews of all available drugs. The first review of all available agents included four RCTs of olanzapine, six RCTs of quetiapine, nine RCTs of risperidone, and two RCTs of sertindole (Leucht *et al.*, 1999a). The authors concluded that there was evidence that sertindole and quetiapine appeared to be indistinguishable from haloperidol in terms of efficacy and that risperidone and olanzapine appeared to be slightly more effective. All SGAs were less likely to be associated with antiparkinsonian medication, although risperidone perhaps had a less favorable EPS profile than the other SGAs. The authors noted that haloperidol, an FGA especially likely to produce EPS, was usually used as comparator and that the doses used were higher than considered optimal at the time, and that caution was needed in interpreting the results.

In a further systematic review and meta-analysis, Geddes *et al.* (2000) identified 52 RCTs, including 12 649 participants, which compared SGAs with FGAs. This review replicated but extended the results of Leucht *et al.* (1999a). Although the trials seemed to suggest small, but worthwhile, advantages in terms of symptom reduction in favor of the SGAs, the authors noted a number of limitations in the trials which seriously limited their ability to reliably inform clinical practice. These included their very short-term nature, the supraoptimal dosing of comparator drugs (especially haloperidol), and the (probably consequent) high and differential withdrawal rates. There was also significant statistical heterogeneity between trials comparing the same experimental and investigational drugs; in other words, the results of the individual trials varied more than could be explained by chance variation alone. Moreover, most patients participating in these trials had been previously exposed to an FGA (only a small subgroup were first-episode cases) with varying degrees of lack of response.

For example, in the large trial of olanzapine *versus* haloperidol (Tollefson *et al.*, 1997), the eligibility criteria were:

"Male and female inpatients and outpatients at least 18 years of age who met the DSM-III-R criteria for schizophrenia, schizophreniform disorder, or schizoaffective disorder were randomly assigned to treatment. Patients were required to have a minimum Brief Psychiatric Rating Scale (BPRS) score of 18 (items extracted from the Positive and Negative Syndrome Scale and scored 0–6) and/or be intolerant of current antipsychotic therapy (excluding haloperidol)."

This clearly suggests that the trial would be likely to include patients who had already been found to be unable to tolerate FGA drugs.

Investigating variations between trials: role of meta-regression

An important role of meta-analysis is to investigate observed heterogeneity in the effects of the drugs estimated by individual primary trials (Thompson, 1994). For example, are SGAs more efficacious in patients with treatment-resistant illness? Or does the relative effect depend on methodological decisions made in the trials, such as the dose of comparator drug used? The most powerful way of investigating heterogeneity between the trials in the context of heterogeneity is *meta-regression*, a technique in which the treatment effect is related to study-level characteristics. Geddes *et al.* (2000) conducted a meta-regression analysis to explore the observed heterogeneity between the trials. A powerful relationship was observed between the dose of FGA comparator drug and the odds of SGA being superior to FGA in both efficacy and tolerability (as estimated by total drop-out rate from the trials). In separate analyses for trials using both chlorpromazine and those using haloperidol, a highly significant association was identified between the dose of comparator drug and the outcome of the trials. Specifically, the higher the dose of FGA comparator, the more likely was the trial to favor SGA (Fig. 25.2).

Although this analysis included all the SGAs, this was a "multivariate" analysis in which variation between the individual SGAs was investigated but not found. It could, therefore, be concluded that the dose effect was a general feature of SGA trials.

This association between the dose of the comparator FGA used in the trial and the tendency of the trial to demonstrate apparent superiority of SGAs indicates that the design of the trials may have been biased in favor of the SGA. This is because the dose of FGA might have been higher than necessary, increasing the risk of EPS and therefore withdrawal, leading to poorer outcomes.

Further, this analysis was one of the first reported uses of the technique of "indirect meta-analysis" (Glenny *et al.*, 2005) in which the comparative efficacy of the SGAs was

a

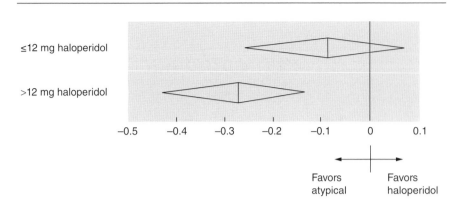

b

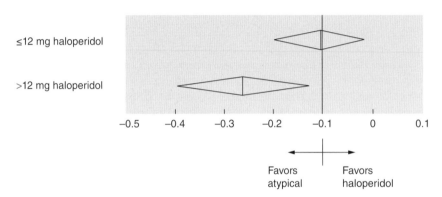

Fig. 25.2 Dose effect in both (a) efficacy and (b) tolerability in meta-regression analysis comparing FGAs and SGAs. Note: to illustrate the dose relationship, these figures dichotomize doses at 12 mg haloperidol—the primary analysis investigated the effect of haloperidol as a continuous explanatory variable (reproduced from Geddes *et al.*, 2000 with permission from BMJ Publishing Group Ltd.)

estimated in the absence of reliable comparative trials by comparing the efficacy of the drugs to the common FGA comparator. The analysis reported that indirect comparison in meta-regression models did not identify any individual atypical antipsychotic as more or less effective when dose of comparator drug was taken into account.

Although the quantitative results of the Geddes *et al.* review were comparable to previous meta-analysis, the results of the meta-regression led the authors to be more cautious than previous authors in their estimation of the relative benefits of the SGAs, particularly in view of the increased acquisition costs and also the emerging evidence of metabolic adverse effects with some of the SGAs. The review was heavily criticized by some, although the criticisms could not dispel the fundamental conclusion that SGAs had not been shown to be unequivocally superior to FGAs (Geddes, 2003; Geddes *et al.*, 2001).

Davis *et al.* (2003) conducted a further review of the SGA *versus* FGA trials, including the additional trials. The

authors conducted several subanalyses, including an attempt to replicate the Geddes *et al.* (2003) meta-regression analysis regarding the effect of comparator dose. They were not able to replicate the results of Geddes *et al.*, although this may have been because they used different methods. In particular, they do not seem to have used multivariate meta-regression. These minor inconsistencies should not obscure the fact that the pooled results of all three meta-analyses were actually very similar (Geddes *et al.*, 2000; Leucht *et al.*, 1999b; Davis *et al.*, 2003): the differences were mainly in the degree to which the reviewers were willing to overlook the clear flaws and biases in the primary RCTs. Practically, there were material differences in the degree to which the review authors concluded that the data were robust enough to support a conclusion that SGAs were more efficacious and better tolerated than FGAs, with one review (Davis *et al.*, 2003) in particular appearing to be more supportive than the others.

Relapse prevention: efficacy and safety compared to first-generation antipsychotics

SGAs appear to be more effective than placebo in the prevention of relapse in schizophrenia (Leucht *et al.*, 2003). However, there have been very few properly conducted, long-term trials comparing SGAs with FGAs and focused on preventing relapse in schizophrenia. In addition, many of the methodological flaws in these trials were overlooked in systematic reviews (Leucht *et al.*, 2003). For example, most of the trials of olanzapine followed up only patients who had responded in the short-term (Tran *et al.*, 1998) without re-randomization. One long-term trial of risperidone *versus* haloperidol appeared to show benefits for risperidone (Csernansky *et al.*, 2001), although the dose of haloperidol was supraoptimal (Geddes, 2002). Furthermore, the trial provided no good evidence that treatment with haloperidol was more likely to lead to tardive dyskinesia than risperidone, although creative use of the available data provided some support that this might be the case (Correll *et al.*, 2004).

Summary of conclusions from industry-sponsored Phase III acute phase and relapse prevention trials

Although the trials conducted for regulatory purposes suggested that SGAs were more effective than FGAs in the treatment of acute-phase schizophrenia, the methodological shortcomings of the trials made it impossible to draw firm conclusions about their relative efficacy and tolerability either in the shorter or longer term. This uncertainty and continuing equipoise (Freedman, 1987) created the basis for the next generation of trials which were conducted independent of commercial interest.

Pragmatic trials comparing first- and second-generation antipsychotics

The short-term nature, and other methodological limitations, of most of the industry-sponsored Phase III trials inevitably left unanswered questions about the comparative efficacy, tolerability, and cost-effectiveness of the SGAs compared to the FGAs over a more clinically meaningful time horizon (Geddes *et al.*, 2000). Several trials were therefore initiated, independent of commercial organizations and aimed at answering some of these questions using more pragmatic, or practical, designs (Stroup & Geddes, 2008). These trials are methodologically and clinically heterogeneous in design and are described individually below.

The Clinical Antipsychotic Trials of Intervention Effectiveness (CATIE) study

CATIE was a large double-blind trial conducted in the US and funded by the National Institute for Mental Health (NIMH) to compare the efficacy and safety of the then available SGAs with each other and with the FGA, perphenazine (Lieberman *et al.*, 2005). The CATIE study was conducted between January 2001 and December 2004 at 57 clinical sites in the US, and included patients aged between 18 and 65 years with a diagnosis of schizophrenia according to DSM-IV. Patients were randomly allocated to perphenazine, olanzapine, quetiapine, risperidone or ziprasidone and followed for up to 18 months (Fig. 25.3). This longer duration of follow-up contrasts with the

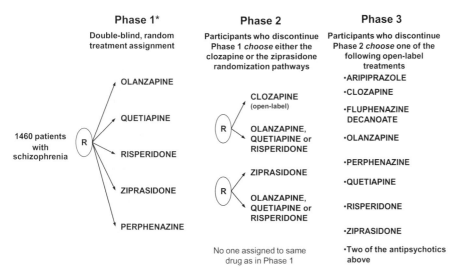

Fig. 25.3 Schematic of CATIE. *Phase IA, patients with tardive dyskinesia were not randomized to perphenazine; Phase IB, participants who fail perphenazine were randomized to olanzapine, quetiapine or risperidone before eligibility for Phase II.

short-term nature of the industry Phase III trials, which was typically 6 weeks in, for example, the olanzapine *versus* placebo/haloperidol trials (Beasley *et al.*, 1997). The primary outcome in CATIE was the discontinuation of treatment for any cause, which was chosen because it integrates a treatment's effectiveness and tolerability from both the patient's and the clinician's point of view. Secondary outcomes included discontinuation due to inadequate efficacy and to intolerability as judged by the treating clinician. Additional secondary outcomes included adverse events (weight gain, EPS, etc.), neurocognitive functioning, quality of life, and efficacy outcomes, including the Positive and Negative Symptom Scale (PANSS) and the Clinical Global Impressions scale (CGI) .

In the primary analysis of CATIE, olanzapine was found to be superior to risperidone and quetiapine on the main effectiveness measure, although the advantage was modest. Olanzapine was not more effective than perphenazine and ziprasidone, but the power to detect such differences was low. Olanzapine was superior to perphenazine, quetiapine, and risperidone in terms of rates of discontinuation due to inadequate efficacy. There were no differences in the rates of discontinuation due to intolerability, or in the effects of the drugs on neurocognition or quality of life.

Although olanzapine had some advantages over other treatments with regard to overall effectiveness and efficacy in reducing symptoms, this advantage was mitigated by findings that olanzapine was associated with more weight gain and other adverse metabolic effects than the other medications (see Chapter 28). The most surprising result of CATIE to many observers was that perphenazine performed very similarly to most of the other medications in overall effectiveness, efficacy, and tolerability. Because of its much lower cost, it was the most cost-effective of the medications studied.

Methodological aspects

CATIE stands out as the largest and most comprehensive direct comparison of antipsychotic medications since the atypical medications were marketed. As a double-blinded RCT, it provided a rigorous comparison of the study treatments. However, CATIE has a number of limitations worth noting. Because the double-blinded design required the investigators to make choices about dose equivalence of the drugs, these choices are open to criticism (Tandon *et al.*, 2008). Many critics have asserted that the dosing of olanzapine was more aggressive than that of other medications, perhaps giving it an advantage. Another common criticism is that the complicated design led to diminished statistical power. Because individuals with tardive dyskinesia could not be assigned to perphenazine due to ethical considerations, and because ziprasidone was added late to the protocol, fewer participants were assigned to these medications. The result was that although perphenazine and ziprasi-

done performed similarly to quetiapine and risperidone, reduced power to detect the difference made interpretation of the results confusing to some observers.

Cost Utility of the Latest Antipsychotic Drugs in Schizophrenia Study (CUtLASS 1)

CUtLASS 1 was a pragmatic, randomized trial comparing FGAs and SGAs in patients with schizophrenia who required a change of treatment (Jones *et al.*, 2006). Two hundred and twenty-seven participants were recruited from 14 community mental health services in the UK. The trial was funded by the UK National Health Services and the primary outcome was quality of life with secondary outcomes, including symptoms, adverse effects, participant satisfaction, and costs of care over 1 year. Treatment was open but outcome assessment was masked to treatment allocation. CUtLASS found no evidence that treatment with SGAs led to improved quality of life compared to FGAs. There was no clear difference in patient preferences for FGAs or SGAs and costs were similar.

Methodological aspects

CUtLASS has a substantially different design from other trials in that it compared SGAs with FGAs as classes. Clinicians could choose which drug to use from these groups. Of the 227 participants in the trial, 109 were randomized to receive an SGA and, of those patients, 50 were prescribed olanzapine, 22 risperidone, 23 quetiapine, and 13 amisulpride. Of the 118 patients randomized to the FGA arm, 58 were prescribed sulpiride (one of 11 FGAs prescribed in the study). The results were, perhaps, therefore more applicable to olanzapine and sulpiride than to other antipsychotic drugs. This design is perhaps more intended to answer the needs of policymakers that clinicians or patients, and interpretation is made more difficult in that choice between heterogeneous drugs was allowed in the classes.

As with all the independent trials, there were difficulties in the recruitment of participants. CUtLASS 1 enrolled far fewer participants than intended, in part because a secular trend strongly favoring the use of FGAs before and during the study appeared to limit the willingness of clinicians and patients to agree to participate. The relatively small sample size meant that power to detect differences between FGAs and SGAs was small; however, the trend on the primary outcome strongly favored FGAs, suggesting that even a more powerful study would not have found an advantage with SGA on quality of life.

Department of Veterans Affairs Co-operative Study on the Cost-Effectiveness of Olanzapine

This was a double-blind, RCT comparing olanzapine (5–20 mg/day; 159 patients) and haloperidol (5–20 mg/day) in combination with prophylactic benztropine (1–4 mg/day; 150 patients) in the treatment of schizophrenia over 12 months (Rosenheck *et al.*, 2003). This trial found "no statistically or clinically significant advantages of olanzapine for schizophrenia on measures of compliance, symptoms, or overall quality of life, nor did it find evidence of reduced inpatient or total cost". Olanzapine caused fewer EPS but more weight gain than haloperidol. It led to small but statistically significant improvements in measures of memory and motor function. The authors concluded that olanzapine did not demonstrate advantages compared with haloperidol (in combination with prophylactic benztropine) in compliance, symptoms, EPS, or overall quality of life, and its benefits in reducing akathisia and improving cognition must be balanced with the problems of weight gain and higher cost (Rosenheck *et al.*, 2003).

Methodological aspects

This study had several advantages over other independent trials. It was conducted reasonably soon after the introduction of the newer agents (recruiting between June 1998 and June 2000), which possibly helped recruitment, and the doses of drugs used were clinically representative. There have been two main criticisms of this trial, neither of which, in our view, substantially limits the validity of the results. The first concern is that all patients allocated to haloperidol were also treated with benztropine, an anticholinergic agent. The concern is that this does not reflect established clinical practice (many reserve anticholinergics for patients who suffer EPS rather than using them routinely) and also potentially reduces the rate of EPS in patients treated with haloperidol, hence obscuring the inherent advantage of olanzapine. The second concern is that the sample size was smaller than originally planned and this limits the confidence in the results.

European First-Episode Schizophrenia Trial (EUFEST)

EUFEST was an open-label randomized trial that compared haloperidol, amisulpride, olanzapine, quetiapine or ziprasidone in the treatment of first-episode schizophrenia (Kahn *et al.*, 2008). Between December 2002 and January 2006, EUFEST recruited patients aged 18–40 who were within 2 years of diagnosis of schizophrenia, schizophreniform or schizoaffective disorder according to DSM-IV from 50 sites in Europe and Israel. The primary outcome was all-cause discontinuation at 12 months; a number of secondary outcomes of efficacy and safety were also measured. All SGAs were superior to haloperidol in terms of the primary outcome but there was no difference on other key outcomes such as symptomatic status or hospital admission. EPS were more common with haloperidol and weight gain was more common with olanzapine.

Methodological aspects

A key feature of the EUFEST trial was that it was conducted as an open trial; in other words, patients and clinicians knew which drug they had been allocated, and treatment and outcome assessment were not conducted blind to treatment assignment. Open trials are susceptible to performance bias (patients in the trial groups are treated differently depending on the allocated treatment) and ascertainment bias (assessment of outcome is biased by knowledge of the treatment assignment). These biases are likely to be substantial if clinicians and patients have preferences about the treatments at the beginning of the trial. In EUFEST, we know that the coordinators (and presumably the investigators) were not all in equipoise at the beginning of the trial; the authors report that 11 (34%) site coordinators expected haloperidol to lead to the worst outcome, and 21 (66%) of them thought that it would be no worse than the SGAs (i.e., none of the coordinators expected haloperidol to outperform the SGAs). These prior expectations would make it more likely that patients allocated to haloperidol would be switched off allocated treatment earlier, leading to a higher rate of discontinuation—and this was the primary outcome. The survival plots show that almost half of patients allocated haloperidol were switched to another therapy within the first month post-randomization—the most common reason given was insufficient efficacy. Further, the trial report suggests that the discontinuation rate in the haloperidol arm was non-significantly higher in the sites that believed that haloperidol was the worst option.

This potential (and probable) bias is one of the main reasons that, despite the apparent clear-cut result in favor of the SGAs over haloperidol, the EUFEST report states, "it cannot be concluded that second-generation antipsychotic drugs are more efficacious than is haloperidol in the treatment of these patients". The other reason for this statement was that there was no difference between the drugs in terms of symptomatic improvement on the PANSS (although there was a significant difference in global status measured by the CGI scale). In retrospect, the open-label design of EUFEST, though pragmatic, led to great doubt about the validity of the primary analysis. The striking absence of any difference in efficacy between drugs as measured by the PANSS is at odds with the observed (and probably biased) differences in discontinuation rates.

Summary of conclusions from independent pragmatic trials

Taken together, the independent clinical trials were unable to show that SGAs were clearly superior to FGAs to a clinically meaningful extent. Even when an agent appears to demonstrate some advantage in terms of efficacy, e.g., olanzapine, this needs to be balanced against the higher risk of metabolic adverse effects (Lieberman *et al.*, 2005). This conclusion appears to be at odds with the views of some of the earlier proponents of the SGAs. Such was the extent of the prior belief that SGAs were superior to FGAs that some questioned if the field would be able to accept the accumulating new evidence (Lewis & Lieberman, 2008). While some of the initial uncritical enthusiasm for SGAs was probably driven by the marketing efforts of the drug companies, it is instructive to consider the impact of the heterogeneous trial designs deployed at different stages of the development of the SGAs (Geddes, 2009).

Antipsychotics: clinical trial design and data interpretation

Methodological issues in the design of clinical trials

The apparently discrepant findings between the industry-sponsored trials and independently-conducted trials of SGAs *versus* FGAs reviewed above require some comment (Fleischhacker & Goodwin, 2009). RCTs remain the most reliable way of estimating the efficacy of treatments. Although the general design of an RCT is constant, i.e., random allocation between treatments, the methods deployed depend on the nature of the primary research question and the phase of development of the treatment (Schwartz & Lellouch, 1967; Geddes, 2005, 2009; Stroup, 2005). The conventional approach to describing drug development is according to several phases:

Phase I: Clinical pharmacology in healthy volunteers (first in man);

Phase II: Clinical pharmacology in patients to establish preliminary efficacy and safety and dose. Frequently subdivided into Phase IIa (to estimate clinically effective dosage) and IIb (preliminary test of efficacy);

Phase III: Formal therapeutic trials to provide pivotal evidence of efficacy and safety;

Phase IV: Post licensing studies to establish broader efficacy and safety.

There is often a degree of overlap between these putative phases and it is increasingly common for a trial to be conducted to meet the needs of multiple phases of development, particularly Phase II and III. For example, a trial may randomize patients between placebo, multiple doses of the investigational drug, and an active comparator. Another way of classifying RCTs is the extent to which they maximize internal or external validity. *Efficacy* trials (sometimes called *explanatory*, or *therapeutic confirmatory*) have the objective of assessing if a drug can work; the design is therefore driven by the need to establish if a drug can work under ideal, highly controlled, circumstances (Geddes, 2005, 2009). The major goals in the design of efficacy trials is to make sure that any treatment effect is likely to be picked up and to reduce the background "noise" caused

particularly by interrater variation in the assessment of outcomes and the presence of comorbidity. The aim here is to maximize the signal-to-noise ratio. To reduce variability and noise, these trials use trained personnel with high interrater reliability, specialized settings, and highly selected compliant participants. They use rating scales of symptoms that are highly sensitive to drug effects, rather than clinical events, as they study primary outcomes (Geddes, 2005). A potential antipsychotic drug is usually compared both to placebo and to a known antipsychotic; this procedure helps to confirm "assay sensitivity", or that the study design and procedures were adequate to detect a difference between a drug known to be effective and placebo.

In an efficacy trial, trained research personnel recruit patients experiencing an acute episode of schizophrenia and ensure that diagnostic and severity of illness criteria are met using standardized and comprehensive assessment procedures. Most individuals with medical illnesses, substance use disorders, or additional psychiatric diagnoses are excluded both to reduce the likelihood of serious adverse events and limit the variance in outcomes. To protect against ascertainment and performance biases, treatments are assigned randomly under double-blind conditions, so that neither the patient nor the research team providing clinical care and conducting outcome assessments knows the treatment assignment. Typical efficacy trials are designed to follow the clinical course of participants for 6–8 weeks. Follow-up is by trained personnel who conduct frequent assessments of symptoms and side effects using psychometrically validated instruments. The primary outcome is typically improvement on a symptom rating scale, such as the PANSS. Response, or improvement by 30% or some other pre-specified amount on a symptom rating scale, is a common secondary outcome. Known side effects and common laboratory parameters are measured systematically, while other adverse events are reported spontaneously if and when they occur.

Efficacy trials efficiently meet the requirements of drug licensing and regulatory agencies. They work well for drug developers who want to complete trials rapidly, because the high costs of using many highly trained and geographically dispersed research centers can be offset against the reduced time to market and profitability. However, efficacy trials do not reveal much about how a new drug works in typical settings, with patients who may have medical and psychiatric comorbidities and who may take other medications. They do not tell us about longer-term safety issues or about the effects of drug therapies on mortality, ability to work, or other issues that are important to patients.

By contrast, *practical* (also called *pragmatic* trials) have the objective of providing independent evidence to inform decision-makers about clinical and policy choices related to the risks and benefits of approved treatments. Researchers design practical trials to provide high-quality evidence, with high internal and external validity, regarding the everyday effectiveness of clinically relevant alternative interventions (Tunis *et al.*, 2003). To do this, researchers include a heterogeneous population of patients and collect data on a broad range of meaningful health outcomes in many types of practice settings intended to represent usual treatment (Tunis *et al.*, 2003).

Practical trials use broad patient inclusion criteria and minimal exclusion criteria to enhance external validity and thus enhance the believability of study results for clinicians and patients in typical treatment settings (Stroup, 2005). Practical trials compare treatments about which there is clinical uncertainty about the outcome at the individual patient level, and use randomization to protect against selection biases (March *et al.*, 2005). Not all practical trials conceal the treatment assignment from patients and study clinicians, but for subjective outcomes determined by raters blinding is necessary. The training and personnel requirements of rater blinding places burdens on sites that make it less likely that typical clinical sites, rather than research sites, can participate in these trials. In addition, a desire to examine "a broad range of meaningful health outcomes", often including service utilization to allow estimation of cost-effectiveness, is at variance with a desire to limit participant and researcher burden. To some extent, practical trials can be conceptualized as hybrids of efficacy and large simple trials with the main trade-offs being in internal validity and the potential for a low signal-to-noise ratio.

A further category of trial is the *large simple trial* (LST) which focuses narrowly on clearly defined, patient-oriented outcomes (Yusuf *et al.*, 1984; Stroup & Geddes, 2008). A typical LST outcome, mortality, is discrete and meaningful. In designing an LST, the desire to collect information on a wide array of outcomes is resisted and resources are used to enroll large numbers of participants to provide sufficient power to detect relatively small but clinically important differences. LSTs are conducted at typical treatment settings with usual clinical personnel. Study procedures are simple so that the need for specialized research training and interference with routine clinical care is minimized. Inclusion criteria are broad and exclusion criteria are minimal. The key criterion for study entry is uncertainty about which treatment option is best for the individual participant (Peto & Baigent, 1998). Treatments are randomly assigned to avoid selection bias.

The key features of the different approaches to clinical trial design are shown in Table 25.1.

Summarizing the totality of the randomized evidence

The thorough assessment of any health technology, including pharmaceuticals, should include a systematic appraisal of all the available randomized evidence. The confidence that we can have that a drug is likely to be effective in the real world will be increased if a comparable treatment effect is observed in pragmatic practical trials as well as in highly controlled efficacy trials. For example, the treatment effect on cognition observed in the large pragmatic AD2000 trial comparing donepezil with placebo (AD 2000 Collaborative Group 2105–15) was comparable to that estimated in the shorter-term efficacy trials conducted by the manufacturer (Whitehead *et al.*, 2004). However, what can we conclude when trials with different design characteristics differ in their results? We would argue that it cannot be concluded that the results from one kind of trial are necessarily "true" and the results from the other trials are "wrong". Rather, reasons for the apparent heterogeneity between trials should be sought by examining the clinical and design differences between the trials. If the trials are judged reasonably similar in terms of design and participants, meta-analysis may be possible, in which case it is simple enough to determine whether the differences between trials are likely to be real or simply due to the play of chance. The reasons for any material differences between trials can be assessed using meta-regression, a technique which statistically compares the results of trials according to trial-level characteristics (Thompson & Higgins, 2002). For example, a systematic review of industry-sponsored trials of SGAs compared to FGAs found a number of methodological weaknesses in the trials and, furthermore, a meta-regression strongly suggested that the substantial statistical heterogeneity between trials could be explained by differences in the dose of the FGA used in the trial (Geddes *et al.*, 2000). The use of a higher dose of FGA was more likely to produce a result favoring the atypical antipsychotic drug. The design of CATIE, a practical trial (see above), was informed by these findings, among other considerations, with particular attention paid to the doses of the investigational drugs. CATIE largely confirmed the conclusion that there were probably no major differences between drugs selected from both available FGAs and SGAs on a broad range of clinically relevant outcomes and cost-effectiveness (Lieberman *et al.*, 2005). This example demonstrates the particular usefulness of practical trials in situations where there is substantial residual uncertainty about the comparative effectiveness of drugs, even in the presence of a large body of efficacy trials. As in this case, the reason for the uncertainty will often be concerns about the design or applicability of the efficacy trials. The different objectives of efficacy and practical trials should be considered in the interpretation of the complete body of randomized evidence: this may make simple pooling of the results of the trials in a standard meta-analysis inappropriate.

Leucht *et al.* (2009) reported an extensive overview of all the available evidence (with key omissions, including EUFEST) in an attempt to draw conclusions about the relative safety and efficacy of FGAs and SGAs. Their broad

Table 25.1 Typical features of different clinical trial designs used to investigate the efficacy and safety of antipsychotic drugs.

	Efficacy trials	Practical trials	Large simple trials
Goal	To achieve regulatory approval to market drug	To inform decision-makers about clinical and policy choices	To compare treatment options to examine small but potentially important differences
Specific aims	To establish short-term efficacy and safety of a new drug	To examine relative benefits and risks of available treatments	To determine comparative longer-term safety or effectiveness
Primary outcome	Improvement of target symptoms	A discrete and clinically meaningful outcome	A discrete and clinically meaningful outcome
Secondary outcomes	Safety measures; response rates	Often many health-related outcomes, including health economic measures	
Timing	Before a drug is marketed	Post-market	Post-market
Funding	Drug maker	Varies; drug manuafacturer, government agency, foundation	Varies; drug manufacturer, government agency, foundation
Diagnosis	Diagnosis by structured interview	Clinical diagnosis or structured interview	Clinical diagnosis or structured interview
Sample size	A few hundred	Hundreds to thousands	Thousands
Comparisons	Placebo and an active comparator	One or more active comparators; clinical equipoise	One or more active comparators; clinical equipoise
Dosing	Fixed dosing	Flexible dosing in clinically used range	Flexible dosing in clinically used range
Blinding	Double-blinded	Open label, single or double blinded	Open label, single or double blinded
Duration	6 weeks	1 year or longer	1 year or longer for primary outcome
Research sites	Experienced research sites capable of specialized procedures: number variable but usually <100	Sites are typical treatment settings, may need capacity to measure many outcomes: often hundreds of sites	Sites are typical treatment settings: often hundreds of sites
Protocol	Strictly defined research protocol with frequent research assessments and procedures	Protocol designed to mimic usual decision-making for antipsychotic drugs; many research procedures may be included	Protocol very similar to usual practice; minimal additional assessments or procedures
Comorbid medical and psychiatric conditions	Excluded to isolate the effects of the drug	Included except for specific contraindications to examine effects in typical patient populations	Included except for specific contraindications to examine effects in typical patient populations
Adjunctive and concomitant treatments	Excluded except specific drugs for limited time	Allowed as in usual practice; some exclusions depending on study aims	Allowed as in usual practice

conclusions were that it is not valid to conclude that, overall, SGAs are superior to FGAs and the compounds are heterogeneous in terms of pharmacology, efficacy, and safety. Although some SGAs appeared to have some degree of superior efficacy across all domains of symptoms, this is of unclear clinical relevance (Fig. 25.4).

Conclusions

At the time of writing, the evidence does not unequivocally suggest that one or other antipsychotic, or indeed that one or other "class" of antipsychotic, should be preferred to another. The characteristics of individual drugs and the

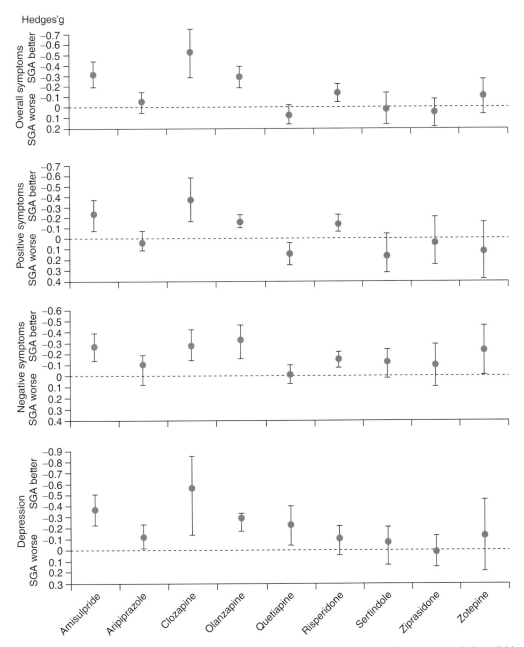

Fig. 25.4 Relative safety and efficacy of first- and second-generation antipsychotics: overview of all available evidence. The results are significant at p < 0.05 if the 95% CI does not overlap the x axis. SGA, second-generation antipsychotic drug (reproduced from Leucht *et al.*, 2009 with permission from Elsevier).

clinical situation and preferences of individual patients seem to be the most important factors when choosing an antipsychotic medication. Several lessons should, however, be drawn from the development and introduction of the SGAs over the past two decades. First, Phase III trials conducted by industry for regulatory purposes should not be relied upon to provide reliable evidence to guide clinical practice. Such trials will usually be designed to optimize the performance of the new agent(s) and may not provide

a fair test of the efficacy and acceptability compared to existing treatments. Second, independent, non-commercial trials should be initiated early following the emergence of novel treatments that promise greatly enhanced benefits. Third, clinical interpretation of, and recommendations based on, early evidence should not exaggerate benefits. Premature acceptance of marketing claims can make it much harder to recruit to, and distort, subsequent independent trials due to lack of equipoise (Geddes, 2003).

References

Adams, C.E., Awad, G., Rathbone, J. & Thornley, B. (2007) Chlorpromazine versus placebo for schizophrenia. *Cochrane Database Systematic Reviews* CD000284.

Agid, O., Kapur, S., Arenovich, T. & Zipursky, R.B. (2003) Delayed-onset hypothesis of antipsychotic action, a hypothesis tested and rejected. *Archives of General Psychiatry* **60**, 1228–1235.

Alvir, J.M., Lieberman, J.A., Safferman, A.Z., Schwimmer, J.L. & Schaaf, J.A. (1993) Clozapine-induced agranulocytosis. Incidence and risk factors in the United States. *New England Journal of Medicine* **329**, 162–167.

Antman, E.M., Lau, J., Kupelnick, B., Mosteller, F. & Chalmers, T.C. (1992) A comparison of results of meta-analyses of randomized control trials and recommendations of clinical experts. Treatments for myocardial infarction [see comments]. *JAMA* **68**, 240–248.

Baldessarini, R.J. & Viguera, A.C. (1995) Neuroleptic withdrawal in schizophrenic patients. *Archives of General Psychiatry* **52**, 189–192.

Beasley, C.M., Jr., Hamilton, S.H., Crawford, A.M. *et al.* (1997) Olanzapine versus haloperidol, acute phase results of the international double-blind olanzapine trial. *European Neuropsychopharmacology* **7**, 125–137.

Carlsson, A. & Lindqvist, M. (1963) Effect of chlorpromazine or haloperidol on formation of 3-methoxytyramine and normetanephrine in mouse brain. *Acta Pharmacologica et Toxicologica* **20**, 140.

Chakos, M.H., Alvir, J.M., Woerner, M.G. *et al.* (1996) Incidence and correlates of tardive dyskinesia in first episode of schizophrenia. *Archives of General Psychiatry* **53**, 313–19.

Cipriani, A. & Geddes, J.R. (2003) Comparison of systematic and narrative reviews, the example of the atypical antipsychotics. *Epidemiologia e Psichiatrica Sociale* **12**, 146–154.

Correll, C.U., Leucht, S. & Kane, J.M. (2004) Lower risk for tardive dyskinesia associated with second-generation antipsychotics, a systematic review of 1-year studies. *American Journal of Psychiatry* **161**, 414–425.

Csernansky, J.G., Mahmoud, R., Brenner, R., Riseridone Ris-USA-79 Study Group (2001) A comparison of risperidone and haloperidol for the prevention of relapse in patients with schizophrenia. *New England Journal of Medicine* **346**, 16–22.

Davis, J.M., Chen, N. & Glick, I.D. (2003) A Meta-analysis of the Efficacy of Second-Generation Antipsychotics. *Archives of General Psychiatry* **60**, 553–564.

Essali, A., Al-Haj Haasan, N., Li, C., & Rathbone, J. Clozapine versus typical neuroleptic medication for schizophrenia. Cochrane Database of Systematic Reviews 2009, Issue 1. Art. No.: CD000059. DOI: 10.1002/14651858.CD000059.pub2.

Fleischhacker, W.W. & Goodwin, G.M. (2009) Effectiveness as an outcome measure for treatment trials in psychiatry. *World Psychiatry* **8**, 23–27.

Freedman, B. (1987) Equipoise and the ethics of clinical research. *New England Journal of Medicine* **317**, 141–145.

Geddes, J. (2002) Prevention of relapse in schizophrenia. *New England Journal of Medicine* **346**, 56–58.

Geddes, J. (2003) Generating evidence to inform policy and practice, the example of the second generation "atypical" antipsychotics. *Schizophrenia Bulletin* **29**, 105–114.

Geddes, J.R. (2005) Large simple trials in psychiatry, providing reliable answers to important clinical questions. *Epidemiologia e Psichiatrica Sociale* **14**, 122–126.

Geddes, J.R. (2009) Clinical trial design, horses for courses. *World Psychiatry* **8**, 28–29.

Geddes, J., Freemantle, N., Harrison, P. & Bebbington, P. (2000) Atypical antipsychotics in the treatment of schizophrenia, systematic overview and meta-regression analysis. *BMJ* **321**, 1371–1376.

Geddes, J., Harrison, P., Freemantle, N. & Bebbington, P. (2001) Atypical antipsychotics in the treatment of schizophrenia— Reply. *BMJ* **322**, 927–928.

Gilbert, P.L., Harris, M.J., McAdams, L.A., & Jeste, D.V. (1995) Neuroleptic withdrawal in schizophrenic patients. A review of the literature. *Archives of General Psychiatry* **52**, 173–188.

Glenny, A.M., Altman, D.G., Song, F. *et al.* (2005) Indirect comparisons of competing interventions. *Health Technol Assess* **9**, i–iv.

Hippius, H. (1989) The history of clozapine. *Psychopharmacology (Berlin)* **99** (Suppl), S3–S5.

Huston, P. & Moher, D. (1996) Redundancy, disaggregation, and the integrity of medical research. *Lancet* **347**, 1024–1026.

Jones, P.B., Barnes, T.R.E., Davies, L. *et al.* (2006) Randomized controlled trial of the effect on quality of life of second- vs first-generation antipsychotic drugs in schizophrenia, Cost Utility of the Latest Antipsychotic Drugs in Schizophrenia Study (CUtLASS 1). *Archives of General Psychiatry* **63**, 1079–1087.

Joy, C.B., Adams, C.E. & Lawrie, S.M. (2001) Haloperidol versus placebo for schizophrenia. *Cochrane Database of Systematic Reviews* **4**.

Kahn, R.S., Fleischhacker, W.W., Boter, H. *et al.* (2008) Effectiveness of antipsychotic drugs in first-episode schizophrenia and schizophreniform disorder, an open randomised clinical trial. *Lancet* **371**, 1085–1097.

Kane, J., Honigfeld, G., Singer, J. & Meltzer, H. (1988) Clozapine for the treatment-resistant schizophrenic. A double-blind comparison with chlorpromazine. *Archives of General Psychiatry* **45**, 789–796.

Kapur, S. & Seeman, P. (2000) Does fast dissociation from the dopamine D2 receptor explain the action of atypical antipsychotics? A new hypothesis. *American Journal of Psychiatry* **158**, 360–369.

Leucht, S., Pitschel, W.G., Abraham, D. & Kissling, W. (1999a) Efficacy and extrapyramidal side-effects of the new antipsychotics olanzapine, quetiapine, risperidone, and sertindole compared to conventional antipsychotics and placebo. A meta-analysis of randomized controlled trials. *Schizophrenia Research* **35**, 51–68.

Leucht, S., Pitschel, W.G., Abraham, D. & Kissling, W. (1999b) Efficacy and extrapyramidal side-effects of the new antipsychotics olanzapine, quetiapine, risperidone, and sertindole compared to conventional antipsychotics and placebo. A meta-analysis of randomized controlled trials. *Schizophrenia Research* **35**, 51–68.

Leucht, S., Barnes, T.R., Kissling, W., Engel, R.R., Correll, C. & Kane, J.M. (2003) Relapse prevention in schizophrenia with new-generation antipsychotics, a systematic review and exploratory meta-analysis of randomized, controlled trials. *American Journal of Psychiatry* **160**, 1209–1222.

Leucht, S., Corves, C., Arbter, D., Engel, R.R., Li, C. & Davis, J.M. (2009) Second-generation versus first-generation antipsychotic drugs for schizophrenia, a meta-analysis. *Lancet* **373**, 31–41 .

Lewis, S. & Lieberman, J. (2008) CATIE and CUtLASS, can we handle the truth? *British Journal of Psychiatry* **192**, 161–163.

Lieberman, J.A., Mailman, R.B., Duncan, G. *et al.* (1998) Serotonergic basis of antipsychotic drug effects in schizophrenia. *Biological Psychiatry* **44**, 1099–1117.

Lieberman, J.A., Phillips, M., Gu, H. *et al.* (2003) Atypical and conventional antipsychotic drugs in treatment-naive first-episode schizophrenia, a 52-week randomized trial of clozapine vs chlorpromazine. *Neuropsychopharmacology* **28**, 995–1003.

Lieberman, J.A., Stroup, T.S., McEvoy, J.P. *et al.*, the Clinical Antipsychotic Trials of Intervention Effectiveness (CATIE) Investigators (2005) Effectiveness of antipsychotic drugs in patients with chronic schizophrenia. *New England Journal of Medicine* **353**, 1209–1223.

March, J.S., Silva, S.G., Compton, S., Shapiro, M., Califf, R. & Krishnan, R. (2005) The case for practical clinical trials in psychiatry. *American Journal of Psychiatry* **162**, 836–846.

Marques, L.O., Lima, M.S. & Soares, B.G. (2004) Trifluoperazine for schizophrenia. *Cochrane Database Systematic Review* CD003545.

McEvoy, J.P., Lieberman, J.A., Stroup, T.S. *et al.*, for the CATIE Investigators (2006) Effectiveness of clozapine versus olanzapine, quetiapine, and risperidone in patients with chronic schizophrenia who did not respond to prior atypical antipsychotic treatment. *American Journal of Psychiatry* **163**, 600–610.

Meltzer, H.Y., Alphs, L., Green, A.I. *et al.* (2003) Clozapine treatment for suicidality in schizophrenia, International Suicide Prevention Trial (InterSePT). *Archives of General Psychiatry* **60**, 82–91.

Peto, R. & Baigent, C. (1998) Trials, the next 50 years. Large scale randomised evidence of moderate benefits. *BMJ* **317**, 1170–1171.

Rosenheck, R., Perlick, D., Bingham, S. *et al.* (2003) Effectiveness and cost of olanzapine and haloperidol in the treatment of schizophrenia, a randomized controlled trial. *JAMA* **290**, 2693–2702.

Schwartz, D. & Lellouch, J. (1967) Explanatory and pragmatic attitudes in therapeutic trials. *Journal of Chronic Diseases* **20**, 637–648.

Seeman, P., Lee, T., Chau-Wong, M. & Wong, K. (1976) Antipsychotic drug doses and neuroleptic/dopamine receptors. *Nature* **261**, 717–719.

Streiner, D.L. (2002) The case of the missing data, methods of dealing with dropouts and other research vagaries. *Canadian Journal of Psychiatry* **47**, 68–75.

Stroup, S. (2005) Practical clinical trials for schizophrenia. *Epidemiologia e Psichiatrica Sociale* **14**, 132–136.

Stroup, T.S. & Geddes, J.R. (2008) Randomized controlled trials for schizophrenia, study designs targeted to distinct goals. *Schizophrenia Bulletin* **34**, 266–274.

Tandon, R, Belmaker, RH, Gattaz, WF et al. (2008) World Psychiatric Association Pharmacopsychiatry Section statement on comparative effectiveness of antipsychotics in the treatment of schizophrenia. *Schizophrenia Research* **100**, 20–38.

Thompson, S.G. (1994) Why sources of heterogeneity in meta-analysis should be investigated. *BMJ* **309**, 1351–1355.

Thompson, S.G. & Higgins, J.P.T. (2002) How should meta-regression analyses be undertaken and interpreted? *Statistics in Medicine* **21**, 1559–1573.

Tollefson, G.D., Beasley, C.M., Tran, P.V. *et al.* (1997) Olanzapine versus haloperidol in the treatment of schizophrenia and schizoaffective and schizophreniform disorders, results of an international collaborative trial. *American Journal of Psychiatry* **154**, 457–465.

Tran, P.V., Dellva, M.A., Tollefson, G.D., Wentley, A.L. & Beasley, C.M., Jr. (1998) Oral olanzapine versus oral haloperidol in the maintenance treatment of schizophrenia and related psychoses. *British Journal of Psychiatry* **172**, 499–505.

Tunis, S.R., Stryer, D.B. & Clancy, C.M. (2003) Practical clinical trials, increasing the value of clinical research for decision making in clinical and health policy. *JAMA* **290**, 1624–1632.

van Putten, T., Marder, S.R., May, P.R., Poland, R.E. & O'Brien, R.P. (1985) Plasma levels of haloperidol and clinical response. *Psychopharmacology Bulletin* **21**, 69–72.

van Putten, T., Marder, S.R. & Mintz, J. (1987) The therapeutic index of haloperidol in newly admitted schizophrenic patients. *Psychopharmacology Bulletin* **23**, 201–205.

van Putten, T., Marder, S.R. & Mintz, J. (1990) A controlled dose comparison of haloperidol in newly admitted schizophrenic patients. *Archives of General Psychiatry* **47**, 754–758.

van Putten, T., Marder, S.R., Mintz, J. & Poland, R.E. (1992) Haloperidol plasma levels and clinical response, a therapeutic window relationship. *American Journal of Psychiatry* **149**, 500–505.

Whitehead, A., Perdomo, C., Pratt, R.D., Birks, J., Wilcock, G.K. & Evans, J.G. (2004) Donepezil for the symptomatic treatment of patients with mild to moderate Alzheimer's disease, a meta-analysis of individual patient data from randomised controlled trials. *International Journal of Geriatric Psychiatry* **19**, 624–633.

Yusuf, S., Collins, R. & Peto, R. (1984) Why do we need some large, simple randomized trials? *Statistics in Medicine* **3**, 409–422.

CHAPTER 26

Approaches to treatment-resistant patients

Stephan Leucht[1], Christoph U. Correll[2], and John M. Kane[2]

[1]Technische Universität München, Mnich, Germany
[2]The Zucker Hillside Hospital, Glen Oaks, NY, USA

Introduction

Resistance to antipsychotic drugs is frequent and one of the most serious problems in the treatment of schizophrenia. In this chapter we first discuss critical concepts and definitions in this context. We then describe the epidemiology of the phenomenon. Regarding management, we describe factors that need to be ruled out before non-response should be assumed. Here, we focus particularly on the appropriate duration of an antipsychotic drug trial. Thereafter we present the evidence on key clinical strategies in cases of initial non-response to antipsychotic drugs; in particular, should the dose be increased or the antipsychotic drug be changed? The section on treatments for persistently treatment-resistant patients covers clozapine, the evidence for other second-generation antipsychotics (SGAs) in this indication, and the numerous adjuncts that have been tried to alleviate refractory symptoms. The last section is devoted to the treatment of treatment-resistant childhood schizophrenia.

Conceptual issues: definitions of response to treatment, remission, and treatment resistance

A major problem in this research area is the lack of uniformly accepted definitions of "response, remission, and

treatment resistance". Below we discuss important issues around these concepts.

Response to treatment

Response to treatment can be designated as a clinically significant improvement of the psychopathology of a patient, irrespective of whether the person is still ill or not. In clinical trials, cut-off values in the sense of a minimum percentage reduction from the initial score on a scale such as the Brief Psychiatric Rating Scale (BPRS; Overall & Gorham, 1962) or the Positive and Negative Syndrome Scale (PANSS; Kay et al., 1987) are used for this purpose. The problem is that there is no agreement as to which cut-off should be used. In the literature, at least 20%, 30%, 40%, 50%, and 60% reduction from the initial score have all been applied, but the clinical meaning of the cut-offs is unclear. Four publications using data of several thousand participants who were rated simultaneously with the BPRS/PANSS and the Clinical Global Impression scale (CGI; Guy, 1976) provided some insights to this question (Leucht et al., 2005b,c, 2006; Leucht & Kane, 2006; Levine et al., 2007). Equipercentile linking of percentage improvement of the BPRS/PANSS with CGI improvement score showed that a 25% reduction of the BPRS/PANSS baseline score corresponded roughly to a minimal improvement according to the CGI, while a 50% reduction corresponded to "much improved". As "typical", acutely ill patients with schizophrenia often respond well to therapy, we concluded that for such patients the 50% cut-off would be a more

Schizophrenia, 3rd edition. Edited by Daniel R. Weinberger and Paul J Harrison © 2011 Blackwell Publishing Ltd.

clinically meaningful criterion than lower cut-offs. On the other hand, in very chronic or treatment-resistant patients, even a slight improvement might represent a clinically significant effect, justifying the use of the 25% cut-off in treatment-refractory patients. Interestingly, the 20% cut-off was indeed initially used in a study of refractory patients (Kane *et al.*, 1988), but was subsequently widely applied in studies of non-refractory subjects. We also suggested displaying the results on response to treatment in 25% quartiles (Table 26.1; Leucht *et al.*, 2007c). A table such as Table 26.1 covers the extreme ranges of patients whose symptoms did not change or worsened during a trial (≤0% BPRS/PANSS reduction), patients who responded at least minimally (25% BPRS/PANSS reduction), patients who were at least much improved (50% BPRS/PANSS reduction), and patients who had exceptionally good responses compared to other participants in such studies (>75% BPRS/PANSS reduction). Table 26.1 also gives the results based on remission criteria which have recently been presented (Andreasen *et al.*, 2005;, see below). Many assume that greater than or equal to 75% BPRS/PANSS reduction is rare in schizophrenia. Nevertheless, in an analysis of 1870 patients in randomized amisulpride trials, approximately 25% reached at least 75% BPRS reduction (Leucht *et al.*, 2007c). The advantage of such a presentation is that the reader gets an impression of the *distribution* of the response. Presenting results based on only one cut-off cannot provide such information and the choice of the cut-off remains somewhat arbitrary. It should be noted that when 1–7 scaling of the BPRS/PANSS is used, the 18/30 minimum score needs to be subtracted when calculating percentage reduction from baseline (Leucht *et al.*, 2007c). For the statistical analysis of a clinical trial, it is important to choose a primary cut-off *a priori* to avoid problems of multiple testing. Finally, in the event that the CGI is used as a response criterion, the results could be shown in a similar fashion, presenting the number of participants who were unchanged, minimally improved and much improved; or not ill, mildly ill, severely ill, etc. (Table 26.2). A new version of the CGI that is specific for schizophrenia has recently been developed. This version uses the same items and scores, but provides clear anchors as to what "mildly ill" or "moderately ill" means. Furthermore, there are subscales for positive, negative, depressive, and cognitive symptoms using the same scoring system. In contrast to the original CGI, the psychometric properties of the new

Table 26.1 Suggested presentation of responder and remission rates based on percentage Positive and Negative Syndrome Scale (PANSS) or Brief Psychiatric Rating Scale (BPRS) reduction in clinical trials (modified from Leucht *et al.*, 2007c; Leucht *et al.*, 2009d).

	PANSS/BPRS reduction						
	≤0%	>0–24%	25–49%	50–74%	75–100%	Remission*	Total n
Intervention group	n (%)	n (%)	n (%)	n (%)	n (%)	n (%)	n
Control group	n (%)	n (%)	n (%)	n (%)	n (%)	n (%)	n

*Based on Andreasen *et al.* (2005).

Table 26.2 Suggested presentation of responder rates based on the Clinical Global Impressions (CGI) improvement scale in clinical trials (modified from Leucht *et al.*, 2007c; Leucht *et al.*, 2009d).

CGI improvement score	Very much worse	Much worse	Mini mally worse	Unchanged	Minimally better	Much better	Very much better	Total n
Score	7	6	5	4	3	2	1	
Intervention group	n (%)	n (%)	n (%)	n (%)	n (%)	n (%)	n (%)	n
Control Group	n (%)	n (%)	n (%)	n (%)	n (%)	n (%)	n (%)	n

CGI severity score	Extremly ill	Severely ill	Mar kedly ill	Modera-tely ill	Mildly ill	Borderline mentally ill	Normal, not at all ill	Total n
Score	7	6	5	4	3	2	1	
Intervention group	n (%)	n (%)	n (%)	n (%)	n (%)	n (%)	n (%)	n
Control group	n (%)	n (%)	n (%)	n (%)	n (%)	n (%)	n (%)	n

version have been examined and found to be sufficient (Haro *et al.*, 2003).

Remission

Remission can be defined as a state of *absence of significant symptoms*. Similarly to the variety of available response criteria, clinical and epidemiological studies on the frequency of remission in schizophrenia have been hampered by the lack of a uniformly accepted definition. For example, a series of long-term studies suggested that many patients may be in remission or even recover in the long run (for a survey, see Leucht & Lasser, 2006), but any comparison is difficult due to the variety of definitions used. In 2005, American and European expert groups suggested a remission definition for schizophrenia, which is likely to be adopted in future trials (Andreasen *et al.*, 2005; van Os *et al.*, 2006). According to these criteria, a patient is in remission if eight items of the PANSS are rated as "mildly present" or better (Table 26.3). In addition to this severity criterion, there is a time component which requires that this low level of symptoms must persist for at least 6 months, although short-term trials may only apply the severity criterion. The rationale for the selection of the eight

Table 26.3 Proposed items for remission criteria as defined by the Remission in Schizophrenia Working Group (reproduced with permission from Andreasen *et al.* 2005).[a] Copyright @ 2005 American Medical Association. All rights reserved.

Dimension of psychopathology	DSM-IV criterion	Scale for Assessment of Positive Symptoms (SAPS) and Scale for Assessment of Negative Symptoms (SANS) items		Positive and Negative Syndrome Scale (PANSS) items		Brief Psychiatric Rating Scale (BPRS) items	
		Criterion	Global rating item number	Criterion	Item number	Criterion[b]	Item number
Psychoticism (reality, distortion)	Delusions	Delusions (SAPS)	20	Delusions	P1	Grandiosity	8
						Suspiciousness	11
				Unusual thought content	G9	Unusual thought content	15
	Hallucinations	Hallucinations (SAPS)	7	Hallucinatory behavior	P3	Hallucinatory behavior	12
Disorganization	Disorganized speech	Positive formal thought disorder (SAPS)	34	Conceptual disorganization	P2	Conceptual disorganization	4
	Grossly disorganized or catatonic behavior	Bizarre behavior (SAPS)	25	Mannerisms/ posturing	G5	Mannerisms/ posturing	7
Negative symptoms (psychomotor poverty)	Negative symptoms	Affective flattening (SANS)	7	Blunted effect	N1	Blunted affect	16
		Avolition-apathy (SANS)	17	Social withdrawal	N4	No clearly related symptom	
		Anhedonia-asociality (SANS)	22				
		Alogia (SANS)	13	Lack of spontaneity	N6	No clearly related symptom	

[a]For symptomatic remission, maintenance over a 6-month period of simultaneous ratings of mild or less on all items is required. Rating scale items are listed by item number.
[b]Use of BPRS criteria may be complemented by use of the SANS criteria for evaluating overall remission. The PANSS scale is the simplest instrument on which a definition of symptom remission can be practically based.

PANSS items was that they reflect key symptoms that are required according to DSM-IV for the diagnosis of schizophrenia. The rationale for the severity threshold "mildly present at worst" was that such mild symptoms would not interfere with a patient's psychosocial functioning. This definition is also a compromise accounting for the reality of clinical trials. Two analyses of large databases of double-blind trials showed that very few patients reach the clinical state of being fully free of symptoms (Beitinger *et al.*, 2008; Leucht *et al.*, 2007a), so that a more stringent threshold ("not more than questionable symptoms" or "no symptoms at all") would not have been clinically realistic. Finally, it should also be taken into consideration that there is a dimensional distribution of mild and quasi-psychotic symptoms in a subgroup of the general population, and that—for similar reasons—the remission criteria of other chronic illnesses, e.g., polyarthritis, also do not require the complete absence of symptoms.

Pros and cons of response and remission criteria

The difference between response and remission is that response based on a percentage BPRS/PANSS reduction from baseline does not provide information on how symptomatic the patient is at endpoint. A reduction on the PANSS from 120 to 60 points is a 50% reduction, as is a change from 80 to 40 points; however the patient with a score of 60 is far more symptomatic than the patient with a score of 40, although they had an absolute change score of 60 as compared to 40 points. The remission criteria provide information as to where patients end up, i.e., are they still symptomatic? At the same time, the remission criteria do not reflect the amount of change. For example, if at baseline the participants are on average only mildly ill, many will be in remission at the end of the trial, although there will have been little reduction of symptoms (Leucht & Kane, 2006). We believe that often the best way of reporting symptomatic outcome in schizophrenia trials would be to display both measures, as is current practice in depression and bipolar mania trials, e.g., by applying the methodology summarized in Table 26.1.

Definitions of treatment resistance

Compared to simple "non-response", treatment resistance/refractoriness implies a more persistent lack of improvement despite adequate treatment. The definition is at least as complex as that of (non-)response and remission. Numerous criteria have been used (Table 26.4 provides a small selection). Often, such criteria focus on positive symptoms, but in a broader sense negative symptoms, affective symptoms, disturbed behavior, and cognitive dysfunction also play a role, because they lead to social

Table 26.4 Proposed criteria for treatment-resistant schizophrenia.

Reference	Criteria
Kane *et al.* (1988)	*Historical*: no period of good functioning or significant symptomatic relief within preceding 5 years despite at least two courses of antipsychotics (doses: ≥1000 mg/day chlorpromazine) for 6 weeks *Cross-sectional*: BPRS score ≥45, score of ≥4 on at least two of the following factors: conceptual disorganization, suspiciousness, hallucinatory behavior, unusual thought contents, CGI score of ≥-4 *Prospective*: 6-week trial of haloperidol- (60mg/day) fails to reduce BPRS by 20% or to below 35, or fails to reduce CGI to below 3
Brenner *et al.* (1990)	Seven levels of treatment response incorporating evaluation of *symptomatology, personal and social adjustment*: Level 1: clinical remission Level 2: partial remission Level 3: slight resistance Level 4: moderate resistance Level 5; severe resistance Level 6; refractory Level 7: severely refractory
Meltzer (1990)	At least in theory every patient who has not fully recovered to their premorbid level of functioning should be regarded as treatment refractory

BPRS, Brief Psychiatric Rating Scale; CGI, Clinical Global Impression scale.

dysfunction. From a conceptual point of view, such definitions can span a wide range. One extreme may be that any patient who has not achieved their level of functioning before the onset of psychosis is considered treatment resistant (Meltzer, 1990). At the other extreme are very stringent definitions that may combine historical, cross-sectional, and prospective aspects. Such definitions are often used in research. A good example is the criteria applied in a landmark study demonstrating clozapine's superiority compared to chlorpromazine in treatment-refractory patients (Kane *et al.*, 1988). Historically, patients had received in the preceding 5 years three antipsychotics from two different classes at a dosage of at least 1000 mg/day chlorpromazine equivalents for at least 6 weeks without significant clinical improvement, and without good functioning in the last 5 years. Cross-sectionally, the patients had a BPRS total score greater than or equal to 45, were at least moderately ill according to the CGI, and exhibited four at least moderately pronounced BPRS positive symptoms. Prospectively, the patients had not responded to a 6-week trial with haloperidol of up to 60 mg/day (non-response was defined as <20% BPRS reduction, BPRS total score >35, and CGI severity score >3). Also noteworthy is the attempt of an international study group which described treatment resistance by combining symptoms and social functioning on a scale from 1 (complete remission) to 7 (severe therapy resistance; Brenner *et al.*, 1990).

The choice of the specific criteria may depend on the situation. For example, the extremely stringent criteria in the Kane *et al.* (1988) study were necessary in the context of the reintroduction of an antipsychotic with potentially life-threatening side-effects (i.e., clozapine and its risk for agranulocytosis). Nevertheless, at least in schizophrenia practice guidelines a certain consensus seems to emerge. For example, the guideline of the American Psychiatric Association (APA) (Lehman *et al.*, 2004) defines treatment resistance as "little or no symptomatic response to multiple (at least two) antipsychotic trials of an adequate duration (at least 6 weeks) and dose (therapeutic range)". Other important guidelines such as those by the National Institute for Clinical Excellence (2003), the World Association of Societies of Biological Psychiatry (Falkai *et al.*, 2005), or other national psychiatric associations present similar definitions (Table 26.5).

Epidemiology

While there is no doubt that many patients do not respond sufficiently to antipsychotic drugs, the exact epidemiology is unclear. This deficiency is at least in part due to the above described lack of consensus about the definitions. The treatment guideline of the APA states that "10–30% of patients have little or no response to antipsychotic medications" (Lehman *et al.*, 2004), but no reference is given. A similarly vague statement is indicated in the Australian schizophrenia guideline: "About 10–15% of first-episode schizophrenia will develop early treatment resistance, however with sample selection and passage of time this proportion cumulatively increases to 30–50% in standard services" (McGorry, 2005). In a previous edition of this book, Schulz and Buckley (1995) stated that "some 20–40% of patients will prove resistant to standard antipsychotic treatments," but they argued that such numbers depend strongly on the definition used.

The best available data for first-episode patients come from two prospective 1-year studies. Robinson *et al.* (1999) studied 118 first-episode patients who were treated according to an algorithm in which flufenazine (up to 20 mg/day) was given for 6 weeks, followed by a dose increase to 40 mg/day for 4 weeks, haloperidol (up to 20 mg/day) for 6 weeks, increased to 40 mg/day for 4 weeks, then haloperidol plus lithium, a third antipsychotic of a different biochemical class, and finally clozapine up to 900 mg/day. Twenty percent of the participants had not achieved rela-

Table 26.5 Criteria for treatment resistance according to a selection of guidelines.

Guideline	Definition
American Psychiatric Association (Lehman *et al.*, 2004, p. 24)	Treatment resistance is defined as little or no symptomatic response to multiple (at least two) antipsychotic trials of an adequate duration (at least 6 weeks) and dose (therapeutic range)
National Institute for Clinical Excellence (2003, p. 46)	Treatment resistance is suggested by a lack of satisfactory clinical improvement despite the sequential use of the recommended doses for 6–8 weeks of at least two antipsychotic drugs, at least one of which should be an atypical
World Federation of Societies of Biological Psychiatry (Falkai *et al.*, 2005, p. 163)	Treatment resistance is assumed if there is either no improvement at all or only insufficient improvement in the target symptoms, despite treatment at the recommended dosage for a duration of at least 6–8 weeks with at least two antipsychotics, one of which should be an atypical antipsychotic
Royal Australian and New Zealand College of Psychiatrists (McGorry, 2005, p. 22)	Two adequate trials (at least 6 weeks of 300–1000 mg in chlorpromazine equivalents) of antipsychotic medication, of which at least one agent should be atypical, should have been conducted

tively stringent response criteria, including a CGI of at least much improved and not more than mild positive symptoms (Fig. 26.1). In the second study, Chinese patients with a first episode of schizophrenia were randomized to treatment with either chlorpromazine (up to 600 mg/day) or clozapine (up to 400 mg/day) in a double-blind study (Lieberman *et al.*, 2003). At 1 year, 13% had not met stringent response criteria that were similar to those used by Robinson *et al.* (1999). In another large study of a median duration of 205 days in 555 first-episode participants, 70% reached the severity component of the above-mentioned new remission criteria (Emsley *et al.*, 2006).

Concerning multiepisode patients, a number of *post-hoc* analyses of the new remission criteria have been published. As expected, the remission rates were lower than those in the first-episode samples. A pooled analysis of two randomized amisulpride studies (n = 748) suggested that 73% (worst case) and 48% (completer analysis) did not achieve a remission according to the Andreasen *et al.* (2005) criteria at 1 year. Similarly, in a 1-year, double-blind study, 68% (intent-to-treat analysis) and 23% (completer analysis) of

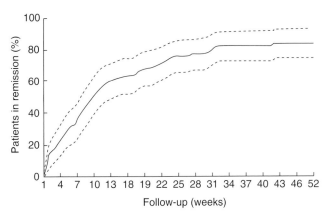

Fig. 26.1 Sustained response after 1-year treatment of patients with a first-episode of schizophrenia (n = 118) . Within 1 year, 87% reached a sustained response, defined as a Clinical Global Impressions scale (CGI) rating of "much" or "very much" improved and a rating of 3 (mild) or less on all the following Schedule for the Assessment of Affective Disorders and Schizophrenia—Change Version with Psychosis and Disorganisation Rating Scale (SADS-C) + PDI items: severity of delusions, severity of hallucinations, impaired understandability, derailment, illogical thinking, and bizarre behaviour; this level of improvement had to be sustained for 8 consecutive weeks. Dotted lines are confidence intervals (reproduced from Robinson *et al.*, 1999, with permission). Copyright @ 2005 American Medical Association. All rights reserved.

participants treated with aripiprazole (n = 853) did not achieve remission (Kane *et al.*, 2007a). The discrepancy of the intent-to-treat and completer results of these studies is explained by the very high drop-out rates in modern trials, which limit the interpretation. In a large, naturalistic sample from Belgium (De Hert *et al.*, 2007), the authors reported that 71% of 422 inpatients did not achieve a remission (time and severity criteria). Similarly, in a cross-sectional study from Sweden, 62% of 243 participants did not meet the severity criteria (Helldin *et al.*, 2007).

We hope that in future the general application of the above described definitions of remission, response, and treatment resistance will allow for more precise statements about the epidemiology of treatment response in schizophrenia.

Management and treatment

What should be checked before insufficient response to the treatment is assumed?

Before assuming non-response and introducing a major change in treatment, the following items should be clarified. These are pragmatic, logical considerations, not evidence-based facts.

Is the diagnosis of schizophrenia correct?

Before changing the therapy, it may be indicated to reconsider the diagnosis. For example, a psychotic depression or severe personality disturbance can sometimes be difficult to distinguish from a schizophrenic episode, but they require a different treatment.

Do side effects mask a response?

Side effects—especially those of high-potency conventional antipsychotic drugs—can mask a response. They can induce secondary negative symptoms via parkinsonism or the inner restlessness of akathisia that can resemble psychotic agitation. Depending on their nature, such side effects need to be stringently treated with dose reduction, anticholinergics, beta-blockers or a change of medication.

Did the patient receive a sufficient dose?

It is an advantage of the SGAs that dose-finding studies have been carried out right from the start: The APA guideline (Lehman *et al.*, 2004) recommends the following dose ranges: aripiprazole 10–30 mg/day, clozapine 150–600 mg/day, olanzapine 10–30 mg/day, quetiapine 300–800 mg/day, risperidone 2–8 mg/day, and ziprasidone 120–160 mg/day. According to the guideline of the World Federation of Societies of Biological Psychiatry (WFSBP) the target dose range of zotepine in patients with multiple episode is 150–250 mg/day (Falkai *et al.*, 2005). The optimum amisulpride dose is 400–800 mg/day for patients with predominant positive symptoms and 50–-300 mg/day for patients with predominant negative symptoms. The dose ranges for first-generation antipsychotics (FGAs) are less well defined. The APA guideline recommends 300–1000 mg/day for chlorpromazine and 5–20 mg/day for haloperidol, although two studies suggest that 4 mg/day for haloperidol (Zimbroff *et al.*, 1997) and neuroleptic threshold doses (2–3 mg/day) may be sufficient (McEvoy *et al.*, 1991). In addition, a Cochrane review on the optimum haloperidol dose concluded that in uncomplicated patients doses higher than 7.5 mg/day for haloperidol do not bring about more efficacy (Waraich *et al.*, 2002).

Was the patient adherent in taking the medication?

Adherence problems are so frequent that they should always be considered in the case of an insufficient response to treatment (Leucht & Heres, 2006). In inpatient settings, a change to a liquid mode of administration or to rapidly dissolving tablets can be helpful. In outpatients, a trial of depot medication can help to rule out non-adherence. Plasma levels and sometimes also the determination of a patient's cytochrome P450 status are useful to distinguish between poor adherence or genetically determined excessive metabolism of medication (ultra-rapid metabolizers). In addition, some medications, such as ziprasidone, must be taken together with food to assure that they are adequately absorbed.

Has the patient developed a sufficient plasma level?

Although studies of the relationship between plasma levels and efficacy and side effects have been carried out for a large number of antipsychotic drugs (a good review is provided by Baumann *et al.*, 2004), the establishment of therapeutic level ranges has proven difficult. Ideally, patients would have to be randomized to different target plasma level ranges and the efficacy of these ranges would have to be compared. There are, however, very few such studies. Many studies only compared the mean plasma levels of responders and non-responders. Haloperidol and clozapine may be the best investigated compounds. Table 26.6 lists the current recommendations by a therapeutic drug monitoring expert group. Due to these limitations, the evidence base is not sufficient to allow for a titration of antipsychotics guided by therapeutic drug monitoring. Rather, plasma level measurements are only indicated in the following situations:

- Suspicion of *non-adherence*.
- *Lack of response in spite of taking doses which are as a rule sufficient*. Excessive metabolization as a result of a polymorphism of the cytochrome P450 enzyme system in which too much enzyme is produced ("ultra-rapid metabolizer"; in the case of cytochrome P4502D6, approximately 1% of the Caucasian population) leads to spuriously low plasma

levels and consequently insufficient response. A polymorphism of this kind can be detected by a gene test, but other causes must be considered, such as smoking, which induces CYP1A2 and can accelerate the metabolism of certain antipsychotic drugs (especially clozapine and olanzapine) via enzyme induction. Table 26.7 is not complete, but it displays some classically relevant interactions. In addition, websites, where the current knowledge about medication interactions is regularly updated, may need to be consulted (e.g., www.drug-interactions.com or http://www.genemedrx.com/).

- *Pronounced side effects* despite the administration of a usual dose. In this situation, it is possible that a gene defect leads to too slow metabolism of the medication ("poor metabolizer"; approximately 5% of Caucasians produce too little CYP2D6), which results in disproportionately increased plasma levels and side effects. Again, drug–drug interactions can be the cause as well.
- *Known polymorphism of the cytochrome P450 enzyme system* ("ultra-rapid or poor metabolizers"). Here, serum level measurements are indicated to avoid too high or too low doses from the outset.
- *Medication interactions* can also lead to elevated or lowered plasma levels via similar or opposing effects on the cytochrome P450 system.

Table 26.6 Recommended plasma level ranges for different antipsychotic drugs (modified from Baumann *et al.*, 2004).

Antipsychotic drug and active metabolite	Degree of recommendation[b]	Recommended therapeutic range (ng/ml; trough level in steady state)
Amisulpride	3	100–400
Aripiprazole	3	150–300[a]
Benperidol	3	2–10
Chlorpromazine	2	30–300
Chlorprothixene	3	20–200
Clozapine	1	350–600
Flufenazine	1	0.5–2
Flupentixol	2	>2
Haloperidol	1	5–17
Levomepromazine	3	15–60
Olanzapine	1	20–80
Perazine	2	100–230
Perfenazine	2	0.6–2.4
Pimozide	4	15–20
Quetiapine	3	70–170
Risperidone plus9-hydroxyrisperidone	2	20–60
Sulpiride	3	200–1000
Thioridazine	2	200–2000
Zotepine	3	12–120
Ziprasidone	4	50–120
Zuclopentixol	3	4–50

[a]Data from Kirschbaum *et al.* (2008).
[b]Degree of recommendation: 1, strongly recommended; 2, recommended; 3, useful; 4, probably useful.

Table 26.7 Key cytochrome P450 enzymes involved in the metabolism of second-generation antipsychotics (modified from Conley & Kelly, 2007).

Second- generation antipsychotic	Key metabolizing P450 enzymes		Drugs/substances potentially leading to clinically relevant metabolic interactions upon coadministration	
			Inducers	Inhibitors
Amisulpride	Almost entirely excreted via the kidney	—	—	—
Aripiprazole	Major	CYP2D6 CYP3A4	Carbamazepine, rifampin	Ketoconazole, grapefruit juice, fluoxetine, erythromycine
Clozapine	Major Minor	CYP1A2 CYP3A4 CYP2D6	Carbamazepine, smoking, omeprazole, rifampin	Caffeine, fluvoxamine, ciprofloxacine, norfloxacine, fluoxetine, nortriptyline, erythromycin, levomepromazine
Olanzapine	Major Minor	CYP1A2 CYP2D6	Carbamazepine, smoking, omeprazole	Caffeine, fluvoxamine, ciprofloxacine, norfloxacine, fluoxetine, nortriptiline, levomepromazine
Quetiapine	Major Minor	CYP3A4 CYP2D6	Thioridazin, phenytoin, rifampin	Divalproex, ketoconazole, cimetidine, fluoxetine, grapefruit juice, protease inhibitors, erythromycine, nefazodon
Paliperidone extended release	Not metabolized via CYP	—	—	—
Risperidone	Major	CYP2D6 CYP3A4	Carbamazepine, rifampin	Fluoxetine, paroxetine, thioridazine, reboxetine, fluvoxamine, ketoconazole, grapefruit juice, erythromycine
Sertindole	Major	CYP2D6 CYP3A4	Carbamazepine, phenytoin, phenobarbital, rifampin	Fluoxetine, paroxetine, erythromycine, calcium antagonists, ketoconazole, grapefruit juice
Ziprasidone[a]	Major Minor	— CYP3A4 CYP1A2	Carbamazepine	Ketoconazole, grapefruit juice
Zotepine	Major	CYP1A2 CYP3A4	Carbamazepine, smoking, omeprazole, rifampin, phenobarbital	Fluvoxamine, cimetidine, ciprofloxacine, enoxacine, lomefloxacine, mexiletine, norfloxatine, propafenone, erythromycine, ketoconazole, calcium antagonists

CYP = cytochrome P450.
[a]Less than a third of ziprasidone is metabolized by CYP, two-thirds are metabolized by aldehydoxidase.
Information on amisulpride, sertindole and zotepine from Benkert and Hippius (2005) and the German product information.

Has the patient been treated sufficiently long?

Time course of the antipsychotic drug effect
A crucial question in clinical routine practice is the duration of an appropriate antipsychotic drug trial. How long should one continue an antipsychotic drug before inefficacy is assumed and a switch to another medication is made? Generally, the response to medication varies considerably from patient to patient. In some patients a significant improvement appears after several hours; for other patients it can take weeks. Textbooks suggested that the treatment effect of antipsychotic drugs only shows up with a delay of several weeks (Gelder *et al.*, 2000; Marder & van Kammen, 2000). Recent work has refuted the theory of a delayed onset of action. In a meta-analysis of 53 studies with 8177 patients (Agid *et al.*, 2003) found that in a 4-week course the greatest symptom reduction occurred within the first week. The additional change between the end of week 1 and the end of week 2 was less than that in the first week, the additional change between weeks 2 and 3 yet lower, and between weeks 3 and 4 was similar to that between weeks 2 and 3. This result was repeated for the positive symptoms as well

as after subtraction of the placebo response. Therefore, the delay of onset of antipsychotic drug action hypothesis was clearly refuted. Leucht *et al.* (2005a) replicated these results in a large database of 1708 individual patients from antipsychotic drug trials. Individual patient data have the advantage compared to conventional meta-analyses that they allow for a better modeling of the data. Namely, there was an important potential source of bias in the meta-analysis by Agid *et al.* (2003) in that most of the studies included were industry sponsored. In such trials the baseline score may sometimes be artificially inflated to make a patient meet the study's inclusion criteria. Leucht *et al.*, (2005a) could rule out this potential bias by analyzing a subgroup of patients who were so severely ill that any artificial inflation was unlikely, and, again, there was no delay of onset of action. The early onset of the antipsychotic drug effect was also shown for the single drugs available in the database. Furthermore, in two studies the analysis could be extended to 1 year and showed that most of the 1-year drug effect occurred in the first 4 weeks (Leucht *et al.*, 2005a). *Post-hoc* analyses of two further studies demonstrated that the effects of olanzapine, haloperidol, and ziprasidone on positive symptoms can be disentangled from those of placebo as early as 24 h after the initiation of treatment (Agid *et al.*, 2008; Kapur *et al.*, 2005).

Consequences of the refutation of the delay of onset hypothesis for the appropriate length of an antipsychotic drug trial

The refutation of the theory of delayed antipsychotic drug action has consequences for clinical treatment, in particular for what is considered an appropriate duration of an antipsychotic drug trial. The early onset of the antipsychotic drug effect and the strong initial reduction of symptoms, which decreases over time, suggest that it may be possible to detect non-responders very early. As a consequence, the medication of those patients who are unlikely to respond to it could be changed early on. A series of studies since the 1980s has shown that a degree of initial response correlates well with the degree of response after 4–6 weeks (Bartko *et al.*, 1987; Gaebel *et al.*, 1988; Nedopil *et al.*, 1983; Stern *et al.*, 1993; Zemlan *et al.*, 1990). The main limitation of these studies was that they were all of a correlative nature but did not provide cut-offs of the degree of initial non-response, which predicts future response or remission. Correll *et al.* (2003) were the first to attempt to predict non-response at 4 weeks from the change of symptoms at 1 week using a sensitivity–specificity analysis in 131 patients treated with flufenazine. Less than 20% BPRS reduction best predicted non-response at 4 weeks. Leucht *et al.*, (2007b) applied a more sophisticated receiver–operator curve approach to examine this question. Their conclusion was that a 0% BPRS total score reduction at week 2 strongly predicted non-response, defined as a less than 25% BPRS

reduction at week 4. The same group essentially replicated this finding in 1996 patients from an olanzapine study (Leucht *et al.*, 2008). Lin *et al.* (2007) showed that a reduction of the BPRS positive subscore by 6 points at 2 weeks was the best predictor of non-response at week 4. Chang *et al.* (2006) developed an algorithm that included several possible predictors at one timepoint, including the degree of early response, which yielded high specificity and sensitivity in 123 patients treated with risperidone. In a randomized naturalistic cost-effectiveness study (n = 443), more than 20% PANSS reduction at week 2 predicted more than 40% PANSS reduction at week 8 with a specificity of 89%, sensitivity of 42%, and positive predictive value of 67%. Early non-response doubled the cost of care, and functional outcome was much worse (Ascher-Svanum *et al.*, 2007). Kinon *et al.* (2008b) undertook a *post-hoc* analysis of 1077 patients in five randomized double-blind studies comparing olanzapine with other SGAs. More than 20% PANSS reduction at week 2 predicted less than 40% PANSS reduction at week 12 with a specificity of 80%, sensitivity of 60%, and positive predictive value of 54%. Early non-responders discontinued treatment more frequently.

Summary

In summary, while the exact results of the studies varied, there is increasing evidence that patients with little to no response at 2 weeks are unlikely to respond at later stages. However, it needs to be clarified by randomized trials whether this means that changing medication at 2 weeks leads to better outcome. The alternative hypothesis is that early non-responders have a poor outcome, irrespective of whether they stay on the same drug or are switched to another drug. The design of such explanatory studies would require that early non-responders at 2 weeks are randomized to either staying on the same drug (control group) or switching to another compound or an augmentation strategy. The first trial of this kind has recently been completed (Kinon *et al.*, 2010). Patients with an acute exacerbation of schizophrenia were treated for 2 weeks with risperidone 2–6 mg/day. The 192 non-responders (defined as <20% PANSS total score reduction) were then randomized to an additional 10 weeks' treatment with either continuation of risperidone 2–6 mg/day or olanzapine 10–20 mg/day. As in the previous *post-hoc* analyses, the initial degree of response predicted the later degree of response. The non-responders who were switched to olanzapine had a better outcome than those who stayed on risperidone. The overall effect was small, but was more pronounced in the more severely ill patients. The main limitation of the study was that the design could not clarify whether the better outcome of the switch group was due to the switching to a drug with a different receptor binding profile or whether it was due to a generally better efficacy of olanzapine (Leucht *et al.*, 2009a). In addition, studies in which the initial drug is switched to an antipsychotic drug with a more different receptor binding profile (e.g., amisulpride, sulpiride or a high-potency typical antipsychotic) or other strategies (e.g., combination treatment, early switch to clozapine, adding an adjunct) are required. These studies could clarify what the best strategy is and whether the currently recommended length of an antipsychotic drug trial in guidelines (usually 4–6 weeks; Gaebel et al., 2006; Lehman et al., 2004; McGorry, 2005; National Institute for Clinical Excellence, 2003)) can be shortened.

Strategies in the case of initial non-response to an antipsychotic

Increasing the dose or switching to a different compound

If in spite of ruling out the above factors, a patient has not responded sufficiently to the treatment, the question arises whether the dose should be increased significantly or a switch made to another antipsychotic. A further possibility is an augmentation strategy (see below). Only a few randomized studies have addressed the first question.

Kinon et al. (1993) treated 115 patients with schizophrenia for 4 weeks with flufenazine 20 mg/day. The 47 non-responders at 4 weeks were randomized to either double-blind continuation with flufenazine 20 mg/day (control group), flufenazine 80 mg/day (dose increase group) or haloperidol 20 mg/day (switching group). The result was sobering, since only four (9%) of the patients responded, with no difference between the treatment strategies. However, the treatment had been switched from one high-potency conventional antipsychotic (flufenazine) to another high-potency conventional antipsychotic (haloperidol), both of which have a similar receptor binding profile in that they have a high affinity to dopamine receptors. The study needs to be replicated with SGAs.

Shalev et al. (1993) randomized 60 patients with acute schizophrenia to eitherhaloperidol, perfenazine or chlorpromazine. Non-responders after 4 weeks' treatment were randomized to open treatment with one of the other two antipsychotics; after a further 4 weeks non-responders received the remaining antipsychotic. After the first 4 weeks 67% of patients had responded (defined as at least 30% BPRS reduction from baseline); after the second 4 weeks 55% of the remaining 20 patients had responded and after the third 4 weeks 67% of the remaining patients had. The high response rate (defined as at least 30% BPRS reduction and readiness for discharge) of overall 95% was discussed as an argument for the efficacy of the switching treatment. Although the study is encouraging, it lacked the crucial control group of patients who stayed on the initial drug to rule out that the improvement was not simply an effect of time, rather than due to switching the drug.

McEvoy et al. (1991) randomized patients who did not respond to neuroleptic threshold doses of haloperidol to either continuation of threshold doses or to 2–10 times higher dosages. The increased dose led to no better efficacy in comparison with a continuation of the threshold dose.

Louwerens and van der Meij (2000) randomized 36 patients who did not respond to the initially administered conventional antipsychotic into three groups: continuation of the initial antipsychotic, change to another conventional antipsychotic, or change to clozapine. Both change strategies were significantly more effective than the continuation of the initial medication. But the authors discuss their results very cautiously, since of an initial 146 patients who fulfilled the inclusion criteria, only 36 could be randomized.

Suzuki et al. (2007) randomized 78 patients with schizophrenia to open-label treatment with olanzapine, quetiapine, and risperidone; non-responders to treatment of up to 8 weeks' duration were rerandomized twice to the other compounds. Sixteen patients did not respond to any of the three antipsychotic drugs and seven dropped out. Although the results support that switching may be effective, there were the following limitations: the drugs were only switched after treatment of up to 8 weeks' duration; this was a single-center study and open label trial; the sample size was small; and the study lacked the crucial control group of patients who stayed on the initial drug to rule out that the improvement is not simply an effect of time, rather than due to switching the drug.

It is astonishing how few studies have investigated these essential questions about antipsychotic treatment strategies in view of the considerable non-response rate. Nevertheless, if the drug is switched, a medication with a different receptor binding profile should be chosen. Stroup et al. (2007) presented a post-hoc analysis of the clinical antipsychotic treatment effectiveness study (CATIE; Lieberman et al., 2005), which also provided some indirect evidence that switching to an antipsychotic drug with a different receptor binding profile may be an effective strategy. Those participants (n = 114) who had been treated unsuccessfully with perfenazine in CATIE's Phase I responded better (i.e., they had a longer mean time to study discontinuation) if they were randomized to quetiapine or olanzapine than to risperidone. This effect was explained by the fact that risperidone resembles perfenazine most in terms of affinity to dopamine D_2 receptors.

Clozapine in the case of therapy resistance

A landmark study demonstrated the superiority of clozapine in comparison with chlorpromazine for treatment-resistant patients (Kane et al., 1988). This led to its reintroduction in the US despite increased risk of agranulocytosis. Nevertheless, clozapine can only be administered under specific precautions, most importantly, regular differential blood counts. Furthermore, patients must have been either intolerant or have insufficiently responded to at least two other antipsychotic drugs (for details see package inserts). The superior efficacy of clozapine for treatment-resistant patients has been replicated in several studies (Kane *et al.*, 2001; Rosenheck *et al.*, 1997), although the effect sizes were usually not as high as in the original trial (Kane *et al.*, 1988). Various meta-analyses have also confirmed clozapine's superiority in treatment-resistant patients (Chakos *et al.*, 2001; Essali *et al.*, 2009; Wahlbeck *et al.*, 1999).

Whether clozapine is also superior to the other SGAs can at present not be definitively confirmed. Two recent industry-independent studies showed a superiority but in one of them (CATIE Phase II) clozapine was the only open-label arm (McEvoy *et al.*, 2006), and the CUtLASS study compared clozapine with the group of other SGAs (Lewis *et al.*, 2006). In a meta-analysis of 28 randomized head-to-head comparisons of clozapine with other SGAs, clozapine was only superior to zotepine in a small single trial, and to risperidone in terms of drop-outs due to inefficacy of treatment (Leucht *et al.*, 2009c). Several limitations of the available evidence base were discussed: most studies used low or very low clozapine dosages. The mean doses in some studies were below 200 mg/day, and several studies had an upper limit of 400 mg/day. This contrasts with two pivotal studies (Kane *et al.*, 1988; Rosenheck *et al.*, 1997) which showed clozapine's superiority to FGAs when the mean doses were 600 mg/day and 523 mg/day. A dose-finding study found 600 mg/day to be best (Simpson *et al.*, 1999), and a review of clozapine plasma-level studies (Davis & Chen, 2004) showed that low clozapine dosages produce worse results than high dosages. The patients in these recent head-to-head trials may not have been as refractory as those in the pivotal studies (Kane *et al.*, 1988; Rosenheck *et al.*, 1997). Hardly any studies had a run-in phase to confirm refractoriness. A reasonable evidence base is only available for the comparison of clozapine with risperidone and olanzapine, both of which turned out to be among the more efficacious SGAs (Leucht *et al.*, 2009a). Importantly, as only two of 22 individual studies found clozapine to be superior (Azorin *et al.*, 2001; Lin *et al.*, 2003), a narrative review would have reached similar conclusions. Nevertheless, a conclusive, sufficiently dosed, double-blind trial is needed to demonstrate whether clozapine truly is a more efficacious SGA (Leucht *et al.*, 2009c).

Other second-generation antipsychotic drugs in treatment-resistant schizophrenia

The evidence base for the efficacy of other SGAs in treatment-resistant patients is much weaker than that for clozapine. A meta-analysis published in 2001 concluded that only clozapine has been convincingly shown to be superior to FGAs in treatment-resistant patients (Chakos

et al., 2001). These results for treatment-resistant patients have not really changed since the publication of this meta-analysis.

First, it should be noted that systematic reviews found a consistent superiority only for amisulpride, clozapine, olanzapine, and risperidone (Davis *et al.*, 2003; Geddes *et al.*, 2000; Leucht *et al.*, 2002b, 2009a,b)). Nevertheless, these meta-analyses did not restrict their inclusion criteria to treatment-refractory patients.

According to the meta-analysis by Leucht *et al.* (2009a), there is no randomized controlled trial comparing amisulpride, sertindole or zotepine with FGAs in schizophrenia. Kane *et al.* (2007b) randomized 300 participants who had not responded to a 4-week trial with olanzapine or risperidone to aripiprazole or perfenazine, but did not find any difference in efficacy. A *post-hoc* analysis of a large olanzapine *versus* haloperidol trial (Tollefson *et al.*, 1997) confirmed olanzapine's superiority in a treatment-resistant subgroup (Breier & Hamilton, 1999). Four smaller studies did not find a clear superiority of olanzapine compared to FGAs in treatment-resistant schizophrenia (Altamura *et al.*, 2002; Buchanan *et al.*, 2005; Conley *et al.*, 1998; Smith *et al.*, 2001). Volavka *et al.* (2002) found olanzapine to be superior to haloperidol, but the limitation of this study was that it was conducted in non-responders to typical antipsychotics. Two studies on quetiapine are available. Conley *et al.* (2005) found no difference compared to flufenazine. Emsley *et al.* (2000) treated 228 patients for 4 weeks with flufenazine and randomized the partial non-responders to 600 mg/day quetiapine or 20 mg/day haloperidol. Quetiapine reduced symptoms significantly more than haloperidol. Wirshing *et al.* (1999) found risperidone to be superior to haloperidol only in the first 4 study weeks. See *et al.* (1999), Conley *et al.* (2005), and Volavka *et al.* (2002) found no clear superiority of risperidone compared to haloperidol in resistant patients. Finally, Kane *et al.* (2006) treated patients for 6 weeks with haloperidol and randomized the 306 non-responders to ziprasidone or chlorpromazine. At endpoint, there was no significant difference in overall and psychotic symptoms, but ziprasidone was superior in terms of negative symptoms.

In summary, the effects of SGAs compared to FGAs in treatment-resistant patients are less consistent than those for clozapine. This explains why, according to treatment guidelines, clozapine remains the gold standard (Lehman *et al.*, 2004; McGorry, 2005; National Institute for Clinical Excellence, 2003), although a recent meta-analysis could not demonstrate clozapine's superiority in head-to-head comparisons that were not restricted to treatment-resistant patients (Leucht *et al*, 2009c).

Augmentation strategies

Numerous augmentation strategies have been investigated in the last decades. Nevertheless, for none of these strategies is the supporting evidence so robust that it can be generally recommended. Therefore, treatment guidelines recommend antipsychotic monotherapy as a matter of principle (Lehman *et al.*, 2004; McGorry, 2005; National Institute for Clinical Excellence, 2003). Important reasons are:

• Combinations of medications increase the risk of side effects;
• Combinations of medications increase the risk of drug–drug interactions;
• If two medications are administered at the same time, it is often not clear which of them has finally led to success and which should be discontinued;
• Adherence, which is often difficult for patients with schizophrenia due to cognitive deficits and lack of insight, is made more difficult when several medications are to be taken at the same time;
• As the mechanism of action of many adjuncts is not well understood, the rationale for adding a given compound is often unclear;
• The evidence base is lacking, mixed or too incomplete to recommend specific augmentation treatments.

Benzodiazepines

A narrative review from the end of the 1980s, which considered not only randomized, double-blind studies, but also case series, came to the conclusion that benzodiazepines could have an effect in the treatment of positive symptoms (Wolkowitz & Pickar, 1991). A Cochrane review based on 34 randomized studies with 2454 participants could not confirm this conclusion (Volz *et al.*, 2007). Nevertheless, a number of methodological problems, such as insufficient presentation of the results in the individual studies or the use of different outcome criteria, often made a meta-analytic combination of the trials impossible. The sedative effects of benzodiazepines in schizophrenia could be shown, but there is much room for randomized studies on the decisive question whether benzodiazepines improve or, at least, hasten the amelioration of positive symptoms.

Mood stabilizers

Mood stabilizers are frequently used in people with schizophrenia. For example, Citrome *et al.* (2000) showed that in 1998, 43.4% of all patients with schizophrenia in New York's state hospitals received a mood stabilizer. The authors also documented a shift over time from lithium to the more recent mood stabilizers, especially valproate.

Lithium

Studies in the 1970s and 1980s showed that lithium is not efficacious as a monotherapy in schizophrenia (Dube & Sethi, 1981; Johnstone *et al.*, 1988; Prien *et al.*, 1972), but several small early randomized studies suggested that lithium may be effective as an adjunct to antipsychotic drugs (Growe *et al.*, 1979; Small *et al.*, 1975). Some of these

studies, however, investigated patients who were schizoaffective or schizophrenic with pronounced affective symptoms (Biederman *et al.*, 1979). A series of studies on treatment-resistant patients was then carried out which, considered individually, all yielded negative results. Likewise, a Cochrane review of 11 studies and 244 participants found no clear proof of efficacy (Leucht *et al.*, 2007d). Only for one of three response cut-offs (at least 50% reduction of the BPRS total score from baseline) was a significant superiority of the combination therapy found, but not for the cut-offs of at least 20% and 80% BPRS reduction, not for the mean BPRS at endpoint, and not when patients with prominent affective symptoms were excluded. Moreover, significantly more patients in the lithium augmentation group dropped out of the studies, probably due to side effects.

Carbamazepine

A systematic review that included 10 studies with 258 participants found no evidence that augmentation of antipsychotic drugs with carbamazepine is effective (Leucht *et al.*, 2002a). In addition carbamazepine is an inducer of cytochrome P450 enzymes. This can lead to a drop in the plasma levels of antipsychotic drugs, e.g., haloperidol. Therefore, this combination is often not suitable.

Valproate

According to a Cochrane review only five randomized studies with 379 participants have been carried out. The meta-analysis did not find a significant benefit of augmentation with valproate (Schwartz *et al.*, 2008). The largest study (249 participants; addition of valproate or placebo to risperidone or olanzapine) showed a more rapid onset of improvement in the augmentation group at 2 weeks. This superiority was lost, however, at the end of the 4-week study (Casey *et al.*, 2003). A large replication study (n = 402), which has not yet been included in the Cochrane review, did not even find any superiority at 2 weeks (Casey *et al.*, 2009).

Lamotrigine

Recent evidence from five lamotrigine augmentation studies (537 participants) was summarized in a Cochrane review (Premkumar & Pick, 2006). Some indications of efficacy on positive and negative symptoms were found, but the results were not designated as robust. Another meta-analysis specifically examined lamotrigine added to clozapine in resistant patients and found a significant effect (five trials, n = 161; Tiihonen *et al.*, 2009)). However, patients for this meta-analysis were drawn from individual trials where a mixture of baseline antipsychotics were allowed and clozapine treatment was not used as a stratification factor, which is why the included patients were not perfectly randomly assigned to clozapine or placebo. Overall, lamotrigine appears to be a promising adjunct, but the evidence base needs to be extended.

Beta-blockers

A Cochrane review currently includes five studies with 117 patients and does not support the efficacy of augmentation with beta-blockers (Cheine *et al.*, 2003).

Antidepressants for the treatment of negative symptoms and depression

Antidepressants are added to antipsychotics above all for two indications. First, they are given for patients who in addition to schizophrenia also suffer from *pronounced depressive symptoms*. A Cochrane review analyzed 11 small randomized studies, each with fewer than 30 participants. The addition of antidepressants was efficacious, but due to the limited data available the conclusions of the authors were cautiously expressed. Furthermore, since most of the studies used tricyclic antidepressants, the evidence base on selective serotonin reuptake inhibitors (SSRIs) and other new antidepressants is small (Whitehead *et al.*, 2003). Second, antidepressants are also frequently administered for the *treatment of negative symptoms*. As it is a general methodological problem in this area to disentangle the effects of antidepressants on negative symptoms from those on depression, a Cochrane review restricted its inclusion criteria to participants with predominant negative symptoms. It found significant positive effects (five studies with 190 participants), but drew its conclusions with restraint due to the limited evidence; again most of the studies examined tricyclic antidepressants (Rummel *et al.*, 2006). Another meta-analysis did not restrict its inclusion criteria to predominant negative symptoms, but only addressed studies using SSRIs as antidepressants (11 included studies; Sepehry *et al.*, 2007). A significant effect was only found in a subgroup of studies in chronic patients. The authors, therefore, concluded that the meta-analysis did not provide global support for an improvement in negative symptoms with SSRI augmentation. The latest meta-analysis included 23 trials (n = 819 participants) of SSRIs and other antidepressants; it found a significant benefit of moderate effect size (Singh *et al.*, 2010).

Acetylcholinesterase inhibitors for the improvement of cognitive deficits

Several small randomized studies (6–40 participants; Freudenreich *et al.*, 2005; Friedman *et al.*, 2002; Nahas *et al.*, 2003; Schubert *et al.*, 2006; Sharma *et al.*, 2006; Tugal *et al.*, 2004) and one large study (250 participants; Keefe *et al.*, 2008)) found no positive effects of the addition of acetylcholinesterase inhibitors on the cognitive deficits of patients with schizophrenia. These negative results were confirmed by a systematic review and meta-analysis (Stip *et al.*, 2007).

Combinations of antipsychotic drugs

There are numerous publications showing a high prevalence of antipsychotic combinations in clinical practice (for

a review, see Correll & Kane, 2004). A number of meta-analyses on this issue have recently been conducted and have come up with similar conclusions.

Correll *et al.* (2009) identified 19 randomized controlled trials with 1216 participants, which overall suggested a better response in the combination group compared to monotherapy. The interpretation of the review was limited by the high number of different combinations, leaving it unclear exactly which strategy was effective. There were also a number of significant moderators: antipsychotic combinations were more effective when they were administered right from the start rather than added only in the case of non-response (which is current practice), in trials lasting longer than 10 weeks (supporting a smaller review by Paton *et al.*, 2007, but not that of Taylor & Smith 2009), when clozapine was part of the combination treatment, and in Chinese studies. Furthermore, there was also a possibility of publication bias.

Barbui *et al.* (2009) focused on combinations including clozapine and identified 21 studies. A significant superiority was only found in randomized open studies, but not in double-blind studies. They therefore concluded that the evidence base supporting a second antipsychotic in addition to clozapine in partially responsive patients with schizophrenia is weak, indicating modest to absent benefit.

However, two recent randomized augmentation studies where aripiprazole or placebo was added to clozapine confirmed several open-label studies in that at least a reduction in weight and lipid abnormalities was observed in the augmentation group, even without dose reduction of clozapine (Chang *et al.*, 2008; Fleischhacker *et al.*, 2008). Moreover, in the Korean study (n = 62) augmentation with aripiprazole (dose: 5–30 mg) led to a significantly greater reduction in negative symptoms (p < 0.01; Chang *et al.*, 2008). In the other study, where aripiprazole was only dosed up to 15 mg/day, positive or negative symptoms were not significantly different, but CGI improvement scores were reduced significantly more in the aripiprazole compared to the placebo augmentation group (p = 0.037; Fleischhacker *et al.*, 2010).

In summary, these data and reviews show that combinations of antipsychotics may be effective in certain situations and patients, but that there are methodological issues and, if there are positive effects, they are small. The available data therefore do not allow for a recommendation of combining antipsychotic drugs. A major limitation is the lack of clarity concerning which exact combinations are useful, because there have been a plethora of different strategies. From a theoretical point of view, it may make sense to combine drugs with relatively different receptor binding profiles, e.g., drugs with relatively little antidopaminergic effects, such as clozapine, with selective dopamine receptor antagonists, such as amisulpride, sulpiride or the partial agonist, aripiprazole.

Electroconvulsive therapy

Prior to the introduction of antipsychotics, electroconvulsive therapy (ECT) was a standard treatment for schizophrenia. A Cochrane review identified 26 randomized controlled trials with over 798 participants (Tharyan & Adams, 2005). In 10 short-term studies (n = 392) ECT was more efficacious than sham-ECT. However, in another 10 short-term studies (n = 443) ECT was less efficacious than antipsychotic drugs. There was very limited evidence on the effects of ECT added to antipsychotic drugs, but one small study (n = 40) showed a more pronounced symptom reduction, and another small study (n = 30) found positive effects when continuation ECT was added to antipsychotic drugs compared to antipsychotic medication or ECT alone.

A number of methodological problems limited the interpretation of the review: there were many differences in the ways ECT was administered; diagnostic criteria varied strongly in the course of the years; only six studies explicitly included only treatment resistant patients; and combinations of ECT with atypical antipsychotics are lacking with the exception of clozapine.

In this context it is understandable that ECT is currently only recommended as a last resort. A point in favor of ECT is its efficacy as monotherapy, while for most of the other augmentation strategies listed above efficacy as monotherapy has not been shown. Furthermore, the mechanism of action is different from that of antipsychotic drugs, possibly making augmentation effects more likely.

Repetitive transcranial magnetic stimulation

In repetitive transcranial magnetic stimulation (rTMS) a magnetic field is applied to the cranial dome to stimulate the brain areas lying below it. It is assumed that effects similar to those of ECT can thereby be produced. Several randomized studies have been performed; in most the rTMS was applied over the temporo-parietal cortex of the dominant hemisphere with the goal of reducing positive symptoms. A meta-analysis of 10 randomized controlled trials (n = 232) found a medium effect size for adding rTMS to antipsychotic drugs (Tranulis et al., 2008; see also Aleman et al., 2007)). Less often, rTMS has been applied over frontal areas in order to influence negative symptoms with equivocal results (Hajak et al., 2004; Klein et al., 1999).

Cognitive–behavioral therapy

Most systematic reviews support the efficacy of cognitive–behavioral therapy in treatment-resistant schizophrenia (Gould et al., 2001; Pilling et al., 2002a,b; Wykes et al., 2008), although the Cochrane review is more critical (Jones et al., 2004). This strategy is thoroughly reviewed in Chapter 32.

Miscellaneous treatments

The effects of *polyunsaturated fatty acids* (omega-3 and -6 fatty acids) have been investigated in a large number of illnesses. It is hypothesized that in schizophrenia they can have an effect on neuronal membranes or their metabolism. The results of six studies (five of which were on omega-3 fatty acids) included in a Cochrane review were partly contradictory, and the authors concluded that this treatment is still in an experimental stage (Joy et al., 2006).

Glutamate antagonists such as PCP (phencyclidin, "angel dust") or ketamine can produce psychotic symptoms. Derived from these findings, the glutamate hypothesis of schizophrenia suggests that glutamatergic agents could be effective in its treatment (see Chapter 21). The Cochrane review on glycine, D-serine, D-cycloserine or ampakine included 18 randomized studies with 358 participants. D-cycloserine, a partial N-methyl-D-aspartate (NMDA) agonist, did not appear to have any effect. The NMDA-receptor co-agonists glycine and D-serine showed significant effects on schizophrenic negative symptoms as adjuvant therapy (Tuominen et al., 2006). In a new study by the National Institute of Mental Health (NIMH), however, the largest yet performed, no conclusive proof of efficacy resulted (Buchanan et al., 2007). While at least two small, placebo-controlled trials of a glutamate transporter inhibitor, N-methylglycine, have been encouraging (Tsai et al., 2004; Lane et al., 2005), medications with this mechanism of action require further study. To our knowledge glutamate agonists have not yet been approved as a treatment for schizophrenia in any country.

It is well known that the average onset of schizophrenia is later in women than in men, and that there is a second frequency peak for women after age 40. These effects are attributed to the higher estrogen levels in women, stimulating research on the addition of *estrogens*. In a recent study of 100 women with schizophrenia, the addition of 100 µg of transdermal estradiol to ongoing antipsychotic treatment significantly reduced positive (p < 0.05) and general psychopathological (p < 0.05) symptoms during the 28-day trial period compared to antipsychotic treatment alone (Kulkarni et al., 2008). In an earlier, placebo-controlled study of 32 women of childbearing age with schizophrenia, ethinyl estradiol 0.05 mg/day added to haloperidol 15 mg/day showed significant superiority over haloperidol alone for the treatment of positive and general psychopathology symptoms, as well as Positive and Negative Syndrome Scale (PANSS) total scores (Akhondzadeh et al., 2003). However, there have also been studies that do not show significant benefits from estrogen augmentation on symptomatic change or relapse rates (Bergemann et al., 2005; Louzã et al., 2004), and in a Cochrane review that summarized four studies with a total of 105 women, no conclusive proof of efficacy could be achieved (Chua et al., 2005).

Even fewer controlled studies exist for the addition of male hormones in schizophrenia. *Dehydroepiandrosterone (DHEA)* is a precursor of estrogens and androgens, which also develops androgenic and anabolic effects itself. Three randomized studies (n = 100) found significant effects, above all on negative symptoms (Strous *et al.*, 2003, 2007). However, a Cochrane review and meta-analysis that pre-dated the two latest positive trials concluded that the findings available up to January 2007 required confirmation and were not strong or consistent enough to recommend DHEA/testosterone augmentation in patients with schizophrenia at this point (Elias & Kumar, 2007).

Amphetamine preparations are sometimes administered in the case of therapy-refractory negative symptoms. A Cochrane review identified four studies with 85 participants but allowed no clear conclusions (Nolte *et al.*, 2004). Based on immunological theories, double-blind studies found significant effects for the addition of the cyclooxygenase-2 (COX-2) inhibitor celecoxib (Akhondzadeh *et al.*, 2007, Müller *et al.*, 2002, Müller *et al.*, 2010), but it would be premature to generally recommend this augmentation strategy.

Another new experimental approach is to enhance oxygenation by coadministration of *erythropoietin*. One study found a specific improvement of cognitive symptoms without simultaneous effects on the symptoms of the schizophrenia (Ehrenreich *et al.*, 2007).

Summary

On the whole, despite enormous research efforts, there is little evidence supporting the use of pharmacological augmentation strategies. Correspondingly, if addressed, all these augmentation strategies were only ranked at best as strategies of second choice by 50 American experts in schizophrenia (Kane *et al.*, 2003). Clozapine remains the gold standard. Should one nevertheless decide on combinations, the interactions and side effects should be considered and the target symptoms taken into account. For example, the administration of mood stabilizers for manic symptoms can be reasonable, but according to currently available data an effect on positive symptoms is unlikely.

Childhood-onset schizophrenia

Childhood- or early-onset schizophrenia is usually considered to begin before age 17, whereas very early-onset schizophrenia has its onset prior to age 13 (see Chapter 3). Although this condition is relatively rare, these individuals often have severe and disabling symptoms which respond poorly to medication. This form of schizophrenia is generally believed to be clinically and neurobiologically continuous with adult-onset cases; however, treatment response is often suboptimal (Kumra *et al.*, 2008). In recent years this special population has received increasing attention and a number of clinical trials have been conducted in treatment-resistant subjects.

The first study to focus on this population (Kumra *et al.*, 1996) enrolled 21 childhood-onset (before age 12; 11 males

and 10 females) subjects (mean age 14; SD 2.3) in a 6-week double-blind inpatient trial comparing clozapine to haloperidol. Patients had been non-responsive, intolerant or both to at least two different antipsychotics. The mean final dose of clozapine was 176 mg/day (SD 149) and haloperidol 16 mg/day (SD 8). Clozapine was superior to haloperidol on all measures of psychosis (p < 0.04). Both positive and negative symptoms improved.

Shaw *et al.* (2006) compared the efficacy and safety of olanzapine and clozapine in a double-blind controlled trial lasting 8 weeks, with a 2-year open-label follow-up. Subjects were included if they experienced an onset of schizophrenia before age 13 and failed to respond to two antipsychotic medications (typical or atypical), given in doses greater than 100 mg chlorpromazine equivalents for at least 4 weeks (unless terminated due to intolerable side effects). Twenty-five subjects were randomized (mean age at study entry was 25; 15 males and 10 females). Twelve patients received clozapine with a mean final dose of 327 mg (SD 113) and a mean plasma concentration of 715 mg/ml. For the 13 patients randomized to olanzapine, the final mean dose was 18.1 mg (SD 4.3). Clozapine was associated with a significant reduction in all outcome measures whereas olanzapine showed a less consistent clinical improvement. However, given the small sample size, only alleviation of negative symptoms was statistically significant (p = 0.04; effect size 0.89) in favor of clozapine. Clozapine was associated with more overall adverse effects. At 2-year follow-up, 15 patients (some of whom were switched from olanzapine to clozapine) were still receiving clozapine with evidence of sustained clinical improvement, but additional adverse effects (predominantly metabolic) had emerged.

Kumra *et al.* (2008) identified patients aged 10(SD 149) 18 with a diagnosis of schizophrenia who had documented treatment failure of at least two prior antipsychotics, had a score of at least 35 on the BPRS and a score of at least "moderate" on one or more of its psychotic items. Patients who had previously failed clozapine or olanzapine were excluded. Participants were randomly assigned, under double-blind conditions, to clozapine (18 patients) or "high-dose" olanzapine (i.e., up to 30 mg/day; 21 patients) for 12 weeks. The mean dose of clozapine at endpoint was 403 mg (SD 201) and the mean serum concentration 514 ng/dL (SD 284). For olanzapine the mean endpoint dose was 26 mg (SD 6.5) and the mean serum concentration 74 ng/dL (SD 42). An *a priori* response criterion of a 30% or more decrease in the total BPRS from baseline to endpoint and a CGI improvement rating of "much improved" or "very much improved" was the primary outcome variable. A significantly greater proportion of clozapine-treated subjects (66%) in comparison to olanzapine-treated subjects (33%) met these response criteria (p = 0.04). The changes from baseline in rating scale scores between the two groups was similar with the exception of negative symptoms, where clozapine was associated with significantly greater improvement. Both treatments were associated with significant weight gain and related metabolic abnormalities (see Chapter 28).

Children with treatment-refractory schizophrenia are a rare, but very vulnerable population. These data support the potential value of clozapine; however, like in adults, it is associated with a variety of potential adverse effects which must be appropriately managed.

References

Agid, O., Kapur, S., Arenovich, T. & Zipursky, R.B. (2003) Delayed-onset hypothesis of antipsychotic action—A hypothesis tested and rejected. *Archives of General Psychiatry* **60**, 1228–1235.

Agid, O., Kapur, S., Warrington, L., Loebel, A. & Siu, C. (2008) Early onset of antipsychotic response in the treatment of acutely agitated patients with psychotic disorders. *Schizophrenia Research* **102**, 241–248.

Akhondzadeh, S., Nehatusafa, A.A., Amini, H. *et al.* (2003) Adjunctive estrogen treatment in women with chronic schizophrenia: a double-blind, randomized, and placebo controlled trial. *Progress in Neuropsychopharmacology and Biological Psychiatry* **27**, 1007–1012.

Akhondzadeh, S., Tabatbaee, M., Amini, H., Ahmadi Abhari, S.A., Abbasi, S. H. & Behnam, B. (2007) Celecoxib as adjunctive therapy in schizophrenia: A double-blind, randomized and placebo-controlled trial. *Schizophrenia Research* **90**, 179–185.

Aleman, A., Sommer, I.E. & Kahn, R.S. (2007) Efficacy of slow repetitive transcranial magnetic stimulation in the treatment of resistant auditory hallucinations in schizophrenia: a meta-analysis. *Journal of Clinical Psychiatry* **68**, 416–421.

Altamura, A.C., Velona, I., Curreli, R., Mundo, E. & Bravi, D. (2002) Is olanzapine better than haloperidol in resistant schizophrenia? A double-blind study in partial responders. *International Journal of Psychiatric Clinical Practice* **6**, 107–111.

Andreasen, N., Carpenter, W., Kane, J., Lasser, R., Marder, S. & Weinberger, D. (2005) Remission in schizophrenia: proposed criteria and rationale for consensus. *American Journal of Psychiatry* **62**, 441–449.

Ascher-Svanum, H., Nyhuis, A.W., Faries, D.E., Kinon, B.J., Baker, R.W. & Shekhar, A. (2007) Clinical, functional, and economic ramifications of early nonresponse to antipsychotics in the naturalistic treatment of schizophrenia. *Schizophrenia Bulletin* **34**, 1163–1171.

Azorin, J.M., Spiegel, R., Remington, G., Vanelle, J.M. *et al.* (2001) A double-blind comparative study of clozapine and risperidone in the management of severe chronic schizophrenia. *American Journal of Psychiatry* **158**, 1305–1313.

Barbui, C., Signoretti, A., Mule, S., Boso, M. & Cipriani, A. (2009) Does the addition of a second antipsychotic drug improve clozapine treatment? *Schizophrenia Bulletin* **35**, 458–468.

Bartko, G., Herczeg, I. & Bekesy, M. (1987) Predicting outcome of neuroleptic treatment on the basis of subjective response and early clinical improvement. *Journal of Clinical Psychiatry* **48**, 363–365.

Baumann, P., Hiemke, C., Ulrich, S. *et al.* (2004) The AGNP-TDM expert group consensus guidelines: therapeutic drug monitoring in psychiatry. *Pharmacopsychiatry* **37**, 243–265.

Beitinger, R., Lin, J., Kissling, W. & Leucht, S. (2008) Comparative remission rates of schizophrenic patients using various remission criteria. *Progress in Neuropsychopharmacology and Biological Psychiatry* **32**, 1643–1651.

Benkert, O. & Hippius, H. (2005) *Kompendium der Psychiatrischen Pharmakotherapie.* Heidelberg: Springer.

Bergemann, N., Mundt, C., Parzer, P. *et al.* (2005) Estrogen as an adjuvant therapy to antipsychotics does not prevent relapse in women suffering from schizophrenia: results of a placebo-controlled double-blind study. *Schizophrenia Research* **74**, 125–134.

Biederman, J., Lerner, Y. & Belmaker, R.H. (1979) Combination of lithium carbonate and haloperidol in schizo-affective patients. *Archives of General Psychiatry* **36**, 327–333.

Breier, A. & Hamilton, S.H. (1999) Comparative efficacy of olanzapine and haloperidol for patients with treatment-resistant schizophrenia. *Biological Psychiatry* **45**, 403–411.

Brenner, H.D., Dencker, S.J., Goldstein, M.J. *et al.* (1990) Defining treatment refractoriness in schizophrenia. *Schizophrenia Bulletin* **16**, 551–561.

Buchanan, R.W., Ball, M.P., Weiner, E. *et al.* (2005) Olanzapine treatment of residual positive and negative symptoms. *American Journal of Psychiatry* **162**, 124–129.

Buchanan, R.W., Javitt, D.C., Marder, S.R. *et al.* (2007) The Cognitive and Negative Symptoms in Schizophrenia, Trial (CONSIST): The efficacy of glutamatergic agents for negative symptoms and cognitive impairments. *American Journal of Psychiatry* **164**, 1593–1602.

Casey, D.E., Daniel, D.G., Wassef, A.A., Tracy, K.A., Wozniak, P. & Sommerville, K.W. (2003) Effect of divalproex combined with olanzapine or risperidone in patients with an acute exacerbation of schizophrenia. *Neuropsychopharmacology* **28**, 182–192.

Casey, D.E., Daniel, D.G., Tamminga, C. *et al.* (2009) Divalproex ER combined with olanzapine or risperidone for treatment of acute exacerbations of schizophrenia. *Neuropsychopharmacology* **34**, 1330–1338.

Chakos, M., Lieberman, J., Hoffman, E., Bradford, D. & Sheitman, B. (2001) Effectiveness of second generation antipsychotics for treatment-resistant schizophrenia: A review and meta-analysis of randomized trials. *American Journal of Psychiatry* **158**, 518–526.

Chang, Y.C., Lane, H.Y., Yang, K.H. & Huang, C.L. (2006) Optimizing early prediction for antipsychotic response in schizophrenia. *Journal of Clinical Psychopharmacology* **26**, 554–559.

Chang, J.S., Ahn, Y.M., Park, H.J. *et al.* (2008) Aripiprazole augmentation in clozapine-treated patients with refractory schizophrenia: an 8-week, double-blind, placebo-controlled trial. *Journal of Clinical Psychiatry* **69**, 720–731.

Cheine, M., Ahonen, J., & Wahlbeck, K. (2003) Beta-blocker supplementation of standard drug treatment for schizophrenia (Cochrane Review). *The Cochrane Library* Issue 1, CD000234.

Chua, W.L., Santiago, A.D., Kulkarni, J. & Mortimer, A. (2005) Estrogen for schizophrenia. *Database of Systematic Reviews* Issue 4, CD004719.

Citrome, L., Levine, J. & Allingham, B. (2000) Changes in use of valproate and other mood stabilizers for patients with schizophrenia from 1994 to 1998. *Psychiatric Services* **51**, 634–638.

Conley, R.R. & Kelly, D.L. (2007) Drug-drug interactions associated with second-generation antipsychotics: considerations for clinicians and patients. *Psychopharmacology Bulletin* **40**, 77–97.

Conley, R.R., Tamminga, C.A., Bartko, J.J. *et al.* (1998) Olanzapine compared with chlorpromazine in treatment-resistant schizophrenia. *American Journal of Psychiatry* **155**, 914–920.

Conley, R.R., Kelly, D.L., Nelson, M.W. *et al.* (2005) Risperidone, quetiapine, and fluphenazine in the treatment of patients with therapy-refractory schizophrenia. *Clinical Neuropharmacology* **28**, 163–168.

Correll, C.U., Malhotra, A.K., Kaushik, S., McMeniman, M. & Kane, J.M. (2003) Early prediction of antipsychotic response in schizophrenia. *American Journal of Psychiatry* **160**, 2063–2065.

Correll, C.U. & Kane, J.M. (2004) Is there a rationale for antipsychotic polypharmacy in schizophrenia? In: Fleischhaker, W.W. & Hummer, M., eds. *Schizophrene Störungen—State of the Art III*. Insbruck: Verlag integrative Psychiatrie, pp. 95–112.

Correll, C.U., Rummel-Kluge, C., Corves, C., Kane, J.M. & Leucht, S. (2009) Antipsychotic combinations vs monotherapy in schizophrenia: A meta-analysis of randomized controlled trials. *Schizophrenia Bulletin* **35**, 443–457.

Davis, J.M. & Chen, N. (2004) Dose-response and dose equivalence of antipsychotics. *Journal of Clinical Psychopharmacology* **24**, 192–208.

Davis, J.M., Chen, N., & Glick, I.D. (2003) A meta-analysis of the efficacy of second-generation antipsychotics. *Archives of General Psychiatry* **60**, 553–564.

De Hert, M., van Winkel, R., Wampers, M., Kane, J., van Os, J. & Peuskens, J. (2007) Remission criteria for schizophrenia: Evaluation in a large naturalistic cohort. *Schizophrenia Research* **92**, 68–73.

Dube, S. & Sethi, B.B. (1981) Efficacy of lithium in schizophrenia. *Indian Journal of Psychiatry* **23**, 193–199.

Ehrenreich, H., Hinze-Selch, D., Stawicki, S. *et al.* (2007) Improvement of cognitive functions in chronic schizophrenic patients by recombinant human erythropoietin. *Molecular Psychiatry* **12**, 206–220.

Elias, A. & Kumar, A. (2007) Testosterone for schizophrenia. *Cochrane Database Systematic Review* Issue 3, CD006197.

Emsley, R.A., Raniwalla, J., Bailey, P.J. & Jones, A.M. (2000) A comparison of the effects of quetiapine ("Seroquel") and haloperidol in schizophrenic patients with a history of and a demonstrated, partial response to conventional antipsychotic treatment. *International Clinical Psychopharmacology* **15**, 121–131.

Emsley, R., Oosthuizen, P., Koen, L., Niehaus, D., Lex, A. & Medori, R. (2006) Remission in schizophrenia: Results from a 12-month analysis of long-acting risperidone in patients with first-episode psychosis. *Schizophrenia Research* **86**, S131.

Essali, A., Al-Haj, H.N., Li, C. & Rathbone, J. (2009) Clozapine versus typical neuroleptic medication for schizophrenia. *Cochrane Database Systematic Reviews* Issue 1, CD000059.

Falkai, P., Wobrock, T., Lieberman, J., Glenthoj, B., Gattaz, W.F. & Moller, H. J. (2005) World Federation of Societies of Biological Psychiatry (WFSBP)—Guidelines for biological treatment of schizophrenia, part 1: Acute treatment of schizophrenia. *World Journal Biological Psychiatry* **6**, 132–191.

Fleischhacker, W.W., Heikkinen, M.E., Olie, J.P. *et al.* (2010) Effects of adjunctive treatment with aripiprazole on body weight and clinical efficacy in schizophrenia patients treated with clozapine: a randomized, double-blind, placebo-controlled trial. *International Journal of Neuropsychopharmacology* **13**, 1115–1125.

Freudenreich, O., Herz, L., Deckersbach, T., Evins, A.E., Henderson, D.C., Cather, C. & Goff, D.C. (2005) Added donepezil for stable schizophrenia: a double-blind, placebo-controlled trial. *Psychopharmacology* **181**, 358–363.

Friedman, J.I., Adler, D.N., Howanitz, E. *et al.* (2002) A double blind placebo controlled trial of donepezil adjunctive treatment to risperidone for the cognitive impairment of schizophrenia. *Biological Psychiatry* **51**, 349–357.

Gaebel, W., Pietzcker, A., Ulrich, G., Schley, J. & Mueller-Oerlinghausen, B. (1988) Predictors of neuroleptic treatment response in acute schizophrenia: results of a treatment study with perazine. *Pharmacopsychiatry* **21**, 384–386.

Gaebel, W., Falkai, P., Weinmann, S., & Wobrock, T. (2006) *Behandlungsleitlinie Schizophrenie*. Darmstadt: Steinkopff.

Geddes, J., Freemantle, N., Harrison, P. & Bebbington, P. (2000) Atypical antipsychotics in the treatment of schizophrenia: systematic overview and meta-regression analysis. *BMJ* **321**, 1371–1376.

Gelder, M.G., Lopez-Ibor, J.J. & Andreasen, N. (2000) *New Oxford Textbook of Psychiatry*. New York: Oxford University Press.

Gould, R.A., Mueser, K.T., Bolton, E., Mays, V. & Goff, D. (2001) Cognitive therapy for psychosis in schizophrenia: an effect size analysis. *Schizophrenia Research* **48**, 335–342.

Growe, G.A., Crayton, J.W., Klass, D.B., Evans, H. & Strizich, M. (1979) Lithium in chronic schizophrenia. *American Journal of Psychiatry* **136**, 454–455.

Guy, W. (1976) Clinical Global Impression. In: *ECDEU Assessment Manual for Psychopharmacology, revised (DHEW Publ No ADM 76-338)*. Rockville, MD: National Institute of Mental Health, pp. 218–222.

Hajak, G., Marienhagen, J., Langguth, B., Werner, S., Binder, H. & Eichhammer, P. (2004) High-frequency repetitive transcranial magnetic stimulation in schizophrenia: a combined treatment and neuroimaging study. *Psychological Medicine* **34**, 1157–1163.

Haro, J.M., Kamath, S.A., Ochoa, S. *et al.* (2003) The Clinical Global Impression-Schizophrenia scale: a simple instrument to measure the diversity of symptoms present in schizophrenia. *Acta Psychiatrica Scandinavica* **107**, 16–23.

Helldin, L., Kane, J.M., Karilampi, U., Norlander, T. & Archer, T. (2007) Remission in prognosis of functional outcome: A new dimension in the treatment of patients with psychotic disorders. *Schizophrenia Research* **93**, 160–168.

Johnstone, E.C., Crow, T.J., Frith, C.D. & Owens, D. (1988) The Northwick Park "functional" psychosis study: diagnosis and treatment response. *Lancet* **2**, 119–125.

Jones, C., Cormac, I., Silveira da Mota Neto, J.I. & Campbell, C. (2004) Cognitive behaviour therapy for schizophrenia

(Cochrane review). *Cochrane Database Systematic Reviews* Issue 4, CD000524.

Joy, C.B., Mumby-Croft, R. & Joy, L.A. 92006) Polyunsaturated fatty acid supplementation for schizophrenia. *Cochrane Database of Systematic Reviews* Issue 3, CD001257.

Kane, J.M., Honigfeld, G., Singer, J., Meltzer, H. & and the Clozaril Collaborative Study Group (1988) Clozapine for the treatment-resistant schizophrenic. A double-blind comparison with chlorpromazine. *Archives of General Psychiatry* **45**, 789–796.

Kane, J.M., Marder, S.R., Schooler, N.R. *et al.* (2001) Clozapine and haloperidol in moderately refractory schizophrenia—A 6-month randomized and double-blind comparison. *Archives of General Psychiatry* **58**, 965–972.

Kane, J.M., Leucht, S., Carpenter, D. & Docherty, J.P. (2003) Optimising pharmacologic treatment of psychotic disorders. *Journal of Clinical Psychiatry* **64** (Suppl. 12), 1–100.

Kane, J. M., Khanna, S., Rajadhyaksha, S. & Giller, E. (2006) Efficacy and tolerability of ziprasidone in patients with treatment-resistant schizophrenia. *International Clinical Psychopharmacology* **21**, 21–28.

Kane, J.M., Crandall, D.T., Marcus, R.N. *et al.* (2007a) Symptomatic remission in schizophrenia patients treated with aripiprazole or haloperidol for up to 52 weeks. *Schizophrenia Research* **95**, 143–150.

Kane, J.M., Meltzer, H.Y., Carson, W.H., McQuade, R.D., Marcus, R.N. & Sanchez, R. (2007b) Aripiprazole for treatment-resistant schizophrenia: Results of a multicenter, randomized, double-blind, comparison study versus perphenazine. *Journal of Clinical Psychiatry* **68**, 213–223.

Kapur, S., Arenovich, T., Agid, O., Zipursky, R., Lindborg, S. & Jones, B. (2005) Evidence for onset of antipsychotic effects within the first 24 hours of treatment. *American Journal of Psychiatry* **162**, 939–946.

Kay, S.R., Fiszbein, A. & Opler, L.A. (1987) The positive and negative syndrome scale (PANSS) for schizophrenia. *Schizophrenia Bulletin* **13**, 261–275.

Keefe, R.S., Malhotra, A.K., Meltzer, H.Y. *et al.* (2008) Efficacy and safety of donepezil in patients with schizophrenia or schizoaffective disorder: significant placebo/practice effects in a 12-week, randomized, double-blind, placebo-controlled trial. *Neuropsychopharmacology* **33**, 1217–1228.

Kinon, B.J., Kane, J.M., Johns, C. *et al.* (1993) Treatment of neuroleptic-resistant schizophrenic relapse. *Psychopharmacology Bulletin* **29**, 309–314.

Kinon, B.J., Chen, L., Ascher-Svanum, H. *et al.* (2008) Predicting response to atypical antipsychotics based on early response in the treatment of schizophrenia. *Schizophrenia Research* **102**, 230–240.

Kinon, B.J., Chen, L., Ascher-Svanum, H., Stauffer, V.L., Kollack-Walker, S., Zhou, W., Kapur, S., Kane, J.M. (2010) HYPERLINK "http://www.ncbi.nlm.nih.gov/pubmed/19890258" Early response to antipsychotic drug therapy as a clinical marker of subsequent response in the treatment of schizophrenia. *Neuropsychopharmacology.* **35**(2), 581–590.

Kirschbaum, K.M., Muller, M.J., Malevani, J. *et al.* (2008) Serum levels of aripiprazole and dehydroaripiprazole, clinical response and side effects. *World Journal of Biological Psychiatry* **9**, 212–218.

Klein, E., Kolsky, Y., Puyerovsky, M., Koren, D., Chistyakov, A. & Feinsod, M. (1999) Right prefrontal slow repetitive transcranial magnetic stimulation in schizophrenia: A double-blind sham-controlled pilot study. *Biological Psychiatry* **46**, 1451–1454.

Kulkarni, J. de Castella, A., Fitzgerald, P.B. *et al.* (2008) Estrogen in severe mental illness: a potential new treatment approach. *Archives of General Psychiatry* **65**, 955–960.

Kumra, S., Frazier, J.A., Jacobsen, L.K. *et al.* (1996) Childhood-onset schizophrenia—A double-blind clozapine-haloperidol comparison. *Archives of General Psychiatry* **53**, 1090–1097.

Kumra, S., Kranzler, H., Gerbino-Rosen, G. *et al.* (2008) Clozapine and "high-dose" olanzapine in refractory early-onset schizophrenia: A 12-week randomized and double-blind comparison. *Biological Psychiatry* **63**, 524–529.

Lane, H.Y., Chang, Y.C., Liu, Y.C,, Chiu, C.C. & Tsai, G.E. (2005) Sarcosine or D-serine add-on treatment for acute exacerbation of schizophrenia: a randomized, double-blind, placebo-controlled study. *Archives of General Psychiatry* **62**, 1196–1204.

Lehman, A.F., Lieberman, J.A., Dixon, L.B. *et al.* (2004) Practice guideline for the treatment of patients with schizophrenia, second edition. *American Journal of Psychiatry* **161**, 1–56.

Leucht, S. & Heres, S. (2006) Epidemiology, clinical consequences, and psychosocial treatment of nonadherence in schizophrenia. *Journal of Clinical Psychiatry* **67**, 3–8.

Leucht, S. & Kane, J.M. (2006) Measurement based psychiatry: definitions of response, remission, stability and relapse in schizophrenia. *Journal of Clinical Psychiatry* **67**, 1813–1814.

Leucht, S. & Lasser, R. (2006) The concepts of remission and recovery in schizophrenia. *Pharmacopsychiatry* **39**, 161–170.

Leucht, S., McGrath, J., White, P. & Kissling, W. (2002a) Carbamazepine augmentation for schizophrenia: how good is the evidence? *Journal of Clinical Psychiatry* **63**, 218–224.

Leucht, S., Pitschel-Walz, G., Engel, R. & Kissling, W. (2002b) Amisulpride—an unusual atypical antipsychotic. A meta-analysis of randomized controlled trials. *American Journal of Psychiatry* **159**, 180–190.

Leucht, S., Busch, R., Hamann, J., Kissling, W. & Kane, J.M. (2005a) Early onset of antipsychotic drug action: a hypothesis tested, confirmed and extended. *Biological Psychiatry* **57**, 1543–1549.

Leucht, S., Kane, J.M., Kissling, W., Hamann, J., Etschel, E. & Engel, R.R. (2005b) Clinical implications of BPRS scores. *British Journal of Psychiatry* **187**, 363–371.

Leucht, S., Kane, J. M., Kissling, W., Hamann, J., Etschel, E. & Engel, R.R. (2005c) What does the PANSS mean? *Schizophrenia Research* **79**, 231–238.

Leucht, S., Kane, J.M., Etschel, E., Kissling, W., Hamann, J. & Engel, R.R. (2006) Linking the PANSS, BPRS, and CGI: Clinical implications. *Neuropsychopharmacology* **31**, 2318–2325.

Leucht, S., Beitinger, R. & Kissling, W. (2007a) On the concept of remission in schizophrenia. *Psychopharmacology* **194**, 453–461.

Leucht, S., Busch, R., Kissling, W. & Kane, J.M. (2007b) Early prediction of antipsychotic non-response. *Journal of Clinical Psychiatry* **68**, 352–360.

Leucht, S., Davis, J.M., Engel, R.R., Kane, J.M. & Wagenpfeil, S. (2007c) Defining "response" in antipsychotic drug trials: recommendations for the use of scale-derived cutoffs. *Neuropsychopharmacology* **32**, 1903–1910.

Leucht, S., Kissling, W., & McGrath, J. (2007d) Lithium for schizophrenia. *Cochrane Database of Systematic Reviews* Issue 3, CD003834.

Leucht, S., Shamsi, A.S., Busch, R., Kissling, W. & Kane, J.M. (2008) Early prediction of antipsychotic response. Replication and six weeks extension. *Schizophrenia Research* **101**, 312–319.

Leucht, S., Corves, C., Arbter, D., Engel, R.R., Li, C. & Davis, J.M. (2009a) Second-generation versus first-generation antipsychotic drugs for schizophrenia: a meta-analysis. *Lancet* **373**, 31–41.

Leucht, S., Kissling, W. & Davis, J.M. (2009b) Second-generation antipsychotic drugs for schizophrenia: can we resolve the conflict? *Psychological Medicine* **39**, 1591–1602.

Leucht, S., Komossa, K., Rummel-Kluge, C. *et al.* (2009c) A meta-analysis of head to head comparisons of second generation antipsychotics in the treatment of schizophrenia. *American Journal of Psychiatry* **166**, 152–163.

Leucht, S., Davis, J.M., Engel, R.R., Kissling, W., Kane, J.M. (2009d). HYPERLINK "http://www.ncbi.nlm.nih.gov/pubmed/19132961" Definitions of response and remission in schizophrenia: recommendations for their use and their presentation. *Acta Psychiatrica Scandinavica* Supplement **438**, 7–14.

Levine, S.Z., Rabinowitz, J., Engel, R., Etschel, E. & Leucht, S. (2007) Extrapolation between measures of symptom severity and change: An examination of the PANSS and CGI. *Schizophrenia Research* **98**, 318–322.

Lewis, S.W., Barnes, T.R., Davies, L. *et al.* (2006) Randomized controlled trial of effect of prescription of clozapine versus other second-generation antipsychotic drugs in resistant schizophrenia. *Schizophrenia Bulletin* **32**, 715–723.

Lieberman, J.A., Phillips, M., Gu, H. *et al.* (2003) Atypical and conventional antipsychotic drugs in treatment-naive first-episode schizophrenia: a 52-week randomized trial of clozapine vs chlorpromazine. *Neuropsychopharmacology* **28**, 995–1003.

Lieberman, J.A., Stroup, T.S., McEvoy, J.P. *et al.* (2005) Effectiveness of antipsychotic drugs in patients with chronic schizophrenia. *New England Journal of Medicine* **353**, 1209–1223.

Lin, C.C., Bai, Y.M., Chen, J.Y. *et al.* (2003) Switching from clozapine to zotepine in schizophrenic patients. A randomised single blind controlled study. *European Neuropsychopharmacology* **13**, 318.

Lin, C.H., Chou, L.S., Lin, C.H. *et al.* (2007) Early prediction of clinical response in schizophrenia patients receiving the atypical antipsychotic zotepine. *Journal of Clinical Psychiatry* **68**, 1522–1527.

Louwerens, J.W. & van der Meij, A.P.M. (2000) Therapy resistance: the effectiveness of the second antipsychotic drug, a multicentric double-blind comparative study ('switch study'). *Schizophrenia Research* **41**, 183–184.

Louzã, M.R., Marques, A.P., Elkis, H., Bassitt, D., Diegoli, M. & Gattaz, W.F. (2004) Conjugated estrogens as adjuvant therapy in the treatment of acute schizophrenia: a double-blind study. *Schizophrenia Research* **66**, 97–100.

Marder, S.R. & van Kammen, D.P. (2000) Dopamine receptor antagonists. In: Kaplan, H.I. & Saddock, B.J., eds. *Comprehensive Textbook of Psychiatry*, 7th edn. Baltimore: Lippincott Williams and Wilkins, pp. 2356–2377.

McEvoy, J.P., Hogarty, G.E. & Steingard, S. (1991) Optimal dose of neuroleptic in acute schizophrenia. *Archives of General Psychiatry* **48**, 740–745.

McEvoy, J.P., Lieberman, J.A., Stroup, T.S. *et al.* (2006) Effectiveness of clozapine versus olanzapine, quetiapine, and risperidone in patients with chronic schizophrenia who did not respond to prior atypical antipsychotic treatment. *American Journal of Psychiatry* **163**, 600–610.

McGorry, P.D. (2005) Royal Australian and New Zealand College of Psychiatrists clinical practice guidelines for the treatment of schizophrenia and related disorders. *Australian and New Zealand Journal of Psychiatry* **39**, 1–30.

Meltzer, H.Y. (1990) Commentary: defining treatment refractoriness in schizophrenia. *Schizophrenia Bulletin* **16**, 563–565.

Müller, N., Riedel, M., Scheppach, C. *et al.* (2002) Beneficial antipsychotic effects of celecoxib add-on therapy compared to risperidone alone in schizophrenia. *American Journal of Psychiatry* **159**, 1029–1034.

Müller, N., Krause, D., Dehning, S., Musil, R., Schennach-Wolff, R., Obermeier, M., Möller, H.J., Klauss, V., Schwarz, M.J., Riedel, M. (2010). HYPERLINK "http://www.ncbi.nlm.nih.gov/pubmed/20570110" Celecoxib treatment in an early stage of schizophrenia: results of a randomized, double-blind, placebo-controlled trial of celecoxib augmentation of amisulpride treatment. *Schizophrenia Research* **121**, 118–124.

Nahas, Z., George, M.S., Horner, M.D. *et al.* (2003) Augmenting atypical Antipsychotics with a cognitive enhancer (donepezil) improves regional brain activity in schizophrenia patients: A pilot double-blind placebo controlled BOLD fMRI study. *Neurocase* **9**, 274–282.

National Institute for Clinical Excellence (2003) *Schizophrenia: Full National Guideline on Core Interventions in Primary and Secondary Care*. London: Royal College of Psychiatrists.

Nedopil, N., Pflieger, R. & Ruether, E. (1983) The prediction of acute response, remission and general outcome of neuroleptic treatment in acute schizophrenic patients. *Pharmacopsychiatria* **16**, 201–205.

Nolte, S., Wong, D., & Latchford, G. (2004) Amphetamines for schizophrenia. *Cochrane Database of Systematic Reviews* Issue 3, CD004964.

Overall, J.E. & Gorham, D.R. (1962) The Brief Psychiatric Rating Scale. *Psychology Reports* **10**, 790–812.

Paton, C., Whittington, C. & Barnes, T.R. (2007) Augmentation with a second antipsychotic in patients with schizophrenia who partially respond to clozapine—A meta-analysis. *Journal of Clinical Psychopharmacology* **27**, 198–204.

Pilling, S., Bebbington, P., Kuipers, E. *et al.* (2002a) Psychological treatments in schizophrenia: II. Meta-analyses of randomized controlled trials of social skills training and cognitive remediation. *Psychological Medicine* **32**, 783–791.

Pilling, S., Bebbington, P., Kuipers, E. *et al.* (2002b) Psychological treatments in schizophrenia: I. Meta-analysis of family intervention and cognitive behaviour therapy. *Psychological Medicine* **32**, 763–782.

Premkumar, T.S. & Pick, J. (2006) Lamotrigine for schizophrenia. *Cochrane Database of Systematic Reviews* Issue. 4, CD005962.

Prien, R., Caffey, E. J. & Klett, C. (1972) A comparison of lithium carbonate and chlorpromazine in the treatment of excited schizo-affectives. Report of the Veterans Administration and National Institute of Mental Health collaborative study group. *Archives of General Psychiatry* **27**, 182–189.

Robinson, D.G., Woerner, M.G., Alvir, J.M.J. *et al.* (1999) Predictors of treatment response from a first episode of schizophrenia or schizoaffective disorder. *American Journal of Psychiatry* **156**, 544–549.

Rosenheck, R., Cramer, J., Xu, W.C. *et al.* (1997) A comparison of clozapine and haloperidol in hospitalized patients with refractory schizophrenia. *New England Journal of Medicine* **337**, 809–815.

Rummel, C., Kissling, W., & Leucht, S. (2006) Antidepressants for the negative symptoms of schizophrenia. *Cochrane Database of Systematic Reviews* Issue 3, CD005581.

Schubert, M.H., Young, K.A., & Hicks, P.B. (2006) Galantamine improves cognition in schizophrenic patients stabilized on risperidone. *Biological Psychiatry* **60**, 530–533.

Schulz, S.C. & Buckley, P.F. (1995) Treatment resistant schizophrenia. In: Hirsch, S.T. & Weinberger, D.R., eds. *Schizophrenia.* Oxford: Blackwell Science, pp. 469–484.

Schwartz, C., Volz, A., Li, C. & Leucht, S. (2008) Valproate for schizophrenia. *Cochrane Database of Systematic Reviews* Issue 3, CD004028.

See, R.E., Fido, A.A., Maurice, M., Ibrahim, M.M. & Salama, G.M.S. (1999) Risperidone-induced increase of plasma norepinephrine is not correlated with symptom improvement in chronic schizophrenia. *Biological Psychiatry* **45**, 1653–1656.

Sepehry, A.A., Potvin, S., Elie, R. & Stip, E. (2007) Selective serotonin reuptake inhibitor (SSRI) add-on therapy for the negative symptoms of schizophrenia: a meta-analysis. *Journal of Clinical Psychiatry* **68**, 604–610.

Shalev, A., Hermesh, H., Rothberg, J. & Munitz, H. (1993) Poor neuroleptic response in acutely exacerbated schizophrenic patients. *Acta Psychiatrica Scandinavica* **87**, 86–91.

Sharma, T., Reed, C., Aasen, I., & Kumari, V. (2006) Cognitive effects of adjunctive 24-weeks Rivastigmine treatment to antipsychotics in schizophrenia: A randomized, placebo-controlled, double-blind investigation. *Schizophrenia Research* **85**, 73–83.

Shaw, P., Sporn, A., Gogtay, N., Overman, G.P. *et al.* (2006) Childhood-onset schizophrenia: A double-blind, randomized clozapine-olanzapine comparison. *Archives of General Psychiatry* **63**, 721–730.

Simpson, G.M., Josiassen, R.C., Stanilla, J.K. *et al.* (1999) Double-blind study of clozapine dose response in chronic schizophrenia. *American Journal of Psychiatry* **156**, 1744–1750.

Singh, S.P., Singh, V., Kar, N. & Chan, K. (2010) Efficacy of antidepressants in treating the negative symptoms of schizophrenia: meta-analysis. *British Journal of Psychiatry* **197**, 174–179.

Small, J.G., Kellams, J.J., Milstein, V. & Moore, J. (1975) A placebo-controlled study of lithium combined with neuroleptics in chronic schizophrenic patients. *American Journal of Psychiatry* **132**, 1315–1317.

Smith, R.C., Infante, M., Singh, A. & Khandat, A. (2001) The effects of olanzapine on neurocognitive functioning in medication-refractory schizophrenia. *International Journal of Neuropsychopharmacology* **4**, 239–250.

Stern, R.G., Kahn, R.S., Harvey, P.D., Amin, F., Apter, S.H. & Hirschowitz, J. (1993) Early response to haloperidol treatment in chronic schizophrenia. *Schizophrenia Research* **10**, 165–171.

Stip, E., Sepehry, A.A. & Chouinard, S. (2007) Add-on therapy with acetylcholinesterase inhibitors for memory dysfunction in schizophrenia: a systematic quantitative review, part 2. *Clinical Neuropharmacology* **30**, 21–229.

Stroup, T.S., Lieberman, J.A., McEvoy, J.P. *et al.* (2007) Effectiveness of olanzapine, quetiapine, and risperidone in patients with chronic schizophrenia after discontinuing perphenazine: A CATIE study. *American Journal of Psychiatry* **164**, 415–427.

Strous, R.D., Maayan, R., Lapidus, R. *et al.* (2003) Dehydroepiandrosterone augmentation in the management of negative, depressive, and anxiety symptoms in schizophrenia. *Archives of General Psychiatry* **60**, 133–141.

Strous, R.D., Stryjer, R., Maayan, R. *et al.* (2007) Analysis of clinical symptomatology, extrapyramidal symptoms and neurocognitive dysfunction following dehydroepiandrosterone (DHEA) administration in olanzapine treated schizophrenia patients: A randomized, double-blind placebo controlled trial. *Psychoneuroendocrinology* **32**, 96–105.

Suzuki, T., Uchida, H., Watanabe, K. *et al.* (2007) How effective is it to sequentially switch among olanzapine, quetiapine and risperidone?—A randomized, open-label study of algorithm-based antipsychotic treatment to patients with symptomatic schizophrenia in the real-world clinical setting. *Psychopharmacology (Berlin)* **195**, 285–295.

Taylor, D.M. & Smith, L. (2009) Augmentation of clozapine with a second antipsychotic—a meta-analysis of randomized, placebo-controlled studies. *Acta Psychiatrica Scandinavica* **119**, 419–425.

Tharyan, P. & Adams, C.E. (2005) Electroconvulsive therapy for schizophrenia. *Cochrane Database of Systematic Reviews* Issue 2, CD000076.

Tiihonen, J., Wahlbeck, K. & Kiviniemi, V. (2009) The efficacy of lamotrigine in clozapine-resistant schizophrenia: A systematic review and meta-analysis. *Schizophrenia Research* **109**, 10–14.

Tollefson, G.D., Beasley, C.M., Tran, P.V. *et al.* (1997) Olanzapine versus haloperidol in the treatment of schizophrenia and schizoaffective and schizophreniform disorders: results of an international collaborative trial. *American Journal of Psychiatry* **154**, 457–465.

Tranulis, C., Sepehry, A.A., Galinowski, A. & Stip, E. (2008) Should we treat auditory hallucinations with repetitive transcranial magnetic stimulation? A metaanalysis. *Canadian Journal of Psychiatry* **53**, 577–586.

Tsai, G., Lane, H.Y., Yang, P,, Chong, M.Y. & Lange, N. (2004) Glycine transporter I inhibitor, N-methylglycine (sarcosine), added to antipsychotics for the treatment of schizophrenia. *Biological Psychiatry* **55**, 452–456.

Tugal, O., Yazici, K.M., Yagcioglu, A.E.A. & Gogus, A. (2004) A double-blind, placebo controlled, cross-over trial of adjunctive donepezil for cognitive impairment in schizophrenia. *International Journal of Neuropsychopharmacology* **7**, 117–123.

Tuominen, H.J., Tiihonen, J. & Wahlbeck, K. (2006) Glutamatergic drugs for schizophrenia. *Cochrane Database of Systematic Reviews* Issue 2, CD003730.

van Os, J., Burns, T., Cavallaro, R. *et al.* (2006) Standardized remission criteria in schizophrenia. *Acta Psychiatrica Scandinavica* **113**, 91–95.

Volavka, J., Czobor, P., Sheitman, B. *et al.* (2002) Clozapine, olanzapine, risperidone, and haloperidol in the treatment of patients with chronic schizophrenia and schizoaffective disorder. *American Journal of Psychiatry* **159**, 255–262.

Volz, A., Khorsand, V., Gillies, D. & Leucht, S. (2007) Benzodiazepines for schizophrenia. *The Cochrane Library* [1]. Chichester: Wiley & Sons.

Wahlbeck, K., Cheine, M., Essali, A., & Adams, C. (1999) Evidence of clozapine's effectiveness in schizophrenia: A systematic review and meta-analysis of randomized trials. *American Journal of Psychiatry* **156**, 990–999.

Waraich, P., Adams, C., Hammill, K., Marti, J. & Roque, M. (2002) Haloperidol dose for the acutely ill phase of schizophrenia. *Cochrane Database Systematic Reviews* Issue 2, CD001951.

Whitehead, C., Moss, S., Cardno, A. & Lewis, G. (2003) Antidepressants for the treatment of depression in people with schizophrenia: a systematic review. *Psychological Medicine* **33**, 589–599.

Wirshing, D.A., Marshall, B.D., Green, M.F., Mintz, J., Marder, S.R. & Wirshing, W.C. (1999) Risperidone in treatment-refractory schizophrenia. *American Journal of Psychiatry* **156**, 1374–1379.

Wolkowitz, O.M. & Pickar, D. (1991) Benzodiazepines in the treatment of schizophrenia: a review and reappraisal. *American Journal of Psychiatry* **148**, 714–726.

Wykes, T., Steel, C., Everitt, B. & Tarrier, N. (2008) Cognitive behavior therapy for schizophrenia: effect sizes, clinical models, and methodological rigor. *Schizophrenia Bulletin* **34**, 523–537.

Zemlan, F.P., Thienhaus, O.J. & Garver, D.L. (1990) Length of psychiatric hospitalization and prediction of antipsychotic response. *Progress in Neuropsychopharmacology and Biological Psychiatry* **14**, 13–24.

Zimbroff, D.L., Kane, J.M., Tamminga, C.A. *et al.* (1997) Controlled, dose response study of sertindole and haloperidol in the treatment of schizophrenia. *American Journal of Psychiatry* **154**, 782–791.

CHAPTER 27

Neurological complications of antipsychotic drugs

Peter M. Haddad[1] and Venkata S. Mattay[2]

[1]University of Manchester, Manchester, UK
[2]National Institute of Mental Health, Bethesda, MD, USA

Introduction

This chapter reviews the key neurological complications seen with antipsychotic drugs. Some of these syndromes can occur with other medications; e.g., antidepressants can lower the seizure threshold and a wide range of drugs have been causally linked to neuroleptic malignant syndrome. The neurological adverse effects of antipsychotics can be severe and in extreme cases can prove fatal. However, simple strategies can reduce the risk of their occurrence. These include ensuring that the lowest effective dose of medication is used, that dosages are titrated upward gradually, that unnecessary polypharmacy is avoided, and that the potential for drug interactions is considered prior to prescribing. In addition, antipsychotics should be chosen so that patients at high risk for a specific side effect are treated with a drug that has less risk of causing that adverse effect. During treatment, health professionals should enquire about common adverse effects using language that patients can understand. It is insufficient to simply rely on patients' spontaneous reports of adverse effects. If adverse effects develop, they should be managed promptly and effectively. When considering adverse effects, it is important to consider the severity of the illnesses for which antipsychotics are indicated and their benefits when prescribed appropriately. Schizophrenia and bipolar disorder cause great suffering to patients and their families, impair quality of life, and are associated with an increased risk of suicide. Both rank among the leading causes of disability in the world (Murray & Lopez, 1996). Antipsychotic drugs, when prescribed appropriately, can bring benefits to patients in terms of symptom reduction and improved quality of life.

Acute extrapyramidal syndromes

Four key extrapyramidal syndromes (EPS) are recognized with antipsychotic drugs; parkinsonism, akathisia, acute dystonia, and tardive dyskinesia. The first three usually occur early in antipsychotic treatment and are considered as "acute EPS". Tardive dyskinesia occurs after months or years of antipsychotic treatment and is dealt with separately. This separation in terms of onset is not absolute. For example, akathisia can start during long-term antipsychotic treatment without any change in antipsychotic or dose. Conversely, tardive dyskinesia occasionally appears early in antipsychotic treatment.

Schizophrenia, 3rd edition. Edited by Daniel R. Weinberger and Paul J Harrison © 2011 Blackwell Publishing Ltd.

Clinical presentation

Parkinsonism

Drug-induced and idiopathic parkinsonism are phenomenologically identical; both include the classical triad of tremor, rigidity, and bradykinesia. The features may be unilateral, symmetrical or asymmetrically bilateral. Parkinsonism tends to emerge insidiously after several weeks of antipsychotic treatment (Ayd, 1961). The tremor is worse at rest, of low frequency and wide amplitude, and primarily affects the hands, which show a rhythmical to-and-fro motion, but other parts of the body, including the head, can be affected. Rigidity can be "cog-wheel" or "lead pipe" in nature and is most evident in the upper limbs. Bradykinesia, or akinesia, refers to a reduction in spontaneous movement. It manifests as decreased arm swing during walking, reduced ability to initiate movement, and a reduction in facial expression and the blink rate, leading to the characteristic mask-like facial appearance and "staring" expression. Other features of parkinsonism include seborrhea, sialorrhea, and changes to the pitch and power of the voice. Speech tends to become quieter as well as deeper and monotonous in tone, sometimes making it difficult to understand what the patient is saying.

Bradykinesia needs to be distinguished from negative symptoms of schizophrenia or psychomotor retardation in depression. This can be difficult and may not be fully achievable until the suspected causal antipsychotic drug has been discontinued for several weeks or months. If this is not possible, then a trial of an antiparkinsonian drug may be warranted.

Acute dystonia

Acute dystonia usually appears in the first week after starting or increasing the dose of an antipsychotic and is more common in younger patients and with higher doses of antipsychotics (Singh et al., 1990). The syndrome consists of the contraction of a voluntary muscle to its maximal degree that is sustained and so leads to a postural distortion. The contraction may last from minutes to hours and is highly distressing for the patient. The muscles of the neck are most commonly affected (torticollis) though any part of body can be involved, including the tongue, trunk, limbs, and pharyngeal and laryngeal muscles (Swett, 1975). Examples of muscle contractions that can occur include hyperpronation of the arms, wrist flexion, plantar flexion of the feet, adductor spasm of the thighs, protrusion of the tongue, and contraction of the extraocular muscles (oculogyric crisis). Because dystonia often leads to bizarre postures, it can be misdiagnosed as malingering, hysteria or seizures, particularly by inexperienced staff (Casey, 1991).

Akathisia

Akathisia is characterized by subjective feelings of restlessness or distress accompanied by objective signs of restlessness. Patients may describe akathisia as anxiety, an inability to relax, feeling uptight or jittery. Objective signs of restlessness include pacing, rocking back and forth while sitting or standing, lifting the feet repeatedly as if marching on the spot, crossing and uncrossing the legs when sitting, or other repetitive purposeless actions. Many patients with classic objective signs of restlessness do not describe subjective experiences. This may reflect their absence or the patient being unable to give an accurate report.

Akathisia may be misdiagnosed as psychotic agitation, which can lead to an increase in antipsychotic dosage and worsening of akathisia. The likelihood of misdiagnosis is increased as psychotic patients often have great difficulty communicating their feelings of restlessness and discomfort, and may describe their feelings with bizarre and delusional statements. Akathisia often begins within days of starting or switching antipsychotic drugs (Adler et al., 1989). When it is persistent, the term "chronic akathisia" is sometimes applied (Barnes & Braude, 1985). There are no major differences in the motor phenomena of acute and chronic akathisia, although the subjective sense of restlessness may be less intense in the latter.

Consequences

Acute EPS can cause distress, impair quality of life, cause stigma, and in severe cases, lead to secondary morbidity and even mortality. For example, parkinsonism can cause muscle aching, weakness, and impairment of dexterity, which may impinge on a wide range of occupational and social tasks. Severe parkinsonism can result in a festinant gait that leads to falls and injuries, particularly in the elderly. Occasional reports document antipsychotic-induced dystonia of the laryngeal and pharyngeal muscles causing asphyxia and choking, respectively (Newton-John, 1988; Norton, 2001; Stones et al., 1990). Both may be rare causes of sudden unexpected death in those treated with antipsychotics. Anecdotal reports have linked akathisia to suicide attempts and violence, though it is impossible to categorically prove either association (Hansen, 2001). Akathisia is cited as a common cause of poor adherence with medication.

EPS often go undiagnosed and untreated (Weiden et al., 1987; Mitra & Haddad, 2007). This partly reflects the fact that screening for EPS is not routine despite being recommended (American Psychiatric Association, 1997; National Institute for Clinical Excellence, 2009). Possible explanations for the neglect of EPS in clinical practice include clinicians lacking the knowledge, skills, and confidence to assess and manage EPS, being too time-pressured to address this aspect of care, and underestimating the distress that antipsychotic side effects cause (Day *et al.*, 1998).

Pathophysiology

Antipsychotic blockade of dopamine D_2 receptors of the basal ganglia is the most commonly proposed mechanism to explain acute EPS. Positron emission tomography (PET) studies suggest that EPS occur when D_2 occupancy exceeds a threshold of 75–80% (Farde *et al.*, 1992). The reciprocal balance between dopamine and acetylcholine in the basal ganglia and the efficacy of anticholinergic drugs in reversing and mitigating EPS support a role for acetylcholine in mediating EPS. Several antipsychotics with a low risk of EPS have a relatively high affinity for muscarinic receptors, lending further support to this mechanism. Examples include thioridazine, clozapine, quetiapine, and olanzapine. The high ratio of serotonin 5-HT_{2A} to D_2 receptor blockade seen with the atypical antipsychotics has also been proposed to account for their relatively low risk of EPS (Bersani *et al.*, 1990; Pehek, 1996; see also Chapter 23).

In some patients, susceptibility to drug-induced parkinsonism may reflect subclinical Parkinson disease (Rajput *et al.*, 1982; Brooks, 1991, 1993). Some, but not all studies, find that women are at increased risk of drug-induced parkinsonism and tardive dyskinesia, possibly reflecting estrogen-related dopamine receptor blockade (Glazer *et al.*, 1983).There are many unanswered questions about the pathophysiology of EPS. For example, parkinsonism usually commences several days after antipsychotics are initiated, which is not compatible with the mechanism of acute D_2 blockade that takes place within hours after antipsychotic administration. In some patients partial or complete tolerance to antipsychotic drug-induced parkinsonism may evolve over several months, even though antipsychotic treatment remains stable, and the compensatory processes which underlie this are unclear (Casey, 1991).

Epidemiology

The prevalence of EPS is strongly influenced by patient, drug, and time characteristics explaining the wide variation in reported rates (Casey & Keepers, 1988). Young age and high doses of high-potency compounds are predictors of acute dystonia (Singh *et al.*, 1990; Boyer *et al.*, 1989). Drug-induced parkinsonism occurs more often in older patients. A history of prior EPS predicts vulnerability to future EPS if a similar drug and dosage are represcribed. In patients prescribed conventional antipsychotics, recurrence of EPS could be predicted with approximately 80% accuracy if prior history of EPS is known (Keepers & Casey, 1987, 1991). A recent meta-analysis concluded that bipolar patients, especially those with a depressive syndrome,

were more at risk of developing acute antipsychotic-induced EPS than those with schizophrenia (Gao *et al.*, 2008). First-episode patients also appear more vulnerable to develop EPS than patients with chronic schizophrenia, at least when treated with high-potency antipsychotics, including haloperidol. The EPS risk of antipsychotics has been attributed to various factors, including D_2 occupancy, 5-HT_2 receptor occupancy, α_1 adrenergic antagonism, involvement of D_4 receptor, and antimuscarinic activity (M_1). Kapur and Seeman (2001) proposed that the key factor was blockade of the D_2 receptor, which may be influenced by the kinetics of occupancy and the relationship of peak-to-trough occupancy. According to their model, all antipsychotics, conventional or atypical, give rise to EPS only when they exceed 78–80% D_2 occupancy. An inverted U-shaped function between drug dose and EPS has been reported with some typical antipsychotic drugs, i.e., lower doses produce fewer EPS than moderate to high doses, but very high doses or megadoses also produce fewer EPS than moderate to high doses (Keepers *et al.*, 1983; Casey & Keepers, 1988).

The relative risk of EPS between conventional and atypical drugs has caused much debate. Several meta-analyses show that atypical antipsychotics are associated with a lower incidence of EPS than conventional antipsychotics (Geddes *et al.*, 2000; Bagnall *et al.*, 2003). However, most randomized controlled trials in these meta-analyses (Geddes *et al.*, 2000; Bagnall *et al.*, 2003) used haloperidol as the conventional comparator, leading to the criticism that the trials had a design bias that favored the atypical antipsychotic in terms of EPS. This also raised the question of whether atypicals would have an EPS advantage if compared to low-potency conventional drugs, e.g. chlorpromazine and thioridazine.

Leucht *et al.* (2009) have carried out the most recent meta-analysis comparing atypical and conventional drugs and this included the CATIE data. They found that all atypical antipsychotics had a lower liability to cause EPS than haloperidol, but only olanzapine, clozapine, and risperidone caused less EPS than low-potency conventional antipsychotics. These results are consistent with individual typical and atypical agents having different EPS profiles and emphasize the importance of considering the EPS liability of individual drugs rather than broad classes, i.e., a simplistic distinction between atypical and conventional drugs in terms of EPS risk is of little practical use. This applies to many other adverse effects, including weight gain, prolactin elevation, and QTc prolongation (Haddad & Sharma, 2007). Among the atypical agents, clozapine has the lowest EPS potential, probably due to its low D_2 occupancy—less than 60% 12 h after administration (Kapur *et al.*, 1999; Tauscher *et al.*, 1999), and its anticholinergic properties.

Management

General issues

Management for EPS can be divided into the management of specific EPS and prophylactic treatment to prevent EPS from occurring. The algorithm outlined in Figure 27.1 for managing EPS offers a balanced strategy to obtain the most benefit with the least risk. Avoiding the routine use of high-dose antipsychotics is an important strategy to reduce the risk of EPS, especially as there is no compelling evidence that high antipsychotic doses routinely produce more benefit than standard doses (Baldessarini *et al.*, 1988). The risk of EPS should not be the sole determinant in deciding which antipsychotic to use. Other side effects also need to be considered when selecting an antipsychotic, as does the overall effectiveness. Where possible, selection should be made on an individual basis in discussion with the patient.

Prophylaxis

Prophylactic treatment for EPS with anticholinergic drugs is controversial. Proponents argue that prophylaxis

prevents dystonic episodes, which are potentially dangerous, and automatically treats subtle forms of bradykinesia that may be unrecognized. Opponents argue that anticholinergic drugs have their own side effects, including autonomic nervous system dysfunction, memory impairment, and delirium. Rather than dogmatically applying either approach to all patients, we recommend an individual approach that considers risk factors on an individual patient basis (Fig. 27.1).

In most patients treated with atypical antipsychotics or low-potency conventional agents, the risk of EPS is fairly low and initial prophylaxis with anti-EPS medication is not required and is not recommended. This is because the risk of anticholineric side effects outweighs the potential benefit of reduced EPS. In contrast, initial prophylaxis is justified when there is a high risk of EPS (e.g., a young patient who is to be treated with a high-potency drug), documented predisposition to EPS, and anticipated detrimental consequences of EPS (Casey & Keepers, 1988). For example, acute dystonic reactions can have long-term effects on future drug adherence and a patient who

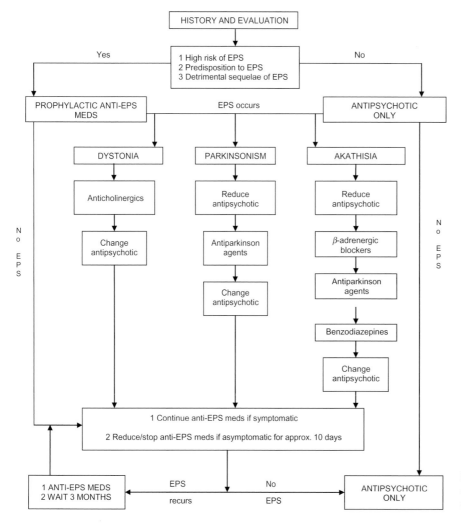

Fig. 27.1 Algorithm for managing extrapyramidal syndromes (EPS) (adapted from Casey, 1995).

is psychotic and believes that external forces are controlling them may further solidify these beliefs when an acute dystonic reaction develops without warning. There is also a stronger case for prophylaxis in a patient who has a prior history of non-adherence related to EPS. Conversely avoiding the adverse effects of anticholinergic drugs is more important in elderly patients. In most practices, only a small proportion of patients are likely to fall into a high-risk EPS group and be candidates for prophylaxis.

Initial prophylaxis can be rationally employed for the first 7–10 days of antipsychotic treatment in high-risk patients. The anticholinergic drug may be gradually decreased and discontinued if no EPS develop. The efficacy for initial prophylaxis in reducing the rates of acute dystonia and other EPS is well established (Sramek et al., 1986; Casey & Keepers. 1988; Boyer et al.. 1989). If prophylactic anticholinergic medication is continued long term, the prescription should be regularly reviewed as tolerance to EPS can develop, allowing the dose of the anticholinergic to be reduced or the prescription stopped.

Management of specific syndromes

Reducing the antipsychotic dose is the preferred approach to managing parkinsonism. If this risks causing a psychotic exacerbation, then an anticholinergic agent can be used or the patient switched to an antipsychotic with less propensity to cause EPS. Acute dystonia is usually treated with anticholinergic agents which can be administered orally, by intramuscular (IM) injection or intravenously (IV) depending on the severity of symptoms and the anticholinergic in question. Response to IM administration will usually be seen in 20 min and to IV administration within 5 min. If there is no improvement, then a further injection can be given. Akathisia is the most difficult EPS to manage. Like drug-induced parkinsonism, the preferred strategy is to reduce the antipsychotic dose and one can also consider switching to an antipsychotic with a lower risk of causing akathisia. If this is not possible on clinical grounds, beta-adrenergic blockers which penetrate the blood–brain barrier, such as propranolol (Inderal) 30–120 mg/day, are often effective (Miller & Fleischhacker, 2000). Benzodiazepines may help for some patients, though caution is warranted as long-term use of benzodiazepines may lead to dependence and abuse. Although there is no high-quality trial data to support their use, anecdotally some patients with akathisia respond to anticholinergic agents or antihistaminic agents, including diphenhydramine (Vinson, 2004).

Tardive dyskinesia

Clinical features

Tardive dyskinesia (TD) usually commences during long-term antipsychotic treatment, but is sometimes precipi-

tated by stopping long-term antipsychotic treatment. The condition was first described in the German literature in 1957 (Schonecker, 1957), soon after cases appeared in the French literature (Sigwald et al., 1959), and the first English language report appeared in 1960 (Uhrbrand & Faurbye, 1960). Descriptive terms such as "buccolinguomasticatory syndrome" appeared in the early literature and the term "tardive dyskinesia" was proposed in 1964 (Faurbye et al., 1964). TD is characterized by repetitive involuntary hyperkinetic movements of the choreiform type. These usually begin in the tongue, lips, and mouth, but with continuing antipsychotic treatment any part of body can be affected and a wide range of movements can occur, including myoclonic jerks, tics, chorea, and dystonia. External and internal stimuli can influence the clinical picture; the abnormal movements increase with stress, decrease with relaxation, disappear during sleep, and can be voluntarily suppressed for a short time (Baldessarini et al., 1980). Table 27.1 lists

Table 27.1 Examples of abnormal movements that can occur in tardive dyskinesia.

Region of body	Movements
Tongue	Tongue rolling, "worm-like" movements on surface of tongue, arrhythmic tongue protrusions (fly catching sign), tongue producing a bulge in the cheek (bon-bon sign)
Lips	Pouting, smacking, puckering, sucking, clicking noises
Jaws	Chewing movements, grinding of teeth
Facial and periorbital area	Grimacing, rapid eye blinking, moving eye brows up and down, blepharospasm
Neck	Arrhythmic head nodding, dystonic movements of neck
Trunk	Irregular rocking movements of the upper torso, truncal dystonia (e.g., "Pisa" syndrome)
Upper limbs	Abnormal stereotypic movements of fingers (as if patient is playing an invisible piano or guitar), myoclonic jerks, dystonias
Lower limbs	Dystonias (e.g., flexion/rotation of ankles, retroflexion of toes), involuntary stamping movements, myoclonic jerks
Laryngopharyngeal, diaphragmatic and intercostal musculature	Irregular breathing or swallowing that causes aerophagia, irregular respiratory rate, belching and grunting noises, dysarthria

some of the abnormal movements that can occur in TD (Marsalek, 2000).

The Abnormal Involuntary Movement Scale (AIMS) is the most commonly used rating tool for assessing TD (Guy, 1976). It is useful to re-emphasize that rating scales have been developed to characterize the nature and severity of abnormal movements and are not diagnostic instruments. A diagnosis requires a thorough clinical evaluation.

Tardive akathisia and tardive dystonia

Tardive dystonia (Burke *et al.*, 1982) and tardive akathisia (Barnes & Braude, 1985) usually begin after months or years of antipsychotic treatment. Both may occur alone or in combination with the typical orofacial and choreoathetoid signs of TD. It is unclear whether these different tardive syndromes represent unique and different pathophysiological mechanisms, or are better explained by a unitary underlying pathophysiology that is expressed in different symptom clusters in different patients.

Tardive dystonia consists of a sustained abnormal posture or position, e.g., torticollis, retrocollis, anterocollis, blepharospasm, grimacing, and torsion of the trunk or limbs. It may persist for months or years after antipsychotics have been discontinued (Burke *et al.*, 1982; Gardos *et al.*, 1987). Discerning whether a dystonia is a result of antipsychotic treatment or idiopathic can be very difficult. One feature in the differentiation is that when antipsychotics are discontinued, tardive dystonia should remain stable or gradually improve, whereas idiopathic dystonias will usually slowly progress in severity. Unfortunately, the response of tardive dystonia to pharmacological interventions does not help to distinguish it from idiopathic dystonia. Some patients with either diagnosis may benefit from treatment with a dopamine-depleting agent, dopamine antagonist or anticholinergic drug, but both syndromes show a poor response to treatment.

Complications

Most patients with TD have a relatively mild form of the disorder and may be unaware of its presence. In these cases, TD is an esthetic problem and may impair social relationships and impede employment. A small percentage of patients have additional complications. Orofacial dyskinesia may lead to dental problems, traumatic ulceration of the tongue and lips, difficulty in eating leading to weight loss and cachexia, and, rarely, degenerative changes of the temporo-mandibular joints. Pharyngeal involvement may sometimes cause aspiration pneumonia. Respiratory dysfunction and speech abnormalities, although rare, may result from diaphragmatic involvement. TD is associated with higher mortality and higher rates of respiratory tract infection (Youssef & Waddington, 1987). Involvement of the limbs and trunk may interfere with ambulation and cause falls, with consequent trauma. Cognitive impairment

is associated with TD (Casey, 1997), but it is unclear whether the cognitive dysfunction precedes the onset of TD (Waddington *et al.*, 1993).

Differential diagnosis

Idiopathic syndromes

At the turn of the 20th century, long before the introduction of antipsychotic drugs, Kraepelin and Bleuler described spontaneous dyskinesias in psychotic patients (Kraepelin, 1907; Bleuler, 1950; Casey, 1985), including "grimacing" and "irregular movements of the tongue and lips". More recently, spontaneous abnormal movements, including dyskinesias and parkinsonism, have been reported in a proportion of antipsychotic-naïve patients with chronic schizophrenia (e.g., McCreadie *et al.*, 1996) and first-episode psychosis (Pappa & Dazzan, 2008). These observations suggest that neurodysfunction of key motor areas is part of the underlying pathophysiology of schizophrenia. Other disorders that must be differentiated from TD include dental problems; stereotypic behavior (repetitive and seemingly purposeless and meaningless actions) and mannerisms (peculiar ways of completing normal actions), which are frequently associated with psychoses, spontaneous hyperkinetic dyskinesias, and simple or complex motor tics (Smith & Baldessarini, 1980; Casey, 1981); Tourette syndrome, characterized by involuntary tics and vocalizations that begin before the age of 18 years, is differentiated from TD by occurring early in life and by the waxing and waning course throughout a patient's lifetime.

Antipsychotic-induced acute extrapyramidal syndromes

Some patients may have more than one antipsychotic-induced movement disorder at the same time, and these must be distinguished from each other. Approximately one-third of patients who have TD and continue antipsychotic therapy have acute EPS (Casey, 1981; Richardson & Craig, 1982). Parkinsonism responds to anticholinergic drugs, whereas TD usually remains unchanged or worsens with these agents. However, some patients with tardive dystonia may improve with anticholinergic drugs (Burke *et al.*, 1982).

Other drug-induced dyskinesias

Several drugs can produce symptoms similar to TD. Some drugs that antagonize dopamine receptors, but are not classified as antipsychotics, can produce TD with extended use. These include the antiemetic drugs prochlorperazine and metoclopramide, and the antidepressant amoxapine. Dopamine agonists, such as bromocriptine and pergolide, and the dopamine precursor L-dopa can all produce hyperkinetic dyskinesias in patients with idiopathic parkinsonism. Chorea and stereotyped behavior can occur during acute use of, and withdrawal from, amphetamine and other stimulants. Chronic use of anticholinergics and antihistamines has rarely been associated with TD-like movements. Anticonvulsant agents at therapeutic or higher levels can produce hyperkinetic dyskinesias similar to TD. Oral contraceptives and chloroquine-based antimalarial agents can produce chorea and hyperkinetic dyskinesias. Lithium carbonate and tricyclic antidepressants may aggravate existing TD, but there is no convincing evidence that these agents by themselves produce TD. There are several reports of TD associated with the use of selective serotonin reuptake inhibitors (SSRIs), some of which were persistent even after discontinuation of the drug (Leo, 1996).

Hereditary and systemic illnesses

Huntington disease is characterized by choreoathetosis and dementia, which may be preceded, accompanied or followed by psychotic symptoms. If patients have received antipsychotics before the onset of chorea, the differential diagnosis becomes more complicated. A thorough family history, progression of symptoms, and development of dementia can help to clarify the diagnosis. Genetic testing for the Huntington gene is available. Wilson disease (hepatolenticular degeneration), a disorder of copper metabolism, can be distinguished from TD on the basis of clinical signs, laboratory tests, and family history. The disease of iron metabolism, Hallervorden–Spatz disease, usually has its onset during childhood and is predominated by symptoms of dystonia and bradykinesia. Other medical conditions that can produce dyskinesias include hyperthyroidism, hypoparathyroidism, severe hyperglycemia, chorea of pregnancy (chorea gravidarum), space-occupying lesions of the central nervous system, and inflammatory or immune disorders, such as lupus erythematosus, Henoch–Schönlein purpura, and Sydenham chorea.

Pathophysiology

The pathophysiology of TD is incompletely understood with neurotransmitter and neurodegeneration theories being proposed. The dopamine supersensitivity hypothesis, proposed by Klawans and Rubovits (1972), implicated an overactivity of the striatal dopaminergic system as being responsible for TD. Gunne and Haggstrom (1985) have proposed that TD is caused by an abnormality of GABA-related striatal neurones. Recent interest has focused on oxidative stress, production of free radicals, and excitotoxic mechanisms leading to neurodegeneration. Sachdev (2000) has proposed a model that encompasses several mechanisms, namely that high levels of catecholamine turnover and oxidative metabolism in the striatum lead to neurotoxicity and cell death, particularly in the gamma-aminobutyric acid (GABA)ergic striatal neurones via free radical and excitatory mechanisms. There are no characteristic patho-

logical findings in patients with TD. Many of these theories are undoubtedly oversimplified and no one theory or set of data offers a succinct explanation to understanding TD.

Epidemiology and risk factors

Incidence/prevalence and antipsychotic use

There is a wide variation in the prevalence of TD, ranging from 0.5% to more than 70% (Baldessarini et al., 1980; Kane & Smith, 1982; Kane et al., 1984a,b). This variation partly reflects methodological differences in the studies, e.g., differences in the characteristics of patients studied, prescribed antipsychotic, duration of antipsychotic exposure, and criteria for the diagnosis of TD.

Both dose and duration of treatment are directly associated with TD risk. The greater the total drug intake, the greater the likelihood of developing TD (Kane et al., 1984b). In two prospective studies of patients treated with conventional antipsychotics, Kane et al. (1986, 1988) found that the cumulative incidence of TD was 5%, 19%, and 26% after 1, 4, and 6 years, respectively. These studies showed that the incidence of TD increased linearly, at least for the first 5 years of antipsychotic treatment. In high-risk subjects, the incidence increased more markedly. For example, in a cohort of older patients, the incidence was 26%, 52%, and 60% after 1, 2, and 3 years, respectively (Jeste et al., 1995).

Correll et al. (2004) conducted a meta-analysis of studies of atypical antipsychotics (risperidone, olanzapine, quetiapine, amisulpride or ziprasidone) conducted over at least 1 year and reported on new cases of TD. Three of the eleven included studies had a haloperidol comparator arm. In young and middle-aged adults (<54 years old), the weighted mean annual incidence of TD for the atypical antipsychotics was 0.8% (range: 0.0–1.5%) compared to 5.4% (range: 4.1–7.4%) for those treated with haloperidol. In older patients (>54 years) treated with atypical antipsychotics, the incidence was 5.3% (range: 0.0–13.4%) which, although higher than the risk in younger adults, remains approximately five times less than that reported with conventional antipsychotic in this age group (Saltz et al., 1991). This meta-analysis indicates that atypical drugs have a reduced risk of TD compared to haloperidol and that this benefit extends to elderly patients. Two important provisos are that (1) the mean haloperidol doses in the three comparator studies in the meta-analysis were relatively high (>10 mg/day) and that (2) the weighted median duration of antipsychotic exposure was 306 days, indicating that most patients did not complete 1 year of treatment.

Age, sex, and psychiatric diagnosis

The prevalence and incidence of TD are positively correlated with increasing age (Smith & Baldessarini, 1980; Jeste et al., 1995). Women have a greater risk of TD compared with men at a ratio of 1.7:1 in most, but not all, studies

(Morgenstern & Glazer, 1993). While it is unclear why women are more susceptible to TD, proposed contributory factors include estrogen status, higher antipsychotic drug dosing per kilogram body weight, and the greater prevalence of affective disorders.

Retrospective (Gardos & Cole, 1997) and prospective studies (Kane *et al.*, 1986) suggest that affective disorders, primarily unipolar depression, are a risk factor for TD. Changes in norepinephrinergic or serotonergic mechanisms (Marsalek, 2000) may explain these findings. Patients with schizophrenia with predominant negative symptoms, evidence of cognitive impairment and neurological deficits, appear more vulnerable to TD (Waddington *et al.*, 1987).

Acute extrapyramidal syndromes

Several prospective studies indicate that early acute drug-induced EPS is a risk factor for developing TD (Kane *et al.*, 1986; Saltz *et al.*, 1991; Jeste *et al.*, 1995). Conversely patients with TD may have a vulnerability to developing acute EPS.

Other factors

Diabetes mellitus (DM) is a risk factor for TD (Ganzini *et al.*, 1992) and preliminary data suggest that phenylketonuria is also a risk factor (Richardson *et al.*, 1986, 1989). Several studies suggest that patients with schizophrenia and comorbid alcohol or drug misuse are at high risk of TD (Dixon *et al.*, 1992; Bailey *et al.*, 1997; van Os *et al.*, 1997). Higher rates of TD have been reported in African–Americans and people from the Dutch Antilles, and lower rates in Chinese and other Asian populations in comparison to white patients (Morgenstern & Glazer, 1993; Pandurangi & Aderibigbe, 1995). The basis of this racial difference is unclear and may reflect differences in therapeutic strategies and/or genetic differences.

Management

General principles

The primary strategy in managing TD is prevention. When antipsychotics are deemed necessary, patients should be given the lowest doses possible. During long-term antipsychotic therapy, patients should be periodically evaluated for the early features of TD. If features suggestive of TD appear, then the clinical strategy for management is presented in the algorithm shown in Figure 27.2. The first step is to confirm the diagnosis. A thorough medical evaluation, including a physical and neurological examination, laboratory testing, and a review of the differential diagnosis, should be performed. If the diagnosis of TD is confirmed, the next step is to evaluate current antipsychotic treatment. If antipsychotic treatment is not clinically required, it should be stopped. If continuing antipsychotic treatment is required, then attempts should be made to minimize the

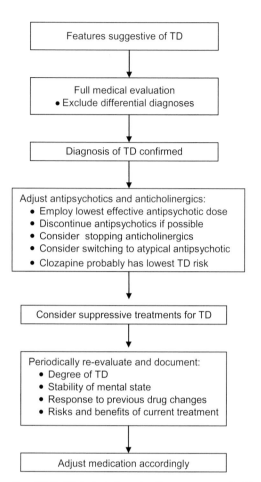

Fig. 27.2 Clinical strategy for the management of tardive dyskinesia (TD) (adapted from Casey, 1999).

severity of TD and to reduce the risk of it worsening over time. To this end, the options are to reduce the antipsychotic dose, switch to an antipsychotic with less propensity to cause TD or to employ specific treatments. Whatever treatment is adopted, it is helpful to monitor the course of TD using a rating scale such as the AIMS (Guy, 1976).

Switching antipsychotics

Several studies have reported an improvement in TD after patients are switched from a conventional to an atypical antipsychotic drug, including clozapine (Bassitt & Louza Neto, 1998; Lieberman *et al.*, 1991; Spivak *et al.*, 1997), olanzapine (Kinon *et al.*, 2004), quetiapine (Emsley *et al.*, 2004), and risperidone (Bai *et al.*, 2003). Whether this reflects certain atypical drugs having a specific antidyskinetic effect or simply having less propensity to cause TD is unclear. Bai *et al.* (2003) used a randomized design to compare risperidone to placebo in the treatment of patients with schizophrenia and TD. After 12 weeks, the mean AIMS total score showed a significantly greater decrease in the risperidone group than in the placebo group. This could indicate that risperidone has an antidyskenesia effect, but an alternative explanation is that a withdrawal effect from the original antipsychotic led to an exacerbation of TD in the placebo arm, inflating the difference between the placebo and risperidone arms. Several reports have described improvement in tardive dystonia after a switch to clozapine (Adityanjee & Estrera, 1996; van Harten & Kahn, 1999).

Switching antipsychotics when a patient develops TD raises several issues. The new antipsychotic may not be as effective as the previous drug in symptom control and a lower TD risk with the new agent may be counteracted by a worsening mental state or an increased risk of another side effect.

Specific treatments

A wide range of treatments have been proposed for TD but there is no strong evidence base to support any of them. Proposed treatments include dopamine-depleting drugs such as reserpine, tetrabenazine, and oxypertine; dopamine agonists (direct agonists such as apomorphine and bromocriptine, and the indirect agonists such as amantadine and levodopa); norepinephrenergic agonists such as clonidine; anticholinergics such as benztropine; GABA agonists such as valproate, diazepam, clonazepam, and baclofen; and miscellaneous agents including calcium-channel blockers, botulinum toxin, and vitamin E. Of all these agents the evidence is probably best for tetrabenazine, which has both presynaptic depleting and postsynaptic dopamine receptor blockade activity. While anticholinergic agents can temporarily aggravate TD, they may be beneficial in high doses in some patients with tardive dystonia. Benzodiazepines help some patients, although it is unclear whether this is via a specific or a non-specific sedative effect and long-term use carries the risk of dependence or abuse.

Botulinum toxin (type A) injection, primarily designed for idiopathic dystonia, has been successfully applied in the treatment of tardive dystonia, including blepharospasm, laryngeal dystonia, hemifacial spasm, and torticollis (Tarsy et al., 1997). It blocks acetylcholine release at the neurochemical junction and produces a chemical denervation with focal muscle paralysis that persists for up to 4 months (Hughes, 1994).

Invasive measures such as deep brain stimulation and pallidotomy have been reported to be beneficial (Wang et al., 1997; Weetman et al., 1997) in some patients with severe and refractory TD. The effect of electroconvulsive therapy, although reported to be variable, has had a dramatic effect in a few patients (Hay et al., 1990).

Long-term outcome

TD improvement rates vary widely across studies from 0% to 92% (Casey & Gerlach, 1986). The multiple contributions of patient, drug, and temporal factors undoubtedly influence this outcome range. Younger patients are the most likely to improve and elderly patients are the least likely to do so (Smith & Baldessarini, 1980). Discontinuing antipsychotic drugs is positively correlated with a favorable outcome in most, but not all, studies (Quitkin et al., 1977; Casey, 1985; Casey & Gerlach, 1986; Kane et al., 1986; Gardos et al., 1987). When antipsychotics can be discontinued, TD spontaneously resolves in some patients (Baldessarini et al., 1980), transiently worsens in others, and persists in some. Improvement may continue for many years after cessation of antipsychotic treatment. Approximately one-third of cases with TD remit within 3 months of discontinuation of antipsychotics, though resolution can occur as long as 5 years after stopping antipsychotics (Klawans & Tanner, 1983). Resolution of TD is more likely if antipsychotics are discontinued soon after the onset of the dyskinesias and patients are under the age of 60.

Long-term follow-up studies show that the course of TD can be fluctuating, with spontaneous remissions (Gardos et al., 1988), when lower doses of antipsychotics are maintained for a long time. Some patients show complete remission despite continued therapy (Gardos et al., 1994).

Neuroleptic malignant syndrome

Clinical features

Neuroleptic malignant syndrome (NMS) was first described in the French language by Delay and colleagues in 1960 who referred to it as "akinetic hypertonic syndrome" (Delay et al., 1960). The first report in the English language was in 1968 (Delay & Deniker, 1968). Most cases involve high-potency conventional antipsychotic drugs, in particular haloperidol, but NMS has been reported with all the atypical antipsychotics. A review by Ananth et al. (2004) identified 68 published cases of NMS associated with atypical antipsychotic drugs (21 for clozapine; 23 for risperidone; 19 for olanzapine; 5 for quetiapine). Other reports have involved amisulpride (Bottlender et al., 2002) and aripiprazole (Chakraborty & Johnston, 2004). NMS has been reported with non-antipsychotic drugs, including lithium, antidepressants of various classes, and metoclopramide, and also following sudden withdrawal of dopamine agonists in Parkinson disease (Haddad, 1994).

NMS is twice as common in men as in women, and 80% of cases occur in patients under the age of 40 years (Caroff, 1980). The incidence is often quoted as 0.2% (Caroff & Mann, 1993) but it appears to be decreasing. This may reflect the use of lower doses of antipsychotics, less frequent antipsychotic polypharmacy, and the introduction of the atypical antipsychotics. Shalev et al. (1989) reviewed over 200 published case reports of NMS and concluded that the mortality had decreased significantly since 1984. This may reflect better recognition and management.

Various diagnostic criteria have been proposed, including those by Pope *et al.* (1986), DSM-IV, and Mathews and Aderibigbe (1999). The four key features of NMS are:

1. *Muscle rigidity*—can be generalized or in milder forms can be localized to the tongue, facial or masticatory muscles, leading to dysarthria or dysphagia;
2. *Pyrexia*—can vary from a mild pyrexia to temperatures above 42°C.
3. *Change in consciousness level*—can range from mild confusion to coma;
4. *Autonomic disturbance*—can manifest as diaphoresis, tachycardia, labile blood pressure, and hypersalivation.

Most cases of NMS occur within days of starting a new antipsychotic, particularly if it is rapidly increased in dose. Symptoms typically develop over 24–72 h, but their evolution can be more insidious. When the condition is severe, patients are usually mute and akinetic, but diagnosing milder forms of the syndrome can be problematic, particularly as symptoms can fluctuate over hours or days. A spectrum concept has been proposed with severe NMS at one end of the spectrum, mild EPS at the other end, and intermediate forms occurring at the mid-point. The diagnosis of early or mild NMS in patients receiving clozapine is complicated by the benign fever and tachycardia commonly encountered during the early stage of clozapine treatment.

Serum creatine phosphokinase (CPK) is elevated (>100 IU/dL) reflecting sustained muscle contraction causing myonecrosis. Leukocytosis, ranging from a slight elevation to 30 000/mm^3, is frequently seen. Other non-specific laboratory abnormalities have been reported, including mildly elevated hepatic enzymes. NMS is not associated with specific structural brain changes and so the brain computerized tomographic (CT) scan is normal.

Differential diagnosis

Lethal catatonia

This was first reported by Kahlbaum in 1874. It is clinically identical to NMS but occurs independent of exposure to antipsychotics (Weller, 1992; White, 1992). It is possible that some cases of NMS are actually lethal catatonia, or represent an interaction between lethal catatonia and antipsychotic drugs (White & Robins, 1991).

Heat exhaustion and heat stroke

Heat exhaustion and heat stroke are part of a continuum of heat-related illness with heat stroke representing the severe end of the spectrum. In both conditions heat gain from metabolism and the environment exceeds heat loss by evaporation and convection, leading to a rise in body temperature. In heat exhaustion the body temperature is between 37°C and 40°C, and symptoms include dizziness, thirst, weakness, headache, and malaise. Heat stroke is a medical emergency and is divided into classic and exertional forms. Classic heat stroke occurs in hot weather, primarily affects the elderly and those with chronic illness, and often develops slowly over several days with symptoms including delirium, convulsions, and coma, though the temperature may be only slightly elevated. Exertional heat stroke primarily affects younger, active persons. It has a rapid onset, developing in hours, and is associated with marked pyrexia (>40°C). Some drugs can predispose to heat stoke by interfering with temperature regulation and so clinicians may encounter antipsychotic-induced heat stoke (Mann & Bolger, 1978). Both NMS and heat stoke can present with the sudden onset of pyrexia and altered consciousness.

In heat stroke the muscles are flaccid and the skin is dry whereas NMS is characterized by rigidity and sweating. Also, heat stroke will be suggested by a person working or exercising strenuously in hot and humid weather conditions and often neglecting fluid intake.

Serotonin toxicity

Symptoms of serotonin toxicity lie on a spectrum of severity and the term "serotonin syndrome" is usually used to refer to the severe end of the spectrum. Serotonin toxicity is characterized by altered mental state, neuromuscular hyperactivity, and autonomic overactivity. Several features can assist differentiation from NMS. Rigidity is only present in very severe serotonin toxicity, whereas rigidity is a cardinal feature of NMS. The patient with serotonin toxicity is usually restless and agitated whereas akinesia is characteristic in NMS. Gastrointestinal features (diarrhea, nausea, vomiting) are common in serotonin toxicity but not in NMS. Serotonin syndrome has a rapid onset over 24 h (Mason *et al.*, 2000) whereas NMS often develops over several days. Recent drug history may assist diagnosis. NMS is usually caused by antipsychotics whereas serotonin toxicity is due to drugs that increase serotonergic transmission. Severe cases of serotonin toxicity are usually due to the coprescription of drugs that increase serotonergic transmission via different mechanisms, e.g., a monoamine-oxidase inhibitor (MAOI) and an SSRI.

Anticholinergic toxicity

Anticholinergic toxicity can occur when a patient takes an overdose of medication that has an anticholinergic action or when patients are prescribed several medications with anticholinergic effects. It is characterized by confusion and pyrexia, hence the potential for misdiagnosis with NMS. However, in anticholinergic toxicity, the skin is dry and the muscles are not rigid; in contrast sweating and rigidity are usually present in NMS. Dilated pupils and urinary retention are common in anticholinergic toxicity. Physostigmine may induce a resolution of symptoms in anticholinergic toxicity but not in NMS.

Pathophysiology

The pharmacological basis of NMS is uncertain and various theories have been proposed, including the view that NMS results from drugs causing central dopamine receptor blockade. According to the dopaminergic hypothesis, NMS is due to a sudden drop in dopamine levels, which in the hypothalamus affects thermoregulation and in the striatum leads to rigidity, which in turn will cause peripheral heat production and contribute to pyrexia. Support for this theory comes from several sources. Dopamine is known to play a role in central thermoregulation in mammals. Injecting dopamine into the preoptic–anterior hypothalamus of rats causes a reduction in core temperature (Cox et al., 1978). Antipsychotics are the drugs most commonly associated with NMS and all block dopamine receptors. The hypodopaminergic mechanism also explains the observation that some patients with Parkinson disease develop an NMS-like syndrome when dopamine agonists are abruptly discontinued (Friedman et al., 1985). Finally, some dopaminergic drugs, including bromocriptine and amantadine (McCarron et al., 1992), have shown efficacy in treating NMS.

Management

If NMS is suspected, one should stop all antipsychotic medication and ideally other prescribed drugs that can cause the syndrome, e.g., antidepressants and lithium. Other dopamine antagonists, such as metoclopramide, should be avoided. A medical opinion should be obtained and transfer to a medical bed considered. This is essential if more specialized treatment is needed. General supportive measures should be instigated, including rehydration, cooling, and the treatment of any intercurrent infection. Secondary complications, such as hypoxia, acidosis, and renal failure, require aggressive treatment. Severe NMS can lead to rhabdomyolysis, myoglobinuria, renal failure, and long-term neuropsychiatric sequelae (Adityanjee et al., 2005). The clinical course should be monitored by means of regular physical observations and daily serum CPK levels.

The benefit of adding specific therapies to supportive measures remains debated. There are conflicting reports of benefit of using dopamine agonists (bromocriptine, amantadine) and the muscle relaxant dantrolene to treat NMS (Susman, 2001; Reulbach et al., 2007). Hypotension can be a limiting side effect when using bromocriptine. Dantrolene inhibits calcium release from the sarcoplasmic reticulum, decreasing available calcium for ongoing muscle contracture. High doses can lead to hepatic toxicity. Benzodiazepines have been used to facilitate muscle relaxation (Susman, 2001).

There are reports of the beneficial effect of electroconvulsive therapy (ECT) in treating NMS, particularly in improving fever, sweating, and level of consciousness (Hermesh et al., 1987). There is no evidence that patients with a history of NMS are more vulnerable to developing malignant hyperthermia as a complication of general anesthesia (Hermesh et al., 1988).

Rechallenge

A previous episode of NMS is not an absolute contraindication to further antipsychotic treatment. Estimates of the risk of recurrence of NMS following rechallenge with antipsychotic medication vary. There were 13 recurrences in 29 rechallenges (48%) reviewed by Olmsted (1998) with two fatalities. Rosebush et al. (1989) reported that 13 of 15 patients with NMS (87%) were eventually able to take antipsychotics again. After a case of NMS one should not automatically restart antipsychotic treatment but rather weigh the potential benefits and risks of antipsychotic treatment for that individual and the possibility of alternative treatments. For example, if a patient develops NMS during antipsychotic treatment for mania, one should consider whether the mania could subsequently be managed using a mood stabilizer, such as valproate or lithium, rather than an antipsychotic drug.

If the clinical need warrants further antipsychotic treatment, then several factors can reduce the risk of a recurrence of NMS. Duration of time between the resolution of NMS and restarting antipsychotic medication appears to be an important determinant of the risk for relapse (Rosebush et al., 1989). Consequently one should wait 2–4 weeks after NMS has resolved before restarting antipsychotic treatment. A different antipsychotic to that implicated in the original episode should be chosen and ideally this should be an atypical. Depot antipsychotics should not be used. To help identify the early reappearance of NMS, the patient should be monitored closely; this includes monitoring for pyrexia, autonomic instability, mental state changes, and rigidity, and taking serial measurements of the white cell count and serum CPK. These recommendations are not based on systematic studies, as none exists, but on reviews of anecdotal reports (e.g., Olmsted, 1998; Rosebush et al., 1989) and clinical and theoretical knowledge about risk factors for NMS.

Seizures

Most antipsychotic drugs lower the seizure threshold though the underlying mechanism remains unclear. In general, the most sedating agents appear to be the most likely to produce seizures (Itil & Soldatos, 1980). Among the conventional antipsychotics the risk of seizures appears highest with chlorpromazine. Chlorpromazine had been marketed for less than 1 year before a case of seizure was associated with its use (Anton-Stephens, 1953). Logothetis (1967) studied 859 patients treated with phenothiazines over 5 years and found a 1.2% risk for seizures. The risk for seizures was strongly related to dosage, and approached 10% in patients treated with more than 1000 mg/day chlorpromazine. Rapid increases in dose and the presence of organic brain disease also increased the risk for seizures. Other surveys have supported the relationship between seizures and higher dosage of phenothiazines (Schlichther et al., 1956; Messing et al., 1984).

Among the atypical antipsychotics the risk of seizures is greatest with clozapine, reaching an estimated frequency of 10% in patients receiving the drug for 3.8 years (Devinsky et al., 1991). The risk of clozapine-associated seizures increases with dose and speed of dose escalation. The risk of seizures is estimated at approximately 1% with doses of clozapine below 300 mg/day and 4.4% with doses above 600 mg/day (Devinsky et al., 1991). Severe myoclonus may precede seizures during clozapine treatment. Most patients can continue treatment with clozapine after a seizure, with addition of an anticonvulsant or dose reduction (Devinsky et al., 1991). Of the other atypical antipsychotics, zotepine has been reported to carry a relatively high risk of seizures (Zoleptil Summary of Product Characteristics, 2002).

Antipsychotics should be used with caution in patients with a history of seizures or in those vulnerable to seizures, e.g., those with dementia or brain injury. Depot antipsychotics should be avoided in patients with epilepsy, not because they are of high epileptogenic risk, but because if seizures occur then the antipsychotic cannot be quickly withdrawn. For antipsychotic agents other than clozapine and zotepine, the risk of provoking seizures in patients with epilepsy appears to be quite small. One study found that the addition of psychotropic medication, including antipsychotics, was generally associated with improved seizure control (Ojemann et al., 1987). Some authorities recommend considering prophylactic valproate to prevent seizures if patients are prescribed high-dose clozapine or if plasma clozapine levels are high (>50 μg/dL; Taylor et al., 2007). If a seizure occurs on clozapine, it is advisable to withhold clozapine for 1 day and then restart it at a lower dose.

Cerebrovascular events

Until fairly recently, antipsychotics were often used to treat elderly patients with behavioral and psychological symptoms of dementia (BPSD) though none is licensed for this indication. A meta-analysis of placebo-controlled trials of four atypical antipsychotics (aripiprazole, olanzapine, quetiapine, risperidone) in patients with dementia showed a significantly increased risk for cerebrovascular events (including stroke and transient ischemic attacks) associated with atypical drug use (Schneider et al., 2006a) and a small but significant increase in overall mortality (3.5% with drug versus 2.3% with placebo; Schneider et al., 2005). Regulatory authorities in the UK and US have issued warnings that specific atypical antipsychotics should not be used to treat BPSD due to this risk (e.g., Food and Drug Administration, 2003; Committee on Safety of Medicines, 2004). The lack of placebo-controlled data with specific older conventional antipsychotics in patients with dementia does not indicate that they are without similar risks. Three cohort studies have compared the risk of death or stoke in elderly patients (>65 years) treated with conventional antipsychotic versus atypical antipsychotics (Gill et al., 2005; Herrmann et al., 2004; Wang et al., 2005). Two studies found no significant difference in risk of stroke between the two groups (Gill et al., 2005; Herrmann et al., 2004), while the third found that conventional antipsychotics were associated with significantly higher adjusted mortality (Wang et al., 2005). A recent large randomized controlled trial found that the adverse effects of atypical antipsychotics offset their advantages in terms of efficacy when treating behavioral and psychiatric symptoms of Alzheimer disease (Schneider et al., 2006b).

In summary, meta-analyses (Schneider et al., 2005, 2006a) show that atypical antipsychotics are associated with a higher risk of stroke or death than placebo in elderly patients with dementia. Cohort studies suggest that conventional drugs carry at least the same risk. At present there is no evidence of a differential risk between individual antipsychotics in their association with cerebrovascular events. The mechanism by which antipsychotics increase the risk of stroke is unclear. As the risk is seen in 6–12 weeks in clinical trials, it is unlikely to be mediated through effects on vascular risk factors such as glucose or lipid metabolism. One potential mechanism is that antipsychotics cause orthostatic hypotension, which in patients with pre-existing cerebrovascular disease leads to "watershed" strokes (Smith & Beier, 2004). Alternatively, antipsychotics may promote platelet aggregation (Smith & Beier, 2004), though some data suggest the opposite effect (Harrison-Woolrych & Clark, 2004).

When treating elderly patients with BPSD, clinicians should consider these risks on an individual patient basis, taking into account the medical needs of the patient, the efficacy of antipsychotics in specific symptom domains, pre-existing cerebrovascular risk factors, and the efficacy and safety of alternative treatments. The latter include psychosocial interventions and eliminating any factors that may inadvertently exacerbate cognitive impairment and BPSD, e.g., drugs with anticholinergic properties. If antipsychotics are used to treat BPSD, then treatment should be kept short-term whenever possible.

References

Adityanjee & Estrera A.B. (1996) Successful treatment of tardive dystonia with clozapine. *Biological Psychiatry* **39**, 1064–1065.

Adityanjee, Sajatovic, M. & Munshi, K.R. (2005) Neuropsychiatric sequelae of neuroleptic malignant syndrome. *Clinical Neuropharmacology* **28**, 197–204.

Adler, L., Angrist, B., Reiter, S. & Rotrosen, J. (1989) Neuroleptic-induced akathisia: a review. *Psychopharmacology* **97**, 1–11.

American Psychiatric Association (1997) American Psychiatric Association: Practice Guideline for the Treatment of Patients with Schizophrenia. *American Journal of Psychiatry* **154** (Suppl.), 1–63

Ananth, J., Parameswaran, S., Gunatilake, S., Burgoyne, K. & Sidhom, T. (2004) Neuroleptic malignant syndrome and atypical antipsychotic drugs. *Journal of Clinical Psychiatry* **65**, 464–470

Anton-Stephens, D. (1953) Preliminary observations on the psychiatric use of chlorpromazine. *Journal of Mental Science* **100**, 543–547.

Ayd, F. (1961) A survey of drug-induced extrapyramidal reactions. *Journal of the American Medical Association* **175**, 1054–1060.

Bagnall, A.M., Jones, L, Ginnelly, L. *et al* (2003) A systematic review of atypical antipsychotic drugs in schizophrenia. *Health Technology Assessement* **7**, 1–193.

Bai, Y.M., Yu, S.C. & Lin, C.C. (2003) Risperidone for severe tardive dyskinesia: a 12-week randomized, double-blind, placebo-controlled study. *Journal of Clinical Psychiatry* **64**, 1342–1348.

Bailey, L., Maxwell, S. & Brandabur, M. (1997) Substance abuse as a risk factor for tardive dyskinesia: a retrospective analysis of 1027 patients. *Psychopharmacological Bulletin* **33**, 177–181.

Baldessarini, R., Cole J., Davis, J. *et al.* (1980) Tardive dyskinesia: summary of a task force report of the American Psychiatric Association. *American Journal of Psychiatry* **137**, 1163–1172.

Baldessarini, R., Cohen, B. & Teicher, M. (1988) Significance of neuroleptic dose and plasma level in pharmacological treatment of psychosis. *Archives of General Psychiatry* **45**, 79–91.

Barnes, T. & Braude, W. (1985) Akathisia variants and tardive dyskinesia. *Archives of General Psychiatry* **42**, 874–878.

Bassitt, D.P. & Louza Neto, M.R. (1998) Clozapine efficacy in tardive dyskinesia in schizophrenic patients. *European Archives of Psychiatry Clinical Neuroscience* **248**, 209–211.

Bersani, G., Grispini, A., Marini, S. *et al.* (1990) 5-HT2 antagonist ritanserin in neuroleptic-induced parkinsonism: a double-blind comparison with orphenadrine and placebo. *Clinical Neuropharmacology* **13**, 125–137.

Bleuler, E. (1950) *Dementia Praecox or the Group of Schizophrenias.* New York: International Universities Press.

Bottlender, R., Jager, M., Hofschuster, E., Dobmeier, P. & Moller, H.J. (2002) Neuroleptic malignant syndrome due to atypical neuroleptics: three episodes in one patient. *Pharmacopsychiatry* **35,** 119–121.

Boyer, W., Bakalar, N. & Lake, C. (1989) Anticholinergic prophylaxis of acute haloperidol-induced dystonic reactions. *Journal of Clinical Psychopharmacology* **7**, 164–166.

Brooks, D. (1991) Detection of preclinical Parkinson's disease with PET. *Neurology* **41** (Suppl. 2), 24–27.

Brooks, D.J. (1993) Functional imaging in relation to parkinsonian syndromes. *Journal of Neurological Science* **115**, 1–17.

Burke, R.E., Fahn, S. & Jankovic, J. (1982) Tardive dystonia: late-onset and persistent dystonia caused by antipsychotic drugs. *Neurology* **32**, 1335–1346.

Caroff, S.N. (1980) The neuroleptic malignant syndrome. *Journal of Clinics in Psychiatry* **41**, 79–83.

Caroff, S.N. & Mann, S.C. (1993) Neuroleptic malignant syndrome. *Medical Clinics of North America* **77**, 185–202

Casey, D. (1981) The differential diagnosis of tardive dyskinesia. *Acta Psychiatrica Scandinavica* **63** (Suppl. 291), 71–87.

Casey, D. (1985) Spontaneous and tardive dyskinesias: clinical and laboratory studies. *Journal of Clincal Psychiatry* **46**, 42–47.

Casey, D. (1991) Neuroleptic drug-induced extrapyramidal syndromes and tardive dyskinesia. *Schizophrenia Research* **4**, 109–120.

Casey, D. (1995) Neuroleptic-induced acute extrapyramidal syndromes and tardive dyskinesia. In: Hirsch, S.R. & Weinberger, D.R., eds. *Schizophrenia.* Oxford: Blackwell Science, pp. 546–565.

Casey, D. (1997) The relationship of pharmacology to side effects. *Journal of Clinical Psychiatry* **58** (Suppl. 10), 55–62.

Casey, D. (1999) Tardive dyskinesia and atypical antipsychotic drugs. *Schizophrenia Research* **35**, S61–S66.

Casey, D. & Gerlach, J. (1986) Tardive dyskinesia: what is the long-term outcome? In: Casey, D. & Gardos, G., eds. *Tardive Dyskinesia and Neuroleptics: From Dogma to Reason.* Washington, DC: American Psychiatric Press, pp. 76–97.

Casey, D. & Keepers, G.A. (1988) Neuroleptic side effects: acute extrapyramidal syndromes and tardive dyskinesia. In: Casey, D. & Christensen, A., eds. *Psychopharmacology: Current Trends.* Berlin: Springer-Verlag, pp. 74–93.

Chakraborty, N. & Johnston, T. (2004) Aripiprazole and neuroleptic malignant syndrome. *International Clinical Psychopharmacology* **19**, 351–353.

Committee on Safety of Medicines (2004) Atypical antipsychotic drugs and stroke: message from Professor Gordon Duff, Chairman, Committee on Safety of medicines (CEM/CMO/200401).

Correll, C.U., Leucht, S. & Kane, J.M. (2004) Lower risk for tardive dyskinesia associated with second generation antipsychotics: a systematic review of one year studies. *American Journal of Psychiatry* **161**, 414–425.

Cox, B., Kerwin, R. & Lee, T.E. (1978) Dopamine receptors in the central thermoregulatory pathways of the rat. *Journal of Physiology (London)* **282**, 471–483.

Day, J.C., Kinderman, P. & Bentall, R. (1998) A comparison of patients' and prescribers' beliefs about neuroleptic side-effects: prevalence, distress and causation. *Acta Psychiatrica Scandinavica* **97**, 93–97.

Delay, J. & Deniker, P. (1968) Drug-induced extra-pyramidal syndromes. In: Vinken, P.S. & Bruyn, G.W., eds. *Handbook of Clinical Neurology, Vol. 6. Diseases of the Basal Ganglia.* New York: Elsevier North-Holland, pp. 248–266.

Delay, J., Pichot, P., Lempiere, T., Blissalde, B. & Peigne, F. (1960) Un neuroleptique majeur non phenothiazinique et non réserpinique, l'halopéridol, dans le traitement des psychoses. *Annals of Medical Psychology* **18**, 145–152.

Devinsky, O., Honigfeld, G. & Patin, J. (1991) Clozapine-related seizures. *Neurology* **41**, 369–371.

Dixon, L., Weiden, P., Haag, G., Sweeney, J. & Frances, A. (1992) Increased tardive dyskinesia in alcohol-abusing schizophrenic patients. *Comparative Psychiatry* **33**, 121–122.

Emsley, R., Turner, H.J., Schronen, J., Botha, K., Smit, R. & Oosthuizen, P.P. (2004) A single-blind randomised trial comparing quetiapine and haloperidol in the treatment of tardive dyskinesia. *Journal of Clinical Psychiatry* **65**, 696–701.

Farde, L., Nordstrom, A., Wiesel, F. *et al.* (1992) Positron emission tomographic analysis of central D1-dopamine and D2-dopamine receptor occupancy in patients treated with classical neuroleptics and clozapine: relation to extrapyramidal side-effects. *Archives of General Psychiatry* **49**, 538–544.

Faurbye, A., Rasch, P., Bender Peterson, P., Brandenborg, G. & Pakkenberg, H. (1964) Neurological symptoms in the pharmacotherapy of psychoses. *Acta Psychiatrica Scandinavica* **40**, 10–26.

Food and Drug Administration (2003) Safety alert: RISPERDAL (risperidone). Washington, DC: US Food and Drug Administration; 1 Mar 2004. www.fda.gov/medwatch/SAFETY/2003/risperdal.htm (accessed 15 Nov 2004).

Friedman, J.H., Feinberg, S.S. & Feldman, R.G. (1985) A neuroleptic malignant-like syndrome due to levodopa therapy withdrawal. *Journal of the American Medical Association* **254**, 2792–2795.

Ganzini, L., Casey, D., Hoffman, W. & Heintz, R. (1992) Tardive dyskinesia and diabetes mellitus. *Psychopharmacology Bulletin* **23**, 281–286.

Gao, K., Kemp, D.E., Ganocy, S.J., Gajwani, P., Xia, G. & Calabrese, J.R. (2008). Antipsychotic-induced extrapyramidal side effects in bipolar disorder and schizophrenia: a systematic review. *Journal of Clinical Psychopharmacology* **28**, 203–209.

Gardos, G. & Cole. (1997) Tardive dyskinesia and affective disorder, In: Yassa, R., Nair, N. & Jeste, D., eds. *Neuroleptic-Induced Movement Disorders*. Cambridge: Cambridge University Press, pp. 69–81.

Gardos, G., Cole, J., Salomon, M. & Schniebolk, S. (1987) Clinical forms of severe tardive dyskinesia. *American Journal of Psychiatry* **144**, 895–902.

Gardos, G., Cole, J., Haskell, D. *et al.* (1988) The natural history of tardive dyskinesia. *Journal of Clinical Psychopharmacology* **8** (Suppl. 4), 31S–37S.

Gardos, G., Casey, D.E., Cole, J.O. *et al.* (1994) Ten-year outcome of tardive dyskinesia. *American Journal of Psychiatry* **151**, 836–841.

Geddes, J., Freemantle, N., Harrison, P. & Bebbington, P. (2000) Atypical antipsychotics in the treatment of schizophrenia: systematic overview and meta-regression analysis. *BMJ* **321**, 1371–1376.

Gill, S.S., Rochon, P.A., Herrmann, N. *et al.* (2005) Atypical antipsychotic drugs and risk of ischaemic stroke: population based retrospective cohort study. *British Medical Journal* **330**, 445–448.

Glazer, W., Naftolin, F., Moore, D.C., Bowers, M.B. & MacLusky, N.J. (1983) The relationship of circulating estradiol to tardive dyskinesia in men and post-menopausal women. *Psychoneuroendocrinology* **8**, 429–434.

Gunne, L. & Haggstrom, J. (1985) Pathophysiology of tardive dyskinesia. *Psychopharmacology* **232**, 191–193.

Guy, W. (1976) ECDEU Assessment Manual for Psychopharmacology (revised 1976), pp. 534–537. United Staes Government Printing Office Washington, DC.

Haddad PM (1994) Neuroleptic malignant syndrome. May be caused by other drugs. *BMJ* **308**, 200.

Haddad, P.M. & Sharma, S.G. (2007) Adverse effects of atypical antipsychotics: differential risk and clinical implications. *CNS Drugs* **21**, 911–936.

Hansen, L. (2001) A critical review of akathisia, and its possible association with suicidal behaviour. *Human Psychopharmacology* **16**, 495–505.

Harrison-Woolrych, M. & Clark, D.W.J. (2004) Nose bleeds associated with use of risperidone. *BMJ* **328**, 1416.

Hay, D., Hay, L., Blackwell, B. & Spiro, H. (1990) ECT and tardive dyskinesia. *Journal of Geriatric Psychiatry and Neurology* **3**, 106–109.

Hermesh H, Aizenberg D, Weizman A (1987) A successful electroconvulsive treatment of neuroleptic malignant syndrome. *Acta Psychiatrica Scandinavica* **75**, 237–239.

Hermesh H, Aizenberg D, Lapidot M, Munitz H (1988) Risk of malignant hyperthermia among patients with neuroleptic malignant syndrome and their families. *American Journal of Psychiatry* **145**, 1431–1434.

Herrmann, N., Mamdani, M. & Lanctôt, K.L. (2004) Atypical antipsychotics and risk of cerebrovascular accidents. *American Journal of Psychiatry* **161**, 1113–1115.

Hughes, A. (1994) Botulinum toxin in clinical practice. *Drugs* **48**, 888–893.

Itil, T. & Soldatos, C. (1980) Epileptogenic side effects of psychotropic drugs. *Journal of the American Medical Association* **244**, 1460–1463.

Jeste, D., Caligiuri, M., Paulsen, J. *et al.* (1995) Risk of tardive dyskinesia in older patients. *Archives of General Psychiatry* **52**, 756–765.

Kane, J. & Smith, J. (1982) Tardive dyskinesia: prevalence and risk factors, 1959–79. *Archives of General Psychiatry* **39**, 473–481.

Kane, J., Woerner, M., Weinhold, P. *et al.* (1984a) Incidence and severity of tardive dyskinesia in affective illness. In: *Tardive Dyskinesia and Affective Illness*. American Psychiatric Press, Washington, DC, pp. 22–28.

Kane, J., Woerner, M., Weinhold, P. *et al.* (1984b) Incidence of tardive dyskinesia: five year data from a prospective study. *Psychopharmacology Bulletin* **20**, 39–40.

Kane, J., Woerner, M., Borenstein, M., Wegner, J. & Lieberman, J. (1986) Integrating incidence and prevalence of tardive dyskinesia. *Psychopharmacological Bulletin* **22**, 254–258.

Kane, J., Woerner, M. & Lieberman, J. (1988) Tardive dyskinesia: prevalence, incidence, and risk factors. *Journal of Clinical Psychopharmacology* **8** (Suppl.), 52S–56S.

Kapur, S. & Seeman, P. (2001) Does fast dissociation from the dopamine D(2) receptor explain the action of atypical antipsychotics? A new hypothesis. *American Journal of Psychiatry* **158**, 360–369.

Kapur, S., Zipursky, R. & Remington, G. (1999) Clinical and theoretical implications of 5-HT2 and D2 receptor occupancy of clozapine, risperidone, and olanzapine in schizophrenia. *American Journal of Psychiatry* **156**, 286–293.

Keepers, G. & Casey, D. (1987) Prediction of neuroleptic-induced dystonia. *Journal of Clinical Psychopharmacology* **7**, 342–344.

Keepers, G. & Casey, D. (1991) Use of neuroleptic-induced extrapyramidal symptoms to predict future vulnerability to side effects. *American Journal of Psychiatry* **148**, 85–89.

Keepers, G., Clappison, V. & Casey, D. (1983) Initial anticholinergic prophylaxis for neuroleptic–induced extrapyramidal syndromes. *Archives of General Psychiatry* **40**, 1113–1117.

Kinon, B.J., Jeste, D.V., Kollack-Walker, S., Stauffer, V. & Liu-Seifert, H. (2004) Olanzapine treatment for tardive dyskinesia in schizophrenia patients: a prospective clinical trial with patients randomized to blinded dose reduction periods. *Progress in Neuropsychopharmacology Biological Psychiatry* **28**, 985–996.

Klawans, H. & Rubovits, R. (1972) An experimental model of tardive dyskinesia. *Journal of Neural Transmission* **33**, 235–246.

Klawans, H. & Tanner, C. (1983) The reversibility of permanent tardive dyskinesia. *Neurology* **33** (Suppl. 2), 163.

Kraepelin, E. (1907) *Clinical Psychiatry.* New York: MacMillan.

Leo, R. (1996) Movement disorders associated with serotonin selective reuptake inhibitors. *Journal of Clinical Psychiatry* **57**, 449–454.

Leucht, S., Corves, C., Arbter, D., Engel, R.R., Li, C. & Davis, J.M. (2009) Second-generation versus first-generation antipsychotic drugs for schizophrenia: a meta-analysis. *Lancet* **373**, 31–41.

Lieberman, J.A., Saltz, B.L., Johns, C.A., Pollack, S., Borenstein, M. & Kane, J. (1991) The effects of clozapine on tardive dyskinesia. *British Journal of Psychiatry* **58**, 503–510.

Logothetis, J. (1967) Spontaneous epileptic seizures and electroencephalographic changes in the course of phenothiazine therapy. *Neurology* **17**, 869–877.

Mann, S.C. & Bolger, W.P. (1978) Psychotropic drugs, summer heat and humidity, and hyperpyrexia: a danger restated. *American Journal of Psychiatry* **135**, 1097–1100.

Marsalek, M. (2000) Tardive drug-induced extrapyramidal syndromes. *Pharmacopsychiatry* **33**, 14–33.

Mason, P.J., Morris, V.A. & Balcezak, T.J. (2000) Serotonin syndrome. Presentation of 2 cases and review of the literature. *Medicine (Baltimore)* **79**, 201–209.

Mathews, T. & Aderibigbe, Y.A. (1999) Proposed research diagnostic criteria for neuroleptic malignant syndrome. *International Journal of Neuropsychopharmacology* **2**, 129–144

McCarron, M.M., Boettger, M.L. & Peck, J.I. (1992) A case of neuroleptic malignant syndrome successfully treated with amantadine. *Journal of Clinical Psychiatry* **43**, 381–382.

McCreadie, R.G., Thara, R., Kamath, S. *et al.* (1996). Abnormal movements in never- medicated Indian patients with schizophrenia. *British Journal of Psychiatry* **168**, 221–226.

Messing, R.O., Closson, R.G. & Simon, R.P. (1984) Drug-induced seizures: a 10 year experience. *Neurology* **17**, 869–877.

Miller, C.H. & Fleischhacker, W.W. (2000) Managing antipsychotic-induced acute and chronic akathisia. *Drug Safety* **22**, 73–81.

Mitra, S. & Haddad, P.M. (2007) Documentation of extrapyramidal symptoms. *Psychiatric Bulletin* **31**, 76–77.

Morgenstern, H. & Glazer, W. (1993) Identifying risk factors for tardive dyskinesia among long-term outpatients maintained with neuroleptic medications. *Archives of General Psychiatry* **50**, 723–733.

Murray, C.J., Lopez, A.D. (1996) The Global Burden of Disease: a comprehensive assessment of mortality and disability from diseases, injuries and risk factors in 1990 and projected to 2020. Cambridge, MA, Harvard School of Public Health, (Global Burden of Disease and Injury Series, vol. I), 1996.

National Institute for Clinical Excellence (2009) Core interventions in the treatment and management of schizophrenia in primary and secondary care. Clinical Guideline 82. March 2009. London: NICE. www.nice.org.uk

Newton-John, H. (1988) Acute upper airway obstruction due to supraglottic dystonia induced by a neuroleptic. *BMJ* **297**, 964–965.

Norton, J. (2001) Laryngeal dystonia in psychiatry. *Canadian Journal of Psychiatry* **46**, 453.

Ojemann, L.M., Baugh-Bookman, C. & Dudley, D.L. (1987) Effect of psychotropic medications on seizure control in patients with epilepsy. *Neurology* **37**, 1525–1527.

Olmsted, T.R. (1998) Neuroleptic malignant syndrome: guidelines for treatment and reinstitution of neuroleptics. *South Medical Journal* **81**, 888–891.

Pandurangi, A. & Aderibigbe, Y. (1995) Tardive dyskinesia in non-western countries: a review. *European Archives of Psychiatry and Clinical Neuroscience* **246**, 47–52.

Pappa, S. & Dazzan, P. (2008) Spontaneous movement disorders in antipsychotic-naive patients with first-episode psychoses: a systematic review. *Psychological Medicine* **12**, 1–12

Pehek, E. (1996) Local infusion of the serotonin antagonist ritanserin or ICS 205,930 increases *in vivo* dopamine release in the rat medial prefrontal cortex. *Synapse* **24**, 12–18.

Pope, H.G., Keck, P.E. & McElroy, S.L. (1986) Frequency and presentation of neuroleptic malignant syndrome in a large psychiatric hospital. *American Journal of Psychiatry* **143**, 1227–1233.

Quitkin, F., Rifkin, A., Gochfeld, L. & Klein, D. (1977) Tardive dyskinesia: are first signs reversible? *American Journal of Psychiatry* **134**, 84–87.

Rajput, A., Rozdilsky, B., Hornykiewicz, O. *et al.* (1982) Reversible drug-induced parkinsonism: clinicopathologic study of two cases. *Archives of Neurology* **39**, 644–646.

Reulbach, U., Dütsch, C., Biermann, T. *et al.* (2007) Managing an effective treatment for neuroleptic malignant syndrome. *Critical Care* **11**, R4.

Richardson, M. & Craig, T. (1982) The coexistence of parkinsonism-like symptoms and tardive dyskinesia. *American Journal of Psychiatry* **139**, 341–343.

Richardson, M., Haugland, M., Pass, R. & Craig, T. (1986) The prevalence of tardive dyskinesia in a mentally retarded population. *Psychopharmacological Bulletin* **22**, 243–249.

Richardson, M., Suckow, R., Whittaker, R. *et al.* (1989) The plasma phenylalanine/large neutral amino acid ratio: a risk factor for tardive dyskinesia. *Psychopharmacological Bulletin* **25**, 47–51.

Rosebush, P.I., Stewart, T.D. & Gelenberg, A.J. (1989) Twenty neuroleptic rechallenges after neuroleptic malignant syndrome in 15 patients. *Journal of Clinical Psychiatry* **50**, 295–298.

Sachdev, P. (2000) The current status of tardive dyskinesia. *Australian and New Zealand Journal of Psychiatry* **34**, 355–369.

Saltz, B.L., Woerner, M.G., Kane, J.M. et al. (1991) Prospective study of tardive dyskinesia incidence in the elderly. *Journal of the American Medical Association* **266**, 2402–2406.

Schlichther, W., Bristow, M.E., Schultz, S. & Henderson, A.C. (1956) Seizures occurring during intensive chlorpromazine therapy. *Canadian Medical Association Journal* **74**, 364–366.

Schneider, L.S., Dagerman, K.S. & Insel, P. (2005) Risk of death with atypical antipsychotic drug treatment for dementia: meta-analysis of randomized placebo-controlled trials. *JAMA* **294**, 1934–1943.

Schneider, L.S., Dagerman, K. & Insel, P.S. (2006a) Efficacy and adverse effects of atypical antipsychotics for dementia: meta-analysis of randomized, placebo-controlled trials. *Amerian Journal of Geriatric Psychiatry* **14**, 191–210.

Schneider, L.S., Tariot, P.N., Dagerman, K.S. et al. (2006b) Effectiveness of atypical antipsychotic drugs in patients with Alzheimer's disease. *New England Journal of Medicine* **355**, 1525–1538.

Schonecker, M. (1957) Ein eigentumliches Syndrom im oralen Bereich bei Megaphenapplikation. *Nervenaerzt* **28**, 35–36.

Shalev, A., Hermesh, H. & Munitz, H. (1989) Mortality from neuroleptic malignant syndrome. *Journal of Clinical Psychiatry* **50**, 18–25.

Sigwald, J., Bouttier, D. & Raymondeaud, C. (1959) Quatre cas de dyskinesie facio-bucco-lingua-masticatrice a l'evolution prolongee secondaire a un traitement par les neuroleptiques. *Revue Neurologique* **100**, 751–755.

Singh, H., Levinson, D.F., Simpson, G.M., Lo, E.S. & Friedman, E. (1990) Acute dystonia during fixed-dose neuroleptic treatment. *Journal of Clinical Psychopharmacology* **10**, 389–396.

Smith, J. & Baldessarini, R. (1980) Changes in prevalence, severity and recovery in tardive dyskinesia with age. *Archives of General Psychiatry* **37**, 1368–1373.

Smith, D.A. & Beier, M.T. (2004) Association between risperidone treatment and cerebrovascular adverse events: examining the evidence and postulating hypotheses for an underlying mechanism. *Journal of the American Medical Directors Association* **5**, 129–132.

Spivak, B., Mester, R., Abesgaus, J. et al. (1997) Clozapine treatment for neuroleptic-induced tardive dyskinesia, parkinsonism, and chronic akathisia in schizophrenic patients. *Journal of Clinical Psychiatry* **58**, 318–322.

Sramek, J., Simpson, G., Morrison, R. & Heiser, J. (1986) Anticholinergic agents for prophylaxis of neuroleptic-induced dystonic reactions: a prospective study. *Journal of Clinical Psychiatry* **47**, 305–309.

Stones, M., Kennie, D.C. & Fulton, J.D. (1990) Dystonic dysphagia associated with fluspirilene. *BMJ* **301**, 668–669.

Susman, V.L. (2001) Clinical management of neuroleptic malignant syndrome. *Psychiatric Quarterly* **72**, 325–336.

Swett, C. (1975) Drug-induced dystonia. *American Journal of Psychiatry* **132**, 532–534.

Tarsy, D., Kaufman, D., Sethi, K.D., Rivner, M.H., Molho, E. & Factor, S. (1997) An open-label study of botulinum toxin A for treatment of tardive dystonia. *Clinical Neuropharmacology* **20**, 90–93.

Tauscher, J., Kufferle, B., Asenbaum, S. et al. (1999) *In vivo* [123]I IBZM SPECT imaging of striatal dopamine-2 receptor occupancy in schizophrenic patients treated with olanzapine in comparison to clozapine and haloperidol. *Psychopharmacology (Berlin)* **141**, 175–181.

Taylor, D., Paton, C. & Kerwin, R. (2007) *The Maudsley Prescribing Guidelines*, 9th edn. South London and Maudsley NHS Foundation Trust & Oxleas NHS Foundation Trust, Informa Healthcare.

Uhrbrand, L. & Faurbye, A. (1960) Reversible and irreversible dyskinesia after treatment with perphenazine, chlorpromazine, reserpine, and electroconvulsive therapy. *Psychopharmacoligia* **1**, 408–418.

van Harten, P.N. & Kahn, R.S. (1999) Tardive dystonia. *Schizophrenia Bulletin* **25**, 741–748.

van Os, J., Fahy, T., Jones, P. et al. (1997) Tardive dyskinesia: who is at risk? *Acta Psychiatrica Scandinavica* **96**, 206–216.

Vinson, D.R. (2004) Diphenhydramine in the treatment of akathisia induced by prochlorperazine. *Journal of Emergency Medicine* **26**, 265–270.

Waddington, J., Youssef, H., Dolphin, C. & Kinsella, A. (1987) Cognitive dysfunction, negative symptoms, and tardive dyskinesia in schizophrenia. *Archives of General Psychiatry* **44**, 907–912.

Waddington, J.L., O'Callaghan, E., Larkin, C. & Kinsella, A. (1993) Cognitive dysfunction in schizophrenia: organic vulnerability factor or state marker for tardive dyskinesia? *Brain and Cognition* **23**, 56–70.

Wang, Y., Turnbull, I., Calne, S., Stoessl, A. & Calne, D. (1997) Pallidotomy for tardive diskinesia. *Lancet* **349**, 777–778.

Wang P.S., Schneeweiss S., Avorn J. et al. (2005) Risk of death in elderly users of conventional vs. atypical antipsychotic medications. *New England Journal of Medicine* **353**, 2335–2341.

Weetman, J., Anderson, I., Gregory, R. & Gill, S. (1997) Bilateral posteroventral pallidotomy for severe antipsychotic induced tardive dyskinesia and dystonia [letter]. *Journal of Neurology, Neurosurgery, and Psychiatry* **63**, 554–556.

Weiden, P.J., Mann, J.J., Haas, G., Mattson, M. & Frances, A. (1987) Clinical non-recognition of neuroleptic-induced movement disorders: a cautionary study. *American Journal of Psychiatry* **144**, 1148–1153.

Weller, M. (1992) NMS and lethal catatonia. *Journal of Clinical Psychiatry* **53**, 294.

White, D.A.C. (1992) Catatonia and the neuroleptic malignant syndrome: a single entity? *British Journal of Psychiatry* **161**, 558–560.

White, D.A.C. & Robins, A.H. (1991) Catatonia: harbinger of the neuroleptic syndrome. *British Journal of Psychiatry* **158**, 419–421.

Youssef, H. & Waddington, J. (1987) Mortality and morbidity in tardive dyskinesia: association in chronic schizophrenia. *Acta Psychiatrica Scandinavica* **75**, 74–77.

Zoleptil Summary of Product Characteristics (2002) Newbury: Orion Pharma (UK) Ltd.

CHAPTER 28

Metabolic adverse effects associated with antipsychotic medications

John W. Newcomer[1] and Stefan Leucht[2]

[1]Washington University School of Medicine, Department of Psychiatry, St Louis, MO, USA
[2]Department of Psychiatry and Psychotherapy, Technische Universität München, Munich, Germany

Introduction

Antipsychotic medications offer essential benefits for individuals with schizophrenia, as discussed in other chapters. However, they can also induce increases in body weight and adiposity, decreases in insulin sensitivity, and adverse changes in plasma lipids. Drugs with the largest adverse metabolic effects produce measurable increases in risk for Type 2 diabetes mellitus and cardiovascular disease [CVD; i.e., coronary heart disease (CHD), cerebrovascular disease, and peripheral vascular disease; Newcomer, 2005b]. Metabolic effects (e.g., on diabetes risk) are also seen with some drugs in other therapeutic classes (e.g., thiazide diuretics, beta-blockers, antidepressants; Yood *et al.*, 2009; Andersohn *et al.*, 2009), but the action of antipsychotics is notable because patients with schizophrenia often take the drugs for decades, and because the magnitude of the adverse effects can be greater.

In general, patients with schizophrenia have elevated rates of medical comorbidity from a variety of conditions

(Leucht *et al.*, 2007), including CVD and Type 2 diabetes (Casey *et al.*, 2004), with significant reductions in life-expectancy due primarily to premature CHD (Colton & Manderscheid, 2006). While there has been speculation, based on limited evidence, that genetic factors may play a role in the increased risk (Dynes, 1969; Mukherjee *et al.*, 1989; Cheta *et al.*, 1990; Lamberti *et al.*, 2003; Shiloah *et al.*, 2003), it is likely that environmental factors such as reduced activity, poor nutrition, reduced access to quality prevention efforts and medical care, as well as the adverse cardiometabolic effects of medications used to treat schizophrenia may all play a major role (Newcomer & Hennekens, 2007). Primary and secondary prevention targeting risk factors for these conditions is particularly important in the population with schizophrenia, but major limitations in the effectiveness of such prevention efforts are now well documented, as discussed below. Efforts are currently underway in many countries to address this problem (American Diabetes Association, 2004; De Hert *et al.*, 2009; Institute of Medicine, 2005; NASMHPD Medical Directors Council, 2006; Fleischhacker *et al.*, 2008). This chapter provides a review of the increased prevalence of CVD, diabetes, and other major medical conditions in patients with schizophrenia, explains the role of cardiovascular and metabolic risk factors in contributing to their development, and provides an overview of the range of evidence indicating that antipsychotic medications can induce adverse cardiometabolic effects. It also highlights the importance of recommended prevention approaches and summarizes emerging research on the effects of recent warnings and guidelines on prevention efforts in this population.

Morbidity and mortality in schizophrenia

The life-expectancy of patients with schizophrenia and other major mental disorders is substantially reduced compared with the general population (Brown, 1997; Lutterman *et al.*, 2003; Colton & Manderscheid, 2006; Saha *et al.*, 2007; Tiihonen *et al.*, 2009, see also Chapters 7 and 31). One study indicated that patients with schizophrenia had a 20% shorter life-expectancy compared with the general population (Harris & Barraclough, 1998). A more recent US study indicated even greater reductions in life-expectancy (Colton & Manderscheid, 2006). It examined age-adjusted death rates, standardized mortality ratios, and years of potential life lost for mental health patients in the public sector, compared with the general population within several US states over a period of several years. For those states in which both inpatient and outpatient data were available, allowing appropriate comparisons, the median number of potential years of life lost in these patients with major mental illness ranged from 25 to 30 years (Newcomer & Hennekens, 2007; Druss & Bornemann, 2010).

The causes of this premature mortality have varied, largely as a function of the "developed" *versus* "developing" public health status of the countries of origin of the studies (Leucht *et al.*, 2007). Early reports indicate increased mortality from various medical conditions, including infectious diseases and common mortality from "unnatural causes" (accidents, suicide, etc.). More recent reports indicate that suicide, sudden death, pulmonary disease, stroke, and diabetes continue to account for many deaths, but CVD has emerged as the leading contemporary cause of the excess mortality (Allebeck, 1989; Brown *et al.*, 2000; Lutterman *et al.*, 2003; Colton & Manderscheid, 2006; Leucht *et al.*, 2007). While this leading role is similar to the ranking of CVD in the general population in virtually all developed nations, the observation of substantially earlier CVD-related death in the mentally ill is important for clinicians, researchers, and policy-makers (Newcomer & Hennekens, 2007; Druss & Bornemann, 2010).

Leucht *et al.* (2007) conducted a careful survey of the literature regarding morbidity, rather than mortality, in patients with schizophrenia. They noted that there are high quality population-based studies of the association between schizophrenia and conditions like cancer or CVD, but limited data for some other diseases. With respect to CVD,

the 19 studies reviewed (e.g., Hennessy *et al.*, 2002; Cohn *et al.*, 2004; Curkendall *et al.*, 2004; Kilbourne *et al.*, 2005; Goff *et al.*, 2005; McDermott *et al.*, 2005) confirmed that cardiovascular conditions are more frequent in schizophrenia compared to control populations. Some studies have reported that hypertension is less frequent in individuals with schizophrenia (e.g., Silver *et al.*, 1990), perhaps explained by the blood-pressure-lowering effects of some antipsychotic drugs. Any such benefits are likely offset by the high rates of smoking (de Leon & Diaz, 2005), obesity (Allison *et al.*, 1999a), diabetes (Dixon *et al.*, 2000), dyslipidemia (Heiskanen *et al.*, 2003), and lack of exercise (Daumit *et al.*, 2005), all of which may contribute to the higher rates of cardiovascular morbidity in schizophrenia.

Risk factors

Underlying their increased morbidity and premature mortality from CVD and diabetes, individuals with major mental disorders like schizophrenia have an increased prevalence of modifiable risk factors such as obesity, dyslipidemia, hyperglycemia, and smoking (Newcomer & Hennekens, 2007). The increased prevalence is explained in large part by relative failures in primary and secondary prevention, as discussed below (Newcomer & Hennekens, 2007). These modifiable "cardiometabolic" risk factors can all lead to reduced insulin sensitivity, an effect associated with risk for both CVD and diabetes. The American Diabetes Association (ADA) recently launched the Cardiometabolic Risk Initiative, an educational effort to improve awareness in this area (see diabetes.org/CMR).

A particularly important contributor to excess morbidity and mortality is excess adiposity (American Heart Association, 2006; Despres *et al.*, 2008), which can be estimated using body mass index [BMI; weight in $kg/(height in m)^2$]. Increasing BMI (>25) is associated with increasing risk of morbidity and mortality (Calle *et al.*, 1999). Of note, not all adipose tissue deposits confer the same degree of metabolic risk; increases in visceral abdominal adiposity are especially associated with decreases in insulin sensitivity (Banerji *et al.*, 1997; Despres *et al.*, 2008). Importantly, becoming overweight or obese earlier in life leads to more substantial reductions in life-expectancy (Fontaine *et al.*, 2003), but even obesity and weight gain later in life is associated with an increased risk of diabetes (Biggs *et al.*, 2010).

Obesity is up to twice as prevalent in individuals with mental illnesses such as schizophrenia, in comparison to the general population (Allison *et al.*, 1999b; 2009; Susce *et al.*, 2005). Numerous studies illustrate this. For example, in a study of 102 Scottish patients with schizophrenia, 73% were overweight, including 86% of the women (McCreadie, 2003). Of 240 Canadian patients with schizophrenia or schizoaffective disorder, 31% of the men and 43% of the women were obese (Cohn *et al.*, 2004). A study of 214 psychiatric inpatients with schizophrenia indicated that the rate of obesity was 36% in men and 75% in women *versus* 17% and 22%, respectively, in the reference population (Cormac *et al.*, 2005).

Obesity and weight gain are major risk factors for insulin resistance, a state of reduced tissue sensitivity to insulin actions that increases risk for Type 2 diabetes (Pi-Sunyer, 1993). Insulin resistance is associated with impaired glucose homeostasis, an atherogenic dyslipidemia with increased fasting plasma triglyceride and more highly oxidized low-density lipoprotein (LDL) particles, increased blood pressure, and prothrombotic and proinflammatory states, all of which are associated with an increased risk for CVD and diabetes (Casey *et al.*, 2004; Grundy, 2002; Willett *et al.*, 1999). Increases in insulin resistance and free fatty acid levels may be detected clinically as an increase in fasting plasma triglyceride levels, and there has been recent interest in the use of the latter as a useful indicator of insulin resistance. About 50% of overweight or obese individuals (BMI ≥ 25) have clinically significant insulin resistance, rising to 70% in those who additionally have fasting plasma triglyceride levels greater than 130 mg/dL (McLaughlin *et al.*, 2003). As discussed below, substantial adverse effects on this lipid fraction are seen during treatment with some but not all agents.

As an example of public health efforts in this area, the US National Cholesterol Education Program, Adult Treatment Panel III (ATP III) guidelines (National Cholesterol Education Program, 2002) considers a patient with any three of the following to have the "metabolic syndrome", a constellation of insulin resistance-related risk factors for Type 2 diabetes (Lorenzo *et al.*, 2003) and CVD (Sattar *et al.*, 2003): (1) obesity (defined as a waist circumference >102 cm for men, 88 cm for women); (2) low levels of high-density lipoprotein (HDL) cholesterol (<40 mg/dL for men, 50 mg/dL for women); (3) high triglyceride levels (≥150 mg/dL); (4) elevated blood pressure (≥130 mmHg systolic or 85 mmHg diastolic); and (5) increased fasting blood glucose levels (≥100 mg/dL). However, the metabolic syndrome construct has been criticized from the public health perspective as suggesting that individuals with fewer than three criteria are somehow not worthy of attention, when each one of the criteria is itself an important risk factor that may require intervention (Kahn *et al.*, 2005).

Reductions in insulin sensitivity, from obesity and other factors, can initially be compensated for by increases in pancreatic beta-cell secretion of insulin, as well as reductions in insulin clearance. However, in individuals at risk for diabetes, this compensation is time limited, with progressive reductions in insulin secretory capacity and increases in plasma glucose beginning usually within a decade of the onset of significant insulin resistance. Failures in glucose homeostasis are usually initially manifested by

reductions in glucose tolerance and eventually by elevations in fasting plasma glucose. Data from the Framingham Heart Study can be used to estimate the number of excess cases of diabetes that can be anticipated over a 10-year period based on initial BMI and the magnitude of weight gain over the observation period (Fontaine *et al.*, 2001). A population who at baseline has a BMI less than 23 and then gains, for example, 22 lb (9.25 kg), will develop 610 excess cases of diabetes per 100 000 people. Those with baseline BMIs between 23 and 27 and the same weight gain develop 1403 excess cases, and those with a baseline BMI greater than 27 develop 3166 excess cases. The last group is probably most representative of Western patients with schizophrenia who take antipsychotics, many of whom are overweight or obese at the start of a treatment trial.

Long-term risks of hyperglycemia and diabetes include microvascular disease (retinopathy, nephropathy, and neuropathies) and macrovascular or atherosclerosis-related CVD. Diabetes is considered a CVD "risk equivalent" condition from a public health perspective, meaning that having diabetes is equivalent to having established CVD (e.g., a prior myocardial infarction), with respect to predicting risk for subsequent myocardial infarction (Haffner *et al.*, 1998). Diabetes is also associated with a risk of short-term complications, including diabetic ketoacidosis (DKA) and non-ketotic hyperosmolar states (Harris, 2000; American Diabetes Association, 2003). The mortality risk of DKA is approximately 2% in optimal clinical settings, rising as high as 20% in the elderly, with mortality risk increasing with age, intercurrent illness, and delay in the initiation of insulin therapy (Koller *et al.*, 2001a).

Impact of reduced primary and secondary prevention

The ideal public health approach to prevention is to establish a screening and intervention plan for the overall population, and then to target high-risk subpopulations with additional primary and secondary prevention efforts. However, patients with schizophrenia are less, not more, likely to receive screening and preventative measure. Patients have less access to high-quality general medical care, receive less preventative care and fewer medications for the treatment of risk factors, and have decreased adherence to medical pharmacotherapies (Newcomer & Hennekens, 2007). A review of community-based mental healthcare of patients with schizophrenia and other psychiatric disorders found significant limitations in their medical treatment (Kohn *et al.*, 2004). The reduced availability of healthcare services, combined with socioeconomic factors that make it difficult for some patients to work, retain healthcare insurance, and pursue care, complicate the identification and treatment of comorbid medical conditions. In addition, psychiatrists may neglect physical health issues in their patients, and physicians may pay less attention to patients with a psychiatric history. In the US, for example, individuals with schizophrenia are less likely to be screened, diagnosed or treated for dyslipidemia, hyperglycemia, and hypertension than the general population (Newcomer & Hennekens, 2007). An important large study of elderly Medicare patients following acute myocardial infarctions indicated that patients with mental disorders were less likely than those without to subsequently receive appropriate treatments like reperfusion, aspirin, beta-blockers, or angiotensin-converting enzyme (ACE) inhibitors; the presence of any mental disorder was associated with a 19% increased risk of mortality within a year, with a 34% increase in those with schizophrenia (Druss et al., 2001). In this context, the potential adverse metabolic effects of treatment can be challenging to manage. It is important therefore, from the primary prevention perspective, to be well aware of potential metabolic effects that can be associated with antipsychotic treatment. Evidence is reviewed below that antipsychotic drugs can increase risk for weight gain, insulin resistance, diabetes, and dyslipidemia.

Weight gain during antipsychotic treatment

Treatment with antipsychotic medication can cause clinically significant weight gain, which is a key risk factor for insulin resistance that in turn increases risk for diabetes (Pi-Sunyer, 1993). While it has been suggested that this relationship might not apply to the weight gain caused by antipsychotic treatment (Boehm et al., 2004), this hypothesis would seem to depend on the existence of unknown protective factors in patients with schizophrenia that might block the adverse effects of adiposity. Given clear evidence for the higher prevalence of diabetes in psychiatric populations (Mukherjee et al., 1996; Brown, 1997; Dixon et al., 2000; Okamura et al., 2000; Mokdad et al., 2001; Haupt & Newcomer, 2002; Regenold et al., 2002; Ryan et al., 2003), it seems rather unlikely that such protective factors are operational. In the absence of evidence to the contrary, it is prudent to assume that antipsychotic-induced weight gain will be associated with the same adverse physiological effects established in the general population.

Short-term studies

A review of placebo-controlled trials and head-to-head comparisons indicates that the relative incidence and magnitude of weight gain is not equal among individual antipsychotic medications (Newcomer, 2005b). Short-term treatment with various agents has been reported to produce increases in body weight ranging from less than 1 kg to more than 4 kg (Allison et al., 1999a,c; Leucht et al., 2004).

This spectrum of effect on body weight can be observed within both the first- and second-generations of antipsychotic drugs (FGAs and SGAs), with lower and higher risk agents identifiable in both groups. Medications at the lower end of the risk spectrum include high-potency FGAs (e.g., haloperidol and fluphenazine) and some SGAs (e.g., ziprasidone and aripiprazole); those at the higher end of the risk spectrum include low-potency FGAs (e.g., chlorpromazine) and SGAs (e.g., olanzapine and clozapine). In terms of the biological basis of this variability, the vast majority of the variance between individual medications is attributed to their antagonism of H_1 receptors (Kroeze et al., 2003) and downstream effects on hypothalamic H_1 signalling (Kim et al., 2007), with additional contributions from other receptors (e.g., serotonin 2C receptors) and from pharmacogenetic factors (Harrison, 2005; Nasrallah, 2008; Adkins et al., 2010).

The results of prospective randomized controlled trials (RCTs) comparing antipsychotic drugs have been generally consistent with the early estimates that came from pivotal placebo-controlled trials, particularly with respect to preserving the rank order of weight gain risk. For example, a 6-week study comparing olanzapine and ziprasidone therapy in 269 inpatients with acute exacerbations of schizophrenia or schizoaffective disorder reported a median body weight increase of 3.3 kg with olanzapine compared with 0.5 kg with ziprasidone, along with a significantly higher median body weight in the olanzapine group at endpoint (p < 0.0001; Glick et al., 2001). Cutler et al. (2008) conducted a 4-week RCT comparing iloperidone (n = 295), ziprasidone (n = 149), and placebo (n = 149). The mean weight changes were 2.8 kg, 1.1 kg, and 0.5 kg, respectively. In a 4-week RCT of ziprasidone (n = 127) at an average dose of 149 mg/day and aripiprazole (n = 129) at 20 mg/day, Zimbroff et al. (2007) found a mean weight change of 0.45 kg with both drugs. In a 6-week study, Davidson et al. (2007) compared placebo, paliperidone (3, 6 or 9 mg/day), and olanzapine (10 mg/day). The observed change in weight (mean, with standard deviation in parentheses) was −0.8 (4.2) kg for placebo, 0.6 (2.8) kg, 1.5 (3.1) kg, and 1.9 (3.6) kg for paliperidone 3 mg, 6 mg, and 9 mg, respectively, and 2.2 (3.9) kg for olanzapine. Similarly, Kane et al. (2007) reported on a 6–week, RCT comparing paliperidone 6, 9 or 12 mg/day with olanzapine 10 mg/day or placebo (n = 122–129 per group). The observed mean change in weight for the respective arms was 0.2 (2.4) kg, 0.6 (2.7) kg, 0.9 (3.3) kg, 1.3 (2.8) kg, and −0.7 (2.4) kg. As a final example of another recent short-term study, demonstrating the variability that can be observed across different study cohorts, Marder et al. (2007) reported another 6-week RCT comparing paliperidone (6 or 12 mg/day), olanzapine (10 mg/ day), and placebo (n = 110–112 per group). The weight change in the respective groups was 1.0 (3.9) kg, 2.0 (3.5) kg, 2.7 (4.4) kg, and 0.4 (3.6) kg.

Long-term studies

While short-term treatment studies are more common and short-term weight gain is therefore better quantified, the long-term effects of antipsychotic drugs on weight are more relevant to clinical practice in the treatment of schizophrenia (Newcomer, 2005b). Though the rank order of weight gain effects is preserved in longer-term studies, weight gain is generally greater overall, and those medications with the largest effects generally take longer to arrive at their maximum effect. The net result is a greater separation between mean weight changes from baseline observed over longer periods of observation on lower- *versus* higher-risk drugs. Pooling multiple doses assessed in clinical trials programs shows weight gains of about 1 kg for, aripiprazole (Marder *et al.*, 2003; Kasper *et al.*, 2003; Pigott *et al.*, 2003; McQuade *et al.*, 2003) and ziprasidone (Allison *et al.*, 1999a; Daniel *et al.*, 2004; Hirsch *et al.*, 2002); 1.5 kg for amisulpride (Leucht *et al.*, 2004); 1.8 kg for paliperidone (Kramer *et al.*, 2007); 2–3 kg for quetiapine and risperidone (Jones *et al.*, 2000; Csernansky *et al.*, 2002); and greater than 6 kg for olanzapine (Nemeroff, 1997; Kinon, 1998).

Other long-term studies comparing antipsychotic drugs head to head have helped to estimate the range of potential effects on weight (examples are summarized in Table 28.1). In addition, and deserving special mention, is the NIMH Clinical Antipsychotic Trials of Intervention Effectiveness (CATIE; see Chapter 25), designed to assess the effectiveness of the olanzapine, quetiapine, risperidone, ziprasidone, and the FGA perphenazine. The trial included 1493 patients with schizophrenia, and the secondary outcome measures included quantification of weight gain and changes in plasma glucose and lipids, with comparisons of estimated monthly changes in body weight made in all three phases of the trial (Lieberman *et al.*, 2005; Stroup *et al.*, 2006, 2009). The results of the main trial (Phase I)

provided metabolic results consistent with the other evidence in this area (see above; Lieberman *et al.*, 2005): patients in the olanzapine group gained more weight than patients in any of the other assigned treatment groups, with a mean increase of 0.9 kg/month. Overall, 30% of patients in the olanzapine group gained 7% or more of their baseline body weight (*vs.* 7–16% in the other groups; p < 0.001). In all three phases of the study, patients assigned to olanzapine gained weight. In Phase III, patients who chose clozapine gained the most weight, followed by those given olanzapine (Stroup *et al.*, 2009).

A general principle observed in clinical trials and in clinical practice is that while initial courses of treatment are almost always associated with weight gain of some magnitude, chronically-treated patients do not always gain weight during a new course of treatment. Indeed, if treatment with a medication that generally produces less weight gain is used after a course of treatment with a medication that generally produces more, mean reductions in weight may occur. For example, in the CATIE Phase I analysis, perphenazine and ziprasidone treatment yielded mean decreases in weight per month of treatment, likely related to the high frequency of prior treatment with olanzapine in the cohort of patients entering the trial. The greatest monthly weight losses in CATIE were associated with aripiprazole and ziprasidone, medications chosen in Phase III by patients with the highest BMI.

Factors affecting the magnitude of weight gain with a given antipsychotic drug

Limited evidence supports a possible dose-dependence for the weight gain. In a review of AstraZeneca's pooled registration trial database for quetiapine (Brecher *et al.*, 2007), doses less than 200 mg/day were generally associated with approximately half the weight gain seen at higher doses. A

Table 28.1 Long-term studies comparing weight gain between antipsychotic drugs.

Study	Duration	Drugs studied (sample size)	Weight gain in kg (SD)
Mortimer *et al.* (2004)	6 months	AMI (189), OLZ (188) OLZ > AMI, p < 0.01	OLZ 3.9; AMI 1.6
Hardy *et al.* (2003)/ Breier *et al.* (2005)	28 weeks	OLZ (277), ZIP (271) OLZ > ZIP, p < 0.001	OLZ 3.1 (6.9); ZIP −1.1 (4.7); 35% in OLZ group gained >7% *vs.* 5% on ZIP
Kinon *et al.* (2006)	24 weeks	OLZ (202), ZIP (192) OLZ > ZIP, p < 0.05	OLZ 2.5 (1.9); ZIP −1.6 (4.2)
Kane *et al.* (2008)	46 weeks	ILO (371), HAL (118)	ILO 3.8 (7.0); HAL 2.3 (6.2)
Kahn *et al.* (2008)	1 year	HAL (103), AMI (104), OLZ (105) QUE (104), ZIP (82) Overall p < 0.0001	HAL 7.3 (1.8); AMI 9.7 (1.7); OLZ 13.9 (1.7); QUE 10.5 (1.8); ZIP 4.8 (1.9)
Bushe *et al.* (2010)	6 months	OLZ (171), QUE (175) NS (p = 0.18)	OLZ 1.0 (5.8); QUE 0.4 (4.7); 19% in OLZ group gained >7% *vs.* 13% on QUE

AMI, amisulpride; HAL, haloperidol; ILO, iloperidone; OLZ, olanzapine; QUE, quetiapine; ZIP, ziprasidone.

report by Kinon *et al.* (2008) concerned an 8–week, double-blind study comparing olanzapine at 10, 20 or 40 mg/day in patients with schizophrenia or schizoaffective disorder; the change in weight (±SD) for 10 mg/day was 1.9 (3.5) kg, for 20 mg/day was 2.3 (4.2) kg, and for 40 mg/day was 3.0 (4) kg. Similar trends for paliperidone were evident in the short-term studies summarized above.

Important individual factors that increase the magnitude of weight gain, in both short- and longer-term trials, are the baseline level of adiposity and the amount of previous treatment exposure to weight gain-inducing medications. Lean drug-naïve patient populations (i.e., usually first episode) generally demonstrate greatest weight gain. Perez-Iglesias *et al.* (2007) reported on an open-label, 12-week study in drug-naïve first-episode psychosis, with patients receiving haloperidol (n = 40), olanzapine (n = 41) or risperidone (n = 47). The mean changes in weight in the three groups were 3.8 (4.9) kg, 7.5 (5.1) kg, and 5.6 (4.5) kg, respectively (cf. the data in the comparable trials of mostly chronic patients summarized above). Similarly, Saddichha *et al.* (2008) reported on a 6-week trial in drug-naïve patients with schizophrenia, with randomization to olanzapine (n = 35), risperidone (n = 33) or haloperidol (n = 31), and an untreated healthy control group also followed up (n = 51). Mean weight changes were 5 kg on olanzapine, 4.2 kg on risperidone, 2.4 kg on haloperidol, and 0.1 kg in the controls. In longer-term exposures, the vulnerability of treatment-naïve patients becomes more evident. For example, haloperidol produced a mean increase of 4 kg in a large study of first-episode patients over a year, with a 15 kg mean increase with olanzapine (Zipursky *et al.*, 2005). A larger effect on body weight during initial exposures to medications was also noted in the Comparison of Antipsychotics in the First Episode of Schizophrenia study (CAFÉ; McEvoy *et al.*, 2007), where patients needing an initial or early course of antipsychotic treatment were randomized to olanzapine, quetiapine or risperidone. These agents, typically associated with 2–3 kg mean increases in body weight over 52 weeks in previous reports from chronically-treated samples (Brecher *et al.*, 2007), produced mean increases of 6 kg at 52 weeks in CAFÉ.

Finally, a small but evolving literature of randomized trials in children with schizophrenia indicates a similar pattern of effects of antipsychotic treatment on body weight (Correll *et al.*, 2009). There is some indication of greater adverse weight changes, but this is consistent with the larger effects seen in first-episode adults. In a 12-week, double-blind study of children with treatment-refractory schizophrenia or schizoaffective disorder, weight gain was 4.5 kg in those randomized to clozapine (n = 18) and 3.6 kg with olanzapine (n = 21; Kumra *et al.*, 2008). Sikich *et al.* (2008) reported results of an 8-week RCT of early-onset schizophrenia, testing the effects of molindone (n = 40), olanzapine (n = 35), and risperidone (n = 41). The weight changes (±SD) in the respective groups were 0.3 (2.9) kg, 6.1 (3.6) kg, and 3.6 (4.0) kg.

Metabolic effects of antipsychotic treatment

Treatment with some antipsychotic medications is associated with an increased risk for insulin resistance, hyperglycemia, and Type 2 diabetes, compared with no treatment or treatment with alternative antipsychotics (Koro *et al.*, 2002b; Newcomer, 2005b; Casey *et al.*, 2004; Yood *et al.*, 2009). Interpretation of this literature has been complicated by reports that patients with major mental disorders such as schizophrenia have an increased prevalence of abnormalities in glucose regulation (e.g., insulin resistance), initially observed in the preneuroleptic era (e.g., Kasanin, 1926). However, early and even many contemporary studies have not controlled for age, ethnicity, diet, adiposity, pre-existing hyperglycemia or dyslipidemia.

The interaction between schizophrenia and diabetes is complex, and remains incompletely understood (Bushe & Holt, 2004; Peet, 2004), but parsimony suggests that the well-documented prevalence of a number of risk factors in this population may fully explain the observed increase in disease prevalence. Relevant risk factors include poverty, urbanization, crowding, psychological stress, obesity, as well as hypothesized but so far unidentified genetic factors (Bushe & Holt, 2004; Haupt & Newcomer, 2002; Newcomer, 2005a). Limited data from drug-naïve acutely ill patients with schizophrenia suggest that increases in plasma cortisol related to increased activation of the hypothalamic–pituitary–adrenal (HPA) axis and the sympathetic nervous system may contribute to hyperglycemia (Ryan & Thakore, 2002; Ryan *et al.*, 2003). However, the finding of increased adiposity or glucoregulatory impairments in unmedicated patients is not consistently observed (Reynolds, 2006). HPA activation is only variably associated with schizophrenia (Newcomer *et al.*, 2002), and HPA activity and plasma cortisol levels are reduced rather than increased by antipsychotic treatment. Therefore, samples like the one studied by Ryan and colleagues may overestimate the degree of insulin resistance and hyperglycemia that persists past the acute psychotic episode. In addition, "matching" groups on measures such as waist circumference or BMI may not accurately capture true group differences in total or intra-abdominal adiposity, so higher levels of unmeasured adiposity could explain observed differences in laboratory parameters. Indeed, the same research group has also reported increases in intra-abdominal fat in drug-naïve patients, in contrast to other larger samples that have reported no differences (Ryan *et al.*, 2004; Arranz *et al.*, 2004; Zhang *et al.*, 2004). Further, the unmedicated patient sample in which hyperglycemia was observed had a longer duration of illness and was older than most reported samples of first-episode patients, suggesting a possible explanation for why an increase in metabolic risk prior to treatment has not been detected in other untreated first-episode samples (Reynolds, 2006). If there is a true predisposition of patients with schizophrenia to diabetes, then familial, possibly genetic but likely shared environmental, factors may play a role, as one report found that 18–19% of individuals with schizophrenia had a family history of Type 2 diabetes mellitus (Dixon *et al.*, 2000). However, the dominant thesis continues to be that the increased prevalence of diabetes in schizophrenia can be fully explained by the elevated prevalence of overweight and obesity, reductions in the overall level of physical fitness, and other secondary effects related to lifestyle (Allison *et al.*, 1999a; Newcomer, 2005b; Newcomer & Hennekens, 2007).

We now review the evidence associating certain antipsychotic medications with adverse metabolic events. The evidence comes from a range of sources, including case reports and uncontrolled prospective observational studies, retrospective database analyses, and controlled experimental studies including RCTs (Casey *et al.*, 2004; Newcomer, 2005b). These three types of study are considered in turn.

Case reports and uncontrolled observational studies

Case reports of adverse effects on glucose and lipid metabolism have been most frequently associated with clozapine and olanzapine, followed by risperidone and quetiapine (Newcomer *et al.*, 2005; American Diabetes Association, 2004a; Koller *et al.*, 2001b; 2003, 2004; Koller & Doraiswamy, 2002), with much sparser data for ziprasidone, amisulpride, or aripiprazole (Casey *et al.*, 2004; American Diabetes Association, 2004; Haupt & Newcomer, 2001; Yang & McNeely, 2002).

The US Food and Drug Administration (FDA) MedWatch Drug Surveillance System has provided data on the numbers of cases of various metabolic complications associated with antipsychotic drugs. For clozapine, a case series (for the period 1990–2001) identified 384 cases of hyperglycaemia, accompanied by metabolic acidosis or ketosis in 80 cases, 73 of which were new-onset diabetes. There were 25 deaths during hyperglycemic episodes; acidosis or ketosis was reported in 16 of these (Koller *et al.*, 2001b). For olanzapine, 237 cases of diabetes or hyperglycemia were reported (1994–2001; Koller & Doraiswamy, 2002), with metabolic acidosis or ketosis in 80 cases. The proportion of fatalities among the cases of DKA was high (11.3%) relative to the optimal outcome reported in non-psychiatric samples (e.g., 3–5%). In an addendum to the paper, the authors reported an additional 52 cases of hyperglycemia, including 20 with DKA and 10 deaths, identified by extending the MedWatch search to February 2002. For risperidone (1993–2002), there were 131 cases of diabetes or hypergly-

cemia, with metabolic acidosis or ketosis in 26 patients, mostly in those with new-onset diabetes. There were four deaths, with three associated with acidosis or ketosis (Koller *et al.*, 2003). Finally, for quetiapine, 46 cases of diabetes or hyperglycemia, with 21 cases of metabolic acidosis or ketosis, and 11 deaths were identified (1997–2002); extending the search until November 2003, identified an additional 23 cases of diabetes, with eight associated with acidosis or ketosis, two reports of pancreatitis, and three deaths.

There have been few case reports of DKA associated with aripiprazole, and none for amisulpride or ziprasidone with DKA (Church *et al.*, 2005), although one case of rhabdomyolysis, hyperglycemia, and pancreatitis has been associated with the latter (Yang & McNeely, 2002).

Importantly, the MedWatch data indicate that approximately 25% of cases of diabetes and hyperglycemia occurred in the absence of substantial weight gain or obesity, and as many as half of cases involved individuals with no reported family history of diabetes. Thus, an absence of weight gain or family history in no way precludes the occurrence of metabolic complications with antipsychotic drugs, nor the need for monitoring. The MedWatch analyses also suggested that most new-onset cases of diabetes occurred within the first 6 months after initiation of treatment, although this may be explained by a reporting bias. In general, case reports can be difficult to interpret due to the lack of control data, such as the number of treated patients who did not experience the event, as well as the high likelihood of reporting bias.

While some reviewers have suggested that the relatively high rates of DKA in the setting of "new-onset" diabetes in these case series should be interpreted as evidence that antipsychotics can adversely impact pancreatic beta-cell function, this conclusion is not supported by available evidence. DKA not uncommonly occurs in advanced cases of Type 2 diabetes (Newton & Raskin, 2004) when the remaining capacity for insulin secretion is so limited that even the small amounts needed to shut off lipolysis can no longer be secreted. The presentation of patients to an emergency room in DKA with new-onset diabetes on antipsychotic treatment was reviewed in a case series (Henderson *et al.*, 2007). All had glycated hemoglobin (HbA$_{1c}$) values greater than 10%, suggesting that they may have had a prolonged period of undiagnosed diabetes. Further controlled study results, detailed below, support the conclusion that some antipsychotic treatment conditions can indeed increase risk for incident diabetes, or a worsening of pre-existing diabetes, but this appears to occur primarily through reductions in insulin sensitivity rather than through any large changes in insulin secretion.

The types of study described in this section are difficult to interpret due to the lack of control data, such as the number of treated patients who did *not* experience the event, as well as the high likelihood of reporting bias, notably underreporting. For example, only 1–10% of adverse events are reported to MedWatch. With respect to the number of patients who had to be exposed to a given drug in order to observe the reported adverse events, the higher number of adverse events reported for clozapine and olanzapine in comparison with risperidone cannot be explained by a larger number of patient-years of drug exposure with either of the former agents.

Controlled observational database studies

Analyses of diabetes risks

Consistent with the above data, pharmacoepidemiological studies in healthcare databases suggest an increased risk for diabetes, with a variable pattern of differential risk across individual medications in the different studies, but relatively consistent evidence of increased risk associated with treatment with clozapine and olanzapine (Newcomer, 2005b). These observational analyses have used large administrative or health plan databases to test the association between treatment with specific antipsychotic medications and the prevalence or incidence of diabetes (Lund et al., 2001; Caro et al., 2002; Gianfrancesco et al., 2002, 2003; Koro et al., 2002b; Sernyak et al., 2002; Wang et al., 2002; Buse et al., 2003; Fuller et al., 2003; Citrome et al., 2004; Lambert et al., 2005b; Leslie & Rosenheck, 2004; Sumiyoshi et al., 2004; Yood et al., 2009). The approach taken by these studies is to measure the association within a database between the use of specific antipsychotic medications and the presence of one or more surrogate indicators of diabetes [e.g., diagnostic codes or prescription of an antidiabetic medication). The majority of these studies suggest that the drugs associated with greater weight gain are also associated with an increased risk of diabetes compared to either no treatment or to antipsychotics associated with less weight gain; a minority have detected no difference in risk for diabetes between medications or a non-specific increase in diabetes risk for all SGA-treated groups compared with one or more controls. However, although explicit tests of the relationship between diabetes risk and weight gain are not possible in these studies, none of the reports provides any compelling evidence to indicate the opposite relationship, i.e., that medications with greater weight-gain potential are associated with a *lower* risk for diabetes. This is consistent with well-established evidence that a substantial increase in mean body weight in any population, especially in cohorts that are already overweight (i.e., already more likely to be insulin resistant), is associated with an increased risk of diabetes (Mokdad et al., 1999, 2001; Fontaine et al., 2001).

The use of medical claims databases has a number of methodological limitations, including lack of diagnostic verification, uncertainty whether treatments were actually received, high rates of polypharmacy, and limited if any knowledge of earlier treatment conditions that may have affected adiposity and insulin resistance extant during the period of study. Most importantly, these studies lack direct measures of metabolism, relying on surrogate markers which require the successful diagnosis of diabetes in the study sample; however, underdiagnosis of diabetes is common. The ADA has estimated that approximately one-third of cases of diabetes were undiagnosed in the US during the period when many of these studies were run (Harris et al., 1998). Given that these database studies may involve samples that underestimate the prevalence of diabetes, and that the hypothesized difference in prevalence rates across treatment conditions may be less than the prevalence of undiagnosed diabetes, this type of retrospective database analysis may face serious signal-to-noise challenges. This problem and others may explain some of the variability in studies of this kind.

To clarify the evidence from these large datasets, Newcomer (2005b) conducted a meta-analytic review to quantify the relationship between different antipsychotic treatments and risk for diabetes, for all relevant publications from 1990 to 2004. Fourteen primary studies were analyzed, including 11 retrospective cohorts (n = 232 871 patients) and five case–control analyses (n = 4084). The study settings were primarily healthcare plans (Medicaid, Blue Cross/Blue Shield, Veterans Affairs, etc.). Six studies (n = 122 270) selected only patients with a diagnosis of schizophrenia, while 10 studies included patients receiving antipsychotic treatment for various psychoses (n = 150 685). Data were available for clozapine, olanzapine, quetiapine, and risperidone. Random effects models were applied. Meta-analyses on the association of diabetes incidence among patients treated with atypical antipsychotics were performed using conventional antipsychotics or no antipsychotic treatment as the comparator. All estimates were adjusted for a variety of covariates, most commonly treatment duration, age, and gender. The results are shown in Table 28.2, which gives the odds ratios (ORs) and 95% confidence intervals (CIs) for the main comparisons. Clozapine and olanzapine, but not risperidone and quetiap-

Table 28.2 Odds ratios for risk of diabetes: data from a meta-analysis of controlled observational databases (Newcomer et al., 2005).

	Versus typical antipsychotics	Versus no treatment
Clozapine	1.37 (1.25–1.52)	7.44 (1.59–34.75)
Olanzapine	1.26 (1.10–1.46)	2.31 (0.98–5.46)
Risperidone	1.07 (1.00–1.13)	1.20 (0.51–2.85)
Quetiapine	1.22 (0.92–1.61)	1.00 (0.83–1.20)

ine, were found to be significantly associated with an increase in risk of incident diabetes. The meta-analysis confirms that the risk varies between atypical antipsychotics, ranging from increases in diabetes risk relative to multiple comparators to no increase in risk relative to any tested comparator.

The observational database studies reviewed above could not include the more recently approved SGAs, such as ziprasidone and aripiprazole, which have a lower weight gain propensity. This has now been remedied by a recent large observational database study that has provided estimates of relative risk for diabetes for all available SGAs (Yood et al., 2009). This study identified two overlapping cohorts, a simple cohort (all antipsychotic users) and an inception cohort (new users), using data from three US sites (60.4 million covered lives). In the 55 287-member inception cohort, 357 cases of newly-treated diabetes were identified. Compared with current use of typical antipsychotics, there was no increased risk of diabetes among current users of aripiprazole [adjusted hazard ratio (aHR) 0.93; 95% CI 0.50–1.76], quetiapine (aHR 1.04; 95% CI 0.67–1.62), risperidone (aHR 0.85; 95% CI 0.54–1.36), and ziprasidone (aHR 1.05; 95% CI 0.54–2.08). Patients exposed to olanzapine did have an increased risk of diabetes (aHR 1.71; 95% CI 1.12–2.61), and although the effect estimate was imprecise, this was also seen with clozapine (aHR 2.58; 95% CI 0.76–8.80). Results for the simple cohort were similar. The results provide further evidence that some antipsychotics, unlike olanzapine and clozapine, are not associated with a higher relative risk of diabetes compared to other "low-risk" FGAs.

Analyses of dyslipidemia

Lambert et al. (2005a) examined the risk of hyperlipidemia among people with schizophrenia exposed to clozapine, olanzapine, quetiapine or risperidone compared to those exposed to typical agents. A case–control study of MediCal claims data was conducted within a monotherapy inception cohort of 12 weeks' exposure. Hyperlipidemia was defined by diagnostic claim or prescription claim for antilipemic agents, with cases matched on gender and age to patients who did not develop hyperlipidemia. Conditional logistic regression was used, controlling for various confounders. Analyses were repeated using a 24- and 52-week retrospective exposure period. For the 12-week exposure period, olanzapine increased the risk of developing hyperlipidemia compared to other SGAs (OR 1.20; 95% CI 1.08–1.33), whereas clozapine (OR 1.16; 95% CI 0.99–1.37), risperidone (OR 1.00; 95% CI 0.90–1.12), and quetiapine (OR 1.01; 95% CI 0.78–1.32) did not. Tests comparing the four SGAs revealed that the OR for olanzapine was greater than that for risperidone (p = 0.002). Results for 24 and 52 weeks' exposure were similar, except that the OR for clozapine became significant at 24 weeks (OR 1.22; 95% CI 1.03–

1.45). The authors concluded that, compared to conventional antipsychotics, exposure to olanzapine and perhaps clozapine increased the risk of hyperlipidemia.

The UK General Practice Research Database, which includes over 6% of the total UK population, was used to assess the risk of hyperlipidemia with risperidone, olanzapine, and typical antipsychotics (Koro et al., 2002a). Using data collected between June 1997 and September 2000, 1268 cases of hyperlipidemia were identified among 18 309 patients with schizophrenia. The incidence rate for hyperlipidemia among all patients receiving antipsychotic therapy was 17.0 per 1000 person-years. The incidence rate for olanzapine was 26.6 per 1000 person-years (95% CI 17.2–41.2), compared with 18.5 per 1000 person-years for typical antipsychotics (95% CI 17.3–19.8), and 11.5 per 1000 person-years for risperidone (95% CI 7.4–17.8). Patients treated with olanzapine had a 40% increase in the risk of developing hyperlipidemia compared to those treated with typical antipsychotics. Nested case–control analysis, involving 7598 matched control subjects with schizophrenia but no hyperlipidemia, was also used to determine the risk of hyperlipidemia with olanzapine therapy. Logistic regression analysis, adjusted for age, gender, other medications, and disease conditions affecting lipid levels, demonstrated a significant increased risk for olanzapine compared with no antipsychotic therapy (OR 4.6; 95% CI 2.4–8.8; p < 0.001) and with typical antipsychotic treatment (OR 3.4; 95% CI 1.8–6.4; p < 0.001). In contrast, there was no increase in risk of hyperlipidemia for patients treated with risperidone compared with either typical antipsychotic treatment (OR 0.8; 95% CI 0.4–1.5) or no antipsychotic therapy (OR 1.1; 95% CI 0.6–2.1). This result supports the hypothesis that different antipsychotic medications are associated with different levels of risk for adverse effects on lipid metabolism that could in turn increase risk for diabetes or CVD.

Controlled experimental studies (including randomized clinical trials)

The final level of evidence for an association between antipsychotic medication and adverse metabolic outcomes is derived from controlled experimental studies and RCTs, with a relatively large body of data now supporting the key observation that treatments producing the greatest increases in body weight and adiposity are also associated with a consistent pattern of adverse effects on markers of insulin resistance and changes in blood glucose and lipid levels. An increasing proportion of RCTs now include measures of fasting or post-load plasma glucose, plasma lipids, and other indicators of insulin resistance. The experimental studies use sensitive techniques to estimate insulin resistance, such as a frequently sampled oral glucose tolerance test, or use direct measures, such as minimal model

(MINMOD)-derived insulin sensitivity values from frequently sampled intravenous glucose tolerance tests or measurements based on gold-standard hyperinsulinemic euglycemic clamp techniques. This section summarizes key and representative studies of both kinds. It should be noted in advance that correlations between change in weight and change in plasma glucose values during the time frame of RCTs are often weak compared to correlations between weight change and change in markers of insulin sensitivity (e.g., fasting insulin or triglyceride), because compensatory hyperinsulinemia routinely buffers changes in plasma glucose when insulin resistance increases with increasing adiposity. Thus, unchanged plasma glucose levels within a study do not provide a reliable indication of whether treatment-related changes in insulin sensitivity were occurring.

Data on lipids and glucose from short-term randomized controlled trials

A review of measured changes in metabolic variables in placebo-controlled trials and head-to-head comparisons indicates that the relative incidence and magnitude of change in insulin sensitivity as well as plasma glucose and lipids is not equal among individual antipsychotic medications (Newcomer, 2005b). The results of prospective randomized comparisons of individual agents over short treatment durations illustrate the generally consistent rank order of risk for changes in fasting plasma triglyceride, insulin when measured, and to a lesser extent plasma glucose. For example, an early study using fasting laboratory measures was the RCT comparing olanzapine and ziprasidone mentioned above (Glick et al., 2001). During olanzepine treatment, increases from baseline in median fasting plasma insulin levels (p < 0.0001) and homeostasis model assessment of insulin resistance (p < 0.0001) were observed. In this relatively young patient sample, plasma glucose in the olanzapine-treated subjects did not increase, due to significant compensatory hyperinsulinemia. Cutler et al. (2008) reported on a 4-week, RCT comparing iloperidone (n = 295), ziprasidone (n = 149), and placebo (n = 149). Reported changes in random plasma triglyceride were 0.8 mg/dL for iloperidone, 4.6 mg/dL for ziprasidone, and 19.5 mg/dL for placebo, illustrating the challenge of interpreting non-fasting triglyceride (where the fat content of the last meal can significantly impact values). The changes in fasting glucose level were 7.9 mg/dL for iloperidone, 4.7 mg/dL for ziprasidone, and 3.2 mg/dL for placebo. Highlighting the importance of previous treatment in explaining potential improvement in metabolic parameters that can occur during some studies, a non-blinded, crossover study of 15 previously treated patients with schizophrenia examined the effects of olanzapine and risperidone on fasting lipid profiles after 3 months of treatment (Su et al., 2005). Plasma triglycerides decreased from 212 ± 135

mg/dL to 126 ± 91 mg/dL in patients switched to risperidone, but increased from 112 ± 76 mg/dL to 197 ± 155 mg/dL in patients switched to olanzapine (p = 0.001). A double-blind RCT involving 157 patients with schizophrenia treated with 8 weeks of fixed-dose and 6 weeks of variable-dose clozapine, olanzapine, risperidone or haloperidol (Lindenmayer et al., 2003) reported a trend-level difference in mean glucose levels between treatments at the end of the 8-week fixed-dose period (p = 0.06) but not the 6-week variable-dose phase. There were significant increases from baseline in cholesterol (p < 0.01) and glucose (p < 0.02) at the end of the 6-week variable-dose period in 22 patients who received olanzapine. Interpretation of the results was complicated by baseline and endpoint body weights in some groups that were not consistent with those seen in clinical practice or clinical trials.

Zimbroff et al. (2007) reported on a 4-week RCT comparing ziprasidone (n = 127) and aripiprazole (n = 129). The change in fasting triglyceride level was a modest 6.0 mg/dL for both drugs, and in fasting glucose was a modest 2.0 mg/dL for ziprasidone and 3.0 mg/dL for aripiprazole. In an RCT also described above, Davidson et al. (2007) reported on the metabolic effects of placebo, paliperidone (3, 6 or 9 mg/day), and olanzapine (10 mg/day). The mean changes in fasting triglyceride level were –0.2 (±1.1) mmol/L for placebo, –0.2 (±0.9) mmol/L for paliperidone 3 mg, –0.1 (±0.9) mmol/L for paliperidone 6 mg, 0.0 (±0.7) mmol/L for paliperidone 9 mg, and 0.3 (±0.8) mmol/L for olanzapine. The respective changes in fasting glucose level were 0.0 (±1.6) mmol/L, 0.0 (±1.6) mmol/L, 0.1 (±1.2) mmol/L, 0.0 (±0.9) mmol/L, and 0.0 (±1.2) mmol/L. Similarly, Kane et al. (2007) reported on a 6-week RCT comparing paliperidone 6 mg/day (n = 123), paliperidone 9 mg/day (n = 122), paliperidone 12 mg/day (n = 129), olanzapine (n = 128), and placebo (n = 126). The changes in fasting triglyceride level in the respective arms were –0.2 (±0.9) mmol/L, –0.1 (±0.7) mmol/L, –0.3 (±0.8) mmol/L, 0.1 (±1.2) mmol/l, and –0.3 (±0.7) mmol/L; the respective changes in fasting blood glucose were 0.0 (±1.0) mmol/L, 0.1 (±1.0) mmol/L, 0.1 (±0.9) mmol/L, 0.0 (±0.9) mmol/L, and 0.1 (±1.0) mmol/L. A final example of a short-term study demonstrates the variability that can be observed across different study cohorts. Marder et al. (2007) compared paliperidone 6 mg/day (n = 112), paliperidone 12 mg/day (n = 112), olanzapine 10 mg/day (n = 110), and placebo. The changes in fasting triglyceride for these groups over the 6-week trial were 5.4 (±1.8) mmol/L, 5.3 (±0.9) mmol/L, 5.2 (±1.0) mmol/L, and 5.8 (±1.8) mmol/L, respectively; the changes in fasting blood glucose were 0.0 (±1.3) mmol/L, 0.4 (±1.2) mmol/L, 0.5 (±1.7) mmol/L, and 0.1 (±1.5) mmol/L, respectively. Illustrating the value of a placebo control, a 6-week study of aripiprazole treatment in patients with schizophrenia measured changes in fasting blood glucose (Marder et al., 2003). Data pooled from three aripiprazole groups (10, 15 or 20 mg/day) indicated minimal mean changes in blood glucose from baseline (–0.4 mg/dL; n = 120), but these were numerically larger than the effect observed with placebo (–5.0 mg/dL; n = 34).

Data on lipids and glucose from long-term randomized controlled trials

The available long-term RCTs have generally confirmed the rank order of metabolic risk with antipsychotics seen in shorter-term studies and help to estimate the range of potential effects over longer-term treatment. For example, the effects of olanzapine and ziprasidone were compared in a 28–week RCT (Breier *et al.*,2005). The change in plasma triglyceride from baseline was 0.39 (±1.2) mmol/L for olanzapine and –0.2 (±1.1) mmol/L for ziprasidone, and in blood glucose was 0.3 (±1.7) mmol/L and –0.0 (±1.2) mmol/L, respectively. A similar result was observed in a 24-week, trial Kinon *et al.*, 2006), which showed a mean change in fasting triglyceride level with olanzapine of 13.6 (±192.7) mg/dL and –9.5 (±130.1) mg/dL with ziprasidone; the mean changes in fasting blood glucose were 2.9 (±37.8) mg/dL and 0.1 (±36.3) mg/dL, respectively. Sacchetti *et al.* (2008) showed an increase in fasting triglyceride of 10 mg/dL for clozapine compared to –15 mg/dL for ziprasidone over 18 weeks; blood glucose level rose by 6 mg/dL for clozapine but was unchanged in the ziprasidone arm. Pigott *et al.* (2003) reported on a 26–week RCT comparing olanzapine (n = 85), aripiprazole (n = 148), and placebo (n = 149). Mean change in fasting triglyceride was –37.2 mg/dL for aripiprazole and –2.9 mg/dL for placebo (no value was given for olanzapine), while the mean change in fasting glucose was 1.4 mg/dL for olanzapine, 0.1 mg/dL for aripiprazole, and 2.1 mg/dL for placebo. Bushe *et al.* (2010) compared treatment with quetiapine (n = 175) and olanzapine (n = 171) over 6 months. The mean change in triglyceride level was 0.5 (±2.4) mmol/L for quetiapine and 0.4 (±2.3) mmol/L for olanzapine, and for fasting glucose was 0.8 (±2.5) mmol/L and 0.1 (±2.4) mmol/L, respectively. Kane *et al.* (2008) reported on a 46-week, double-blind study comparing iloperidone (n = 371) and haloperidol (n = 118). The mean change in fasting triglyceride was 6.8 (±95.2) mg/dL for iloperidone and 12.1 (±112.2) mg/dL for haloperidol, with mean changes in fasting glucose of 2.7 (±2.4) mg/dL and –0.5 (±19.9) mg/dL, respectively. A 26-week, multicenter trial of olanzapine (n = 161) and aripiprazole (n = 156) showed significant differences between the groups in mean change from baseline in fasting triglyceride (+79.4 mg/dL *vs.* –6.5 mg/dL, respectively; p < 0.05) and HDL levels (–3.4 mg/dL *vs.* +3.6 mg/dL, respectively; p < 0.05; McQuade *et al.*, 2004). Of patients with normal baseline lipids, 47% of the olanzapine-treated patients at endpoint had total cholesterol values greater than 200 mg/dL, *versus* 17% of the aripiprazole-treated patients. Similar differences in the change from baseline, among patients

with normal baseline lipids, were seen for LDL levels greater than 130 mg/dL at endpoint (38% with olanzapine *versus* 19% with aripiprazole) and triglyceride levels greater than 150 mg/dL at endpoint (50% with olanzapine *versus* 18% with aripiprazole).

The CATIE study (see Long-term studies above) also collected data in each phase on metabolic indices, which provide further evidence of significant metabolic risk with olanzapine. In Phase I, olanzapine-treated patients showed the greatest increases in total cholesterol (+9.7 ± 2.1 mg/dL), triglycerides (+42.9 ± 8.4 mg/dL), and glycosylated hemoglobin (+0.4 ± 0.1 mg/dL), with statistically significant differences between treatment groups in each of these indices (Lieberman *et al.*, 2005). A small decrease in mean plasma triglyceride levels occurred in patients treated with ziprasidone, presumably as a result of the lower risk of weight gain, insulin resistance, and triglyceride elevation with ziprasidone compared to the drugs which patients were taking before being switched into this treatment arm. In Phase IIT, olanzapine-treated patients again showed the greatest exposure-adjusted mean increases in total cholesterol (17.5 ± 5.2 mg/dL), triglyceride (94.1 ± 21.8 mg/dL), and HbA$_{1c}$ (0.97 ± 0.3%), with significant differences between treatment groups in each of these indices (Stroup *et al.*, 2006). Risperidone showed mean exposure-adjusted increases in blood glucose (6.9 ± 5.8 mg/dL) and HbA$_{1c}$ (0.49%), with mean exposure-adjusted decreases in triglycerides (–5.2 ± 21.6 mg/dL) and total cholesterol (–3.1 ± 5.2 mg/dL). Quetiapine showed mean exposure-adjusted increases in blood glucose (1.2 ± 6.0 mg/dL), HbA$_{1c}$ (0.6 + 0.3%), triglycerides (39.3 ± 22.1 mg/dL), and total cholesterol (6.5 ± 5.3 mg/dL). Ziprasidone showed mean exposure-adjusted increases in blood glucose (0.8 ± 5.6 mg/dL) and HbA1c (0.5 ± 0.3%), and mean exposure-adjusted decreases in triglycerides (–3.5 ± 20.9 mg/dL) and total cholesterol (–10.7 ± 5.1 mg/dL). Of the 99 patients in Phase IIE, changes in total cholesterol, triglycerides, and HbA$_{1c}$ were not significantly different across treatment groups (Stroup *et al.*, 2006), perhaps attributable to the small sample sizes and/or a selection bias toward patients with a history of extensive previous treatment, including treatment with a high weight-gain agent, such as olanzapine, given that this arm of the study was intended for those who had experienced insufficient treatment efficacy. In Phase III (Stroup *et al.*, 2009), decreases in triglyceride levels were noted in patients who chose ziprasidone or fluphenazine decanoate, while levels rose to varying degrees in those taking the other medications.

Measurements of insulin, insulin resistance, and metabolic syndrome

Five early studies reported statistically significant increases in plasma insulin levels during olanzapine treatment compared with various control conditions (Cuijpers & Smit,

2002; Sikich *et al.*, 2004; Visser *et al.*, 2003; Gallagher *et al.*, 2000; Barak *et al.*, 2002), with two also reporting an increase in calculated insulin resistance (p < 0.05; Gallagher *et al.*, 2000; Visser *et al.*, 2003). The results are consistent with the evidence from population samples (Resnick *et al.*, 1998; Montague & O'Rahilly, 2000), suggesting that any condition that increases adiposity tends to be associated with increases in insulin resistance. Using data pooled from two 26-week RCTs mentioned earlier (Pigott *et al.*, 2003; McQuade *et al.*, 2003), the effects of aripiprazole, olanzapine, and placebo on the incidence of worsening metabolic syndrome in 624 subjects were observed (L'Italien, 2003). The cumulative incidence varied significantly (p = 0.003) between treatments, from a mean (SEM) of 19% (4%) for olanzapine, 13% (4%) for placebo and 8% (2%) for aripiprazole, with a 69% relative risk reduction for aripiprazole *versus* olanzapine (L'Italien, 2003; Casey *et al.*, 2003b).

Insulin resistance can lead to compensatory insulin secretion in persons with pancreatic beta-cell reserve or to hyperglycemia in individuals with relative beta-cell failure. A study of healthy participants taking olanzapine for 2 weeks indicated increased insulin response and decreased insulin sensitivity with both olanzapine and risperidone compared to placebo (Sowell *et al.*, 2002). These changes in insulin response were associated with changes in BMI. Adjusting for the effects of weight gain, no significant change in insulin response or sensitivity was detected with olanzapine or risperidone therapy, suggesting that the adverse effects are largely related to changes in adiposity. A later study using two-step, hyperinsulinemic euglycemic clamp methodology in healthy volunteers receiving olanzapine (n = 22), risperidone (n = 14) or placebo (n = 19) for 3 weeks, with restricted access to food, showed no statistically significant changes in the insulin sensitivity index from baseline during either clamp stage (Sowell *et al.*, 2003). However, fasting insulin and glucose levels both increased significantly in the olanzapine group, but decreased slightly in the risperidone group. Relevant to the interpretation of results, restricted access to food is not a condition that generalizes to most patients with schizophrenia, underscoring the potential for adiposity-related reductions in insulin sensitivity during real-world treatment. Another study in patients with schizophrenia showed no significant changes in insulin resistance after 2 or more months of olanzapine treatment (Kurt & Oral, 2002). Berry and Mahmoud (2002) reported significant improvements in insulin resistance and beta-cell function in patients following a change from olanzapine to risperidone. Finally, a careful study by Sacher *et al.* (2008) investigated the acute effects of oral olanzapine and ziprasidone on whole-body insulin sensitivity in healthy subjects using the standardized hyperinsulinemic euglycemic clamp technique in 29 healthy male volunteers after either olanzapine (10 mg/day) or ziprasidone (80 mg/day) for 10 days. A decrease in whole-body insulin sensitivity after olanzapine (p < 0.001) but not ziprasidone was seen, accompanied by a small mean increase in BMI on olanzapine but not ziprasidone.

The case of quetiapine

Results for quetiapine deserve separate mention, because RCTs rather consistently indicate increases in fasting triglyceride levels, which are less than those observed with olanzapine but greater than would be expected from an agent with a relatively modest risk for weight gain (see above). Proportionally greater increases in triglyceride might be interpreted as evidence of greater effects on insulin sensitivity, but the available evidence, again reviewed earlier, suggests that quetiapine is not associated with a disproportionate increase in the risk for diabetes above that observed for other agents with the same weight gain potential. A 6-week RCT of atypical antipsychotics in schizophrenia (clozapine, olanzapine, quetiapine, and risperidone; each n = 14) found significant increases from baseline in triglyceride levels with quetiapine therapy (11.6 mg/dL; p < 0.05; Atmaca *et al.*, 2003), which was approximately three times less than that observed with clozapine (36.3 mg/dL; p < 0.01) or olanzapine (31.2 mg/dL; p < 0.01), but contrasted with the lack of increase from baseline in triglyceride levels observed with risperidone (p = 0.76). In an example of studies using more sensitive measures of glucose metabolism and insulin sensitivity, Newcomer *et al.* (2009) recently reported the results of a randomized, 24-week, flexible-dose study that compared changes in glucose metabolism in patients with schizophrenia receiving their initial exposure to olanzapine, quetiapine or risperidone. Using data from 395 patients [quetiapine n = 115 (mean 607 mg/day), olanzapine n = 146 (15 mg/day), and risperidone n = 134 (5 mg/day)], the change in area under the curve (AUC) 0–2 h glucose (mg/dL x h) at week 24 was lower for quetiapine compared to olanzapine (p < 0.05). Increases in AUC 0–2 h glucose were significant with olanzapine (+22 mg/dL; 95% CI 11–32) and risperidone (+19, 95% CI 8–29), but not with quetiapine (+9 mg/dL; 95% CI −2–20). AUC 0–2 h insulin increased significantly with olanzapine, but not with quetiapine or risperidone. Reductions in insulin sensitivity were significant with olanzapine and risperidone, but not with quetiapine. Mean weight changes over 24 weeks were +3.7 kg (quetiapine), +4.6 kg (olanzapine), and +3.6 kg (risperidone). Total cholesterol and LDL increased significantly with olanzapine and quetiapine, but not with risperidone; significant increases in triglycerides, and cholesterol:HDL and triglyceride:HDL ratios were observed with olanzapine only. The results indicate a difference in the change in glucose tolerance during 6 months' treatment with different antipsychotics, with changes largely explained by reductions in insulin sensitivity and the largest adverse effects associated with olanzapine. The results also suggest that the intermediate effect of quetiapine on the change in fasting triglyceride from baseline is not due to intermediate effects on insulin sensitivity, which remained the same or less than changes seen with risperidone, which produced a similar change in weight.

Metabolic effects of antipsychotics independent of changes in adiposity

The studies reviewed above show that the relative risk for Type 2 diabetes mellitus appears to match the rank order of weight gain potential for the different antipsychotic drugs. Haupt *et al.* (2007) showed that adiposity levels are highly predictive of insulin sensitivity, with readily available measures of adiposity like waist circumference and BMI significantly ($p < 0.0001$) predicting insulin sensitivity, as measured during frequently sampled intravenous glucose tolerance tests, in antipsychotic-treated patients with schizophrenia as well as in untreated healthy controls. Higher levels of adiposity are associated with lower levels of insulin sensitivity, with adiposity explaining more than 30% of the variance. However, a significant minority of patients can experience glucose dysregulation temporally or statistically independent of weight change or adiposity differences (Koller *et al.*, 2001ba, 2003; Newcomer *et al.*, 2002; Koller & Doraiswamy, 2002; Kemner *et al.*, 2002; Ebenbichler *et al.*, 2003), suggesting that at least some antipsychotic medications may have a direct effect on insulin sensitivity or secretion. A study using euglycemic hyperinsulinemic clamps in freely roaming Wistar rats found a highly significant dose-dependent reduction in insulin sensitivity within 2 h of initial exposure to clozapine or olanzapine, but not ziprasidone or risperidone (Houseknecht *et al.*, 2005).

Two cross-sectional studies support the possibility that weight gain may not explain all the observed metabolic adverse effects. Newcomer *et al.* (2002) examined the effects of antipsychotics on glucose regulation in chronically-treated non-diabetic patients with schizophrenia, compared with untreated healthy control subjects matched for adiposity and age. Using a modified oral glucose tolerance test, patients receiving olanzapine (n = 12) and clozapine (n = 9) had higher fasting and post-load plasma glucose values compared with patients receiving typical (high-potency) antipsychotics (n = 17) and untreated healthy control subjects (n = 31; $p < 0.001$ for all comparisons). The risperidone group did not differ from the conventional antipsychotics group, but did have higher post-load glucose levels as compared to controls ($p < 0.01$). Patients who received olanzapine and clozapine also had higher calculated insulin resistance compared with those who received conventional agents ($p < 0.05$ and $p < 0.08$, respectively), whereas those who received risperidone or typical

antipsychotics did not differ from controls. Similar findings were reported by Henderson *et al.* (2005) using frequently-sampled intravenous glucose tolerance tests to study non-diabetic patients chronically treated with clozapine, olanzapine, or risperidone, where the treatment groups were matched for adiposity, age, gender, and ethnicity: patients treated with clozapine or olanzapine showed significant insulin resistance, as measured by MINMOD-derived insulin sensitivity, compared with subjects treated with risperidone. There was no significant difference in insulin resistance between the clozapine and olanzapine treated groups. Both of these studies were limited by adiposity matching that relied on BMI values, which can fail to capture the full extent of group-related differences in abdominal fat mass, leading to differences in insulin sensitivity that might actually be driven by differences in fat mass rather than a true adiposity-independent mechanism.

Changes in metabolic risk associated with switching antipsychotic treatment

Recent studies analyzing the effects of switching antipsychotics suggest the clinical utility of switching from a medication with higher weight gain risk to one with lower weight gain risk. Two studies indicate statistically significant reductions in body weight and BMI over periods of 6–8 weeks after a switch from risperidone or olanzapine to either aripiprazole (Casey *et al.*, 2003a) or ziprasidone (Weiden *et al.*, 2003). The study involving the switch to ziprasidone further detected a significant reduction in non-fasting total plasma cholesterol and triglycerides.

The effects of treatment switch on weight change and psychiatric status were first formally tested in a 16-week, multicenter, double-blind RCT of overweight patients initially taking olanzapine (n = 173). The primary outcome variable was the difference in change in weight between patients randomly assigned to continue olanzapine *versus* a group randomized to switch to aripiprazole (Newcomer *et al.*, 2008). In this study, patients who switched to aripiprazole experienced a significant mean weight decrease [–4.0 lb (1.7 kg)] compared with those who continued olanzapine [+3.1 lb (1.3 kg)]. Fasting plasma triglyceride levels decreased from baseline in the aripiprazole group and increased from baseline in the olanzapine group ($p = 0.002$). Of note, while there was statistical advantage for "stayers" compared to "switchers" in Clinical Global Impression Improvement (CGI-I) scale scores ($p = 0.02$), CGI-I ratings for both groups remained in the range of "minimal improvement" to "no change". A recent *ad hoc* but nevertheless important analysis of CATIE Phase I results further confirmed that switching from olanzapine to any of the other antipsychotics resulted in no weight gain or weight loss, whereas continued use of olanazapine was associated with weight gain (Rosenheck *et al.*, 2009). Weight loss was also found in patients switching from olanzapine to ziprasidone (Weiden *et al.*, 2008).

Even when studies do not formally aim to test the effect of medication switches from higher to lower risk agents, the characteristics of commonly tested study populations are such that many patients historically entering recent trials have been on agents with higher risk for weight gain at the outset. The results from CATIE Phase I demonstrated that randomized treatment with ziprasidone produced statistically significant weight loss (0.73 kg, SE 0.5), and similar weight reductions have been reported with aripiprazole (1.37 kg loss after 26 weeks of treatment; McQuade *et al.*, 2004). It is important to note that medications like aripiprazole and ziprasidone, while associated with weight loss in this particular clinical context, routinely induce at least small amounts of mean weight gain in other contexts and in large unselected patient samples. There is no indication that any currently available antipsychotic drug is generally associated with mean weight reductions.

Weight changes in these studies approximate a 10% reduction in body weight, an effect that matches or betters well-studied behavioral or pharmacological weight loss approaches that have been tested in large non-psychiatric obese patient samples. All available results in patients with schizophrenia suggest that switching from an antipsychotic with high weight-gain risk, like olanzapine, to a medication with lower risk can help to achieve weight loss, with no large or readily detected group differences in psychiatric outcome.

Recommendations to reduce cardiometabolic risk

An ADA Consensus Development Report, co-sponsored by the American Psychiatric Association, the American Association of Clinical Endocrinologists, and the North American Association for the Study of Obesity (American Diabetes Association, 2004), noted that clozapine and olanzapine treatment are associated with the greatest potential weight gain among SGAs, and with consistent evidence for an increased risk of Type 2 diabetes mellitus and dyslipidemia. The report emphasized that physicians should consider multiple factors, including the presence of medical and psychiatric conditions, when evaluating the risks and benefits of prescribing specific antipsychotic agents, and that the potential benefits of drugs with metabolic liabilities might under certain circumstances outweigh the potential risks (e.g., use of clozapine therapy in patients with treatment-resistant schizophrenia).

A recent European Psychiatric Association statement, co-sponsored by the European Society of Cardiology and the European Association for the Study of Diabetes (De Hert *et al.*, 2009) has similarly called for monitoring and interventions to manage risk for patients during treatment.

Both the US and European groups, and other international expert panels (e.g., Fleischhacker *et al.*, 2008), have produced guidelines and recommendations as to the indices that should be monitored, and their frequency. For example, the ADA recommends weight monitoring at 4, 8, and 12 weeks after initiating a change in antipsychotic therapy, and quarterly thereafter. A weight gain of 5% or greater of baseline weight may signal the need to switch to a different atypical antipsychotic agent. In addition to monitoring by physicians, patients should be encouraged to track their own weight and waist circumference (American Diabetes Association, 2004).

However, despite the increasing call for action, little change has been demonstrated in large administrative datasets that track clinician behavior. For example, in the US, although the likelihood of glucose testing increased two-fold between 1998 and 2003, a large Medicaid patient population who received index prescriptions for SGAs demonstrated that it is still a small percentage of patients who receive any testing (Morrato *et al.*, 2008). Over the period examined, less than 20% of patients received baseline glucose testing and less than 10% received baseline lipid testing. With medication initiation, the rates increased slightly (glucose testing increased 7–11%; lipids, 2–3%). Patients with pre-existing diabetes or dyslipidemia were about two to three times more likely to receive baseline testing than those without these conditions, but only a small percentage were tested within 14 days before or 28 days after starting antipsychotic medication. Another illustration is provided by the fact that since the 2004 ADA report and the FDA recommendation (US Food and Drug Administration, 2004) to modify package inserts for atypical antipsychotics with a warning about hyperglycemia and diabetes risk, awareness of the need for glucose and lipid testing has increased (Ketter & Haupt, 2006), but actual screening and monitoring rates for glucose and lipids have shown only limited improvement (Haupt *et al.*, 2009; Morrato *et al.*, 2009).

This state of affairs represents a missed opportunity. Compared with secondary prevention, early screening and identification of risk offer a substantial opportunity to impact the course of cardiometabolic disease for the largest number of patients (Grundy *et al.*, 1998). Even small reductions in any one of the modifiable risk factors for cardiometabolic diseases can lead to large payoffs over the long term. For example, a 10% reduction in blood cholesterol can result in a 30% decrease in 10-year risk of CHD; a 6 mmHg decrease in diastolic pressures greater than 90 mmHg can result in a 16% decrease in 10-year risk for CHD and a 42% reduction in 10-year risk for stroke (Hennekens, 1998). Maintaining an ideal BMI of 18.5–25 and an active lifestyle by walking about 30 min/day can reduce 10-year risk of CHD by between 35% and 55% (Bassuk & Manson, 2005). A range of strategies are available to manage cardiovascular risk. Behavioral interventions such as healthy food choices, physical activity increases, and smoking cessation are standard approaches that are appropriate for patients with major mental disorders (De Backer *et al.*, 2003). Managing treatment-related risk is also critical.

Conclusions

Patients with schizophrenia are at elevated risk for overall medical morbidity and mortality, particularly CVD-related mortality. Modifiable cardiometabolic risk factors are prevalent in patients with major mental disorders. Antipsychotic medications are associated with different levels of risk for weight gain, insulin resistance, dyslipidemia, and hyperglycemia. Clinicians can beneficially modify patient risk through medication choice, regular monitoring of weight, BMI, waist circumference, fasting plasma glucose level, and lipid profiles, with active interventions for identified risk, including ongoing encouragement of healthy lifestyle choices.

Conflict of interest

John W. Newcomer MD has no significant financial conflict of interest in compliance with the Washington University Conflict of Interest Policy. Dr Newcomer has received research grant support from The National Institute of Mental Health (NIMH), NARSAD, Bristol-Myers Squibb, Janssen Pharmaceutica, Pfizer, Inc., and Wyeth; he has served as a consultant to AstraZeneca Pharmaceuticals, Bristol-Myers Squibb, BioVail, H. Lundbeck, Janssen Pharmaceutica, Obecure, Otsuka Pharmaceuticals, Pfizer, Inc., Sepracor, Inc., Solvay Pharma, Inc., Vanda Pharmaceutica, and Wyeth Pharmaceuticals; he has been a consultant to litigation; he has been a member of Data Safety Monitoring Boards for Dainippon Sumitomo Pharma America, Inc., Organon Pharmaceuticals USA Inc., Schering-Plough/Merck, and Vivus, Inc; finally he has received royalties from Compact Clinicals/Jones and Bartlett Publishing for a metabolic screening form.

References

Adkins, D.E., Aberg, K., McClay, J.L. *et al.* (2010) Genomewide pharmacogenic study of metabolic side effects to antipsychotic drugs. *Molecular Psychiatry* (in press).

Allebeck, P. (1989) Schizophrenia: a life-shortening disease. *Schizophrenia Bulletin* **15**, 81–89.

Allison, D.B., Fontaine, K.R., Heo, M. *et al.* (1999a) The distribution of body mass index among individuals with and without schizophrenia. *Journal of Clinical Psychiatry*, **60**, 215–220.

Allison, D.B., Fontaine, K.R., Manson, J.E., Stevens, J. & Vanitallie, T.B. (1999b) Annual deaths attributable to obesity in the United States. *JAMA* **282**, 1530–1538.

Allison, D.B., Mentore, J.L., Heo, M. *et al.* (1999c) Antipsychotic-induced weight gain: a comprehensive research synthesis. *American Journal of Psychiatry* **156**, 1686–1696.

Allison, D.B., Newcomer, J.W., Dunn, A.L. *et al.* (2009) Obesity among those with mental disorders: a National Institute of Mental Health meeting report. *American Journal of Preventive Medicine* **36**, 341–350.

American Diabetes Association (2003) Standards of medical care for patients with diabetes mellitus. *Diabetes Care* **26**, S33–S50.

American Diabetes Association (2004) Consensus development conference on antipsychotic drugs and obesity and diabetes. *Diabetes Care* **27**, 596–601.

American Heart Association (2006) Metabolic syndrome. Available at: http://www.americanheart.org/presenter. jhtml?identifier=4756. [Accessed 10 October 2006].

Andersohn, F., Schade, R., Suissa, S. & Garbe, E. (2009) Long-term use of antidepressants for depressive disorders and the risk of diabetes mellitus. *American Journal of Psychiatry* **166**, 591–598.

Arranz, B., Rosel, P., Ramirez, N. *et al.* (2004) Insulin resistance and increased leptin concentrations in noncompliant schizophrenia patients but not in antipsychotic-naive first-episode schizophrenia patients. *Journal of Clinical Psychiatry* **65**, 1335–1342.

Atmaca, M., Kuloglu, M., Tezcan, E. & Ustundag, B. (2003) Serum leptin and triglyceride levels in patients on treatment with atypical antipsychotics. *Journal of Clinical Psychiatry* **64**, 598–604.

Banerji, M.A., Lebowitz, J., Chaiken, R.L., Gordon, D., Kral, J.G. & Lebovitz, H.E. (1997) Relationship of visceral adipose tissue and glucose disposal is independent of sex in black NIDDM subjects. *American Journal of Physiology* **273**, E425–432.

Barak, Y., Shamir, E. & Weizman, R. (2002) Would a switch from typical antipsychotics to risperidone be beneficial for elderly schizophrenic patients? A naturalistic, long-term, retrospective, comparative study. *Journal of Clinical Psychopharmacology* **22**, 115–120.

Bassuk, S.S. & Manson, J.E. (2005) Epidemiological evidence for the role of physical activity in reducing risk of type 2 diabetes and cardiovascular disease. *Journal of Applied Physiology* **99**, 1193–1204.

Berry, S. & Mahmoud, R. (2002) Improvement of insulin indices after switch from olanzapine to risperidone. *European Neuropsychopharmacology* **12**, S316.

Biggs, M.L., Mukamal, K.J., Luchsinger, J.A. IX, *et al.* (2010) Association between adiposity in midlife and older age and risk of diabetes in older adults. *JAMA* **303**, 2504–2512.

Boehm, G., Racoosin, J.A., Laughren, T.P. & Katz, R. (2004) Consensus development conference on antipsychotic drugs and obesity and diabetes: response to consensus statement. *Diabetes Care* **27**, 2088–2089; author reply 2089–2090.

Brecher, M., Leong, R.W., Stening, G., Osterling-Koskinen, L. & Jones, A.M. (2007) Quetiapine and long-term weight change: a comprehensive data review of patients with schizophrenia. *Journal of Clinical Psychiatry* **68**, 597–603.

Breier, A., Berg, P.H., Thakore, J.H. *et al.* (2005) Olanzapine versus ziprasidone: results of a 28-week double-blind study in patients with schizophrenia. *American Journal Psychiatry* **162**, 1879–1887.

Brown, S. (1997) Excess mortality of schizophrenia. A meta-analysis. *British Journal of Psychiatry* **171**, 502–508.

Brown, S., Inskip, H. & Barraclough, B. (2000) Causes of the excess mortality of schizophrenia. *British Journal of Psychiatry* **177**, 212–217.

Buse, J.B., Cavazzoni, P., Hornbuckle, K., Hutchins, D., Breier, A. & Jovanovic, L. (2003) A retrospective cohort study of diabetes mellitus and antipsychotic treatment in the United States. *Journal of Clinical Epidemiology* **56**, 164–170.

Bushe, C. & Holt, R. (2004) Prevalence of diabetes and impaired glucose tolerance in patients with schizophrenia. *British Journal of Psychiatry* **47** (Suppl.), S67–71.

Bushe, C., Sniadecki, J., Bradley, A. & Poole Hoffmann, V. (2010) Comparison of metabolic and prolactin variables from a six-month randomised trial of olanzapine and quetiapine in schizophrenia. *Journal of Psychopharmacology* **24**, 1001–1009.

Calle, E.E., Thun, M.J., Petrelli, J.M., Rodriquez, C. & Heath, C.W. Jr (1999) Body-mass index and mortality in a prospective cohort of U.S. adults. *New England Journal of Medicine* **341**, 1097–1105.

Caro, J.J., Ward, A., Levinton, C. & Robinson, K. (2002) The risk of diabetes during olanzapine use compared with risperidone use: a retrospective database analysis. *Journal of Clinical Psychiatry* **63**, 1135–1139.

Casey, D.E., Carson, W.H., Saha, A.R. *et al.* (2003a) Switching patients to aripiprazole from other antipsychotic agents: a multicenter randomized study. *Psychopharmacology (Berlin)* **166**, 391–399.

Casey, D.E., L'Italien, G.J., Waldeck, R., Cislo, P. & Carson, W.H. (2003b) Metabolic syndrome comparison between olanzapine, aripiprazole, and placebo. Poster presented at the American Psychiatric Association, San Francisco.

Casey, D.E., Haupt, D.W., Newcomer, J.W. *et al.* (2004) Antipsychotic-induced weight gain and metabolic abnormalities: implications for increased mortality in patients with schizophrenia. *Journal of Clinical Psychiatry* **65**, 4–18.

Cheta, D., Dumitrescu, C., Georgescu, M. *et al.* (1990) A study on the types of diabetes mellitus in first degree relatives of diabetic patients. *Diabetes Metabolism* **16**, 11–15.

Church, C.O., Stevens, D.L. & Fugate, S.E. (2005) Diabetic ketoacidosis associated with aripiprazole. *Diabetes Medicine* **22**, 1440–1443.

Citrome, L., Jaffe, A., Levine, J., Allingham, B. & Robinson, J. (2004) Relationship between antipsychotic medication treatment and new cases of diabetes among psychiatric inpatients. *Psychiatric Services* **55**, 1006–1013.

Cohn, T., Prud'homme, D., Streiner, D., Kameh, H. & Remington, G. (2004) Characterizing coronary heart disease risk in chronic schizophrenia: high prevalence of the metabolic syndrome. *Canadian Journal of Psychiatry* **49**, 753–760.

Colton, C.W. & Manderscheid, R.W. (2006) Congruencies in increased mortality rates, years of potential life lost, and causes of death among public mental health clients in eight states. *Prevention of Chronic Diseases* **3**, A42.

Cormac, I., Ferriter, M., Benning, R. & Saul, C. (2005) Physical health and health risk factors in a population of long-stay psychiatric patients. *Psychiatric Bulletin* **29**, 18–20.

Correll, C.U., Manu, P., Olshankiy, V. *et al.* (2009) Cardiometabolic risk of second-generation antipsychotic medications during first-time use in children and adolescents. *JAMA* **302**, 1765–1773.

Csernansky, J.G., Mahmoud, R. & Brenner, R. (2002) A comparison of risperidone and haloperidol for the prevention of relapse in patients with schizophrenia. *New England Journal of Medicine* **346**, 16–22.

Cuijpers, P. & Smit, F. (2002) Excess mortality in depression: a meta-analysis of community studies. *Journal of Affective Disorders* **72**, 227–236.

Curkendall, S.M., Mo, J., Glasser, D.B., Rose Stang, M. & Jones, J.K. (2004) Cardiovascular disease in patients with schizophrenia in Saskatchewan, Canada. *Journal of Clinical Psychiatry* **65**, 715–720.

Cutler, A.J., Kalali, A.H., Weiden, P.J., Hamilton, J. & Wolfgang, C.D. (2008) Four-week, double-blind, placebo- and ziprasidone-controlled trial of iloperidone in patients with acute exacerbations of schizophrenia. *Journal of Clinical Psychopharmacology* **28**, S20–28.

Daniel, D.G., Zimbroff, D.L., Swift, R.H. & Harrigan, E.P. (2004) The tolerability of intramuscular ziprasidone and haloperidol treatment and the transition to oral therapy. *International Clinical Psychopharmacology* **19**, 9–15.

Daumit, G.L., Goldberg, R.W., Anthony, C. *et al.* (2005) Physical activity patterns in adults with severe mental illness. *Journal of Nervous and Mental Diseases* **193**, 641–646.

Davidson, M., Emsley, R., Kramer, M. *et al.* (2007) Efficacy, safety and early response of paliperidone extended-release tablets (paliperidone ER): results of a 6-week, randomized, placebo-controlled study. *Schizophrenia Research* **93**, 117–130.

De Backer, G., Ambrosioni, E., Borch-Johnsen, K. *et al.* (2003) European guidelines on cardiovascular disease prevention in clinical practice. Third Joint Task Force of European and Other Societies on Cardiovascular Disease Prevention in Clinical Practice. *European Heart Journal* **24**, 1601–1610.

De Hert, M., Dekker, J.M., Wood, D., Kahl, K.G., Holt, R.I. & Moller, H.-J. (2009) Cardiovascular disease and diabetes in people with severe mental illness position statement from the European Psychiatric Association (EPA), supported by the European Association for the Study of Diabetes (EASD) and the European Society of Cardiology (ESC). *European Psychiatry* **24**, 412–424.

De Leon, J. & Diaz, F.J. (2005) A meta-analysis of worldwide studies demonstrates an association between schizophrenia and tobacco smoking behaviors. *Schizophrenia Research* **76**, 135–157.

Despres, J.-P., Lemieux, I. & Bergeron, J. (2008) Abdominal obesity and the metabolic syndrome: contribution to global cardiometabolic risk. *Arteriosclerosis, Thrombosis, and Vascular Biology* **28**, 1039–1049.

Dixon, L., Weiden, P., Delahanty, J. *et al.* (2000) Prevalence and correlates of diabetes in national schizophrenia samples. *Schizophrenia Bulletin* **26**, 903–912.

Druss, B.G. & Bornemann, T.H. (2010) Improving health and health care for persons with serious mental illness: the window for US federal policy change. *JAMA* **303**, 1972–1973.

Druss, B.G., Bradford, W.D., Rosenheck, R.A., Radford, M.J. & Krumholz, H.M. (2001) Quality of medical care and excess mortality in older patients with mental disorders. *Archives of General Psychiatry* **58**, 565–572.

Dynes, J.B. (1969) Diabetes in schizophrenia and diabetes in nonpsychotic medical patients. *Diseases of the Nervous System* **30**, 341–344.

Ebenbichler, C.F., Laimer, M., Eder, U. *et al.* (2003) Olanzapine induces insulin resistance: results from a prospective study. *Journal of Clinical Psychiatry* **64**, 1436–1439.

Fleischhacker, W.W., Cetkovich-Bakmas, M., De Hert, M. *et al.* (2008) Comorbid somatic illnesses in patients with severe mental disorders: clinical, policy, and research challenges. *Journal of Clinical Psychiatry* **69**, 514–519.

Fontaine, K.R., Heo, M., Harrigan, E.P. *et al.* (2001) Estimating the consequences of anti-psychotic induced weight gain on health and mortality rate. *Psychiatry Research* **101**, 277–288.

Fontaine, K.R., Redden, D.T., Wang, C., Westfall, A.O. & Allison, D.B. (2003) Years of life lost due to obesity. *JAMA* **289**, 187–93.

Fuller, M.A., Shermock, K.M., Secic, M. & Grogg, A.L. (2003) Comparative study of the development of diabetes mellitus in patients taking risperidone and olanzapine. *Pharmacotherapy* **23**, 1037–1043.

Gallagher, D., Ruts, E., Visser, M. *et al.* (2000) Weight stability masks sarcopenia in elderly men and women. *American Journal of Physiology and Endocrinology Metabolism* **279**, E366–375.

Gianfrancesco, F.D., Grogg, A.L., Mahmoud, R.A., Wang, R.H. & Nasrallah, H.A. (2002) Differential effects of risperidone, olanzapine, clozapine, and conventional antipsychotics on type 2 diabetes: findings from a large health plan database. *Journal of Clinical Psychiatry* **63**, 920–930.

Gianfrancesco, F., White, R., Wang, R.H. & Nasrallah, H.A. (2003) Antipsychotic-induced type 2 diabetes: evidence from a large health plan database. *Journal of Clinical Psychopharmacology* **23**, 328–335.

Glick, I.D., Romano, S.J., Simpson, G. *et al.* (2001) Insulin resistance in olanzapine- and ziprasidone-treated patients: results of a double-blind, controlled 6-week trial. Presented at: Annual Meeting of the American Psychiatric Association, May 5–10, 2001, New Orleans, LA.

Goff, D.C., Sullivan, L.M., McEvoy, J.P. *et al.* (2005) A comparison of ten-year cardiac risk estimates in schizophrenia patients from the CATIE study and matched controls. *Schizophrenia Research* **80**, 45–53.

Grundy, S.M. (2002) Obesity, metabolic syndrome, and coronary atherosclerosis. *Circulation* **105**, 2696–2698.

Grundy, S.M., Balady, G.J., Criqui, M.H. *et al.* (1998) Primary prevention of coronary heart disease: guidance from Framingham: a statement for healthcare professionals from the AHA Task Force on Risk Reduction. American Heart Association. *Circulation* **97**, 1876–1887.

Haffner, S.M., Lehto, S., Ronnemaa, T., Pyorala, K. & Laakso, M. (1998) Mortality from coronary heart disease in subjects with type 2 diabetes and in nondiabetic subjects with and without prior myocardial infarction. *New England Journal of Medicine* **339**, 229–234.

Hardy, T.A., Poole-Hoffmann, V., Lu, Y. *et al.* (2003) Fasting glucose and lipid changes in patients with schizophrenia treated with olanzapine or ziprasidone. Poster presented at the 42nd Annual Meeting of the American College of Neuropsychopharmacology, December 7–11, 2003, San Juan, Puerto Rico.

Harris, M.I. (2000) Health care and health status and outcomes for patients with type 2 diabetes. *Diabetes Care* **23**, 754–758.

Harris, E.C. & Barraclough, B. (1998) Excess mortality of mental disorder. *British Journal of Psychiatry* **173**, 11–53.

Harris, M.I., Flegal, K.M., Cowie, C.C. *et al.* (1998) Prevalence of diabetes, impaired fasting glucose, and impaired glucose tolerance in U.S. adults. The Third National Health and Nutrition Examination Survey, 1988–1994. *Diabetes Care* **21**, 518–524.

Harrison, P.J. (2005) Weight gain and antipsychotic drugs: the role of the 5-HT$_{2c}$ receptor (HTR2C) and other genes. *Pharmacogenetics and Genomics* **15**, 518–524.

Haupt, D.W. & Newcomer, J.W. (2001) Hyperglycemia and antipsychotic medications. *Journal of Clinical Psychiatry* **62** (Suppl. 27), 15–26; discussion 40–41.

Haupt, D.W. & Newcomer, J.W. (2002) Abnormalities in glucose regulation associated with mental illness and treatment. *Journal of Psychosomotor Research* **53**, 925–933.

Haupt, D.W., Fahnestock, P.A., Flavin, K.A. *et al.* (2007) Adiposity and insulin sensitivity derived from intravenous glucose tolerance tests in antipsychotic-treated patients. *Neuropsychopharmacology* **32**, 2561–2569.

Haupt, D.W., Rosenblatt, L.C., Kim, E., Baker, R.A., Whitehead, R. & Newcomer, J.W. (2009) Prevalence and predictors of lipid and glucose monitoring in commercially insured patients treated with second-generation antipsychotic agents. *American Journal of Psychiatryi* **166**, 345–353.

Heiskanen, T., Niskanen, L., Lyytikainen, R., Saarienen, P.I. & Hintikka, J. (2003) Metabolic syndrome in patients with schizophrenia. *Journal of Clinical Psychiatry* **64**, 575–579.

Henderson, D.C., Cagliero, E., Copeland, P.M. *et al.* (2005) Glucose metabolism in patients with schizophrenia treated with atypical antipsychotic agents: a frequently sampled intravenous glucose tolerance test and minimal model analysis. *Archives of General Psychiatry* **62**, 19–28.

Henderson, D.C., Cagliero, E., Copeland, P.M. *et al.* (2007) Elevated hemoglobin A1c as a possible indicator of diabetes mellitus and diabetic ketoacidosis in schizophrenia patients receiving atypical antipsychotics. *Journal of Clinical Psychiatry* **68**, 533–541.

Hennekens, C.H. (1998) Increasing burden of cardiovascular disease: current knowledge and future directions for research on risk factors. *Circulation* **97**, 1095–1102.

Hennessy, S., Bilker, W.B., Knauss, J.S. *et al.* (2002) Cardiac arrest and ventricular arrhythmia in patients taking antipsychotic drugs: cohort study using administrative data. *BMJ* **325**, 1070.

Hirsch, S.R., Kissling, W., Bauml, J., Power, A. & O'Connor, R. (2002) A 28-week comparison of ziprasidone and haloperidol in outpatients with stable schizophrenia. *Journal of Clinical Psychiatry* **63**, 516–523.

Houseknecht, K.L., Robertson, A.S., Johnson, D.E. & Rollema, H. et al. (2005) Diabetogenic effects of some atypical antipsychotics: Rapid, whole body insulin resistance following a single dose. *Diabetologia* **48** (Suppl. 1), A212.

Institute of Medicine (2005) *Improving Quality of Health Care for Mental and Substance-Use Conditions: Quality Chasm Series.* Executive summary available at: http://www.nap.edu/catalog/11470.html. National Academy of Sciences. [Accessed April 18, 2006].

Jones, A.M., Rak, I.W. & Raniwalla, J. (2000) Weight changes in patients treated with quetiapine. Poster presented at the 153rd Annual Meeting of the American Psychiatric Association May 13–18, 2000 Chicago, IL.

Kahn, R., Buse, J., Ferrannini, E. & Stern, M. (2005) The metabolic syndrome: time for a critical appraisal. Joint statement from the American Diabetes Association and the European Association for the Study of Diabetes. *Diabetologia* **48**, 1684–1699.

Kahn, R.S., Fleischhacker, W.W., Boter, H. et al. (2008) Effectiveness of antipsychotic drugs in first-episode schizophrenia and schizophreniform disorder: an open randomised clinical trial. *Lancet* **371**, 1085–1097.

Kane, J., Canas, F., Kramer, M. et al. (2007) Treatment of schizophrenia with paliperidone extended-release tablets: a 6-week placebo-controlled trial. *Schizophrenia Research* **90**, 147–161.

Kane, J.M., Lauriello, J., Laska, E., Di Marino, M. & Wolfgang, C.D. (2008) Long-term efficacy and safety of iloperidone: results from 3 clinical trials for the treatment of schizophrenia. *Journal of Clinical Psychopharmacology* **28**, S29–35.

Kasanin, J. (1926) The blood sugar curve in mental disease. *Archives of Neurological Psychiatry* **16**, 414–419.

Kasper, S., Lerman, M.N., McQuade, R.D. et al. (2003) Efficacy and safety of aripiprazole vs. haloperidol for long-term maintenance treatment following acute relapse of schizophrenia. *International Journal of Neuropsychopharmacology* **6**, 325–337.

Kemner, C., Willemsen-Swinkels, S.H., De Jonge, M., Tuynman-Qua, H. & Van Engeland, H. (2002) Open-label study of olanzapine in children with pervasive developmental disorder. *Journal of Clinical Psychopharmacology* **22**, 455–460.

Ketter, T.A. & Haupt, D.W. (2006) Perceptions of weight gain and bipolar pharmacotherapy: results of a 2005 survey of physicians in clinical practice. *Current Medical Research and Opinion* **22**, 2345–2353.

Kilbourne, A.M., Cornelius, J.R., Han, X. et al. (2005) General-medical conditions in older patients with serious mental illness. *American Journal of Geriatric Psychiatry* **13**, 250–254.

Kim, S.F., Huang, A.S., Snowman, A.M., Teuscher, C. & Snyder, S.H. (2007) Antipsychotic drug-induced weight gain mediated by histamine H-1 receptor-linked activation of hypothalamic AMP-kinase. *Proceedings of the National Academy of Sciences USA* **104**, 3456–3459.

Kinon, B.J. (1998) The routine use of atypical antipsychotic agents: maintenance treatment. *Journal of Clinical Psychiatry* **59** (Suppl. 19), 18–22.

Kinon, B.J., Lipkovich, I., Edwards, S.B., Adams, D.H., Ascher-Svanum, H. & Siris, S.G. (2006) A 24-week randomized study of olanzapine versus ziprasidone in the treatment of schizophrenia or schizoaffective disorder in patients with prominent depressive symptoms. *Journal of Clinical Psychopharmacology* **26**, 157–162.

Kinon, B.J., Volavka, J., Stauffer, V. et al. (2008) Standard and higher dose of olanzapine in patients with schizophrenia or schizoaffective disorder: a randomized, double-blind, fixed-dose study. *Journal of Clinical Psychopharmacology* **28**, 392–400.

Kohn, R., Saxena, S., Levav, I. & Saraceno, B. (2004) The treatment gap in mental health care. *Bulletin of the World Health Organization* **82**, 858–866.

Koller, E.A. & Doraiswamy, P.M. (2002) Olanzapine-associated diabetes mellitus. *Pharmacotherapy* **22**, 841–852.

Koller, E., Malozowski, S. & Doraiswamy, P.M. (2001a) Atypical antipsychotic drugs and hyperglycemia in adolescents. *JAMA* **286**, 2547–2548.

Koller, E., Schneider, B., Bennett, K. & Dubitsky, G. (2001b) Clozapine-associated diabetes. *American Journal of Medicine* **111**, 716–723.

Koller, E.A., Cross, J.T., Doraiswamy, P.M. & Schneider, B.S. (2003) Risperidone-associated diabetes mellitus: a pharmacovigilance study. *Pharmacotherapy* **23**, 735–744.

Koller, E.A., Weber, J., Doraiswamy, P.M. & Schneider, B.S. (2004) A survey of reports of quetiapine-associated hyperglycemia and diabetes mellitus. *Journal of Clinical Psychiatry* **65**, 857–863.

Koro, C.E., Fedder, D.O., L'Italien, G.J. et al. (2002a) An assessment of the independent effects of olanzapine and risperidone exposure on the risk of hyperlipidemia in schizophrenic patients. *Archives of General Psychiatry* **59**, 1021–1026.

Koro, C.E., Fedder, D.O., L'Italien, G.J. et al. (2002b) Assessment of independent effect of olanzapine and risperidone on risk of diabetes among patients with schizophrenia: population based nested case-control study. *BMJ* **325**, 243.

Kramer, M., Simpson, G., Maciulis, V. et al. (2007) Paliperidone extended-release tablets for prevention of symptom recurrence in patients with schizophrenia: a randomized, double-blind, placebo-controlled study. *Journal of Clinical Psychopharmacology* **27**, 6–14.

Kroeze, W.K., Hufeisen, S.J., Popadak, B.A. et al. (2003) H1-histamine receptor affinity predicts short-term weight gain for typical and atypical antipsychotic drugs. *Neuropsychopharmacology* **28**, 519–526.

Kumra, S., Kranzler, H., Gerbino-Rosen, G. et al. (2008) Clozapine and "high-dose" olanzapine in refractory early-onset schizophrenia: a 12-week randomized and double-blind comparison. *Biological Psychiatry* **63**, 524–529.

Kurt, E. & Oral, E.T. (2002) Antipsychotics and glucose, insulin, lipids, prolactin, uric acid metabolism in schizophrenia. *European Neuropsychopharmocology* **12**, S276.

Lambert, B.L., Chang, K.Y., Tafesse, E. & Carson, W. (2005a) Association between antipsychotic treatment and hyperlipidemia among California Medicaid patients with schizophrenia. *Journal of Clinical Psychopharmacology* **25**, 12–18.

Lambert, B.L., Chou, C.H., Chang, K.Y., Tafesse, E. & Carson, W. (2005b) Antipsychotic exposure and type 2 diabetes among patients with schizophrenia: a matched case-control study of California Medicaid claims. *Pharmacoepidemiology and Drug Safety* **14**, 417–425.

Lamberti, J., Crilly, J., Maharaj, K., Olson, D. & Costea, O. (2003) Prevalence of adult-onset diabetes among outpatients receiving antipsychotic drugs. *Schizophrenia Research* **60**, 360.

Leslie, D.L. & Rosenheck, R.A. (2004) Incidence of newly diagnosed diabetes attributable to atypical antipsychotic medications. *American Journal of Psychiatry* **161**, 1709–1711.

Leucht, S., Wagenpfeil, S., Hamann, J. & Kissling, W. (2004) Amisulpride is an "atypical" antipsychotic associated with low weight gain. *Psychopharmacology (Berlin)* **173**, 112–115.

Leucht, S., Burkard, T., Henderson, J., Maj, M. & Sartorius, N. (2007) Physical illness and schizophrenia: a review of the literature. *Acta Psychiatrica Scandinavica* **116**, 317–333.

Lieberman, J.A., Stroup, T.S., McEvoy, J.P. *et al.* (2005) Effectiveness of antipsychotic drugs in patients with chronic schizophrenia. *New England Journal of Medicine* **353**, 1209–1223.

Lindenmayer, J.P., Czobor, P., Volavka, J. *et al.* (2003) Changes in glucose and cholesterol levels in patients with schizophrenia treated with typical or atypical antipsychotics. *American Journal of Psychiatry* **160**, 290–296.

L'Italien, G.J. (2003) Pharmacoeconomic impact of antipsychotic-induced metabolic events. *American Journal of Management and Care* **3**, S38–S42.

Lorenzo, C., Okoloise, M., Williams, K., Stern, M.P. & Haffner, S.M. (2003) The metabolic syndrome as predictor of type 2 diabetes: the San Antonio heart study. *Diabetes Care* **26**, 3153–3159.

Lund, B.C., Perry, P.J., Brooks, J.M. & Arndt, S. (2001) Clozapine use in patients with schizophrenia and the risk of diabetes, hyperlipidemia, and hypertension: a claims-based approach. *Archives of General Psychiatry* **58**, 1172–1176.

Lutterman, T., Ganju, V., Schacht, L. *et al.* (2003) *Sixteen State Study on Mental Health Performance Measures.* DHSS Publication No. (SMA) 03-3835. Rockville, MD: Center for Mental Health.

Marder, S.R., McQuade, R.D., Stock, E., *et al.* (2003) Aripiprazole in the treatment of schizophrenia: safety and tolerability in short-term, placebo-controlled trials. *Schizophrenia Research* **61**, 123–136.

Marder, S.R., Kramer, M., Ford, L. *et al.* (2007) Efficacy and safety of paliperidone extended-release tablets: results of a 6-week, randomized, placebo-controlled study. *Biological Psychiatry* **62**, 1363–1370.

McCreadie, R.G. (2003) Diet, smoking and cardiovascular risk in people with schizophrenia: descriptive study. *British Journal of Psychiatry* **183**, 534–539.

McDermott, S., Moran, R., Platt, T., Isaac, T., Wood, H. & Dasari, S. (2005) Heart disease, schizophrenia, and affective psychoses: epidemiology of risk in primary care. *Community Mental Health Journal* **41**, 747–755.

McEvoy, J.P., Lieberman, J.A., Perkins, D.O. *et al.* (2007) Efficacy and tolerability of olanzapine, quetiapine, and risperidone in the treatment of early psychosis: A randomized, double-blind 52-week comparison. *American Journal of Psychiatry* **164**, 1050–1060.

McLaughlin, T., Abbasi, F., Cheal, K., Chu, J., Lamendola, C. & Reaven, G. (2003) Use of metabolic markers to identify overweight individuals who are insulin resistant. *Annals of Internal Medicine* **139**, 802–809.

McQuade, R.D., Jody, D., Kujawa, M., Carson, W.H. & Iwamoto, T. (2003) Long-term weight effects of aripiprazole versus olanzapine. Poster presented at the American Psychiatric Association (APA) Annual Meeting. San Francisco, CA.

McQuade, R.D., Stock, E., Marcus, R. *et al.* (2004) A comparison of weight change during treatment with olanzapine or aripiprazole: results from a randomized, double-blind study. *Journal of Clinical Psychiatry* **65** (Suppl. 18), 47–56.

Mokdad, A.H., Serdula, M.K., Dietz, W.H., Bowman, B.A., Marks, J.S. & Koplan, J.P. (1999) The spread of the obesity epidemic in the United States, 1991–1998. *JAMA* **282**, 1519–1522.

Mokdad, A.H., Bowman, B.A., Ford, E.S., Vinicor, F., Marks, J.S. & Koplan, J.P. (2001) The continuing epidemics of obesity and diabetes in the United States. *JAMA* **286**, 1195–1200.

Montague, C.T. & O'Rahilly, S. (2000) The perils of portliness: causes and consequences of visceral adiposity. *Diabetes* **49**, 883–888.

Morrato, E.H., Newcomer, J.W., Allen, R.R. & Valuck, R.J. (2008) Prevalence of baseline serum glucose and lipid testing in users of second-generation antipsychotic drugs: a retrospective, population-based study of Medicaid claims data. *Journal of Clinical Psychiatry* **69**, 316–322.

Morrato, E.H., Newcomer, J.W., Kamat, S., Baser, O., Harnett, J. & Cuffel, B. (2009) Metabolic screening after the American Diabetes Association's consensus statement on antipsychotic drugs and diabetes. *Diabetes Care* **32**, 1037–1042.

Mortimer, A., Martin, S., Loo, H. & Peuskens, J. (2004) A double-blind, randomized comparative trial of amisulpride versus olanzapine for 6 months in the treatment of schizophrenia. *International Clinical Psychopharmacology* **19**, 63–69.

Mukherjee, S., Schnur, D.B. & Reddy, R. (1989) Family history of type 2 diabetes in schizophrenic patients. *Lancet* **1**, 495.

Mukherjee, S., Decina, P., Bocola, V., Saraceni, F. & Scapicchio, P.L. (1996) Diabetes mellitus in schizophrenic patients. *Comprehensive Psychiatry* **37**, 68–73.

NASMHPD Medical Directors Council (2006) *Morbidity and Mortality in People with Serious Mental Illness.* Thirteenth in a series of technical reports. Editors: Joe Parks, MD; Dale Svendsen, MD; Patricia Singer, MD; Mary Ellen Foti, MD. Technical Writer Barbara Mauer, MSW, CMC. Alexandria, VA: National Association of State Mental Health Program Directors (NASMHPD) Medical Directors Council.

Nasrallah, H.A. (2008) Atypical antipsychotic-induced metabolic side effects: insights from receptor-binding profiles. *Molecular Psychiatry* **13**, 27–35.

National Cholesterol Education Program (2002) Third Report of the National Cholesterol Education Program (NCEP) Expert Panel on Detection, Evaluation, and Treatment of High Blood Cholesterol in Adults (Adult Treatment Panel III) final report. *Circulation* **106**, 3143–3421.

Nemeroff, C.B. (1997) Dosing the antipsychotic medication olanzapine. *Journal of Clinical Psychiatry* **58** (Suppl. 10), 45–49.

Newcomer, J.W. (2005a) Clinical considerations in selecting and using atypical antipsychotics. *CNS Spectrum* **10**, 12–20.

Newcomer, J.W. (2005b) Second-generation (atypical) antipsychotics and metabolic effects: a comprehensive literature review. *CNS Drugs* **19** (Suppl. 1), 1–93.

Newcomer, J.W. & Hennekens, C.H. (2007) Severe mental illness and risk of cardiovascular disease. *JAMA* **298**, 1794–1796.

Newcomer, J.W., Haupt, D.W., Fucetola, R. *et al.* (2002) Abnormalities in glucose regulation during antipsychotic treatment of schizophrenia. *Archives of General Psychiatry* **59**, 337–345.

Newcomer, J.W., Rasgon, N., Craft, S. & Reaven, G. (2005) Insulin resistance and metabolic risk during antipsychotic treatment. Presented at the Annual American Psychiatric Association Symposium entitled Insulin Resistance and Metabolic Syndrome in Neuropsychiatry, Atlanta, GA.

Newcomer, J.W., Campos, J.A., Marcus, R.N. *et al.* (2008) A multicenter, randomized, double-blind study of the effects of aripiprazole in overweight subjects with schizophrenia or schizoaffective disorder switched from olanzapine. *Journal of Clinical Psychiatry* **69**, 1046–1056.

Newcomer, J.W., Ratner, R.E., Eriksson, J.W. *et al.* (2009) A 24-week, multicenter, open-label, randomized study to compare changes in glucose metabolism in patients with schizophrenia receiving treatment with olanzapine, quetiapine, or risperidone. *Journal of Clinical Psychiatry* **70**, 487–499.

Newton, C.A. & Raskin, P. (2004) Diabetic ketoacidosis in type 1 and type 2 diabetes mellitus: clinical and biochemical differences. *Archives of Internal Medicine* **164**, 1925–1931.

Okamura, F., Tashiro, A., Utumi, A. *et al.* (2000) Insulin resistance in patients with depression and its changes during the clinical course of depression: minimal model analysis. *Metabolism* **49**, 1255–1260.

Peet, M. (2004) Diet, diabetes and schizophrenia: review and hypothesis. *British Journal of Psychiatry* **47** (Suppl.), S102–105.

Perez-Iglesias, R., Crespo-Facorro, B., Amado, J.A. *et al.* (2007) A 12-week randomized clinical trial to evaluate metabolic changes in drug-naive, first-episode psychosis patients treated with haloperidol, olanzapine, or risperidone. *Journal of Clinical Psychiatry* **68**, 1733–1740.

Pi-Sunyer, F.X. (1993) Medical hazards of obesity. *Annals of Internal Medicine* **119**, 655–660.

Pigott, T.A., Carson, W.H., Saha, A.R., Torbeyns, A.F., Stock, E.G. & Ingenito, G.G. (2003) Aripiprazole for the prevention of relapse in stabilized patients with chronic schizophrenia: a placebo-controlled 26-week study. *Journal of Clinical Psychiatry* **64**, 1048–1056.

Regenold, W.T., Thapar, R.K., Marano, C., Gavirneni, S. & Kondapavuluru, P.V. (2002) Increased prevalence of type 2 diabetes mellitus among psychiatric inpatients with bipolar I affective and schizoaffective disorders independent of psychotropic drug use. *Journal of Affective Disorders* **70**, 19–26.

Resnick, H.E., Valsania, P., Halter, J.B. & Lin, X. (1998) Differential effects of BMI on diabetes risk among black and white Americans. *Diabetes Care* **21**, 1828–1835.

Reynolds, G.P. (2006) Metabolic syndrome and schizophrenia. *British Journal of Psychiatry* **188**, 86; author reply 86–87.

Rosenheck, R.A., Davis, S., Covell, N. *et al.* (2009) Does switching to a new antipsychotic improve outcomes? Data from the CATIE Trial. *Schizophrenia Research* **107**, 22–29.

Ryan, M.C. & Thakore, J.H. (2002) Physical consequences of schizophrenia and its treatment: the metabolic syndrome. *Life Science*, **71**, 239–257.

Ryan, M.C., Collins, P. & Thakore, J.H. (2003) Impaired fasting glucose tolerance in first-episode, drug-naive patients with schizophrenia. *American Journal of Psychiatry* **160**, 284–289.

Ryan, M.C., Flanagan, S., Kinsella, U., Keeling, F. & Thakore, J.H. (2004) The effects of atypical antipsychotics on visceral fat distribution in first episode, drug-naive patients with schizophrenia. *Life Science* **74**, 1999–2008.

Sacchetti, E., Valsecchi, P. & Parrinello, G. (2008) A randomized, flexible-dose, quasi-naturalistic comparison of quetiapine, risperidone, and olanzapine in the short-term treatment of schizophrenia: the QUERISOLA trial. *Schizophrenia Research* **98**, 55–65.

Sacher, J., Mossaheb, N., Spindelegger, C. *et al.* (2008) Effects of olanzapine and ziprasidone on glucose tolerance in healthy volunteers. *Neuropsychopharmacology* **33**, 1633–1641.

Saddichha, S., Manjunatha, N., Ameen, S. & Akhtar, S. (2008) Diabetes and schizophrenia – effect of disease or drug? Results from a randomized, double-blind, controlled prospective study in first-episode schizophrenia. *Acta Psychiatrica Scandinavica* **117**, 342–347.

Saha, S., Chant, D. & McGrath, J. (2007) A systematic review of mortality in schizophrenia—is the differential mortality gap worsening over time? *Archives of General Psychiatry* **64**, 1123–1131.

Sattar, N., Gaw, A., Scherbakova, O. *et al.* (2003) Metabolic syndrome with and without C-reactive protein as a predictor of coronary heart disease and diabetes in the West of Scotland Coronary Prevention Study. *Circulation* **108**, 414–419.

Sernyak, M.J., Leslie, D.L., Alarcon, R.D., Losonczy, M.F. & Rosenheck, R. (2002) Association of diabetes mellitus with use of atypical neuroleptics in the treatment of schizophrenia. *American Journal of Psychiatry* **159**, 561–566.

Shiloah, E., Witz, S., Abramovitch, Y. *et al.* (2003) Effect of acute psychotic stress in nondiabetic subjects on beta-cell function and insulin sensitivity. *Diabetes Care* **26**, 1462–1467.

Sikich, L., Hamer, R.M., Bashford, R.A., Sheitman, B.B. & Lieberman, J.A. (2004) A pilot study of risperidone, olanzapine, and haloperidol in psychotic youth: a double-blind, randomized, 8-week trial. *Neuropsychopharmacology* **29**, 133–145.

Sikich, L., Frazier, J.A., McClellan, J. *et al.* (2008) Double-blind comparison of first- and second-generation antipsychotics in early-onset schizophrenia and schizo-affective disorder: Findings from the Treatment of Early-Onset Schizophrenia Spectrum Disorders (TEOSS) Study. *American Journal of Psychiatry* **165**, 1420–1431.

Silver, H., Kogan, H. & Zlotogorski, D. (1990) Postural hypotension in chronically medicated schizophrenics. *Journal of Clinical Psychiatry* **51**, 459–462.

Sowell, M.O., Mukhopadhyay, N., Cavazzoni, P. *et al.* (2002) Hyperglycemic clamp assessment of insulin secretory responses in normal subjects treated with olanzapine, risperidone, or placebo. *Journal of Clinical Endocrinology and Metabolism* **87**, 2918–2923.

Sowell, M., Mukhopadhyay, N., Cavazzoni, P. *et al.* (2003) Evaluation of insulin sensitivity in healthy volunteers treated with olanzapine, risperidone, or placebo: a prospective, randomized study using the two-step hyperinsulinemic, euglycemic clamp. *Journal of Clinical Endocrinology and Metabolism* **88**, 5875–5880.

Stroup, T.S., Lieberman, J.A., McEvoy, J.P. *et al.* (2006) Effectiveness of olanzapine, quetiapine, risperidone, and ziprasidone in patients with chronic schizophrenia following discontinuation of a previous atypical antipsychotic. *American Journal of Psychiatry* **163**, 611–622.

Stroup, T.S., Lieberman, J.A., McEvoy, J.P. *et al.* (2009) Results of phase 3 of the CATIE schizophrenia trial. *Schizophrenia Research* **107**, 1–12.

Su, K.P., Wu, P.L. & Pariante, C.M. (2005) A crossover study on lipid and weight changes associated with olanzapine and risperidone. *Psychopharmacology (Berlin)* **183**, 383–386.

Sumiyoshi, T., Roy, A., Anil, A.E., Jayathilake, K., Ertugrul, A. & Meltzer, H.Y. (2004) A comparison of incidence of diabetes mellitus between atypical antipsychotic drugs: a survey for clozapine, risperidone, olanzapine, and quetiapine. *Journal of Clinical Psychopharmacology* **24**, 345–348.

Susce, M.T., Villanueva, N., Diaz, F.J. & De Leon, J. (2005) Obesity and associated complications in patients with severe mental illnesses: a cross-sectional survey. *Journal of Clinical Psychiatry* **66**, 167–173.

Tiihonen, J., Lonnqvist, J., Wahlbeck, K. *et al.* (2009) 11-year follow-up of mortality in patients with schizophrenia: a population-based cohort study (FIN11 study). *Lancet* **320**, 620–627.

US Food and Drug Administration (2004) Warning about hyperglycemia and atypical antipsychotic drugs. FDA Patient Safety News. June 2004. Available at http://www.accessdata.fda.gov/scripts/cdrh/cfdocs/psn/transcript.cfm?show=28

Visser, M., Pahor, M., Tylavsky, F. *et al.* (2003) One- and two-year change in body composition as measured by DXA in a population-based cohort of older men and women. *Journal of Applied Physiology* **94**, 2368–2374.

Wang, P.S., Glynn, R.J., Ganz, D.A., Schneeweiss, S., Levin, R. & Avorn, J. (2002) Clozapine use and risk of diabetes mellitus. *Journal of Clinical Psychopharmacology* **22**, 236–243.

Weiden, P.J., Daniel, D.G., Simpson, G. & Romano, S.J. (2003) Improvement in indices of health status in outpatients with schizophrenia switched to ziprasidone. *Journal of Clinical Psychopharmacology* **23**, 595–600.

Weiden, P.J., Newcomer, J.W., Loebel, A.D., Yang, R. & Lebovitz, H.E. (2008) Long-term changes in weight and plasma lipids during maintenance treatment with ziprasidone. *Neuropsychopharmacology* **33**, 985–994.

Willett, W.C., Dietz, W.H. & Colditz, G.A. (1999) Guidelines for healthy weight. *New England Journal of Medicine* **341**, 427–434.

Yang, S.H. & McNeely, M.J. (2002) Rhabdomyolysis, pancreatitis, and hyperglycemia with ziprasidone. *American Journal of Psychiatry* **159**, 1435.

Yood, M.U., Delorenze, G., Quesenberry, C.P. Jr *et al.* (2009) The incidence of diabetes in atypical antipsychotic users differs according to agent – results from a multisite epidemiologic study. *Pharmacoepidemiology and Drug Safety* **18**, 791–799.

Zhang, Z.J., Yao, Z.J., Liu, W., Fang, Q. & Reynolds, G.P. (2004) Effects of antipsychotics on fat deposition and changes in leptin and insulin levels. Magnetic resonance imaging study of previously untreated people with schizophrenia. *British Journal of Psychiatry* **184**, 58–62.

Zimbroff, D., Warrington, L., Loebel, A., Yang, R. & Siu, C. (2007) Comparison of ziprasidone and aripiprazole in acutely ill patients with schizophrenia or schizoaffective disorder: a randomized, double-blind, 4-week study. *International Clinical Psychopharmacology* **22**, 363–370.

Zipursky, R.B., Gu, H., Green, A.I. *et al.* (2005) Course and predictors of weight gain in people with first-episode psychosis treated with olanzapine or haloperidol. *British Journal of Psychiatry* **187**, 537–543.

PART 4

Psychosocial Aspects

CHAPTER 29

Schizophrenia and psychosocial stresses

Paul E. Bebbington[1] and Elizabeth Kuipers[2]

[1]University College London, London, UK
[2]Institute of Psychiatry, King's College London, London, UK

Since the last version of this chapter was written, our conceptualization of schizophrenia has altered appreciably. This shift has had three main drivers. The first is that the genetic enterprise in schizophrenia now seems less secure, particularly since the arrival of genome-wide studies (see Chapter 13). Second, there has been more evidence linking *early* adversity with the risk of schizophrenia (see also Chapters 10 and 11). Finally, it is much more accepted that the phenomena of schizophrenia are more widespread than the prevalence of the clinical disorder would suggest. As a consequence of these developments, it has become apparent that a major problem in establishing a convincing etiology of schizophrenia is that all the factors implicated are more represented in people without the disorder than in those with it. This applies to genetic, biological, and social factors alike.

The result has been an elaboration of the stress–vulnerability model of schizophrenia: in addition to putative biological mechanisms, the modern *cognitive models* encompass cognitive and emotional pathways linking the social context to the generation of specific symptoms of psychosis (Garety *et al.*, 2001, 2007; Bentall *et al.*, 2001; Morrison, 2001; Birchwood, 2003; Broome *et al.*, 2005).

The concept of psychosocial stress nevertheless remains central to an understanding of the impact of the social environment on schizophrenia. It can take several forms. One comprises sudden changes in the individual's psychosocial milieu, so-called life events. The social, emotional, cognitive, and behavioral consequences of such changes may dissipate fairly rapidly, or they may persist. Another form of psychosocial stress is characterized rather by an absence of change. This would include persistent poverty, for example, or the daily stresses of a difficult urban environment, where the effects are likely to be gradually cumulative. Yet other types of stress take the form of an insistent repetitiveness. The repeated experience of sexual abuse in childhood and the serial insults experienced by immigrants are examples of this.

As we emphasized in the original version of this chapter (Bebbington *et al.*, 1995), the idea that schizophrenia is, at least in part, a socially reactive condition has gradually gained acceptance in clinical psychiatry over the last 50 years. In the first edition, we focused on research into certain specific potential psychosocial influences on schizophrenia. Thus, we covered in detail studies linking the

Schizophrenia, 3rd edition. Edited by Daniel R. Weinberger and Paul J Harrison © 2011 Blackwell Publishing Ltd.

emergence of schizophrenic symptoms with: (1) antecedent life events and (2) family atmosphere as detected by the expressed emotion (EE) measure.

The 2003 revision of the chapter (Bebbington & Kuipers, 2003) took a broader view of the psychosocial reactivity of psychotic symptoms. It included the issues of psychogenic psychosis and of schizophrenic symptoms in the context of post-traumatic stress disorder (PTSD). The revisions at that time were driven partly by the emergence of cognitive–behavioral therapy (CBT) for psychosis, with its focus on the meaning of clients' symptoms: in the process of therapy, the sheer salience of past trauma and of the psychosocial environment over the whole lifespan often becomes convincingly apparent.

Since then, the study of the impact of events has broadened to include considerations of early trauma, the investigation of links between PTSD and symptoms of schizophrenia, and attempts to demonstrate specificity in the relationship between events and the onset of schizophrenic episodes. Papers have continued to appear examining the impact of family life on schizophrenia. Several of these have sought to discover how relationship difficulties may be linked to psychological and attitudinal processes in both patients and carers, and these will be described below.

Psychosocial stress and the definition of psychotic disorders

Psychiatric classification has always been based primarily on the clinical features of individual disorders. Attempts to base classification on etiological principles have been successful in very few psychiatric conditions. Perhaps because of the medical basis of psychiatry, the etiological hypotheses favored over the last century and a half have tended to involve organic causes, although the attempt to identify such causes has gone relatively unrewarded. However, it has resulted in deliberate and particular refinements of classification. Thus, in order to further the search for organic causation, early psychiatrists set about separating off those cases of symptom-defined disorder which appeared to have a social etiological origin.

The psychogenic element in psychiatric disorders was recognized early by psychiatrists, certainly by the mid-19th century (Griesinger, 1861). Having made the decision to do so, it was easy to differentiate conditions such as bereavement responses from depressive disorders "proper", but by the early 20th century similar attempts were also being made to separate off so-called "reactive psychoses". This strategy results in a core group of disorders covertly defined by *not* having an ostensible and intimate relationship to a social causation.

This has not, however, prevented researchers from continuing to tease out social influences on these ring-fenced

disorders, and they have, perhaps ironically, been rather successful in this. This is particularly so in the case of depressive disorder, although the relation of stressful life events to the onset of those depressive disorders defined by the exclusion of cases immediately and intimately related to social causes tends to mean that the social causation in the remaining disorders is more subtle.

A similar pattern is apparent in psychosis. The search for a social etiology of psychosis has tended to follow the exclusion of those cases in which social causes appear paramount. These disorders have been characterized as reactive psychoses, and their manifestations are held to be typically florid and short-lived. The development of the idea of reactive psychosis had the inevitable result that cases where social reactivity was not completely salient came to be regarded as essentially biological in origin. It is our view that a more productive strategy would involve the examination of factors at every level in relation to the whole range of clinical pictures, including subclinical variants. Nevertheless, much of the evidence reviewed in this chapter must concern the social reactivity of schizophrenic psychoses defined in ways that do tend to exclude immediate and salient social causes. We see this as a major problem for this area of research, as it posts a false dichotomy between biological and social causation.

If we consider psychosis as a psychological process rather than a set of diagnostic categories, the process may be illuminated by the study of reactive psychoses. Nearly half the cases of psychosis in Scandinavia have traditionally been diagnosed as reactive. Although first noted because of its relation to stress, reactive psychosis is defined by characteristic symptoms and a characteristic course (Ungvari & Mullens, 2000). It is typified by perplexity, a pleomorphic clinical picture, a considerable affective component, and an acute onset. It also has a relatively benign and episodic course. Defined in this way, it is certainly more likely to be linked to a precipitating stress than so-called process schizophrenia (Stephens *et al.*, 1982).

Separating off a diagnosis of reactive psychosis should thus reduce the association of the left-over group of psychoses with antecedent stressful events. While the definitions in the American Diagnostic and Statistical Manual (DSM; American Psychiatric Association, 1987, 1994) do not lend themselves to the diagnosis of reactive psychosis (Jauch & Carpenter, 1998), the DSM duration criterion probably constrains the demonstration of the social reactivity of schizophrenia.

Setting the agenda for a social etiology

The earliest demonstrations of the social reactivity of schizophrenia using modern standards of scientific inference leant heavily on the work of George Brown and John Wing.

They established a clear relationship between the poverty of the social environment and the prevalence of negative symptoms in schizophrenia (Wing & Brown, 1970). However, they were also aware that trying to overcome negative symptoms by providing a more stimulating environment carried the opposite risk: too much pressure placed on patients in rehabilitation programs sometimes led to the re-emergence of positive florid symptoms of schizophrenia (Wing *et al.*, 1964).

It was against this background that Brown and Birley (1968) carried out their seminal study into the effects of life events in schizophrenia. The same group also developed the hypothesis that stresses within the families of patients sometimes provoke relapse, testing it by measuring EE (Brown *et al.*, 1972). The importance of these early empirical studies should not be underestimated: the social reactivity of the condition is nowadays generally accepted, where before schizophrenia was thought of as an intractably deteriorating biological condition.

Some of the strongest evidence for the social reactivity of schizophrenia has come from the explosion of EE research in the last 30 years. In contrast, the findings concerning life events remain less robust. Few recent studies have examined the relationship between life events and schizophrenia episodes directly, but our knowledge has been extended by other research strategies.

Expressed emotion and schizophrenia

One of the most compelling indications of the social reactivity of schizophrenia is the large body of work detailing the impact of family atmosphere on its course. The main impetus for this has been studies based on measuring EE; Brown & Rutter, 1966; Brown *et al.*, 1972).

Measurement of EE typically involves rating individual relatives' behavior elicited in a structured interview, the Camberwell Family Interview, to predict the likelihood of subsequent relapse in patients with whom the relatives live. It is presumed that it can do this because it reflects some significant and enduring aspect of the interplay between patient and relative, or the ability of relatives to cope with crises (Kuipers, 1979). Of the various components of the EE rating, critical comments, hostility, and over-involvement have turned out to be the most predictive of relapse. EE is probably dimorphic, given that hostility and criticism are clearly related to each other but less so to over-involvement.

In previous versions of this chapter (Bebbington *et al.*, 1995; Bebbington & Kuipers, 2003), we covered methodological aspects of the measurement of EE, the existing literature demonstrating the predictive capacity of EE in schizophrenia, and the evidence supporting the influence of the family on the course of the disorder. We also discussed the links between EE and the processes presumed to be reflected by the measure. We will now update and refocus this review.

There are currently around 30 prospective studies of the role of EE as a risk factor for relapse in schizophrenia (Table 29.1). Fifteen years ago, we carried out an aggregate analysis of the 25 studies of EE then available, covering over 1300 patients (Bebbington & Kuipers, 1994). Where possible, data on individual cases were obtained from the original authors. Altogether 15 studies showed an association beyond the 5% level, two just failed to reach this level, five showed a non-significant trend, and three either no trend or a small trend in the reverse direction. However, the overall relapse rate for high-EE cases in these studies was 50%, whereas that for low-EE cases was 21%. This result was overwhelmingly significant. The aggregate analysis found that the effect of EE was actually stronger than that of medication. The strength of the association of relapse with EE was virtually identical in medicated and non-medicated groups. It was greater where contact was high, whereas living in high contact with a low-EE relative was, if anything, protective. The lowest rates of EE have been detected in developing countries, notably in India (Wig *et al.*, 1987), China (Maosheng *et al.*, 1998), and Bali (Kurihara *et al.*, 2000). However, the highly significant association of relapse with high EE was unaffected by the location of the study.

Our conclusions were essentially confirmed by a later meta-analysis by Butzlaff and Hooley (1998), based on 27 studies. There has been little recent research into the predictive capacity of EE in psychosis, probably because the finding is so well-established.

While the EE measure is established by expert raters, there is mounting evidence that people with psychosis themselves perceive accurately that they are being criticized (Scazufca *et al.*, 2001; Onwumere *et al.*, 2009). This is a useful development, suggesting as it does that questioning patients directly about their relationships has validity and predictive power that could be used in a therapeutic context.

Inferences from family intervention in schizophrenia

The acknowledgement that family atmosphere has a role in relapse in schizophrenia has led to a considerable number of randomized controlled family intervention (FI) studies. These have been reviewed in various meta-analyses (Pilling *et al.*, 2002; National Institute for Clinical Excellence, 2003, revised 2009; Pfammatter *et al.*, 2006; Pharoah *et al.*, 2006). Pfammatter *et al.* (2006) reviewed 31 randomized controlled trials, and confirmed that, following FI, patients with psychosis had significantly less relapse and hospital admission during follow-up. They concluded there was "considerable shift from high to low EE, a substantial

Table 29.1 Predictive studies of expressed emotion in schizophrenia.

Study	Country	N
Brown et al. (1962)	England	97
Brown et al. (1972)	England	91
Leff & Vaughn (1976)	England	37
Leff et al. (1982)	England	12
Vaughn et al. (1984)	California	36
Moline et al. (1985)	Illinois	16
MacMillan et al. (1986)	England	73
Nuechterlein et al. (1986)	California	36
Karno et al. (1987)	California	43
Leff et al. (1987); Wig et al. (1987)	India	77
McCreadie & Phillips (1988); McCreadie et al. (1991)	Scotland	59
Parker et al. (1988)	Australia	57
Bertrando et al. (1992)	Italy	9
Gutiérrez et al. (1988)	Spain	32
Tarrier et al. (1988a)	England	37
Budzyna-Dawidowski et al. (1989)	Poland	36
Arévalo & Vizcaro (1989)	Spain	31
Barrelet et al. (1990)	Switzerland	42
Buchkremer et al. (1991)	Germany	99
Stirling et al. (1991)	England	33
Možný & Votpkova (1992)	Czechoslovakia	82
Montero et al. (1992)	Spain	60
Vaughan et al. (1992)	Australia	89
Niedermeier et al. (1992)	Germany	48
Ivanović et al. (1994)	Yugoslavia	60
Tanaka et al. (1995)	Japan	52
Linszen et al. (1996)	Netherlands	76
King & Dixon (1999)	Canada	69
Kopelowicz et al. (2002)	US	17 WA, 44 MA
Lopez et al. (2004)	US	54 WA, 44 MA
Rosenfarb et al. (2006)	US	31 WA, 40 AA

WA, white Americans; MA, Mexican Americans; AA, African Americans.

improvement in social adjustment of the patients, a decline in inpatient treatment, and an overall reduction in psychopathology during the follow up" (p. 571). The revised National Institute of Clinical Excellence (NICE) guidelines now list 38 randomized controlled trials of FI (National Institute for Clinical Excellence, 2009).

These trials strongly support the argument that elements of family atmosphere are causally related to relapse in schizophrenia, in that outcomes can be improved when these elements are changed: the reduction in relapse appears to be mediated by the improvement in family atmosphere.

A number of studies have addressed the question of what high EE scores mean in practice about relationships between carers and their relatives with schizophrenia. This has important implications for the mechanisms that mediate the effect of family stress in engendering relapse in psychosis. Measures of EE tap into the quality and style of interactions within family systems that are necessarily complex. Living with a high-EE relative represents a chronic stress. However, it is very likely that low-EE relationships are not merely neutral, in the sense of representing an absence of stress, but actually have positive and beneficial effects on patients. Thus, Hubschmid and Zemp (1989) found that low-EE relatives made significantly more emotionally positive and supportive statements during interactions with patients. This could explain why high contact with low-EE relatives appears to be protective for patients not on medication; in other words, vulnerable patients do better with a larger "dose" of their low-EE (warm) relatives (Bebbington & Kuipers, 1994).

It has long been known that relatives who make frequent critical comments when alone with an interviewer behave similarly in the presence of the patient, albeit usually with more restraint (Brown & Rutter, 1966). This view is supported by the complementary work on Negative Affective Style. This is a coding system used to assess families taking part in a standardized task designed to recreate everyday interaction in a laboratory setting (Goldstein et al., 1968; Doane et al., 1981). Negative Affective Style in these direct interactions was highly correlated with EE measured in the usual way (Strachan et al., 1986; Miklowitz et al., 1989).

Rosenfarb et al. (1995; Woo et al., 1997) used a direct interaction task, and demonstrated not only that people with schizophrenia with high-EE relatives exhibited more subclinical odd and sometimes hostile behaviors, but that the relatives responded very quickly to these in a way that led to further odd behavior. This suggests strongly that a bidirectional interaction underlies the predictive capacity of EE. Bentsen et al. (1996) reported that emotional overinvolvement (EOI) was characteristic of relatives who spent a lot of time with the patients. Patients who lived with EOI relatives actually showed less difficult behavior, but tended to be anxious and depressed.

Birchwood and Smith (1987) put forward a model whereby families' coping style develops over time. There is little to argue with in this. It is difficult to see how the characteristics of high EE might arise *except* from an interaction between the relative and the patient. However, this does not mean that particular responses on the part of the relatives have no influence on the subsequent course of the disorder. This is why intervention studies are so useful in supporting an etiological role for EE-related behaviors, whatever their origins. Nonetheless, there is evidence that, even at first episode, some relatives exhibit both high-EE attitudes and high burden, suggesting that its development is often rapid (Raune *et al.*, 2004).

Other characteristics of carers and patients are of possible importance. Experimental tests suggest people with schizophrenia are poorer judges of affect (Bell *et al.*, 1997), and they rate high-EE carers as particularly inscrutable (Stark & Siol, 1994). However, patients living with critical relatives are quite capable of perceiving their criticality (Tompson *et al.*, 1995; Scazufca *et al.*, 2001; Onwumere *et al.*, 2009). Such perceptions are adversely associated with outcome. However, this may work in both directions; bad memories of the interaction with relatives may increase the readiness to perceive criticism. Thus, Cutting and Docherty (2000) found that patients with schizophrenia and with high-EE relatives recounted fewer happy memories and more stressful memories than those with low-EE relatives. Some relatives may themselves be poor at judging patients' moods, and Giron and Gomez-Beneyto (1998) showed this too was related to relapse, and was seemingly independent of their levels of criticism.

Some studies have addressed the idea that high-EE relatives make *attributions* that distinguish them from low-EE relatives, and that these may be linked to higher relapse rates. High-EE relatives seem to make relatively more attributions about illness, and attribute more causes as internal to the patient and controllable by them (Barrowclough *et al.*, 1994; Weisman *et al.*, 1998). Moreover, these attributional differences distinguish even high- and low-EE relatives living in the same household (Weisman *et al.*, 2000). Harrison *et al.* (1998) found that critical attitudes on the part of carers towards people with schizophrenia were associated with a tendency to attribute negative symptoms to the patient's personality rather than to the illness. Attributions of controllability are related to outcome. (Lopez *et al.*, 1999). The attribution of symptoms to illness (i.e., external to the patient) increased as criticism and overinvolvement fell in the course of family treatment (Brewin, 1994).

The attributions of relatives may also be directed towards themselves. Docherty *et al.* (1998) showed that low-EE parents of people with schizophrenia were less self-critical than high-EE parents, while Bentsen *et al.* (1998) found overinvolved relatives were very prone to guilt. Carers who were critical typically had low self-esteem (Kuipers *et al.*, 2006).

Illness perceptions also involve attributions, have been investigated in a wide range of physical health conditions, and can predict wellbeing (Haggar & Orbell, 2003). In psychosis, Barrowclough *et al.* (2003) showed that critical carers saw themselves as having less control over the illness, thought it would last for longer, and perceived a greater number of symptoms. Lobban *et al.* (2006) reported that when carer–patient dyads diverged in their illness perceptions, carers were also more likely to be high EE and to envisage negative outcomes for patients. Fortune *et al.* (2005) found that carer perceptions of illness in psychosis were related to their level of distress. Kuipers *et al.* (2007) found that carers were more pessimistic about consequences than the patients were themselves. When the views of carers and patients about the illness diverged, this was related to low mood in both carers and patients, but not to the EE status of carers. Recently, we have integrated findings about the attributes of EE to create a cognitive model, designed to drive future investigation (Kuipers *et al.*, 2010).

Conclusions

The more recent research on EE has confirmed its predictive value for poor outcomes in patients, and generated ideas about mechanisms. Probably the most productive areas have been in the utility of EE in identifying therapeutic (or otherwise) aspects of relationships, and the contribution of this information to the improvement of family interventions in psychosis. Overall, psychosocial influences on psychosis have been corroborated by such studies. The pattern of high-EE-related behaviors and frequent relapses represents a vicious cycle rather than linear causality. If this cycle is entered, high EE can be an extremely persistent characteristic of relatives (Favre *et al.*, 1989; McCreadie *et al.*, 1993). However, it is clear that such factors, while powerful, are amenable to change, to the benefit of both carers and patients.

Life events and schizophrenia

Life events classically refer to a somewhat restricted category of sudden changes that have social and psychological implication. As such, they are a subset of the broader concept of psychosocial stress. In the first version of this chapter, we dealt with methodological issues at length (Bebbington *et al.*, 1995). The key issue is dating: to evaluate the temporal relationship between events and any kind of psychiatric disorder, both the event and the disorder must be dated, and this can be difficult.

Concept of triggering

Several authors have claimed that life events "trigger" episodes of schizophrenia. This term has two separate and unconnected meanings. One is that the stress of the life event merely adds the final impetus toward illness in somebody already strongly predisposed because of an underlying diathesis (Brown et al., 1973). This is another way of saying that, in comparison with other factors, the role of life events is not very important. This can be tested by examining the strength of the association between events and onset or relapse.

The other meaning of the "triggering" hypothesis concerns the length of the causal period in which life events are thought to operate. Events would be seen as having a triggering role in this sense if they occurred in close proximity to the onset or relapse of disorder. It has generally been held that a 6-month period should be sufficient to cover all events that might have a role in engendering relapse. However, the length of this critical period is an empirical question, with a corresponding methodological implication: it is important that the antecedent period chosen for canvassing a life-event history should be at least as long as the causal period.

Life-event studies

In the last version of this chapter, we listed 17 studies from a wide range of cultural settings that examined the effect of life events on the etiology or course of schizophrenia (Table 29.2). No similar studies have been reported in the succeeding interval. Overall, the results are somewhat inconsistent. The seminal early study of Brown and Birley (1968) found a significantly raised rate of life events limited to the 3 weeks before the onset or relapse of schizophrenic illness. Most subsequent studies have used similar retrospective designs, although prospective studies have been reported more recently. Some have found an increased rate of events over longer periods of time, even up to a year preceding relapse or illness onset (Dohrenwend et al., 1987; Bebbington et al., 1993; Hirsch et al., 1996). Others yielded negative results (Jacobs & Myers, 1976; Malzacher et al., 1981; Al Khani et al., 1986; Chung et al., 1986; Gureje & Adewumni, 1988; Malla et al., 1990). Some of the negative studies did find non-significant patterns of elevation of life-event rates preceding illness onset. While prospective life-event studies in the field of schizophrenia suffer from few of the important methodological problems of retrospective studies, they have again offered inconsistent support for the triggering hypothesis.

Increased sensitivity to stress

The evidence from the EE literature and life-event studies suggests that stressful social circumstances have an asso-
ciation with the emergence of schizophrenic symptoms. If so, there are two possibilities linking stress and psychosis. One is that there are two distinct types of disorder, one in which psychosocial factors predominate etiologically, the other in which the neurobiological predisposition is salient. Under these circumstances, the two postulated etiological domains would segregate, and it might be expected that the clinical features would also differ. Thus, because the impact of most life events is likely eventually to dissipate, it could be argued that episodes provoked by events would be relatively benign. Patients with event-associated episodes may require less antipsychotic medication despite spending more time in remission that those with unassociated episodes (van Os et al., 1994). Such differences drive the conceptual separation of psychogenic from nuclear schizophrenia.

However, the evidence currently favors the alternative, viz, that psychosis is a special vulnerability to the effects of stress. People with schizophrenia may be abnormally sensitive to events. If so, this would increase the difficulty of demonstrating event–relapse relationships using the methods we have described. This is because comparisons between cases and controls might show no excess of events in the case group, the emergence of psychotic symptoms arising instead from an increased vulnerability to events occurring at a normal rate. This might account for the rather inconsistent results linking stressful life events to the emergence of psychotic symptoms. It would also explain the findings of Horan et al. (2005) that, overall, patients with schizophrenia had significantly lower rates of life events than non-psychiatric controls. What evidence is there for increased sensitivity and what form might it take?

Some of the most persuasive research comes from the use of the experience sampling method (ESM) by the Maastricht group (Myin-Germeys & van Os, 2007). This allows the assessment of emotional reactivity to stressors as they arise in normal daily life. Participants are asked to make contemporaneous ratings of stress and their response to it, prompted by a wrist-watch alarm programmed to go off at randomly varying intervals. These authors used ESM to compare patients with psychotic illness and a group of control subjects (Myin-Germeys et al., 2001). The patients reacted with more intense emotions to subjective appraisal of stress than the control subjects. The authors also studied subjects vulnerable to psychosis, who also showed elevated emotional reactivity to stress (Myin-Germeys et al., 2005). Not only was there a clear affective response to small stressors, but this was paralleled by moment-to-moment variation in subtle positive psychotic experiences. Interestingly, Myin-Germeys & Krabbendam (2004) found that emotional reactivity to daily life stress is stronger in women with psychotic disorder than in men. This parallels their increased response to more severe stress (Fisher et al., 2006; Olff et al., 2007), and thus suggests that sex differences may

Table 29.2 Studies of independent life events in schizophrenic illness.

Study	Country	Period/method	Patient sample	n	Significant results for time period	
					3–5 weeks	>3/12
Retrospective						
Brown & Birley (1968)	UK	12 weeks	Broad group: 30% first onset	50	Yes, for 3 weeks	Not addressed
Jacobs & Myers (1976)	UK	1 year: not LEDS	Narrow definition: all first onset	62	Not addressed	NS
Malzacher et al. (1981)	Germany	6 months	First onset	90	Not addressed	NS
Canton & Fraccon (1985)	Italy	6 months: not LEDS	24 first onset	54	Not addressed	Possible support
Chung et al. (1986)	USA	6 months	Narrow definition: some first onset	15	NS	NS
Al Khani et al. (1986)	Saudi Arabia	1 year	Narrow definition: recent onset	48	Small subgroups only	NS
Day et al. (1987) WHO	10 centers worldwide	12 weeks	Broad definition: some first onset	13–67	Yes for 5 of 6 analyzed fully	NS
Dohrenwend et al. (1987)	USA	6 months: not LEDS	21 first onset	66	NS	Yes, for "non-fateful" events
Gureje & Adewumni (1988)	Nigeria	6 months: not LEDS	All first onset: RDC definition	42	NS	NS
Bebbington et al. (1993)	UK	6 months	Narrow definition	52	Yes	Yes, for up to 6 months
Hultman et al. (1997)	Sweden	9 months after discharge or at relapse	DSM-III schizophrenia	25	Excess of life events 3 weeks before relapse	NS
Prospective						
Leff et al. (1973)	UK	Clinical trial	9 on medication relapsed	116	For medicated only (5 weeks)	NS
Hardesty et al. (1985)	USA	1 year	2–3 years in remission	36	NS (morbidity 3 weeks post LE)	Not addressed
Ventura et al. (1989)	USA	1 year on medication (see Ventura et al., 1992)	Recent onset: 11/30 relapsers		Yes for 4 weeks	NS
Malla et al. (1990)	Canada	1 year	7 relapsed	22	Not addressed	NS unless trivial events included
Ventura et al. (1992)	USA	1 year off medication (see Ventura et al., 1989)	Recent onset: off medication	13	NS for those off medication	NS
Hirsch et al. (1996)	UK	1 year on/off medication	Narrow Relapses: off medication 21/35; on medication 5/36	71	NS for both on and off medication groups	Yes, for up to 1 year

Recent onset, illness history <2 years.
DSM, Diagnostic and Statistical Manual; LEDS, Life Events and Difficulties Schedule; RDC, Research Diagnostic Criteria; WHO, World Health Organization.

not be limited to the characteristics of psychosis, but are perhaps also reflected in underlying etiological mechanisms.

Distal social adversity in people who develop schizophrenia

The stress–vulnerability paradigm in schizophrenia has usually been applied with the implicit view that the vulnerability is genetic, or perhaps related to the early physical environment. This was reflected in a reluctance to attribute to social factors significant effects that could not easily be subsumed under mere triggering. However, biological indicators of vulnerability are by no means universal in individuals with schizophrenia. There is no logical reason why vulnerability should not in some cases be psychological, arising from early social experiences (Read et al., 2001).

Childhood adversity may include actual abuse, whether physical, sexual or emotional, and whether perpetrated by members of the family or by outsiders. Such abuse is now acknowledged to be quite frequent. A recent UK survey estimated a prevalence of childhood physical abuse of around 24% and sexual abuse of about 11% (May-Chahal & Cawson, 2005); higher estimates have been reported from the US (Friedman et al., 2002), and the available studies have been comprehensively reviewed by Pereda et al. (2009). The estimates depend on the definition and on how many types of events are used as prompts. Increasing attention is also being paid to the serious effects of bullying, whether inside or outside school. Bullying may be physical, it is frequently emotional, and these days it may be carried out using texts and pictures on mobile phones. Approximately 17% of children from a nationally representative birth cohort in the UK reported being bullied by the age of 7 years (Arseneault et al., 2006).

The deleterious effects of childhood trauma are now well established. They are non-specific, and include increased risk of adult depression, personality disorder, PTSD, drug and alcohol abuse, and suicide (Bebbington et al., 2009; Jonas et al., 2010). However, there is now increasing evidence of particularly strong links with psychosis. While there are concerns about the reliability of reports of abuse in people whose mental state is affected by schizophrenia, Goodman et al. (1999) showed that accounts are consistent over time, and concluded that the information obtained is sufficiently reliable to allow research in this area. Ellason and Ross (1997) found a significant association of child physical and sexual abuse with psychotic symptoms, confirmed by Mueser et al. (1998). Lysaker et al. (2001) found a level of child sexual abuse in people with schizophrenia of over 40%. Ucok and Bikmaz (2007) provide evidence that childhood sexual abuse is associated with increased prominence of positive symptoms during a first episode of schizophrenia. In the British National Psychiatric Morbidity Survey, Bebbington et al. (2004) found relative odds of psychosis of around 12 in people who had experienced sexual abuse.

Janssen et al. (2004) assessed childhood abuse in non-psychotic members of the general population, and showed it predicted the development of new positive psychotic symptoms at 2-year follow-up. Childhood bullying and sexual trauma were associated in an adolescent population with non-clinical psychotic experiences that might indicate risk of later conversion to frank psychotic disorder (Lataster et al., 2006; Schreier et al., 2009). Reviewing the literature relating childhood trauma to psychosis, Read et al. (2005) concluded the link was now well established. Morgan and Fisher (2007) were more cautious in their conclusions. Although accepting that recent population-based studies provide quite robust evidence of an association, they drew attention to several conceptual and methodological issues.

Home environments can of course be an adverse factor in other ways, including exposure to violence between other members of the family and separation from one or both parents. Thus, early parental loss was found to be more common in people with psychiatric diagnoses (Agid et al., 1999). This applied to people with schizophrenia as much as to those with bipolar disorder and major depressive disorder. The odds ratio comparing patients with schizophrenia with controls was 3.8. Separation from parents was associated with a high risk of psychosis in a recent first-episode study (Morgan et al., 2007). Separation is usually a marker for a plethora of other potentially adverse circumstances in childhood.

One of the attributes of childhood adversity is that its various forms tend to cluster (Bebbington et al., 2004). Some families experience instability in the form of rapid change in structure and composition. Fuchs (1999) compared patients with late paraphrenia and with severe late-onset depression. He found more discriminatory, humiliating or threatening experiences in early life in the first group, and more early loss in the second. Children may also suffer from living in families with considerable socioeconomic difficulties.

The evidence from the prospective study of Myhrman et al. (1994) for a link between an adverse environment in childhood and later psychosis is striking because the authors used a very simple marker of such environments. Mothers taking part in the Finnish 1966 birth cohort study were asked before the birth if the child was wanted, wanted but mistimed, or unwanted. At follow-up, the prevalence of schizophrenia was twice as high (1.5% vs. 0.7%) in those offspring who had been unwanted babies. After correction for sociodemographic variables, the odds ratio was 2.4. Unwantedness might act as a prenatal stress, or as a marker of behaviors associated with risk in either the mother or child.

Another Finnish study (Tienari *et al.*, 1994, 2004) compared adopted children of mothers with a diagnosis of schizophrenia with a group of adopted children of control mothers. As expected, the first group was found to contain more people with severe mental illness, including schizophrenia. However, all children did well in "healthy" adoptive families. Differences were only found where the adoptive families were rated as "disturbed". It remains possible, if rather unlikely, that the adoptive families might equally have been disturbed in response to odd presymptomatic behavior on the part of the adopted child. Nevertheless, both of these Finnish studies suggest a role for distal social factors.

In addition to its effect on the emergence of psychotic symptoms, an adverse early environment may lead to chronicity and poor outcome in people who later develop psychosis. Fowler (1999) found that severe distal trauma histories are particularly common in those with chronic psychosis, less so among those in their first episode (who include a proportion heading for a good outcome). In a German multivariate study of schizophrenia, traumatic experiences and adverse circumstances in childhood were related to the frequency of relapse and rehospitalization (Doering *et al.*, 1998). Non-clinical symptoms of psychosis may also become abnormally persistent if combined with earlier trauma (Cougnard *et al.*, 2007; van Os *et al.*, 2009).

Finally, individual attributes may interact with factors operating at the societal level to increase risk. Thus the risk of psychosis in people from ethnic minorities is increased when they live in areas where there are few representatives from their ethnic group (Boydell *et al.*, 2001; Veling *et al.*, 2008). Other important features of people's area of residence include social cohesion and fragmentation.

Social defeat and schizophrenia

Recently, Selten and Cantor-Graae (2007) have argued that many of the effects of adversity can be integrated through the concept of social defeat. Birchwood *et al.* (2000) has put forward a similar formulation centering on the loss of social rank and stigma in psychosis. Social defeat is characteristic of people with a subordinate position or outsider status. Selten and Cantor-Graae (2007) suggest that the chronic experience of social defeat increases the risk of developing a psychotic disorder. Adverse social environments may be particularly frequent in people from particular ethnic groups, in those who have migrated to their current location, and in those brought up in cities. Rates of psychosis are high in first-generation immigrants, and even higher in their children (Cantor-Graae & Selten, 2005; Veling *et al.*, 2006). The increased risk in second-generation immigrants is difficult to explain except on social grounds, and Cantor-Graae and Selten (2005) discard drug abuse as a predominant explanation. The increased rate of psychosis in immigrants is also reflected in an increased frequency of non-clinical psychosis-like symptoms (Vanheusden *et al.*, 2008). In general, the rates of psychosis in immigrants is greatest in those who are the least successful. Cantor-Graae and Selten (2005) also suggested that social defeat might explain increased rates of psychosis in people living in dense urban areas (Krabbendam & van Os, 2005) and in people with a history of sexual abuse in childhood (Bebbington *et al.*, 2004; Read *et al.*, 2005).

The trauma/post-traumatic stress disorder/schizophrenia triad

Evidence is accumulating of a close relationship between PTSD and psychotic symptoms. This is worth examining in some detail, as it would have obvious implications for the role of stress in the etiology of schizophrenia.

Psychotic symptoms in response to combat trauma were reported by Paster as long ago as 1948, and are not uncommon. Forty percent of one sample of Vietnam veterans had experienced psychotic symptoms in the 6 months before assessment (David *et al.*, 1999). Calhoun *et al.* (2007) provide evidence that PTSD is highly prevalent and underdiagnosed in war veterans with schizophrenia. Schizophrenia associated with PTSD is very similar to schizophrenia without PTSD in the form and intensity of the psychotic features, both positive and negative (Hamner *et al.*, 2000).

Mueser *et al.* (1998) studied 275 patients with a range of severe mental disorders, largely psychosis. Forty-three percent had PTSD as a result of a severe trauma at some stage of their lives, often in childhood. However, only 2% of these had the diagnosis recorded in their notes. Ninety-eight percent of the sample had been exposed to at least one severe trauma. Mueser *et al.* (2002) argue that PTSD may mediate the negative effects of trauma on the course of severe mental illness. This could operate both directly, through the capacity of PTSD to affect symptom generation and psychosis, and indirectly, through retraumatization, substance abuse, and social difficulties. The second channel is probably important. Traumatic early life experiences predispose individuals both to psychosis and to substance abuse. The substance abuse often affects outcome adversely. Scheller-Gilkey *et al.* (2004) showed that patients with the dual diagnosis had a greater history of childhood trauma and more PTSD. Gearon *et al.* (2003) found very high rates of traumatic life events in women with psychosis and comorbid substance abuse. Revictimization was common, and rates of concurrent PTSD were particularly high.

Seedat *et al.* (2003) systematically reviewed the association between PTSD and psychosis. High rates of PTSD were common in people with psychosis, and psychotic phenomena were relatively common in patients with chronic PTSD. The actual figures vary with the method of assessment. Resnick *et al.* (2003) found that 74% of people with schizophrenia had experienced major trauma, although only 13% had full PTSD, and past trauma was associated with current levels of distress. In patients experiencing a first psychiatric admission for psychosis, Neria *et al.* (2002) found a similar prevalence of trauma exposure of nearly 70%, although only 14% had PTSD. Shevlin *et al.* (2007) similarly reported that while many people with schizophrenia have a history of trauma, the prevalence of actual PTSD is rather less. Priebe *et al.* (1998) found that half (51%) of their community patients with schizophrenia also met criteria for PTSD. In another large sample of patients with severe mental illness, the overall rate of current PTSD was 35%, although the rate of PTSD was higher in people with major mood disorders than in those with psychotic disorders (Mueser *et al.*, 2004). Rates of trauma and PTSD were particularly high in a forensic sample of patients with paranoid schizophrenia (Sarkar *et al.*, 2005). Kilcommons and Morrison (2005) found a very high lifetime prevalence of trauma in their patients with psychosis, and over half had current PTSD. The severity of trauma is associated with the severity of PTSD and of psychotic symptoms, with current levels of distress, and with poor psychosocial functioning (Resnick *et al.*, 2003; Lysaker *et al.*, 2001; Kilcommons & Morrison, 2005). Thus, early trauma appears to create a nexus of interacting adverse consequences.

PTSD is a condition defined essentially by an intimate relationship between the content of symptoms and the experience of strongly traumatic events, in particular the phenomenon of re-experiencing. One possibility is that some people who have been exposed to extreme trauma develop psychotic symptoms (delusions, hallucinations) whose content is also closely related to the details of the traumatic experience. If this happens, it may come about by a totally different process from the genesis of symptoms in the majority of cases of schizophrenia, or it may not. The situation is analogous to the relationship between depressive bereavement reactions—in which the event is clearly in the forefront of the thinking of sufferers, and the generality of depressive disorders—where the link between a depressogenic event and the mood disorder may be much less apparent to sufferers. However, most authorities from Freud (1917) onwards have tended to think that the psychosocial processes involved in depression and bereavement responses are quite similar.

Some might argue that florid symptoms in PTSD merely mimic psychotic symptoms. Thus, re-experiencing may have a compelling visual or auditory quality that might be mistaken for hallucinations. However, even in veterans exposed to extreme combat stress, the distinction between flashbacks and psychotic symptoms can be clearly made (Ivezić *et al.*, 1999).

Nevertheless, it is interesting that hallucinations seem to be particularly frequent in psychosis associated with trauma. Thus, in all but one case of Vietnam veterans with psychosis studied by David *et al.* (1999), their symptoms included auditory hallucinations. Read *et al.* (2003) found that child sexual abuse was particularly associated with hallucinations in people with schizophrenia, although adult sexual assault was related equally to delusions and thought disorder. Kilcommons and Morrison (2005) found that sexual abuse appeared specifically related to hallucinations. Moreover, the trauma–hallucination link does not appear to be restricted to schizophrenia. Hammersley *et al.* (2003) found trauma was also associated with auditory hallucinations in bipolar disorder. This was particularly strong for child sexual abuse.

However, Hardy *et al.* (2005) found that in many cases where trauma precedes hallucinations, the hallucinations are only thematically related to the trauma—they did not often involve actual recapitulation of the traumatic event. In other studies as well, the meaningful connection between the characteristics of trauma and the content of symptoms is not always apparent. Thus, Butler *et al.* (1996) felt that, in their series, the psychotic symptoms associated with PTSD were not themselves linked to re-experiencing the trauma. Likewise, in another study, the severity of psychotic symptoms associated with combat-related PTSD correlated with the severity of PTSD symptoms, but there seemed to be no link between psychotic symptoms and re-experiencing the traumatic event *per se* (Hamner *et al.*, 1999). It appeared almost as though the psychotic symptoms were an alternative way of re-experiencing.

Another aspect of the PTSD–psychosis link concerns the salience of dissociative processes. Glaslova *et al.* (2004) suggest that traumatic stress exerts its influence on schizophrenia precisely by increasing the tendency to dissociative processes. Holowka *et al.* (2003) certainly found that childhood trauma was associated with the significant presence of dissociative symptoms in people with schizophrenia. Kilcommons and Morrison (2005) also found that dissociative processes consequent upon trauma were associated with psychotic experiences and with hallucinations in particular.

However, the association is not universally accepted: Brunner *et al.* (2004) in particular have contested the link between dissociative symptoms and schizophrenia. They found an increased frequency of dissociative experiences in a group of patients with borderline personalities, but their group of patients with schizophrenia did not differ from normal volunteers. Irwin (2001) suggested that the link between dissociative experiences and PTSD might arise because both were associated with childhood trauma. However, controlling for childhood trauma did not remove the association. Nevertheless, childhood trauma may explain part of the link between dissociative symptoms and schizotypy (Giesbrecht *et al.*, 2007).

Part of the problem with investigations of this type, relying as they do on retrospective questionnaire measures, is that the process of dissociation is not well specified, and the instruments assessing it may be picking up the tendencies towards anomalous experience and unusual beliefs that form the basis of recognizing both schizotypy and psychosis itself.

Mechanisms

Stress almost certainly operates at more than one level in the origination of psychosis. It appears to act as a trigger to the emergence of psychotic symptoms, and people with psychosis may in any case have a particular vulnerability to stress. However, this vulnerability in turn may be the consequence of earlier stresses. There has been considerable speculation and some research into the mechanism by which triggering, vulnerability, and early adversity exert their effects. This triangulates the stress–psychosis relationship in a way that increases its plausibility.

Mechanism of triggering

It is not impossible to imagine mechanisms by which stress might induce psychotic symptoms in someone with no specific vulnerability. However, the emergence of psychotic symptoms is a relatively unusual response to stress: the more accepted response involves affective symptoms. Explaining the triggering of psychosis without a pre-existing personal vulnerability is thus difficult. It would rely on the postulation of a normal individual facing an abnormal concatenation of circumstances, perhaps invoking affective changes and specific appraisals. The current cognitive models of psychosis emphasize both the person's appraisal of the impact of stress and the ensuing cognitions and emotions, and how they might interact with perceptual abnormalities (Fowler, 2000; Garety et al., 2001, 2007; Bentall et al., 2001; Morrison, 2001; Broome et al., 2005; Birchwood, 2003).

There is appreciable evidence that individuals with a prior history of psychotic symptoms do respond to stressful circumstances with normal anxiety and depression. Such affective changes are also seen in the prodromal period before the emergence or re-emergence of psychotic symptoms. Ventura et al. (2000) showed that the recurrence of psychotic symptoms is not the only response to stressful life events in people who have experienced prior episodes of schizophrenia. In many instances, the response stops with the development of non-psychotic depressive symptoms. This links into the literature on affective prodromes of relapse (Birchwood et al., 1992), not all of which lead to the re-emergence of psychotic symptoms (Yung & McGorry, 1996). Myin-Germeys et al. (2005) were able to show that the clear affective response to small stressors was paralleled by moment-to-moment variation in subtle positive psychotic experiences.

Affective changes clearly accompany exposure to a high-EE environment. Not surprisingly, perceiving that relatives are critical has a negative impact on patients' mood. Renshaw (2007) argued that the link between EE and the recurrence of psychotic symptoms might be mediated by the depressogenic effect of criticism. Kuipers et al. (2006) found that patients with a recent relapse who lived with high-EE relatives also had higher levels of anxiety and depression, independently of levels of psychotic symptoms. Patients whose views about the consequences of their psychotic illness diverged from those of their relatives were more depressed (Kuipers et al., 2007).

Mood and cognitive attributes seem to be independently associated with psychotic and psychotic-like symptoms in clinical and non-clinical populations (Fowler et al., 2006; Smith et al., 2006; Bentall et al., 2009; Freeman et al., 2010). In these studies, a combination of anxiety and schematic views of the self as weak, vulnerable, and inadequate, and of other people as devious, threatening, and bad, was found to be specifically associated with paranoia. High EE has also been shown to affect the cognitions of patients. Thus, Barrowclough et al. (2003) found that criticism by carers was related both to low self-esteem in patients, and to higher positive symptoms.

There is some corroboration from electrophysiological studies suggesting that the presence of low-EE relatives actually serves to reduce arousal (Tarrier et al., 1988b; Tarrier, 1989; Hegerl et al., 1990). However, work by Dixon et al. (2000) goes against this. The authors attempted to test directly the idea that high-EE relatives provide a stressful environment for people with schizophrenia. They argued that memory-loaded vigilance tests are stress-sensitive, and that the presence of a high-EE relative would therefore reduce the patient's performance. In fact the reverse was true, leading them to conclude that patients in the presence of low-EE relatives were actually under-aroused. These results could, however, also be interpreted in terms of the role of anxiety in improving performance, and may therefore not reflect an adverse level of under-arousal.

What of the biological correlates of triggering in schizophrenia? At one level these correspond to the stress responses in normal people, although as we shall see researchers always have a tendency to adduce a modifying vulnerability. In patients newly admitted with an acute episode of psychosis, the severity of recent life stressors was associated with the degree of increase in serum cortisol (Mazure et al., 1997). People with first-episode psychosis may display increased hypothalamic–pituitary–adrenal (HPA) axis activation (Ryan et al., 2004). There is even some evidence that the onset of psychosis may be associated with actual pituitary enlargement (Pariante et al., 2005).

Jones and Fernyhough (2007) incorporated the modulation of cortisol production by stress into their neural diathesis–stress model of schizophrenia. They suggest, further, that cortisol is most strongly produced in response to situations that imply uncontrollable threats to social evaluation or to important goals.

While cortisol metabolism is central to the normal stress response, the predominant explanation of the anomalies of schizophrenia has been couched in terms of the dopamine theory. There is converging evidence from animal research and clinical studies supporting a role for dopamine dysregulation in the prefrontal cortex in schizophrenia (e.g., Goldman-Rakic *et al.*, 2004; Kapur *et al.*, 2005). However, dopamine release is also a recognized response to stress in non-psychotic individuals (Adler *et al.*, 2000; Pruessner *et al.*, 2004). For this reason it remains possible that schizophrenic symptoms might arise in the absence of vulnerability, for instance, if the degree of stress were overwhelming, as in psychosis following war trauma. Nevertheless, most accounts of the effects of stress in schizophrenia do adduce a special susceptibility.

Vulnerability

There are several levels at which vulnerability to stress can be characterized. Genetic, neurophysiological, affective, cognitive, and behavioral abnormalities may be demonstrable, and may interact. Current models of vulnerability include much speculation and rather less evidence, but are nonetheless valuable if they direct and drive future research.

Genetic vulnerability

There are some reports suggesting that life events are more effective in inducing symptoms in people in whom there are genetic indicators of heightened vulnerability. Upsetting life events were associated with the first appearance of psychotic symptoms in people at *increased risk* of developing psychosis, largely because of a family history of the disorder (Miller *et al.*, 2001). Likewise, a small longitudinal study reported by Norman and Malla (2001) suggested a stronger relation between stress and positive symptoms of psychosis in people with a family history. Myin-Germeys *et al.* (2001) used ESM to show that, in terms of the intensity of their emotional response to subjective appraisal of stress, the first-degree relatives of patients with psychotic illness fell between the patients and a group of control subjects. Others have speculated that gene–environment interactions in this condition actually take the form of sensitization to environmental stress (van Os & Marcelis, 1998).

Neurobiological vulnerability

There are certainly indications of a reduction in the normal biological mechanisms for dealing with stress in people with schizophrenia (Jansen *et al.*, 1998; Sumiyoshi *et al.*, 1999). This is reflected in abnormalities of cortisol metabolism. Phillips *et al.* (2006) and Jones and Fernyhough (2007) have proposed similar modifications to the neural diathesis–stress model of schizophrenia. The former argued that abnormalities in the HPA axis in schizophrenia and abnormalities in the hippocampus may be linked to the capacity of stress to precipitate psychotic episodes. Myin-Germeys *et al.* (2005) have speculated that behavioral sensitization to environmental stress might be a vulnerability marker for schizophrenia reflecting dopaminergic hyperresponsivity to environmental stimuli. Neuroreceptor imaging studies suggest that there are increased synaptic dopamine levels in the striatum in schizophrenia (Abi-Dargham *et al.*, 2000), probably indicating increased baseline activity of the meso-limbic dopamine system. Likewise there is an increase in amphetamine-induced dopamine release in people with schizophrenia (Laruelle *et al.*, 2003).

Jay *et al.* (2004) have reviewed synaptic plasticity in the direct links between the hippocampus and prefrontal cortex. Long-term potentiation of this pathway appears to be driven by the level of meso-cortical dopaminergic activity. Moreover, stress appears to be an environmental determinant of this process: acute stress appears to cause a remarkable and long-lasting inhibition of long-term potentiation. Thus, acute events may result in relatively prolonged effects, a potential mechanism for a psychosocially-induced vulnerability. These processes are modified by antipsychotic medication.

Vulnerability, affect, cognition, and behavior

Mood may have persistent as well as temporary effects on the propensity to develop schizophrenic symptoms. Dinzeo *et al.* (2004) suggest that trait arousability is increased in people with schizophrenia, and that this may be related to stress responsiveness and symptom presentation.

Vulnerability at the behavioral level may involve impaired coping mechanisms and ineffective ways of accessing support (Hultman *et al.*, 1997; MacDonald *et al.*, 1998). Pallanti *et al.* (1997) provide evidence of sensitivity to events in terms of coping deficits. Patients whose relapse did not follow a life event in the month before relapse showed less effective coping and poorer information processing capacity. The implication is that patients who have good coping resources (including cognitive capacity) will only be unsettled by events of considerable threat, in contrast to those without. Horan *et al.* (2005) showed that, compared with controls, patients with schizophrenia appraised events as less controllable and thought they had handled them less well. They also down-rated positive events. The same research group compared the responses to the 1994 Californian earthquake of people with schizophrenia, people with bipolar disorder, and healthy controls

(Horan *et al.*, 2007). Both patient groups reported a high level of avoidant symptoms on the Impact of Events Scale. Moreover, avoidant coping was associated with higher residual stress symptoms in the schizophrenia group at follow-up. Using a role play test, Horan and Blanchard (2003) showed that patients with schizophrenia responded with more negative mood if they had maladaptive coping styles and trait negative affectivity.

The ability to access social support may represent a behavioral component of vulnerability. There is an extensive literature in the study of depression directed at the stress-buffering function of social support (Alloway & Bebbington, 1987). Hultman *et al.* (1997) have investigated schizophrenia in similar terms, and made the interesting finding that the time between events and relapse was increased in people with better social support and a coping strategy characterized by active support seeking. Penn *et al.* (2004) have suggested a role for social support in maintaining recovery. The psychological mediation of vulnerability to stress may also involve hopelessness. This is very common in people who have newly developed schizophrenia, and appears to be linked to poor outcome (Aguilar *et al.*, 1997).

Vulnerability to stress may vary over time, and there have been suggestions that the experience of an episode of psychosis may itself alter sensitivity, a sort of scarring process. In bipolar disorder, it has been suggested that life events may only be in excess in early episodes, and that later episodes appear less associated with events because of the process of kindling (Ramana & Bebbington, 1995). There has been little examination of this possibility in schizophrenia; in a small study (n = 32) of American veterans, life events were more likely to be associated with earlier episodes of schizophrenia (Castine *et al.*, 1998), although Bebbington *et al.* (1996) did not find this.

Psychosocial determinants of vulnerability

Life events themselves may modulate the increased sensitivity of patients with psychosis to day-to-day stress (Read *et al.*, 2001; Myin-Germeys *et al.*, 2003). Moreover the risk may accumulate over time as more adverse experiences occur (Myin-Germeys & van Os, 2007). Myin-Germeys *et al.* (2003) found that the increased sensitivity of patients with psychosis to day-to-day stress assessed using ESM was markedly modulated by the background life-event rate. They took this as evidence for a separate affective route to symptom formation in psychosis, characterized by a more episodic reactive type of psychosis with a relatively good outcome.

If early adversity is indeed linked to the later development of psychosis, how might the link work? Part of the mechanism could be gene–environmental. Thus, Kinderman & Cooke (2000) interpreted the Finnish study of Tienari

et al. (1994) as indicating that the family environment was playing a crucial part in moderating genetic risk.

Read *et al.* (2001), however, argued for a direct biological effect of adverse life events in early life on the diathesis underlying psychosis, thus positing a traumagenic neurodevelopmental model of schizophrenia. There is some suggestion that patients with a history of childhood trauma have reduced hippocampal volume (Driessen *et al.*, 2000); this is also seen in people experiencing a first episode of psychosis (Shenton *et al.*, 2001; Lappin *et al.*, 2006). Childhood adversity may also induce lasting effects on the main hormonal stress response system, the HPA axis (Read *et al.*, 2005: Spauwen *et al.*, 2006). Abused girls and women physically or sexually abused in childhood both show HPA dysregulation (Heim *et al.*, 2000). It is of interest that patients with PTSD who also have psychotic symptoms may display reduced plasma dopamine hydroxylase, a biological marker indicative of increased vulnerability to stress (Hamner & Gold, 1998).

Selten and Cantor-Graae (2007) propose a specific mechanism for the effects of their concept of social defeat, *viz*, that it may operate through a restriction in the availability of dopamine (D_2) receptors (Morgan *et al.*, 2002). Animals lower in the pecking order have high synaptic dopamine levels indicative of dopaminergic hyperactivity. Other research has suggested that the requirement to display submissive behavior leads to a sensitization to amphetamine (de Jong *et al.*, 2005).

Trauma may exert its effect on vulnerability through the induction of persistent affective changes. The role of affect in the production of psychotic symptoms in war veterans is clear, and a majority of such cases also met criteria for major depressive disorder (David *et al.*, 1999; Hamner *et al.*, 1999); anxiety is also likely to be an important link. It is of interest that people with PTSD and those with schizophrenia both display abnormal startle responses (Howard & Ford, 1992). Priebe *et al.* (1998) found that PTSD in community patients with schizophrenia was related to levels of neurotic symptoms. Crittendon and Ainsworth (1989) demonstrated that children who have been abused or bullied are hypervigilant to hostile cues in their environment. This may lead such children to make hostile attributions about the intentions of others, and they may have a more general negative set of beliefs about the behavior of other people. Lysaker and Salyers (2007) used cluster analysis to examine links between trauma history and symptoms in schizophrenia. They found that self-report of sexual trauma predicted high levels of anxiety, and severe anxiety was particularly associated with severe hallucinations.

However, the effect of a stressful early environment may equally be mediated through enduring cognitive predispositions, that is to say, a mechanism at the psychological level. Bak *et al.* (2005) examined the link between childhood trauma and incident psychosis. Trauma was associated with a greater degree of distress in response to symptoms, and poorer coping responses. The authors conclude that the early experience of trauma may create lasting cognitive and affective vulnerabilities for the development of clinical symptoms.

Gracie *et al.* (2007) found support for the prediction that there may be two routes linking trauma and the pre-disposition to psychosis. One of these routes involves mediation by negative beliefs about the self and others. However, there may also be a direct association between re-experiencing symptoms and hallucinations.

Schizotypy as vulnerability

Schizophrenia, and psychosis in general, is increasingly seen as the extreme end of abnormalities distributed continuously in the general population (Freeman *et al.*, 2005). Both paranoid ideation of a mild degree and schizotypy are regarded as minor variants of the full form of the disorder. There is also evidence that the determinants of the non-clinical disorders are similar to those of the full form. Thus, Berenbaum *et al.* (2003) found that women with a history of trauma had elevated levels of schizotypal symptoms.

People can be conceived as moving along continuous distributions at different times, moving far enough on occasion to develop the full syndrome. This makes it appropriate to regard schizotypy itself as a vulnerability state, and therefore likely to yield insights into the causation of schizophrenia.

Marzillier and Steel (2007) reported that people seeking help to deal with a traumatic event who scored high on schizotypy had more frequent trauma-related intrusions and worse symptoms of PTSD in general. The authors suggest that certain information processing styles associated with schizotypy may account for vulnerability to trauma-related intrusions.

Steel *et al.* (2005) emphasize the possible role of contextual integration on the development of trauma-related intrusions in psychosis. Schizotypal personality traits are associated with the degree of contextual integration. These traits are also related to trauma-related intrusions. In a large population sample, non-psychotic delusional experiences were more frequent in people who had experienced trauma (Scott *et al.*, 2007). A diagnosis of PTSD further increases the endorsement of delusional experiences. There seemed to be a dose–response relationship between the numbers of traumatic events and the likelihood of such experiences. Holmes and Steel (2004) used a trauma video to elicit trauma intrusions in a normal sample. People who scored high on schizotypy reported more intrusive experiences as a result of this. The authors link this propensity with the influence of trauma on psychotic disorders.

Overview

The findings surveyed in this chapter are wide-ranging and complex. What can be made of them? The EE studies suggest a large and robust effect of a predictor that is now known to reflect stressful aspects of the home environment. On this basis, social factors appear to be important. Why is it that the life-event research does not corroborate the EE research in a more convincing manner? One possibility is that the relatively abrupt changes represented by life events may not be so important in producing relapse as the continuing, albeit perhaps relatively low, levels of stress occasioned by living with a high-EE family member. Another explanation is that the rating of life events is essentially derived from research concerned mainly with depressive disorders. In consequence, the ratings may be set at the wrong threshold for picking up the life events important in schizophrenia. If people with schizophrenia are unnaturally sensitive to life events, it is possible that the relapse is brought about by events that on the surface would seem incapable of provoking an emotional response. One study (Malla *et al.*, 1990) only found a significant effect of events on relapse if trivial events or "hassles" were included in the analysis. Other research has suggested that events of mild threat were in excess in schizophrenia, as in other psychoses (Bebbington *et al.*, 1993). This would certainly tie in with the experience of many service users, who find it important to minimize even minor changes in daily routines.

It is also possible that events are rated along dimensions of reduced relevance for schizophrenia, and there is preliminary evidence that intrusiveness may be an important concept in this context (Harris, 1987; Raune *et al.*, 2006, 2009). Likewise, Rooke and Birchwood (1998; Birchwood *et al.*, 2005) have examined the relationship between humiliating, entrapping, and defeating life events and depression in schizophrenia.

The evidence concerning the psychosocial reactivity of schizophrenia may be important because it reflects the nature of the condition. If we take psychotic experience as a whole, it is clear there is a spectrum of reactivity: the most reactive conditions tend to have a greater admixture of affective symptoms in the clinical picture. This is true whether we define schizophrenia quite narrowly, or whether we also include schizoaffective disorder and affective psychosis. It is also true of psychotic conditions defined closely in relation to psychosocial stress, that is, reactive psychosis and the psychotic features associated with PTSD.

However, affective symptoms are less rare in schizophrenia than once thought—indeed, they are widespread, and are often linked with prodromes of psychotic relapse (Birchwood *et al.*, 2005). It appears that both life events and high EE may be associated with an increase in affective symptoms in people with schizophrenia, and one could postulate that the emergence of psychotic symptoms in response to psychosocial stress represents a further stage in a continuous process that is initially restricted to symptoms of anxiety and depression. It is apparent that this final stage is not necessarily reached in all circumstances (Yung & McGorry, 1996).

Obviously not every member of the general population responds to stress by developing symptoms of psychosis. Thus, there must be something unusual about the people who do react in this way, in their biogenetic make-up, in their circumstances, or in both. The circumstances, biological or social, adhering at the time of relapse must similarly be unusual. The concept of psychosis has drawn its strength from a sense that the mental experiences it expresses are so bizarre and unusual that they represent a categorical separation from the normal. This was very much the position of the influential psychopathologist Karl Jaspers (1913), who used it to argue for biological causation.

However, in recent years this view has been changing, at least in some quarters. Modern cognitive models of psychosis actually start by postulating continuities between psychosis and normal experience. In the past, the urge to make a categorical distinction between psychosis and normality almost certainly led to a Procrustean tendency to discount unusual beliefs and experiences in people we would be reluctant to see as undergoing a psychosis. By the late 1980s though, it became apparent that paranoid ideation and anomalous experiences, such as hearing voices, were not confined to clinical groups. Around 4% of the general population admit to hallucinatory experiences (Johns et al., 2002; Wiles et al., 2006), and the capacity for psychotic experience of this sort may not be at all uncommon. Moreover, intensive studies of delusional thinking suggest that it cannot be categorically separated from the illogicalities of most normal thinking, and that it is best distinguished in dimensional terms (Garety & Hemsley, 1994; Appelbaum et al., 1999).

The effect of these developments has been to normalize our conceptualizations of psychotic experience, and this in turn suggests that "normal" psychosocial processes have more of a part to play in its origins. Few adherents of psychosocial explanations would go so far as to exclude all possibility of genetic or physical environmental causes; most argue only for a shift in balance.

The success of CBT in people with psychosis has implications for the psychosocial reactivity of schizophrenia. Even apparently intractable delusions can be modified to some extent. In the process, the conceptualization of delusions as categorically distinct is weakened. Moreover, this comes about by changing the social context of the person with schizophrenia. This is done by introducing a new social relationship—the therapist uses their relationship with the patient to offer alternative views of their experiences in a way that normalizes them (Sensky et al., 2000). In the

process, not only are delusions modified, but hallucinations also (Kuipers et al., 1998). Our own cognitive model of psychosis, which was developed in relation both to the practice and to the practical experience of cognitive therapy, includes psychosocial elements (Garety et al., 2001). The model was new, in that it incorporated disruptions in automatic cognitive processes and maladaptive conscious appraisals; it covered delusions and hallucinations in one framework; and it accorded a central role to emotion. It has driven a considerable amount of research, largely corroborative (Garety et al., 2007). An integral part of the model is the consideration of how social factors contribute to the origins, maintenance, and recurrence of symptoms. The work on the impact of early loss and trauma on the later development of schizophrenia can certainly be interpreted in this way. We suggest that an early adverse experience such as social trauma may create an enduring cognitive vulnerability reflected in negative schemata, of the self and of the world, that facilitate external attributions and low self-esteem. Pre-existing schemata also affect the content of psychotic attributions (Bowins & Sugar, 1998). Implicit in these ideas is the possibility that social circumstances may influence both the content and the fact of psychotic experience. Evidence consistent with a role for such negative schemata in the development of psychosis has now been summarized (Garety et al., 2007).

Adversity can be seen as having a dual role. It may act as a priming agent, either by inculcating characteristic appraisals, of the self, of other people, and of the way the world generally works, or by inducing a tendency to anomalous experience. Events of this sort are quite likely to occur at a young age, but may happen in adulthood, particularly if the associated trauma is both overwhelming and difficult to process within existing schemata (e.g., rape). For instance, in the UK and Europe, asylum seekers with psychosis have had experiences of this type. The second role of adversity, usually in the form of discrete life events, is as a triggering agent. Events may be particularly likely to do this if they have characteristics ("demand characteristics") that tend to elicit the typical responses of thinking in schizophrenia. It is clear that some events are particularly likely to elicit ideas of persecution. Kaffman (1984) demonstrated that the delusional symptoms of 34 patients with paranoid disorder had a basis in truth. Harris (1987) used this idea in developing the concept of intrusiveness, arguing that this was a characteristic of events associated with psychotic relapse. Raune et al. (2006, 2009) have obtained some corroboration of this. The narrative reviews of life circumstances undertaken in CBT afford compelling examples fulfilling both priming and triggering functions.

Social experiences that do not necessarily raise the idea of adversity may also be important. One such example is social isolation. This may contribute to the patient's acceptance of psychotic appraisal by reducing access to other, more normalizing, explanations. Exposure to alternative views may be particularly important at crucial stages in the development of delusional thinking (exposure to therapists in the course of CBT is a special example of this; Penn *et al.*, 2004). White *et al.* (2000) found that insight in schizophrenia is greater in people with larger social networks.

These ideas linking social factors with cognitive models of schizophrenia require sophisticated methods of research to substantiate them and to elucidate mechanisms (Bebbington *et al.*, 2008). Nevertheless, such research should enhance our understanding of the social reactivity of psychosis, and improve both the treatment and long-term management of schizophrenia.

References

Abi-Dargham, A., Rodenhiser, J., Printz, D. *et al.* (2000) Increased baseline occupancy of D2 receptors by dopamine in schizophrenia. *Proceedings of the National Academy of Science USA* **97**, 8104–8109.

Adler, C.M., Elman, I., Weisenfeld, N., Kestler, L., Pickar, D. & Breier, A. (2000) Effects of acute metabolic stress on striatal dopamine release in healthy volunteers. *Neuropsychopharmacology* **22**, 545–550.

Agid, O., Shapira, B., Zislin, J. *et al.* (1999) Environment and vulnerability to major psychiatric illness: a case–control study of early parental loss in major depression, bipolar disorder and schizophrenia. *Molecular Psychiatry* **4**, 163–172.

Aguilar, E.J., Haas, G., Manzanera, F.J. *et al.* (1997) Hopelessness and first-episode psychosis: a longitudinal study. *Acta Psychiatrica Scandinavica* **96**, 25–30.

Al Khani, M.A.F., Bebbington, P.E., Watson, J.P. & House, F. (1986) Life events and schizophrenia: a Saudi Arabian study. *British Journal of Psychiatry* **148**, 12–22.

Alloway, R. & Bebbington, P.E. (1987) The buffer theory of social support: a review of the literature. *Psychological Medicine* **17**, 91–108.

American Psychiatric Association (1987) *Diagnostic and Statistical Manual of Mental Disorders*, 3rd edn. Revised. Washington, DC: American Psychiatric Association.

American Psychiatric Association (1994) *Diagnostic and Statistical Manual of Mental Disorders*, 4th edn. Washington: American Psychiatric Association.

Appelbaum, P.S., Robbins, P.C. & Roth, L.H. (1999) Dimensional approach to delusions: comparison across types and diagnoses. *Americal Journal of Psychiatry* **156**, 1938–1943.

Arévalo, J. & Vizcaro, C. (1989) "Emocion expresada" y curso de la esquizofrenia en una muestra espanola. *Analisis y Modificacion de Conducta* **15**, 3–23.

Arseneault, L., Walsh, E., Trzesniewski, K., Newcombe, R., Caspi, A. & Moffitt, T.E. (2006) Bullying victimization uniquely contributes to adjustment problems in young children: a nationally representative cohort study. *Pediatrics* **118**, 130–138.

Bak, M., Krabbendam, L., Janssen, I., de Graaf, R., Vollebergh, W. & van Os, J. (2005) Early trauma may increase the risk for psychotic experiences by impacting on emotional response

and perception of control. *Acta Psychiatrica Scandinavica* **112**, 360–366.

Barrelet, L., Ferrero, F., Szigetty, L., Giddey, C. & Pellizzer, G. (1990) Expressed emotion and first admission schizophrenia: nine month follow-up in a French cultural environment. *British Journal of Psychiatry* **156**, 357–362.

Barrowclough, C., Johnston, M. & Tarrier, N. (1994) Attributions, expressed emotion, and patient relapse: an attributional model of relatives' response to schizophrenic illness. *Behavior Therapy* **25**, 67–88.

Barrowclough, C., Tarrier, N., Humphreys, L., Ward, J., Gregg, L. & Andrews, B. (2003) Self-esteem in schizophrenia: relationships between self-evaluation, family attitudes, and symptomatology. *Journal of Abnormal Psychology* **112**, 92–99.

Bebbington, P. & Kuipers, L. (1994) The predictive utility of expressed emotion in schizophrenia: an aggregate analysis. *Psychological Medicine* **24**, 707–718.

Bebbington, P.E. & Kuipers, L. (2003) Schizophrenia and psychosocial stresses. In: Hirsch, S.R. & Weinberger, D., eds. *Schizophrenia*. Oxford: Blackwell Science, pp. 611–634.

Bebbington, P.E., Wilkins, S., Jones, P. *et al.* (1993) Life events and psychosis: initial results from the Camberwell Collaborative Psychosis study. *British Journal of Psychiatry* **162**, 72–79.

Bebbington, P.E., Bowen, J., Hirsch, S.R. & Kuipers, L. (1995) Schizophrenia and psychosocial stressors. In: Hirsch, S.R. & Weinberger, D., eds. *Schizophrenia*. Oxford: Blackwell Science, pp. 587–604.

Bebbington, P.E., Wilkins, S., Sham, P. *et al.* (1996) Life events before psychotic episodes: do clinical and social variables affect the relationship? *Social Psychiatry and Psychiatric Epidemiology* **31**, 122–128.

Bebbington, P.E., Bhugra, D., Brugha, T. *et al.* (2004) Psychosis, victimisation and childhood disadvantage: evidence from the Second British National Survey of Psychiatric Epidemiology. *British Journal of Psychiatry* **185**, 220–226.

Bebbington, P.E., Cooper, C., Minot, S. *et al.* (2009) Suicide attempts, gender and sexual abuse: Data from the British psychiatric morbidity survey 2000. *American Journal of Psychiatry* **166**, 1135–1140.

Bebbington, P., Fowler, D., Garety, P., Freeman D. & Kuipers, E. (2008) Theories of cognition, emotion, and the social world: missing links in psychosis. In: Morgan, C., McKenzie, K. & Fearon, P., eds. *Society and Psychosis*. Cambridge: Cambridge University Press, 219–237.

Bebbington, P.E., Jonas, S., Brugha, T. *et al.* (2010) Child sexual abuse reported by an English national sample: characteristics and demography. *Social Psychiatry and Psychiatric Epidemiology* (Epub ahead of print).

Bell, M., Bryson, G. & Lysaker, P. (1997) Positive and negative affect recognition in schizophrenia: a comparison with substance abuse and normal control subjects. *Psychiatry Research* **73**, 73–82.

Bentall, R.P., Corcoran, R., Howard, R., Blackwood, N. & Kinderman, P. (2001) Persecutory delusions: a review and theoretical integration. *Clinical Psychological Review* **21**, 1143–1192.

Bentall, R.P., Rowse, G., Shryane, N. *et al.* (2009) The cognitive and affective structure of paranoid delusions: a transdiagnostic investigation of patients with schizophrenia spectrum disorders and depression. *Archives of General Psychiatry* **66**, 236–247.

Bentsen, H., Boye, B., Munkvold, O.G. *et al.* (1996) Emotional overinvolvement in parents of patients with schizophrenia or related psychosis: demographic and clinical predictors. *British Journal of Psychiatry* **169**, 622–630.

Bentsen, H., Notland, T.H., Munkvold, O.G. *et al.* (1998) Guilt proneness and expressed emotion in relatives of patients with schizophrenia or related psychoses. *British Journal of Medical Psychology* **71**, 125–138.

Berenbaum, H., Valera, E.M. & Kerns, J.G. (2003) Psychological trauma and schizotypal symptoms. *Schizophrenia Bulletin* **29**, 143–152.

Bertrando, P., Beltz, J., Bressi, C. *et al.* (1992) Expressed emotion and schizophrenia in Italy: a study of an urban population. *British Journal of Psychiatry* **161**, 223–229.

Birchwood, M. (2003) Pathways to emotional dysfunction in first-episode psychosis. *British Journal of Psychiatry* **182**, 373–375.

Birchwood, M. & Smith, J. (1987) Schizophrenia in the family. In: Orford, J., ed. *Coping with Disorder in the Family*. London: Croom-Helm, pp. 7–38.

Birchwood, M., McMillan, F. & Smith, J. (1992) Early intervention. In: Birckwood, M. & Tarrier, N., eds. *Innovations in the Psychological Managment of Schizophrenia*. Chichester: Wiley, pp. 115–146.

Birchwood, M., Meaden, A., Trower, P., Gilbert, P. & Plaistow, J. (2000) The power and omnipotence of choices: subordination and entrapment by voices and by significant others. *Psychological Medicine* **30**, 337–344.

Birchwood, M., Iqbal, Z. & Upthegrove, R. (2005) Psychological pathways to depression in schizophrenia: studies in acute psychosis, post psychotic depression and auditory hallucinations. *European Archives of Psychiatry & Clinical Neurosciences* **255**, 202–212.

Bowins, B. & Sugar, G. (1998) Delusions and self-esteem. *Canadian Journal of Psychiatry* **43**, 154–158.

Boydell, J., van Os, J., McKenzie, K. *et al.* (2001) Incidence of schizophrenia in ethnic minorities in London: ecological study into interactions with environment *British Medical Journal* **323**, 1336–1338.

Brewin, C.R. (1994) Changes in attribution and expressed emotion among the relatives of patients with schizophrenia. *Psychological Medicine* **24**, 905–911.

Broome, M.R., Woolley, J.B., Tabraham, P. *et al.* (2005) What causes the onset of psychosis? *Schizophrenia Research* **79**, 23–34.

Brown, G.W. & Birley, J.L.T. (1968) Crises and life changes and the onset of schizophrenia. *Journal of Health and Social Behavior* **9**, 203–214.

Brown, G.W. & Rutter, M.L. (1966) The measurement of family activities and relationships. *Human Relations* **19**, 241–263.

Brown, G.W., Monck, E.M., Carstairs, G.M. & Wing, J.K. (1962) Influence of family life on the course of schizophrenic illness. *British Journal of Preventive and Social Medicine* **16**, 55–68.

Brown, G.W., Birley, J.L.T. & Wing, J.K. (1972) Influence of family life on the course of schizophrenic disorders: a replication. *British Journal of Psychiatry* **121**, 241–258.

Brown, G.W., Harris, T.O. & Peto, J. (1973) Life events and psychiatric disorders. II. Nature of causal link. *Psychological Medicine* **3**, 159–176.

Brunner, R., Parzer, P., Schmitt, R. & Resch, F. (2004) Dissociative symptoms in schizophrenia: a comparative analysis of patients with borderline personality disorder and healthy controls. *Psychopathology* **37**, 281–284.

Buchkremer, G., Stricker, K., Holle, R. & Kuhs, H. (1991) The predictability of relapses in schizophrenic patients. *European Archives of Psychiatry and Clinical Neuroscience* **240**, 292–300.

Budzyna-Dawidowski, P., Rostworowska, M. & de Barbaro, B. (1989) Stability of Expressed Emotion: a 3 year follow-up study of schizophrenic patients. Paper presented at the 19th Annual Congress of the European Association of Behavior Therapy, Vienna, September 10–24.

Butler, R.W., Mueser, K.T., Sprock, J. & Braff, D.L. (1996) Positive symptoms of psychosis in post-traumatic stress disorder. *Biological Psychiatry* **39**, 839–844.

Butzlaff, R.L. & Hooley, J.M. (1998) Expressed emotion and psychiatric relapse: a meta-analysis. *Archives of General Psychiatry* **55**, 547–552.

Calhoun, P.S., Stechuchak, K.M., Strauss, J., Bosworth, H.B., Marx, C.E. & Butterfield, M.I. (2007) Interpersonal trauma, war zone exposure, and posttraumatic stress disorder among veterans with schizophrenia. *Schizophrenia Research* **91**, 210–216.

Canton, G. & Fraccon, I.G. (1985) Life events and schizophrenia: a replication. *Acta Psychiatrica Scandinavica* **71**, 211–216.

Cantor-Graae, E. & Selten, J.P. (2005) Schizophrenia and migration: a meta-analysis and review. *American Journal of Psychiatry* **162**, 12–24.

Castine, M.R., Meador-Woodruff, J.H. & Dalack, G.W. (1998) The role of life events in onset and recurrent episodes of schizophrenia and schizoaffective disorder. *Journal of Psychiatric Research* **32**, 283–288.

Chung, R.K., Langeluddecke, P. & Tennant, C. (1986) Threatening life events in the onset of schizophrenia, schizophreniform psychosis and hypomania. *British Journal of Psychiatry* **148**, 680–686.

Cougnard, A., Marcelis, M., Myin-Germeys, I. *et al.* (2007) Does normal developmental expression of psychosis combine with environmental risk to cause persistence of psychosis? A psychosis proneness-persistence model. *Psychological Medicine* **37**, 513–527.

Crittendon, P.M., & Ainsworth, M.D.S. (1989) Child maltreatment & attachment theory. In: Cicchetti, D. & Carlson, V., eds. *Childhood Maltreatment: Theory and Research on the Causes and Consequences of Child Abuse and Neglect*. Cambridge: Cambridge University Press.

Cutting, L.P. & Docherty, N.M. (2000) Schizophrenia outpatients' perceptions of their parents: is expressed emotion a factor? *Journal of Abnormal Psychology* **109**, 266–272.

David, D., Kutcher, G.S., Jackson, E.I. & Mellman, T.A. (1999) Psychotic symptoms in combat-related post-traumatic stress disorder. *Journal of Clinical Psychiatry* **60**, 29–32.

Day, R., Neilsen, J.A., Korten, A. *et al.* (1987) Stressful life events preceding the acute onset of schizophrenia: a cross national study from the World Health Organization. *Culture, Medicine and Psychiatry* **11**, 123–206.

de Jong, J.G., Wasilewski, M., van der Vegt, B.J., Buwalda, B. & Koolhaas, J.M. (2005) A single social defeat induces short-lasting behavioral sensitization to amphetamine. *Physiology and Behavior* **83**, 805–811.

Dinzeo, T.J., Cohen, A.S., Nienow, T.M. & Docherty, N.M. (2004) Stress and arousability in schizophrenia. *Schizophrenia Research* **71**, 127–135.

Dixon, M.J., King, S., Stip, E. & Cormier, H. (2000) Continuous performance test differences among schizophrenic outpatients living in high and low expressed emotion environments. *Psychological Medicine* **30**, 1141–1153.

Doane, J.A., West, K.L., Goldstein, M.J., Rodnick, E.H. & Jones, J.E. (1981) Parental communication deviance and affective style: predictors of subsequent schizophrenia spectrum disorders in vulnerable adolescents. *Archives of General Psychiatry* **38**, 679–685.

Docherty, N.M., Cutting, L.P. & Bers, S.A. (1998) Expressed emotion and differentiation of self in the relatives of stable schizophrenia outpatients. *Psychiatry* **61**, 269–278.

Doering, S., Muller, E., Kopcke, W. *et al.* (1998) Predictors of relapse and rehospitalization in schizophrenia and schizoaffective disorder. *Schizophrenia Bulletin* **24**, 87–98.

Dohrenwend, B.P., Levav, I., Shrout, P.E. *et al.* (1987) Life stress and psychopathology: progress with research begun with Barbara Snell Dohrenwend. *American Journal of Community Psychology* **15**, 677–713.

Driessen, M., Herrmann, J., Stahl, K. *et al.* (2000). Magnetic resonance imaging volumes of the hippocampus and the amygdala in women with borderline personality disorder and early traumatization. *Archives of General Psychiatry* **57**, 1115–1122.

Ellason, J.E. & Ross, C.A. (1997) Childhood trauma and psychiatric symptoms. *Psychological Reports* **80**, 447–450.

Favre, S., Gonzales, C., Lendais, G. *et al.* (1989) Expressed Emotion (EE) of schizophrenic relatives. Poster presented at VIIIth World Congress of Psychiatry, Athens, 12–19 October.

Fisher, H., Morgan, C., Fearon, P. *et al.* (2006) Childhood maltreatment as a risk factor for psychosis. *Schizophrenia Research* **86**, S48–S49.

Fortune, D.G., Smith, J.V. & Garvey, K. (2005) Perceptions of psychosis, coping, appraisals, and psychological distress in the relatives of patients with schizophrenia: an exploration using self-regulation theory. *British Journal of Clinical Psychology* **44**, 319–331.

Fowler, D. (1999) The relationship between trauma and psychosis. Paper Presented at the Merseyside Psychotherapy Institute, Liverpool, May 1999.

Fowler, D. (2000) Cognitive behavior therapy for psychosis: from understanding to treatment. *Psychiatric Rehabilitation Skills* **4**, 199–215.

Fowler, D., Freeman, D., Smith, B. *et al.* (2006) The Brief Core Schema Scales (BCSS): Psychometric properties and associations with paranoia and grandiosity in non-clinical and psychosis samples. *Psychological Medicine* **36**, 749–759.

Freeman, D., Garety, P.A., Bebbington, P.E. *et al.* (2005) Psychological investigation of the structure of paranoia in a non-clinical population. *British Journal of Psychiatry* **186**, 427–435.

Freeman, D., Brugha, T., Meltzer, H., Jenkins, R., Stahl, D. & Bebbington, P. (2010) Persecutory ideation and insomnia: findings from the second British National Survey of Psychiatric Morbidity. *Journal of Psychiatric Research* [Epub ahead of print].

Freud, S. (1917) Mourning and melancholia. In: *Collected Papers*, Vol. **IV**. London: Hogarth.

Friedman, S., Smith, L., Fogel, D. *et al.* (2002) The incidence and influence of early traumatic life events in patients with panic disorder: a comparison with other psychiatric outpatients. *Journal of Anxiety Disorders* **16**, 259–272.

Fuchs, T. (1999) Life events in late paraphrenia and depression. *Psychopathology* **32**, 60–69.

Garety, P.A. & Hemsley, D.R. (1994) *Delusions: Investigations into the Psychology of Delusional Reasoning.* Oxford: Oxford University Press.

Garety, P., Kuipers, E., Fowler, D., Freeman, D. & Bebbington, P. (2001) Theoretical paper: a cognitive model of the positive symptoms of psychosis. *Psychological Medicine* **31**, 189–195.

Garety, P.A., Bebbington, P., Fowler, D., Freeman, D. & Kuipers, E. (2007) Implications for neurobiological research of cognitive models of psychosis: a theoretical paper. *Psychological Medicine* **37**, 1377–1391.

Gearon, J.S., Kaltman, S.I., Brown, C. & Bellack, A.S. (2003) Traumatic life events and PTSD among women with substance use disorders and schizophrenia. *Psychiatric Services* **54**, 523–528.

Giesbrecht, T., Merckelbach, H., Kater, M. & Sluis, A.F. (2007) Why dissociation and schizotypy overlap: the joint influence of fantasy proneness, cognitive failures, and childhood trauma. *Journal of Nervous and Mental Disease* **195**, 812–818.

Giron, M. & Gomez-Beneyto, M. (1998) Relationship between empathic family attitude and relapse in schizophrenia: a 2-year follow-up prospective study. *Schizophrenia Bulletin* **24**, 619–627.

Glaslova, K., Bob, P., Jasova, D., Bratkova, N. & Ptacek, R. (2004) Traumatic stress and schizophrenia. *Neurology Psychiatry and Brain Research* **11**, 205–208.

Goldman-Rakic, P.S., Castner, S.A., Svensson, T.H., Siever, L.J. & Williams, G.V. (2004) Targeting the dopamine D1 receptor in schizophrenia: insights for cognitive dysfunction. *Psychopharmacology (Berlin)* **174**, 3–16.

Goldstein, M., Judd, L.L., Rodnick, E.H., Alkire, A. & Gould, E. (1968) A method for studying social influence and coping patterns within families of disturbed adolescents. *Journal of Nervous and Mental Disease* **147**, 233–251.

Goodman, L.A., Thompson, K.M., Weinfurt, K. *et al.* (1999) Reliability of reports of violent victimization and posttraumatic stress disorder among men and women with serious mental health. *Journal of Trauma and Stress* **12**, 587–599.

Gracie, A., Freeman, D., Green, S. *et al.* (2007) The association between traumatic experience, paranoia and hallucinations: a test of the predictions of psychological models. *Acta Psychiatrica Scandinavica* **116**, 280–289.

Griesinger, W. (1861) Die Pathologie und Therapie der Psychischen Krankheiten., 2nd edn. Braunschweig. Wreden (translated as *Mental Pathology and Therapeutics* by Robertson, C.L. & Rutherford, J.). London: New Sydenham Society.

Gutiérrez, E., Escudero, V., Valero, J.A. *et al.* (1988) Expresión de emociones y curso de la esquizofrenia. II. Expresión de emociones y curso de la esquizofrenia en pacientes en remisión. *Análisisy Modificación de Conducta* **14**, 275–316.

Gureje, O. & Adewumni, A. (1988) Life events in schizophrenia in Nigerians: a controlled investigation. *British Journal of Psychiatry* **153**, 367–375.

Haggar, M. & Orbell, S. (2003) A meta-analytic review of the common-sense model of illness representations. *Psychology and Health* **18**, 141–184.

Hammersley, P., Dias, A., Todd, G., Bowen-Jones, K., Reilly, B. & Bentall, R.P. (2003) Childhood trauma and hallucinations in bipolar affective disorder: preliminary investigation. *British Journal of Psychiatry* **182**, 543–547.

Hamner, M.B. & Gold, P.B. (1998) Plasma dopamine β-hydroxylase activity in psychotic and non-psychotic post-traumatic stress disorder. *Psychiatry Research* **77**, 174–181.

Hamner, M.B., Frueh, B.C., Ulmer, H.G. & Arana, G.W. (1999) Psychotic features and illness severity in combat veterans with chronic post-traumatic stress disorder. *Biological Psychiatry* **45**, 846–852.

Hamner, M.D., Frueh, B.C., Ulmer, H.G. *et al.* (2000) Psychotic features in chronic posttraumatic stress disorder and schizophrenia: comparative severity. *Journal of Nervous and Mental Disease* **188**, 217–221.

Hardesty, J., Falloon, I.R.H. & Shirin, K. (1985) The impact of life events, stress and coping on the morbidity of schizophrenia. In: Falloon, I.R., ed. *Family Management of Schizophrenia.* Baltimore: Johns Hopkins University Press.

Hardy, A., Fowler, D., Freeman, D. *et al.* (2005) Trauma and hallucinatory experience in psychosis. *Journal of Nervous and Mental Disease* **193**, 501–507.

Harris, T.O. (1987) Recent developments in the study of life events in relation to psychiatric and physical disorders. In: Cooper, B., ed. *Psychiatric Epidemiology: Progress and Prospects.* London: Croom-Helm, pp. 81–100.

Harrison, C.A., Dadds, M.R. & Smith, G. (1998) Family caregivers' criticism of patients with schizophrenia. *Psychiatric Services* **49**, 918–924.

Hegerl, U., Priebe, S., Wildgrube, C. & Muller-Oerlinghausen, B. (1990) Expressed emotion and auditory evoked potentials. *Psychiatry* **53**, 108–114.

Heim, C., Newport, D.J., Miller, A.H. & Nemeroff, C.B. (2000) Long-term neuroendocrine effects of childhood maltreatment. *JAMA* **284**, 2321.

Hirsch, S., Bowen, J., Emami, J. *et al.* (1996) A one year prospective study of the effects of life events and medication in the etiology of schizophrenic relapse. *British Journal of Psychiatry* **168**, 49–56.

Holmes, E.A. & Steel, C. (2004) Schizotypy: a vulnerability factor for traumatic intrusions. *Journal of Nervous and Mental Disease* **192**, 28–34.

Holowka, D.W., King, S., Saheb, D., Pukall, M. & Brunet, A. (2003) Childhood abuse and dissociative symptoms in adult schizophrenia. *Schizophrenia Research* **60**, 87–90.

Horan, W.P. & Blanchard, J.J. (2003) Emotional responses to psychosocial stress in schizophrenia: the role of individual differences in affective traits and coping. *Schizophrenia Research* **60**, 271–283.

Horan, W.P., Ventura, J., Nuechterlein, K.H., Subotnik, K.L., Hwang, S.S. & Mintz, J. (2005) Stressful life events in recent-onset schizophrenia: reduced frequencies and altered subjective appraisals. *Schizophrenia Research* **75**, 363–374.

Horan, W.P., Ventura, J., Mintz, J. *et al.* (2007) Stress and coping responses to a natural disaster in people with schizophrenia. *Psychiatry Research* **151**, 77–86.

Howard, R. & Ford, R. (1992) From the jumping Frenchmen of Maine to post-traumatic stress disorder: the startle response in neuropsychiatry. *Psychological Medicine* **22**, 695–707.

Hubschmid, T. & Zemp, M. (1989) Interactions in high- and low-EE families. *Social Psychiatry and Psychiatric Epidemiology* **24**, 113–119.

Hultman, C.M., Wieselgren, I.M. & Ohman, A. (1997) Relationships between social support, social coping and life events in the relapse of schizophrenic patients. *Scandinavian Journal of Psychology* **38**, 3–13.

Irwin, H.J. (2001) The relationship between dissociative tendencies and schizotypy: an artifact of childhood trauma? *Journal of Clinical Psychology* **57**, 331–342.

Ivanović, M., Vuletić, Z. & Bebbington, P.E. (1994) Expressed Emotion in the families of patients with schizophrenia and its influence on the course of illness. *Social Psychiatry and Psychiatric Epidemiology* **29**, 61–65.

Ivezić, S., Oruć, L. & Bell, P. (1999) Psychotic symptoms in post-traumatic stress disorder. *Military Medicine* **164**, 73–75.

Jacobs, S. & Myers, J. (1976) Recent life events and acute schizophrenic psychosis: a controlled study. *Journal of Nervous and Mental Disease* **162**, 75–87.

Jansen, L.M.C., Gispen-De-Wied, C.C., Gademan, P.J. *et al.* (1998) Blunted cortisol response to a psychosocial stressor in schizophrenia. *Schizophrenia Research* **33**, 87–94.

Janssen, I., Krabbendam, L., Bak, M. *et al.* (2004) Childhood abuse as a risk factor for psychotic experiences. *Acta Psychiatrica Scandinavica* **109**, 38–45.

Jaspers, K. (1913) Kausale and verständliche Zusammenhänge zwischen Schicksal und Psychose bei der Dementia Praecox (Schizophrenia). *Zeitschrift Neurologie* **14**, 158–263.

Jauch, D.A. & Carpenter, W.T. Jr (1998) Reactive psychosis I. Does the pre-DSM-IIIR concept define a third psychosis? *Journal of Nervous and Mental Disease* **176**, 82–86.

Jay, T.M., Rocher, C., Hotte, M., Naudon, L., Gurden, H. & Spedding, M. (2004) Plasticity at hippocampal to prefrontal cortex synapses is impaired by loss of dopamine and stress: importance for psychiatric diseases. *Neurotoxicity Research* **6**, 233–244.

Johns, L.C., Nazroo, J.Y., Bebbington, P. & Kuipers, E. (2002) Occurrence of hallucinatory experiences in a community sample and ethnic variations. *British Journal of Psychiatry* **180**, 174–178.

Jonas, S., Bebbington, P.E., McManus, S. *et al.* (2010) Sexual abuse and psychiatric disorder in England: Results from the 2007 Adult Psychiatric Morbidity Survey. *Psychological Medicine* (Epub ahead of print).

Jones, S.R. & Fernyhough, C. (2007) A new look at the neural diathesis—stress model of schizophrenia: the primacy of social-evaluative and uncontrollable situations. *Schizophrenia Bulletin*, **33**, 1171–1177.

Kaffman, M. (1984) Paranoid disorders: the core of truth behind the delusional system. *International Journal of Family Therapy* **6**, 220–232.

Kapur, S., Mizrahi, R. & Li, M. (2005) From dopamine to salience to psychosis–linking biology, pharmacology and phenomenology of psychosis. *Schizophrenia Research* **79**, 59–68.

Karno, M., Jenkins, J.H., de la Selva, A. *et al.* (1987) Expressed emotion and schizophrenic outcome among Mexican-American families. *Journal of Nervous and Mental Disease* **175**, 143–151.

Kilcommons, A.M. & Morrison, A.P. (2005) Relationships between trauma and psychosis: an exploration of cognitive and dissociative factors. *Acta Psychiatrica Scandinavica* **112**, 351–359.

Kinderman, P. & Cooke, A. (2000) *Recent Advances in Understanding Mental Illness and Psychotic Experiences. A report by the British Psychological Society Division of Clinical Psychology.* Leicester: British Psychological Society.

King, S. & Dixon, M.J. (1999) Expressed emotion and relapse in young schizophrenia outpatients. *Schizophrenia Bulletin* **25**, 377–386.

Kopelowicz, A., Zarate, R., Gonzalez, V. *et al.* (2002). Evaluation of expressed emotion in schizophrenia: a comparison of Caucasians and Mexican-Americans. *Schizophrenia Research* **55**, 179–186.

Krabbendam, L. & van Os, J. (2005) Schizophrenia and urbanicity: a major environmental influence — conditional on genetic risk. *Schizophrenia Bulletin* **31**, 795–799.

Kuipers, L. (1979) Expressed Emotion: a review. *British Journal of Social and Clinical Psychology* **18**, 237–243.

Kuipers, E., Fowler, D., Garety, G. *et al.* (1998) The London–East Anglia randomised controlled trial of cognitive behavior therapy for psychosis. III. Follow up and economic evaluation at 18 months. *British Journal of Psychiatry* **173**, 61–68.

Kuipers, E., Bebbington, P., Dunn, G. *et al.* (2006) Influence of carer expressed emotion and affect on relapse in non-affective psychosis. *British Journal of Psychiatry* **188**, 173–179.

Kuipers, E., Watson, P., Onwumere, J. *et al.* (2007) Discrepant illness perceptions affect and expressed emotion in people with psychosis and their carers. *Social Psychiatry and Psychiatric Epidemiology* **42**, 277–283.

Kuipers, E., Onwumere, J. & Bebbington, P. (2010) Cognitive model of care-giving in psychosis. *British Journal of Psychiatry* **196**, 259–264.

Kurihara, T., Kato, M., Tsukahara, T., Takano, Y. & Reverger, R. (2000) The low prevalence of high levels of expressed emotion in Bali. *Psychiatry Research* **17**, 229–238.

Lappin, J.M., Morgan, K., Morgan, C. *et al.* (2006) Gray matter abnormalities associated with duration of untreated psychosis. *Schizophrenia Research* **83**, 145–153.

Laruelle, M., Kegeles, L. S. & Abi-Dargham, A. (2003) Glutamate, dopamine, and schizophrenia: from pathophysiology to treatment. *Annals of the New York Academy of Science* **1003**, 138–158.

Lataster T., van Os J., Drukker M. *et al.* (2006) Childhood victimisation and developmental expression of non-clinical delusional ideation and hallucinatory experiences: victimisation

and non-clinical psychotic experiences. *Social Psychiatry and Psychiatric Epidemiology* **41**, 423–428.

Leff, J.P. & Vaughn, C. (1976) Schizophrenia and family life. *Psychology Today* **10**, 13–18.

Leff, J.P., Hirsch, S.R., Gaind, R., Rohde, P.D. & Stevens, B.C. (1973) Life events and maintenance therapy in schizophrenic relapse. *British Journal of Psychiatry* **123**, 659–660.

Leff, J.P., Kuipers, L., Berkowitz, R., Eberlein-Fries, R. & Sturgeon, D. (1982) A controlled trial of intervention in the families of schizophrenic patients. *British Journal of Psychiatry* **141**, 121–134.

Leff, J.P., Wig, N., Ghosh, A. *et al.* (1987) Influence of relatives' Expressed Emotion on the course of schizophrenia in Chandigarh. *British Journal of Psychiatry* **151**, 166–173.

Linszen, D., Dingemans, P., Van-der-Does, J.W. *et al.* (1996) Treatment, expressed emotion and relapse in recent onset schizophrenic disorders. *Psychological Medicine* **26**, 333–342.

Lobban F., Barrowclough C., Jones S. (2006) Does Expressed Emotion need to be understood within a more systemic framework? An examination of discrepancies in appraisals between patients diagnosed with schizophrenia and their relatives. *Social Psychiatry Psychiatric Epidemiology* **41**, 50–55.

Lopez, S.R., Nelson, K.A., Snyder, K.S. & Mintz, J. (1999) Attributions and affective reactions of family members and course of schizophrenia. *Journal of Abnormal Psychology* **108**, 307–314.

Lopez, S.R., Hipke, K.N., Polo, A.J. & Jenkins, J.H. (2004) Ethnicity, expressed emotion, attributions, and course of schizophrenia: Family warmth matters. *Journal of Abnormal Psychology* **113**, 428–439.

Lysaker, P.H. & Salyers, M.P. (2007) Anxiety symptoms in schizophrenia spectrum disorders: associations with social function, positive and negative symptoms, hope and trauma history. *Acta Psychiatrica Scandinavica* **116**, 290–298.

Lysaker, P.H., Meyer, P.S., Evans, J.D., Clements, C.A. & Marks, K.A. (2001) Childhood sexual trauma and psychosocial functioning in adults with schizophrenia. *Psychiatric Services* **52**, 1485–1488.

MacDonald, E.M., Pica, S., McDonald, S., Hayes, R.L. & Baglioni, A.J. Jr (1998) Stress and coping in early psychosis: role of symptoms, self-efficacy, and social support in coping with stress. *British Journal of Psychiatry* **172** (Suppl. 33), 122–127.

MacMillan, J.F., Gold, A., Crow, T.J., Johnson, A.L. & Johnstone, E.C. (1986) The Northwick Park study of first episodes of schizophrenia. IV. Expressed emotion and relapse. *British Journal of Psychiatry* **148**, 133–143.

Malla, A.K., Cortese, L., Shaw, T.S. & Ginsberg, B. (1990) Life events and relapse in schizophrenia: a one year prospective study. *Social Psychiatry and Psychiatric Epidemiology* **25**, 221–224.

Malzacher, M., Merz, J. & Ebnother, D. (1981) Einschneidende Lebensereignisse im Vorfeld akuter schizophrener Episoden: Erstmals erkrankte Patienten im Vergleich mit einer Normalstichprobe. *Archiv Fur Psychiatrie und Nervenkrankheiten* **230**, 227–242.

Maosheng, R., Zaijin, H. & Mengze, S. (1998) Emotional expression among relatives of schizophrenic patients. *Chinese Journal of Psychiatry* **31**, 237–239.

Marzillier, S.L. & Steel, C. (2007) Positive schizotypy and trauma-related intrusions. *Journal of Nervous and Mental Disease* **195**, 60–64.

May-Chahal, C. & Cawson, P. (2005) Measuring child maltreatment in the United Kingdom: a study of the prevalence of child abuse and neglect. *Child Abuse and Neglect* **29**, 969–984.

Mazure, C.M., Quinlan, D.M. & Bowers, M.B., Jr. (1997) Recent life stressors and biological markers in newly admitted psychotic patients. *Biological Psychiatry* **41**, 865–870.

McCreadie, R.G. & Phillips, K. (1988) The Nithsdale Schizophrenia Survey. VII. Does relatives' high Expressed Emotion predict relapse? *British Journal of Psychiatry* **152**, 477–481.

McCreadie, R.G., Phillips, K., Harvey, J.A. *et al.* (1991) The Nithsdale Schizophrenia Surveys. VIII. Do relatives want family intervention and does it help? *British Journal of Psychiatry* **158**, 110–113.

McCreadie, R.G., Robertson, L.J., Hall, D.J. & Berry, I. (1993) The Nithsdale Schizophrenia Surveys. XI. Relatives' expressed emotion: stability over five years and its relations to relapse. *British Journal of Psychiatry* **162**, 393–397.

Miklowitz, D.J., Goldstein, M.J., Doane, J.A. *et al.* (1989) Is expressed emotion an index of a transactional process. I. Parent's affective style. *Family Process* **28**, 153–167.

Miller, P., Lawrie, S.M., Hodges, A., Clafferty, R., Cosway, R. & Johnstone, E.C. (2001) Genetic liability, illicit drug use, life stress and psychotic symptoms: preliminary findings from the Edinburgh study of people at high risk for schizophrenia. *Social Psychiatry and Psychiatric Epidemiology* **36**, 338–342.

Moline, R.A., Singh, S., Morris, A. & Meltzer, H.Y. (1985) Family expressed emotion and relapse in schizophrenia in 24 urban American patients. *American Journal of Psychiatry* **142**, 1078–1081.

Montero, I., Gomez-Beneyto, M., Ruiz, I., Puche, E. & Adam, A. (1992) The influence of family Expressed Emotion on the course of schizophrenia in a sample of Spanish patients: a two year follow-up study. *British Journal of Psychiatry* **161**, 217–222.

Morgan, C. & Fisher, H. (2007) Environment and schizophrenia: environmental factors in schizophrenia: childhood trauma—critical review. *Schizophrenia Bulletin* **33**, 3–10.

Morgan, D., Grant, K.A., Gage, H.D. *et al.* (2002) Social dominance in monkeys: dopamine D2 receptors and cocaine self-administration. *Nature Neuroscience* **5**, 169–174.

Morgan, C., Kirkbride, J., Leff, J. *et al.* (2007) Parental separation, loss and psychosis in different ethnic groups: a case-control study. *Psychological Medicine* **37**, 495–503.

Morrison A.P. (2001) The interpretation of intrusions in psychosis: an integrative cognitive approach to hallucinations and delusions. *Behavioural & Cognitive Psychotherapy* **29**, 257–276.

Možný, N.P. & Votpkova, P. (1992) Expressed emotion, relapse rate and utilisation of psychiatric inpatient care in schizophrenia: a study from Czechoslovakia. *Social Psychiatry and Psychiatric Epidemiology* **27**, 174–179.

Mueser, K.T., Goodman, L.B., Trumbetta, S.L. *et al.* (1998) Trauma and post-traumatic stress disorder in severe mental illness. *Journal of Consulting and Clinical Psychology* **66**, 493–499.

Mueser, K.T., Rosenberg, S.D., Goodman, L.A. & Trumbetta, S.L. (2002) Trauma, PTSD, and the course of severe mental illness: an interactive model. *Schizophrenia Research* **53**, 123–143.

Mueser, K.T., Salyers, M.P., Rosenberg, S.D. *et al.* (2004) Interpersonal trauma and posttraumatic stress disorder in patients with severe mental illness: demographic, clinical, and health correlates. *Schizophrenia Bulletin* **30**, 45–57.

Myhrman, A., Rantakallio, P., Isohanni, M., Jones, P. & Partanen, U. (1994) Unwantedness of a pregnancy and schizophrenia in the child. *British Journal of Psychiatry* **169**, 637–640.

Myin-Germeys, I. & Krabbendam L. (2004) Sex differences in emotional reactivity to daily life stress in psychosis. *Journal of Clinical Psychiatry* **65**, 805–809.

Myin-Germeys, I. & van Os, J. (2007) Stress-reactivity in psychosis: evidence for an affective pathway to psychosis. *Clinical Psychology Review* **27**, 409–424.

Myin-Germeys, I., van Os, J., Schwartz, J.E., Stone, A.A. & Delespaul, P.A. (2001) Emotional reactivity to daily life stress in psychosis. *Archives of General Psychiatry* **58**, 1137–1144.

Myin-Germeys, I., Krabbendam, L., Delespaul, P. & van Os, J. (2003) Can cognitive deficits explain differential sensitivity to life events in psychosis? *Social Psychiatry and Psychiatric Epidemiology* **38**, 262–268.

Myin-Germeys, I., Delespaul, P. & van Os, J. (2005) Behavioural sensitization to daily life stress in psychosis. *Psychological Medicine* **35**, 733–741.

Neria, Y., Bromet, E.J., Sievers, S., Lavelle, J. & Fochtmann, L.J. (2002) Trauma exposure and posttraumatic stress disorder in psychosis: findings from a first-admission cohort. *Journal of Consulting and Clinical Psychology* **70**, 246–251.

National Institute for Clinical Excellence (2003) Schizophrenia: core interventions in the treatment and management of schizophrenia in primary and secondary care (full guideline). London: Gaskell and The British Psychological Society.

National Institute for Clinical Excellence (2009) Schizophrenia: core interventions in the treatment and management of schizophrenia in adults in primary and secondary care: update. http://www.nice.org.uk/nicemedia/pdf/CG82Full Guideline.pdf

Niedermeier, T., Watzl, H. & Cohen, R. (1992) Prediction of relapse of schizophrenic patients: Camberwell Family Interview versus content anlysis of verbal behavior. *Psychiatry Research* **41**, 275–282.

Norman, R.M. & Malla, A.K. (2001) Family history of schizophrenia and the relationship of stress to symptoms: preliminary findings. *Australian and New Zealand Journal of Psychiatry* **35**, 217–223.

Nuechterlein, K.H., Snyder, K.S., Dawson, M.E. *et al.* (1986) Expressed emotion, fixed-dose fluphenazine decanoate maintenance, and relapse in recent onset schizophrenia. *Psychopharmacology Bulletin* **22**, 633–639.

Olff, M., Langeland, W., Draijer, N., & Gersons, B.P.R. (2007) Gender differences in posttraumatic stress disorder. *Psychological Bulletin* **133**, 183–204.

Onwumere, J., Kuipers, E., Bebbington, P. *et al.* (2009) Patient perceptions of caregiver criticism in pychosis. *Journal of Nervous and Mental Disease* **197**, 85–91.

Pallanti, S., Quercioli, L. & Pazzagli, A. (1997) Relapse in young paranoid schizophrenic patients: a prospective study of stressful life events. *American Journal of Psychiatry* **154**, 792–298.

Pariante C.M., Dazzan P., Danese A. *et al.* (2005) Increased pituitary volume in antipsychotic-free and antipsychotic-treated patients of the AEsop first-onset psychosis study. *Neuropsychopharmacology* **30**, 1923–1931.

Parker, G., Johnston, P. & Hayward, L. (1988) Parental "expressed emotion" as a predictor of schizophrenic relapse. *Archives of General Psychiatry* **45**, 806–813.

Paster, S.J. (1948). Psychotic reactions among soldiers of World War II. *Journal of Nervous and Mental Disease* **108**, 54–66.

Penn, D. L., Mueser, K. T., Tarrier, N. *et al.* (2004) Supportive therapy for schizophrenia: possible mechanisms and implications for adjunctive psychosocial treatments. *Schizophrenia Bulletin* **30**, 101–112.

Pereda, N., Guilera, G., Forns, M. & Gómez-Benito, J. (2009) The international epidemiology of child sexual abuse: a continuation of Finkelhor (1994). *Child Abuse and Neglect* **33**, 331–342.

Pfammatter, M., Junghan, U.M. & Brenner, H.D. (2006) Efficacy of psychological therapy in schizophrenia: conclusions from meta-analyses. *Schizophrenia Bulletin* **32** (Suppl. 1), S64–S80.

Pharoah, F., Mari, J., Rathbone, J. & Wong, W. (2006) Family intervention for schizophrenia. *Cochrane Database Systematic Reviews* CD000088.

Phillips, L.J., McGorry, P.D., Garner, B. *et al.* (2006) Stress, the hippocampus and the hypothalamic-pituitary-adrenal axis: implications for the development of psychotic disorders. *Australian and New Zealand Journal of Psychiatry* **40**, 725–741.

Pilling, S., Bebbington, P., Kuipers, E. *et al.* (2002) Psychological treatments in schizophrenia. I. Meta-analysis of family intervention and cognitive behaviour therapy. *Psychological Medicine* **32**, 763–782.

Priebe, S., Broker, M. & Gunkel, S. (1998) Involuntary admission and post-traumatic stress disorder symptoms in schizophrenia patients. *Comprehensive Psychiatry* **39**, 220–224.

Pruessner, J.C., Champagne, F., Meaney, M.J. & Dagher, A. (2004) Dopamine release in response to a psychological stress in humans and its relationship to early life maternal care: a positron emission tomography study using [11C]raclopride. *Journal of Neuroscience* **24**, 2825–2831.

Ramana, R. & Bebbington, P. (1995) Social influences on bipolar affective disorders. *Social Psychiatry and Psychiatric Epidemiology* **30**, 152–160.

Raune, D., Kuipers, E. & Bebbington, P.E. (2004) Expressed emotion at first-episode psychosis: investigating a carer appraisal model. *British Journal of Psychiatry* **184**, 321–326.

Raune, D., Bebbington, P., Dunn, G.D. & Kuipers, E. (2006) Event attributes and the content of psychotic experiences in first episode psychosis. *Psychological Medicine* **188**, 221–230.

Raune, D., Bebbington, P.E. & Kuipers, E.A. (2009) Stressful and intrusive life events preceding first episode psychosis. *Epidemiologia e Psichiatria Sociale* **18**, 221–228.

Read, J., Perry, B.D., Moskowitz, A. & Connolly, J. (2001) The contribution of early traumatic events to schizophrenia in some patients: a traumagenic neurodevelopmental model. *Psychiatry* **64**, 319–345.

Read, J., Agar, K., Argyle, N. & Aderhold, V. (2003) Sexual and physical abuse during childhood and adulthood as predictors of hallucinations, delusions and thought disorder. *Psychology and Psychotherapy-Theory Research and Practice* **76**, 1–22.

Read, J., van Os, J., Morrison, A.P. & Ross, C.A. (2005) Childhood trauma, psychosis and schizophrenia: a literature review with theoretical and clinical implications. *Acta Psychiatrica Scandinavica* **112**, 330–350.

Renshaw, K.D. (2007) Perceived criticism only matters when it comes from those you live with. *Journal of Clinical Psychology* **63**, 1171–1179.

Resnick, S.G., Bond, G.R. & Mueser, K.T. (2003) Trauma and posttraumatic stress disorder in people with schizophrenia. *Journal of Abnormal Psychology* **112**, 415–423.

Rooke, O. & Birchwood, M. (1998) Loss, humiliation and entrapment as appraisals of schizophrenic illness: a prospective study of depressed and non-depressed patients. *British Journal of Clinical Psychology* **37**, 259–268.

Rosenfarb, I.S., Goldstein, M.J., Mintz, J. & Nuechterlein, K.H. (1995) Expressed emotion and subclinical psychopathology observable within the transactions between schizophrenic patients and their family members. *Journal of Abnormal Psychology* **142**, 259–267.

Rosenfarb, I.S., Bellack, A.S. & Aziz, N. (2006) Family interactions and the course of schizophrenia in African American and White patients. *Journal of Abnormal Psychology* **115**, 112–120.

Ryan, M.C., Sharifi, N., Condren, R. & Thakore, J.H. (2004) Evidence of basal pituitary-adrenal overactivity in first episode, drug naive patients with schizophrenia. *Psychoneuroendocrinology* **29**, 1065–1070.

Sarkar, J., Mezey, G., Cohen, A., Singh, S.P. & Olumoroti, O. (2005) Comorbidity of post traumatic stress disorder and paranoid schizophrenia: A comparison of offender and non-offender patients. *Journal of Forensic Psychiatry & Psychology* **16**, 660–670.

Scazufca, M., Kuipers, E. & Menezes, P. (2001) Perception of negative emotions in close relatives by patients with schizophrenia. *British Journal of Clinical Psychology* **40**, 167–175.

Scheller-Gilkey, G., Moynes, K., Cooper, I., Kant, C. & Miller, A.H. (2004) Early life stress and PTSD symptoms in patients with comorbid schizophrenia and substance abuse. *Schizophrenia Research* **69**, 167–174.

Schreier, A., Wolke, D., Thomas, K. *et al.* (2009) Prospective study of bullying victimisation in childhood and psychosis-like symptoms in a non-clinical population at 12 years of age. *Archives of General Psychiatry* **66**, 527–536.

Scott, J., Chant, D., Andrews, G., Martin, G. & McGrath, J. (2007) Association between trauma exposure and delusional experiences in a large community-based sample. *British Journal of Psychiatry* **190**, 339–343.

Seedat, S., Stein, M.B., Oosthuizen, P.P., Emsley, R.A. & Stein, D.J. (2003) Linking posttraumatic stress disorder and psychosis: a look at epidemiology, phenomenology, and treatment. *Journal of Nervous and Mental Disease* **191**, 675–681.

Selten, J.P. & Cantor-Graae, E. (2007) Hypothesis:social defeat is a risk factor for schizophrenia. *British Journal of Psychiatry* **51**, 9–12.

Sensky, T., Turkington, D., Kingdon, D. *et al.* (2000) A randomized controlled trial of cognitive behavioural therapy for persistent symptoms in schizophrenia resistant to medication. *Archives of General Psychiatry* **57**, 165–172.

Shenton, M.E., Dickey, C.C., Frumin, M. & McCarley, R.W. (2001) A review of MRI findings in schizophrenia. *Schizophrenia Research* **49**, 1–52.

Shevlin, M., Dorahy, M. & Adamson, G. (2007) Childhood traumas and hallucinations: an analysis of the National Comorbidity Survey. *Journal of Psychiatric Research* **41**, 222–228.

Smith, B., Fowler, D.G., Freeman, D. *et al.* (2006) Emotion and psychosis: Links between depression, self-esteem, negative schematic beliefs and delusions and hallucinations. *Schizophrenia Research* **86**, 181–188.

Spauwen, J., Krabbendam, L., Lieb, R., Wittchen, H.U. & van Os, J. (2006) Impact of psychological trauma on the development of psychotic symptoms: relationship with psychosis proneness. *British Journal of Psychiatry* **188**, 527–533.

Stark, F.M. & Siol, T. (1994) Expressed emotion in the therapeutic relationship with schizophrenic patients. *European Psychiatry* **9**, 299–303.

Steel, C., Fowler, D. & Holmes, E.A. (2005) Trauma-related intrusions and psychosis: An information processing account. *Behavioural and Cognitive Psychotherapy* **33**, 139–152.

Stephens, J.H., Shaffer, J.W. & Carpenter, W.T. (1982) Reactive psychoses. *Journal of Nervous Mental Disorder* **170**, 657–663.

Stirling, J., Tantam, D., Thomas, P., Newby, D. & Montague, L. (1991) EE and early onset schizophrenia: a one year follow-up. *Psychological Medicine* **21**, 675–685.

Strachan, A.M., Leff, J.P., Goldstein, M.J., Doane, A. & Burrt, C. (1986) Emotional attitudes and direct communication in the families of schizophrenics: a cross-national replication. *British Journal of Psychiatry* **149**, 279–287.

Sumiyoshi, T., Saitoh, T., Yotsutsuji, T. *et al.* (1999) Differential effects of mental stress on plasma homovanillic acid in schizophrenia and normal controls. *Neuropsychopharmacology* **20**, 365–369.

Tanaka, S., Mino, Y. & Inoue, S. (1995) Expressed emotion and the course of schizophrenia in Japan. *British Journal of Psychiatry* **167**, 794–798.

Tarrier, N. (1989) Electrodermal activity, expressed emotion and outcome in schizophrenia. *British Journal of Psychiatry* **155** (Suppl. 5), 51–56.

Tarrier, N., Barrowclough, C., Vaughan, C. *et al.* (1988a) The community management of schizophrenia: a controlled trial of a behavioural intervention with families to reduce relapse. *British Journal of Psychiatry* **153**, 532–542.

Tarrier, N., Barrowclough, C., Porceddu, K. & Watts, S. (1988b) The assessment of psychophysiological reactivity to the expressed emotion of the relatives of schizophrenic patients. *British Journal of Psychiatry* **152**, 618–624.

Tienari, P., Wynne, L.C., Moring, J. *et al.* (1994) The Finnish adoptive family study of schizophrenia: implications for family research. *British Journal of Psychiatry* **23** (Suppl.), 20–26.

Tienari, P., Wynne, L.C., Sorri, A. *et al.* (2004) Genotype-environment interaction in schizophrenia-spectrum disorder. Long-term follow-up study of Finnish adoptees. *British Journal of Psychiatry* **184**, 216–222.

Tompson, M.C., Goldstein, M.J., Lebell, M.B. *et al.* (1995) Schizophrenic patients' perceptions of their relatives' attitudes. *Psychiatry Research* **57**, 155–167.

Ucok, A. & Bikmaz, S. (2007) The effects of childhood trauma in patients with first-episode schizophrenia. *Acta Psychiatrica Scandinavica* **116**, 371–377.

Ungvari, G.S. & Mullens, P.E. (2000) Reactive psychosis revisited. *Australian and New Zealand Journal of Psychiatry* **34**, 458–467.

van Os, J. & Marcelis, M. (1998) The ecogenetics of schizophrenia. *Schizophrenia Research* **23**, 127–135.

van Os, J., Fahy, T.A., Bebbington, P. *et al.* (1994) The influence of life events on the subsequent course of psychotic illness: a prospective follow-up of the Camberwell Collaborative Psychosis Study. *Psychological Medicine* **24**, 503–513.

van Os J., Linscott, R.J., Myin-Germeys, I., Delespaul, P. & Krabbendam, L. (2009) A systematic review and meta-analysis of the psychosis continuum: evidence for a psychosis proneness-persistence-impairment model of psychotic disorder. *Psychological Medicine* **39**, 179–195.

Vanheusden , K., Mulder, C.L., van der Ende, J. *et al.* (2008) Associations between ethnicity and self-reported hallucinations in a population sample of young adults in The Netherlands. *Psychological Medicine* **38**, 1095–1102.

Vaughan, K., Doyle, M., McConathy, N. *et al.* (1992) The relationship between relatives' EE and schizophrenic relapse: an Australian replication. *Social Psychiatry and Psychiatric Epidemiology* **27**, 10–15.

Vaughn, C.E., Snyder, K.S., Jones, S., Freeman, W.B. & Falloon, I.R.H. (1984) Family factors in schizophrenic relapse: replication in California of British research in expressed emotion. *Archives of General Psychiatry* **41**, 1169–1177.

Veling, W., Selten, J.P., Veen, N., Laan, W., Blom, J.D. & Hoek, H.W. (2006) Incidence of schizophrenia among ethnic minorities in the Netherlands: a four-year first-contact study. *Schizophrenia Research* **86**, 189–193.

Veling, W., Susser, E., van Os, J., Mackenbach, J.P., Selten, J-P. & Hoek, H.W. (2008) Ethnic density of neighborhoods and incidence of psychotic disorders among immigrants. *American Journal of Psychiatry* **165**, 66–73.

Ventura, J., Nuechterlein, K.H., Lukoff, D. & Hardisty, J.P. (1989) A prospective study of stressful life events and schizophrenic relapse. *Journal of Abnormal Psychology* **98**, 407–404.

Ventura, J., Nuechterlein, K.H., Hardisty, J.P. & Gitlin, M. (1992) Life events and schizophrenic relapse after withdrawal of medication: a prospective study. *British Journal of Psychiatry* **161**, 615–620.

Ventura, J., Nuechterlein, K.H., Subotnik, K.L., Hardesty, J.P. & Mintz, J. (2000) Live events can trigger depressive exacerbation in the early course of schizophrenia. *Journal of Abnormal Psychology* **109**, 139–144.

Weisman, A.G., Nuechterlein, K.H., Goldstein, M.J. & Snyder, K.S. (1998) Expressed emotion, attributions, and schizophrenia symptom dimensions. *Journal of Abnormal Psychology* **107**, 355–359.

Weisman, A.G., Nuechterlein, K.H., Goldstein, M.J. & Snyder, K.S. (2000) Controllability perceptions and reactions to symptoms of schizophrenia: a within-family comparison of relatives with high and low expressed emotion. *Journal of Abnormal Psychology* **109**, 167–171.

White, R., Bebbington, P., Pearson, J., Johnson, S. & Ellis, D. (2000) The social context of insight in schizophrenia. *Social Psychiatry and Psychiatric Epidemiology* **35**, 500–507.

Wig, N.N., Menon, D.K., Bedi, H. *et al.* (1987) The distribution of Expressed Emotion components among relatives of schizophrenic patients in Aarhus and Chandigarh. *British Journal of Psychiatry* **151**, 160–165.

Wiles, N. J., Zammit, S., Bebbington, P., Singleton, N., Meltzer, H., and Lewis, G. (2006) Self-reported psychotic symptoms in the general population: results from the longitudinal study of the British National Psychiatric Morbidity Survey. *British Journal of Psychiatry* **188**, 519–526.

Wing, J.K. & Brown, G.W. (1970) *Institutionalism and Schizophrenia. A Comparative Study of Three Mental Hospitals 1960–68.* Cambridge: Cambridge University Press.

Wing, J.K., Monck, E., Brown, G.W. & Carstairs, G.M. (1964) Morbidity in the community of schizophrenic patients discharged from London mental hospitals in 1959. *British Journal of Psychiatry* **110**, 10–21.

Woo, S.M., Goldstein, M.J. & Nuechterlein, K.H. (1997) Relatives' expressed emotion and non-verbal signs of subclinical psychopathology in schizophrenia patients. *British Journal of Psychiatry* **170**, 58–61.

Yung, A.R. & McGorry, P.D. (1996) The initial prodrome in psychosis: descriptive and qualitative aspects. *Australian and New Zealand Journal of Psychiatry* **30**, 587–599.

CHAPTER 30

Mental health services for patients with schizophrenia

Tom Burns[1] and Bob Drake[2]

[1]Warneford Hospital, Oxford, UK
[2]Dartmouth Psychiatric Research Center, Lebanon, New Hampshire, USA

Introduction

Schizophrenia's role in shaping mental health services

Schizophrenia has been at the center of psychiatry's development throughout its short history (see Chapter 1). The severity of the disabilities associated with schizophrenia, in both its acute and more long-term stable phases, has ensured that it is impossible to ignore in service planning. The self-neglect, apathy, and disability arising from the negative symptoms and cognitive dysfunction of the disorder have obliged social care and support to form a central part of services. It has recently been suggested that the dominance of this comprehensive and integrated psycho-social approach has been to the detriment of the profession's image and potential (Goodwin & Geddes, 2007).

Goodwin and Geddes (2007) believe that schizophrenia's influence has distracted psychiatry from a pragmatic and flexible medical model that better accommodates the full range of disorders we face. This perspective finds echo in some European systems, such as traditional "social psychiatry" in Germany where long-term psychosis community care was culturally separated from the medically dominated hospital settings, and was often led by social workers. Sweden has radically transformed its mental health provision with the funding stream and responsibility for long-term psychosis (read schizophrenia) care located in local social services and the rest of psychiatry remaining with the regional health boards. The establishment of "Social and Healthcare" partnership Trusts in the UK with nominal equality of both partners has led to some tensions, but in most services medicine continues to take the lead. Whether this will continue to be the case long into

Schizophrenia, 3rd edition. Edited by Daniel R. Weinberger and Paul J Harrison © 2011 Blackwell Publishing Ltd.

the 21st century remains to be seen. In the US, mental healthcare is provided in a two-tiered system: the public sector, which is paid by government to care for patients who are disabled by mental illness (two-thirds of whom have psychotic illnesses), and the private sector, which is paid by private insurance and private income and offers services to all others. The majority of services for people with schizophrenia across Europe are free at the point of delivery and provided by a network of non-profit organizations regulated by the state or by directly state-run organizations. These are funded through social and health budgets (the latter often via health insurers).

For practical purposes this means that the history and configuration of psychiatric services is broadly equivalent to the history and configuration of schizophrenia services. There is evidence of some specialization and divergence more recently in higher income countries, but this is the exception rather than the rule. This chapter will, therefore, focus substantially on general services (albeit through the lens of schizophrenia care), as well as giving consideration to tailored services. As most of current care is conducted by multidisciplinary community teams, they will dominate the descriptions; however, the contributions from traditional outpatient clinics, inpatient, residential and day care remain essential to most services, and will be outlined.

The 19th century and the asylum movement

Up to the late 18th century most care for the mentally ill was supplied by families, but the wealthy also used private mad houses (to protect or hide the patient). The indigent severely mentally ill were accommodated in a variety of almshouses and workhouses along with other social "undesirables" (vagrants, the feeble-minded, drunks, and the demented). Specialist provision, such as the Bethlem Hospital established in London in 1403 and the insane ward in Boston's Almshouse in 1729, were exceptions. The asylum movement gathered momentum after the French Revolution and the York Retreat was opened in 1796 by the Quaker family, the Tukes. This became the international model for "moral treatment" emphasizing kindness, education, patience, and respect for the patient, shifting the focus from physical treatments to meaningful activity and the development of self-control. Asylums were soon established throughout Europe and the US and in their dominions. Over the 19th century they grew rapidly in number and size, and early optimism dwindled as they became overwhelmed with severe and resistant cases.

Psychiatry as we would recognize it (emphasizing careful observation, reliable categorization, and a methodological search for etiology) took off in the second half of the 19th century. Initially a competition between the French and the Germans, Germany soon forged ahead; the first Professor of Psychiatry in Germany was Heinroth in Leipzig in 1813, and the first chair in 1864, Griesinger appointed in Berlin in 1865, and six in post by 1882, ushering in a remarkably productive era. Schizophrenia, initially called dementia praecox, was identified and described by Emil Kraepelin in 1896 and was renamed schizophrenia in 1911 by Eugen Bleuler in Zurich. It was the dominant functional disorder (as distinct from the great number with organic disorders such as general paralysis of the insane, senile dementia, and epilepsy) in asylums of the time and, in many ways, one of the most challenging.

This period was characterized by a degree of therapeutic nihilism, in part because of the rise of the "degeneracy" model of mental illness. Psychiatrists observed the course and psychopathology of schizophrenia, but did not anticipate influencing it. The main function of asylums became the humane residential care of long-stay patients (which several strikingly failed to deliver). Therapeutic stasis, increasing overcrowding, and indifference witnessed a steady decline in the status of asylums and psychiatry until the First World War. The clear association of trauma and shell-shock challenged current degeneracy theories. This and the dramatically effective malaria treatment for general paralysis of the insane, introduced by Wagner-Jauregg in 1917, initiated a reappraisal of psychiatry's possibilities and ushered in the "first medical model" in the 1920s and 1930s.

The optimism of the 1930s was further increased by the introduction of electroconvulsive therapy and improved techniques for sedation. In the UK, the terms "patient" and "mental hospital" had replaced lunatic and asylum, and voluntary care was both permitted and increasingly common. In the US, this optimism was colored by the dominance of both general hospital psychiatry and psychoanalysis. The influence of long-term psychoanalytic treatment in a number of prestigious private hospitals, such as the McLean in Boston, the Yale Psychiatric Institute in New Haven, and the Sheppard Pratt Hospital, profoundly influenced practice and, more significantly, thinking. Adolph Meyer's (1922) emphasis on a broad psychosocial approach to psychiatry, reflecting the power of US general hospital psychiatry, had only limited effects on schizophrenia care.

Despite these developments and some welcome contacts with general medicine, however, the mental hospitals remained generally isolated, both geographically and intellectually. They continued to expand with ever-increasing numbers of mostly chronic patients. Of these the two main groups were those with disabling schizophrenia and the growing number of elderly demented patients. By 1954 psychiatric inpatient care reached its zenith with over 500000 patients in the US and over 160000 in the UK. This number has declined, more or less rapidly, with the respective figures today less than 100000 and 30000.

Move into the community

It is customary to attribute the reduction in the mental hospital population to the introduction of chlorpromazine in the mid-1950s (Brill & Patton, 1962), but it is clear that far-reaching changes were afoot in psychiatry from the end of the Second World War. Change was, of course, in the air generally, which resonated with professional aspirations. Many countries returned reforming governments after the war, questioning old certainties with an enthusiasm for a fairer, more inclusive society.

Some of the psychiatric changes stemmed from greater attention to the course of schizophrenia and an increased understanding of the influences on the observed disabilities. The open-door movement gathered momentum in the late 1940s—Dingleton Hospital in Scotland started the process in 1945 and unlocked its last ward in 1948 (Ratcliffe, 1962), soon to be followed by Mapperly Hospital in Nottingham and Warlingham Park Hospital in Croydon. Dingleton remained a totally open-door hospital until its final closure in 2004. Rehabilitation gained enormous impetus from the work of individuals such as Russell Barton who coined the term "institutional neurosis" to describe the apathy and self-neglect of so many patients with chronic schizophrenia (Barton, 1959). Barton's idea gained empirical support from the influential Three Hospitals study, which demonstrated the impact of the social environment on schizophrenia (Wing & Brown, 1970). The therapeutic potential of social factors in mental illness was simultaneously energetically explored and developed also in the Therapeutic Community movement (Jones, 1952).

Parallel with these pioneering initiatives, a growing and sophisticated critique of psychiatry was developing, drawing on the sociology of deviance and social control. Goffman's (1960) *Asylums* provided an unsettling exposure of the workings of a large mental hospital, and thinkers such as Laing (1960), Foucault (1965), and Szasz (1972) questioned the very validity of the profession. A series of reports detailing serious abuses of patients (Committee of Inquiry, 1969) increased the clamor for radical reform or closure of mental hospitals (National Association for Mental Health, 1961). Much of the later momentum behind deinstitutionalization (as it came to be known) reflected cost-cutting in mental health services ("… an unholy alliance between therapeutic liberals and fiscal conservatives …"; Bachrach, 1997). However, it should be recalled that the process originated within the professions.

Deinstitutionalization and "trans-institutionalization"

The process of the running down and closure of mental hospitals has varied between different countries and cultures and is well documented (Leff *et al.*, 2000). It has been essentially worldwide in developed countries, although there are some notable exceptions, such as Belgium which has maintained its institutions and Japan which has continued to build new mental hospitals throughout this period. Similar phenomena have been observed, although at different times. The early phases, characterized by the reduction of over-crowding and improvement of staffing, were marked by service improvements but no cost savings and often cost increases (particularly per capita cost increases).

As mental hospitals shrank, so did the morale of their staff, and well-planned closure processes had to be expedited and rushed because of staffing difficulties. In London, for instance, despite an explicit early undertaking never to do so, long-stay patients were transferred from one mental hospital to another prior to their permanent resettlement as the critical masses of staff in adjacent hospitals collapsed. Often new facilities were built in the grounds of the old mental hospitals which compromised the sense of a fresh start. Most countries are left with a sprinkling of mental hospitals, but generally these are much smaller than previously and have an emphasis on acute care. In the US, deinstitutionalization and community services vary widely from state to state because state per capita costs for serious mental illness vary 10-fold. Thus, in some states, there is little development of community mental health services and the great majority of individuals with schizophrenia are in hospitals, jails, prisons, nursing homes, and homeless shelters; in other states, community services are better funded and more highly developed, resulting in less trans-institutionalization, although there are no good data on these issues.

The main response to deinstitutionalization has been the development of community services, but the picture is not straightforward. As mental hospitals have shrunk and closed, so the number of persons who are severely mentally ill in prisons has risen (Draine *et al.*, 2002; Fisher *et al.*, 2006) and there has been an enormous growth in forensic facilities for offenders who are mentally disordered (Priebe *et al.*, 2005). The number of mentally ill in prisons has become as great a challenge to modern psychiatry as neglect and homelessness in the large cities. Initially, some of these developments were responses to the reluctance of community psychiatric services to fully engage with difficult and resistant patients, but increasingly they reflect a societal preoccupation with risk avoidance. Specialist long-term care for difficult and offender patients is a legitimate component of schizophrenia care and will be dealt with in this chapter. However, the decreased tolerance both within the wider society and also within general psychiatric service for psychotic patients with behavioral disturbances is an ethical challenge to all involved with these issues and goes beyond the technicalities of service structures.

Limitations of mental health services research

The more scientifically inclined reader is likely to look to research findings when considering how to develop their services. The last 30 years has witnessed a massive increase in mental health services research (Catty *et al.*, 2002; Mueser *et al.*, 1998) and there is a series of service structures and provisions which have become established as "evidence-based care" for psychotic individuals. These range from assertive community treatment (ACT; Marshall & Lockwood, 1998; Stein & Test, 1980) and acute day hospitals (Marshall, 2003) to specific forms of vocational rehabilitation (Bond *et al.*, 2001) and substance abuse management (Drake *et al.*, 1998). The rigor and quality of these studies has steadily improved and there is broad support for most of their findings. However, their findings are increasingly cited in partial and simplistic ways that go far beyond their legitimate conclusions to support policy changes. Caution is still indicated and judgment required when introducing and developing services, even when drawing on evidence. This is not a simple "cookbook" procedure.

Experience with ACT research has been the most extensive, and reveals that its application in very different health and social care systems results in strikingly conflicting results. For instance, the substantial reduction in bed usage (and presumably improved community stability) demonstrated in the early studies (Marshall & Lockwood, 1998; Stein & Test, 1980) failed to transfer to European settings (Burns *et al.*, 1999; Thornicroft *et al.*, 1998). This has now been shown to be a consequence of greater integration of health and social care (Wright *et al.*, 2004) in European systems practices and their routine multidisciplinary team practice, generally sparing use of beds (Burns *et al.*, 2007b).

The main lesson from careful interpretation of the ACT literature is that in mental health services research there is never a placebo condition; developments do not happen in a service vacuum and the results that can be anticipated depend very much on what is currently in operation. This is not to suggest that evidence cannot be carried over from one healthcare system to another, but simply that an informed judgment has to be made about the relative independence of that development from local factors. For example, we have recently tested the effect of Individual Placement and Support (IPS) as a vocational rehabilitation service for patients with schizophrenia in Europe (Burns *et al.*, 2007a). While it is sensitive to local factors such as welfare benefit and unemployment levels, it still maintains its status as a markedly superior intervention than traditional, stepwise rehabilitation.

Despite steady improvement in the rigor of mental health services research, the application of evidence-based medicine with its established hierarchy of evidence from case studies up to randomized controlled trials and meta-analyses is much less secure. Service structure studies are much more costly and difficult to conduct than more simple interventions. They can rarely if ever be blinded, control services are particularly difficult to standardize, the healthcare agenda and practice rarely stand still, practical considerations often force trials at the start-up phases of services when staff competence may be suboptimal, and the non-specific effects of enthusiasm and charismatic leadership are enormous. The sustainability of experimental services can be in doubt (Wright *et al.*, 2004) and is rarely reported. The choice of what to study, because it can be studied, can result in anomalies such as the apparently stronger evidence for schizophrenia care in acute day hospitals than of depot antipsychotics, and no systematic evidence for acute inpatient care.

Developing and running good services for individuals with severe mental illnesses requires an awareness of the best research evidence, but also knowledge of what is practical and sustainable, and what is acceptable to the staff who will have to deliver these services. There is a broader consensus on the components of care that have been found to be useful or essential than can be obtained simply from research studies. Above we have outlined the main components of such care, citing the relevant evidence where it exists. The second part of this chapter dwells not on these care structures and the evidence for them, but on the underlying principles of care (access, equity, continuity, etc.) that need to be considered when choosing between and balancing components.

Components of mental health services for schizophrenia

Most patients with schizophrenia are treated within public mental health services. Whether these services dominate their care or areonly part of it depends on the extent of parallel services (usually private or insurance based). Most mental healthcare occurs in interactions between staff and patients and families, and does not require that much by way of equipment or buildings. So the "components" of mental healthcare outlined here generally reflect how staff organize their work. The balance of these components in any given service will vary and reflect local practice and need, and often just historical circumstances. If an area has a very prestigious and well-functioning day center, emergency clinic or admissions unit, this will inevitably influence the complexion of local community service development. There is no rigid template.

Few patients with schizophrenia need long-term institutional care and most care is in the community with only brief acute admissions. However, psychiatry is still judged to a significant extent on the quality of its inpatient care. This remains an integral part of even the most sophisticated community service and is the starting point of this overview.

Inpatient beds

Access is needed to 24-h nursing supervision for acute episodes of severe illness. For patients with schizophrenia this includes those at risk from neglect or suicide, and particularly for those who refuse treatment and may need it initiated under compulsion. Wards generally accommodate 10–20 patients and most inpatient units consist of at least three to four such wards. Ward size is a trade-off between privacy and domesticity against effective supervision. Single rooms are initially expensive, but improve flexibility, reduce conflict, and are more acceptable to patients. In first-episode services particularly, smaller "crisis houses" with 24-h care complement inpatient wards, but are not an adequate replacement. Ward design, staffing, and management are increasingly stressed with higher concentrations of involuntary and disturbed inpatients.

The question, "How many beds are needed for patients with schizophrenia in the local population?" has no reliable or precise answer. Over-provision is costly and undermines investment in community services (beds are rarely left empty despite enormous variation in their availability), while under-provision drains time and energy searching for available beds and risks tragedies being attributed to it. National or international figures are generally difficult to interpret and unhelpful because of different reporting with a profusion of terms (e.g., night hospitals, crisis homes, step-down wards) and lack of clarity about public/private provision. European public sector acute beds in 2000 ranged from 128 per 100 000 in the Netherlands to 6 per 100 000 in Northern Italy. The UK has little parallel private care and acute beds needed for a population of 250 000 have been estimated to range from 50 to 150 plus five to 20 secure or intensive care beds (Strathdee & Thornicroft, 1992), dependent on morbidity (generally much higher in large urban settings). The need for beds should reduce as community services become more comprehensive and robust. US figures are more difficult to obtain because of wide interstate variation and the range of provision. Data are reliably available on Veteran's Administration (VA) and State hospitals, but rarely on county, city, private, general or forensic hospitals. In New Hampshire, for example, there are 120 state hospital beds for a population of 1.2 million, but many patients in the state are hospitalized in local hospitals and VA hospitals.

Current bed usage in the UK is closer to 50 per 250 000, with about 50% being occupied by patients with schizophrenia in stable communities and up to 80% in deprived inner-city areas. Admissions have been getting shorter over the last three decades. With an uncomplicated psychotic relapse, it is likely to be between 3 and 6 weeks.

Longer inpatient care

A significant proportion of patients with schizophrenia have complex and resistant disorders and need longer care. Such provision is scarce and expensive, and only patients with very severe illnesses or those posing substantial risks are likely to find a place. Modern rehabilitation practice restricts longstay wards to patients whose behavior is persistently unacceptable to local communities. Forensic and secure services are usually a regional or national rather than local responsibility.

Daycare (partial hospitalization)

Daycare (partial hospitalization) is provided either in day hospitals or day centers. There is little consistency in terminology or in practice. Patients attend usually from 1 to 5 days a week for a half or whole day before returning to their homes in the evening. It is particularly valuable when families are out at work but can offer support in the evenings and at weekends, or for very isolated or self-neglecting patients.

Generally day hospitals are provided by health services, include medical and nursing staff, and can offer treatments (e.g., the prescription and monitoring of medication, psychotherapies). Day hospitals occupied a prominent place in the UK's planned move from mental hospitals to general hospitals, but never fulfilled their promise. They rarely offered much for patients with schizophrenia and their less ill patients have been increasingly well provided for by community teams.

Day centers, provided by social care organizations, rarely employ clinical staff. Unlike day hospitals which aimed to provide specific interventions and treatments, they generally provide long-term social support (Catty et al., 2005). Patients with schizophrenia are probably their main clientele, and they welcome the low-key, non-pressurized, and accepting environment. The "Club House" is a specialized rehabilitation day center, popularized in the US, which emphasizes useful normal work and where members take responsibility for running the center with minimal supervision. Daycare services are often idiosyncratic and specific to local context (e.g., a drop-in day center may be the main provider of psychiatric assessment and treatment in areas of high social mobility and homelessness).

Acute day hospitals in Europe and partial hospitalization in the US have recently been energetically proposed as alternatives to inpatient care in schizophrenia (Marshall, 2003). While they have performed well in randomized clinical trials, they have rarely persisted and have had little impact beyond demonstration sites. Daycare is problematic in rural settings, but adaptations such as travelling day centers (i.e., a team that moves from setting to setting on specific days) or a weekly open day run by the community team may be worth considering. In the US, as in much of Europe, the common observation is that partial hospitalization and daycare drift to more long-term social support, whatever the original intentions.

Supported accommodation and residential care

Many patients with schizophrenia require ongoing support outside hospital. Supervision (provided by voluntary agencies, social services or health services) ensures self-care, continued medication, and the spotting and defusing of crises. On balance, voluntary agencies are more efficient providers of long-term residential care (Knapp *et al.*, 1999) but may be wary of patients with a history of violence or substance abuse. A mixed economy works best, and promoting vigorous voluntary as well as social services pays off. Most accommodation is in shared adapted houses to promote integration and reduce stigma.

The terminology for differing types of accommodation is confusing, but generally spans four basic forms:
1. *Group homes*: no regular staff, relatively independent patients, visits from community team staff;
2. *Day-staffed hostels*: one or two staff during the day support and monitor patients (encouraging cooking, cleaning, etc.), usually no specific treatment but liaison with community team staff;
3. *Night-staffed hostels*: non-clinical staff sleep over, greater safety and availability;
4. *24-h-staffed/nursed hostels*: on-site clinical staff available overnight (sleeping-in, sometimes awake). These expensive hostels are generally restricted to long-term severe illnesses (including compulsory detained) and tend to be larger (10–20 residents as opposed to four to eight in day-staffed hostels).

In the UK, most comprehensive local services provide levels 1 and 2 and most social services undertake to provide level 3. Level 4 is relatively rare and would usually serve a population of 500 000–1 000 000. The situation is quite different in the US. Patient preferences and economics have influenced a strong shift toward "supported housing". This refers to independent apartments on the open market, rented by the patient, and unconnected with mental health; mental health staff often provide support as requested by the patient. While encouraging increased empowerment, there are concerns that this development may increase the risk for homelessness and incarceration (especially for patients with comorbid substance use disorders; Drake *et al.*, 1991).

Office-based care and outpatient clinics

Office-based care is increasingly rare for patients with schizophrenia, although not as rare as the research literature would suggest. In insurance-based systems, many psychiatrists run individual office practices and manage patients on their own, referring to hospitals for admission during relapses. It tends to be narrow in remit (usually either psychotherapy or pharmacotherapy), is poorly equipped for managing severe disorders such as schizophrenia, and is generally discouraged.

In outpatient clinics ("polyclinics" or "dispensaries") psychiatrists and psychologists may still operate independently, but with easy and frequent collaboration. In the public sector, outpatient clinics may operate either alongside community mental health teams (CMHTs) or as part of them; the latter works better for severe illness (Wright *et al.*, 2004). They provide an efficient, predictable format for assessments, treatment, and monitoring for relatively stable patients.

Multidisciplinary community teams

With the advent of deinstitutionalization, outpatient clinics took on new and expanded roles (e.g., depot clinics, daycare, psychotherapy) and were housed in community mental health centers (CMHCs). The earliest and most ambitious development of CMHCs was in the US, introduced by President Kennedy (US Congress, 1963). These ran into early problems with staffing but also, more significantly, with a drift away from the care of individuals with severe mental illness, and schizophrenia particularly. This approach demonstrated the limitations of relying on very ill patients to attend and failed to engage them. A rejection of a medical role in the services made it impossible to recruit psychiatrists and consequently to treat psychotic patients.

Case management

Community-based mental health professionals who keep in contact with patients with schizophrenia and try to ensure they stay well have evolved in several guises in different countries. "Community psychiatric nurses (CPNs)" evolved from two nurses working out of a London mental hospital in 1953, and by the 1980s this professional group outnumbered psychiatrists in the UK. Case management (Intagliata, 1982) developed in the US, initially provided by a non-clinician responsible solely for coordination of care ("brokerage case management"). This was rapidly superseded by "clinical case management" where the case manager is a mental health clinician who both provides and coordinates care for the patient. The literature on case management is extensive and many of the earlier studies compared "stand alone" case managers with different forms of multidisciplinary teams and found them wanting (e.g. the Cochrane Reviews contrasting ACT and case management; Marshall *et al.*, 1997; Marshall & Lockwood, 1998). Rapp and Goscha (2004) found a hierarchy of case-management effectiveness in the US. Brokered case management was ineffective, clinical case management and particularly strength-based clinical case management were effective, and more intensive forms of case management were effective for patients with special needs.

Individual case managers are no longer a feature of most mental health services. The term, however, survives to describe the role of professionals within teams who carry responsibility for ongoing care for patients (although drawing on the team's resources). In the UK, the term "care manager" (Department of Health and Social Services Inspectorate, 1991) was absorbed into social services, emphasizing the persisting brokerage function in that role. Within mental healthcare the term "case manager" has persisted globally as a label for an immediately understandable and recognizable role.

Community mental health teams

Most case managers find themselves working in CMHTs. Varied forms of multidisciplinary CMHT consisting of psychiatrists, nurses, social workers, and often psychologists and occupational therapists are the backbone of most community mental health services. The staffing of these teams will vary, but their strength lies in regular meetings to assess and review individual patient care which benefits from their varied professional perspectives; tasks can be distributed according to skills and needs. The CMHT originated in France and the UK, was refined in Italy, and further developed in North America and Australia. The CMHT originated when mental hospital catchment areas were subdivided from whole cities into sectors of 50 000–100 000 inhabitants. Small sectors reduce traveling time but, more importantly, make it possible for team members to know most of their complex and long-term patients. Team members can also establish personal relationships with local referrers and community resources. Sector size in Western Europe ranges from 20 to 100 000 population, and varies according to resources (shrinking as investment increases) and parallel provision. Conversely, as more specialized teams are established, the CMHT's remit shrinks and the sector size may increase while keeping its caseload about the same. Caseloads need to be limited (200–250 is generally considered the maximum) if they are to benefit fully from multidisciplinary working. The number is often significantly less if restricted to complex and difficult patients.

CMHTs assess and care for patients referred to them from primary care or the private sector and those discharged from psychiatric units. While they should prioritize severe mental illnesses (e.g., psychoses and severe affective disorders), diagnosis is not all; social adversity, personality difficulties or substance abuse can make secondary mental healthcare necessary even for ostensibly "minor" disorders. Diagnosis related groups (DRGs) and threshold definitions (Slade et al., 2000, 2001) are of limited use and most teams rely on clinical assessments. Where private care is limited, CMHTs also treat mild and transient disorders. For CMHTs to work well, there needs to be agreement on their purpose, clientele, and systems; they have often suffered from lack of clarity and leadership and require at least a minimum of active management.

Staffing and management

There is no uniform model for CMHT staffing. With fewer than six full-timers it is difficult to provide comprehensive care and cross-cover, while more than about 12–15 can become unwieldy, overwhelmed with structure and information transfer. Skill-sharing, generic working, and an informal, democratic style (Burns, 2004) can generate uncertainty about clinical leadership (originally provided informally by senior medical staff). Disputes about leadership (often unacknowledged) are probably the most common cause of dysfunctional CMHTs. Team managers now coordinate most CMHTs. Their role varies from purely administrative to clinical responsibility and staff supervision. Clarity of clinical leadership (without stifling initiative or creativity) is essential. Where doctors provide leadership, their role, and that of the manager, needs to be clear and their relationships respectful. Well-functioning and well-coordinated teams are particularly important for long-term complex conditions like schizophrenia.

Assessments

A comprehensive and accurate assessment is essential to effective management. Psychiatrists have a central role in assessment, but generally involve other team members both in the details of the assessment and in treatment. Where establishing the diagnosis is the first requirement, then psychiatrists need to shoulder most of the responsibility, but where a patient with an established diagnosis is referred for ongoing management, the assessment can be more structured and prolonged. With severely ill patients, home-based assessments pay considerable dividends (Burns et al., 1993a; Stein & Test, 1980).

Case management

As outlined above, most CMHT staff act as clinical case managers (Holloway et al., 1995; Intagliata, 1982), taking responsibility for coordination, delivery, and review of care for their patients. The caseloads of staff members should be explicitly limited (usually 15–30) and reviews recorded and systematic. In the UK, this is formalized in the care programme approach (CPA; Department of Health, 1990). Figure 30.1 shows a care plan; this indicates a patient's problems ("needs") and the treatment and care offered. It also indicates who is responsible and who is informed, together with an agreed date for review. Such

---

ENHANCED CPA/SECTION 117(2) REVIEW (delete as applicable)

Patient's name:	CMHT: ACT TEAM
	Phone:
Address:	New patient: YES/NO
Phone:	If NO, date of review: ....
Date of birth:	Diagnosis:
GP:	1... F __ __ . __
Phone:	2... F __ __ . __

You must consider the following:

1) Mental health, including indicators of relapse

2) Physical health

3) Medication

4) Daytime activity

5) Personal care/living skills

6) Carers, family, children and social network

7) Forensic history

8) Alcohol or substance misuse

9) Cultural factors

10) Housing/finances/legal issues <u>and</u>

a) make sure a **risk assessment** is done;

b) include: **i) a crisis plan; ii) a contingency plan**

i.e., what should be done if part of the careplan can't
be provided (e.g., the care coordinator is on leave or ill)

Assessed needs or problem	Intervention	Resp.of

Professionals involved in care: Dr Psychologist CPN OT SW Ward Nurse ACT Support worker Other

Present at planning meeting: Dr Psychologist CPN OT SW Ward Nurse ACT Support worker Other

Plan discussed with the patient? YES/NO Copy given to patient? YES/NO Copy sent to GP? **YES/NO**

Care coordinator (print): Phone

Care coordinator (signature): .... Date of next review: ....

Job title: Patient's signature: ....

| On supervision Register? **YES/NO** | Care management? **YES/NO** | Risk history completed? **YES/NO** |
| On supervised discharge? **YES/NO** | Section 117(2)? **YES/NO** | Relapse + risk plan required? **YES/NO** |

Fig. 30.1 Care plan for summarizing current care.

```
┌─────────────────────────────────────────────────────────────┐
│         CONFIDENTIAL:  RELAPSE AND RISK MANAGEMENT PLAN       │
├─────────────────────────────────────────────────────────────┤
│ Name:                                                         │
├─────────────────────────────────────────────────────────────┤
│ Categories of risk identified:                               │
│                                                               │
│ Aggression and violence      YES/NO   Severe self-neglect          YES/NO │
│ Exploitation (self or others) YES/NO  Risk to children & young adults YES/NO │
│ Suicide and self-harm        YES/NO   Other (please specify) ........... │
├─────────────────────────────────────────────────────────────┤
│ Current factors which suggest there is significant apparent risk: │
│ (For example: alcohol or substance misuse; specific threats; suicidal ideation; violent fantasies; anger; suspiciousness; persecutory beliefs; │
│ paranoid feelings or ideas about particular people)           │
├─────────────────────────────────────────────────────────────┤
│ Clear statement of anticipated risk(s):                      │
│ (Who is at risk; how immediate is that risk; how severe; how ongoing) │
├─────────────────────────────────────────────────────────────┤
│ Action plan:                                                 │
│ (Including names of people responsible for each action and steps to be taken if plan breaks down) │
├─────────────────────────────────────────────────────────────┤
│ Date completed:    xx/xx/xx        Review date: xx/xx/xx     │
└─────────────────────────────────────────────────────────────┘
```

Fig. 30.2 Risk management and contingency plan.

concise structured paperwork (as with the risk assessment and contingency plan; Fig. 30.2) can be adapted to any service, coordinates the complex care required in schizophrenia, and ensures regular clinical reviews.

Team meetings
CMHTs need to meet regularly if they to share perspectives, enrich understanding, and coordinate care. How often meetings are held and in what form varies enormously, but the more responsibility for acute care the more frequent the meetings. Care has to be taken to avoid meetings taking up too much clinical time. Generally one to two regular meetings per week (each usually 1.5–2h long) are devoted to both clinical and administrative business. The degree of structure depends on team style and remit, but the following tasks need to be covered:

1. *Allocation of referrals*: Either on availability or by matching the clinical needs with individual skills and training. Long discussions before assessment are generally best avoided with a simple allocation system.

2. *Patient reviews*: Reviews are needed for new patients, routine monitoring, and important transitions and discharge. Reviews can range from simply reporting the problem and proposed treatment in uncomplicated cases through to detailed, structured, multidisciplinary case conferences including other services (e.g., primary care, housing, child protection). *New patient* reviews are an excellent opportunity for providing a broad, experienced overview and ensuring balanced caseloads. *Routine monitoring* is often overlooked but, systematically conducted, it shapes treatment and identifies patients ready for transitions or discharge, as well as monitoring staff burden. It is a legal requirement of the UK CPA and good practice in all case management. *Discharge reviews* are especially useful for audit and learning within the team.

3. *Managing waiting lists and caseloads*: Effective CMHTs need to balance the long-term needs of their patients with schizophrenia against prompt access. *Routine assessments* should be within 2–4 weeks. Sooner is rarely productive and delays above 3 weeks result in a rapidly rising rate of failed appointments (Burns *et al.*, 1993b). *Urgent assessments* (most psychotic episodes) need to be seen within a week, usually within a couple of days. *Emergency assessments* are for those associated with immediate risk (e.g., hostile behavior or suicidal intent) and these patients need to be seen the same day.

A simple system for calculating assessment capacity is to count the new patients in the preceding year and allocate routine appointments for 20% more. Thus, a team with 300 assessments the preceding year allocating seven slots a week will have one available weekly for emergencies. Rapid routine assessment reduces pressure for urgent and emergency referrals more efficiently than emergency rotas and allows a team to protect time for long-term work.

Communication and liaison

CMHTs need good links with a wide network of professional colleagues. In many systems, primary care led by family physicians (general practitioners) is responsible for a significant part of mental healthcare and effective coordination is essential. General practitioner liaison systems range from informal contact through to shared care and co-location of CMHTs in general practice health centers (Burns & Bale, 1997). An optimal system requires regular, timetabled meetings between the two teams or a "link" CMHT member attending the general practice health center. Such meetings about shared and complex patients save more time than they take. Liaison should not be confused with fudging responsibilities, which is particularly risky in patients with schizophrenia.

Liaison with other agencies (social services, housing, charitable and voluntary sector providers) is equally important, but whether regular meetings are cost-effective will depend on the volume of shared work. Showing up and meeting people (even just once) pays enormous dividends in improved relationships and understanding,

although confidentiality and information sharing is more sensitive.

Specialized teams

The extent to which the varied specialist aspects of schizophrenia care are coordinated and delivered from within a single team or whether separate teams or services evolve to provide them varies enormously. This variation is essentially a cultural and resource issue, although often argued in intense ideological terms.

Rehabilitation teams developed to provide stable, long-term care and support for severely disabled individuals discharged from long-term care. More recently, as noted earlier, ACT teams have spread worldwide (Stein & Test, 1980), targeting so-called "revolving door" patients who are psychotic and hard to engage with services. ACT is often referred to as intensive case management (ICM) or assertive outreach (AO) in Europe. Their differences are often contested, but both types of team are well established and generally recognizable, and will be outlined here.

Two further teams which have received recent attention are early intervention services (EIS) and crisis resolution/home treatment (CR/HT) teams. Both of these have been mandated in the UK NHS Plan (Department of Health, 2000). CR/HT teams are peripheral to the care of schizophrenia and will not be addressed here, but EIS services will. Whether a local service needs either or both is a practical decision dependent as much on resources and local provision as on theory.

Assertive community treatment team

The ACT team is the most replicated and researched of any model of community care (Mueser *et al.*, 1998). Stein and Test's original study showed improved clinical and social outcomes with substantially reduced hospitalization at slightly lower cost (Test & Stein, 1980; Weisbrod *et al.*, 1980). Reduced hospital care is the common factor in all of these outcomes, and meta-analyses of ACT and of case management (Marshall *et al.*, 2001; Marshall & Lockwood, 1998) have confirmed this. This confirmation has led to their wholesale adoption throughout much of the Anglophone psychiatric community, where they are central components of government policy in several countries (Department of Health, 1999; US Department of Health and Human Services, 1999). These bed reductions have, however, never been replicated in Europe (Burns *et al.*, 1999; Thornicroft *et al.*, 1998) and there is now convincing evidence that ACT has little to offer over well-functioning CMHTs in this respect (Wright *et al.*, 2004; Burns *et al.*, 2007a,b). However, ACT benefits from the precision of its description and the clarity of its focus, and continues to be adopted as a model for services to care for patients with schizophrenia. It is particularly valuable in helping change the focus of more diffuse services to the care of the severely ill, and its "evidence base" can overcome strong professional resistance.

ACT teams are very similar in practice to the generic CMHT outlined above, but usually have much smaller caseloads (traditionally stated as 1:10, but more usually up to 1:15) and aim to keep more regular contact, even when patients are clinically stable. They exploit the small caseloads to ensure comprehensive and accessible care spanning medical and social inputs. They are very resource intensive and generally reserved for the most difficult ("hard to engage" or "revolving door") patients who are psychotic with frequent, often dangerous, relapses and poor medication adherence plus alcohol or drug abuse, significant personality difficulties, and offending behavior. The clinical practice has been extensively described (Burns & Firn, 2002) and is based on outreach-visiting patients at home even when they are reluctant. Team working is emphasized with daily handover meetings and several members of the team will be actively involved with most patients. This is both for safety considerations, but also to address patients' extensive needs. The approach involves very practical work (taking patients shopping, sorting out accommodation, delivering medicines daily if needs be) and regularly strays well beyond traditional boundaries. The core principles and practices of ACT teams are outlined in Tables 30.1 and 30.2.

Rehabilitation and recovery teams

Rehabilitation teams evolved in response to the need to re-provide in the community comprehensive care, in

Table 30.1 Assertive community treatment (ACT) program principles. Provision of material resources for patients.

- Fostering patient coping skills
- Supporting patient motivation to persevere
- Freeing patient from pathological dependency relationships
- Support and education for those involved with the patient

Table 30.2 Assertive community treatment (ACT) core components.

- Assertive follow-up
- Small caseloads (1:10)
- Increased frequency of contact (weekly to daily)
- *In-vivo* practice (care delivered at home or in neighborhood)
- Emphasis on medication
- Emphasis on engagement
- Support for family and carers
- Provision of services within the team whenever possible
- Liaison with other services when necessary
- Crisis stabilization and availability 24/7

particular support and social care for patients being discharged from down-sizing and closing mental hospitals. Many of the patients discharged in the early phases of deinstitutionalization had significant social deficits (particularly in self-care and managing their time and relationships with the outside world), but relatively stable clinical conditions. This has, of course, changed over time as more and more unwell patients have been discharged. A service dichotomy into patients needing only social care and support with minimal psychiatric input *versus* those with unstable mental states is an oversimplification in most places now.

Supporting severely disabled patients over long periods is routine in most generic services and many rehabilitation services increasingly focus on very challenging patients. This shift in focus reflects the rapidly shrinking service needs of the old long-stay patients and the rise of a very different group of "new long-stay" patients (Hirsch, 1988). These are predominantly young patients with schizophrenia (disproportionately men) who have poor treatment compliance, comorbid drug and alcohol abuse, and often behavioral disturbance. The two defining characteristics of separate rehabilitation services are predominantly their access to more long-term inpatient care for such individuals or a commitment to a defined patient group in long-term supported residential care.

Such an administrative distinction does not do justice to the extensive rehabilitation literature and accumulated clinical skills (Corrigan *et al.*, 2007). Anthony (1979) defined the goal of rehabilitation as helping disabled individuals to establish the emotional, social, and intellectual skills needed to live, learn, and work in the community with the least amount of professional support. The *New Freedom Commission Report* on mental health in the US specifies that patients should "live, learn, work and participate fully" in their communities (New Freedom Commission on Mental Health, 2003). Rehabilitation then focuses on enabling patients to manage their own illnesses, determine their own recovery goals, and acquire the skills and support they need to succeed in achieving their goals. The target patient group is that with persistent psychopathology, marked instability characterized by frequent relapse and persisting social maladaption.

Rehabilitation programs are, by their nature, varied, but share common features to improve performance in the main adult social roles (Corrigan *et al.*, 2007). Aspects of care that are more highly developed in rehabilitation teams include social skills training to help patients manage their own survival (Liberman *et al.*, 1998). These are highly structured, modular approaches focusing on very basic skills, which include extensive *in-vivo* training, homework, and booster courses. They include communication skills and medication management. Attempts at ameliorating the disabling cognitive impairments in schizophrenia have included Brenner *et al.*'s (1992) "integrated psychological therapy" and more recently cognitive remediation (Pilling *et al.*, 2002). However, these highly structured modularized approaches and highly structured social skills training approaches are currently losing influence and being replaced by supported housing, education, employment, and socialization, together with self-help and consumer-run programs in response to user preferences.

Rehabilitation teams have always stressed the importance of meaningful activity and the value of a structured day. They may make extensive use of day centers (see above) and also of vocational rehabilitation (see below) in varied forms. Whether these are delivered within a rehabilitation team, some other team or a separate, dedicated team follows no discernable pattern.

Recovery

The service user movement has steadily argued that the goal of mental health services should be to help people with schizophrenia and other serious mental illnesses to pursue "recovery", which is variably defined, but refers to a process of developing hope, learning to manage one's illness, and pursuing a meaningful life in the community apart from the role of mental patient (Bellack, 2006; Deegan, 1988; Jacobson, 2004; Onken *et al.*, 2007).

Recovery ideology emphasizes optimism, education, self-agency, peer supports, choice, personal goals, and independence. Thus, for many service users, quality of life and personal control of one's life are more important than symptom management and stability, and recovery endorses these personal goals. Promoting recovery is said to involve shifting the mental health system to "recovery-oriented" services, which might be described as being more patient-centered with less coercion, less emphasis on medication adherence, and greater attention to shared decision-making and personal goals. Recovery also involves decreasing stigma, creating opportunities for housing and jobs in the community, and pursuing basic civil rights for persons with disabilities—all laudatory goals, but largely outside of the purview of the mental health system. In this sense, recovery ideology extends considerably beyond mental health treatment.

Recovery is controversial in many ways. The general ideology has been inspirational to patients, advocates, and providers. However, the term has been inconsistently defined and has resisted a consensus. Recovery-oriented services, which are also inconsistently defined, may represent little more than high-quality, patient-centered services. Recovery does not specify how to handle dangerousness, legal issues, decisional incapacity, and other complex problems. Recovery introduces a new piece of jargon into a jargon-filled arena, and the non-standard terminology once again confuses those outside of mental health and separates mental health from other areas of medical care.

A recovery approach may mean tolerating greater risks such as an increased frequency of relapse in exchange for lower doses of a maintenance antipsychotic. It is difficult to be clear if there is any real point of difference between the recovery approach and good quality rehabilitation practice. It is probably very important for all mental health practitioners, and rehabilitation team members most of all, to be regularly reminded that patients with schizophrenia do recover (Harding *et al.*, 1987), and the insistence on accepting the primacy of the patient's experienced quality of life and personal goals is always beneficial. The useful distinction is made between "recovery from" mental illness, which implies complete cure, and "being in recovery", which indicates pursuing meaningful life activities, often despite residual symptoms of illness.

Early intervention services/first-episode psychosis teams

Separate teams for first-episode care in schizophrenia are a relatively new development, championed in Australia and the UK (Birchwood *et al.*, 1997; Edwards *et al.*, 2000; McGorry & Jackson, 1999), but now established internationally. EIS vary in the extent of their remit. The most basic approach is to ensure that all patients with a first-episode of psychosis are treated in a dedicated team that is readily accessible and welcoming (these teams often have an expressly "youth service" approach) and which, as well as ensuring early effective treatment, works hard to protect social and family supports and networks.

A strong case for the establishment of EIS is that outcome is poorer if the duration of untreated psychosis is prolonged (Marshall *et al.*, 2005; see Chapter 6). This basic EIS is closely modeled on ACT (Department of Health, 1999; Edwards *et al.*, 2000), but with an explicit time limit (varying from 18 months to 5 years) for involvement before handing on to routine services. A core feature of EIS is trying to stabilize the situation and avoiding pessimism. These teams prioritize work with families and an avoidance of obtaining extensive welfare benefits to emphasize the goal of rapid return to work or study. They strive to reduce inpatient care and there is some tentative evidence that they may achieve this (Craig *et al.*, 2004; Petersen *et al.*, 2005). They are certainly appreciated by patients and families.

More ambitious EIS services aim to reduce the duration of untreated psychosis further by outreach work to schools and colleges, raising awareness of early psychosis in high-risk groups (where it might otherwise be dismissed as adolescent rebellion or drug taking). More controversially there have been some attempts to identify ultra high-risk individuals (usually those with strong family histories and bizarre but non-psychotic behavior or experiences) and encourage them to take treatment to avoid progression to frank psychosis (McGorry *et al.*, 2002). These studies are encouraging, but such practice is still some distance from regular provision for patients with schizophrenia. EIS are currently evolving rapidly (and often in very different ways), so detailed descriptions of what they offer beyond an intensive ACT approach is unlikely to be helpful. Time will tell which aspects add value to the care of first-episode patients.

Specialist teams or specialist functions?

Whether specific functions require individual teams will depend on the overall level of integration of mental health services and also on judgments about the importance and difficulty of the interventions. The trend in well-funded service areas in the US is increasingly toward specialty teams: young adult teams, dual diagnosis teams, geriatric teams, dialectical behavior therapy teams, forensic mental health teams, etc.

Dual diagnosis services

Drug and alcohol abuse are no longer an exotic rarity in schizophrenia care. Indeed, in most settings, particularly in metropolitan ones, they are the norm rather than the exception. In the US specific services have been developed to deal with substance misuse in severe mental illness; in Europe there are well-developed drug and alcohol services both within statutory healthcare and in the voluntary sector, but they rarely deal with patients with dual diagnosis psychosis. In European addiction services (various terms are used and there is little consistency on whether drugs and alcohol are dealt with by one or two services), "dual diagnosis" or comorbidity are more likely to refer to depression, personality disorder or physical illnesses than to psychoses.

In both the US and Europe there is an emerging consensus that delivering substance abuse treatments separately from routine mental health care to patients with schizophrenia is not successful. The care needs to be integrated and the preferred location is the multidisciplinary CMHT. This reflects the fundamental importance of engagement and an effective therapeutic relationship with this group if any treatments are to work. Mental health staff are generally more experienced and skilled in establishing and maintaining this with psychotic individuals and it is easier to teach them substance abuse skills than *vice versa*. In such integrated services, specified substance abuse workers can be responsible for this care or efforts can be made to skill-up most or all of the case managers. As research and services have evolved over 20 years, several points have become clear (Drake *et al.*, 2006, 2007, 2008). Because substance abuse is ubiquitous, all teams rather than just specialty teams need to be prepared to address substance use disorders that are comorbid with mental disorders. These patients often need engagement and motivational interven-

tions before they are prepared to pursue abstinence, which may require months or years of effort. The most consistently effective interventions for helping dually diagnosed patients to attain abstinence are dual diagnosis groups led by professionals and long-term dual diagnosis residential services. Finally, to maintain abstinence, patients generally need meaningful supports and activities that substitute for substance abuse: stable housing, employment, and relationships with non-substance abusers.

Vocational services

Therapeutic aims in the care of schizophrenia go beyond simple symptom control and focus on enhancing the quality of life of patients and promoting social inclusion (Morgan *et al.*, 2007; Priebe 2007). Returning to work is probably one of the most effective means of radically improving quality of life and social inclusion. Many rehabilitation services include extensive provision for prevocational training, ranging from highly structured approaches to specific skills such as information technology, or interview training. Several have sheltered work environments. This structured approach to vocational rehabilitation reflects the evolution of rehabilitation thinking (Corrigan *et al.*, 2007) with a distinction between impairment, disability, and handicap (World Health Organization, 1988). Many of these vocational services are run by the voluntary sector or social services with minimal healthcare involvement. There is overwhelming evidence, however, that standardized supported employment, also called IPS, mentioned earlier, is more effective in helping patients with severe mental illnesses to achieve competitive employment (Bond *et al.*, 2007, 2008).

Unlike traditional "train and place" vocational rehabilitation where disabilities and deficits are addressed in structured training programs, the "place and train" IPS approach does not require extensive resources or facilities. IPS involves a vocational councilor acting as a "job coach" and, having discussed the patient's preferences and abilities, actively helping them in seeking, obtaining, and sustaining employment. US evidence indicates that IPS is best provided from within the routine mental health services and not as a separate team (Cook *et al.*, 2005). This way the IPS worker can remain focused on their principal goal of supporting the patient at work and rely (with easy, informal liaison) on the CMHT to address issues of psychopathology.

Physical healthcare

Whether the physical healthcare of individuals with schizophrenia belongs in primary care or with mental health services will depend on local and national policies. The strikingly increased standardized mortality in schizophrenia (particularly for cardiovascular and respiratory disorders; Kendrick, 1996) means that their life-expectancy is about 20 years less than the general population. Many factors contribute to this reduced life-expectancy—excess smoking, poor diet, inactivity, and metabolic side effects of antipsychotic drugs (see Chapters 7, 28 and 31). Almost invariably specialist mental health teams pick up much of the responsibility for the most severely ill patients (Saha *et al.*, 2007).

In community care it can be argued that encouraging primary care responsibility for the physical healthcare of patients with schizophrenia both acts against stigma and also ensures these patients receive their general healthcare from those best equipped to provide it (family physicians). In the UK a specific payment is now made to general practitionerss who conduct regular structured healthcare checks for their patients with psychosis. This issue lies outside the scope of this chapter, but pragmatic decisions have to be made to ensure that patients with schizophrenia receive the best possible comprehensive medical care. How the responsibility for this is distributed remains open to debate.

Controversies and ethics in schizophrenia care

Coercion in community mental healthcare

Balancing patients' welfare with their autonomy and their rights with those of their families and the wider community are brought into sharp focus in schizophrenia care. Teams regularly visit patients who vigorously and clearly reject them and may be quite unaware that they are ill, far less that they need treatment. When does intensive support become intrusion? When does professional persistence tip over into coercion or disrespect?

Compulsion was traditionally identified with admission to the old asylums or left to the family (as it still is in many parts of the world). Most compulsory care is inpatient care for obvious reasons. The grounds for compulsory treatment vary internationally, but most are based on clinical evidence of risk to the patient or those around them. Risk is interpreted across a broad range from immediate life-threatening circumstances to a risk to the patient's health (that it will deteriorate or even that it will fail to improve). Similarly, the mechanisms to monitor compulsion vary from the highly legal to those vesting much of the responsibility in clinicians with relatively superficial scrutiny of paperwork.

Community treatment orders and outpatient commitment

With expanded community care, compulsion and coercion (either explicitly in the form of legal requirements or informally through professional or social pressure; Monahan *et al.*, 2005) are now a pervasive feature of practice.

Improved legal and professional scrutiny makes compulsory treatment possible in the community. Most developed common law countries have enacted forms of community treatment order (CTO; "mandated community treatment"', "outpatient committal"; Dawson, 2005). These are mainly applied in the care of established schizophrenia with high levels of self-neglect, poor treatment compliance, and frequent relapse (Gibbs *et al.*, 2005a; Swartz *et al.*, 1999). The introduction of these provisions has often been controversial (Kisely & Campbell, 2007) and the evidence base for them is limited (Churchill *et al.*, 2007). There is evidence that clinicians use and value them (Dawson, 2005; Swartz *et al.*, 2003) and that families (Mullen *et al.*, 2006) and, to some extent, patients (Gibbs *et al.*, 2005b) appreciate them. However, the only successful randomized clinical trial produced equivocal results (Swartz *et al.*, 1999), although the subgroup of patients who received extended CTOs and regular care did appear to benefit. Despite continuing concerns about the absence of a definitive clinical trial, the orders appear to be rapidly accepted by the clinical community, although the frequency with which they are used varies widely and inexplicably (Lawton-Smith, 2005).

CTOs vary in their duration and in their powers. Most require the patient to reside at an agreed address and to accept visits from the clinical team or attend appointments. There is variation in the rights to enter private property, but all empower the clinical team to return the patient to some safe clinical environment for reassessment and theadministration of treatment. None permits the forcible treatment of patients in their own home and in truth it is the "threat" of recall rather than frequent use of CTOs that seems to work.

Informal coercion

CTOs have the advantage of legal scrutiny. Work by the MacArthur Group in the US demonstrates that about half of all long-term psychiatric patients feel that they have been coerced in some form or other to comply with treatment (Monahan *et al.*, 2005); pilot work in the UK indicates very similar rates, although with somewhat different patterns. Few experienced clinicians feel too much discomfort about the judicious use of encouragement and persuasion in the patients' best interests. The informality of such coercion means that there is no external scrutiny and little attention paid to evolving best practice or to ensuring that abuses do not occur. The power imbalance between long-term dependent patients with schizophrenia and their professional carers inevitably poses continuous ethical challenges for which little guidance is currently available.

Practical ethics in schizophrenia care

Dependency

The care of very ill patients with schizophrenia poses many ethical dilemmas beyond that of coercion. Long-term work with severely disabled individuals often involves asymmetrical relationships with a high degree of dependency to which professionals can become blind. Just as in old mental hospitals, professionals may become so used to these relationships and expectations that they cease to recognize that they are not the norm in society. Their expectations of patients and their aspirations for them may become distorted by familiarity and be driven by a very laudable tolerance. Generic teams, with regular contact with brief and moderate mental illness, defend against this, as does a teaching commitment (medical and nursing students are potent reminders of what is normally expected). For teams with less variety or intrusion issues, the complex issues of dependency need to be regularly discussed.

When is dependency healthy and when not? Most mental health staff recognize pathological dependency and many strive to avoid dependency at almost all costs. The avoidance of "pathological dependency" underlay the early ACT insistence on the "whole-team approach", downplaying individual relationships (Stein & Test, 1980). Dependency was seen as undermining autonomy and self-realization. On the other hand, some would argue that dependency is an essential step towards independence and it may contribute to a strong and productive therapeutic alliance. Most teams do not have protracted philosophical debates about dependency, but the issues surface around such actions as giving patients lifts to appointments or helping them with practical tasks and leisure pursuits, when they might be able to do these themselves. Staff vary in seeing this as being over-protective and indulgent or friendly and humane.

The same boundary issue arises in another form, usually expressed in concerns about the proper extent of professional roles. Is it stepping too far outside the traditional professional role to give the patient a lift to the shops when it is raining? Even more controversial is the debate about whether it is right or wrong to send birthday and Christmas cards to patients who the professional knows will get them from nobody else. There is often a strong gender divide within staff on these issues. While there is greater consensus about what constitutes unprofessional boundary violations, there are no hard and fast rules for these minor routine variations. What is important is for teams to take these issues seriously and ensure a culture where they are regularly and frankly discussed. Where possible, such discussion should fully involve patients to ensure proper attention to independence, individual preferences, and respectful interactions.

Confidentiality

Confidentiality and sharing of information is another area where practice has moved faster than established professional guidance. Most Western cultures prioritize patient confidentiality, whereas many Eastern cultures routinely involve families in all decisions. Formal professional guidelines emphasize patient autonomy and the right to deny contact or information sharing. In most instances this presents no problems. The family relationships of severely ill young patients may be fraught and even hostile despite their parents remaining key careers. Overriding patient denial of information sharing when there is immediate risk is generally accepted, but it is clear that this is often interpreted very liberally. Information sharing between professionals within the same team is routine and often this is extended to other professionals—housing agencies, social services, even the police on occasions.

Risk of being assaulted or of being evicted are serious issues and few professionals will simply refuse to share vital information without further thought. In extreme situations even neighbors may need to know. There is a risk that in an overly-defensive environment these practices (like the informal leverage which is known to be widespread) are left to the individual professional to decide for themselves with no reference group to discuss it with or gain advice. It is unhelpful to simply state that the guidelines are well established and clear. In the US, new privacy laws (Health Insurance Portability and Accountability Act of 1996) mandate extremes regarding confidentiality, probably because of possible prejudice from insurance companies. However, if guidelines and directives are too far removed from current practice, they will be of little value in the inevitable gray areas where sensitivity and balance are needed.

Squalor, self-neglect, and stigma

Just as with dependency, services need to have a culture of openness and tolerance, encouraging discussion of these issues. Many patients with schizophrenia will choose to live lives that seem undignified and even risky compared to those which we would wish for them. How much self-neglect and how much squalor can we, should we, tolerate? Clearly we need to protect our patients from abuse—their high rates of victimization are repeatedly recorded (Dean et al., 2007; see Chapter 31). Similarly squalor that leads to eviction or self-neglect that leads to exploitation or bullying need to be prevented. But what of lesser degrees? Team discussions help staff check that they still broadly reflect good current practice.

Multidisciplinary team working

Caring for individuals with disorders as persistent, variable, and complex as schizophrenia inevitably requires close working across a number of disciplines. Generally, this works best in a single multidisciplinary team where the broad range of the patient's needs can be addressed without too much cross-referring (Liberman et al., 2001; Wright et al., 2004). Multidisciplinary team working, while optimal, is not stress free or without controversy.

There is an inherent tension between generic and specialist working—how much overlap should there be between what the different team members do? Clearly there is no point in having a multidisciplinary team unless the members bring different skills. On the other hand, is it a team if there is no substantial degree of shared activity? Where the clinical condition is stable and relatively predictable, multidisciplinary teams tend to emphasize specialism. Where there is unpredictability and fluctuation, then flexible generic working may be more prominent. Personal continuity is a vital component of good quality schizophrenia care which presupposes a significant degree of flexibility and generic working. This is an area of strong opinions and little evidence (Burns *et al.*, 2007a).

Intimately tied up with styles of multidisciplinary working are the issues of team leadership and there are several approaches to this (from relatively democratic matrix models through to differing types of hierarchy) with a range of opinions on the value of senior medical staff or pure managers. What is vital is that there is agreement. Patients with schizophrenia are likely to fare badly if there is chronic discord in teams and also to suffer if there are too many incomprehensible or abrupt changes.

Conclusions

There is no single service structure that best suits schizophrenia care. There appear to be some robust basic principles. The care is inevitably multidisciplinary to reflect the complexity of the patients' needs and their variation over time, and the weight of evidence suggests these varied professionals need to work together in a multidisciplinary team. This team needs to draw on a range of perspectives and skills and will have to address social as well as medical needs if patients are to be effectively engaged over the long periods that are required. Roles and responsibilities in these teams will remain in a dynamic equilibrium—each development in treatment (e.g., better, more complex psychopharmacology, cognitive–behaviorl therapy for delusions, improved structured rehabilitation) will affect the balance of power and specialization within the team. While there needs to be clarity of purpose, it should be obvious that good care is dependent on honest interprofessional relationships that permit the discussion of uncertainty, and structures that are sufficiently flexible to permit the necessary changes over time.

The care of schizophrenia now is unrecognizable compared to that of 50 years ago when it was dominated by large asylums. We are currently going through a period of clinical realism after two decades of intense innovation and change. The roles of inpatient care, daycare, and community care are less the subject of heated polemic than of balancing resources and needs. We would anticipate that schizophrenia care in 50 years' time will be as different from that currently as it is now from 50 years ago.

References

Anthony, W.A. (1979) *The Principles of Psychiatric Rehabilitation.* Baltimore: University Park Press.

Bachrach, L.L. (1997) Lessons in the American experience in providing community-based services. In: Leff, J., ed. *Care in the Community: Illusion or Reality?* Chichester: John Wiley & Sons.

Barton, R. (1959) *Institutional Neurosis.* Bristol: John Wright.

Bellack, A.S. (2006) Scientific and consumer models of recovery in schizophrenia: concordance, contrasts, and implications. *Schizophrenia Bulletin* **32**, 432–442.

Birchwood, M., McGorry, P. & Jackson, H. (1997) Early intervention in schizophrenia. *British Journal of Psychiatry* **170**, 2–5.

Bond, G.R., Becker, D.R., Drake, R.E. *et al.* (2001) Implementing supported employment as an evidence-based practice. *Psychiatric Services* **52**, 313–322.

Bond, G.R., Xie, H., & Drake, R.E. (2007) Can SSDI and SSI beneficiaries with mental illness benefit from evidence-based supported employment? *Psychiatric Services* **58**, 1412–1420.

Bond, G.R., Drake, R.E. & Becker, D.R. (2008) An update on randomized controlled trials of evidence-based supported employment. *Psychiatric Rehabilitation Journal* **31**, 280–290.

Brenner, H.D., Hodel, B., Roder, V. & Corrigan, P. (1992) Treatment of cognitive dysfunctions and behavioral deficits in schizophrenia. *Schizophrenia Bulletin* **18**, 21–26.

Brill, H. & Patton, R.E. (1962) Clinical-statistical analysis of population changes in New York state mental hospitals since the introduction of psychotropic drugs *American Journal of Psychiatry* **119**, 20.

Burns, T. (2004) *Community Mental Health Teams.* Oxford: Oxford University Press.

Burns, T. & Bale, R. (1997) Establishing a mental health liaison attachment with primary care. *Advances in Psychiatric Treatment* **3**, 219–224.

Burns, T. & Firn, M. (2002) *Assertive Outreach in Mental Health: A Manual for Practitioners.* Oxford: Oxford University Press.

Burns, T., Beadsmoore, A., Bhat, A.V. *et al.* (1993a) A controlled trial of home-based acute psychiatric services. I: Clinical and social outcome. *British Journal of Psychiatry* **163**, 49–54.

Burns, T., Raftery, J., Beadsmoore, A. *et al.* (1993b) A controlled trial of home-based acute psychiatric services. II: Treatment patterns and costs *British Journal of Psychiatry* **163**, 55–61.

Burns, T., Creed, F. & Fahy, T. (1999) Intensive versus standard case management for severe psychotic illness: a randomised trial. *Lancet* **353**, 2185–2189.

Burns, T., Catty, J., Becker, T. *et al.* (2007a) The effectiveness of supported employment for people with severe mental illness: a randomised controlled trial. *Lancet* **370**, 1146–1152.

Burns, T., Catty, J. & Dash, M. (2007b) Use of intensive case management to reduce time in hospital in people with severe mental illness: systematic review and meta-regression. *BMJ* **335**, 336.

Catty, J., Burns, T., Knapp, M. *et al.* (2002) Home treatment for mental health problems: A systematic review. *Psychological Medicine* **32**, 383–401.

Catty, J., Goddard, K. & Burns, T. (2005) Social Services Day Care and Health Services Day Care in Mental Health: Do they differ? *International Journal of Psychoanalysis* **51**, 151–161.

Churchill, R., Owen, G., Singh, S. & Hotopf, M. (2007) *International Experiences of Using Community Treatment Orders*. London: Institute of Psychiatry.

Committee of Inquiry (1969) *Report of the Committee of Inquiry into Allegations of Ill-Treatment of Patients and Other Irregularities at the Ely Hospital, Cardiff, Presented to Parliament by the Secretary of State of the Department of Health and Social Security*. London: Department of Health.

Cook, J.A., Lehman, A.F., Drake, R.E. *et al.* (2005) Integration of psychiatric and vocational services: a multi-site randomized implementation effectiveness trial of supported employment. *American Journal of Psychiatry* **162**, 1948–1956.

Corrigan, P.W., Mueser, K.T., Bond, G.R. *et al.* (2007) *The Principles and Practice of Psychiatric Rehabilitation*. New York: Guildford Press.

Craig, T.K.J., Garety, P., Power, P. *et al.* (2004) The Lambeth Early Onset (LEO) Team: randomised controlled trial of the effectiveness of specialised care for early psychosis. *BMJ* **329**, 1067–1070.

Dawson, J. (2005) *Community Treatment Orders: International Comparisons*. Dunedin: Otago University.

Dean, K., Moran, P., Fahy, T. *et al.* (2007) Predictors of violent victimization amongst those with psychosis. *Acta Psychiatrica Scandanavica* **116**, 345–353.

Deegan, P. (1988) Recovery: The lived experience of rehabilitation. *Psychosocial Rehabilitation Journal* **11**, 11–19.

Department of Health (1990) *The Care Programme Approach for People with a Mental Illness Referred to the Special Psychiatric Services*. Joint Health/Social Services Circular HC (90) 23/LASS (90) 11. London: Department of Health.

Department of Health (1999) *Modern Standards and Service Models: National Service Framework for Mental Health*. London: Department of Health.

Department of Health (2000) *The NHS Plan—A Plan for Investment, a Plan for Reform*. London: Department of Health.

Department of Health and Social Services Inspectorate (1991) *Care Management and Assessment: Summary of Practice Guidelines*. London: HMSO.

Draine, J., Salzer, M.S., Culhane, D.P. & Hadley, T.R. (2002) Role of social disadvantage in crime, joblessness and homelessness among persons with serious mental illness. *Psychiatric Services* **53**, 565–573.

Drake, R.E., Osher, F.C. & Wallach, M.A. (1991) Homelessness and Dual Diagnosis. *American Psychologist* **46**, 1149–1158.

Drake, R.E., McHugo, G.J., Clark, R.E. *et al.* (1998) Assertive community treatment for patients with co-occurring severe mental illness and substance use disorder: A clinical trial. *American Journal of Orthopsychiatry* **68**, 201–215.

Drake, R.E., McHugo, G.J., Xie, H. *et al.* (2006) Ten-year recovery outcomes for clients with co-occurring schizophrenia and substance use disorders *Schizophrenia Bulletin* **32**, 464–473.

Drake, R.E., Mueser, K.T., & Brunette, M.F. (2007) Management of persons with co-occurring severe mental illness and substance use disorder: programme implications. *World Psychiatry* **6**, 131–136.

Drake, R.E., O'Neal, E.L. & Wallach, M.A. (2008) A systematic review of psychosocial interventions for people with co-occurring substance use and severe mental disorders. *Journal of Substance Abuse Treatment* **34**, 123–138.

Edwards, J., McGorry, P.D. & Pennell, K. (2000) Models of early intervention in psychosis: an analysis of service approaches. In: Birchwood, M., Fowler, D. & Jackson, C., eds. *Early Intervention in Psychosis: A Guide to Concepts, Evidence and Interventions*. New York: John Wiley & Sons, pp. 281–314.

Fisher, W.H., Roy-Bujnowski, K.M., Grudzinskas, A.J. *et al.* (2006) Patterns and prevalence of arrest in a statewide cohort of mental health care consumers, *Psychiatric Services* **57**, 1623–1628.

Foucault, M. (1965) *Madness and Civilisation: A History of Insanity in the Age of Reason*. New York: Random House Inc.

Gibbs, A., Dawson, J. & Mullen, R. (2005a) Community Treatment Orders for People with serious mental illness: a New Zealand study. *British Journal of Social Work* **36**, 1085–1100.

Gibbs, A., Dawson, J., Ansley, C. & Mullen, R. (2005b) How patients in New Zealand view community treatment orders. *Journal of Mental Health* **14**, 357–368.

Goffman, I. (1960) *Asylums: Essays on the Social Situation of Mental Patients and Other Inmates*. Harmondsworth: Penguin Books.

Goodwin, G.M. & Geddes, J.R. (2007) What is the heartland of psychiatry? *British Journal of Psychiatry* **191**, 189–191.

Harding, C.M., Brooks, G.W., Ashikaga, T. *et al.* (1987) The Vermont longitudinal study of persons with severe mental illness, II: Long-term outcome of subjects who retrospectively met DSM-III criteria for schizophrenia. *American Journal of Psychiatry* **144**, 727–735.

Hirsch, S. (1988) *Psychiatric Beds and Resources: Factors Influencing Bed Use and Service planning*. London: Gaskell (Royal College of Psychiatrists).

Holloway, F., Oliver, N., Collins, E. & Carson, J. (1995) Case management: a critical review of the outcome literature. *European Psychiatry* **10**, 113–128.

Intagliata, J. (1982) Improving the quality of community care for the chronically mentally disabled: the role of case management. *Schizophrenia Bulletin* **8**, 655–674.

Jacobson, N. (2004) *In Recovery*. Nashville: Vanderbilt University Press.

Jones, M. (1952) *Social Psychiatry: A Study of Therapeutic Communities*. London: Tavistock.

Kendrick, T. (1996) Cardiovascular and respiratory risk factors and symptoms among general practice patients with long-term mental illness. *British Journal of Psychiatry* **169**, 733–739.

Kisely, S. & Campbell, L.A. (2007) Does compulsory or supervised community treatment reduce "revolving door" care? *British Journal of Psychiatry* **191**, 373–374.

Knapp, M., Hallam, A., Beecham, J. & Baines, B. (1999) Private, voluntary or public? Comparative cost-effectiveness in community mental health care. *Policy and Politics* **27**, 25–41.

Laing, R. D. (1960) *The Divided Self*. London: Tavistock.

Lawton-Smith, S. (2005) *A Question of Numbers. The Potential Impact of Community-Based Treatment Orders in England and Wales*. London: King's Fund.

Leff, J., Trieman, N., Knapp, M. & Hallam, A. (2000) The TAPS Project: A report on 13 years of research, 1985–1998. *Psychiatric Bulletin* **24**, 165–168.

Liberman, R.P., Wallace, C.J., Blackwell, G. *et al.* (1998) Skills training versus psychosocial occupational therapy for persons with persistent schizophrenia. *American Journal of Psychiatry* **155**, 1087–1091.

Liberman, R.P., Hilty, D.M., Drake, R.E. & Tsang, H.W. (2001) Requirements for multidisciplinary teamwork in psychiatric rehabilitation. *Psychiatric Services* **52**, 1331–1342.

Marshall, M. (2003) Acute psychiatric day hospitals. *BMJ* **327**, 116–117.

Marshall, M. & Lockwood, A. (1998) Assertive Community Treatment for people with severe mental disorders (Cochrane Review). *The Cochrane Library* 3, CD00050.

Marshall, M., Gray, A., Lockwood, A. & Green, R. (1997) Case management for people with severe mental disorders. *The Cochrane Collaboration*, Issue 2, CD00050.

Marshall, M., Gray, A., Lockwood, A. & Green, R. (2001) Case management for severe mental disorders (Cochrane Review). *The Cochrane Library* 1.

Marshall, M., Lewis, S., Lockwood, A. *et al.* (2005) Association between duration of untreated psychosis and outcome in cohorts of first-episode patients: a systematic review. *Archives of General Psychiatry* **62**, 975–983.

McGorry, P. & Jackson, H. (1999) *Recognition and Management of Early Psychosis. A Preventative Approach*. Cambridge: Cambridge University Press.

McGorry, P.D., Yung, A.R., Phillips, L.J. *et al.* (2002) Randomized controlled trial of interventions designed to reduce the risk of progression to first-episode psychosis in a clinical sample with subthreshold symptoms. *Archives of General Psychiatry* **59**, 921–928.

Meyer, A. (1922) Constructive formulation of Schizophrenia *American Journal of Psychiatry* **78**, 355–364.

Monahan, J., Redlich, A.D., Swanson, J. *et al.* (2005) Use of leverage to improve adherence to psychiatric treatment in the community. *Psychiatric Services* **56**, 37–44.

Morgan, C., Burns, T., Fitzpatrick, R. *et al.* (2007) Social exclusion and mental health. Conceptual and methodological review. *British Journal of Psychiatry* **191**, 477–483.

Mueser, K.T., Bond, G.R., Drake, R.E. & Resnick, S.G. (1998) Models of community care for severe mental illness: a review of research on case management. *Schizophrenia Bulletin* **24**, 37–78.

Mullen, R., Gibbs, A. & Dawson, J. (2006) Family perspective on community treatment orders: a New Zealand study. *International Journal of Social Psychiatry* **52**, 469–478.

National Association for Mental Health (1961) Emerging patterns for the mental health services and the public: "Mental health is everybody's business". Proceedings of a conference held at Church House, Westminster, London, on 9th and 10th March 1961 Welbeck, Leeds.

New Freedom Commission on Mental Health (2003) *Achieving the Promise: Transforming Mental Health Care in America. Final Report*. Rockville, MD: DHHS.

Onken, S.J., Craig, C.M. & Ridgway, P. (2007) An analysis of the definitions and elements of recovery: a review of the literature. *Psychiatric Rehabilitation Journal* **31**, 9–22.

Petersen, L., Jeppesen, P., Thorup, A. *et al.* (2005) A randomised multicentre trial of integrated versus standard treatment for patients with a first episode of psychotic illness. *BMJ* **331**, 602.

Pilling, S., Bebbington, P., Kuipers, E. *et al.* (2002) Psychological treatments in schizophrenia: II. Meta-analyses of randomized controlled trials of social skills training and cognitive remediation. *Psychological Medicine* **32**, 783–791.

Priebe, S. (2007) Social outcomes in schizophrenia. *British Journal of Psychiatry* **191**, s15–s20.

Priebe, S., Badesconyi, A., Fioritti, A. *et al.* (2005) Reinstitutionalisation in mental health care: comparison of data on service provision from six European countries. *BMJ* **330**, 123–126.

Rapp, C.A. & Goscha, R.J. (2004) The principles of effective case management of mental health services. *Psychiatric Rehabilitation Journal* **27**, 319–333.

Ratcliffe, R.A.W. (1962) The open door: ten years' experience in Dingleton. *Lancet* **ii**, 188–190.

Saha, S., Chant, D. & McGrath, J. (2007) A systematic review of mortality in schizophrenia: is the differential mortality gap worsening over time? *Archives of General Psychiatry* **64**, 1123–1131.

Slade, M., Powell, R., Rosen, A. & Strathdee, G. (2000) Threshold Assessment Grid (TAG): the development of a valid and brief scale to assess the severity of mental illness. *Social Psychiatry & Psychiatric Epidemiology* **35**, 78–85.

Slade, M., Cahill, S., Kelsey, W. *et al.* (2001) Threshold 3: the feasibility of the Threshold Assessment Grid (TAG) for routine assessment of the severity of mental health problems. *Social Psychiatry & Psychiatric Epidemiology* **36**, 516–521.

Stein, L.I. & Test, M.A. (1980) Alternative to mental hospital treatment. I. Conceptual model, treatment program, and clinical evaluation. *Archives of General Psychiatry* **37**, 392–397.

Strathdee, G. & Thornicroft, G. (1992) Community sectors of need-lead mental health services. In: Thornicroft, G., Brewin, C.R. & Wing, J., eds. *Measuring Mental Health Needs*. London: Gaskell.

Swartz, M.S., Swanson, J.W., Wagner, H.R. *et al.* (1999) Can involuntary outpatient commitment reduce hospital recidivism?: Findings from a randomized trial with severely mentally ill individuals. *American Journal of Psychiatry* **156**, 1968–1975.

Swartz, M.S., Swanson, J.W., Wagner, H.R. *et al.* (2003) Assessment of four stakeholder groups' preferences concerning outpatient commitment for persons with schizophrenia. *American Journal of Psychiatry* **160**, 1139–1146.

Szasz, T.S. (1972) *The Myth of Mental Illness: Foundations of a Theory of Personal Conduct*. London: Paladin.

Test, M.A. & Stein, L.I. (1980) Alternative to mental hospital treatment. III. Social cost. *Archives of General Psychiatry* **37**, 409–412.

Thornicroft, G., Wykes, T., Holloway, F. *et al.* (1998) From efficacy to effectiveness in community mental health services. PRiSM Psychosis Study 10. *British Journal of Psychiatry* **173**, 423–427.

US Congress (1963) Public Law 88-164, 88th Congress, S-1576.

US Department of Health and Human Services (1999) *Mental Health: A Report of the Surgeon General*. Rockville, MD: DHSS.

Weisbrod, B.A., Test, M.A. & Stein, L.I. (1980) Alternative to mental hospital treatment. II. Economic benefit-cost analysis. *Archives of General Psychiatry* **37**, 400–405.

Wing, J.K. & Brown, G.W. (1970) *Institutionalism and Schizophrenia*. Cambrdige: Cambridge University Press.

World Health Organization (1988) *Disability Assessment Schedule*. Geneva: World Health Organization.

Wright, C., Catty, J., Watt, H. & Burns, T. (2004) A systematic review of home treatment services. Classification and sustainability. *Social Psychiatry and Psychiatric Epidemiology* **39**, 789–796.

CHAPTER 31

Societal outcomes in schizophrenia

Iain Kooyman[1] and Elizabeth Walsh[2]

[1]Institute of Psychiatry, London, UK
[2]South London and Maudsley NHS Trust, London, UK

Introduction

Research into schizophrenia management has traditionally focused on reducing symptoms of the illness, or reducing the need for service input, such as inpatient care (see Chapter 30). Recently there has been a shift towards including psychological and social outcomes. However, societal outcomes—which are those impacting on or arising from an interaction with society as a whole—remain rarely considered. This is despite a growing literature highlighting their prevalence and damaging effects. Societal outcomes may have become more apparent since the process of deinstitutionalization and community care, which led to society being re-exposed to people with schizophrenia. *Violence* perpetrated by people with schizophrenia is a matter of widespread public and political concern; although often exaggerated by the media, a link between schizophrenia and violence is undeniable. However, *suicide* and *self-harm* are much more common outcomes, and *victimization* of people with schizophrenia is an especially neglected topic.

Schizophrenia, 3rd edition. Edited by Daniel R. Weinberger and Paul J Harrison © 2011 Blackwell Publishing Ltd.

Substance misuse is overrepresented in schizophrenia and commonly complicates treatment. *Unemployment* rates remain dismally low and *homelessness* is more commonly experienced by people with schizophrenia. As a result of all these adverse outcomes, on top of illness, treatment, and lifestyle factors, it is not surprising that *mortality* is increased in schizophrenia and life-expectancy markedly reduced.

This chapter will first review epidemiological findings for these societal outcomes, paying attention to their methodological limitations. The etiology of each outcome will be considered, through examination of identified risk factors. The secondary outcomes, many of which are harmful for both the individual and for society, will be examined. Finally, a brief review of available prevention and treatment options will be presented. It will become clear that each societal outcome acts as a risk factor for several others, and that the early targeting of a broad range of problems is thus crucial to prevent a domino-like societal decline.

Violence and schizophrenia

The past three decades have seen a surge in epidemiological research which has lain to rest longstanding claims that people with schizophrenia are no more likely to behave violently. Although not all violence can be predicted or prevented, routine risk assessment and risk management can reduce this outcome. The relationship between schizophrenia and violence is complex and only partly driven by symptoms; thus, clinicians and service planners should appreciate the importance of targeting coexistent risk factors for violence, including criminal attitudes, substance misuse, and a number of social factors.

Measurement and limitations

Measurement of violent behavior has relied upon various single or combined sources of information (self-report, informant, case notes, official records). All single sources bias towards underreporting: self-report from a desire for social acceptability or fear of adverse consequences of reporting; informants being unreliable or unaware; case notes being usually incomplete. The proportion of violent acts leading to arrest, prosecution, and conviction vary with the intensity and quality of policing, behavior of the suspect, availability of diversion to the mental health system, and the severity of offence. Most violent individuals are not convicted. Only the more serious violent acts lead to conviction; the association between schizophrenia and more minor forms of violence is impossible to estimate from official sources.

The recent use of multiple combined measures has improved detection. For example, Steadman *et al.* (1998) showed that detection of violence increased steadily as methods were combined, and reached six times the rate of official convictions alone. Multiple measures require judgments about what constitutes a single violent event and in handling inconsistencies between reports.

The definition of violence varies enormously between studies, sometimes including verbal threats. Mostly simple measures are recorded, neglecting contextual aspects. The MacArthur Community Violence Interview (Steadman *et al.*, 1998) is an important step towards consistency. It measures life-time violence, and includes information on recent aggressive behavior and victimization. It incorporates a clear and structured definition of different levels of violence and considers the context for each episode. There is also a collateral version. Encouragingly, its use is growing (e.g., Swanson *et al.*, 2006).

Comparison groups are often not used, or comprise of variably selected groups of people, e.g., neighbors, patients with other mental disorders, or general population figures, and are often not demographically matched to the subjects with schizophrenia. Some studies attempt to control for confounders, but these are potentially numerous, difficult to measure, and may not be truly independent from the mental disorder being examined, acting instead as mediators. Schizophrenia and violence are both rare outcomes, thus vast sample sizes are required.

Prevalence

The prevalence of violence by people with schizophrenia has been estimated in various populations and using several methods.

Psychosis is more prevalent within prisons than in the community. A systematic review of 62 surveys in 12 Western countries revealed psychotic illnesses in 3.7% of male and 4% of female prisoners (Fazel & Danesh, 2002). An early, but influential study found that remand prisoners who had been charged with violent offences had much higher rates of psychosis than those charged with non-violent offences (Taylor & Gunn, 1984). Homicide studies have consistently shown a clear over-representation of schizophrenia: the National Confidential Enquiry into Suicides and Homicides in England and Wales found a prevalence of 5% in homicide perpetrators (Shaw *et al.*, 2006), although official rates of homicide due to mental disorder have fallen dramatically since the mid-1970s in England and Wales (Large *et al.*, 2008). Contrary to much expert opinion, schizophrenia has recently been shown to be overrepresented amongst male sexual offenders, with an odds ratio of 4.8 in a Swedish national case–control study (Fazel *et al.*, 2007).

Cross-sectional population studies have shown violence is also more prevalent in people with schizophrenia living in the community. The large Epidemiology Catchment Area (ECA) sample in the US was one of the first to show this (Swanson *et al.*, 1990). A recent UK two-stage household survey repeated this finding (Coid *et al.*, 2006).

The least biased evidence comes from a collection of unselected birth cohorts, carried out in Sweden (Hodgins, 1992), Denmark (Brennan *et al.*, 2000), Finland (Tiihonen *et al.*, 1997), and New Zealand (Arseneault *et al.*, 2000). These have reported relative risks of between two and seven times for serious violence by people with schizophrenia compared to the general population. The largest cohort study (Brennan *et al.*, 2000) was conducted in Denmark, where offenders are arrested regardless of their mental status. It found that by age 43–46, violent convictions in people with schizophrenia were increased fourfold in males and 23–fold in females; these data also highlight the smaller gender gap in violent offending in schizophrenia; that is, psychosis conveys a higher relative risk of violence in women. Nearly a fifth of community-dwelling women with chronic psychosis committed an assault prospectively over 2 years in a UK sample (Dean *et al.*, 2006). Complementing the birth cohorts, retrospective cohorts with case linkage have allowed large numbers of people with schizophrenia to be compared to matched controls, increasing study power. In Victoria, Australia, 2861 people with schizophrenia were found to have an odds ratio of 4 for all criminal offending and 5 for violent offending (Wallace *et al.*, 2004). In Sweden, 644 patients with schizophrenia were four times more likely to have been convicted of a violent offence (Lindqvist & Allebeck, 1990).

As a final point to note, the association between schizophrenia and violence is seen prior to diagnosis, with about 20% of first-contact patients with schizophrenia having already assaulted another person (Volavka *et al.*, 1997).

Cost to society

With most research to date focusing on relative risk, it is encouraging to see estimates of absolute risk emerging in the literature. The population attributable risk (i.e., the fall in levels of violence in society that would occur if violent incidents by people with schizophrenia were prevented) is an approximate calculation, although this approach assumes causality between schizophrenia and violence and fails to take account of associated factors, such as substance misuse and personality disorders. Wallace *et al.* (2004) estimated 6–11% of violent convictions are attributable to schizophrenia, whereas Fazel and Grann (2006) found a population attributable risk for serious violence of just 2.3%, increasing to 5% for psychosis defined more broadly. Friends and relatives represent a larger proportion of the victims of violence by people with mental disorders than they do by people without mental disorders (Coid *et al.*, 2006). Violent offending by people with schizophrenia not only costs individual victims, but also produces an additional financial strain on criminal justice services.

Patterns of offending

The birth cohort studies inform us that approximately two-thirds of offenders with schizophrenia offend before first psychiatric presentation; however, this leaves a significant subgroup who start offending after illness onset. The proposal of a two-type model of offending in people with schizophrenia (Steinert *et al.*, 1998) has become widely accepted. "Early starters" or "Ttype 2 offenders" begin offending in childhood or adolescence, whilst "late starters" or "Type 1 offenders" begin offending after the onset of symptoms: they are a group unparalleled in the general population. A large Swedish sample of male mentally disordered offenders (Tengstrom *et al.*, 2001) revealed several factors able to discriminate between the two groups–early starters were more likely to have misused substances, to have antisocial personality disorder (APD), higher psychopathy scores, poorer employment history, and higher rates of childhood behavioral disturbance.

Explaining the excess violence

Substance misuse

A consistent finding is that substance misuse correlates strongly with both non-violent and violent offending (as in the non-disordered population) in people with schizophrenia (Swanson *et al.*, 1990; Tiihonen *et al.*, 1997; Wallace *et al.*, 2004). Self-reports indicate substance misuse is common immediately before violent offences are committed (Arseneault *et al.*, 2000). The influential MacArthur study noted earlier even suggested that schizophrenia in the absence of substance misuse is protective against violence (Steadman *et al.*, 1998). However, the authors did not control for the mediating effect of personality disorder, which is highly correlated with substance misuse. Subsequent research has mostly shown that substance misuse cannot account for all the association between schizophrenia and violence (Brennan *et al.*, 2000; Wallace *et al.*, 2004), but two recent studies have re-opened the debate, showing that excess violent offending in people with schizophrenia is non-significant after controlling for substance misuse (Elbogen & Johnson,, 2009; Fazel *et al.*, 2009).

Antisocial personality disorder

There is a markedly increased prevalence of antisocial personality disorder in schizophrenia (Robins *et al.*, 1991). Birth and population cohorts have shown higher rates of childhood aggressive behavior among those who develop schizophrenia. Analysis of data from the CATIE trial showed more than two symptoms of conduct disorder was associated with increased aggression in adults with schizophrenia (Swanson *et al.*, 2006). APD diagnosis in adulthood also predicts aggression in schizophrenia (Moran *et al.*,

2003), and Cluster B personality disorder predicts assaults by women with schizophrenia (Dean *et al.* 2006).

Psychopathy

As in the general population, psychopathy predicts violence in those with schizophrenia (Tengstrom *et al.*, 2000). A meta-analysis showed that score on the Psychopathy Check List-Revised (PLC-R) is the best single predictor of future violence, even amongst persons with mental illness (Salekin *et al.*, 1996). However, the superiority of psychopathy as a predictor of violence may be due to a small subgroup with high PCL scores who commit most of the offences (Tengstrom *et al.*, 2000).

Acute symptoms

Although clinical experience dictates that hallucinations and delusions can lead to violence, the evidence linking psychotic symptoms to aggression is surprisingly poor. Symptoms are difficult to quantify and fluctuate rapidly. Perhaps as a result of these methodological obstacles, community studies have struggled to support the link between psychotic symptoms and aggression in people with schizophrenia. One US community study did find an association between positive symptoms and violence, and an inverse association with negative symptoms (Swanson *et al.*, 2006). Inpatient settings have been more successful in linking aggression and psychotic symptoms, but evaluating the precise motive for an aggressive act is extremely problematic, with frequent discrepancy between staff and patient reports and difficulties even when using video-cameras to supplement interviews. A large prospective study found positive symptoms explained assaults more frequently in female than male inpatients (Krakowski & Czobor, 2004).

The role of specific psychotic symptoms in aggression in schizophrenia is not clear, with many conflicting findings. Specific symptoms found to correlate with violence have varied from disorganization symptoms, to thought disorder, delusions, and hallucinations. A systematic review (Bjorkly, 2002) found most support for persecutory delusions associated with emotional distress, and some support for command hallucinations. There may be a dose–response relationship between symptoms of hostility in schizophrenia and violence (Swanson *et al.*, 2006). Lack of insight predicts aggression in psychosis, but this seems mostly confounded by psychopathy and positive symptoms (Lincoln & Hodgins, 2008).

Deinstitutionalization

Deinstitutionalization has been demonized by the press for making the streets more dangerous. There is some evidence from homicide studies to suggest people with schizophrenia have contributed more to homicides post deinstitutionalization (Grunberg *et al.*, 1977). However, violent acts were and are frequent within institutions, and

violent convictions in people with schizophrenia seem to have risen in line with the general population over the past three decades (Wallace *et al.*, 2004). It has been argued that the forte of the large institutions was to care for the harmlessly dysfunctional, rather than containing the antisocial and violent types, who tended to end up in prison (Mullen, 2006).

Neurobiological explanations

Cognitive deficits and birth complications are linked to criminality in the general population and may interact with early environmental experiences (Raine *et al.*, 1994). High rates of neurological problems, particularly poor motor coordination, poor visuo-spatial function, and low IQ, have been found among inpatients with schizophrenia who have a history of violence (Krakowski *et al.*, 1989). Poor educational attainment, poor grades for attention at school, higher birth weight, and larger head circumference were significantly associated with adult criminal offending in a schizophrenia sample (Cannon *et al.*, 2002). There have been many claims that executive deficits are associated with violence in schizophrenia, but the literature is inconsistent (Fullam & Dolan, 2008). Executive dysfunction is more prevalent in those with late-onset offending compared to those with stable, early-onset aggressive behavior (Naudts & Hodgkins, 2006).

Social factors and vulnerabilities

Social risk factors known to increase violence in the general population are over-represented in people with schizophrenia. They often experience housing instability and are housed in high-crime neighborhoods. Unemployment is very high in schizophrenia. Poor family relations are common in schizophrenia and can often precipitate violence. People with schizophrenia are commonly victimized (Teplin *et al.*, 2005) and this could precipitate reactionary aggression.

Violence risk management

Violence prediction

The first step is to identify the subgroup at risk of violent behavior. Unfortunately, predicting violence is harder than measuring it. Assessing the risk of violence has become an increasingly important part of clinical practice in psychiatry, with time and resource implications. The clinical usefulness of specific risk assessment procedures depends on (1) the accuracy of prediction (predictive validity); (2) applicability to the patient group; and (3) ability of clinicians to act on the results to reduce predicted risk.

Predictive validity has been at the heart of the debate on two differing approaches—actuarial *versus* clinical risk assessment. The former relies on the identification of largely static risk factors (defining at-risk groups within populations), while the latter is an individually-focused case formulation, which underpins routine clinical practice. To combine the advantages and minimize the disadvantages of the two, several structured risk assessment instruments have been devised and tested, such as the Historical Clinical Risk assessment (HCR-20; Douglas *et al.*, 2001) and the Violence Risk Scale (VRS; Wong & Gordon, 2000).

A statistical assessment of predictive validity is essential both for considering the clinical value of a particular instrument and for comparing instruments. Receiver operator characteristics (ROCs) integrate the concepts of sensitivity and specificity, and are relatively independent of the population base rate of violence. A recent UK study compared the relative efficacy of the HCR-20, the Psychopathy Checklist Screening Version (PCL:SV; Hart *et al.*, 1995) and the Offender Group Reconviction Scale (OGRS; Copas & Marshall, 1998) prospectively over 2 years in a group of patients discharged from a medium secure unit (Gray *et al.*, 2004). All three were predictive of offending over the follow-up period, but the purely criminogenic scale (OGRS) performed best. This finding that actuarial instruments outperform even structured clinical assessments in mentally disordered populations is consistent across different settings, while both outperform unaided clinical judgment. However, instruments validated in offending populations may have less predictive validity in the general adult psychiatry than the forensic psychiatry setting.

Even instruments with relatively high predictive validity will generate both false-positives and false-negatives, and an elegant demonstration of the potential implications was provided by Buchanan and Leese (2001) who pooled results from 23 studies employing violence risk assessments. They concluded that six people would need to be detained to prevent one violent act. Overemphasis on violence risk assessment may also detract from consideration of other adverse outcomes.

In clinical practice the usefulness of any risk assessment method will also depend on the implications for intervention. Static factors such as gender and past criminal behavior offer limited scope to inform clinical intervention. Despite the finding that the clinical subset is the least predictive part of the HCR-20 (Gray *et al.*, 2008), consideration of dynamic, clinical factors such as active psychotic symptoms and substance misuse may contribute more to the usefulness of a risk assessment instrument in clinical practice, enabling the shift from risk assessment to risk management or risk reduction.

Risk minimization strategies

It is unclear whether risk assessment itself is an effective intervention, but a randomized controlled trial (RCT) in Switzerland recently demonstrated that routine structured risk assessment soon after admission significantly reduced the subsequent incidence of inpatient violence when combined with mandatory consideration of risk reduction strategies (Abderhalden *et al.*, 2008).

First, symptom control should be maximized, using both pharmacological and psychological interventions (see Chapters 25 and 32). The side effects of typical antipsychotics, particularly akathisia and neuroleptic-deficient syndrome, may increase levels of aggression (Leong & Silvia, 2003); thus, atypical antipsychotics have generally been preferred, supported by a few small RCTs of short duration. However, a recent large RCT with 6-month follow-up found that in fact non-clozapine atypicals may be less effective at reducing violence than the typical antipsychotic perphazine (Swanson *et al.*, 2008). Regardless of the choice of antipsychotic, adherence to medication must be ensured: it is well established that non-adherence increases the risk of violence (Swartz et al., 1998). Administering medication in depot form should always be considered: the risks of illness relapse need to be considered when balancing respect for patient autonomy with ensuring adequate treatment.

All too often, however, clinicians focus on treating symptoms and neglect managing the coexistent risk factors. Reducing substance misuse should be a key target and is explored later in this chapter. Psychological treatments are vital if the personality traits and thinking styles, which perpetuate violent and criminogenic behavior, are to be tackled. Targets include enhancing interpersonal skills, instructing anger management, improving victim empathy, and reducing cognitive distortions. Reasoning and rehabilitation ("R and R") therapy is a group-based, cognitive–behavioral training program for offenders, accredited by the UK Home Office for use with offenders in prison. Encouraging results have been seen in a pilot trial in UK mentally disordered offenders (Clarke *et al.*, 2010). High-risk patients should ideally be placed in stable accommodation in low-crime neighborhoods, although this is an even harder goal for the mentally disordered offender. Daytime structured activities should be maximized so as to increase self-esteem, and reduce time spent with delinquent peers and consuming substances. Paid employment should further reduce the economic drive to offend. Follow-up studies of patients discharged from forensic institutions are showing encouraging reductions in aggression, but evaluation of which components of these treatment packages are effective is needed. Furthermore, similar interventions need to be implemented by general psychiatric services, as many forensic patients are managed within this setting (Hodgins & Muller-Isberner, 2004).

At the societal level, continued improved detection and treatment of schizophrenia in prisons, reduced stigmatization of mental illness, and improved access to psychiatric and social care may help reduce so-called "structural violence" in schizophrenia (Kelly, 2005). Restriction of access to weapons is a societal approach to reducing violence in the US, with increasing restrictions on firearm possession for people with mental disorders (Norris *et al.*, 2006).

Victimization

Research on the relationship between violence and schizophrenia has almost solely focused on people with schizophrenia as the perpetrator of violence, but evidence supporting a bidirectional relationship is accumulating. In fact, individuals with schizophrenia are more likely to be victims than perpetrators of violence. One US study found people with schizophrenia or schizoaffective disorder were 14 times more likely to be a victim of violent crime than a perpetrator (Brekke *et al.*, 2001). If the emphasis continues to be on perpetrating violence, the severely mentally ill will continue to be unfairly stigmatized. Self- reported victimization in schizophrenia has been shown to be associated with poorer community functioning (Hodgins *et al.*, 2009) and it is likely that victims with schizophrenia will be particularly vulnerable to a range of adverse outcomes such as homelessness, unemployment, substance misuse, and violent retaliation.

Measurement and limitations

Optimal methods of measurement of victimization in schizophrenia have yet to be established. Two types of instruments have been used. The first are questionnaires designed for use with mentally disordered subjects, but not specifically to examine victimization: the MacArthur Community Violence Interview, for example, includes a number of questions on victimization and its context (Silver, 2002). The Lancashire Quality of Life Profile includes items on victimization experiences, but without detail on the frequency, severity or context (Oliver, 1991). The second are questionnaires designed to examine victimization in the general population. The National Crime Victimization Survey has been applied to a sample of patients with serious mental illnesses (Teplin *et al.*, 2005). The authors described this instrument as the "'most comprehensive instrument available to assess victimization" as it elicits detailed information about each individual event reported. It required some modification for a mentally disordered sample. As many acts of violence are not reported to police (and this may be more likely for victims with mental illnesses), self-report measures will continue to be the best method of obtaining victimization data. Reporting past victimization may be subject to recall difficulties and may not be reliable. Incorporation of "bounding interviews" to establish reference points for future recalling of index events may reduce "telescoping", a phenomenon where incidents occurring prior to the required recall period are reported (Teplin *et al.*, 2005). Collateral sources (family members, key workers or residential support staff), although generally likely to underestimate, may complement subject reporting and enable some assessment of reliability. As with the measurement of all societal outcomes, the use of multiple sources of information is desirable.

Prevalence

Silver (2002) reported that discharged patients with severe mental illness and/or personality disorder were over twice as likely to be the victims of violence than were their neighbors. Another US group has calculated a more alarming relative risk of 11 for people with severe mental illness (Teplin *et al.*, 2005). The few studies examining victimization in pure samples of patients with schizophrenia have consistently found an excess of violent victimization. In the UK, 16% of a community sample with schizophrenia reported having been violently victimized in the past year: over twice that recorded in the general population (Walsh *et al.*, 2003). This rate is similar to the annual prevalence of violent victimization seen in a Los Angeles sample of people with schizophreniform disorder (11–15%), which was also approximately twice the rate in that population (Brekke *et al.*, 2001). A much lower rate of self-reported violent victimization was seen in a Finish cohort, with only 5.6% of a diagnostically pure sample of discharged patients with schizophrenia self-reporting over 3 years: this was still more than twice the rate of self-reported violent perpetration (Honkonen *et al.*, 2004). Over half of those with schizophreniform disorder reported being assaulted in a 12-month period in the Dunedin study in New Zealand (Silver *et al.*, 2005). Men with schizophrenia are at increased risk of dying by homicide (Hiroeh *et al.*, 2001).

Risk factors

As in the general population, victimization in schizophrenia is predicted by young age and male sex (Honkonen *et al.*, 2004). It has been suggested that people with schizophrenia are victimized because they are aggressive. Indeed, being a perpetrator of violence has been shown to increase risk of violent victimization (Walsh *et al.*, 2003; Honkonen *et al.*, 2004), although the increased risk of victimization in psychosis is present independent of the individual's own violent behavior (Silver, 2002).

Substance misuse is a clear risk factor for victimization (Brekke *et al.*, 2001; Honkonen *et al.*, 2004). The relationship with symptomatology is less clear: total symptom scores have been shown to be predictive of violent victimization in some studies (Brekke *et al.*, 2001; Walsh *et al.*, 2003) but not others (Honkonen *et al.*, 2004). Rates of victimization are much increased in the inpatient setting, although this may not be due solely to acute symptoms.

Patients with schizophrenia now live in the community within a variety of social relationships, and Silver (2002) has shown that their violent victimization can be mediated by conflict in such relationships as well as by indices of social deprivation. Poor financial situation predicts victimization independent of confounding factors (Honkonen et al., 2004). Most samples have been too small to reveal homelessness as a significant risk factor, but data from the UK 700 cohort data did reveal this (Walsh et al., 2003). Elevated rates have also been found prospectively to be associated with comorbid personality disorder, young age at onset, previous victimization, and infrequent contact with family members (Dean et al., 2007).

Management

Victimization remains poorly detected, and mental health clinicians need to inquire about both non-violent and violent victimization. Risk factors such as homelessness and substance misuse should be managed. High-risk individuals should be housed in as supportive, low-risk environment as is possible. Counseling should be offered post-victimization; people with schizophrenia may be less likely to utilize generic victim support structures.

Suicide

Prevention of suicide has become a priority for health services worldwide. The widely cited 10% lifetime risk of suicide in schizophrenia may well be an overestimate (see below), but nonetheless suicide remains an all too frequent outcome, and schizophrenia accounts for 20% of suicides in the under 35s in England and Wales (Appleby et al., 1999). Although risk factors are similar to those seen in the general population, there are also notable differences: these reflect psychological and social sequelae of the illness, rather than acute symptoms. Insight is a well recognized risk factor, but should not deter clinicians from treating patients with suicidal ideation.

Measurement and limitations

Accurate estimation of suicide rates is difficult: official statistics and Coroners' reports are known to be underestimates. More recently, research has included *in vivo* assessments of a range of suicide behaviors. The European Parasuicide Study Interview Schedule (EPSIS), for example, has been specifically developed to examine parasuicidal behavior, suicidal thoughts, and associated factors in detail (Kerkhkof et al., 1991), but has only been used to a limited extent in samples with psychotic disorders (Nordentoft et al., 2002). Some guarded patients, of course, will not disclose suicidal thoughts to researchers.

Prevalence

An early review estimated a 10% lifetime risk of suicide in schizophrenia (Miles, 1977). A subsequent review increased this to 10–13% (Caldwell & Gottesman, 1990). However, both of these estimates relied on proportionate mortality (the percentage of those dead who committed suicide). This assumes a constant rate of suicide, which given the increased rates of early suicides in schizophrenia, may lead to an overestimate of the lifetime suicide risk. A more recent review argues for the use of case-fatality rates (the percentage of a sample of patients who will die by suicide) and reduces the estimate to 5.6% (Palmer et al., 2005). Nonetheless, people with schizophrenia who have attempted suicide are more likely to go on to complete suicide than people with unipolar or bipolar disorder (Tidemalm et al., 2008) and suicide accounts for almost 50% of deaths of people with schizophrenia aged 16–39 (Alaraisanen et al., 2009).

The incidence of suicide in schizophrenia may have increased greatly over the past century, with one group estimating (using historical data) the lifetime rate to have been less than 0.5% in North Wales 100 years ago (Healy et al., 2006). Approximately two-thirds of suicides occur during the first 5 years after diagnosis (Harris & Barraclough, 1997). First-admission patients have three times higher rates of suicide than chronic patients (Palmer et al., 2005).

Lifetime risk of non-fatal suicide attempts in schizophrenia is estimated at 20–40% (Pompili et al., 2007). Suicide attempts in schizophrenia appear higher in North America than the rest of the world (Altamura et al., 2007). A significant proportion of patients with schizophrenia attempt suicide before presenting to services, with reported rates of 10–15% (e.g., Addington et al., 2004) and it is sometimes the mode of first presentation. Reported 1-year rates of suicide attempts in patients with first-episode psychosis vary from 2.9% (Addington et al., 2004) to 11% (Nordentoft et al., 2002).

The National Confidential Inquiry into Suicide and Homicide by People with Mental Illness, incorporating a large survey of suicides in England and Wales, revealed that completed suicide is more likely to result from a violent method in people with schizophrenia, with 27% jumping from a height or under a moving vehicle, compared to only 10% of the remaining sample (Hunt et al., 2006); conversely, self-poisoning was significantly less common in people with schizophrenia.

Etiology

The International Suicide Prevention Trial revealed few transcultural variations in risk factors for suicide in patients with schizophrenia (Altamura et al., 2007). A recent meta-analysis incorporating 29 eligible studies identified the following additional risk factors for suicide in schizophrenia: recent loss; fear of mental disintegration; agitation or motor restlessness; poor adherence to treatment; drug misuse; previous depressive disorders (Hawton et al., 2005). This review found that in contrast with the general population, the male excess is less pronounced, being married or cohabiting is not protective, and alcohol consumption does not appear to be a risk factor. Religiousness is another factor which generally protects against suicide, but not in schizophrenia (Huguelet *et al.*, 2007). Other identified risk factors include unemployment (Hunt *et al.*, 2006) and poor quality of life (Xiang *et al.*, 2008). Being white is often claimed to be a risk factor for suicide in schizophrenia, but has only been found in three studies (Hawton *et al.*, 2005), and one large study found an excess of suicide in schizophrenia in ethnic minorities (Hunt *et al.*, 2006).

Some studies have shown positive symptoms are associated with suicide attempts (e.g., Nordentoft *et al.*, 2002) and in early studies cited, command hallucinations were shown to drive suicide. However, the meta-analysis by Hawton *et al.* (2005) found no association between suicide and positive symptoms and, in stark contrast to popular opinion, revealed a significant negative correlation between hallucinations and suicide. The Psychological Prevention of Relapse in Psychosis Trial in the UK found neither auditory hallucinations nor preoccupation with delusions correlated with suicidal ideation, but "positive symptom distress" did, leading to the suggestion that suicidal thinking in psychosis is "understandable and affect-driven, rather than being of psychotic or inexplicable origin" (Fialko *et al.*, 2006). Negative symptoms (in particular emotional withdrawal) have been associated inversely with suicidal behavior. Level of insight has been shown repeatedly to be correlated with suicidal ideation, and insight at the time of first presentation predicted depression and suicide attempts over a 4-year follow-up in an Irish sample (Crumlish *et al.*, 2005).

The introduction of chlorpromazine has been accused of fuelling suicide rises, by leaving patients with continued disability and dependency yet with increased insight and freedom from psychotic experiences (Hesso, 1977). Others have suggested institutionalization in asylums may have protected against suicide (Healy *et al.*, 2006), although a large Finnish register study revealed no increase in suicides in patients with schizophrenia after deinstitutionalization (Pirkola *et al.*, 2007).

Suicide prediction

The low sensitivity and specificity of the risk factors noted above, plus the rarity of suicide, diminish the ability to predict suicide without an unacceptably high false-positive rate. Indeed, only two of 112 psychiatric inpatients had a predicted risk of suicide above 5% (having at least three of five predictive factors) in a case–control study (Powell *et al.*, 2000). Not surprisingly, current suicidal ideation is the best indicator of suicide attempts in psychiatric patients (Mann *et al.*, 2008).

Suicide reduction

Early detection of psychosis

Given the early peak in suicide risk, it is crucial to detect patients as early as possible. An ecological prevention study found lower levels of suicidality in first-episode patients in two areas with early psychosis detection programs, compared to those in two areas without (Melle *et al.*, 2006).

Screening and close supervision

There is some evidence that good community screening and supervision can reduce suicide attempts. Addington *et al.* (2004) suggest the low rate of suicide attempts in a cohort of patients with first-onset psychosis was reflective of the high standard of care, which included assessments of mood and suicidal thinking and access to individual and group therapy. Xiang *et al.* (2008) propose the lifetime suicide attempts in people with schizophrenia are lower in Hong Kong (20%) compared to Beijing (34%) due to the more developed model of healthcare there, with increased detection and management of mental health relapses. However, the UK 700 study, an RCT of intensive *versus* standard case management, found no significant difference in suicidal behavior between the two groups (Walsh *et al.*, 2001).

Medical treatments

The potential benefit of first-generation antipsychotics on suicidal behavior is unclear (Mamo, 2007). Akathisia should be avoided by judicious choice of dose, drug, and anticholinergic coadministration. Although atypical antipsychotics are viewed favorably with regard to suicide risk, only clozapine has an evidence base. InterSePT, a large randomized study, revealed a significantly lower rate of serious suicide attempts in the clozapine group, compared to the group given olanzapine, with a number needed to treat (to reduce one suicide event) of 13 (Meltzer *et al.*, 2003). This led the US Food and Drug Administration to allow suicidal behavior in schizophrenia to become an indication for clozapine treatment. However, sample sizes (and event rates) have not been sufficiently large to definitively confirm that clozapine reduces completed suicide (Mamo, 2007). Given the importance of depressive symptoms in suicidal behavior, treating coexistent depression should be a goal. However, trials of antidepressants in schizophrenia have been inconsistent (Mamo, 2007). Electroconvulsive therapy remains a useful therapeutic option in severe depression.

Psychological treatments

There is a lack of published literature on the efficacy of psychosocial treatments for suicidality in schizophrenia. Clinicians are often wary of improving insight due to fear of intensifying suicidal impulses. However, insight is positively related to adherence with management, which could counterbalance this (Pompili *et al.*, 2007). Cognitive–behavioral therapy (CBT) has been shown to reduce depressive symptoms and increase insight without increasing suicidality in patients with schizophrenia (Turkington *et al.*, 2002), and CBT led to significant reductions (maintained at 9 months) in suicidal ideation, compared to befriended controls in a UK-based randomized trial (Bateman *et al.*, 2007).

Social treatments

Socials skills training, vocational rehabilitation, and supported employment are important, in order to reduce daily problems and increase daily structure, thus improving self-esteem: this is particularly important for people with good premorbid functioning and insight, in order to counterbalance the high levels of hopelessness.

General management guidelines

Findings from the National Confidential Inquiry into Suicide and Homicide by People with Mental Illness led the authors to conclude that measures which may prevent suicide in schizophrenia include: improved ward safety; closer supervision (especially for those with poor medication compliance), multiagency planning, and effective treatment of substance misuse (Hunt *et al.*, 2006).

Substance misuse

Substance misuse in schizophrenia is an increasing comorbid problem, with significant adverse consequences for the patient and their healthcare professionals. Managing "dual diagnosis" or "comorbid substance misusers" in people with schizophrenia is made difficult by the poor motivation of patients to reduce intake. However, they can respond to interventions and should not be immediately "written off" as being treatment resistant.

Measurement and limitations

"Use" of substances can be quantified by frequency, quantity or duration of use and should be differentiated from "misuse" and "dependency", but for convenience, poorly defined pooled categories have been preferred in the literature (e.g. "Problem use"). Studies vary in extent of inclusion, both of legal and of prescribed substances. Substance use diagnoses can refer to current, past (with varying time-frames), or lifetime criteria. Different classes of substances are often grouped together, which may not be legitimate due to the extremely varying psychopharmacological effects and social contexts of use.

Historically, research studies have tended to use either case notes or unstructured interviews. Structured assess-

ment tools minimize information variance and increase reliability. Commonly used structured questionnaires include the Alcohol Use Disorders Identification Test (AUDIT; Saunders *et al.*, 1993) and twinned Drug Use Disorders Identification Test (DUDIT). It should be noted, however, that the only tools which have been validated in the mentally ill are the brief, clinician-rated Alcohol Use Scale (AUS) and Drug Use Scale (DUS; Drake *et al.*, 1990).

Self-report measures are poorly sensitive: patients grossly underreport their use, particularly for stimulants and opiates, when compared to toxicology screens (Swartz *et al.*, 2003). Clinicians and family informants also underestimate substance misuse in the absence of dependency. Staff suspicion and questioning should be combined with toxicology screens, but these require staff training. Saliva tests avoid the risk of subjects corrupting samples and awkward supervision, but it remains unclear whether they are more or less accurate than urine kits. Breathalizers are practical and valid for measuring alcohol intoxication. For detecting more distal substance use, radioimmunoassay of hair specimens is non-intrusive and reliable (Swartz *et al.*, 2003). Encouragingly, multiple measures, incorporating informant history and biological testing in addition to structured interviews and case note reviews, are increasingly being used (Swartz *et al.*, 2006).

Epidemiological findings

Although the absolute number of people with schizophrenia who have comorbid substance misuse varies widely in studies, they consistently use more than geographical controls. The ECA study in the US was one of the first population surveys to reveal the strength of the association: the odds of having past substance misuse was 4.6 times higher in people with schizophrenia (Reiger *et al.*, 1990). Forty-seven percent of people with schizophrenia in this survey had experienced substance misuse of some kind. Rates of active substance misuse in schizophrenia in the UK vary from 9% to 36% (McCreadie, 2002) and have historically been lower than in the US. Lifetime rates are much higher, e.g., the West London first-episode schizophrenia study (Barnes *et al.*, 2006) reported lifetime rates of 27% for alcohol and 68% for substance misuse.

Comorbid substance misuse in schizophrenia has risen dramatically in developed countries over recent decades, proportional to a rise in the general population, and includes all substance classes (Wallace *et al.*, 2004). Alcohol and cannabis are the most commonly abused substances. This is aside from smoking, which had a 74% prevalence in schizophrenia in the National Psychiatric Morbidity Study, compared to only 31% of the general population, and higher than for any other diagnostic group (Duke *et al.*, 2001).

Explaining the correlation between schizophrenia and substance misuse

It is likely that multiple processes are in play, some contributing to the initiation and others to the maintenance of substance misuse in schizophrenia. The same demographic correlates seen in the general population are also seen in schizophrenia: young, male, unemployed, lower social class. The following theories attempt to explain the excess substance use and misuse in schizophrenia.

Substance misuse may contribute to schizophrenia onset

Most people who abuse substances do not develop schizophrenia, but substance use may act as one causal risk factor. Cocaine, amphetamines, and cannabis are widely known to induce acute transient psychotic episodes in healthy controls. However, only cannabis has an evidence base for being on the causal pathway (see Chapter 11). The population attributable fraction of schizophrenia for cannabis use could be as high as 8% (Arseneault *et al.*, 2004), with implications for policy and law makers.

Substance misuse may result from schizophrenia

Hambrecht and Hafner (1996) showed, retrospectively, that only a third of subjects began using substances before the onset of their illness, with a third beginning use around the same time, and a third beginning use later. Clearly, not all of the excess substance misuse in schizophrenia commences premorbidly, suggesting many abuse substances as a consequence of their psychotic illness. This may be in order to self-medicate in an attempt to cope with symptoms or secondary events. Patients with schizophrenia report using street drugs to counter depression and anxiety, to reduce negative symptoms such as apathy and anhedonia, to assist sleeping, and to reduce extrapryramidal side effects. A review of self-report studies (Gregg *et al.*, 2007) found most support for the "alleviation of dysphoria" hypothesis. Evidence that people use street drugs to treat positive symptoms is equivocal. Nicotine may be used to alleviate neurocognitive deficits or increase the metabolism of antipsychotic drugs to reduce side effects. A second contributory factor may be that people with schizophrenia feel alienated from society and, rejected by peers, may drift into networks of drug users, who may be more accepting of them. The choice of drug abused certainly correlates with ambient drug use in the community. An accumulative risk factor hypothesis has been proposed, conceptualizing the cumulative effects of poor cognitive, social, educational and vocational functioning, poverty, and victimization (Mueser *et al.*, 1998). Many have argued that the effects of deinstitutionalization have led to an increase in the prevalence of dual diagnosis.

Confounding due to antisocial personality disorder

APD is associated with both substance misuse (Reiger *et al.*, 1990) and schizophrenia (Robins *et al.*, 1991). Childhood conduct problems are higher in dual diagnosis patients (Swartz *et al.*, 2006). Comorbid schizophrenia and APD is associated with enhanced substance misuse (Moran & Hodgins, 2004).

Shared developmental pathway for both substance misuse and schizophrenia

A proposed shared underlying neurobiological vulnerability for both schizophrenia and substance misuse (Janowsky *et al.*, 1973) remains a popular theory. It inspired the "supersensitivity theory", which proposes that people with schizophrenia are supersensitive to the adverse effects of substances, thus "misuse" arises from lower levels of use (Mueser *et al.*, 1998). Reward circuitry dysfunction is one suggested vulnerability (Green *et al.*, 2007). Psychological and social shared pathways for schizophrenia and substance misuse have also been postulated.

Cost to the individual

Comorbid patients have poorer treatment outcomes for both their illness and substance misuse. "Dual diagnosis" patients present younger and have more globally severe illness (Barnes *et al.*, 2006), are less adherent with medication (Olfson *et al.*, 2000), and have more positive symptoms (Hambrecht & Hafner, 1996). They have higher use of inpatient, outpatient, and emergency care, and more commonly require treatment by assertive outreach teams (Priebe *et al.*, 2003). They have more tardive dyskinesia and parkinsonian symptoms (Duke *et al.*, 2001), and are more likely to commit suicide (Appleby *et al.*, 1999; Hawton *et al.*, 2005) and to die from medical illnesses, especially smoking-related (Brown *et al.*, 2000). These more adverse outcomes are made more striking by the fact that the comorbid patients tend to have had superior premorbid intellectual functioning and socioeconomic status (Sevy *et al.*, 2001).

Cost to society

People with schizophrenia who misuse substances exhibit higher rates of violence (Hodgins, 1992). In a large Finnish birth cohort, men with schizophrenia who misused alcohol were 25 times more likely to be violent than male healthy controls (Rasanen *et al.*, 1998). They cost services more than their non-misusing counterparts (Hoff & Rosenheck, 1999). As will be seen later, they are also more likely to be unemployed and homeless, and create more interpersonal conflict and stress for family members (Barrowclough *et al.*, 2005).

Management

Encouragingly, comorbid patients may have a superior prognosis to non-misusing patients if they quit using (Krystal *et al.*, 1999). Patients with schizophrenia should be routinely screened for substance misuse. The process of change model (Procahaska *et al.*, 1992) allows categorization of the stage of motivation to change.

Patients with comorbid substance misuse are often excluded from both generic and specific psychosocial interventions, despite a wealth of evidence from over 50 controlled trials that dual diagnosis patients do benefit from interventions such as early intervention and assertive outreach, group-based CBT, contingency management, and long-term residential treatment (Drake & Green, 2006). Family intervention has been highlighted for this group, due to the fact that high "expressed emotion" by carers of dual diagnosis individuals are more likely to view the patient's problems in a blaming way (Barrowclough *et al.*, 2005). Specific psychological interventions for substance misuse may require modification for people with schizophrenia due to the presence of cognitive deficits. The current popular approaches are to use motivational interviewing, relapse prevention work, or group therapy. Finally, Swartz *et al.* (2006) stress the importance of reconnecting comorbid substance misusers to non-using peer groups. All too often the opposite is achieved.

Medication also has a role to play. Atypical antipsychotics may be superior at reducing rates of substance use relapse in schizophrenia; the evidence is strongest for clozapine (Brunette *et al.*, 2006). Naltrexone and acamprosate can be used safely in comorbid patients with alcohol dependence, but disulfiram is more controversial, due to its pro-psychotic potential. Atypical antipsychotics, including clozapine, may also improve smoking cessation rates, in combination with nicotine replacement therapy (George *et al.*, 2000). An increased dose of antipsychotic may be required in smokers, due to the induction of cytochrome P450 enzymes in the liver.

Unemployment

Employment is an essential component of social inclusion. It improves quality of life, leads to improved self-esteem, alleviates symptoms and reduces dependency (Crowther *et al.*, 2001). Disappointingly, employment in schizophrenia is the exception in Western countries. This is despite the intended emancipation brought about by deinstitutionalization, antistigma campaigns, and government initiatives, such as the Disability Discrimination Acts (1995 and 2005) in the UK and the Ticket to Work and Work Incentives Improvement Act (1999) in the US, and the recent uptake of the schizophrenia recovery model. In fact, whilst research supporting the effectiveness of supported employment schemes is rapidly accumulating, employment rates are sliding in the opposite direction, to the detriment of individuals with schizophrenia and at a cost to society.

Measurement and limitations

Employment is not an all-or-nothing phenomenon. It should be considered in terms of quantity and quality. Quantity can be recorded by hours worked, income earned or job tenure, i.e., how long each job is maintained. Measuring quality first of all requires classification of employment type. "Open" or "competitive" employment has been defined as a job in which: (1) payment is at least the minimum wage; (2) is not reserved for people with disabilities; and (3) fewer than 50% of the person's coworkers have disabilities. "Sheltered employment", on the other hand, is provided by an employer who has set aside vacancies for people with disabilities. Secondary benefits, such as social contact and quality of life, should also be considered. Most studies use self-report measures, which probably overestimate employment rates due to bias arising from social-desirability and denial. Few studies have included employer interviews. Receiving benefits has been used as a proxy measure for employment, neglecting people who are supported by savings or loved ones, whilst including those who may be working "off the books".

Prevalence

Although figures vary, all studies agree that the employment rate in schizophrenia is dismal, especially in the developed world, and is lower than in any other mental illness (Wewiorski & Fabian, 2004). Employment rates of 10–20% were seen in the UK in the 1990s, a decline since the 1970s despite a rise in population employment (Marwaha & Johnson, 2004). Evidence for a reduction in employment rate in schizophrenia over recent years was also seen in a large, nationally representative Finnish follow-up study examining discharged patients with schizophrenia, which found a decline in rates of competitive employment from 7% in 1989 to 1.5% in 1997, but constant rates of non-competitive employment (Honkonen *et al.*, 2007). The Psychiatric Morbidity in Great Britain Survey revealed 27% employment in schizophrenia, but used wide inclusion criteria (O'Brien *et al.*, 2003), whilst only 12% of the British sample in the European Schizophrenia Cohort were actively employed, despite including sheltered employment (Bebbington *et al.*, 2005). The French rate was similar (13%), but the German much higher (30%). Estimates around 22% have been made in both the US (Mechanic *et al.*, 2002) and Australia (Carr *et al.*, 2004).

The picture is less bleak in developing countries. The International Pilot Study of Schizophrenia reported much higher rates of employment in psychosis in non-Western countries (Sartorius *et al.*, 1977), particularly those under communist rule, with 90% being employed in Moscow, for example, highlighting the importance of political factors. More recent data, from the International Study of Schizophrenia, pooling a mix of deloping and developed countries, found that 37% had received paid work for most of the past 2 years (Harrison *et al.*, 2001), although attrition rates were significant. Other recent data include 53% employment after 10 years of illness in India (Srinivasan & Thara, 1997), 65% at first contact in Trinidad (Bhugra *et al.*, 2000), and 43% after 1 year of illness in Jamaica, compared to 60% in the general population (Hickling *et al.*, 2001). The latter finding contrasts with the significantly lower levels of employment in African-Caribbeans with first-onset schizophrenia in London, compared to their white or Asian counterparts (Bhugra *et al.*, 1997).

Employment rates decline in the years leading up to diagnosis, beginning as long as 15 years before presentation (Agerbo *et al.*, 2004). In the UK, employment rates are lower in those with established schizophrenia than in new-onset cases (Marwaha & Johnson, 2004). Decline in occupation post-onset is also seen in US studies (Mechanic *et al.*, 2002), but a large, Danish retrospective cohort found that rates of employment actually improved to premorbid levels and then stabilized (Agerbo *et al.*, 2004).

Etiology

Demographic factors

Being male and never having married are often but not always found to be associated with unemployment in schizophrenia (Marwaha & Johnson, 2004).

Clinical factors

Hospitalization necessitates taking sick leave if employed. Days spent in hospital have been shown to reduce the probability of gaining competitive employment (Honkonen *et al.*, 2007). Unemployment at illness onset was associated with the duration of untreated psychosis in two UK samples: the small West London first-episode sample (Barnes *et al.*, 2000) and the large ÆSOP sample (Morgan *et al.*, 2006). The role of positive symptoms seems intuitive, e.g., in those who chose to leave their job due to paranoid thoughts or are dismissed for inappropriate behavior. However, the evidence base is surprisingly poor (Marwaha & Johnson, 2004), with one study even finding a positive association with employment (McGurk & Meltzer, 2000). Negative symptoms seem to produce a much larger barrier to employment, impacting on motivation to seek work, personal presentation, interview performance, social skills, and task orientation (Marwaha & Johnson, 2004). Social skills and motivation to work predicted future employment in a large prospective cohort of people with schizophrenia (Mueser *et al.*, 2001).

Cognitive function also influences employment in schizophrenia. An early review found that specific deficits in verbal memory and executive dysfunction (the same deficits linked to unemployment in brain-injured patients) significantly correlated with current and future functional outcomes (Green, 1996). Memory and executive functioning are significant predictors of attaining full-time work for those partaking in a vocational rehabilitation program (McGurk & Meltzer, 2000). Cognitive functioning may have more of a role in job tenure than job attainment, as seen in a controlled trial (Gold *et al.*, 2002). Cognitive impairment and negative symptoms may overlap, but both independently impede obtaining employment (McGurk & Meltzer, 2000).

Educational and employment history

As in the general population, educational attainment protects against unemployment in people with schizophrenia (Mechanic *et al.*, 2002), and previous employment history is also protective (Mueser *et al.*, 2001). However, early onset of illness could confound this association by causing disruption to studies and thus educational underachievement.

Societal factors

Stigmatization of mental illness undoubtedly impacts negatively on both recruitment and retention of employees. The "benefits trap" is often cited as a significant barrier to getting back to work in people with severe mental illness. Rosenheck *et al.* (2006) found a dose–response relationship with amount of benefits received and engagement in competitive employment, although illness severity could confound this relationship. Marwaha and Johnson (2004), who reported declining employment rates in the UK over the past two decades, propose that the generosity of the benefit system over this period may have lowered financial incentives to work; they also suggest that changes in the national labor market, such as increased competitiveness, a reduction in availability of manual work, and the inability to pay workers rates below the minimum wage, have also been to blame.

Health service factors

Low expectations by mental health professionals may be contributing to the problem. The emphasis placed on occupational needs by psychiatric services may have declined since the start of the deinstitutionalization period, when "industrial therapy units" (mostly factory based) were set up in most hospitals (Marwaha & Johnson, 2004).

Cost to the individual

Quality of life is lower in people with schizophrenia who are unemployed, and correlates strongly with job satisfaction (Priebe *et al.*, 1998). Gainful employment improves economic independence, enhanced self-esteem, and overall functioning (Lehman, 1995). A randomized trial of people with serious mental illness found that those assigned to paid work had significantly fewer symptoms and rehospitalizations than the group assigned to non-paid work (Bell *et al.*, 1996). Even in the presence of social benefits, unemployment puts people with mental illness at risk of poverty (Priebe *et al.*, 1998) and poor health habits, with increased physical morbidity and mortality (Roick *et al.*, 2007).

Cost to society

Unemployment has consistently been hailed as the single biggest financial cost to society from schizophrenia, outstripping the direct costs of healthcare. The cost of lost productivity due to unemployment, absence from work, and premature mortality was estimated to be £3.4 billion in England in 2004–05, compared to direct treatment costs of approximately £2 billion (Mangalore & Knapp, 2007). A further £570 million was paid out in benefits. Similarly, in Canada in 2004, employment productivity losses associated with schizophrenia accounted for 70% of the total estimated cost of Canadian $6.85 billion (Goeree *et al.*, 2005). In the US, Wu *et al.* (2005) claimed that unemployment was the largest component of the $32.4 billion of non-direct costs due to schizophrenia in 2002. US recipients of disability benefits for schizophrenia rose by 35% between 1994 and 2003 (Rosenheck, 2006).

Management

In the UK, there is a statutory duty to include employment within care plans for patients on an enhanced "care program approach". There is also evidence that the majority of people with schizophrenia want to work (Bates, 1996).

Claims of enhanced employment outcomes in those taking second-generation antipsychotics have been made, but a review revealed weak evidence only for superiority of clozapine (Percudani *et al.*, 2004). Slade and Salkever (2001) estimated that even a 40% reduction in symptoms of schizophrenia would result in only an 8% rise in employment rates. Thus, psychosocial treatments, aiming specifically to encourage and support employment, are likely to be the most effective way to improve employment rates.

Sheltered workshops providing vocational rehabilitation have been popular for several decades and can reduce psychopathology and lead to higher global functioning and improved self-esteem (Mueser *et al.*, 1997). However, the more socially integrative "competitive employment" is more financially rewarding and has greater effect in raising self-esteem and reducing symptoms (Bond *et al.*, 2001). A

Cochrane review (Crowther *et al.*, 2001) concluded that supported employment schemes are more effective than prevocational training in helping patients obtain competitive employment. A series of recent randomized trials in the US and Canada have provided strong support for efficacy of the Individual Placement and Support (IPS) model, whereby patients are supported in both obtaining and maintaining their choice of employment. Rates of employment gained in IPS groups have averaged around 50–75%, but the type of employment gained is often basic, part-time, and poorly sustained (Lehman *et al.*, 2002). The effectiveness of IPS in Europe has been demonstrated by a six-center RCT which found that IPS doubled access to work for patients with psychosis (Burns *et al.*, 2007). Factors predicting a favorable response included: previous work history and, interestingly, fewer met social needs, which may have increased motivation to find work (Catty *et al.*, 2008). IPS has recently been shown to be very effective in first-episode psychosis (Killackey *et al.*, 2008).

Neurocognitive enhancement therapy (NET) improves executive function and working memory and has been shown to enhance employment outcomes when added to vocational training (Bell *et al.*, 2009).

Homelessness

Homelessness and housing instability are commonly experienced by people with schizophrenia. Being homeless produces a barrier to receiving treatment and gives rise to an array of other adverse outcomes. Studies show that, if given housing, people with schizophrenia can often maintain this, but research evaluating housing intervention effectiveness is scarce. Homeless patients benefit clinically from intensive outreach support, but are often hard to engage with (Rosenheck, 2000).

Measurement and limitations

"Homelessness" can be variably defined. "Rooflessness" refers to those living on the streets and defines the group of most public concern, and which is hardest to locate or follow-up. A looser definition is having no fixed address, including people living in hostels and emergency accommodation. An even wider concept is a spectrum of "housing instability", signifying tenuousness and stressfulness of housing. This group of so-called "sofa-surfers" move frequently between friends, family, and emergency housing.

There are no valid national databases of housing, due to the unofficial rental market, unregistered housing by friends and family, and the rapid movements of individuals. Case manager rating scales of housing instability have been used, such as a five-point scale rating accommodation from "highly supportive" to "highly stressful" (Drake *et al.*, 1991). However, individuals who are living on the streets, especially those with prominent negative symptoms or an itinerant lifestyle, are less likely to be in regular contact with mental health services; thus, rates of literal homelessness in people with schizophrenia may be underestimated. UK surveys have shown that only a minority of people sleeping rough are even registered with a general practitioner.

Epidemiological findings

Homelessness is a well-recognized outcome of schizophrenia. The European Schizophrenia Cohort found 33% of the British sample had experienced homelessness in their lifetime, compared to just 8% in Germany and 13% in France (Bebbington *et al.*, 2005). The London rate was even higher (43%), and 13% of the British sample had experienced rooflessness, despite currently roofless subjects being excluded from the study. The EPSILON project, a multisite study of schizophrenia outcomes and needs that sampled from five European countries, found that 22% of men and 17% of the women had current accommodation needs (Thornicroft *et al.*, 2002). A US community study (Folsom *et al.*, 2005) found that 20% of more than 4000 patients with schizophrenia had no fixed address, 2.4 times higher than for patients with major depression. In the developing world, where housing services are less developed, rates of sleeping rough may be higher, with 8% of community patients with schizophrenia in rural China experiencing literal homelessness over a 10-year period (Ran *et al.*, 2006). Finally, a review of 33 published studies of rates of schizophrenia in homeless populations led the authors to estimate that 11% of homeless people have schizophrenia and that homelessness is experienced up to 10 times more often in people with schizophrenia (Folsom & Jeste, 2002).

Risk factors

Deinstitutionalization, a failure of the community mental healthcare system to meet the needs of people with schizophrenia, and economic forces have been put forward as societal etiological factors to explain homelessness among people with schizophrenia (Bassuk *et al.*, 1984; Bachrach, 1992).

Individual risk factors for homelessness in schizophrenia have mostly been derived from cross-sectional associations, making cause and effect difficult to disentangle. Follow-up studies have mostly been over a short time span, e.g., 3 months (Olfson *et al.*, 1999). Nonetheless, the following associations are seen with homelessness in people with schizophrenia.

Demographic factors
Being male and single has been identified as a risk factor for homelessness in schizophrenia in many studies, includ-

ing a sample of more than 10 000 in the US (Folsom *et al.*, 2005). However, it is not a universal finding.

Clinical factors
Symptom severity is associated with homelessness in schizophrenia and predicts homelessness after hospital discharge (Olfson *et al.*, 1999). Duration of untreated psychosis correlated with higher rates of homelessness and unemployment in the West London first-episode study (Barnes *et al.*, 2000).

Substance misuse
Substance misuse has repeatedly been linked to homelessness in schizophrenia (Folsom *et al.*, 2005; Opler *et al.*, 2001) and has also been shown to prospectively predict homelessness after discharge from hospital (Olfson *et al.*, 1999).

Cognitive impairment
Executive dysfunction (Barnes *et al.*, 2000) and poor global functioning (Folsom *et al.*, 2005) are seen in homeless people with schizophrenia. Level of global functioning also predicts homelessness after hospital discharge (Olfson *et al.*, 1999).

Criminal offending
Offending correlates with homelessness. Nearly half of all clients of a psychiatric probation and parole service had experienced lifetime homelessness in a US study (Solomon & Draine, 1999) and this was even higher in the group with schizophrenia. The number of lifetime arrests correlated with probability of having been homeless.

Financial factors
Lack of income was one of four factors shown to predict homelessness in a 10-year follow-up study in rural China (Ran *et al.*, 2006). A US sample of more than 10 000 people with severe mental illness (Folsom *et al.*, 2005) found that homelessness, present in 15%, was associated (two-fold) with lacking medical insurance.

Cost to the individual

Treatment rates for homeless persons with schizophrenia are poor. The struggle for food and shelter may take priority over mental healthcare and having no fixed address may limit ability to obtain treatment in those who do seek it. Housing instability is associated with non-adherence with treatment and psychosocial problems (Drake *et al.*, 1989) and decreased quality of life (Lehman *et al.*, 1995). Physical and sexual abuse are common (Wenzel *et al.*, 2000). Homelessness further increases the risk of suicide in schizophrenia (Bickley *et al.*, 2006). Overall mortality rates for homeless people with schizophrenia are four times that of the general population (Babidge *et al.*, 2001) and more than twice that of non-homeless people with schizophrenia (Mortensen & Juel, 1990). Outcomes may be poorer for homeless people with schizophrenia in urban compared to rural areas (Drake *et al.*, 1991).

Cost to society

If able to register with mental health services, homeless people have higher mental health treatment costs (Rosenheck & Seibyl, 1998). Housing instability in schizophrenia may predispose to institutionalization in prisons as well as hospitals (Appleby & Desai, 1987).

Prevention and management

Most studies evaluating the effectiveness of interventions have been in the US and have collectively examined people with a range of severe mental illnesses, rather than studying people with schizophrenia specifically.

Housing interventions

People with schizophrenia can be assisted in finding independent accommodation, or can be housed in specialist supported housing, with varying degrees of in-house support up to 24 hour-staffed residential care. People with mental illness stress the autonomy aspect regarding choice of housing, and tend to prefer living both in their own abode and alone, to living in shared accommodation with other people with mental illness (Tanzam, 1993). A Swedish survey found that people with schizophrenia living in independent accommodation reported higher subjective quality of life and better social network (Hansson *et al.*, 2002). Clinicians however mostly feel that patients in supported group homes will fare better, especially for patients with poor daily living skills or who pose risks to themselves or others. Despite the large amounts of money spent on supported and residential accommodation in some countries, including the UK, a Cochrane review found no methodologically robust trials have examined the effectiveness of supported accommodation (Chilvers *et al.*, 2006), let alone examining whether they are cost effective.

Clinical interventions

A review by Morse *et al.* (1998) identified 10 experimental studies of case management programs for homeless people with mental illness: seven showed a reduction in homeless days, but only two showed a significant reduction in symptoms. Subsequently, success has been seen with more intensive outreach programs. The New York Choices Program (Shern *et al.*, 2000) randomized a sample of homeless people with severe mental illness to psychiatric rehabilitation or treatment as usual. The experimental group benefited from outreach, a drop-in center, access to a small respite housing unit, and community-based rehabilitation:

they showed a greater reduction in nights sleeping on the streets (55% *vs.* 28%), improved life satisfaction, and greater reduction in symptoms. The Access to Community Care and Effective Supportive Services Program (Lam & Rosenheck, 1999), an 18-site study of over 5400 clients being case managed, showed improvements in both clinical and housing domains. However, only 34% of clients expressed an interest in the program at first contact and only 19% entered case management. The process of engagement took on average 101 days, revealing strong opposition to treatment in this group of clients. Rosenheck (2000) reviewed the cost-effectiveness of intervention programs for mentally ill homeless people. Some programs found a significant reduction in inpatient costs, which more than offset the additional cost of the treatment, whilst others showed overall increased costs.

Integrated interventions

It may be beneficial to integrate the provision of housing and psychiatric care. Adults with severe mental illness, randomly assigned to integrated housing and clinical management, had more days of stable housing, greater life satisfaction, and less psychiatric symptoms at 18-month follow-up than those assigned parallel housing and clinical management (McHugo *et al.*, 2004).

Mortality

Epidemiological findings

Mortality is a major and neglected adverse outcome of schizophrenia (see Chapters 7 and 28). Having schizophrenia reduces life-expectancy, e.g., in the US, from 76 years to 61 years (Seeman 2007). Standardized mortality ratios (SMRs) compare death rates to those in the general population, matched for age and gender. A meta-analysis of 37 studies calculated a median SMR for people with schizophrenia of 2.6 (Brown, 1997), meaning that the risk of dying over the next year is 2.6 times higher if you have schizophrenia. An SMR of 3.0 was calculated for schizophrenia in Southampton, UK (Brown *et al.*, 2000). Mortality outcomes may be even poorer in developing countries, with an SMR of 4 seen in a prospective cohort in rural China (Ran *et al.*, 2007), but the "mortality gap" in developed countries has increased in recent decades (Saha *et al.*, 2007).

SMR falls with increasing age due to the peak of suicides early in the illness and the gradual rise in general population mortality (Brown *et al.*, 2000). No sex difference for SMRs in schizophrenia is evident (Brown, 1997). Mortality in schizophrenia is higher in urban than non-urban areas in the West (Fors *et al.*, 2007), but the converse may be seen in developing countries (Ran *et al.*, 2007). SMRs for schizophrenia appear even higher in the unmarried, unemployed, and lower social classes (Brown *et al.*, 2000).

Modes of death

As noted above, suicide is markedly increased in schizophrenia and contributes substantially to the excess mortality. Accidents make up another 12% of the mortality excess in schizophrenia (Brown, 1997). In line with the risk of victimization discussed earlier, a UK study reported that men with schizophrenia have an increased risk of dying by homicide, especially when they comorbidly misuse alcohol and drugs (Hiroeh et al., 2001).

Individual SMRs are much lower for natural than for unnatural causes of death in schizophrenia, but in combination make up the majority of the mortality excess, with estimates from 59% (Brown, 1997) to 70% (Osby et al., 2000). Circulatory disease (cardiovascular and cerebrovascular disease) makes up the largest slice of the excess and death from heart disease is nearly three times more common in people with severe mental illness (Laursen et al., 2009). Diabetes mellitus, epilepsy, lung cancer and other respiratory diseases, gastrointestinal disease, and genitourinary and nervous diseases are also significantly increased in schizophrenia (Brown et al., 2000; Osby et al., 2000). The SMR for breast cancer in women with schizophrenia may be as high as 2.8 (Tran et al., 2009).

Several mechanisms have been proposed to explain the increased natural deaths in schizophrenia.

Inadequate treatment

Patients may refuse to seek medical help or may be nonadherent with medical treatments. They may also receive substandard medical care, as was shown for people presenting with a cardiac event (Druss et al., 2000).

Unhealthy lifestyle

People with schizophrenia smoke more, eat less fiber and more fat (Brown et al., 1999). Smoking-related diseases are commoner (Brown et al., 2000). Metabolic syndrome (a combination of abdominal obesity, atherogenic dyslipidemia, hypertension, and elevated fasting glucose) is increased and may be more common than in any other patient group (Ford et al., 2002). Coronary heart disease is twice as common as in the general population (Brown et al., 2000).

Socioeconomic factors

Socioeconomic factors, including homelessness and access to medical care, may contribute (Seeman 2007).

Deinstitutionalization

The rise in rates of cardiovascular deaths, particularly for men, following deinstitutionalization (Hansen et al., 2001) has been blamed on homelessness and lack of supervision and healthcare. A large excess of deaths of natural causes was seen in 6776 long-term psychiatrically ill patients dis-charged into the community in Scotland between 1977 and 1994 (Stark et al., 2003). Mortality increased in young people with schizophrenia in Finland after a sharp reduction in the number of hospital beds (Salokangas et al., 2002).

Antipsychotic medication

There is some evidence that long-term antipsychotic treatment contributes to the excess mortality in schizophrenia (Weinmann et al., 2009), especially through the metabolic syndrome and hyperlipidemia, but also via QTc prolongation (see Chapter 28). A stark example of relative harms and benefits is provided by clozapine, for which the reduction in suicide risk (Meltzer et al., 2003) may be offset by the excess mortality caused by the average 10-kg weight gain (Fontaine et al., 2001).

Strategies for mortality reduction

Suicide prevention programs play an important role and should target individuals early on in their illness, when suicide risk is greatest. Antistigma campaigns are also required, particularly in developing countries (Ran et al., 2007).

Clinicians should routinely assess cardiovascular risk factors, including blood pressure, cholesterol levels, and obesity on a regular basis. A healthy lifestyle should be promoted, especially: smoking cessation, diet, exercise, reduction of alcohol and drugs. Treatment for medical illnesses needs to improve. Doctors should consider regular physical examinations of people who may fail to recognize that they are ill or to seek treatment (Brown et al., 2000). Compliance with medical as well as psychiatric treatments should be targeted. Compulsory treatment should be considered when the patient's mental state is adversely affecting their physical health, although the legal basis for this varies from place to place (Brown et al., 2000), and has bioethical implications concerning the value placed on patient autonomy (Seeman 2007). Unnecessarily high doses of antipsychotics and polypharmacy should be avoided.

Homelessness amongst people with schizophrenia must be reduced, particularly in developing countries where rates are high (Ran et al., 2007). A wide network of foster families to look after vulnerable individuals has also been proposed (Seeman 2007).

References

Abderhalden, C., Needham, I., Dassen, T. et al. (2008) Structured risk assessment and violence in acute psychiatric wards: randomised controlled trial. *British Journal of Psychiatry* **193**, 44–50.

Addington, J., Williams, J., Young, J. & Addington, D. (2004) Suicidal behaviour in early psychosis. *Acta Psychiatrica Scandanavica* **109**, 116–120.

Agerbo, E., Bryne, M., Eaton, W. & Mortensen, P. (2004) Marital and labor market status in the long run in schizophrenia. *Archives of General Psychiatry* **61**, 28–33.

Alaraisanen, A., Miettunen, J., Rasanen, P., Fenton, W., Koivumaa-Honkanen, H.T. & Isohannis, M. (2009) Suicide rate in schizphrenia in Northern Finland 1966 Birth Cohort. *Social Psychiatry & Psyshiatric Epidemiology* **44**, 1107–1110.

Altamura, A., Mundo, E., Bassetti, R. *et al.* (2007) Transcultural differences in suicide attempters: analysis on a high risk population of patients with schizophrenia or schizoaffective disorder. *Schizophrenia Research* **89**, 140–146.

Appleby, L. & Desai, P. (1987) Residential instability: a perspective on system imbalance. *American Journal of Orthopsychiatry* **57**, 515–524.

Appleby, L., Cooper, J., Amos, T. *et al.* (1999) Psychological autopsy study of suicides by people aged under 35. *British Journal of Psychiatry* **175**, 168–174.

Arseneault, L., Moffitt, T.E., Caspi, A. *et al.* (2000) Mental disorders and violence in a total birth cohort: results from the Dunedin study. *Archives of General Psychiatry* **57**, 979–968.

Arseneault, L., Cannon, M., Witton, J. & Murray, R. (2004) Causal association between cannabis and psychosis: examination of the evidence. *British Journal of Psychiatry* **184**, 110–117.

Babidge, N.C., Buhrich, N. & Butler, T. (2001) Mortality among homeless people with schizophrenia in Sydney, Australia. *Acta Psychiatrica Scandanavica* **103**, 105–110.

Bachrach, L.L. (1992) What we know about homelessness among mentally ill persons: an analytical review and commentary. *Hospital & Community Psychiatry* **43**, 453–464.

Barnes, T.R., Hutton, S.B., Chapman, M.J. *et al.* (2000) West London first-episode study of schizophrenia. Clinical correlates of duration of untreated psychosis. *British Journal Psychiatry* **177**, 207–211.

Barnes, T., Mustafa, S., Hutton, S. *et al.* (2006) Comorbid substance use and age at onset of schizophrenia. *British Journal of Psychiatry* **188**, 237–242.

Barrowclough, C., Ward, J., Wearden, A. & Gregg, L. (2005) Expressed emotion and attributions in relatives of schizophrenia patients with and without substance misuse. *Social Psychiatry Psychiatric Epidemiology* **40**, 884–891.

Bassuk, E.L., Rubin, L. & Lauriat, A. (1984) Is homelessness a mental health problem? *American Journal of Psychiatry* **141**, 1546–1550.

Bateman, K., Hansen, L., Turkington, D. & Kingdon, D. (2007) Cognitive behavioural therapy reduces suicidal ideation in schizophrenia: results from a randomized controlled trial. *Suicide and Life-Threatening Behavior* **37**, 284–290.

Bates, P. (1996) Stuff as dreams are made of. *Health Service Journal* **33**, 5497.

Bebbington, P.E., Angermeyer, M., Azorin, J. *et al.* (2005) The European Schizophrenia Cohort: A naturalistic prognostic and economic study. *Social Psychiatry and Pscyhiatric Epidemiology* **40**, 707–717.

Bell, M.D., Lysaker, P.H. & Milstein, R.M. (1996) Clinical benefits of paid work activity in schizophrenia. *Schizophrenia Bulletin* **22**, 51–67.

Bell, M., Zito, W., Greig, T. & Wexler, B. (2009) Neurogcognitive enhancement therapy with vocational services: work outcomes at two-year follow-up. *Schizophrenia Research* **105**, 18–29.

Bhugra, D., Leff, J., Mallett, R. *et al.* (1997) Incidence and outcome of schizophrenia in whites, African-Carribeans and Asians in London. *Psychological Medicine* **27**, 791–798.

Bhugra, D., Hilwig, M., Mallett, R. *et al.* (2000) Factors in the onset of schizophrenia: a comparison between London and Trinidad samples. *Acta Psychaitrica Scandanavica* **101**, 135–141.

Bickley, H., Kapur., N., Hunt, I. *et al.* (2006) Suicide in the homeless within 12 months of contact with mental health services: a national clinical survey in the UK. *Social Psychiatry and Pscyhiatric Epidemiology* **41**, 686–691.

Bjorkly, S. (2002) Psychotic symptoms and violence toward others—A literature review of some preliminary findings. *Aggression and Violent Behaviour* **7**, 605–631.

Bond, G., Resnick, S., Drake R. *et al.* (2001) Does competitive employment improve nonvocational outcomes for people with severe mental illness? *Journal of Consulting and Clinical Psychology* **69**, 489–501.

Brekke, J.S., Prindle, C. *et al.* (2001) Risks for individuals with schizophrenia who are living in the community. *Psychiatric Services* **52**, 1358–1366.

Brennan, P.A., Mednick, S.A. & Hodgins, S. (2000) Major Mental Disorders and Criminal Violence in a Danish Birth Cohort. *Archives of General Psychiatry* **57**, 494–500.

Brown, S. (1997) Excess mortality in schizophrenia. A meta-analysis. *British Journal of Psychiatry* **171**, 502–508.

Brown, S., Birtwistle, J., Roe, L. & Thompson, C. (1999) The unhealthy lifestyle of people with schizophrenia. *Psychological Medicine* **29**, 697–701.

Brown, S., Inskip, H. & Barraclough, B. (2000) Causes of the excess mortality of schizophrenia. *British Journal of Psychiatry* **177**, 212–217.

Brunette, M., Drake, R., Xie, H. *et al.* (2006) Clozapine use and relapses of substance use disorder among patients with co-occurring schizophrenia and substance use disorders. *Schizophrenia Bulletin* **32**, 637–643.

Buchanan, A. & Leese, M. (2001) Detention of people with dangerous severe personality disorders: a systematic review. *Lancet* **358**, 1955–1959.

Burns, T., Catty, J., Becker, T. *et al.* (2007) The effectiveness of supported employment for people with severe mental illness: a randomised controlled trial. *Lancet* **370**, 1146–1152.

Caldwell, C.B. & Gottesman, I.I. (1990) Schizophrenics kill themselves too: a review of risk factors for suicide. *Schizophrenia Bulletin* **16**, 571–589.

Cannon, M., Huttunen, M., Tanskanen, A. *et al.* (2002) Perinatal and childhood risk factors for later criminality and violence in schizophrenia. *British Journal of Psychiatry* **180**, 496–501.

Carr, V.J, Lewin, T.J., Neil, A.L. *et al.* (2004) Premorbid, psychosocial and clinical predictors of the costs of schizophrenia and other psychoses. *British Journal Psychiatry* **184**, 517–525.

Catty, J., Lissouba, P., White, S. *et al.* (2008) Predictors of employment for people with severe metal illness: results of an international six-centre randomised controlled trial. *British Journal of Psychiatry* **192**, 224–231.

Chilvers, R., Macdonald, G.M. & Hayes, A.A. (2006) Supported housing for people with severe mental disorders. *Cochrane Database of Systematic Reviews* Issue 4 CD000453.

Clarke, A., Cullen, A., Walwyn, R. & Fahy, T. (2010) A quasi-experimental pilot study of the Reasoning and Rehabilitation programme with mentally disordered offenders. *Journal of Forensic Psychiatry and Psychology*, **21**, 490–500.

Coid, J., Min, Y., Roberts, A. *et al.* (2006) Violence and psychiatric morbidity in the national household population of Britain: public health implications. *British Journal Psychiatry* **189**, 12–19.

Copas, J. & Marshall, P. (1998) The offender group reconviction scale: A statistical reconviction score score for use by probation officers. *Applied Statistics* **47**, 159–171.

Crowther, R.E., Marshall, M., Bond, G.R. & Huxley P. (2001) Helping people with severe mental illness to obtain work: systematic review. *British Medical Journal* **322**, 204–208.

Crumlish, N., Whitty, P., Kamali, M. *et al.* (2005) Early insight predicts depression and attempted suicide after 4 years in first-onset schizophrenia and schizophreniform disorder. *Acta Psychiatrica Scandanavica* **112**, 449–455.

Dean, K., Walsh, E., Moran, P. *et al.* (2006) Violence in women with psychosis in the community: prospective study. *British Journal of Psychiatry* **188**, 264–270.

Dean, K., Moran, P., Fahy, T. *et al.* (2007) Predictors of violent victimization amongst those with psychoses. *Acta Psychiatrica Scandanavica* **116**, 353.

Douglas, K., Webster, C., Hart, S. *et al.* (2001) *HCR-20 Violence Risk Management Companion Guide.* Mental Health, Law and Policy Institute, Simon Fraser University/Department of Mental Health Law and Policy, University of South Florida.

Drake, R. & Green, A. (2006) Current research on co-occurring substance use disorder in schizophrenia. *Schizophrenia Bulletin* **32**, 616–617.

Drake. R.E., Wallach, M.A. & Hoffman, J.S. (1989) Housing instability and homelessness among aftercare patients of an urban state hospital. *Hospital and Community Psychiatry* **40**, 46–51.

Drake, R., Osher, F., Noordsy, D. *et al.* (1990) Diagnosis of alcohol use disorders in schizophrenia. *Schizophrenia Bulletin* **16**, 57–67.

Drake, R., Wallach, M., Teague, G. *et al.* (1991) Housing instability and homelessness among rural schizophrenic patients. *American Journal of Psychiatry* **148**, 330–336.

Druss, B., Bradford, D., Roseheck, R. *et al.* (2000) Mental disorders and use of cardiovascular procedures after myocardial infarction. *JAMA* **283**, 506–511.

Duke, P., Pantellis C., McPhillips, M. & Barnes, R. (2001) Comorbid non-alcohol substance misuse among people with schizophrenia. *British Journal of Psychiatry* **179**, 509–513.

Elbogen, E. & Johnson, S. (2009) The intricate link between Violence and Mental Disorder: results from the National Epidemiologic Survey on Alcohol and Related Conditions. *Archives of General Psychiatry* **66**, 152–161.

Fazel, S. & Danesh, J. (2002) Serious mental disorder in 23,000 prisoners: a systematic review of 62 surveys. *Lancet* **359**, 545–555.

Fazel, S. & Grann, M. (2006) The population impact of severe mental illness on violent crime. *American Journal of Psychiatry* **163**, 1397–1403.

Fazel, S., Sjostedt, G., Langstrom, N. & Grann, M. (2007) Severe mental illness and risk of sexual offending in men: a case-control study based on Swedish national registers. *Journal of Clinical Psychiatry* **68**, 588–596.

Fazel, S., Langstrom, N., Hjern, A. *et al.* (2009) Schizophrenia, substance abuse, and violent crime. *JAMA* **301**, 2016–2023.

Fialko L., Freeman, D., Bebbington, P. *et al.* (2006) Understanding suicidal ideation in psychosis: findings from the Psychological Prevention of Relapse in Psychosis (PRP) trial. *Acta Psychiatrica Scandanavica* **114**, 177–186.

Folsom, D. & Jeste, D.V. (2002) Schizophrenia in homeless persons: a systematic review of the literature. *Acta Psychiatrica Scandanavica* **105**, 404–413.

Folsom, S., Hawthorne, W., Lindamer, L. *et al.* (2005) Prevalence and risk factors for homelessness and utilization of mental health services among 10,340 patients with serious mental illness in a large public mental health system. *American Journal of Psychiatry* **162**, 370–376.

Fontaine, K.R., Heo, M., Harrigan, E.P. *et al.* (2001) Estimating the consequences of anti-psychotic induced weight gain on health and mortality rate. *Psychiatry Research* **101**, 277–288.

Ford, E.S., Giles, W.H. & Dietz, W.H. (2002) Prevalence of the metabolic syndrome among US adults: findings from the third national health and nutrition examination survey. *JAMA* **287**, 356–359.

Fors, B.M., Isacson, D., Bingefors, K. & Widerlov, B. (2007) Mortality among persons with schizophrenia in Sweden: an epidemiological study. *Nordic Journal of Psychiatry* **61**, 252–259.

Fullam, R. & Dolan, M. (2008) Executive function and in-patient violence in forensic patients with schizophrenia. *British Journal of Psychiatry* **193**, 247–253.

George, T.P., Ziedonis, D.M., Feingold, A. *et al.* (2000) Nicotine transdermal patch and atypical antipsychotic medications for smoking cessation in schizophrenia. *American Journal of Psychiatry* **157**, 1835–1842.

Goeree, R., Farahati, F., Burke, N. *et al.* (2005) The economic burden of schizophrenia in Canada in 2004. *Current Medical Research and Opinion* **21**, 2017–2028.

Gold, J., Godberg, R., McNary, S. *et al.* (2002) Cognitive correlates of job tenure among patients with severe mental illness. *American Journal of Psychiatry* **159**, 1395–1402.

Gray, N.S., Snowden, R.J., MacCulloch, S. *et al.* (2004) Relative efficacy of criminological, clinical, and personality measures of future risk of offending in mentally disordered offenders: a comparative study of HCR-20, PCL:SV, and OGRS. *Journal of Consulting and Clinical Psychology* **72**, 523–530.

Gray, N., Taylor, J. & Snowden, R. (2008) Predicting violent reconvictions using the HCR-20. *British Journal of Psychiatry* **192**, 384–387.

Green, M.F. (1996) What are the functional consequences of neurocognitive deficits in schizophrenia. *American Journal of Psychiatry* **153**, 321–330.

Green, A., Drake, R.E., Brunette, M.F. & Noordsy, D.L. (2007) Schizophrenia and co-occurring substance use disorder. *American Journal of Psychiatry* **164**, 402–408.

Gregg, L., Barrowclough, C. & Haddock, G. (2007) Reasons for increased substance use in psychosis. *Clinical Psychology Review* **27**, 494–510.

Grunberg, F., Klinger, B. & Grumet, B. (1977) Homicide and deinstitutionalisation of the mentally ill. *American Journal of Psychiatry* **134**, 685–687.

Hambrecht, M. & Hafner,H. (1996) Substance abuse and the onset of schizophrenia. *Biological Psychiatry* **40**, 1155–1163.

Hansen, V., Jacobsen, B.K. & Arnesen, E. (2001) Cause-specifc mortality in psychiatric patients after deinstitutionalisation. *British Journal of Psychiatry* **179**, 438–443.

Hansson, L., Middelboe, T., Sorgaard, K.W. *et al.* (2002) Living situation, subjective quality of life and social network among individuals with schizophrenia in community settings. *Acta Psychiatrica Scandanavica* **105**, 343–350.

Harris, E.C. & Barraclough, B. (1997) Suicide as an outcome for mental disorders. A meta analysis. *British Journal of Psychiatry* **170**, 205–228.

Harrison, G., Hopper, K., Craig, T. *et al.* (2001) Recovery from psychotic illness: a 15 and 25 year international follow up study. *British Journal of Psychiatry* **178**, 506–517.

Hart, S.D., Cox, D.N. & Hare, R.D. (1995) *The Hare Psychopathy Checklist—Screening Version (PCL:SV)*. Toronto: Multi-health Systems.

Hawton, K., Sutton, L., Haw, C. *et al.* (2005) Schizophrenia and suicide: systematic review of risk factors. *British Journal of Psychiatry* **187**, 9–20.

Healy, D., Harris, M., Tranter, R. *et al.* (2006) Lifetime suicide rates in treated schizophrenia: 1875–1924 and 1994–1998 cohorts compared. *British Journal of Psychiatry* **188**, 223–228.

Hesso, R. (1977) Suicide in Norwegian, Finnish and Swedish psychiatric hospitals. *Acta Psychiatr Nervenkr* **224**, 119–127.

Hickling, R.W., McCallum, M., Nooks, L. & Rodgers-Johnson, P. (2001) Outcome of first contact schizophrenia in Jamaica. *West Indian Medical Journal* **50**, 194–197.

Hiroeh, U., Appleby L., Mortensen, P. & Dunn, G. (2001) Death by homicide, suicide and other unnatural causes in people with mental illness: a population based study. *Lancet* **358**, 2110–2112.

Hodgins, S. & Muller-Isberner, R. (2004) Preventing crime by people with schizophrenic disorders: the role of psychiatric services. *British Journal of Psychiatry* **185**, 245–250.

Hodgins, S. (1992) Mental disorder, intellectual deficiency and crime:evidence from a birth cohort. *Archives of General Psychiatry* **49**, 476–483.

Hodgins, S., Lincoln, T. & Mak, T. (2009) Experiences of victimisation and depression are associated with community functioning in men with schizophrenia. *Social Psychiatry and Psychiatric Epidemiology* **44**, 448–457.

Hoff, R.A. & Rosenheck, R.A. (1999) The cost of treating substance abuse patients with and without comorbid psychiatric disorders. *Psychiatric Services* **50**, 1309–1315.

Honkonen, T., Henriksson, M., Koivisto, A. *et al.* (2004) Violent victimization in schizophrenia. *Social Psychiatry and Psychiatric Epidemiology* **39**, 606–612.

Honkonen, T., Stengard, E., Virtanen, M. & Salokangas, R. (2007) Employment predictors for discharged schizophrenia patients. *Social Psychiatry and Psychiatric Epidemiology* **42**, 372–380.

Huguelet, P., Mohr, S., Jung, V. *et al.* (2007) Effect of religion on suicide attempts in outpatients with schizophrenia or schizoaffective disorders compared with inpatients with non-psychotic disorders. *European Psychiatry* **22**, 188–194.

Hunt, I., Kapur, N., Windfuhr, K. *et al.* (2006) Suicide in schizophrenia: Findings from a National Clinical Survey. *Journal of Psychiatric Practice* **12**, 139–147.

Janowsky, D.S., El.-Yousef, M.K., Davis, J.M. *et al.* (1973) Provocation of schizophrenic symptoms by intravenous administration of methylphenidate. *Archives of General Psychiatry* **28**, 185–191.

Kelly, B. (2005) Structural violence and schizophrenia. *Social Science & Medicine* **61**, 721–730.

Kerkhkof, A., van Egmond, M. & Bille-Brahe, U. (1991) *WHO/EURO Multicentre Study on Parasuicide. European Parasuicide Interview Schedule (EPSIS): EPSIS II Version 3.2. Follow-up Interview*. Leiden: Department of Clinical, Health and Personality Psychology, University of Leiden.

Killackey, E., Jackson, H. & McGorry, P. (2008) Vocational intervention in frist-episode psychosis: individual placement and support v. treatment as usual. *British Journal of Psychiatry* **193**, 114–120.

Krakowski, M.I., Convit, A., Jaeger, J. *et al.* (1989) Neurological impairment in violent schizophrenic inpatients. *American Journal of Psychiatry* **146**, 849–853.

Krakowski, M. & Czobor, P. (2004) Gender differences in Violent Behaviours: Relationship to clinical symptoms and psychosocial factors. *American Journal of Psychiatry* **161**, 459–465.

Krystal, J.H., D'Souza, D.C., Madonick, S. & Petrakis, I.L. (1999) Towards a rational pharmacotherapy of comorbid substance abuse in schizophrenic patients. *Schizophrenia Research* **35**, S35–S49.

Lam, J.A. & Rosenheck, R.A. (1999) Street outreach for homeless persons with serious mental illness: is it effective? *Medical Care* **37**, 894–907.

Large, M., Smith, G., Swinson, N. *et al.* (2008) Homicide due to mental disorder in England and Wales over 50 years. *British Journal of Psychiatry* **193**, 130–133.

Laursen, T., Munk-Olsen, T., Agerbo, E. *et al.* (2009) Somatic hospital contacts, invasive cardiac procedures and mortality from heart disease in patients with severe mental disorder. *Archives of General Psychiatry* **66**, 713–720.

Lehman, A. (1995) Vocational rehabilitation in schizophrenia. *Schizophrenia Bulletin* **21**, 645–656.

Lehman, A.F., Kernan, E., DeForge, B.R. & Dixon, L. (1995) Effects of homelessness on the quality of life of persons with severe mental illness. *Psychiatric Services* **46**, 922–926.

Lehman, A., Goldberg, R., Dixon, L. *et al.* (2002) Improving employment outcomes for persons with severe mental illnesses. *Archives of General Psychiatry* **59**, 165–172.

Leong, G. & Silvia, J. (2003) Neuroleptic-induced akathisia and violence: a review. *Journal of Forensic Science* **48**, 187–189.

Lincoln, T. & Hodgins, S. (2008) Is lack of insight associated with physically aggressive behaviour among people with schizophrenia living in the community? *Journal of Mental Disorders* **196**, 62–66.

Lindqvist, P. & Allebeck, P. (1990) Schizophrenia and crime. A longitudinal follow-up of 644 schizophrenics in Stockholm. *British Journal Psychiatry* **157**, 345–350.

Mamo, D. (2007) Managing suicidality in Schizophrenia. *The Canadian Journal of Psychiatry* **52**, s59–s70.

Mangalore, R. & Knapp, M. (2007) Cost of Schizophrenia in England. *Journal of Mental Health Policy & Economics* **10**, 23–41.

Mann, J., Ellis, S., Waternaux, C. *et al.* (2008) Classification trees distinguish suicide attempters in major psychiatric disorders. *Journal of Clinical Psychiatry* **69**, 23–31.

Marwaha, S. & Johnson, S. (2004) Schizophrenia and employment. A review. *Social Psychiatry & Psychiatric Epidemiology* **39**, 337–349.

McCreadie, R.G. (2002) Use of drugs, alcohol and tobacco by people with sciizophrenia: case-control study. *British Journal of Psychiatry* **181**, 321–325.

McGurk, S.R. & Meltzer, H.Y. (2000) The role of cognition in vocational functioning in schizophrenia. *Schizophrenia Research* **45**, 175–184.

McHugo, G., Bebout, R., Harris, M. *et al.* (2004) A randomized controlled trial of integrated versus parallel housing services for homeless adults with severe mental illness. *Schizophrenia Bulletin* **30**, 969–982.

Mechanic, D., Blider, S. & McAlpine, D.D. (2002) Employing persons with serious mental illness. *Health Affairs (Milwood)* **21**, 242–253.

Melle, I., Olav-Johannesen, J., Friis, S. *et al.* (2006) Early detection of the first episode of schizophrenia and suicidal behavior. *American Journal of Psychiatry* **163**, 800–804.

Meltzer, H.Y., Alphs, L., Green, A.I. *et al.* (2003) Clozapine treatment for suicidality in schizophrenia: International Suicide Prevention Trial (InterSePT). *Archives of General Psychiatry* **60**, 82–91.

Miles, C.P. (1977) Conditions predisposing to suicide: a review. *Journal of Nervous and Mental Disease* **164**, 231–246.

Moran, P. & Hodgins, S. (2004) The correlates of comorbid antisocial personality disorder in schizophrenia. *Schizophrenia Bulletin* **30**, 791–802.

Moran, P., Walsh, E., Tyrer, P. *et al.* (2003) Impact of comorbid personality disorder on violence in psychosis. Report from the UK700 trial. *British Journal of Psychiatry* **182**, 129–134.

Morgan, C., Abdul-Al, R., Lappin, J.M. *et al.* (2006) Clinical and social determinants of duration of untreated psychosis in the AESOP first-episode psychosis study. *British Journal of Psychiatry* **189**, 446–452.

Morse, G. (1998) A review of case management for people who are homeless: implications for practice, policy and research. In: Fosburg, L.B. & Dennis, D.L., eds. *Practical Lessons: The 1998 National Symposium on Homelessness Research.* Washington, DC: US Department of Housing and Urban Development, US Department of Health and Human Services, pp. 7.1–7.34.

Mortensen, J.B. & Juel, K. (1990) Mortality and causes of death of schizophrenic patients in Denmark. *Acta Psychiatrica Scandanavica* **81**, 372–377.

Mueser, K., Becker, D., Torrey, W.C. *et al.* (1997) Work and nonvocational domains of functioning in persons with severe mental illness: a longitudinal analysis. *Journal of Nervous and Mental Disease* **185**, 419–426.

Mueser, K.T., Drake, R.E. & Wallach M (1998) Dual diagnosis: a review of etiological theories. *Addictive Behavior* **23**, 717–734.

Mueser, K.T., Salyers, M.P. & Mueser, P.R. (2001) A prospective analysis of work in schizophrenia. *Schizophrenia Bulletin* **27**, 281–296.

Mullen, P. (2006) Schizophrenia and vilence: from correlations to preventive strategies. *Advances in Psychiatric Treatment* **12**, 239–248.

Naudts, K. & Hodgkins, S. (2006) Neurobiological correlates of violent behaviour among persons with schizophrenia. *Schizophrenia Bulletin* **32**, 562–572.

Nordentoft, M., Jeppesen, P., Abel, M. *et al.* (2002) OPUS study: suicidal behaviour, suicidal ideation and hopelessness among patients with first-episode psychosis. One-year follow-up of a randomised controlled trial. *British Journal of Psychiatry* **43** (Suppl.), s98–s106.

Norris, D., Price, M., Gutheil, T. & Reid, W. (2006) Firearm laws, patients and the roles of psychiatrists. *American Journal of Psychiatry* **163**, 1392–1396.

O'Brien, M., Singleton, N., Sparks, J. *et al.* (2003) Adults with a psychotic disorder living in private households 2000. National Statistics. London: HMSO.

Olfson, M., Mechanic, D., Hansell, S. *et al.* (1999) Prediction of homelessness within three months of discharge among inpatients with schizophrenia. *Psychiatric Services* **50**, 667–673.

Olfson, M., Mechanic, D., Hansell, S. *et al.* (2000) Predicting medication non-compliance after hospital discharge among patients with schizophrenia. *Psychiatric Services* **51**, 216–222.

Oliver, J. (1991) The social care directive: development of a quality of life profile for use in community services for the mentally ill. *Social Work and Social Sciences Review* **3**, 53–60.

Opler, L., White, L., Caton, C. *et al.* (2001) Gender differences in the relationship of homelessness to symptom severity, substance abuse and neuroleptic noncompliance in schizophrenia. *Journal of Nervous and Mental Disease* **189**, 449–456.

Osby, U., Correia, N., Brandt, L. *et al.* (2000) Mortality and causes of death in schizophrenia in Stockholm county. *Schizophrenia Research* **45**, 21–28.

Palmer, B.A., Pankratz, V.S. & Bostwick, J.M. (2005) The lifetime risk of suicide in schizophrenia: a reexamination. *Archives of General Psychiatry* **62**, 247–253.

Percudani, M., Barbui, C. & Tansella, M. (2004) Effect of second-generation atipsychotics on employment and productivity in individuals with schizophrenia: an economic perspective. *Pharmacoeconomics* **22**, 701–718.

Pirkola, S., Sohlman, B., Heila, H. & Wahlbeck, K. (2007) Reductions in postdischarge suicide after deinstitutionalisation and decetralization: a nationwide register study in Finland. *Psychiatric Services* **58**, 879–880.

Pompili, M., Amador, X., Girardi, P. *et al.* (2007) Suicide risk in schizophrenia: learning from the past to change the future. *Annals of General Psychiatry* **6**, 10–32.

Powell, J., Geddes, J., Deeks, J. *et al.* (2000) Suicide in psychiatric hospital in-patients. Risk factors and their predictive power. *British Journal of Psychiatry* **176**, 266–272.

Priebe, S., Warner, R., Hubschmid, T. & Eckle, I. (1998) Employment , attitudes towards work, and quality of life among people with schizophrenia in three countries. *Schizophrenia Bulletin* **24**, 469–477.

Priebe, S., Fakhoury, W., Watts, J. *et al.* (2003) Assertive outreach teams in London: patient characteristics and outcomes. *British Journal of Psychiatry* **183**, 148–154.

Procahaska, J.O., DiClemente, C.C. & Norcross, J.C. (1992) In search of how people change: applications to addictive disorders. *American Psychology* **47**, 1102–1114.

Raine, A., Brennan, P. & Mednick, S.A. (1994) Birth complications combined with early maternal rejection at age 1 year predispose to violent crime at age 18 years. *Archives of General Psychiatry* **51**, 984–988.

Rasanen, P., Tiihonen, J., Isohanni, M. *et al.* (1998) Schizophrenia, alcohol abuse and violent behaviour: a 26 year followup study of an unselected birth cohort. *Schizophrenia Bulletin* **24**, 437–441.

Ran, M.S., Chan, C.L.W., Chen, E.Y.H. *et al.* (2006) Homelessness among patients with schizophrenia in rural China: a 10-year cohort study. *Acta Psychiatrica Scandanavica* **114**, 118–123.

Ran, M.S., Chen, E.Y., Conwell, Y. *et al.* (2007) Mortality in people with schizophrenia in rural China: a 10-year cohort. *British Journal of Psychiatry* **190**, 237–242.

Reiger, D.A., Farmer, M.E., Rae, D.S. *et al.* (1990) Comorbidity of mental disorders with alcohol and other drug abuse: results from the Epidemiological catchment area (ECA) study. *JAMA* **264**, 2511–2518.

Robins, L.N., Tipp, J. & Przybeck, T. (1991) Antisocial personality. In: Robins, L.N. & Regier, D., eds. *Psychiatric Disorders in America: The Epidemiologica Catchment Area Study*. New York: Macmillan/Free Press, pp. 258–290.

Roick, C., Fritz-Wieacker, A., Matschinger, H. *et al.* (2007) Health habits of patients with schizophrenia. *Social Psychiatry & Psychiatric Epidemiology* **42**, 268–276.

Rosenheck, R. (2000) Cost-effectiveness of services for mentally ill homeless people: The application of research to policy and practice. *American Journal of Psychiatry* **157**, 1553–1570.

Rosenheck, R.A. (2006) Outcomes, costs and policy caution: a commentary on the cost utility of the latest antipsychotic drugs in schizophrenia study. *Archives of General Psychiatry* **63**, 1074–1076.

Rosenheck, R. & Seibyl, C.L. (1998) Homelessness: health service use and related costs. *Medical Care* **36**, 1121–1122.

Rosenheck, R.A., Leslie, D., Keefe, R. *et al.* (2006) Barriers to employment for people with schizophrenia. *American Journal of Psychiatry* **163**, 411–417.

Saha, S., Chant, D. & McGrath, J. (2007) A systematic review of mortality in schizophrenia: is the differential mortality gap worsening over time? *Archives of General Psychiatry* **64**, 1123–1131.

Salekin, R., Rogers, R, & Sewell, K. (1996) A review and meta-analysis of the psychopathy checklist and Psychopathy Checklist—Revised: Predictive validity and dangerousness. *Clinical Psychology: Science and Practice* **3**, 203–215.

Salokangas, R.K., Honoken, T., Stengard, E. *et al.* (2002) Mortality in chronic schizophrenia during decreasing number of psychiatric beds in Finland. *Schizophrenia Research* **54**, 265–275.

Sartorius, N., Jablensky, A. & Shapiro, R. (1977) Two-year follow-up of patients included in the WHO International Pilot Study of Schizophrenia. *Psychological Medicine* **7**, 529–541.

Saunders, J., Aasland, O., Babor, T. *et al.* (1993) Developement of the alcohol use disorders identification test (AUDIT): WHO Collaborative Project on early detection of persons with harmful Alcohol consumption—II. *Addiction* **88**, 791–804.

Seeman, M. (2007) An outcome measure in schizophrenia: Mortality. *The Canadian Journal of Psychiatry* **52**, 55–59.

Sevy, S., Robinson, D.G., Holloway S. *et al.* (2001) Correlates of substance misuse in patients wtih first-episode schizophrenia and schizoaffective disorder. *Acta Pschiatrica Scandanavica* **104**, 367–374.

Shaw, J., Hunt, I.M., Flynn, S. *et al.* (2006) Rates of mental disorder in people convicted of homicide: a national clinical survey. *British Journal of Psychiatry* **188**, 143–147.

Shern, D.L., Tsemberis, S., Anthony, W. *et al.* (2000) Serving street-dwelling individuals with psychiatric disabilities: outcomes of a psychiatric rehabilitation clinical trial. *American Journal of Public Health* **90**, 1873–1874.

Silver, E. (2002) Mental disorder and violent victimization: the mediating role of involvement in conflicted social relationships. *Criminology* **40**, 191–211.

Silver, E., Arseneault, L., Langley, J. *et al.* (2005) Mental disorder and violent victimization in a total birth cohort. *American Journal of Public Health* **95**, 2015–2021.

Slade, E. & Salkever, D. (2001) Symptom effects o employment in a structural model of mental illness and treatment: analysis of patients with schizophrenia. *Journal of Mental Health Policy and Economics* **4**, 25–34.

Solomon, P. & Draine, J. (1999) Using clinical and criminal involvement factors to explain homelessness among clients of a psychiatric probation and parole service. *Psychiatric Quarterly* **70**, 75–87.

Srinivasan, T.N. & Thara, R. (1997) How do men with schizophrenia fare at work? A follow up study from India. *Schziophrenia Research* **25**, 149–154.

Stark, C., Macleod, M., Hall, D. *et al.* (2003) Mortality after discharge form long-term psychiatric care in Scotland, 1977–1994: a retrospective cohort study. *BMC Public Health* **3**, 30.

Steadman, H.J., Mulvey, E.P., Monahan, J. *et al.* (1998) Violence by people discharged from acute psychiatric inpatient facilities and by others in the same neighborhoods. *Archives of General Psychiatry* **55**, 1–9.

Steinert, T., Voellner, A. & Faust, V. (1998) Violence and schizophrenia: two types of criminal offenders. *European Psychiatry* **12**, 153–165.

Swanson, J., Holzer, C., Ganju, V. & Jonjo, R. (1990) Violence and psychiatric disorder in the community: evidence from the Epidemiology Catchment Area Surveys. *Hospital and Community Psychiatry* **41**, 761–770.

Swanson, J., Swartz, M., Van Dorn, R. *et al.* (2006) A national study of violent behaviour in persons with schizophrenia. *Archives of General Psychiatry* **63**, 490–499.

Swanson, J., Swartz, M., Van Dorn, R. *et al.* (2008) Comparison of antipsychotic medication effects on reducing violence in people with schizophrenia. *British Journal of Psychiatry* **193**, 37–43.

Swartz, M.S., Swanson, J.W., Hiday, V.A. *et al.* (1998) Violence and severe mental illness: the effects of substance abuse and nonadherence to medication. *American Journal of Psychiatry* **155**, 226–231.

Swartz, M.S., Swanson, J.W. & Hannon, M.J. (2003) Detection of illicit substance use in persons with schizophrenia. *Psychiatric Services* **54**, 891–895.

Swartz, M.S., Wagner, R., Swanson, J.W. *et al.* (2006) Substance use in persons with schizophrenia. Baseline prevalence and correlates from the NIMH CATIE study. *Journal of Nervous and Mental Disease* **194**, 164–172.

Tanzman, B. (1993) An overview of surveys of mental health consumers' preferences for housing and support services. *Hospital & Community Psychiatry* **44**, 450–455.

Taylor, P. & Gunn, J. (1984) Violence and psychosis;. Risk of violence among psychotic men. *BMJ* **288**, 1945–1949.

Tengstrom, A., Grann, M., Langstrom N. *et al.* (2000) Psychopathy (PCL-R) as a predictor of violent recidivism among criminal offenders with schizophrenia. *Law and Human Behaviour* **24**, 45–48.

Tengstrom, A., Hodgkins, S. & Kullgren, G. (2001) Men with Schizophrenia Who Behave violently: the usefulness of an early- versus late-start offender typology. *Schizophrenia Bulletin* **27**, 205–218.

Teplin, L., McClelland, G., Abram, K. *et al.* (2005) Crime victimization in adults with severe mental illness: comparison with the National Crime Victimization Survey. *Archives of General Psychiatry* **62**, 911–921.

Thornicroft, G., Leese, M., Tansella, M. *et al.* (2002) Gender differences in living with schizophrenia. A cross-sectional European multi-site study. *Schizophrenia Research* **57**, 191–200.

Tidemalm, D., Langstrom, N., Lichtenstein, P. *et al.* (2008) Risk of suicide after suicide attempt according to coexisting psychiatric disorder: Swedish cohort study with long term follow-up. *BMJ* **337**, a2205.

Tiihonen, J., Isohanni, M., Räsänen, P. *et al.* (1997) Specific major mental disorder and criminality: a 26-year prospective study of the 1966 northern Finland birth cohort. *American Journal of Psychiatry* **154**, 840–845.

Tran, E., Rouillon, F., Loze, J. *et al.* (2009) Cancer mortality in patients with schizophrenia: an 11 year prospective study. *Cancer* **115**, 3555–3562.

Turkington, D., Kingdon, D. & Turner, T. (2002) Effectiveness of a brief cognitive-behavioural therapy intervention in treatment of schizophrenia. *British Journal of Psychiatry* **180**, 523–527.

Volavka, J., Lasaka, E., Baker, S. *et al.* (1997) History of violent behaviour and schizophrenia in different cultures. Analyses based on the WHO study on Determinants of Outcome of Severe Mental Disorder. *British Journal of Psychiatry* **171**, 9–14.

Wallace, C., Mullen, P.E. & Burgess, P. (2004) Criminal offending in schizophrenia over a 25-year period marked by deinstitutionalization and increasing prevalence of comorbid substance use disorders. *American Journal of Psychiatry* **161**, 716–727.

Walsh, E., Harvey, K., White, I. *et al.* (2001) Suicidal behaviour in psychosis: prevalence and predictors from a randomised controlled trial of case management: report from the UK700 trial. *British Journal of Psychiatry* **178**, 255–260.

Walsh, E., Moran, P., Scott, C. *et al.* (2003) Prevalence of violent victimisation in severe mental illness. *British Journal of Psychiatry* **183**, 233–238.

Weinmann, S., Read, J. & Aderhold, V. (2009) Influence of antipsychotics on mortality in schizophrenia: Systematic review. *Schizophrenia Research* **113**, 1–11.

Wenzel, S., Koegel, P. & Gelberg, L. (2000) Antecendets of physical and sexual victimisation among homeless women: a comparison to homeless men. *American Journal of Community Psychology* **28**, 367–390.

Wewiorski, N.J. & Fabian, E.S. (2004) Association between demographic and diagnostic factors and employment outcomes for people with psychiatric disabilities: A synthesis of recent research. *Mental Health Services Research* **6**, 9–21.

Wong, S. & Gordon, A. (2000) *Violence Risk Scale*. Saskatoon: Regional Psychiatric Centre.

Wu, E., Birnbaum, H., Shi, L. *et al.* (2005) The economic burden of schizophrenia in the United States in 2002. *Journal of Clinical Psychiatry* **66**, 1122–1129.

Xiang, Y., Weng, Y., Leung, C. *et al.* (2008) Socio-demographic and clinical correlates of lifetime suicide attempts and their impact on quality of life in Chinese schizophrenia patients. *Journal of Psychiatric Research* **42**, 495–502.

CHAPTER 32

Psychological treatment of psychosis

Gillian Haddock[1] and Will Spaulding[2]

[1]University of Manchester, Manchester, UK
[2]University of Nebraska, Lincoln, NE, USA

Introduction

Psychological approaches in the management of mental health problems have become well established for many disorders throughout the developed world. For many disorders, for example, anxiety and depressive disorders, psychological treatments can be first line. Psychological treatment of psychotic disorders has received less attention in the literature, despite being utilized for many years. For example, Bleuler (1911/1950) advocated the use of psychotherapies with people with schizophrenia and this has been supported by a number of other clinicians over the 20th century (e.g., Beck, 1952; Sullivan, 1962). Aaron T. Beck, often described as the "father" of cognitive therapy, published a case study in 1952 describing a successful treat-

ment using psychological approaches of a young man with a delusional disorder. Since that time, there have been a large number of published reports on psychological treatments for psychosis. Initially these tended to be in the form of case study or case series reports rather than controlled trials. However, over the last 20–30 years, there has been a growing body of well carried out, controlled research describing and evaluating psychological treatments for psychosis, suggesting that these have an important place in the management of such disorders. In addition, government legislation is endorsing the use of psychological approaches in the management of psychosis, for example, the National Institute of Clinical Effectiveness (NICE, 2009) in the UK makes the following recommendations:
• Offer CBT to all people with schizophrenia;
• Offer family intervention to families of people with schizophrenia living with or in close contact with the service user;

Schizophrenia, 3rd edition. Edited by Daniel R. Weinberger and
Paul J Harrison © 2011 Blackwell Publishing Ltd.

• Consider offering arts therapies, particularly to help negative symptoms of schizophrenia;
• Start CBT, family intervention or arts therapies either during the acute phase or later, including in inpatient settings.

In the US, a renewed interest in psychological treatments is associated with the recovery movement, a growing consensus that recovery from mental illness must include more than suppression of symptoms. In 2004, a Presidential Commission (President's New Freedom Commission on Mental Health, 2004) sounded a keynote for this movement, setting in motion a massive reform of the federal mental health infrastructure, including the Veterans Administration (one of the largest healthcare organizations in the world) and the Substance Abuse and Mental Health Services Administration (SAMHSA). SAMHSA (2004) has developed a set of "toolkits", packaged materials for disseminating evidence-based treatment and rehabilitation modalities that are largely psychological in nature. The American Psychological Association's Task Force on Serious Mental Illness and Severe Emotional Disturbance (APA/CAPP, 2007) compiled a guide to evidence-based practices pertinent to schizophrenia and related disorders, along with resources for staff training and program development, composed primarily of psychological treatment approaches. In addition, the United States PORT (Patient Outcome Research Team; Dixon *et al.*, 2010) makes specific recommendations about the application of evidence-based psychological approaches for psychosis.

Psychodynamic treatment approaches in schizophrenia

Psychological interventions in psychosis have been influenced by a range of theoretical schools over the past 100 years, such as the psychoanalytical field, the literature on psychopathological processes in schizophrenia, and the behavioral school and learning theory. Psychoanalytical approaches to the treatment of psychosis have not been evaluated widely or systematically, and there is very little evidence that this type of approach can be helpful. Past reviewers of psychodynamic approaches have varied in their conclusions, with some authors suggesting that this type of approach has a place in the treatment of psychosis despite this conclusion being based on very little evidence (Huxley *et al.*, 2000). Other authors have concluded that psychodynamic psychotherapy is clearly not effective in schizophrenia and that it may possibly be unhelpful (Mueser & Berenbaum, 1990). Paley and Shapiro (2002), when discussing the relative merits of different types of therapy in the treatment of psychosis, argue that there may be an "equivalence paradox" in relation to outcome from therapy across disorders, i.e., that different therapies gen-

erally produce equivalent outcomes. They present this as support for the idea that different therapies, for example, psychodynamic psychotherapy, need more evaluation before discounting them as potential treatments for psychosis. However, given that there has been very little pilot evidence to suggest that psychodynamic psychotherapy is helpful in psychosis, there is no good rationale for large investments in evaluation of the approach, particularly as it is unlikely to offer any advantages over other, well-evaluated interventions that are already available (Tarrier *et al.*, 2002).

Due to the limited evidence base for many interventions and the findings that some approaches have limited applicability in this area, the rest of this chapter will focus on the areas where there is a good supporting evidence base. These fall under the following headings, to be discussed in turn:

1. Individual cognitive and behavioral therapies (CBTs) for psychosis;
2. Family interventions for psychosis;
3. Neuropsychological and cognitive remediation approaches;
4. Social skills training and integrated approaches;
5. Contingency management;
6. Dealing with comorbid disorders.

Individual cognitive and behavioral therapies for psychosis

One area that has received much attention in the psychological treatment of psychosis is the CBT approach. This approach has a long history of use in the treatment of psychotic disorders, highlighted by the case study by Beck in 1952 described above. Since that early case study, there has been a wealth of descriptions of interventions, usually focused on the remediation of particular psychotic symptoms, i.e., hallucinations, delusions or negative symptoms. Early approaches were influenced more by the strictly behavioral psychology school, such as the use of contingency or reward approaches for reducing the occurrence of particular target behaviors (Nydegger, 1972; Haynes & Geddy, 1973), distraction procedures (Margo *et al.*, 1981; James, 1983; Nelson *et al.*, 1991), thought stopping (Samaan, 1975; Allen *et al.*, 1983), and the use of aversion therapy (Alford & Turner, 1976; Turner *et al.*, 1977). Whilst successful reduction in the occurrence of target behaviors were frequently reported, there was little evaluation of this type of approach in larger controlled trials and little evidence that the approaches generalized across situations or people (see below, Contingency management). These approaches highlighted researchers' and clinicians' emphasis on the removal of psychotic symptoms and the notion that symptoms of psychosis were "ununderstandable" phenomena and were therefore not likely to respond to reason or discussion (Jaspers, 1963). However, this notion of the "ununderstandability" of psychotic symptoms has been much disputed by both psychopathology researchers and service users in recent years, resulting in a greater understanding of the development and maintenance of psychotic symptoms. For example, the application of effective techniques to help individuals test out the reality of delusional beliefs (e.g., Chadwick & Lowe, 1990) has demonstrated that, contrary to Jaspers' earlier assertion, these beliefs do indeed respond to reason and are often understandable when considered in relation to the individual's beliefs and life experiences (Garety & Hemsley, 1997). In addition, the growing interest in "talking" therapies for the treatment of other disorders, e.g., cognitive therapy for anxiety and depression, as well as the greater interest in understanding the nature of particular psychotic symptoms, led to the development of psychological approaches that involved exploring and treating psychotic phenomena in one-to-one talking therapies. This heralded the development of CBTs for psychotic disorders which lent themselves well to evaluation in controlled trials of their effectiveness. CBT has been applied to all phases of the disorder, i.e., acute and recent-onset psychosis (Lewis *et al.*, 2002; Garety *et al.*, 2007), and chronic and treatment-resistant psychosis (Tarrier *et al.*, 1998; Sensky *et al.*, 2000). In addition, CBT has also been shown to be effective at reducing the transition to full-blown psychosis in those people experiencing prepsychotic or high risk for psychosis states (Morrison *et al.*, 2004), and has been used with people who are experiencing comorbid or dual disorders (see below) and to increase adherence to antipsychotic medication (Kemp *et al.*, 1996).

Cognitive–behavioral therapy treatment program

CBT is a one-to-one therapy, carried out in a collaborative fashion led by a shared agenda agreed between the therapist and individual. The approach assumes that the key problems of the client or patient develop and are maintained by cognitive (thoughts and beliefs), physiological (emotional reactions), and behavioral factors, and that these factors can be modified and influenced using psychological means. The therapy is individualized to the person's needs, although it usually contains some basic, common elements. Therapy typically lasts for between 12 and 30 sessions (although this may need to be longer for some individuals) over a period of 6–12 months. Therapy sessions would usually last for between 30 and 60 min, although flexibility is required to ensure that the session length is matched to the individual's concentration and other cognitive abilities. Therapy tends to consist of four main stages: (1) engagement and socialization into the model; (2) assessment and formulation of key problems;

(3) intervention strategies to reduce severity and distress; and (4) consolidation and generalization of the benefits and strategies to enhance staying well.

Engagement and socialization to the model

The nature of CBT is collaborative and based on a shared agenda between the therapist and individual. As a result, the first part of therapy involves engaging the individual. This phase is crucial to being able to use the approach and is likely to vary from person to person. Many people are keen and interested to engage in an approach which encourages them to discuss and reflect on their psychotic experiences; other therapeutic approaches that they have experienced may have discouraged or even provided negative feedback for doing so. Other individuals may be more skeptical of talking therapies or their symptoms may interfere with their ability to engage. For example, some psychotic experiences may considerably influence an individual's cognitive functioning such that they are unable to concentrate for more than a few moments, or the severity or intrusiveness of their symptoms interferes with their ability to engage in the interpersonal relationships required in therapy, in which case they may be more likely to benefit at a later stage. Nevertheless, there is evidence that people with psychosis can engage in CBT regardless of the stage of illness or the acuteness of their symptoms, so no assumptions should be made about who would be most likely to engage. Several strategies can be taken to maximize the possibility of engagement, such as being cognisant of the cognitive processing difficulties the patient may be experiencing, by being aware of where delusional or other psychotic beliefs may be influencing the person's ability to engage, and by being aware of the possible mismatch between therapist and patient as to whether treatment using this approach is either helpful or necessary. Specific therapeutic strategies can assist with the engagement process. For example, where cognitive processing of information is a problem, the sessions should be short and frequent, and contain multiple summaries to ensure the individual is able to process the information. Where the patient does not recognize the need for, or importance of, treatment, motivational interviewing strategies (Miller & Rollnick, 2002; see also below Comorbid disorders) may be helpful to clarify the patient's key values and goals. This may lead to recognition as to how therapy may help them to realize those goals. This type of approach can also be helpful in addressing issues relating to motivation to adhere to medication and to address problems with substance use (see below).

Until an individual is fully engaged, it is unlikely to be helpful to persist with therapy. A key marker for moving into the assessment phase is when the therapist is aware that the patient is willing to continue with therapy and has identified some key, shared problems and goals to work on in therapy. This will then provide the basis for future therapy sessions.

Assessment and formulation of key problems

These sessions typically involve a therapist assessing and gaining an understanding of the individual's main problems. This may take one or more sessions (typically three to four). It culminates in the therapist and individual producing a shared formulation of the key problems. These are described in relation to the way they have developed and are being maintained in relation to the individual's key thinking patterns and beliefs (cognition), emotional responses, and behavior patterns.

Assessment approaches

The use of assessment tools in psychosis is often, largely, for diagnostic purposes, aimed at eliciting and measuring symptoms in terms of their presence, absence or severity, i.e., different dimensions have been aggregated into a global, unidimensional representation of "severity" (e.g., the Brief Psychiatric Rating Scale; Overall & Gorham, 1962). This type of assessment has been driven by the degree of information which is necessary to establish diagnosis in relation to prescribing drug treatment rather than psychological interventions. CBTs may be directed towards individuals who have a similar diagnosis, such as schizophrenia, but are not generally directed towards treating the whole "syndrome". CBT is usually aimed at eliciting the symptoms associated with a particular diagnosis and assessing the behavioral and cognitive correlates of these symptoms. It is then towards these correlates that treatment is directed. As a result, although diagnostic instruments can be invaluable in improving reliability in diagnosis and for eliciting symptoms, they are not primarily designed to provide sufficient information for cognitive–behavioral therapists to formulate patient's key problems. Nevertheless, these types of instruments can be invaluable as a starting point in therapy.

Instruments which elicit symptoms

As psychotic patients present with multiple and complex problems, a thorough assessment of a range of potential problem areas, in addition to the key psychotic symptoms, is often helpful. Eliciting information on non-psychotic symptoms is important as these may interact with, and impact on, the occurrence of the psychotic symptoms. This can help clinicians and patients to prioritize problems and to ensure that CBT is being applied to other psychotic symptoms appropriately. Instruments such as the Present State Examination (PSE; Wing *et al.*, 1974) can be used to elicit symptoms and rating scales, such as the Positive and Negative Syndrome Scale (PANSS; Kay *et al.*, 1989), can be used to rate the severity of the symptoms. This can provide

a starting point around which a further analysis of the individual experiences can be assessed.

Instruments which measure the severity of the dimensions of psychotic symptoms

Despite the above scales being invaluable as tools to assist clinicians in the early stages of engagement, they are not sufficiently specific to tell us anything about the nature of the individual dimensions of symptoms and how they covary as a result of treatment. This is necessary in CBT to provide information to assist with generating the formulation, but also as a tool for monitoring outcome. For example, a patient who experiences a reduction in the distress caused by their hallucinations as a result of treatment may not show a concurrent change in their frequency or duration; therefore, the improvement will not be picked up on measures of severity such as the Brief Psychiatric Rating Scale (BPRS). This is essential in CBT where treatment might be directed towards reducing the distress or other dimensions associated with a particular symptom rather than at removing or reducing the occurrence or frequency of a symptom. For some people, feeling more positive about the future or being in control of their symptoms is viewed as a good outcome from therapy, and complete removal of the symptom may not be their priority. Scales are available which have been developed to measure the severity of a number of different dimensions of auditory hallucinations and delusions (Psychotic Symptom Rating Scales; PSYRATS; Haddock *et al.*, 1999). Thirteen dimensions of auditory hallucinations (frequency, duration, amount of distress, intensity of distress, location, conviction of beliefs regarding origin, disruption, controllability, loudness, amount of negative content, degree of negative content, number, form) and six dimensions of delusions (amount of preoccupation, duration of preoccupation, amount of distress, intensity of distress, conviction, disruption) are elicited and rated by an interviewer on a five-point scale which has specified anchor points. This type of instrument can be used at the beginning, during, and following treatment to track changes in dimensions over time and to assess specific changes in individual dimensions.

Instruments for carrying out a cognitive–behavioral analysis of symptoms

Instruments as described above allow us to monitor changes in symptoms over time but they are not sufficient to help a therapist to gain a detailed understanding of the variables which are contributing to the occurrence and maintenance of a symptom. This is essential to achieve a working formulation which will direct a psychological intervention. Structured interviews such as the Maudsley Assessment of Delusions Schedule (MADS; Buchanan, 1997) and the Antecedent and Coping Interview (ACI; Tarrier, 1994) are designed to achieve this. For example, the

MADS is a structured interview which is designed to elicit information from the patient about their delusions in terms of a large number of different variables, e.g., the degree of conviction, the behaviors associated with the belief, the evidence which the patient holds which contributes to their conviction, etc. The ACI is a structured interview designed to elicit the behavioral and cognitive antecedents and consequences associated with a symptom. For example, a delusional belief may be maintained by the types of behavior which the patient engages in. A paranoid patient may engage in continual searching for evidence which will confirm their belief that the whole world is against them and ignore disconfirmatory evidence. A detailed analysis of this is required to provide the basis for intervention, which might involve helping the patient to change their interpretation of behavioral evidence.

The above structure can contribute to an overall assessment with a patient, but this also must be carried out in the context of a general assessment of other important need areas. Most patients who have a psychotic illness have multiple needs and it is important to fully assess all areas before intervening with psychotic symptoms. For example, many patients with psychotic symptoms are depressed or anxious (Tarrier, 1987) or are suicidal (Falloon & Talbot, 1981), and these non-psychotic symptoms must be taken into account as removal of psychotic symptoms (especially if they are of a grandiose nature) may be detrimental for a patient if this results in a further increase in depression or anxiety. Likewise, some patients have symptoms which form an important part of their life, e.g., supportive or comforting voices, and their removal may have a negative impact. This is not to say that this person cannot be helped to improve their functioning, but that the focus for intervention may be to enhance that person's access to other support before intervening directly with the symptoms (Yusupoff & Haddock, 1998).

More detailed ratings scales and monitoring tools can be used to explore hypotheses generated by a formulation. For example, initial assessment may reveal that one person's voices appear to be associated with certain types of interactions or events. It may be useful to get the patient to concurrently monitor these types of situations by recording the antecedent and consequential events surrounding a symptom occurring in terms of behavioral, physiological, and cognitive factors. This may help the therapist and patient gain a clear idea of the types of thoughts and emotions which are contributing to symptom occurrence or worsening, and provide an ideal place for intervention. These types of ratings or diaries can be kept by the patient and be made as simple or as complex as appropriate. They may also be an essential part of a treatment intervention, e.g., a patient who expresses paranoid beliefs may utilize this type of monitoring tool to keep a record of the types of evidence collected during times when the belief is held most strongly. This may then be reviewed during therapy sessions.

Monitoring tools may also play an important part in intervention with patients experiencing auditory hallucinations; for example, it has been noted that concurrent monitoring of these types of symptoms may reduce their severity (Haddock *et al.*, 1993). In addition, focusing on the nature of auditory hallucinations may reduce the distress associated with them (i.e., serve a desensitization purpose) and help some patients to explore the content, their respondent thoughts and feelings, as well as explore the patient's underlying beliefs which can add to the distress associated with voices (Chadwick & Birchwood, 1994). Strategies which can aid this type of focusing approach have been described in detail by Haddock and colleagues (Bentall *et al.*, 1994; Haddock *et al.*, 1996), and are designed to help patients to concurrently monitor their voices by gradually exposing themselves to increasingly emotive aspects of them. Monitoring begins by asking the patient to monitor only the physical characteristics of their voices. When the patient feels comfortable with this, they can then move on to monitoring the content and their resultant thoughts, and to focus on the beliefs which are activated as a result of the voices. Verbal and written shadowing (immediately repeating the content out loud or writing it down) can aid focusing on voice content and thoughts, and help the patient to discuss their voices without becoming aroused or distressed.

Assessment is an essential part of treatment for people experiencing psychotic symptoms, and as outlined above, this can form an important component of the therapy itself. As a result, initial assessment may take a number of sessions and some assessment will be ongoing throughout the intervention. Once assessment material is collected, intervention can be informed by a working formulation of the patient's difficulties. This formulation will guide the intervention and help therapist and patient to decide on the priorities for treatment.

Formulation

There are a number of underlying assumptions which should be borne in mind when attempting to formulate an individual's key problems. These apply in psychosis as much as in other disorders. They are: (1) a person's mood/symptoms/problems are affected by their cognitions and beliefs; (2) those cognitions and beliefs are modifiable; and (3) modifying cognitions and beliefs will result in modified symptoms. These assumptions should underpin all of the assessment work which leads towards a preliminary formulation to be shared between therapist and client.

An accurate and concise description of the main symptoms or problems should be made in terms of the presenting symptoms, the related key cognitions, affect, behavior, and specific and general beliefs. This should highlight how the individual's thoughts, feelings, and behaviors may have interacted to contribute to the maintenance and development of symptoms or problems, and how these may be targeted using CBT. This formulation is then used to guide the direction and content of therapy. If possible, this should be generated collaboratively as a summary and reflection of the information that has been elicited and collected during assessment. The impact of presenting the formulation and the complexity required should be considered in advance and should take account of the individual's needs and cognitive ability. For some people, a simple summary of their main problem areas is sufficient. For others, a more complex model can be presented. It is often easier to add to the formulation later rather than present something complex initially. The formulation should be prepared in a way that is easily understandable and can be prepared in a written as well as a verbal form. Written material is useful to allow both therapist and individual to have a record of what has been discussed in therapy. It also encourages feedback and potential for modification. Audio recordings of sessions are also useful and can be used by therapists and individuals to listen to between sessions and/or to keep as a record.

The formulation should be refined and modified, in negotiation with the patient and in the light of evidence. This may be an ongoing process throughout therapy. For some people, the initial part of the intervention process may relate to helping them to generate evidence which supports the formulation. This can serve to highlight how cognitions are affecting behavior and mood, and to help them to pinpoint how particular interventions might be useful. For example, an individual may agree that the formulation reflects certain aspects of their difficulties but believe that it does not account for some occurrences of the problem or that there are parts of the formulation which do not quite fit. The therapist and client can then generate homework tasks designed to test out the formulation in the light of events which occur between sessions. This process helps the client to fine-tune the formulation and to increase their motivation for change.

Figure 32.1 illustrates an example of a formulation of an individual (James) whose main problem relates to hearing derogatory and abusive voices. The formulation highlights how recurrent conflict with his partner increases James's arousal levels and results in intense physical anxiety symptoms and worries which have themes of "inadequacy", "hopelessness", and "fear of being abandoned". These thoughts tend to trigger an exacerbation of voice hearing which he believes are external spirits that are helping him. The "spirits" endorse and confirm the accuracy of his negative thoughts and encourage him to "give up on life by taking an overdose". In the past he had taken an overdose to try to escape from his distress. He is often tempted to do this again as he believes it is his only way out of his torment,

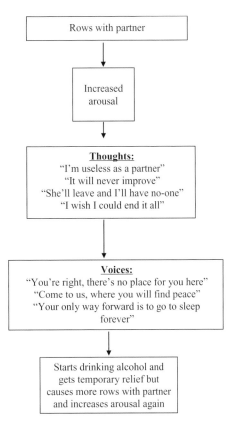

Fig. 32.1 Formulation of "James".

but is stopped by his strong religious belief that the taking of his life is a mortal sin. His most common way of dealing with his anxieties and voices is to drink. This blocks out his worries temporarily but ultimately results in more conflict with his partner and failure to address and challenge his beliefs about his inadequacy, hopelessness, and being abandoned. The formulation highlights how his thinking and behavior contribute to his ongoing problems and suggests that changes in some of these areas may reduce the distress and disruption caused by his voices. For example, James became aware that his alcohol use was actually worsening his situation by reinforcing both his and his partner's views that he could not cope or that he was inadequate. In addition, he was able to notice that his thoughts about himself were very negative and that there may be some virtue in challenging and assessing how accurately these reflected his true self. This also led to the realization that the voices were "extensions of his own thinking" and that by changing the way he thought about himself, he could reduce the strength and impact of the voice content, i.e., if he did not agree with what the voices were saying, he was not so bothered about them being there.

Intervention strategies

Using the information recorded in the formulation, appropriate targets or goals should be prioritized for intervention collaboratively. These should usually be explicit, although it is possible that there may be instances when the therapist may have different or additional goals from the client. The potential outcome of implementing a particular intervention or strategy should be assessed in terms of positive and negative consequences with reference to the formulation. The interventions should be selected in terms of the degree of expected effectiveness with respect to the particular problem area targeted, but should also take into account the client's motivation and ability, and the achievability of the goal. In addition, safety and risk factors should be considered at all times. In the absence of life-threatening difficulties, the initial goals are likely to be focused on symptom reduction or the modification of coping strategies. Underlying core and long-standing beliefs and behavior patterns influencing current problems may to be tackled at a later stage, if appropriate, though there are instances when interventions might be concurrently targeted upon these areas.

Interventions should be directly related to addressing goals which are pin-pointed in the formulation and are likely to cover the following areas: delusions, hallucinations, anxiety, depression, suicide, relapse prevention/ keeping well, schemas, coping strategies, negative symptoms, and medication compliance. However, this list is not exhaustive and interventions may vary considerably from individual to individual.

Commonly used cognitive–behavioral intervention techniques include: ongoing monitoring of key cognitions, behaviors, and feelings, strategies to test out delusional or core beliefs (e.g., behavioral experiments), strategies to challenge and modify negative thoughts, strategies to enhance coping, developing helpful distraction strategies, and motivational work to increase desire to take helpful medication. These approaches will be used collaboratively and will aim to reduce the distress and disruption of the individual's symptoms. They may not result in removal of the symptoms, although for some people this is an outcome from therapy.

Generalization

A key part of a psychological intervention is to ensure that the approaches worked on in therapy generalize beyond the end of therapy and that techniques and strategies used with the therapist can be used by the individual on their own. This can be facilitated by therapist and client developing a keeping well strategy during or at the end of therapy. The aims of this are to help the individual to:
1. Keep as well as possible and to continue to implement helpful strategies;
2. Monitor and detect when things might not be going so well;
3. Have an action plan that enables them to implement strategies to overcome difficult times or situations.

There are a number of ways that this can be achieved. The following example provides a guide to how this can be achieved for an individual.

Example: A guide to staying well. It can be helpful to put together a keeping well plan with your therapist. This may help you to maintain the gains you have made in therapy and help you to keep well in the future. A good place to start is by asking yourself the following questions. You may also want to discuss this with your therapist. Each person is different and individual so not all of the suggestions will apply to you. It's possible that none of them suits you, so please add your own personal suggestions so that you can create your own Keeping Well Manual.
1. *What things have helped me to feel better and overcome my problems? (e.g., relationships, talking over my problems, changing my drinking or eating habits, managing my negative thoughts, challenging my paranoia, etc.)*
2. *What things should I avoid because they are not helpful or make things worse? (e.g., stressful situations, particular people, using drugs, etc.)*
Once you have a good idea of the things that are helpful/ should be avoided, you can start to build up a plan to ensure that you have plans or strategies in place to deal with any future problems. Some people find it useful to put together a folder with useful tips and information that has been discussed in therapy. Some people might file things under the following headings.
1. *The things that keep me well.*
2. *How do I keep a check that things are going OK?*
3. *How do I know when things are starting to deteriorate and what shall I do if I notice this?*
4. *What to do if things get really bad?*

Some people use a personal "traffic light" system to help them to see easily how things need to be/what they should be doing when they are well (green), how they are when things are not so good (amber), and how they are when things have become really bad (red). Figure 32.2 shows an example of this. This way of doing it will not suit everyone; you might want to come up with other strategies or you might find that just going through the above is sufficient.

Ensuring treatment addresses the phase of illness and the individual's developmental needs

The nature of a psychotic illness for many people is that it is long lasting and pervades all areas of their life. The way it influences an individual may be very dependent on their developmental stage. For example, the therapeutic needs of an adolescent experiencing a first episode of psychosis may be very different from that of an older adult who has experienced treatment-resistant symptoms for many years. A number of treatment programs have been developed to meet the needs of the early psychosis group, indicating that it is possible and beneficial to engage young people at very early stages of illness. Indeed, some programs have focused

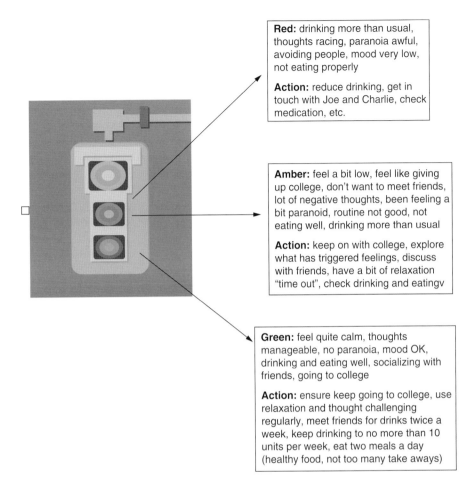

Red: drinking more than usual, thoughts racing, paranoia awful, avoiding people, mood very low, not eating properly

Action: reduce drinking, get in touch with Joe and Charlie, check medication, etc.

Amber: feel a bit low, feel like giving up college, don't want to meet friends, lot of negative thoughts, been feeling a bit paranoid, routine not good, not eating well, drinking more than usual

Action: keep on with college, explore what has triggered feelings, discuss with friends, have a bit of relaxation "time out", check drinking and eatingv

Green: feel quite calm, thoughts manageable, no paranoia, mood OK, drinking and eating well, socializing with friends, going to college

Action: ensure keep going to college, use relaxation and thought challenging regularly, meet friends for drinks twice a week, keep drinking to no more than 10 units per week, eat two meals a day (healthy food, not too many take aways)

Fig. 32.2 Keeping well traffic light.

on engaging those people who are displaying at-risk signs of developing psychosis but who have not yet gone on to develop full-blown psychosis (see Chapter 6). For example, Morrison *et al.* (2004) carried out CBT with a sample of "at-risk" individuals and demonstrated that this could reduce the conversion rate to psychosis. Specific topics that may be particularly pertinent are developmental issues, familial issues, issues in relation to the change from school to university or work, and use of alcohol and cannabis.

Evaluations of the effectiveness of individual cognitive–behavioral therapies

Individual CBT has been subject to much evaluation in controlled and uncontrolled trials. Several trials have demonstrated the superiority of CBT over control treatments and treatment as usual (usually antipsychotic medication and care/case management approaches; see Rector & Beck, 2004; Pfammatter *et al.*, 2006; Jones *et al.*, 2007; Wykes *et al.*, 2008 for reviews). Conclusions differ slightly, probably as a result of the different samples and types of intervention studied. However, it is notable that in a recent meta-analysis, which concluded that CBT consistently showed superiority over control treatments, with an overall mean

weighted effect size, taken from 33 studies, of 0.4, the effect size reduced in proportion to the quality of the methodology employed in the studies (Wykes *et al.*, 2008).

Family interventions for psychosis

A substantial amount of research has demonstrated that providing family interventions can significantly reduce relapse rates of people with psychosis over follow-up periods (Pfammatter *et al.*, 2006; Pharoah *et al.*, 2006). Family interventions are based on the assumption that a stressful interpersonal environment in which an individual lives can exacerbate psychotic symptoms and lead to premature or more frequent relapse of illness. This type of stressful environment is often referred to as being high in "expressed emotion (EE)". This term was first described in relation to families by Brown *et al.*, (1962) following observations that people with schizophrenia who were discharged from hospital to live with parents or close family fared worse than those who lived alone or in hostel accommodation. Brown and colleagues developed a measure of EE that could be used to assess the emotional climate in an individual's home environment. It is characterized as one in which the interpersonal environment is high in critical comments, hostility, and emotional over-involvement. Research showed that those individuals living in environments scoring high on a measure of high EE resulted in significantly higher relapse rates for the individual with schizophrenia than those in low-EE environments (Brown *et al.*, 1962, Vaughn & Leff, 1976). This finding has now been replicated many times in different settings and in different populations. This type of environment is not thought to be a result of relatives or carers deliberately critical or hostile towards their relative. On the contrary, this behavior is generally considered to be a result of a normal reaction to the incredible stress associated with experiencing a relative who has a psychotic illness. For example, it has been shown that relatives who demonstrate high levels of criticism for their relative's behavior often believe that by doing so, they are assisting their relative to get back to their normal premorbid level of functioning (Barrowclough & Hooley, 2003). Those relatives who display high levels of emotional over-involvement have been shown to hold beliefs that their relative's require a high degree of assistance and help to function and that they need to provide this, often at the expense of their own psychosocial functioning.

Family intervention treatment programs

A number of different family approaches have been evaluated (see Pharoah *et al.*, 2006 for review) and although they may differ in the techniques employed, they tend to be cognitive–behavioral in their underpinning therapeutic model and have major aspects in common. They usually focus on attempting to improve the interpersonal environment by providing the following key elements: (1) assessment and problem formulation (as with CBT above); (2) information about the nature of the illness, its prognosis, and treatment; and (3) intervention and problem-solving strategies to address areas of conflict and concern, and goal setting to improve social and interpersonal functioning of all family members.

Family interventions can involve close family members and carers and may also be effective with staff groups for people living in inpatient environments (Oliver & Kuipers, 1996). Interventions are often delivered with single families, although those delivered to groups of families simultaneously have also been shown to be effective (McFarlane *et al.*, 1995). There is no limit to the numbers of family members that can be engaged in the approach, although for practical reasons it is often limited to those living in closest contact with the individual, such as parents, partners, brothers, and sisters. Family interventions typically last for between 6 and 12 months, with sessions weekly or fortnightly. The meetings are flexible with some sessions taking place as a family group with the individual, some with relatives alone, and others with the individual alone.

The exact nature of the sessions will depend on what is collaboratively agreed between all parties during the earlier assessment and formulation sessions. As the approach is collaborative, agreement from all parties as to what takes place is important within the confines of each stage. Further details of these stages are outlined below. However, as many of the principles of family intervention are similar to those required for individual CBT, a detailed description of the characteristics and principles of treatment will not be repeated here.

Assessment of key problems

As each family's needs and problems will be unique to their situation, careful assessment about the nature of these is essential before proceeding to intervene. This may involve meeting with key relatives separately to gain the perspective on their situation, view of their relative's problems, and their own mental health. Structured interviews and questionnaires can be used to assist with this process, e.g., the Relative's Assessment Interview and Knowledge about Schizophrenia Interview (Barrowclough & Tarrier, 1992) and General Health Questionnaire (Goldberg & Williams, 1988).

Information about the nature of the illness, its prognosis, and treatment

Helping relatives and sufferers to gain correct information and understanding about the nature of the psychotic illness, the causes, prognosis, and treatment is often very important and can help correct erroneous beliefs that may have been driving relatives' behavior and can help with the discovery and implementation of more helpful behaviors. It can also reduce the distress and allay any fears that have arisen from erroneous mythical or media sources. It is helpful if information provision is delivered in a way that is "tailored" to the needs of the family members. For example, some people will hold erroneous beliefs about cause of their relative's illness that is making them behave in a way that is not helpful. Believing that their relative's illness is a disability that results in the individual not being able to care for themselves could result in a concerned carer trying hard to provide as much support for their relative as possible. Whilst this is driven by good intentions, this may be at the expense of their needs or mental health, and may actually be unhelpful for their relative as well. It can be useful to specifically target these types of erroneous beliefs when providing information in order that the relative can target their caring efforts more effectively.

Intervention strategies to address areas of conflict and concern, set individual and family goals, and improve functioning

Specific intervention strategies will depend on the needs of the individual patient and their family; however, some common elements are usually involved. For example, most interventions will provide strategies to assist patients and carers to set realistic and achievable goals and provide assistance in achieving these with the intention of improving functioning of family members and patients. Some approaches will include strategies to assist with managing unpleasant affect, distress, and symptoms. Action plans are often used to assist relatives to monitor and detect early signs of relapse and to provide a plan of action should any family member become aware of early signs of relapse. The family intervention may also be delivered in tandem with individual CBT for family members and patients where necessary to deal with any individual problems (see Barrowclough & Tarrier, 1992; Falloon, 1985; Mueser & Glynn, 1995; Kuipers *et al.*, 2002 for detailed descriptions of interventions).

Effectiveness

Family interventions have been rigorously evaluated, indicating consistent superiority of the approach compared to treatment as usual on relapse rates (Pfammatter *et al.*, 2006) with replications in many parts of the world including Eastern and developing countries (Xiong *et al.*, 1994). Recent meta-analyses have varied somewhat in their conclusions, but the recently updated Cochrane systematic review (Pharoah *et al.*, 2006) concluded that family interventions in schizophrenia can reduce the frequency of relapse, reduce hospital admission, and increase adherence to medication.

Neuropsychological and cognitive remediation approaches

In addition to the developments in therapy for people with schizophrenia in individual CBT and family intervention, there have been parallel developments in the neuropsychological domain. Beginning in the 1970s, a set of techniques and supporting principles has evolved that extends the cognitive–behavioral armamentarium for schizophrenia to the neuropsychological level. Not coincidentally, this paralleled the emergence of the hypothesis that schizophrenia is, among other things, a *neurocognitive disorder* (e.g., Green, 1998; see Chapter 8). It is increasingly clear that neurocognitive impairment plays an important role in vulnerability to schizophrenia (e.g., Walker, 1994) and in its course and outcome (e.g. Green, 1996). Neurocognitive impairment compromises social functioning and response to rehabilitation in the short term (Penn *et al.*, 1992, 1993; 1995, 1996); and global recovery in the long term (Green, 1996). The effectiveness of antipsychotic drugs in treating neurocognitive impairment has been generally disappointing. These findings stimulate the hypothesis that psychological approaches to reducing or eliminating neurocognitive impairments might be helpful.

Clinical procedures for assessment and treatment of neurocognitive impairment draw heavily from work in the clinical neuropsychology and experimental psychopathology of psychotic disorders. They are also heavily influenced by familiar principles of CBT as described above. These include the need to quantify and monitor the target of treatment, the need for well-defined and manualized procedures, the need for outcome criteria that reflect significant behavioral dimensions of personal and social functioning, and the importance of scientific support for clinical effectiveness.

Definition of the approach

There is no universally accepted title for this set of techniques and related research. The term *cognitive remediation* often appears in the literature, but is met with the objection that there is no evidence that something gets "remediated" in the course of treatment. *Cognitive therapy* avoids the connotation of a hypothetical treatment mechanism, but does not distinguish from the familiar schematic therapy model described above. *Neuropsychological therapy* is more descriptive, but not widely used, perhaps because of potentially misleading connotations of "neuropsychological". *Neurocognitive therapy* avoids the connotations of "neuropsychological", but does not fully describe the principles involved or the range of techniques. "Rehabilitation" appears interchangeably with "therapy". Arguably, *CBT for neuropsychological functioning* best describes most of the techniques, but many are very different from conventional CBT.

Terminology aside, the common primary principle is that personal and social functioning can be improved by strengthening impaired cognitive processes that normally support that functioning. This is distinct from the CBT principle underpinning the approaches described in the earlier section above, i.e., that behavior change is facilitated by changes in cognition. CBT mostly involves manipulation of declarative and procedural information structures, such as beliefs, attributions, and self-regulation skills. The processes that support or operate upon those structures (perception, attention, memory, etc.) are usually assumed to be more-or-less intact (although CBT does include some manipulation of processes as well as content, and in this sense the two approaches overlap somewhat). In CBT for neuropsychological functioning those processes are known or assumed to be impaired and are therefore the targets of treatment. For the purposes of this chapter, the rhetorically economical and reasonably descriptive term neuropsychological therapy (NPT) will be used to describe the approach.

Neuropsychological therapy: a description of the approach

In practice, NPT consists of therapeutic exercises in which the patient performs tasks that require use of the cognitive processes being treated. The tasks are generally derived from neuropsychological and psychopathological tests that measure those processes. The cognitive constructs reflected in these tasks fall mostly under the categories of attention and executive functioning, e.g., vigilance for signal events, continuous performance of simple motor behaviors, resistance to distraction, concept formation, working memory, and problem solving. The tasks are performed in a range of formats, ranging from dyadic therapy (comparable to the dyadic format in conventional CBT) to group therapy (also comparable to CBT group formats) to occupational/vocational formats (such as used in day programs and therapeutic industrial workshops). The treatment protocol is usually designed to first establish normal performance with simple versions of a task, and then gradually add complications to approximate performance demands in more real-life circumstances. Accordingly, the key outcome measures shift as treatment proceeds, from performance on laboratory tasks or in group therapy exercises to performance of meaningful activities in natural environments. In comprehensive psychiatric rehabilitation programs, there is a natural segue from NPT to social skills training and related modalities (discussed below).

Many NPT exercises have been computerized. These generally resemble comparable tasks developed for rehabilitation following traumatic brain injury, and in fact the latter are often used in cognitive remediation for schizophrenia and related disorders.

The therapist's role in NPT is generally to introduce and explain the tasks, and in some cases provide various kinds of assistance. Assistance ranges from simple social reinforcement (encouragement) to prompting specific behaviors (e.g. "pay attention to the screen") to more complex coaching protocols. Coaching often includes prompting "self-talk" comparable to self-talk techniques of conventional CBT (e.g., Meichenbaum, 1969; Meichenbaum & Cameron, 1973). Coaching may also include procedures intended to help the patient develop a *meta-cognitive* perspective on the task, i.e., analyzing the cognitive abilities and strategies required for task performance, and then using that information to self-prompt acquisition and/or activation of those abilities and strategies. Also, as in conventional self-talk approaches, the therapist prompts self-reinforcement, and as in modern CBT, reinforces the patient's sense of mastery and consequent benefits to self-esteem. The therapist also monitors and evaluates progress. Depending on the particular approach and on individual patient needs, the therapist makes ongoing decisions about adjusting task difficulty or moving on to other exercises.

A few examples are described here to show the range of specific procedures included under the rubric of NPT:

A simple non-verbal vigilance exercise. The patient watches a computer screen showing changing geometric shapes of varying colors. When the colors of two of the figures match, the patient is to respond by pressing a button. This type of task can be made into a working memory exercise by adding more complex stimuli and response contingencies (e.g., "press the button when you see a square preceded by two triangles").

A group-format concept abstraction exercise. A group of patients is dealt special cards that include various combinations of shapes, numbers, and colors. In turn, the group members identify different ways to organize and categorize the cards, and then physically sort them accordingly (neuropsychologists recognize this as an exercise version of the familiar Wisconsin Card Sorting Task).

An attention-focusing distraction resistance task. A patient listens for target words played over earphones to one ear while ignoring various kinds of audio distraction played to the other ear.

An interpersonal verbal perception, concept abstraction, and working memory task. The patient listens to declarative statements and brief narratives spoken by a group partner, then repeats, first verbatim and later for conceptual content.

A group-format concept formation/problem-solving exercise. A group of patients engages in the familiar parlor game "20 questions" with coaching by the therapist that emphasizes use of logical, systematic questioning strategies instead of random guesses.

A social schematization exercise. A group of patients systematically analyzes the stimulus features and then the thematic content of a picture of a complex social situation, while the therapist coaches toward complete and accurate perception and avoiding unwarranted inferences.

It is increasingly practical to implement NPT in real-world clinical settings. Manuals, training materials, and program development consultation are available from a number of the research groups working in this area (Hogarty & Flesher, 1999a,b; Wykes & Reeder, 2005; Brenner *et al.*, 1994; APA/CAPP Task Force, 2007). In some venues NPT is acknowledged and reimbursed as an evidence-based practice for people with chronic psychotic disorders, and this is expected to increase as the technology is further disseminated.

There is a closely related but different approach, *attention shaping* (Silverstein *et al.*, 2000, 2009). Attention shaping is an operant learning procedure, wherein patients in conventional psychoeducational or skill training groups are systematically reinforced with tokens, on a moment-to-moment basis, for engaging in the training process. In contrast to NPT, attention shaping does not rely on cognitive or neuropsychological constructs. The target behavior is behavioral attending (eye contact, attentive posture, etc.) and participation in the group activity. Attention shaping does share an important proximal outcome dimension with NPT, improved performance in psychoeducation, skill training, and related rehabilitation modalities.

Another closely related approach, *errorless learning* (O'Carroll *et al.*, 1999; Kern *et al.*, 2002, 2005), uses learning principles to enhance acquisition of key skills. These skills include elemental abilities such as repeatedly performing work tasks (e.g., as needed in assembly line-type work). However, as with attention shaping, the mechanism of the treatment effect is assumed to be the enhancement of normal learning, not enhancement of impaired cognitive processes.

Outcome research methodology and evidence base

Although a number of randomized controlled trials and meta-analyses (Twamley *et al.*, 2003; Kurtz *et al.*, 2001; Pfammatter *et al.*, 2006; McGurk *et al.*, 2008) support the effectiveness of NPT, its effectiveness is not beyond question. One meta-analysis (Pilling *et al.*, 2002) concluded there are no beneficial effects on ecologically important dimensions of personal or social functioning, although this analysis included a very limited number of original studies. The ambiguity in the findings stems partly from inconsistent and ambiguous definitions of NPT (or whatever else it might be called). The authors of one meta-analysis (Twamley *et al.*, 2003) noted that the techniques they analyzed fell into at least four logically distinct categories. Similarly, outcome measures are diverse and have varying degrees of *a priori* ecological validity (the degree to which the measure has obvious relevance to real-life functioning). Nevertheless, combining all in a single analysis, they computed small-to-medium effect sizes. Considering the heterogeneity of the techniques and outcome measures, a small to medium effect size is quite promising, and probably a conservative estimate of effectiveness when tailored to individual patients with particular profiles of cognitive impairment, or to specific purposes.

Generally, the evidence on cognitive remediation is strongest in demonstrating that people with schizophrenia and related disorders can improve performance on the particular abilities that are exercised in treatment. Although this has limited implications for overall recovery, it is a key research finding. Much skepticism toward NPT is based on the presumption that neuropsychological or neurocognitive impairments in schizophrenia are permanent and immutable. The research evidence also strongly supports effective enhancement of patients' response to other rehabilitation modalities, e.g., social skills training and occupational/vocational programs. There is insufficient evidence concerning highly generalized benefits, e.g.,

improved interpersonal functioning, self-esteem or quality of life. Unless such benefits can be demonstrated independent of other treatments, cognitive remediation will likely become recognized as a useful, sometimes crucial, component of more comprehensive psychiatric rehabilitation, rather than as a stand-alone treatment approach.

One unexpected methodological complication in NPT research is the possible relevance of non-specific treatment effects. Most longitudinal studies of cognitive impairments in schizophrenia suggest they are remarkably stable over time, refractory to "treatment as usual", and persistent between episodes of relapse or exacerbation (e.g., Nuechterlein & Dawson, 1984; Addington & Addington, 1999). These were among the findings that spurred development of NPT in the first place. However, the control conditions in some trials of NPT have been unusually rich, including psychiatric rehabilitation modalities well beyond "treatment as usual". In at least one study that specifically analyzed cognitive changes in an enriched control condition (Spaulding *et al.*, 1999), substantial improvements were observed (although not as great as in the treatment condition). It therefore appears that cognitive recovery may generally be more possible than previously believed, whether or not the treatment and rehabilitation regimen includes modalities that explicitly address cognitive impairments. Accordingly, research on cognitive remediation has shifted from simply demonstrating overall benefits to analyzing the particular dimensions of treatment and rehabilitation that may enhance cognitive recovery in a variety of contexts (for a more extended discussion, see Silverstein & Wilkniss, 2004).

NPT research is thus moving in the direction foreseen by earlier behavior therapy researchers, toward articulating more precisely *which* therapy accomplishes *what* outcome for *whom* under *what* circumstances. The moderating factors for NPT effects are likely to include the severity and profile of neuropsychological impairment, the availability of comprehensive psychiatric rehabilitation and its non-specific cognitive benefits, and the particular purposes to which NPT is applied. In some cases, the most important benefits may be highly generalized, broadly affecting many domains of personal and social functioning, while in others it may be specific to enhancing engagement in other key rehabilitation modalities.

Theory base

Considering the diversity and heterogeneity of neuropsychological and behavioral impairments in severe mental illness, it is unlikely that a single mechanism can account for all NPT treatment effects. The mechanisms that produce cognitive recovery with NPT may be the same, different or overlapping with those that produce non-specific benefits in enriched rehabilitation milieus. Proposed mechanisms tend to fall within five (or so) categories (neither the categories nor the specific proposed mechanisms are mutually exclusive).

Enhanced normal learning

Psychiatric rehabilitation in general, and cognitive remediation in particular, facilitate acquisition of new or lost skills by overcoming barriers to learning created by cognitive impairments. Cognition itself is not changed or "remediated". New skills are acquired that would not be acquired without enhanced learning conditions. This is also the theoretical mechanism for the attention shaping and errorless learning procedures mentioned earlier. Enhanced normal learning could also account for non-specific effects in treatment milieus that explicitly enrich learning conditions, such as in token economies and related contingency management approaches.

Learning compensatory cognitive skills

Cognitive impairments are not "remediated". The patient learns new cognitive skills, including non-verbal procedural skills that neither patient nor therapist can necessarily verbally articulate, that enhance task performance despite the remaining impairment (Kurtz, 2003). This mechanism is related to the enhanced normal learning mechanism above, and is similar to the "self-talk" mechanism historically proposed to account for some of the effects of conventional CBT. In self-talk explanations, individuals learn to verbally prompt themselves to activate key cognitive processes that would normally be automatically activated by eliciting circumstances. The self-prompts acquired in NPT may be non-verbal and procedural, as well as verbal self-talk.

Post-psychotic response repertoire reorganization

Acute psychosis disables a dopaminergic subcortical brain mechanism that normally adjusts the accessibility of elements of a person's response repertoire according to environmental demand (Spaulding *et al.* 2003, Chapter 6). Even after neurophysiological stabilization, environmental input is required to re-establish accessibility of key cognitive abilities, e.g., social perception and problem solving. Post-acute cognitive impairment is a residual inability to activate these abilities when needed. An enriched rehabilitation milieu encourages repertoire reorganization by providing high environmental structure, immediate and concrete response contingencies (e.g., via behavioral contingency programs), and much prompting for adaptive social behavior. Cognitive remediation provides an even more focused regimen for re-establishing the accessibility of key neuropsychological processes and abilities, especially those needed for interpersonal functioning and adaptive problem solving.

Enhancing automatization of cognitive processes

Human cognition involves execution of many processes that operate automatically without conscious or verbal monitoring. Skill acquisition is in large part automatization of specific abilities that would not otherwise operate automatically. Automatization is impaired in severe mental illness. NPT identifies key abilities that need to be automated to perform certain tasks and provides special conditions in which the automatization deficit is overcome. Versions of this explanatory model have been proposed by two groups, one in terms of basic, conventional neuropsychological processes (Wykes & Reeder, 2005), the other in terms of automatic processing of complex social situations not conventionally addressed in neuropsychology (Hogarty & Flesher, 1999a,b).

Neuroendocrine activation

Chronic psychotic disorders compromise the diurnal activation cycle of the hypothalamic–pituitary–adrenal (HPA) regulatory system. One hormone in the HPA system, cortisol, plays a key role in activating cortical neurons for cognitive processing. When the diurnal activating function of cortisol is compromised, the result is cortical hypoactivation and consequent cognitive impairment. A highly structured, enriched rehabilitation milieu provides stimulation sufficient to recover the diurnal activation cycle (Spaulding *et al.*, 2003; note that this mechanism is probably more pertinent to non-specific benefits of a rehabilitation milieu than specific effects of NPT).

Summary

In summary, NPT is promising as a component of comprehensive psychiatric rehabilitation. Its overall benefits have been demonstrated in controlled clinical trials. Further research is expected to identify key moderators of the treatment effect so that treatment can be more precisely tailored to individual needs. Similarly, further research will identify specific purposes, e.g., enhancing response to social or occupational skill training, for which NPT is most effective.

Social skills training and integrated approaches

Social skills training (SST) is one of the oldest and most familiar behavioral therapy approaches applied to schizophrenia. It originated in the 1960s coincident with comparable approaches for other disorders. Its most complete and extensive development is in the work of Robert Liberman and colleagues at UCLA, who have been disseminating manuals and training materials for many years (Liberman, 2008). There are numerous other accessible sources (e.g., Bellack *et al.*, 2004; Pratt & Mueser, 2002; APA/CAPP Task

Force, 2007), and a strong SST program can be developed in real-world settings with a modest amount of administrative and fiscal support. In the context of comprehensive psychiatric rehabilitation, SST is one component that can address specific problems and barriers to recovery. However, the principles of SST complement and extend broader principles of CBT and of psychiatric rehabilitation, and in that sense an SST perspective can pervade all aspects of services for people with severe mental illness.

Definition of social skills training

SST is a structured procedure designed to strengthen the cognitive and behavioral elements that comprise interpersonal functioning. These elements include accurate perception and understanding of interpersonal situations, appropriate choice of behavioral response in specific situations, and competent performance of those behavioral responses. The initial objective of SST is to establish competent interpersonal behavior within the structured therapy situation. The longer-term objective is to generalize those competencies to the natural environment.

To varying degrees, SST approaches include *interpersonal problem solving* as an element of social competence. Interpersonal problem solving is a cognitive construct, in the sense that it can be characterized and taught in terms of specific analytical steps: (1) recognize there is a problem or conflict; (2) articulate the nature of the problem; (3) generate a menu of possible behavioral responses or solutions; (4) choose one solution and implement it; and (5) evaluate the results. However, interpersonal problem-solving cognition does not naturally occur in the way it is structured in SST, and in that sense it is more properly a heuristic model, not a true cognitive construct.

Description of the approach

The version of SST most common in settings that serve people with severe mental illness is a highly structured group modality. The therapist explains that the purpose of the group is to help people become more effective in their social and interpersonal interactions and relationships. In early phases of treatment, there are brief didactic presentations on specific kinds of interactions, e.g., how to strike up a casual conversation, how to make a request, how to express pleasure or displeasure. This is followed by role playing, in which designated members play parts in contrived social situations, and the other group members function as observers. The therapist directs the role play, setting up the situation, sometimes prompting the players, and ending it at an appropriate point. After the role play, the therapist gives feedback to the players, couched as praise and constructive criticism. Further feedback is prompted from the other group members, who follow the same pro-

tocol of first praising the strengths of the role play and then suggesting alternatives for suboptimal responses. The role play is repeated as the players incorporate the feedback and hone the effectiveness of their behavior.

Role plays of simple situations are followed by more complex ones, as skills develop. In later phases, patients are asked to bring their own personal experiences to the group for role playing. When the role play portrays a particular problem or conflict, the patient is prompted to try out the role-played solution in the real world and report back on its effectiveness. In some SST versions, an interpersonal problem-solving model is introduced after the initial phase, and the group members practice applying this model to conflicts and problems they encounter. Some versions of SST are time-limited, identifying specific behavioral competencies as the treatment goal and the criterion for discontinuation. SST is also often used as an open-ended continuing modality, comparable to long-term supportive group therapy but with continuing use of specific role-playing and problem-solving exercises.

Outcome research methodology and evidence base

The effectiveness of SST has been demonstrated in many clinical trials, but meta-analyses yield inconsistent results. Three meta-analyses of SST studies (Benton & Schroeder, 1990; Corrigan, 1991; Dilk & Bond, 1996) found strong evidence for effectiveness in improving social competence, suppressing symptoms, and postponing relapse. A fourth (Pilling *et al.*, 2002) found no evidence for any kind of effectiveness. A broader meta-analysis of SST and related psychosocial treatment (Pfammatter *et al.*, 2006) found qualified evidence for effectiveness. A review of the problem-solving component in SST (Xia & Li, 2007) found insufficient studies to conduct a quantitative meta-analysis, and did not reach conclusions. This confusing picture is at least partially attributable to the remarkable scope of application of SST and to the diversity of outcome criteria. Individual trials show strong benefits for a particular application with particular outcome measures, but questionable comparability of applications and outcome measures across trials undermines the effectiveness of quantitative meta-analyses. As with neuropsychological therapy, the strongest evidence is for effects on the particular abilities that are directly addressed in the group. The evidence becomes weaker for generalization of these effects to natural settings and to domains of functioning beyond social competence.

Some key factors contribute to the popularity of SST despite the mixed evidence base. First, as Pilling *et al.* (2002) pointed out, it has strong *a priori* validity. The relevance of competent interpersonal functioning to recovery from severe mental illness is obvious. Similarly, SST's emphasis on interpersonal functioning and on problems actually encountered by patients is notably complementary to contemporary recovery-oriented perspectives on mental illness. Second, most patients like SST. They have the sense that it is addressing issues that are personally relevant and important. They often experience it as quite distinct from less helpful therapy experiences they have had. Third, the therapy skills involved in providing SST are easily generalized to other skill training applications, such as illness management, occupational and independent living skills (in fact, these are considered by some to simply be variants of SST). Investment in training a cohort of competent SST trainers can return benefits across an entire rehabilitation program.

Integration with other modalities

The close historical relationship between SST and the broader psychiatric rehabilitation paradigm has encouraged integration of SST with other rehabilitation modalities. The first was with the problem-solving model, reflecting the more general integration of behavioral and cognitive approaches in the 1970s and 1980s. More recently, NPT has been integrated with SST. At least two of the manualized NPT systems (Brenner et al, 1994; Hogarty & Flesher, 1999) segue to procedures that are recognizably SST. Both NPT and SST can be applied in occupational/ vocational contexts, further expanding opportunities for integration. In the future, as the active ingredients and optimal applications of NPT and SST are identified, it is likely that both approaches will lose their separate identities, becoming instead specific principles and techniques that can be applied in a variety of ways for a variety of purposes in the context of a broader, unified rehabilitation and recovery enterprise.

Summary

In summary, SST is a structured, evidence-based treatment approach which can be applied in a variety of rehabilitative skill training contexts. SST therapy principles and skills generalize to a range of contexts, and can even serve as a basis for dyadic therapy. The specific benefits of SST depend on the specific application, but improved interpersonal competence is an outcome that permeates most applications.

Contingency management

Contingency management is a genre of techniques that evolved from learning and social-learning theories in the 1960s, and treatment programs based on the principles received particular attention during the 1970s in inpatient settings (see Corrigan & Liberman, 1994). However, as community-based programs for people with severe mental illness have proliferated, the relevance of contingency management has not been widely generalized, particularly in the UK, and contingency management is one of the most underutilized technologies in adult mental health services.

In contingency management approaches, a specific target behavior is identified; whose increase or decrease would have therapeutic benefit. A precise, quantitative record, usually based on systematic staff observation, is kept of the occurrence of the behavior. Following a functional analysis of the environmental events which may prompt or reinforce the behavior of interest, a plan or "program" is developed wherein key people in the patient's social environment deliver or withhold reinforcers contingent on the occurrence or non-occurrence of the behavior. The record is continually re-analyzed to determine whether the behavior responds as desired to the alteration of environmental contingencies.

The earliest applications of contingency management for schizophrenia, in the form of token economies in psychiatric hospitals, provided some empirical evidence of effectiveness in promoting adaptive behavior (Ayllon & Azrin, 1965; Baker et al., 1977). In a 7-year controlled clinical outcome trial (Paul & Lentz, 1977), described at the time as "the largest outcome trial in the history of psychiatry", a rehabilitation program that included contingency management was vastly superior to treatment as usual. However, there have been relatively few controlled trials of the approach (see McMonagle & Sultana, 2000; Dickerson et al., 2005 for reviews of token economy in schizophrenia), although clinical evaluations, case studies, and institutional experience continue to support its effectiveness in suppressing or changing behavior and symptoms (particularly negative symptoms), increasing adaptive behavior, and increasing participation in treatment and rehabilitation (e.g., McMonagle & Sultana, 2000; Paul & Menditto, 1992; Wong et al., 1986). In addition to general effects on maladaptive and adaptive behavior, when combined with other social-learning modalities, contingency management has been shown to be effective with two of the most troublesome and drug-resistant problems encountered in inpatient settings: aggression (Beck et al., 1991; 1997) and polydipsia (Baldwin et al., 1992).

As many of the studies evaluating the approach are not recent, it is uncertain how approaches will perform with patients on contemporary inpatient units, in community settings or other types of residential programs. As a result, there is further need for trials evaluating its effectiveness in different settings. Also, it should be noted that contingency management is often used "informally", without a recognized need for professional supervision (any time a staff person says to a patient "if you do X, I will do Y" it is a form of contingency management, whether therapeutically intended or not). As concern for patients' rights and demand for evidence-based treatments have increased, professionally supervised contingency management may need to be increasingly recognized as a key component in services for people with severe mental illness, especially in inpatient and institutional settings.

Comorbid disorders

Most of the application and evaluation of CBT for psychosis has been carried out with people without comorbid disorders; however, perhaps due to the high proportion of people presenting to services with comorbid disorders, greater attention has been paid to these groups in recent years. Groups for whom particular attention has been paid are people with comorbid substance misuse disorders, those with coexisting problems with violence and aggression, and those with learning difficulties.

Substance use

Comorbid substance use in those people with a diagnosis of schizophrenia is higher than in the non-psychotic population and affects a significant number of sufferers. Estimates of prevalence vary depending on the location and type of participants included however, the widely cited NIMH Epidemiological Catchment Area study (Regier et al., 1990) identified 47% of participants with a diagnosis of schizophrenia to have a lifetime prevalence of some form of substance use. The presence of substance misuse is associated with a range of negative outcomes, such as higher rates of violent and aggressive behavior, more frequent relapse rates, higher suicide rates, and poorer engagement and adherence with services (Maslin, 2003). The reasons for the inflated rates are not clearly elucidated; research suggests a number of contributory factors that vary amongst individuals, e.g., to control unpleasant symptoms, to manage side effects, to cope with unpleasant affect, and to increase social confidence (Gregg et al., 2007).

Although there have been few controlled trials evaluating the effectiveness of treatments for this subgroup of people, service evaluations and evidence from pilot trials suggest that strategies integrated to address both the problems of psychosis and substance use are necessary together with assertive approaches that optimize the engagement of individuals into treatment (Mueser & Drake, 2003; see Chapter 30). Integrated programs have usually consisted of the following elements: (1) motivational interviewing strategies (Miller & Rollnick, 2002) to enhance engagement, to identify important individual goals, and to explore and increase motivation to change substance using behavior; and (2) individual psychological therapy (usually CBT) to implement change in substance using and problems associated with psychosis. The rationale behind this is that the

psychosis and substance use problems are not independent and hence should be addressed simultaneously. Where family members or carers are present, family interventions have also been viewed as important. Evaluations of this type of approach have shown significant benefits over treatment as usual (case management and antipsychotic medication for mental health and substance use services) at the end of a 9-month treatment period and at follow-up (Barrowclough et al., 2001; Haddock et al., 2003).

Violence and aggression

Violence and aggression, when associated with psychosis, causes much media and public concern. However, the actual rate of violent crime associated with schizophrenia is low, attributed to about 5% of all cases of homicide and violent offences (UK National Homicide and Suicide Survey; Meehan et al., 2006). Nevertheless, within mental health services, aggression and violence are seen as significant areas of concern. The reasons for aggression and violence in psychosis are multifactorial and a number of key issues have been implicated (see Chapter 31). For example, the presence of particular types of delusions, such as threat control override symptoms (delusions that contain content associated with perceived threat to the individual or belief that the individual's body or mind is being controlled by outside sources), have been associated with increased rates of violence in retrospective and prospective studies (Swanson et al., 1997; Link & Steuve, 1994), although findings have been inconsistent and other factors such as substance misuse, personality factors, and affective states such as anger have also been implicated (Hodgkins et al., 2003; Applebaum et al., 2000). Treatment programs have been developed to address these issues. For example, CBT programs for anger delivered in a group format reduce the occurrence of violence and aggression at follow-up in forensic samples with psychosis (Renwick et al., 1997; Taylor et al., 2002). To date there has been little published work evaluating CBT in secure or forensic samples and little evaluation of their impact on violence and aggression outcomes, despite this being an area of great concern for both the public and mental health services. However, a recent randomized controlled trial demonstrated that CBT can significantly reduce violence in people with psychosis who are at high risk for aggressive behavior when the intervention is targeted simultaneously on psychotic symptoms and anger (Haddock et al., 2004, 2009) and is preceded by motivational strategies to aid engagement. Further research in this area is warranted.

Learning disabilities

There have been very few controlled trials evaluating psychological treatments for people with psychosis and a coexisting learning disability, although there are some case series and anecdotal data that suggest the approaches can be adapted for this group with beneficial outcomes (Legget *et al.*, 1997; Haddock *et al.*, 2004). However, some modifications are necessary, such as less reliance on written materials, increased use of pictorial and symbolic means for communicating, and particular attention to the cognitive abilities of the client. For example, concentration and understanding of material may be more limited. Shorter sessions, greater use of summaries, and repetition of material can be important. In addition, as CBT approaches rely to a certain extent on an individual's ability to make links between their problems, cognition, emotion, and behavior, assessment of their ability to recognize the links between cognition, feelings, and behavior may be useful precursors to therapy to tailor the intervention to their abilities (Oathamshaw & Haddock, 2006). In addition, a preparatory phase for therapy can be included to enable some training in cognitive approaches to be carried out (Haddock *et al.*, 2004; Taylor *et al.*, 2002).

Implementation and skills needed to deliver psychological therapists

Whilst there is a large evidence base in support of psychological treatments for psychosis and substantial amounts of government guidance advocating their use, their implementation as routine interventions can be limited by the availability of trained therapists to deliver the treatments. The British Association of Behavioural and Cognitive Psychotherapies, European Association of Behavioral and Cognitive Therapies, and the American Association of Behavior Therapy all have minimum training standards and guidelines for the practice of CBT, and there are specialist training courses providing clinicians with the necessary skills for applying the approach. Often these are designed to train mental health professionals who already have some of the skills necessary for engaging psychotic individuals in treatment (such as mental health nurses, clinical psychologists, psychiatrists) and provide training in the supervised practice of CBT over 1–2 years. The training involves face-to-face teaching in the theoretical and evidence base surrounding CBT, and experience and practice of the approach with real clients with supervision from experts. Trainees are usually expected to demonstrate competence in the delivery of the CBT with clients in order to graduate and to continue to receive supervision when practicing.

Conclusions

Psychological treatments are important in the treatment of psychosis and offer significant benefits in a range of areas, particularly in reducing relapse, hospital admission, symptom severity, and distress, and improving cognitive functioning and performance. In addition, wider benefits for the individual and services may be observed, such as reduced violence and aggression, improvements in medication adherence, reductions in substance use, reduced suicide, and benefits for relatives and carers. Further research is necessary to elucidate the exact ingredients for therapy and what treatment is best suited to which individual.

References

Addington, J. & Addington, D. (1999) Neurocognitive and social functioning in schizophrenia. *Schizophrenia Bulletin* **25**, 173–182.

Alford, G.S. & Turner, S.M. (1976) Stimulus interference and conditioned inhibition of auditory hallucinations. *Journal of Behaviour Therapy and Experimental Psychology* **7**, 155–160.

Allen, H.A., Halperin, J. & Friend, R. (1983) Removal and diversion tactics and the control of auditory hallucinations. *Behaviour, Research and Therapy* **23**, 601–605.

APA/CAPP Task Force on Serious Mental Illness and Severe Emotional Disturbance (2007) Best practices for recovery and improved outcomes for people with serious mental illness. www.apa.org/practice/grid.html

Applebaum, S., Robbins, C. & Monahan, J. (2000) Violence and delusions: data from the MacArthur Violence Risk Assessment Study. *Archives of General Psychiatry* **157**, 566–572.

Ayllon, T. & Azrin, N.H. (1965) The measurement and reinforcement of behaviour of psychotics. *Journal of the Experimental Analysis of Behaviour* **8**, 357–383.

Baker, R., Hall, J.N., Hutchinson, K. & Bridge, G. (1977) Symptom changes in chronic schizophrenic patients on a token economy: a controlled experiment. *British Journal of Psychiatry* **131**, 381–393.

Baldwin, L., Beck, N., Menditto, A., Arms, T. & Cormier, J. (1992) Decreasing excessive water drinking by chronic mentally ill forensic patients. *Hospital and Community Psychiatry* **43**, 507–509.

Barrowclough, C. & Hooley J.M. (2003) Attributions and expressed emotion: a review. *Clinical Psychology Review* **23**, 849–880.

Barrowclough. C. & Tarrier, N. (1992) *Families of Schizophrenic Patients: A Cognitive Behavioural Approach*. London: Chapman and Hall.

Barrowclough, C., Haddock, G., Tarrier, N. *et al.* (2001) Randomized controlled trial of motivational intervention, cognitive behavior therapy, and family intervention for patients with co-morbid schizophrenia and substance use disorders. *American Journal of Psychiatry* **158**, 1706–1713.

Beck, A.T. (1952) Successful outpatient psychotherapy of a chronic schizophrenic with a delusion based on borrowed guilt. *Psychiatry* **15**, 305–312.

Beck, N., Greenfield, S., Gotham, H., Menditto, A., Stuve, P. & Hemme, C. (1997) Risperidone in the management of violent, treatment-resistant schizophrenics hospitalized in a maximum security forensic facility. *Journal of the American Academy of Psychiatry and the Law* **25**, 461–468.

Beck, N., Menditto, A., Baldwin, L., Angelone, E. & Maddox, M. (1991) Reduced frequency of aggressive behavior in forensic patients in a social learning program. *Hospital and Community Psychiatry* **42**, 750–752.

Bellack, A., Mueser, K., Gingerich, S. & Agresta, J. (2004) *Social Skills Training for Schizophrenia: A Step-by-Step Guide*, 2nd edn. New York: Guilford Press.

Bentall, R., Kinderman, P. & Kaney, S. (1994) The self, attributional processes and abnormal beliefs: towards a model of persecutory delusions. *Behaviour, Research and Therapy* **32**, 331–341.

Benton, M. & Schroeder, H. (1990) Social skills training with schizophrenics: A meta-analytic evaluation. *Journal of Consulting and Clinical Psychology* **58**, 741–747.

Bleuler, E. (1911/1950) *Demetia Praecox or the Group of Schizophrenias*. New York: International University Press.

Brenner, H., Roder, V., Hodel, B., Kienzle, N., Reed, D. & Liberman, R. (1994) *Integrated Psychological Therapy for Schizophrenic Patients*. Toronto: Hogrefe & Huber.

Brown, G.W., Monck, E.M., Carstairs, G.M. *et al.* (1962) Influences of family life on the course of schizophrenic illness. *British Journal of Preventive and Social Medicine* **16**, 55–68.

Buchanan, A. (1997) The investigation of acting on delusions as a tool for risk assessment in the mentally disordered. *British Journal of Psychiatry* **170** (Suppl. 32), 12–16.

Chadwick, P.D. & Birchwood, M. (1994) The omnipotence of voices. A cognitive approach to auditory hallucinations. *British Journal of Psychiatry* **164**, 190–201.

Chadwick, P.D. & Lowe, C.F. (1990) Measurement and modification of delusional beliefs. *Journal of Consulting and Clinical Psychology* **58**, 225–232.

Corrigan, W. (1991) Social skills training in adult psychiatric populations: a meta-analysis. *Journal of Behavior Therapy and Experimental Psychiatry* **22**, 203–210.

Corrigan, W. & Liberman, R., eds. (1994) *Behavior Therapy in Psychiatric Hospitals*, New York: Springer.

Dickerson, F.B., Tenhula, W.N. & Green-Paden, L.D. (2005) The token economy for schizophrenia: review of the literature and recommendations for future research. *Schizophrenia Research* **75**, 405–416.

Dilk, M.N. & Bond, G.R. (1996) Meta-analytic evaluation of skills training research for individuals with severe mental illness. *Journal of Consulting and Clinical Psychology* **64**, 1337–1346.

Dixon, L.B., Dickerson, F., Bellack, A.S. *et al.* (2010) Schizophrenia Patient Outcomes Research Team (PORT). The 2009 schizophrenia PORT psychosocial treatment recommendations and summary statements. *Schizophrenia Bulletin* **36**, 48–70.

Falloon I.R.H. (1985) *Family Management of Schizophrenia*. Baltimore: John Hopkins University Press.

Falloon, I.R. & Talbot, R.E. (1981) Persistent auditory hallucinations: coping mechanisms and implications for management. *Psychological Medicine* **11**, 329–339.

Garety, A. & Hemsley, D.R. (1997) *Delusions: Investigations into the Psychology of Delusional Reasoning*. Psychology Press Ltd.

Garety, A., Bebbington, P., Fowler, D., Freeman, D. & Kuipers, E. (2007) Implications for neurobiological research of cognitive models of psychosis: a theoretical paper. *Psychological Medicine* **37**, 1377–1391.

Goldberg, D. & Williams, P. (1988) *A User's Guide to the General Health Questionnaire*. Windsor: NFER Nelson.

Green, M. (1996) What are the functional consequences of neurocognitive deficits in schizophrenia? *American Journal of Psychiatry* **153**, 321–330.

Green, M. (1998) *Schizophenia as a Neurocognitive Disorder*. Boston: Ayllon & Bacon.

Gregg, L., Barrowclough, C. & Haddock, G. (2007) Reasons for increased substance use in psychosis. *Clinical Psychology Review* **27**, 494–510.

Haddock, G., Bentall, R. & Slade, D. (1993) Psychological treatment of auditory hallucinations: two case studies. *Behavioural and Cognitive Psychotherapy* **21**, 335–346.

Haddock, G., Bentall, R. & Slade, D. (1996) Focusing versus distraction approaches in the treatment of persistent auditory hallucinations. In: Haddock, G. & Slade, D., eds. *Cognitive-Behavioural Interventions with Psychotic Disorders*. London: Routledge.

Haddock, G., McCarron, J., Tarrier, N. & Faragher, E.B. (1999) Scales to measure dimensions of hallucinations and delusions: the psychotic symptom rating scales (PSYRATS). *Psychological Medicine* **29**, 879–889.

Haddock, G., Barrowclough, C., Tarrier, N. *et al.* (2003) Randomised controlled trial of cognitive-behaviour therapy and motivational intervention for schizophrenia and substance use: 18 month, carer and economic outcomes. *British Journal of Psychiatry* **183**, 418–426.

Haddock, G., Lobban, F., Hatton, C. & Carson, R. (2004) Cognitive-behaviour therapy for people with psychosis and mild learning disability: a case series. *Clinical Psychology and Psychotherapy* **11**, 282–298.

Haddock, G., Barrowclough, C., Shaw, J.J., Dunn, G., Novaco, R.W. & Tarrier, N. (2009) Cognitive-behavioural therapy v. social activity therapyt for people with psychosis and a history of violence: a randomised controlled trial. *British Journal of Psychiatry* **194**, 152–157.

Haynes, S.N. & Geddy (1973) Suppression of psychotic hallucinations through time-out. *Behavior Therapy* **4**, 123–127.

Hodgkins, S, Hiscoke, U.L. & Freese, R. (2003) The antecedents of aggressive behavior among men with schizophrenia: a prospective investigation of patients in community treatment. *Behavioral Sciences and the Law* **21**, 521–546.

Hogarty, G.E. & Flesher, S. (1999a) Developmental theory for a cognitive enhancement therapy of schizophrenia. *Schizophrenia Bulletin* **25**, 677–692.

Hogarty, G. & Flesher, S. (1999b) Practice principles of cognitive enhancement therapy for schizophrenia. *Schizophrenia Bulletin* **25**, 693–708.

Huxley, N.A., Rendall, M. & Sederer, L. (2000) Psychosocial treatments in schizophrenia: A review of the past 20 years. *Journal of Nervous and Mental Disease* **188**, 187–201.

James, D.A. (1983) The experimental treatment of two cases of auditory hallucinations. *British Journal of Psychiatry* **143**, 515–516.

Jaspers, K. (1963) *General Psychopathology* (translated by Hoenig, J. & Hamilton, M.W.). Manchester: Manchester University Press.

Jones, C., Cormac, I., Silveira da Mota Neto J.I. & Campbell, C. (2007) Cognitive behaviour therapy for schizophrenia. *Cochrane Database of Systematic Reviews* Issue 4, CD000524.

Kay, S.R., Opler, L.A. & Lindenmayer, J. (1989) The Positive and Negative Syndrome Scale (PANSS): rationale and standardisation. *British Journal of Psychiatry* **7** (Suppl.), 59–67.

Kemp, R., Hayward, P., Applewhaite, G., Everitt, B. & David, A. (1996) Compliance therapy in psychotic patients: randomised controlled trial. *British Medicine Journal* **10**, 312, 345–349.

Kern, R.S., Liberman, R., Kopelowicz, A., Mintz, J. & Green, M.F. (2002) Applications of errorless learning for improving work performance in persons with schizophrenia. *American Journal of Psychiatry* **159**, 1921–1926.

Kern, R.S., Green, M.F., Mitchell, S., Kopelowicz, A., Mintz, J. & Liberman, R. (2005) Extensions of errorless learning for social problem-solving deficits in schizophrenia. *American Journal of Psychiatry* **162**, 513–519.

Kuipers, E., Leff, J. & Lam, D. (2002) *Family Work for Schizophrenia: A Practical Guide*, 2nd edn. London: Gaskill.

Kurtz, M.M. (2003) Neurocognitive rehabilitation for schizophrenia. *Current Psychiatry Reports* **5**, 303–310.

Kurtz, M.M., Moberg, J., Gur, R.C. & Gur, R.E. (2001) Approaches to cognitive remediation of neuropsychological deficits in schizophrenia: a review and meta-analysis. *Neuropsychology Review* **11**, 197–210.

Legget, J., Hurn, C. & Goodman, W. (1997) Teaching psychological strategies for managing auditory hallucinations: A case report. *British Journal of Learning Disabilities* **25**, 158–162.

Lewis, S., Tarrier, N., Haddock, G. *et al.* (2002) Randomised controlled trial of cognitive-behavioural therapy in early schizophrenia: acute-phase outcomes. *British Journal of Psychiatry* **181** (Suppl. 43), 91–97.

Liberman, R. (2008) *Recovery from Disability: Manual of Psychiatric Rehabilitation*. Arlington, VA: American Psychiatric Publishing.

Link, B.G. & Steuve, A. (1994) Psychotic symptoms and the violent/illegal behavior of mental patients compared to community controls. In: Monahan, J. & Steadman, H.J., eds. *Violence and Mental Disorders*. Chicago: Chicago University Press.

Margo, A., Hemsley, D.R. & Slade, D. (1981) The effects of varying auditory input on schizophrenic hallucinations. *British Journal of Psychiatry* **139**, 122–127.

Maslin, J. (2003) Substance misuse in psychosis: contextual issues. In: Graham, H.L. *et al.*, eds. *Substance Misuse in Psychosis: Approaches to Treatment and Service Delivery*. Chichester: John Wiley & Sons.

McFarlane, W.R., Lukens, E., Link, B. *et al.* (1995) Multiple-family groups and psychoeducation in the treatment of schizophrenia. *Archives of General Psychiatry* **52**, 679–687.

McGurk, S.R., Twamley, E.W., Sitzer, E., McHugo, D.I., Gregory, J. & Mueser, K. (2008) A meta-analysis of cognitive remediation in schizophrenia. *American Journal of Psychiatry* **164**, 1791–1802.

McMonagle, T. & Sultana, A. (2000) Token economy for schizophrenia. *Cochrane Database of Systematic Reviews* Issue 3, CD001473.

Meehan, J., Flynn, S., Hunt, I.M. *et al.* (2006) Perpetrators of homicide with schizophrenia: a national clinical survey in England and Wales. *Psychiatric Services* **57**, 1648–1651.

Meichenbaum, D. (1969) The effects of instructions and reinforcement on thinking and language behavior of schizophrenics. *Behavior Research and Therapy* **7**, 101–114.

Meichenbaum, D.M. & Cameron, R. (1973) Training schizophrenics to talk to themselves: A means of developing attentional controls. *Behavior Therapy* **4**, 515–534.

Miller, W. & Rollnick, S. (2002) *Motivational Interviewing*. New York: Guilford.

Morrison, A.P., French, P., Walford, L. *et al.* (2004) Cognitive therapy for the prevention of psychosis in people at ultra-high risk: randomised controlled trial. *British Journal of Psychiatry* **185**, 291–297.

Mueser, K.T. & Berenbaum, H. (1990) Psychodynamic treatment of schizophrenia: Is there a future. *Psychological Medicine* **20**, 253–262.

Mueser, K.T. & Drake R.E. (2003) Integrated dual diagnosis treatment in New Hampshire (USA). In: Graham, H.L., *et al.*, eds. *Substance Misuse in Psychosis: Approaches to Treatment and Service Delivery*. Chichester: Wiley.

Mueser, K. & Glynn, S. (1995). *Behavioral Family Therapy for Psychiatric Disorders*. Boston: Allyn and Bacon.

National Institute for Clinical Excellence (2007) *Guidelines for Schizophrenia*. London: Department of Health.

Nelson, H., Thrasher, S. & Barnes, T.R.E. (1991) Practical ways of alleviating auditory hallucinations. *British Medical Journal* **302**, 307.

Nuechterlein, K.H. & Dawson, M.E. (1984) A heuristic vulnerability/stress model of schizophrenic episodes. *Schizophrenia Bulletin* **10**, 300–312.

Nydegger R.V. (1972) The elimination of hallucinatory and delusional behaviour by verbal conditioning and assertive training: a case study. *Journal of Behaviour Therapy and Experimental Psychiatry* **3**, 225–227.

Oathamshaw, S. & Haddock, G. (2006) Do people with intellectual disabilities and psychosis have the cognitive skills required to undertake cognitive behavioural therapy? *Journal of Applied Research in Intellectual Disabilities* **19**, 35–46.

O'Carroll, R.E., Russell, H.H., Lawrie, S.M. & Johnstone, E.C. (1999) Errorless learning and the cognitive rehabilitation of memory-impaired schizophrenic patients. *Psychological Medicine* **29**, 105–112.

Oliver, N. & Kuipers, E. (1996) Stress and its relationship to expressed emotion in community mental health workers. *International Journal of Social Psychiatry* **42**, 150.

Overall, J. & Gorham, D. (1962) The Brief Psychiatric Rating Scale. *Psychological Reports* **10**, 799–812.

Paley, G. & Shapiro, D.A. (2002) Lessons from psychotherapy research for psychological interventions for people with schizophrenia. *Psychology and Psychotherapy* **75**, 365–374.

Paul, G.L. & Lentz, R.J. (1977) *Psychosocial Treatment of Chronic Mental Patients: Milieu vs. Social Learning Programs*. Cambridge: Harvard University Press.

Paul, G. & Menditto, A. (1992) Effectiveness of inpatient treatment programs for mentally ill adults in public psychiatric facilities. *Applied and Preventive Psychology* **1**, 41–63.

Penn, D., Hope, D., Spaulding, W., Nelson, C. & Sullivan, M. (1992) Behavioral correlates of ward behavior and symptomatology in schizophrenia. Paper presented at the Association for Advancement of Behavior Therapy, Boston.

Penn, D., Mueser, K., Spaulding, W., Hope, D. & Reed, D. (1995) Information processing and social competence in chronic schizophenia. *Schizophrenia Bulletin* **21**, 269–281.

Penn, D., Spaulding, W., Reed, D., & Sullivan, M. (1996) The relationship of social cognition to ward behavior in chronic schizophrenia. *Schizophrenia Research* **20**, 327–335.

Penn, D., van der Does, J., Spaulding, W., Garbin, C., Linzen, D. & Dingamans (1993) Information processing and social-cognitive problem solving in schizophrenia. *Journal of Nervous and Mental Disease* **181**, 13–20.

Pfammatter, M., Junghan, U.M. & Brenner, H.D. (2006) Efficacy of psychological therapy in schizophrenia: Conclusions from meta-analyses. *Schizophrenia Bulletin* **32** (Suppl.1), S64–S80.

Pharoah, F.M., Mari, J.J. & Streiner, D. (2006) Family interventions in schizophrenia. *Cochrane Database of Systematic Reviews* Issue 4, CD000088.

Pilling, S., Bebbington, , Kuipers, E. *et al.* (2002) Psychological treatments in schizophrenia: II. Meta-analyses of randomized controlled trials of social skills training and cognitive remediation. *Psychology Medicine* **32**, 783–791.

Pratt, S. & Mueser, K. (2002) Social skills training for schizophrenia. In: Hofmann, S. & Tompson, M., eds. *Treating Chronic and Severe Mental Disorders: A Handbook of Empirically Supported Interventions.* New York: Guilford.

President's New Freedom Commission on Mental Health (2004) *Report to the President.* Recovered from the internet 10/15/04 at http://www.mentalhealthcommission.gov/reports/reports.htm.

Rector, A.T. & Beck, N.A. (2004) Cognitive therapy of schizophrenia: a new therapy for the new millennium. *American Journal of Psychotherapy* **54**, 291–300.

Regier, D.A., Farmer, M.F., Rae, D.S. *et al.* (1990) Comorbidity of mental disorders with alcohol and other drug abuse: results from the Epidemiologic Catchment Area (ECA) Study. *Journal of the American Medical Association* **264**, 251–258.

Renwick, S., Black, L., Ramm, M. & Novaco, R. (1997) Anger treatment for forensic hospital patients. *Legal and Criminological Psychology* **2**, 103–116.

Samaan, M. (1975) Thought stopping and flooding in a case of auditory hallucinations, obsessions, and homicidal-suicidal behaviour. *Journal of Behaviour Therapy and Experimental Psychiatry* **6**, 65–67.

Sensky, T., Turkington, D., Kingdon, D. *et al.* (2000) A randomized controlled trial of cognitive-behavioural therapy for persistent symptoms in schizophrenia resistant to medication. *Archives of General Psychiatry* **57**, 165–172.

Silverstein, S.M. & Wilkniss, S.M. (2004) At issue: The future of cognitive rehabilitation of schizophrenia. *Schizophrenia Bulletin* **30**, 679–692.

Silverstein, S., Menditto, A. & Stuve, P. (2000) Shaping procedures as cognitive retraining techniques in individuals with severe and persistent mental illness. *Psychiatric Rehabilitation Skills* **3**, 59–76.

Silverstein, S., Spaulding, W., Menditto, A. *et al.* (2009) Attention shaping: a reward-based learning method to enhance skills training outcomes in schizophrenia. *Schizophrenia Bulletin* **35**, 222–232.

Spaulding, W.D., Reed, D., Sullivan, M., Richardson, C. & Weiler, M. (1999) Effects of cognitive treatment in psychiatric rehabilitation. *Schizophrenia Bulletin* **25**, 657–676.

Spaulding, W.D., Sullivan, M.E. & Poland, J.S. (2003) *Treatment and Rehabilitation of Severe Mental Illness.* New York: Guilford Press.

Substance Abuse and Mental Health Services Administration (SAMHSA) (2004) *Evidence-Based Practices: Shaping Mental Health Services Toward Recovery.* http://mentalhealth.samhsa.gov/cmhs/communitysupport/toolkits.

Sullivan, H.F. (1962) *Schizophrenia as a Human Process.* New York: W.W. Norton.

Swanson, J., Estroff, S., Swartz, M. *et al.* (1997) Violence and severe mental disorder in clinical and community populations: the effects of psychotic symptoms, comorbidity, and lack of treatment. *Psychiatry* **60**, 1–22.

Tarrier, N. (1987) An investigation of residual psychotic symptoms in discharged schizophrenic patients. *British Journal of Clinical Psychology* **26**, 141–143.

Tarrier, N. (1994) Management and modification of residual psychotic symptoms In: Birchwood, M. & Tarrier, N., eds. *Innovations in the Psychological Management of Schizophrenia.* Chichester: Wiley, pp. 147–169.

Tarrier, N., Yusupoff, L., Kinney, C. *et al.* (1998) Randomised controlled trial of intensive cognitive behaviour therapy for patients with chronic schizophrenia. *British Medical Journal* **317**, 303–307.

Tarrier, N., Barrowclough, C., Haddock, G. & Wykes, T. (2002) Are all psychological treatments for psychosis equal? The need for CBT in the treatment of psychosis and not for psychodynamic psychotherapy. *Psychology and Psychotherapy* **75**, 5–17.

Taylor, J., Novaco, R., Gillmere, B. & Thorne, I. (2002) Cognitive-behavioural treatment of anger intensity among offenders with mental retardation. *Journal of Applied Research in Mental Retardation* **15**, 151–165.

Turner, S.M., Hersen, M. & Hellack A.S. (1977) Generalization effects of social skills training in chronic schizophrenics: an experimental analysis. *Behaviour Research and Therapy* **14**, 391–398.

Twamley, E.W., Jeste, D.V. & Bellack, A.S. (2003) A review of cognitive training in schizophrenia. *Schizophrenia Bulletin* **29**, 359–382.

Vaughn C.E. & Leff, J. (1976) The influence of family and social factors on the course of psychiatric illness. *British Journal of Psychology* **129**, 125–137.

Walker, E. (1994). Developmentally moderated expressions of the neuropathology underlying schizophrenia. *Schizophrenia Bulletin* **20**, 453–480.

Wing, J.K., Cooper, J.E. & Sartorius N (1974) *The Description and Classfication of Psychiatric Symptoms. An Instruction Manual for the PSE and CATEGO System.* Cambridge: Cambridge University Press.

Wong, S., Massel, H., Mosk, M. & Liberman, R. (1986) Behavioral approaches to the treatment of schizophrenia. In: Burroughs, G., Norman, T. & Rubenstein, G., eds. *Handbook of Studies on Schizophrenia*. Amsterdam: Elsevier Science Publishers, pp. 79–100.

Wykes, T. & Reeder, C. (2005) *Cognitive Remediation Therapy for Schizophrenia: Theory and Practice*. London: Routledge.

Wykes, T., Steel, C., Everitt, B. & Tarrier, N. (2008) Cognitive behaviour therapy for schizophrenia: Effect sizes, clinical models and methodological rigour. *Schizophrenia Bulletin* **34**, 523–537.

Xia, J. & Li, C. (2007) Problem solving skills for schizophrenia. *Cochrane Database Systematic Reviews* Issue 2, CD006365.

Xiong, W., Phillips, M.R., Hu, X. *et al.* (1994) Family-based intervention for schizophrenic patients in China. A randomised controlled trial. *British Journal of Psychiatry* **165**, 239–247.

Yusupoff, L. & Haddock, G. (1998) Options and clinical decision making in the assessment and psychological treatment of hallucinations and delusions. In: Perris, C. & McGorry, eds. *Cognitively-Oriented Psychotherapy in Psychotic Disorders*. Chichester: Wiley.

33

Economics of the treatment of schizophrenia

Nancy H. Covell[1,2], Susan M. Essock[2], and Linda K. Frisman[1,3]

[1]Conneticut Department of Mental Health and Addition Services, Hartford, CT, USA
[2]Columbia University, New York State Psychiatric Institute, New York, NY, USA
[3]University of Connecticut School of Social Work, West Hartford, CT, USA

Economics of mental health and schizophrenia

Until recently, the economics of mental illness were little understood. For most of the last century, economists paid scant attention to schizophrenia, or indeed to mental health in general (McGuire, 1990). Yet today, with new and expensive medications arriving on the market, and conventional treatments under pressure to meet financial strictures, economic considerations in mental health policy are growing ever more important. This chapter focuses on two aspects of the economics of schizophrenia: the costs of the mental illness and the cost-effectiveness of treatment modalities.

Studies of the cost of mental illnesses appeared before other types of work in the economics of mental health. Early work in the 1980s considered the impact of organization and financing on system efficiency and addressed the supply of personnel in caring for persons with mental illness. One study reviewed the market for psychotherapy and the insurability of mental healthcare (McGuire, 1981), and another examined the supply of psychiatrists (Frank, 1983). The impact of cost sharing on demand for mental healthcare was analyzed by researchers at the RAND Corporation (Manning et al., 1984). The use of diagnosis-related groupings to pay for care under prospective payment was considered (Taube et al., 1984). The impact of various funding mechanisms in public mental health was reviewed by Dickey and Goldman (1986).

More recently, economic analyses have contributed to a range of activities in the field of mental health economics, including the economics of schizophrenia. During the 1990s, studies continued with work on insurance, regulation, and the organization of mental health services. Examination of insurance mandates for mental healthcare, such as simulation of mandates and related costs, provided valuable information to legislators in the US considering such laws (Frank et al., 1991). Advocates for systems change considered major reorganizational efforts, such as those implemented through the Robert Wood Johnson Program on Chronic Mental Illness and other types of organizational reforms (Goldman et al., 1994, 1995; McGuire et al., 1995; Semke et al., 1995; Shepherd et al., 1996). The 1990s also brought analysis of the increasing implementation of managed care with behavioral health carve-outs (Mechanic, 1998). In the current decade, studies have also examined the impact of mental health parity on cost (Barry et al., 2006), the cost implications of implementing evidence-based practices (Goldman et al., 2001), the impact of Medicaid on mental healthcare (Frank et al., 2003), and the increasing costs of psychotropic medications (Frank et al., 2005).

Cost studies lay the foundation for cost-effectiveness and cost–benefit studies because they identify the range of resources that are consumed as a result of an illness.

Schizophrenia, 3rd edition. Edited by Daniel R. Weinberger and Paul J Harrison © 2011 Blackwell Publishing Ltd.

Cost-effectiveness analyses of mental health programs began to appear in the early 1980s with a hallmark study on the cost–benefit of assertive community treatment teams (Weisbrod *et al.*, 1980). Together, studies of costs and cost-effectiveness are perhaps the most important measures of the economics of schizophrenia. First, the sizeable cost to society captures the attention of policy-makers and taxpayers, and convinces them of the huge fiscal impact of schizophrenia. Second, decisions by clinicians, managers, and policy-makers that are informed by research on costs and cost-effectiveness lead to better distribution of the resources available for mental healthcare.

Costs of schizophrenia

Early studies of the costs of mental illness (Cruze *et al.*, 1981; Harwood *et al.*, 1984; Rice *et al.*, 1990) did not distinguish between the costs of different diagnostic categories (McGuire, 1991). Samples that were examined included bipolar disorder and major depression, as well as schizophrenia. More recent studies have estimated specific costs for schizophrenia and other illnesses. Rice estimated the cost of schizophrenia in the US at $32.5 billion in 1990 (Rice 1999a) and $44.9 billion in 1994 (Rice 1999b). Costs in Canada were calculated to be approximately $2.35 billion (Goeree *et al.*, 1999) and in Taiwan to be $112.4 million (Lang & Su, 2004) in 1996, while costs of schizophrenia were estimated to be £2.6 billion in 1992–1993 in the UK (Knapp, 1997) and £6.7 billion in 2004–2005 in England (Mangalore & Knapp, 2007). Some schizophrenia cost studies focus only on service costs, such as Rund and Ruud's (1999) study of costs in Norway and Martin and Miller's (1998) study of Medicaid recipients in Georgia. In contrast, Rice's, Knapp's, and Mangalore's studies included both direct costs, such as treatment and other service costs, and indirect costs, such as lost income. However, no study of the cost of schizophrenia can claim to capture all costs. As noted by McGuire (1991), even comprehensive studies of the cost of schizophrenia often underestimate two types of costs: the costs to families and the costs of publicly owned capital. What does seem to be clear across studies and between countries is that schizophrenia accounts for substantial spending (typically 1.5–3% of total national healthcare expenditures with one-third to two-thirds of this cost attributed to hospitalization), both because of the expense of hospitalizations and because of the long-term nature of the illness (Knapp *et al.*, 2004).

Cost perspective

Cost-effectiveness and cost–benefit analysis should always state the perspective from which the study is undertaken. Cost-of-illness studies, which consider economic costs, typically reflect the perspective of society in general

(Knapp, 1997; Mangalore & Knapp, 2007; Rice, 1999a,b). Economic, or social, costs are the costs of resources consumed because of an illness. Although a societal perspective presumably provides the balanced view of a neutral scientist, it is also helpful to examine costs from perspectives of particular stakeholders. In an analysis of the impact of assertive community treatment in Connecticut, Essock *et al.* (1998) presented costs from the perspectives of society, the state, and the Department of Mental Health. Comparison of the results from multiple perspectives may identify areas of cost-shifting that result from certain programs and policies. For example, a treatment that reduces hospital days may shift costs from state-run inpatient facilities to private non-profit outpatient settings. These shifts in cost may mean that changes within treatment systems that are beneficial to patients and revenue-neutral from a societal perspective may still be more expensive from the vantage point of particular stakeholders. By identifying such stakeholders, policy- makers can identify important potential sticking points to implementing system changes and intervene (e.g., by creating fiscal incentives for the stakeholders who would otherwise be fiscal losers to cooperate).

Cost components

Costs of treatment and other services

The examples provided by Rice, Knapp, and Mangalore are instructive for those conducting cost-of-illness studies and cost-effectiveness studies in the area of schizophrenia. They show that there are many ways in which the illness is associated with costs greater than those found with other illnesses. First are the costs of treatment, including medication. Treatment may be offered by public, private or voluntary sector settings, and many persons with schizophrenia receive care in multiple places. Besides treatment, services such as case management, vocational rehabilitation, and psychosocial clubhouses generate significant costs, though the cost of some services (e.g., supported employment) may be offset by a decreased use of other services (e.g., outpatient mental health services; Bond *et al.*, 2001). Medical and surgical costs also may be relevant in cost-effectiveness analyses, because utilization of these services may vary depending on the adequacy of mental healthcare (Mumford & Schlesinger, 1987; Pallack & Cummings, 1992) and because individuals with schizophrenia are at increased risk for particular other illnesses. For example, compared to the general population, individuals with psychotic disorders are about twice as likely to have Type 2 diabetes (Dixon *et al.*, 2000), about 1.5 times more likely to have coronary heart disease (Goff *et al.*, 2005), eight times more likely to be infected with human immunodeficiency virus (HIV; Rosenberg *et al.*, 2001), five times more likely to be infected with hepatitis B (Rosenberg *et al.*, 2001), and over ten times more likely to be infected with hepatitis C

(Rosenberg *et al.*, 2001). The increased cost of treating these medical conditions can be significant. For example, in 2007, the total cost of treating diabetes in the US was estimated to be $174 billion with healthcare costs for those with diabetes about 2.3 times the healthcare costs for those without diabetes (US Department of Health and Human Services Centers for Disease Control and Prevention, 2007). Additionally, the cost of treating heart disease and stroke in the US is projected to be nearly $503.2 billion in 2010 (Lloyd-Jones *et al.*, 2010).

Lost productivity and family burden

Mental illnesses, like other disorders, cause people to lose work days (Kessler & Frank, 1997) and sometimes even to forfeit aspirations of having any career at all. Comprehensive studies of the costs of schizophrenia may address lost productivity, but because of the high rates of disability in this population, many studies of interventions for persons with schizophrenia ignore productivity losses. However, evidence-based strategies for improving the employment outcomes for persons with serious mental illness, such as individual placement and supportive employment (Bond *et al.*, 2001; Drake *et al.*, 1996), have made employment a realistic goal of rehabilitation. These new successes suggest that loss of productivity should be included when calculating the cost of interventions for persons with schizophrenia. In addition to the productivity losses of the individuals affected, cost studies should attend to the work losses of family members and others who contribute time and in-kind services (Clark, 1994).

Capital costs

Economic cost studies appropriately study the opportunity costs of all resources, i.e., the value of resources in their best alternative use. In a cost-effectiveness study of a new residential model for persons with serious mental illness, Cannon *et al.* (1985) carefully considered the value of capital costs of a public hospital, which would have been underestimated if valued through traditional methods of depreciation. Capital costs can be large enough to change the most basic findings of a cost study, as shown by Rosenheck *et al.* (1994). Public administrators may not consider the value of buildings and property to be part of a cost equation because they are not always part of the operating costs, but the value of the property in alternative use may be considerable. For example, in the US, for the past 20 years states have decreased their reliance on large state hospitals, leaving them with many-acre campuses, many of which are located in areas where the market rate for land is very high.

Other components

It is important to attend to criminal justice costs, especially when an intervention is expected to have an impact on co-occurring substance use disorders (Clark *et al.*, 1999). Another neglected aspect of cost studies is the cost of administering transfer payments (such as social security). Although disability payments themselves do not represent the use of new resources, the cost of administering these payments should be counted, especially if the intervention could change the rate of receipt of disability payments or other public benefits (Frisman & Rosenheck, 1996). An intervention that returns people to work will not only increase their productivity (a benefit), but also decrease disability payments (decrease a cost).

Whether a particular cost is included in a cost-effectiveness study is related to the potential impact of that type of cost on the study findings. The larger the cost per unit, or the more frequently it is used, the more carefully it should be assessed (Hargreaves *et al.*, 1998). But should cost-effectiveness analyses always be conducted? Because of the wide range of costs and cost perspectives that might be included, these studies can be expensive to implement. This expense is further increased because, in order to be able to detect significant differences, a highly variable outcome such as cost may require many more study participants than would be needed for an effectiveness study alone. The usefulness of a cost study depends in large part on the likelihood that the treatment or intervention under study will have an effect on costs—either positive or negative. Cost studies are critical in the analysis of non-clozapine second-generation antipsychotic agents because of the relatively high purchase price of the drugs compared with first-generation (conventional) antipsychotic medications, and because of the potential that these drugs can reduce the number of days that people with schizophrenia are hospitalized (Byrom *et al.*, 1998). On the other hand, because clozapine is available in a generic form (less expensive) and has demonstrated effectiveness over other agents (Lewis *et al.* 2006; McEvoy *et al.* 2006), a cost-effectiveness study comparing clozapine to other second-generation agents may be moot.

Cost-effectiveness

The success of interventions in schizophrenia, whether medications or psychosocial rehabilitation programs, is reflected in multiple domains. An antipsychotic medication may have an impact on cognition, hallucinations, affect, disruptiveness, sexual functioning, extrapyramidal side effects (EPS), weight and employment—the list goes on and on. Some of the measures of the effectiveness of the agent may be positive and some may be negative. Some domains, such as hallucinations and delusions, may be influenced much more directly by the medication than more distal outcomes, such as housing or employment. Different individuals value changes in the domains differently, e.g., eliminating voices that other people do not hear may be much more important to the person troubled by harassing voices than to the person whose voices are good company or connect them to an imagined network of internationally renowned researchers. Similarly, some people are very troubled by changes in weight or sexual functioning (Covell *et al.*, 2007), while such changes may mean little to others.

Hence, much as we would like a composite measure across all effectiveness domains, this reductionistic approach is fraught with untenable compromises. Just as there is variation among different patients, so providers and payers may ascribe different values to the same outcome. Legislators who make funding allocations to public mental health systems may be more concerned about decreases in violence, while patients may be more concerned with increases in quality of life. How much is a symptom-free day worth? It depends on who is asking and who is paying.

Cost-effectiveness analyses have evolved to deal with the multiple domains touched by a single treatment. Such analyses report the change in a given effectiveness measure associated with a particular cost investment in treatment. A medication may be cost-effective with respect to certain outcomes, cost neutral for others, and costly for yet others. In 1999, Lehman reminded us that the current explosion of new knowledge about effective treatments and the advent of evidence-based quality standards for treating schizophrenia come at a time when cost containment is paramount on the health policy agenda; a decade later, this remains a priority. Policy-makers need to know the impact of dollars invested in treatment—but not just in a single domain such as reductions in hospital care. Those who make purchasing decisions for the public systems of care, which fund most treatment for schizophrenia, need information on multiple domains of effectiveness.

An alternative to cost-effectiveness analysis is cost–utility analysis, which calculates a comprehensive outcome indicator as a preference-weighted sum of the outcome measures. This tool is useful in cases as noted above, where different stakeholder groups value outcomes differently. An example of a cost–utility approach is the use of quality-adjusted life years (QALYs; Gold *et al.*, 1996; Drummond *et al.*, 1997). This approach creates an effectiveness metric representative of one stakeholder group; at worst, the resulting metric is representative of no one. Although a QALY representation of different stakeholder groups is elegant, making it is like creating sausages—observing their manufacture may reduce enthusiasm for their use. One must find or create weights to apply to the various effectiveness measures and then choose a combination scheme, deciding, for example, what weight gain is the equivalent of what change in EPS and what change in psychotic symptoms. Typically, one does this either by interviewing individuals representative of the population

under study (e.g., treatment-refractory patients with schizophrenia) or by adopting someone else's measures as "close enough". Because "close enough" is a very subjective call, it is important for researchers to disclose the sources of the weighting estimates so that readers can make their own call. For example, in their report of changes in QALYs among mostly male veterans with schizophrenia, Rosenheck *et al.* (1999) used weights derived as part of a doctoral dissertation where the sample was mainly African-American women (Kleinman, 1995). Only about half of these women (55%) were diagnosed with schizophrenia, and the rest were diagnosed with major depression, bipolar, and other affective disorders. We are unwilling to take the leap of faith needed to generalize from groups this disparate when presenting cost-effectiveness results from our own work (Essock *et al.*, 2000, 2002). Nevertheless, Rosenheck and colleagues are to be commended for providing the information necessary to follow back their methods to see what was used. This is not always the case.

Another type of utility analysis compares interventions with respect to the number of symptom-free days they produce. One such analysis followed the methodology of Lave *et al.* (1998) for calculating depression-free days using scores on depression measures, including partial days for mid-range scores (Simon *et al.*, 2001). Many people with depression, as well as many researchers, would take issue with saying that someone was symptom-free for half a year if they reported having 50% of full symptoms for each day of that year. Symptom-free days may be a poor measure within schizophrenia studies simply because, unlike depression, symptoms and functioning in schizophrenia are poorly correlated, and the likelihood of someone with schizophrenia having a completely symptom-free day may be small.

In a population where individuals may live for a long period of time with a relatively debilitating illness like schizophrenia, measures of mortality alone do not adequately capture the impact of the disability. Disability-adjusted life years (DALYs) can be used to express years lost either to premature death or to disabilities associated with living with schizophrenia (Shore, 1999). In contrast to QALYs, which estimate symptom-free days, 1 DALY equals 1 lost year of healthy life. DALYs are proxies for negative outcomes (Murray & Lopez, 1997), and thus the calculation of cost-effectiveness centers on how many DALYs are saved by using a particular intervention. DALYs are calculated by adding together the number of years between mortality and life-expectancy (years of life lost, YLL) and the number of years lived with a disability (YLD).

Calculating YLDs requires making assumptions about the relative impact of illness onset, duration, and severity on healthy living (e.g., making an assumption that a first psychotic episode at age 15 is worse than a first episode at age 25). As with QALYs, these metrics can be derived by surveying individuals with schizophrenia or their proxies, with the accompanying assumptions that how one weights hypothetical events is the same as the trade-offs one would make if one could trade fewer days of healthy life for more days of life with particular disabilities. Because such ratings are inherently untestable by rigorous methods, whether reliable or not, their validity remains suspect. Further, the calculation of DALYs "presupposes that life years of disabled people are worth less than life years of people without disabilities" (Arneson & Nord, 1999), and may even rank some individuals' lives as worse than death (Rock, 2000). Schizophrenia does bring with it an increased risk of suicide (Radomsky *et al.*, 1999), which is consistent with DALYs ranking some lives as worse than death. However, to assume that person A and person B would in fact make the same choices regarding what fates are worse than death presumes an ecological validity to DALY ratings that may be unwarranted.

Cost–utility measures, such as QALYs, DALYs, and measures like symptom-free days, have enormous appeal because of their ability to reduce multiple effectiveness domains to a single bullet measure. By deriving a single measure, one can compare any treatment approach to any other treatment approach. Where the measure is reduced to dollars (as in QALYs), one may even compare the values of interventions between different conditions, such as whether dollars expended on diabetes reap more benefits than dollars spent on schizophrenia (Drummond *et al.*, 1997). However, the assumptions built into such bullet measures may have limited usefulness for informing decisions at the level of the individual patient, prescriber, or healthcare payer. These individuals weigh their particular circumstances, and may be unwilling to have others' preferences serve as proxies for their own. Instead, these stakeholders ask more specific questions. The mental health commissioner may ask, "If I put an extra 3 million dollars in the pharmacy budget for medication X, what can I expect this to buy me in terms of other program costs? What is the downside risk? What will it buy me in terms of reductions in hospital use, improvements in vocational functioning, reductions in violent episodes, and reductions in side effects?" Similarly, patients and families paying for medications ask, "If I increase or decrease my spending by changing to medication X, what changes may I realize in the voices I hear, in my employability, in my sexual functioning, and in my body movements?" An alternative to composite measures is measures that contrast invested costs to a variety of outcome domains that are more important to some stakeholders than others. An analogy is a proposal for a city park to be funded from multiple sources. The park may or may not be a good idea depending on your perspective—whether you would use the park, and how the park would impact on the value of your property, your safety, your recreational options or what you are

called on to invest. Depending on who is paying for what, and which outcome domains are most important to you, you will stand to get a lot or a little out of your dollars that pay for the park. The challenge in funding the park is to present the data on costs and effects in such a way that the various payers (the city, private foundations, neighborhood organizations, individual contributors) can look from their different perspectives and identify the expected gains and losses in the outcome domains that are relevant to them. Each stakeholder can weigh factors such as less street noise, more open space, more dogs, and more people drawn to the neighborhood, and decide whether or not to support the park.

In contrast to cost–utility analysis, cost-effectiveness analysis does not reduce the impact of an intervention to one measure. Some outcomes, such as lower costs and higher effectiveness, may be clearly preferred or "dominant choices". Other outcomes, such as higher costs and higher effectiveness, are not as clearly dominant. In these cases, it may be useful to show the likely range of cost compared with multiple domains of effectiveness. One method of examining these ranges is to create sampling distributions for costs and effectiveness measures that show the precision of estimates as well as their mean. Bootstrap techniques, for example, create an empirical sampling distribution for every study participant's test data, using incremental cost-effectiveness ratios (ICERs) calculated by dividing the difference in cost (clozapine *vs.* usual care) by the difference in effectiveness (clozapine *vs.* usual care). We used 10 000 bootstrap replications to calculate the numerator and denominator of the ICER, and each of the 10 000 bootstrap replications was plotted as a point on the cost-effectiveness plane (Fig. 33.1). Cost data are often highly positively skewed, and ICERs can be used to provide less biased estimates of confidence intervals (Black, 1990; Pollack *et al.*, 1994; Chaudhary & Stearns, 1996; Briggs & Fenn, 1998; Lave *et al.*, 1998).

Figure 33.1 shows the cost-effectiveness of clozapine compared with first-generation antipsychotic medications among long-stay state hospital patients (Essock *et al.*, 2000). The cluster of points displays the sampling distribution of ICERs. Most of the points fall in the lower right quadrant, indicating that clozapine is most likely to be less costly and more effective than first-generation antipsychotic agents from the cost perspective (total societal cost) and for the effectiveness measure in question (reduction in EPS). This method can be applied to multiple outcomes within any given study. For example, Stant *et al.* (2007) applied ICERs to examine the cost-effectiveness of an intervention for individuals with schizophrenia. Similar to results reported by Essock *et al.* (2000), depending upon the outcome, the intervention would be considered cost-effective or cost neutral; hence, the authors stress the importance of reporting multiple outcomes to provide decision-makers with

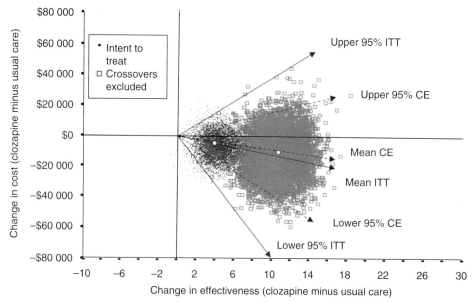

Fig. 33.1 Cost-effectiveness plane: number of extrapyramidal side effect (EPS)-free months. Difference in effectiveness (*x*-axis) compared with difference in cost (*y*-axis) for 10 000 bootstrap replications plotted in the cost-effectiveness plane. The *x* and *y* axes, respectively, show the difference between clozapine and usual-care groups in estimated number of EPS-free months and total cost during a 2-year period, with n = 136 clozapine, intent-to-treat (ITT), and n = 87 usual care, ITT, and with n = 89 clozapine, treatment cross-overs excluded (CE) and n = 30 usual care, CE. The quadrant to the lower right of the origin (0,0) contains those estimates where clozapine was found to be less costly and more effective than usual care (80% of the estimates for the ITT analyses and 81% of the estimates when treatment cross-overs are excluded). The cluster of points displays the sampling distribution of the incremental cost-effectiveness ratio (ICER) (reproduced from Essock *et al.*, 2000, with permission of the American Medical Association). Copyright @ 2000 American Medical Association. All rights reserved.

sufficient information on which to base policy decisions (Stant *et al.*, 2007). Such displays of information give the reader/policy-maker two important pieces of information at a glance:

1. A sense of the precision of the point estimate (a large cloud around the central point indicates great variability in the estimate, whereas a compact cloud means that the central point is a good estimate of what they might expect to see); and

2. The risk of falling into a quadrant other than the one indicating the intervention is dominant (less costly and more effective); the more points outside of the lower right quadrant, the more likely the intervention will be less effective or will be more costly in addition to being more effective.

It is incumbent on mental health services researchers to report their findings in ways that speak to funders and service system managers by providing estimates of the most likely outcome, as well as the likelihood of alternative outcomes. Saul Feldman, formerly head of the National Institute of Mental Health Staff College and chief executive officer of one of the largest managed behavioral healthcare organizations in the US, has been in a position to make policy based on research, and to inform policy-makers with

research. He poses the question, "Is good research good if it does not inform policy and practice?" (Feldman, 1999).

Cost of the newer antipsychotic medications

In general, the purchase price of the newer antipsychotic medications is greater than that of first-generation ones. These costs are reflected in formulary budgets. Once a relatively small component of treatment costs, formulary budgets in psychiatric settings have risen dramatically in the past decade, and the market share of the newer agents has risen as they have replaced the less costly first-generation antipsychotic medications. In less than a decade, Medicaid drug expenditures increased from $8 billion (1994) to $34 billion (2003), with three antipsychotic medications, olanzapine, risperidone, and quetiapine, occupying the top reimbursement slots in 2003 (Lied *et al.*, 2006). Figure 33.2 shows the distribution of antipsychotic prescriptions paid for by Medicaid in 2005 (left) and the dollars that Medicaid paid for these prescriptions (right). These data show that the newer agents account for 65% of all antipsychotic prescriptions paid for by Medicaid, but they represent 92% of the $8.5 billion in Medicaid costs for

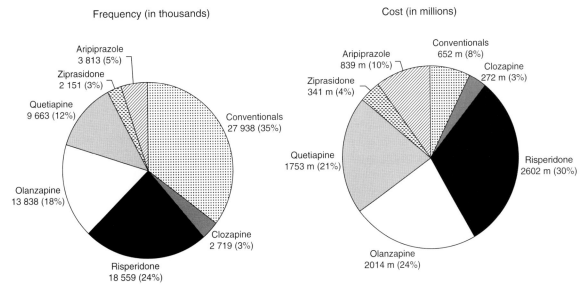

Frequency (in thousands)

Aripiprazole
3 813 (5%)

Ziprasidone
2 151 (3%)

Quetiapine
9 663 (12%)

Conventionals
27 938 (35%)

Olanzapine
13 838 (18%)

Clozapine
2 719 (3%)

Risperidone
18 559 (24%)

Cost (in millions)

Conventionals
652 m (8%)

Aripiprazole
839 m (10%)

Clozapine
272 m (3%)

Ziprasidone
341 m (4%)

Quetiapine
1753 m (21%)

Risperidone
2602 m (30%)

Olanzapine
2014 m (24%)

Fig. 33.2 Antipsychotic prescriptions: 2005, United States Medicaid. Distribution of frequency prescribed (left pie chart) and total dollars paid (right pie chart) by Medicaid for antipsychotic medication prescriptions during 2005. Newer antipsychotic medications represented about two-thirds of the total prescriptions and were responsible for 92% of the total cost. Note: 2 189 000 (12%) of the risperidone prescriptions and $346 million (13%) of the risperidone costs were for long-acting risperidone.

antipsychotic prescriptions. These charts dramatically display the disparity in medication costs associated with the first- *versus* second-generation agents. In the US, the price difference between the first- and second-generation antipsychotic medications can be 100-fold as, for example, when contrasting generic decanoate haloperidol with brand-name long-acting injectable risperidone. Two of the newer antipsychotics, clozapine and risperidone, are available generically; others will remain under patent for the next 3–6 years.

This large price differential has prompted scores of studies that consider more than simply the cost of the medication when determining the cost impact of using the newer medications. For example, let us say that using new and expensive medication X results in fewer days hospitalized than a lower cost alternative. Using X will reduce overall costs as long as the cost savings associated with fewer days in hospital are greater than the cost difference between medication X and the alternative—all else being equal.

Clozapine cost-effectiveness studies as case examples

The rub, of course, is that "all else" is rarely equal in effectiveness or cost-effectiveness studies, and the early cost projections concerning the impact of using clozapine often suffered from faulty assumptions about what was equivalent. Many of these studies were prepost comparisons that examined changes in hospital use but lacked a comparison group (Meltzer *et al.*, 1993; Reid *et al.*, 1994; Jonsson &

Walinder, 1995; Aitchison & Kerwin, 1997; Blieden *et al.*, 1998; Ghaemi *et al.*, 1998; Luchins *et al.*, 1998). The study by Meltzer *et al.* (1993) collected retrospective cost data for 2 years before and after 47 individuals began taking clozapine, and they concluded that clozapine was associated with a 23% drop in treatment costs. This conclusion generated a series of letters criticizing the study's methodology (Essock, 1995; Rosenheck *et al.*, 1995; Schiller & Hargreaves, 1995; response by Meltzer & Cola, 1995). Critics focused on the problem of regression toward the mean that can be expected whenever study participants are enrolled during a low point in their functioning (such as may have prompted the initiation of clozapine). They also noted that, unless there is random assignment to treatment conditions, studies comparing individuals who were and were not selected to begin a new medication are also open to case-mix confounds (differences in the characteristics of people who were and were not selected to receive the new medication).

Two randomized clinical trials of the cost-effectiveness of clozapine each showed much more modest benefits associated with clozapine than predicted by the mirror-image analyses. The first study was a 2-year open-label trial comparing clozapine to the usual care with a range of first-generation antipsychotics among long-term patients in state hospitals (Essock *et al.*, 1996a,b, 2000). The second study was a 1-year, masked (blinded) trial comparing clozapine to haloperidol among veterans hospitalized for a year or less (Rosenheck *et al.*, 1997). Each trial showed clozapine to be somewhat more effective than the comparison agents, and this increase in effectiveness came at no additional cost when costs were viewed from a societal perspective. Each study also showed that clozapine was more effective than usual care in minimizing days hospitalized, enough so that the reduction in hospital days more than covered the increased cost of the medication plus increased outpatient services. If cost-effectiveness studies are to influence planning and policy-making, the perspectives of different payers need to be taken into account. From more narrow perspectives, such as the hospital formulary budget or capitated outpatient service providers, clozapine could be viewed as increasing costs. These local incentives and disincentives must be addressed to be sure that fiscal incentives are lined up to promote good care. If a hospital has a fixed budget (the case with many state hospitals), it would have a great incentive to use clozapine for a heavy user of hospital services, but a hospital that is paid per diem would have no such incentive.

Lengthy randomized clinical trials in routine practice settings, such as the clozapine studies in Connecticut state hospitals and in Department of Veterans Affairs (VA) hospitals, suffer from treatment cross-overs. By the end of 6 months in the Connecticut study, only 11% of the usual care patients had begun a trial on clozapine, but by the end of 24 months 66% had begun such a trial. In the VA clozapine study, 72% of the patients assigned to masked haloperidol had ceased taking that medication by the end of the 1-year study period, with 31% (49 of 157) switching to clozapine and the rest to first-generation antipsychotics, including unmasked haloperidol (Rosenheck et al., 1997). Because of the biases introduced by what is likely to be highly non-random discontinuation of the assigned treatment, the importance of intent-to-treat analyses, and the hazards of unspecified biases in cross-over-excluded analyses, are well documented (Lavori, 1992).

When cross-overs are common, analyses excluding cross-overs may offer a proxy for the best case scenarios for each treatment condition by comparing only those who do well enough on treatment A to stay on it with only those who do well enough on treatment B to stay on it. Figure 33.1 illustrates such an analysis using data from the Connecticut clozapine study. The exclusion of treatment cross-overs increases the apparent effectiveness of clozapine because the cross-overs-excluded cluster is shifted to the right of the intent-to-treat cluster in Figure 33.1. Relative to the intent-to-treat analysis, the cross-overs-excluded analysis has decreased the estimate of the relative costliness of clozapine because the cross-over-excluded cluster is shifted lower by about $5500 (Essock et al., 2000). Clearly, individuals who leave their assigned treatment are different in terms of costs and outcomes from those who remain in their assigned treatment condition.

Another difficulty when trying to assess relative costs is the great variability in costs across patients. For example, in the VA study just cited, healthcare costs in the 6 months prior to randomization were approximately $27 000 with a standard deviation of about $17 000 (Rosenheck et al., 1997). For the Connecticut clozapine study, the 95% confidence interval for patients assigned to clozapine was $96 847–114 308 for year 2, versus $103 665–121 144 for those assigned to usual care. With such variability, cost differences are very difficult to detect, even with the relatively large sample sizes of the VA and Connecticut trials (n = 423 and 227, respectively). Even for individuals who are heavy service users at study entry, mounting a trial powered to detect cost differences requires hundreds of individuals per treatment arm. If the trial were a study of outpatients who are infrequent users of expensive services like hospitals, it would require even larger samples to detect cost differences apart from medication.

From a public health perspective, an emphasis on point estimates of costs and effectiveness is misguided when the confidence intervals are so broad. Economists would call clozapine the dominant alternative in these randomized trials because most of the range spanned by the cost confidence intervals includes the values where clozapine costs less than or the same as usual care, and the effectiveness measures favor clozapine or are neutral (see Chapter 26). The reduction of data to such a point estimate belies the broad distribution of possible outcomes that are likely to occur across patients. Planners and policy-makers, as well as patients and their treating clinicians, need a sense of the range of possible outcomes, as well as the relative likelihood of these outcomes, to inform their decisions about what chances they want to take.

Costs associated with risperidone, olanzapine, quetiapine, ziprasidone, and aripiprazole

Figure 33.3 shows the frequency of prescribing by type of antipsychotic in three large states in different parts of the US among individuals whose medications are paid via Medicaid. Because Medicaid formularies allow unrestricted access to any of these medications, independent of location in the country, and because the same financial incentives apply, one would expect to see similar rates of prescribing these medications. Indeed, the distributions do appear quite similar to each other and to the national data (see Fig. 33.2). That these distributions do not reflect what we know about the relative effectiveness of these agents (see Chapter 25) suggests that other factors are strong influences on medication choice and that these influences combine to create similar patterns of antipsychotic prescribing under Medicaid nationwide. In addition to effectiveness, factors as disparate as patients' past histories of medication use, order of receiving Food and Drug Administration (FDA) approval, convenience of use, purchase price, relative marketing budgets, and side effect profiles may be at play. Figures 33.2 and 33.3 serve as reminders that medications

2005, California Medicaid

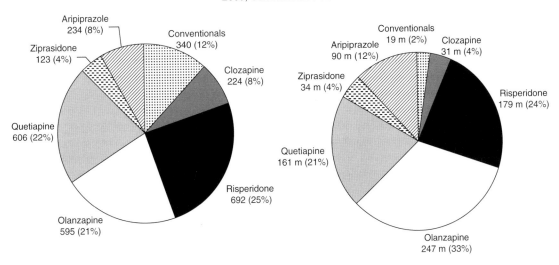

2005, Ohio Medicaid

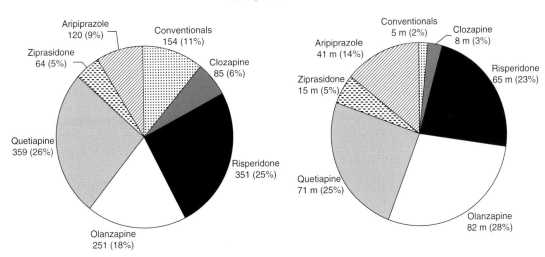

2005, New York Medicaid

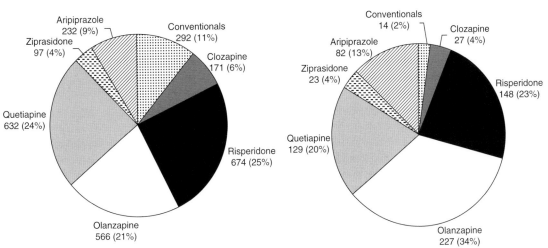

Fig. 33.3 Antipsychotic prescriptions. Distribution of frequency prescribed (left pie charts) and total dollars paid (right pie charts) by Medicaid for antipsychotic medication prescriptions in California, Ohio, and New York during 2005.

are started and discontinued for reasons other than effectiveness. (Data for these pie charts were extracted from the Health Care Financing Administration (HCFA) website at http://www.cms.hhs.gov/MedicaidDrugRebate Program/SDUD/list.asp).

Several studies of risperidone and olanzapine also suggest that the purchase prices of these medications may be offset by the reduction in use of more expensive healthcare services such as inpatient treatment. Many of these studies have methodological shortcomings similar to those of the earlier cost studies of clozapine described above. Another concern is that, because of industry sponsorship of many of these studies, they do not meet the criteria of lack of an incentive for bias set forth by the *New England Journal of Medicine* (Kassirer & Angell, 1994). The editors of that journal noted that opportunities for introducing bias into economic studies are far greater than in studies of biological phenomena. The unusually discretionary nature of model building and data selection in such analyses allows the introduction of bias, and drug costs in particular can be quite arbitrary because they are prices (not costs) set by the manufacturer. Hence, additional work is needed in this area.

In general, studies by pharmaceutical companies show support for cost reductions favoring that manufacturer's medication, such as risperidone (Nightengale *et al.*, 1998) or olanzapine (Hamilton *et al.*, 1999; Tunis *et al.* 1999). Although such studies may form useful starting points for further investigation, they need follow-up by independent investigators to assess how the agents' cost-effectiveness plays out in broader settings with representative patients. Otherwise, best-case examples might be generalized to settings where they are not applicable and used to set policy there. For example, an important follow-up study found that, among 84 treatment-refractory patients randomly assigned to a double-blind 8-week fixed dose trial of either olanzapine or chlorpromazine, olanzapine appeared to have limited efficacy, showing only a 7% response (Conley *et al.*, 1998). Hence, the reduction in treatment costs associated with olanzapine noted in the reviews of Palmer *et al.* (1998) and Foster and Goa (1999) would not be expected among treatment-refractory patients, even though these patients are heavy users of inpatient services. Under other scenarios, these patients are the very ones for whom new interventions produce cost savings because their higher initial rates of utilization allow the potential to show greater savings (Essock *et al.*, 1998; Rosenheck *et al.* 1999). An independent study among outpatients with schizophrenia, using a matched comparison group, compared risperidone with first-generation antipsychotics and found no difference in total treatment costs or effectiveness measures. There was a trend for the risperidone-treated group to have higher costs, attributable to higher medication costs (Schiller *et al.*, 1999). Recently, Polsky *et al.* (2006) reviewed

six clinical trials examining the cost-effectiveness of second-generation compared to first-generation antipsychotic medications and concluded that methodological issues such as measurement of costs and effectiveness, analytic approaches, sample size, missing data, and external validity precluded clear-cut conclusions, although these studies generally reported results favoring second-generation agents (two of the six trials compared clozapine to first-generation antipsychotic medications, and in all but one the comparator was haloperidol). On the other hand, despite similar methodological limitations, two large-scale randomized trials concluded that evidence did not support the cost-effectiveness of second-generation antipsychotic agents compared to either perphenazine (Rosenheck *et al.*, 2006) or a range of first-generation alternatives (Davies *et al.*, 2007). Clearly, well-designed and comprehensive cost studies are needed to address these open questions.

Conclusions and additional resources

The economics of the treatment of mental illness introduce methodological complexities not always present when considering the economics of other medical conditions. We have illustrated the importance of estimating and eliminating bias when constructing studies and reporting results. We especially stress the importance of reporting results from the perspective of different payers and have described how to estimate the variability of any findings when reporting them as point estimates. These factors should be acknowledged and accounted for when addressing treatment costs for schizophrenia. It is important to tell patients, prescribers, and payers not just the best estimate of costs and effectiveness, but the likelihood that their costs and outcomes will fall within the acceptable ranges of what they are willing to pay or risk to achieve a given outcome.

Fortunately, the literature of the economics of schizophrenia is currently evolving. Many active champions in this field now publish widely and lead the way in documenting how fiscal incentives and disincentives, as well as overall societal costs, impact access to treatment, quality of care received, and patient outcomes. Although all of this work cannot be summarized here, useful source books include those by Drummond *et al.* (1997), Frank and Glied (2006), Frank and Manning (1992), Gold *et al.* (1996), and Hargreaves *et al.* (1998). The journals *Health Affairs* and *Schizophrenia Bulletin* continue to be a particularly valuable resource for reports on mental health economics, and contain thoughtful analyses of economic influences on the treatment of individuals with schizophrenia.

Acknowledgements

The material in this chapter is based on a chapter in *Neuropsychopharmacology: The Fifth Generation of Progress*,

2002, edited by Kenneth L. Davis, Dennis Charney, Joseph T. Coyle, and Charles Nemeroff, American College of Neuropsychopharmacology, Lipincott, Williams and Wilkins. This research is the product of the collaboration of many individuals, both within and outside the Connecticut Department of Mental Health and Addiction Services (DMHAS). The research was funded in part by USPHS Grants R01 MH-48830 and R01 MH-52872 and R01 MH-59312 from the National Institute of Mental Health (NIMH) to Susan Essock, Principal Investigator, by R03 MH-71663 from NIMH to Nancy Covell, Principal Investigator, and by DMHAS. This publication does not express the views of the DMHAS or the State of Connecticut. The views and opinions expressed are those of the authors.

References

Aitchison, K.J. & Kerwin, R.W. (1997) Cost-effectiveness of clozapine: a UK clinic-based study. *British Journal of Psychiatry* **171**, 125–130.

Arneson, T. & Nord, E. (1999) The value of DALY life: problems with ethics and validity of disability adjusted life years. *British Medical Journal* **319**, 1423–1425.

Barry, C.L., Frank, R.G. & McGuire, T.G. (2006) The costs of mental health parity: Still an impediment? *Health Affairs* **25**, 623–634.

Black, W.C. (1990) The CE plane: a graphic representation of cost-effectiveness. *Medical Decision Making* **10**, 212–214.

Blieden, N., Flinders, S., Hawkins, K. *et al.* (1998) Health status and health care costs for publicly funded patients with schizophrenia started on clozapine. *Psychiatric Services* **49**, 1590–1593.

Bond, G.R., Becker, D.R., Drake, R.E. *et al.* (2001) Implementing supported employment as an evidence-based practice. *Psychiatric Services* **52**, 313–322.

Briggs, A. & Fenn, P. (1998) Confidence intervals or surfaces? Uncertainty on the cost-effectiveness plane. *Health Economics* **7**, 723–740.

Byrom, B.D., Garratt, C.J. & Kilpatrick, A.T. (1998) Influence of antipsychotic profile on cost of treatment in schizophrenia: a decision analysis approach. *International Journal of Psychiatry in Clinical Practice* **2**, 129–138.

Cannon, N.C., McGuire, T.G. & Dickey, B. (1985) Capital costs in economic program evaluation: the case of mental health services. In: Catterall, J., ed. *Economic Evaluation of Public Programs New Direction for Program Evaluation*, Vol. 26. San Francisco, CA: Jossey-Bass, pp. 69–82.

Chaudhary, M.A. & Stearns, S.C. (1996) Estimating confidence intervals for cost-effectiveness ratios: an example from a randomized trial. *Statistics in Medicine* **15**, 1447–1458.

Clark, R.E. (1994) Family costs associated with severe mental illness and substance use. *Hospital and Community Psychiatry* **45**, 808–813.

Clark, R.E., Ricketts, S.K. & McHugo, G.J. (1999) Legal system involvement and costs for person in treatment for severe mental illness and substance use disorders. *Psychiatric Services* **50**, 641–647.

Conley, R., Tamminga, C. & Group, M.S. (1998) Olanzapine compared with chlorpromazine in treatment-resistant schizophrenia. *American Journal of Psychiatry* **155**, 914–920.

Covell, N.H., Weissman, E.M., Schell, B. *et al.* (2007) Distress with medication side effects among persons with severe mental illness. *Administration and Policy in Mental Health and Mental Health Services Research* **34**, 435–442.

Cruze, A.M., Harwood, H.J., Kristiansen, P.L. *et al.* (1981) *Economic Costs to Society of Alcohol and Drug Abuse and Mental Illness, 1977.* Triangle Park, NC: Research Triangle Institute.

Davies, L.M., Lewis, S., Jones, P.B. *et al.* (2007) Cost-effectiveness of first- v. second-generation antipsychotic drugs: results from a randomized controlled trial in schizophrenia responding poorly to previous therapy. *British Journal of Psychiatry* **191**, 14–22.

Dickey, B. & Goldman, H.H. (1986) Public health care for the chronically mentally ill: financing operating costs. *Administration in Mental Health* **14**, 63–77.

Dixon, L., Weiden, P., Delahanty, J. *et al.* (2000) Prevalence and correlates of diabetes in national schizophrenia samples. *Schizophrenia Bulletin* **26**, 903–912.

Drake, R.E., McHugo, G.J., Becker, D.R. *et al.* (1996) The New Hampshire study of supported employment for people with severe mental illness. *Journal of Consulting and Clinical Psychology* **64**, 391–399.

Drummond, M.F., O'Brien, B., Stoddart, G.L. *et al.* (1997) *Methods for the Economic Evaluation of Health Care Programs*, 2nd edn. New York: Oxford University Press.

Essock, S.M. (1995) Clozapine's cost effectiveness [letter]. *American Journal of Psychiatry* **152**, 152.

Essock, S.M., Hargreaves, W.A., Covell, N.H. *et al.* (1996a) Clozapine's effectiveness for patients in state hospitals: results from a randomized trial. *Psychopharmacological Bulletin* **32**, 683–697.

Essock, S.M., Hargreaves, W.A., Dohm, F.A. *et al.* (1996b) Clozapine eligibility among state hospital patients. *Schizophrenia Bulletin* **22**, 15–25.

Essock, S.M., Frisman, L.K. & Kontos, N.J. (1998) Cost effectiveness of assertive community treatment teams. *American Journal of Orthopsychiatry* **68**, 179–190.

Essock, S.M., Frisman, L.K., Covell, N.H. *et al.* (2000) Cost-effectiveness of clozapine compared to conventional antipsychotic medication for patients in state hospitals. *Archives of General Psychiatry* **57**, 987–944.

Essock, S.M., Frisman, L.K. & Covell, N.H. (2002) The economics of the treatment of schizophrenia. In: Davis, K.L., Charney, D., Charney, J.T. & Nemeroff, C., eds. *Neuropsychopharmacology: the Fifth Generation of Progress American College of Neuropsychopharmacology.* New York: Lippincott, Williams & Wilkins, pp. 809–818.

Feldman, S. (1999) Strangers in the night: research and managed mental health care. *Health Affairs* **18**, 48–51.

Foster, R.H. & Goa, K.L. (1999) Olanzapine: a pharmacoeconomic review of its use in schizophrenia. *Pharmacoeconomics* **15**, 611–640.

Frank, R.G. (1983) Is there a shortage of psychiatrists? *Community Mental Health Journal* **19**, 42–53.

Frank, R.G. & Glied, S.A. (2006) *Better But Not Well: Mental Health Policy in the United States Since 1950.* Baltimore, MD: Johns Hopkins University Press.

Frank, R.G. & Manning, W.G., eds. (1992) *Economics and Mental Health.* Baltimore, MD: Johns Hopkins University Press.

Frank, R.G., McGuire, T.G. & Salkever, D.S. (1991) Benefit flexibility, cost shifting, and mandated mental health coverage. *Journal of Mental Health Administration* **18**, 264–271.

Frank, R.G., Goldman, H.H. & Hogan, M. (2003) Medicaid and mental health: Be careful what you ask for. *Health Affairs* **22**, 101–113.

Frank, R.G., Conti, R.M. & Goldman, H.H. (2005) Mental health policy and psychotropic drugs. *Milbank Quarterly* **83**, 271–298.

Frisman, L. & Rosenheck, R. (1996) How transfer payments are treated in cost-effectiveness and cost-benefit analyses. *Administration and Policy in Mental Health* **23**, 533–545.

Ghaemi, S.N., Ziegler, D.M., Peachey, T.J. *et al.* (1998) Cost-effectiveness of clozapine therapy for severe psychosis. *Psychiatric Services* **49**, 829–831.

Goeree, R., O'Brien, B.J., Goering, P. *et al.* (1999) The economic burden of schizophrenia in Canada. *Canadian Journal of Psychiatry* **44**, 464–472.

Goff, D.C., Sullivan, L.M., McEvoy, J.P. *et al.* (2005) A comparison of ten-year cardiac risk estimates in schizophrenia patients from the CATIE study and matched controls. *Schizophrenia Research* **80**, 45–53.

Gold, M.R., Siegel, J.E., Russell, L.B. *et al.*, eds. (1996) *Cost-Effectiveness in Health and Mental Health.* New York: Oxford University Press.

Goldman, H.H., Morrissey, J.P. & Ridgely, M.S. (1994) Evaluating the Robert Wood Johnson Foundation program on chronic mental illness. *Millbank Quarterly* **72**, 37–47.

Goldman, H.H., Frank, R.G. & Gaynor, M.S. (1995) What level of government? Balancing the interests of the state and the local community. *Administration and Policy in Mental Health* **23**, 127–135.

Goldman, H.H., Ganju, V., Drake, R.E. *et al.* (2001) Policy implications for implementing evidence-based practices. *Psychiatric Services* **52**, 1591–1597.

Hamilton, S.H., Revicki, D.A., Edgell, E.T. *et al.* (1999) Clinical and economic outcomes of olanzapine compared with haloperidol for schizophrenia. *Pharmacoeconomics* **15**, 469–480.

Hargreaves, W.A., Shumway, M., Hu, T. *et al.* (1998) *Cost–Outcome Methods for Mental Health.* New York: Academic Press.

Harwood, H.J., Napolitano, D.M., Kristiansen, P.L. *et al.* (1984) *Economic Costs to Society of Alcohol and Drug Abuse and Mental Illness, 1980.* Research Triangle Park, NC: Research Triangle Institute.

Jonsson, D. & Walinder, J. (1995) Cost-effectiveness of clozapine treatment in therapy-refractory schizophrenia. *Acta Psychiatrica Scandinavica* **92**, 199–201.

Kassirer, J.P. & Angell, M. (1994) Journal's policy on cost-effectiveness analyses. *New England Journal of Medicine* **331**, 669–670.

Kessler, R.C. & Frank, R.G. (1997) The impact of psychiatric disorders on work loss days. *Psychological Medicine* **27**, 861–873.

Kleinmann, L.S. (1995) *Preferences for Outpatient Mental Health Treatment.* PhD dissertation. The Johns Hopkins University, Baltimore, MD.

Knapp, M. (1997) Costs of schizophrenia. *British Journal of Psychiatry* **171**, 509–518.

Knapp, M., Mangalore, R. & Simon, J. (2004). The global costs of schizophrenia. *Schizophrenia Bulletin* **30**, 279–293.

Lang, H. & Su, T. (2004) The cost of schizophrenia treatment in Taiwan. *Psychiatric Services* **55**, 928–930.

Lave, J.R., Frank, R.G., Schulberg, H.C. *et al.* (1998) Cost-effectiveness of treatments for major depression in primary care practice. *Archives of General Psychiatry* **55**, 645–651.

Lavori, P.W. (1992) Clinical trials in psychiatry: should protocol deviation censor patient data? *Neuropsychopharmacology* **6**, 39–48.

Lehman, A.F. (1999) Quality of care in mental health: the case of schizophrenia. *Health Affairs* **18**, 52–70.

Lewis, S.W., Barnes, T.R.E., Davies, L. *et al.* (2006) Randomized controlled trial of effect of prescription of clozapine versus other second-generation antipsychotic drugs in resistant schizophrenia. *Schizophrenia Bulletin* **32**, 715–723.

Lied, T. R., Gonzalez, J., Taparanskas, W. & Shukla, T. (2006) Trends and current drug utilization patterns of Mediciad beneficiaries. *Health Care Financing Review* **27**, 123–132.

Lloyd-Jones, D, Adams, R.J., Brown, T.M. *et al.*, on behalf of the American Heart Association Statistics Committee and Stroke Statistics Subcommittee (2010) Heart Disease and Stroke Statistics 2010 Update: A report from the American Heart Association. *Circulation* **121**, e46–e215.

Luchins, D.J., Hanrahan, P., Shinderman, M. *et al.* (1998) Initiating clozapine treatment in the outpatient clinic: service utilization and cost trends. *Psychiatric Services* **49**, 1034–1038.

Mangalore, R. & Knapp, M. (2007). Cost of schizophrenia in England. *Journal of Mental Health Policy and Economics* **109**, 23–41.

Manning, W.G., Wells, K.B., Duan, N. *et al.* (1984) Cost sharing and the use of ambulatory mental health services. *American Psychologist* **39**, 1077–1089.

Martin, B.C. & Miller, L.S. (1998) Expenditures for treating schizophrenia: a population-based study of Georgia Medicaid recipients. *Schizophrenia Bulletin* **24**, 479–488.

McEvoy, J.P., Lieberman, J.A., Stroup, T.S. *et al.* (2006). Effectiveness of clozapine versus olanzapine, quetiapine, and risperidone in patients with chronic schizophrenia who did not respond to prior atypical antipsychotic treatment. *American Journal of Psychiatry* **163**, 600–610.

McGuire, T.G. (1981) *Financing Psychotherapy: Costs, Effects, and Public Policy.* Cambridge, MA: Ballinger Books.

McGuire, T.G. (1990) Growth of a field in policy research: the economics of mental health. *Administration and Policy in Mental Health* **17**, 165–175.

McGuire, T.G. (1991) Measuring the economic costs of schizophrenia. *Schizophrenia Bulletin* **17**, 375–388.

McGuire, T.G., Hodgkin, D. & Shumway, D. (1995) Managing Medicaid mental health costs: the case of New Hampshire. *Administration and Policy in Mental Health* **23**, 97–117.

Mechanic, D., ed. (1998) Managed behavioral health care: current realities and future potential. *New Directions for Mental Health Services,* no. 78. San Francisco, CA: Jossey-Bass.

Meltzer, H.Y. & Cola, P. (1995) Clozapine's cost effectiveness [reply]. *American Journal of Psychiatry* **152**, 153–154.

Meltzer, H.Y., Cola, P., Way, L. *et al.* (1993) Cost effectiveness of clozapine in neuroleptic-resistant schizophrenia. *American Journal of Psychiatry* **150**, 1630–1638.

Mumford, E. & Schlesinger, H.J. (1987) Assessing consumer benefit: cost offset as an incidental effect of psychotherapy. *General Hospital Psychiatry* **9**, 360–363.

Murray, C.J.L. & Lopez, A.D. (1997) Alternative projections of mortality and disability by cause 1990–2020: global burden of disease study. *Lancet* **349**, 1498–1504.

Nightengale, B.S., Crumly, J.M., Liao, J. *et al.* (1998) Current topics in clinical psychopharmacology. *Psychopharmacological Bulletin* **34**, 373–382.

Pallack, M.S. & Cummings, N.A. (1992) Inpatient and outpatient psychiatric treatment: the effect of matching patients to appropriate level of treatment on psychiatric and medical–surgical hospital days. *Applied and Preventive Psychology* **1**, 83–87.

Palmer, C.S., Revicki, D.A., Genduso, L.A. *et al.* (1998) A cost-effectiveness clinical decision analysis model for schizophrenia. *American Journal of Managment Care* **4**, 345–355.

Pollack, S., Bruce, P., Borenstein, M. *et al.* (1994) The resampling method of statistical analysis. *Psychopharmacological Bulletin* **30**, 227–234.

Polsky, D., Doshi, J.A., Bauer, M.S. & Glick, H.A. (2006) Clinical trial-based cost-effectiveness analyses of antipsychotic use. *American Journal of Psychiatry* **163**, 2047–2056.

Radomsky, E.D., Haas, G.L., Mann, J.J. *et al.* (1999) Suicidal behavior in patients with schizophrenia and other psychotic disorders. *American Journal of Psychiatry* **156**, 1590–1595.

Reid, W.H., Mason, M. & Toprac, M. (1994) Savings in hospital bed-days related to treatment with clozapine. *Hospital and Community Psychiatry* **45**, 261–264.

Rice, D.P. (1999a) The economic impact of schizophrenia. *Journal of Clinical Psychiatry* **60** (Suppl. 1), 4–6.

Rice, D.P. (1999b) Economic burden of mental disorders in the United States. *Economics of Neuroscience* **1**, 40–44.

Rice, D.P., Kelman, S., Miller, L.S. *et al.* (1990) *The Economic Costs of Alcohol and Drug Abuse and Mental Illness: 1985*. Rockville, MD: National Institute of Mental Health, DHHS Publications (ADM), 90–1694.

Rock, M. (2000) Discounted lives? Weighing disability when measuring health and ruling on "compassionate" murder. *Social Science and Medicine* **51**, 407–417.

Rosenberg, S.D., Goodman, L.A., Osher, F.C. *et al.* (2001) Prevalence of HIV, hepatitis B, and hepatitis C in people with severe mental illness. *American Journal of Public Health* **91**, 31–37.

Rosenheck, R.A., Frisman, L.N. & Neale, M. (1994) Estimating the capital component of mental health care costs in the public sector. *Administration and Policy in Mental Health* **21**, 493–509.

Rosenheck, R., Charney, D.S., Frisman, L.K. *et al.* (1995) Clozapine's cost effectiveness [letter]. *American Journal of Psychiatry* **152**, 152–153.

Rosenheck, R.A., Cramer, J., Xu, W. *et al.* (1997) A comparison of clozapine and haloperidol in the treatment of hospitalized patients with refractory schizophrenia. *New England Journal of Medicine* **337**, 451–458.

Rosenheck, R., Cramer, J., Allan, E. *et al.* (1999) Cost-effectiveness of clozapine in patients with high and low levels of hospital use. *Archives of General Psychiatry* **56**, 565–572.

Rosenheck, R. A., Leslie, D. L., Sindelar, J. *et al.* (2006) Cost-effectiveness of second-generation antipsychotics and perphenazine in a randomized trial of treatment for chronic schizophrenia. *American Journal of Psychiatry* **163**, 2080–2089.

Rund, B.R. & Ruud, T. (1999) Costs of services for schizophrenic patients in Norway. *Acta Psychiatrica Scandinavica* **99**, 120–125.

Schiller, M. & Hargreaves, W.A. (1995) Clozapine's cost effectiveness [letter]. *American Journal of Psychiatry* **152**, 151–152.

Schiller, M.J., Shumway, M. & Hargreaves, W.A. (1999) Treatment costs and patient outcomes with use of risperidone in a public mental health setting. *Psychiatric Services* **50**, 228–230.

Semke, J., Fisher, W.H., Goldman, H.H. *et al.* (1995) The evolving role of the state hospital in the care and treatment of older adults: state trends 1984–93. *Psychiatric Services* **47**, 1082–1087.

Shepherd, G., Muijen, M., Hadley, T.R. *et al.* (1996) Effects of mental health services reform on clinical practice in the United Kingdom. *Psychiatric Services* **47**, 1351–1355.

Shore, M.F. (1999) Replacing cost with value. *Harvard Review of Psychiatry* **6**, 334–336.

Simon, G.E., Manning, W.G., Katzelnick, D.J. *et al.* (2001) Cost-effectiveness of systematic depression treatment for high utilizers of general medical care. *Archives of General Psychiatry* **58**, 181–187.

Stant, A.D., Buskens, E., Jenner, J.A., Wiersma, D. & TenVergert, E.M. (2007) Cost-effectiveness analysis in severe mental illness: Outcome measures selection. *Journal of Mental Health Policy and Economics* **10**, 101–108.

Taube, C.A., Lee, E.S. & Forthofer, R.N. (1984) DRGs in psychiatry: an empirical evaluation. *Medical Care* **22**, 597–610.

Tunis, S.L., Bryan, M.J., Gibson, J. *et al.* (1999) Changes in perceived health and functioning as a cost-effectiveness measure for olanzapine versus haloperidol treatment of schizophrenia. *Journal of Clinical Psychiatry* **60** (Suppl.), 38–45.

U.S. Department of Health and Human Services Centers for Disease Control and Prevention (2007) National Diabetes Fact Sheet, 2007. http://www.cdc.gov/diabetes/pubs/pdf/ndfs_2007.pdf.

Weisbrod, B.A., Test, M.A. & Stein, L.I. (1980) Alternative to hospital treatment. II. Economic benefit–cost analysis. *Archives of General Psychiatry* **37**, 400–405.

Index

Page numbers in **bold** refer to information in tables. Page numbers in *italics* refer to information in figures.

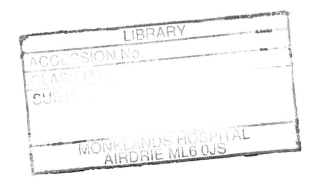